Histology

A Text and Atlas With Cell and Molecular Biology

Fourth Edition

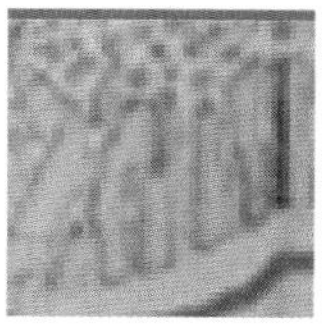
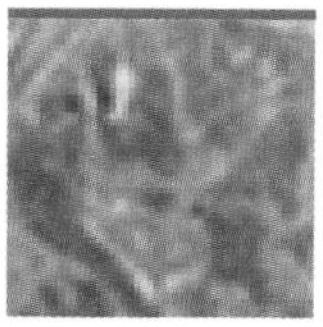
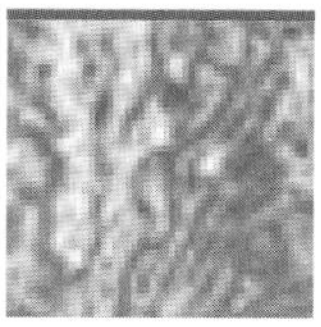

Histology

A Text and Atlas

With Cell and Molecular Biology

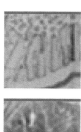

Fourth Edition

Michael H. Ross, PhD
Professor and Chairman Emeritus
Department of Anatomy and Cell Biology
University of Florida College of Medicine
Gainesville, Florida

Gordon I. Kaye, PhD
Alden March Professor Emeritus
Pathology and Laboratory Medicine
Albany Medical College
Albany, New York

Wojciech Pawlina, MD
Associate Professor of Anatomy
Department of Anatomy
Mayo Clinic/Mayo Medical School
Rochester, Minnesota

Lippincott Williams & Wilkins
A **Wolters Kluwer** Company
Philadelphia • Baltimore • New York • London
Buenos Aires • Hong Kong • Sydney • Tokyo

Publisher: Susan Katz
Development Editor: Kathleen H. Scogna
Marketing Manager: Aimee Sirmon
Production Editor: Bill Cady
Designer: Armen Kojoyian
Compositor: Graphic World
Printer: R. R. Donnelley & Sons

351 West Camden Street
Baltimore, MD 21201

530 Walnut St.
Philadelphia, PA 19106

Printed in the United States of America

First Edition, 1985
Second Edition, 1989
Third Edition, 1995

Library of Congress Cataloging-in-Publication Data

Ross, Michael H.
Histology : a text and atlas / Michael H. Ross, Gordon I. Kaye, Wojciech Pawlina.—4th ed.
p. cm.
Includes index.
ISBN 0-683-30242-6
1. Histology. 2. Histology—Atlases. I. Kaye, Gordon I. II. Pawlina, Wojciech. III. Title.

QM551 .R67 2002
611'.018—dc21

2002070243

The publishers have made every effort to trace the copyright holders for borrowed material. If they have inadvertently overlooked any, they will be pleased to make the necessary arrangements at the first opportunity.

To purchase additional copies of this book, call our customer service department at **(800) 638-3030** or fax orders to **(301) 824-7390.** International customers should call **(301) 714-2324.**

Visit Lippincott Williams & Wilkins on the Internet: http://www.LWW.com. Lippincott Williams & Wilkins customer service representatives are available from 8:30 am to 6:00 pm, EST.

03 04 05 06
3 4 5 6 7 8 9 10

This newest edition is dedicated to our wives,
Agnes, Nancy, and Teresa,
whose love, patience, and endurance
created safe havens for us while working on this project.

Preface

This fourth edition of *Histology: A Text and Atlas with Cell and Molecular Biology* continues its tradition of providing medical and health sciences students with a textual and visual introduction to histology. As in previous editions, the book is a combination "text-atlas." It includes a standard textbook description of histologic principles, supplemented by illustrations and photos. In addition, separate atlas sections placed after selected chapters provide large-format, labeled atlas plates with detailed legends that highlight details of microanatomy. *Histology: A Text and Atlas* is therefore "two books in one."

A number of significant changes have been undertaken in this edition to create a more useful and understandable approach to the subject material.

More cell biology information. A major change is the incorporation of more cell biology as it relates to the understanding of histology as well as that of living systems. The additional cell biology has been incorporated in the chapter on the cell as well as in the chapters on tissues and organs.

Reader-friendly innovations. A major attempt in terms of the cell biology as well as new information that can be related to histology has been to limit the amount of text and to underscore pertinent information with the additional use of sentence headings and bulleted lists.

Emphasis on features. Many of the pedagogic features from the last edition have been refined, and some new features have been added.

- To help students preview each chapter and study for exams, an **outline of the major headings** has been provided at the beginning of each chapter.
- More **tables** are included to allow the student to review material without the need for strict memorization of data.
- The "**Clinical Correlations**" and "**Functional Considerations**" **boxes** have been updated and enhanced. While these boxes might be considered ancillary material, it was felt that they provide more relevance to the general subject of histology and its relationship to the understanding of how the body works and its practical significance.

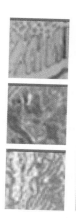

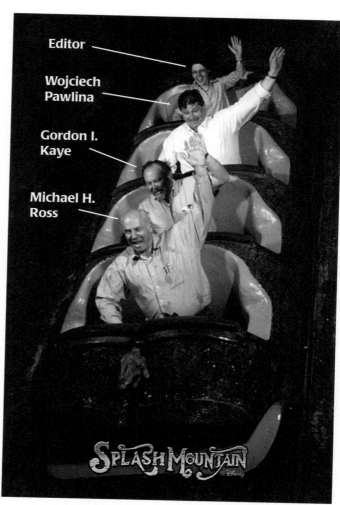

Authors with their editor at work. Fresh specimens, no fixatives, natural colors, ×0.0015. ©Disney Enterprises, Inc.

New Illustrations. Another area of improvement has been in the photos and illustrations. Almost all of the art in this edition has been redrawn for greater clarity and conceptual focus. An important new feature is the use of a consistent color code for all of the illustrations in the book.

For example, all nuclei are blue and all mitochondria are green. Such consistency acts as a visual memory tool that facilitates learning.

Digital photomicrographs. Also in this edition, we have incorporated many high-resolution digital photomicrographs. Many of the black and white photomicrographs in the text chapters have been replaced by color, and many additional photomicrographs have been added to illustrate the text material.

New design. A bright, energetic text design sets off the new illustrations and photos and makes navigation of the text even easier than in previous editions.

Color atlas. The atlas section is now completely in color with a large portion of the plates converted to digital photomicrographs. The legends for the atlas plates have also been reformatted to provide greater facility in correlating the legends with the micrographs.

As in previous editions, all of the changes were undertaken with student needs in mind, namely, to understand the subject matter, to add current information, and to apply it as a base in the understanding of body function.

Michael H. Ross
Gordon I. Kaye
Wojciech Pawlina

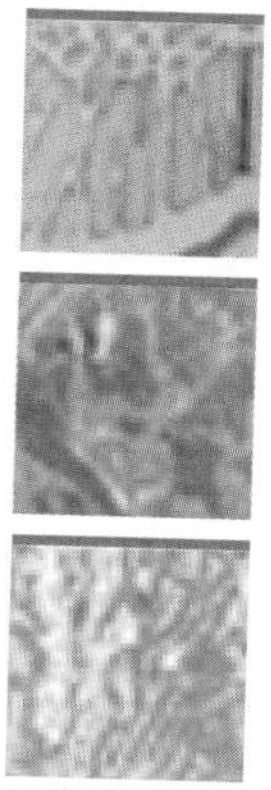

Acknowledgments

This fourth edition of *Histology: A Text and Atlas* reflects considerable change from the previous editions. The changes that have occurred have come largely from comments and suggestions by students who have taken the time and effort to tell us what they liked about the book and, more importantly, how it might be improved to help them better understand the subject material. Their comments and suggestions were, for the most part, incorporated into this new edition.

Many of our colleagues who teach histology and cell biology courses, likewise, were also most helpful in producing this new edition. Many of them suggested increasing clinical relevance. We responded to this as best we could within page limitations. Others were most helpful in providing new micrographs and suggestions for new diagrams and redrawing existing diagrams. Finally, there are many of our colleagues who suggested adding specific new information, particularly as it relates to cell biology and its relation to histology. Our special thanks go to a number of these colleagues including Drs. Johannes Rhodin, Craig C. Tisher, Alvin Telser, Susan Frost, Kevin McCarthy, Jeffrey Salisbury, Wilma Lingle, Larry Baker, Wade Schultz, and Aletta Houwink. We are grateful to Dr. Marshall Lichtman from the University of Rochester School of Medicine and Dentistry for his many valuable suggestions and critical reading of the chapter on blood. Our appreciation goes to Dr. Izabela Maciejewska from the Medical University of Gdansk, Poland, for her critical review of the chapter on the oral cavity. In addition, we are grateful to Dr. Stephen Carmichael for his helpful suggestions relating to the chapters on methods and endocrine glands.

We are also indebted to a number of people who were involved in the technical aspects of producing this book. Todd Barnash provided invaluable assistance in digitizing text and atlas figures as well as in the creation of high-resolution photomicrographs and also doing the seemingly impossible in putting this work together. Thanks also go to Denny Player for his continued superb technical expertise involving electron microscopy.

The authors wish to express special thanks to several people at Lippincott Williams & Wilkins. Jane Velker worked with us for a short time when work on this new edition was initiated. Her ideas and cooperation were highly valued. Kathleen Scogna later worked with us and provided her expertise during the majority of the development process. Her assistance, encouragement, problem solving, and technical expertise were invaluable in bringing this edition to fruition. In essence, she did an incredible job.

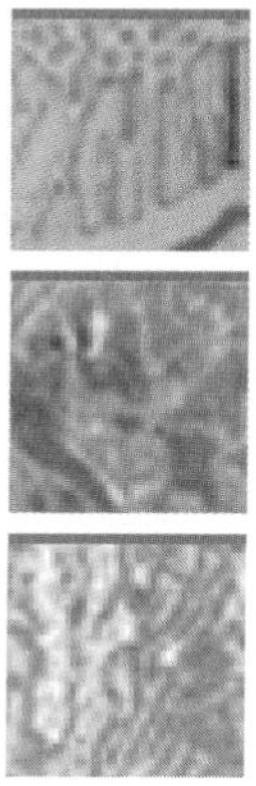

Contents

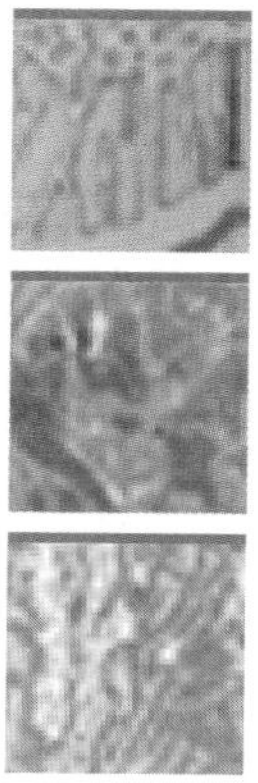

Contents

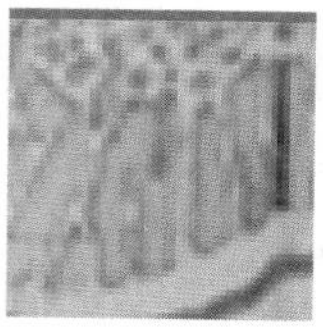
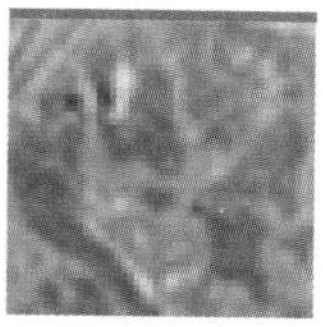
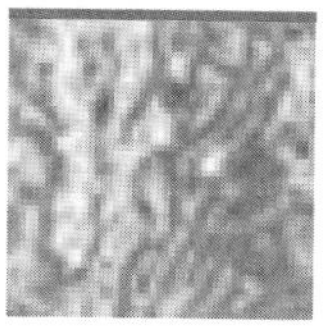

Histology

A Text and Atlas

Fourth Edition

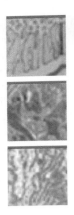

1

Methods

▽ OVERVIEW OF METHODS USED IN HISTOLOGY

The objective of a histology course is to lead the student to understand the microanatomy of cells, tissues, and organs and to correlate structure with function

The methods used by histologists are extremely diverse. Much of the histology course content can be framed in terms of light microscopy, which students use in the laboratory exercises. More detailed interpretation of microanatomy rests with the electron microscope (EM), both the transmission electron microscope (TEM) and the scanning electron microscope (SEM). The EM, because of its greater resolution and useful magnification, is often the last step in data acquisition from many auxiliary techniques of cell and molecular biology. These auxiliary techniques include

- Histochemistry and cytochemistry
- Autoradiography
- Organ and tissue culture

- Cell and organelle separation by differential centrifugation
- Specialized microscopic techniques and microscopes

The student may feel removed from such techniques and experimental procedures because direct experience with them is usually not available in current curricula. Nevertheless, it is important to know something about specialized procedures and the data they yield. *This chapter provides a survey of methods and offers an explanation of how the data provided by these methods can help the student acquire a sound appreciation of histology.*

One problem faced by the student in histology is understanding the nature of the two-dimensional image of a histologic slide or an electron micrograph and how it relates to the three-dimensional structure from which it came. To bridge this conceptual gap, we must first present a brief description of the methods by which slides and electron microscopic specimens are produced.

▼ TISSUE PREPARATION

Hematoxylin and Eosin Staining With Formalin Fixation

The routinely prepared hematoxylin and eosin–stained section is the specimen most commonly studied

The slide set given each student to study with the light microscope consists mostly of formalin-fixed, paraffin-embedded, hematoxylin and eosin (H&E)–stained specimens. Nearly all of the light micrographs in the Atlas section of this book are of slides from actual student sets. Also, most photomicrographs used to illustrate tissues and organs in histology lectures and conferences are taken from such slides. Other techniques are sometimes used to demonstrate specific cell and tissue components; several of these are described below.

The first step in preparation of a tissue or organ sample is fixation to preserve structure

Fixation, usually by a chemical or mixture of chemicals, stops cell metabolism and preserves the tissue structure for subsequent treatments. ***Formalin,*** a 37% aqueous solution of formaldehyde, at various dilutions and in combination with other chemicals and buffers, is the most commonly used fixative. Formaldehyde preserves the general structure of the cell and extracellular components by reacting with the amino groups of proteins; formaldehyde does not react with lipids and, therefore, is a poor fixative of membranes.

In the second step, the specimen is prepared for embedding in paraffin to permit sectioning

To allow the specimen to be examined, it must be infiltrated with an ***embedding*** medium that allows it to be thinly sliced, 5 to 15 μm (1 micrometer [μm] equals 1/1,000th of a millimeter [mm]; see Table 1.1). The specimen is ***washed*** after fixation and ***dehydrated*** in a series of alcohol solutions of ascending concentration up to 100% alcohol to remove water. Organic solvents such as xylol or toluol, which are miscible in both alcohol and ***paraffin,*** are then used to remove the alcohol prior to infiltration of the specimen with melted paraffin.

When the melted paraffin is cool and hardened, it is trimmed into an appropriately sized block. The block is then mounted in a specially designed slicing machine, a microtome, and cut with a steel knife. The resulting sections are then mounted on glass slides, with albumin used as an adhesive.

In the third step, the specimen is stained to permit examination

Because the paraffin sections are colorless, the specimen is not yet suitable for light microscopic examination. To color or stain the tissue sections, the paraffin must be dissolved out, again with xylol or toluol, and the slide must then be rehydrated through a series of solutions of descending alcohol concentration. The tissue on the slides is then stained with ***hematoxylin*** in water. Because the counterstain, ***eosin,*** is more soluble in alcohol than in water, the specimen is again dehydrated through a series of alcohol solutions of ascending concentration and stained with eosin in alcohol. The results of staining with hematoxylin alone, eosin alone, and hematoxylin with counterstain eosin are shown in Figure 1.1. After staining, the specimen is then passed through xylol or toluol to a nonaqueous mounting medium and covered with a coverslip to obtain a permanent preparation. A summary of H&E staining reactions of various cell and tissue components is presented in Table 1.2.

Other Fixatives

Formalin does not preserve all cell and tissue components

Although H&E–stained sections of formalin-fixed specimens are convenient to use because they adequately display general structural features, they are not specific to elucidate the chemical composition of cell components. Also, many components are lost in the preparation of the specimen. To retain these components and structures, other fixation methods must be used. These methods are

TABLE 1.1. **Commonly Used Linear Equivalents**

1 Angstrom (Å)	=	0.1 nanometer (nm)
10 Angstroms	=	1.0 nanometer (formerly millimicron [mμ])
1,000 nanometers	=	1.0 micrometer (μm) (formerly micron [μ])
1,000 micrometers	=	1.0 millimeter (mm)

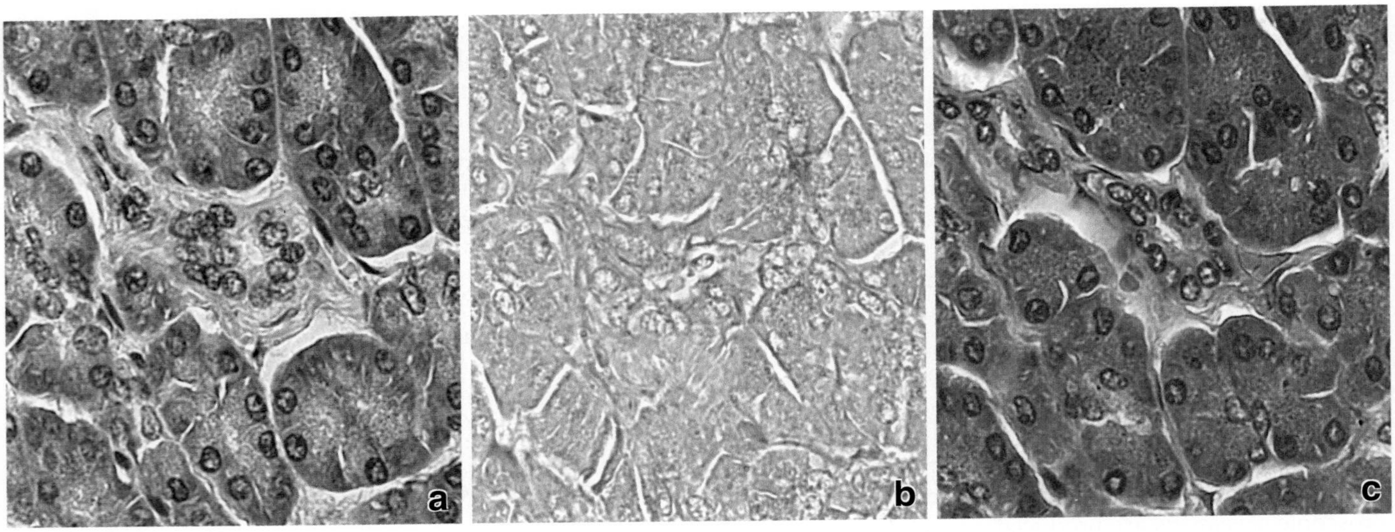

FIGURE 1.1
Hematoxylin and eosin (H&E) staining. The series of specimens from the pancreas shown here are serial (adjacent) sections to demonstrate the effect of hematoxylin and eosin used alone and hematoxylin and eosin used in combination. **a.** This photomicrograph reveals the staining with hematoxylin only. While there is a general overall staining of the specimen, those components and structures that have a high affinity for the dye are most heavily stained, e.g., nuclear DNA and areas of the cell containing cytoplasmic RNA. **b.** In this photomicrograph the counterstain, eosin, likewise has an overall staining effect when used alone. Note, however, that the nuclei are less conspicuous than in the specimen stained with hematoxylin only. After the specimen is stained with hematoxylin and is then prepared for staining with eosin in alcohol solution, the hematoxylin that is not tightly bound is lost, and the eosin then stains those components to which it has a high affinity. **c.** This photomicrograph reveals the combined staining effect of H&E. ×480.

TABLE 1.2. **Summary of Hematoxylin and Eosin (H&E) Staining**

Cell and Extracellular Component	Stain Reaction
Nucleus	
Heterochromatin	Blue
Euchromatin	Negative
Nucleolus	Blue
Cytoplasm	
Ergastoplasm	Blue
General cytoplasm	Pink
Cytoplasmic filaments	Pink
Extracellular material	
Collagen fibers	Pink
Elastic fibers[A]	Pink, but not usually distinguishable from collagen fibers
Reticular fibers[B]	Pink, but not usually distinguishable from collagen fibers
Ground substance	Blue, but only if present in large amounts, as in cartilage matrix
Bone matrix (decalcified)	Pink
Basement membrane[B]	Pink

[A] Special staining procedure used for their demonstration, such as one containing resorcin-fuchsin or orcein.
[B] Special staining procedure used for their demonstration, such as silver impregnation or periodic acid–Schiff (PAS) stain.

generally based on a clear understanding of the chemistry involved. For instance, the use of alcohols and organic solvents in routine preparations removes neutral lipids.

To retain neutral lipids, such as those in adipose cells, frozen sections of formalin-fixed tissue and dyes that dissolve in fats must be used; to retain membrane structures, special fixatives containing heavy metals, such as permanganate and osmium, that bind to the phospholipids must be used. The routine use of osmium tetroxide as a fixative for electron microscopy is the primary reason for the ex-

cellent preservation of membranes in electron micrographs.

Other Staining Procedures

Hematoxylin and eosin are used in histology primarily to display structural features

Despite the merits of H&E staining, the procedure does not adequately reveal certain structural components of histologic sections, including elastic material, reticular fibers, basement membranes, and lipids. When it is desirable to display these components, other staining procedures, most of them selective, can be used. These procedures include the use of orcein and resorcin-fuchsin for elastic material and the use of silver impregnation for reticular fibers and basement membrane material. Although the chemical bases of many staining methods are not always understood, they work. Knowing the components a procedure reveals is more important than knowing precisely how the procedure works.

▽ HISTOCHEMISTRY AND CYTOCHEMISTRY

Specific chemical procedures can provide detailed information about the function of the cells and extracellular components of the tissues

Histochemical and cytochemical procedures may be based on ***specific binding*** of a dye, use of a ***fluorescent dye–labeled antibody*** to a particular cell component, or the ***inherent enzymatic activity*** of a cell component. In addition, many large molecules found in cells can be localized by autoradiography, in which radioactively tagged precursors of the molecule are incorporated by cells and tissues prior to fixation. Many of these procedures can be used with both light microscopic and electron microscopic preparations.

Before discussing the chemistry of routine staining and histochemical and cytochemical methods, it is useful to examine briefly the nature of a routinely fixed and embedded section of a specimen.

Chemical Composition of Histologic Samples

The chemical composition of a tissue ready for routine staining differs greatly from living tissue

The components that remain after fixation consist mostly of large molecules that do not readily dissolve, especially after treatment with the fixative. These large molecules, particularly those that react with other large molecules to form macromolecular complexes, are usually preserved in a tissue section. Examples of such large macromolecular complexes include

- ***Nucleoproteins,*** formed from nucleic acids bound to protein
- ***Intracellular cytoskeletal proteins*** complexed with other proteins
- ***Extracellular proteins*** in large insoluble aggregates, bound to similar molecules by cross-linking of neighboring molecules, as in collagen fiber formation
- ***Membrane phospholipid–protein (or carbohydrate) complexes***

For the most part, these molecules constitute the structure of cells and tissues, in that they make up the formed elements of the tissue. They are the basis for the organization that is seen in tissue with the microscope.

In many cases a structural element is at the same time a functional unit. For example, in the case of proteins that make up the contractile filaments of muscle cells, the filaments are the visible structural components and the actual participants in the contractile process. The RNA of the cytoplasm is visualized as part of a structural component (ergastoplasm of gland cells, Nissl bodies of nerve cells), while being the actual participant in the synthesis of protein.

Many tissue components are lost during the preparation of H&E–stained sections

Despite the fact that nucleic acids, proteins, and phospholipids are mostly retained in tissue sections, many are also lost. Small proteins and small nucleic acids, such as transfer RNAs, are generally lost during the preparation of the tissue. Large molecules also may be lost, for example, by being hydrolyzed because of an unfavorable pH of the fixative solutions. Examples of large molecules lost during routine fixation in aqueous fixatives are

- ***Glycogen*** (an intracellular storage carbohydrate common in liver and muscle cells)
- ***Proteoglycans*** and ***glycosaminoglycans*** (extracellular complex carbohydrates found in connective tissue)

These molecules can be preserved, however, by the use of nonaqueous fixative for glycogen or by the addition to the fixative solution of specific binding agents that preserve extracellular carbohydrate-containing molecules. Also, as described above, neutral lipids are usually dissolved by the organic solvents used in tissue preparation.

Soluble components, ions, and small molecules are also lost during preparation of paraffin sections

Intermediary metabolites, glucose, sodium, chloride, and similar substances are lost during preparation of rou-

tine H&E paraffin sections. Many of these substances can be studied in special preparations, sometimes with considerable loss of structural integrity. These small soluble ions and molecules do not make up the formed elements of a tissue; they participate in synthetic processes or cellular reactions. When they can be preserved and demonstrated by specific methods, they provide invaluable information about cell metabolism, active transport, and other vital cellular processes. Water, a highly versatile molecule, participates in these reactions and processes and contributes to the stabilization of macromolecular structure through hydrogen bonding.

Chemical Basis of Staining

ACIDIC AND BASIC DYES

Hematoxylin and eosin are the most commonly used dyes in histology

An ***acidic dye,*** such as eosin, carries a *net negative charge* on its colored portion and is described by the general formula [Na^+dye^-].

A ***basic dye*** carries a *net positive charge* on its colored portion and is described by the general formula [dye^+Cl^-].

Hematoxylin does not meet the definition of a strict basic dye but has properties that closely resemble those of a basic dye. The color of a dye is not related to whether it is basic or acidic, as can be noted by the examples of basic and acidic dyes listed in Table 1.3.

Basic dyes react with anionic components of cells and tissue (components that carry a net negative charge)

Anionic components include the phosphate groups of nucleic acids, the sulfate groups of glycosaminoglycans, and the carboxyl groups of proteins. The ability of such anionic groups to react with a basic dye is called ***basophilia*** *[Gr., base-loving]*. Tissue components that stain with hematoxylin also exhibit basophilia.

TABLE 1.3. **Some Basic and Acidic Dyes**

Dye	Color
Basic dyes	
Methyl green	Green
Methylene blue	Blue
Pyronin G	Red
Toluidine blue	Blue
Acidic dyes	
Acid fuchsin	Red
Aniline blue	Blue
Eosin	Red
Orange G	Orange

The reaction of the anionic groups varies with pH. Thus

- At a high pH (about 10), all three groups are ionized and available for reaction by electrostatic linkages with the basic dye.
- At a *slightly acidic to neutral pH* (5 to 7), sulfate and phosphate groups are ionized and available for reaction with the basic dye by electrostatic linkages.
- At *low pH* (below 4), only sulfate groups remain ionized and react with basic dyes.

Therefore, staining with basic dyes at a specific pH can be used to focus on specific anionic groups, and because the specific anionic groups are found predominantly on certain macromolecules, the staining serves as an indicator of these macromolecules.

As mentioned, hematoxylin is not, strictly speaking, a basic dye. It is used with a mordant (i.e., an intermediate link between the tissue component and the dye). The mordant causes the stain to resemble a basic dye. The linkage in the tissue–mordant–hematoxylin complex is not a simple electrostatic linkage, and when sections are placed in water, hematoxylin does not dissociate from the tissue. Hematoxylin lends itself to those staining sequences in which it is followed by aqueous solutions of acidic dyes. True basic dyes, as distinguished from hematoxylin, are not generally used in sequences wherein the basic dye is followed by an acidic dye. The basic dye then tends to dissociate from the tissue during the aqueous solution washes between the two dye solutions.

Acidic dyes react with cationic groups in cells and tissues, particularly with the ionized amino groups of proteins

The reaction of cationic groups with an acidic dye is called ***acidophilia*** *[Gr., acid-loving]*. Reactions of cell and tissue components with acidic dyes are neither as specific nor as precise as reactions with basic dyes.

Although electrostatic linkage is the major factor in the primary binding of an acidic dye to the tissue, it is not the only one; because of this, acidic dyes are sometimes used in combinations to color different tissue constituents selectively. For example, three acidic dyes are used in the ***Mallory staining technique***: aniline blue, acid fuchsin, and orange G. These dyes selectively stain collagen, ordinary cytoplasm, and red blood cells, respectively. Acid fuchsin also stains nuclei.

In other multiple acidic dye techniques, hematoxylin is used to stain nuclei first, then acidic dyes are used to stain cytoplasm and extracellular fibers selectively. The selective staining of tissue components by acidic dyes is due to relative factors, such as size and degree of aggregation of the dye molecules and permeability and "compactness" of the tissue.

Basic dyes can also be used in combination or sequentially (e.g., methyl green and pyronin to study protein synthesis and secretion), but these combinations are not as widely used as acidic dye combinations.

A limited number of substances within cells and the extracellular matrix display basophilia

These substances include

- *Heterochromatin* and *nucleoli* of the nucleus (chiefly because of ionized phosphate groups in nucleic acids of both)
- *Cytoplasmic components* such as the ergastoplasm (also because of ionized phosphate groups in ribosomal RNA)
- *Extracellular materials* such as the complex carbohydrates of the matrix of cartilage (because of ionized sulfate groups)

Staining with acidic dyes is less specific, but more substances within cells and the extracellular matrix exhibit acidophilia

These substances include

- Most *cytoplasmic filaments,* especially those of muscle cells
- Most *intracellular membranous components* and much of the otherwise unspecialized cytoplasm
- Most *extracellular fibers* (primarily because of ionized amino groups)

Certain basic dyes react with tissue components that shift their normal color from blue to red or purple; this absorbance change is called metachromasia

The underlying mechanism for *metachromasia* is the presence of polyanions within the tissue. When these tissues are stained with a concentrated basic dye solution, such as toluidine blue, the dye molecules are sufficiently close to form dimeric and polymeric aggregates. The absorption properties of these aggregations differ from those of the individual nonaggregated dye molecules.

Cell and tissue structures that have high concentrations of ionized sulfate and phosphate groups, such as the ground substance of cartilage, heparin-containing granules of mast cells, and rough endoplasmic reticulum of plasma cells, exhibit metachromasia. Therefore, toluidine blue will appear purple to red when it stains these components.

ALDEHYDE GROUPS AND THE SCHIFF REAGENT

The ability of bleached basic fuchsin (Schiff reagent) to react with aldehyde groups results in a distinctive red color and is the basis of the periodic acid–Schiff and Feulgen reactions

The *periodic acid–Schiff (PAS) reaction* stains carbohydrates and carbohydrate-rich macromolecules. It is used to demonstrate glycogen in cells, mucus in various cells and tissues, the basement membrane that underlies epithelia, and reticular fibers in connective tissue. The *Feulgen reaction,* which employs a mild hydrochloric acid hydrolysis, is used to stain DNA.

The PAS reaction is based on the following facts:

- Hexose rings of carbohydrates contain adjacent carbons, each of which bears a hydroxyl (—OH) group.
- Hexosamines of glycosaminoglycans contain adjacent carbons, one of which bears an —OH group, while the other bears an amino (—NH_2) group.
- Periodic acid cleaves the bond between these adjacent carbon atoms and forms aldehyde groups.
- These aldehyde groups react with the Schiff reagent to give a distinctive magenta color.

The PAS staining of basement membrane (Fig. 1.2) and reticular fibers is based on the content or association of proteoglycans (complex carbohydrates associated with a protein core). PAS staining is an alternative to silver impregnation methods, which are also based on reaction with the sugar molecules in the proteoglycans.

The Feulgen reaction is based on cleavage of purines from the deoxyribose of DNA by mild acid hydrolysis; the sugar ring then opens with the formation of aldehyde groups. Again, it is the newly formed aldehyde groups that react with the Schiff reagent to give the distinctive magenta color. The reaction of the Schiff reagent with DNA is *stoichiometric* and can be used, therefore, in spectrophotometric methods to quantify the amount of DNA in the nucleus of a cell. RNA does not stain with the Schiff reagent because it lacks deoxyribose.

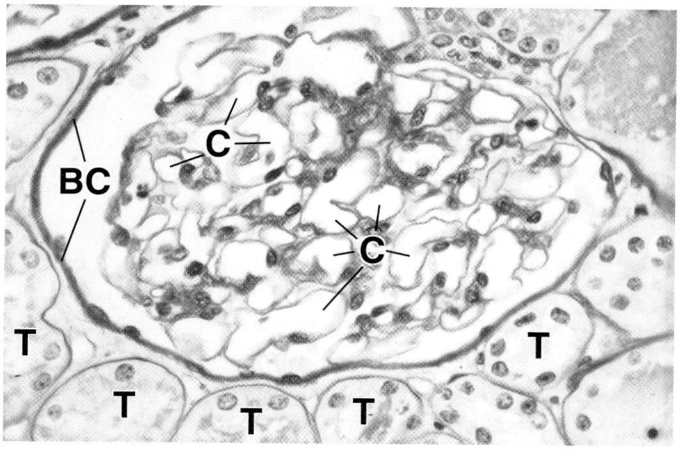

FIGURE 1.2
Photomicrograph of kidney tissue stained by the PAS method. This histochemical method demonstrates and localizes carbohydrate and carbohydrate-rich macromolecules. The basement membranes are PAS positive, as evidenced by the magenta staining of these sites. The kidney tubules *(T)* are sharply delineated by the stained basement membrane surrounding the tubules. The glomerular capillaries *(C)* and the epithelium of Bowman's capsule *(BC)* also show PAS-positive basement membranes. ×360.

BOX 1.1

Functional Considerations: Feulgen Microspectrophotometry

Feulgen microspectrophotometry is a technique that was developed to study DNA increases in developing cells and to analyze ***ploidy,*** i.e., the number of times the normal DNA content of a cell is multiplied (a normal, nondividing cell is said to be ***diploid;*** a sperm or egg cell is ***haploid).*** Recently, it has become a valuable tool for surgical pathologists in evaluating the metastatic potential of a malignant tumor and in making prognostic and treatment decisions. The technique of ***static cytometry*** of Feulgen-stained sections of tumors (contrasted with ***flow cytometry,*** which can only be used on isolated individual cells) uses microspectrophotometry coupled with a digitizing imaging system to measure the absorption of light at 560 nm by cells and cell clusters in Feulgen-stained sections. This technique allows the pathologist to describe ploidy patterns in specific adenocarcinomas (epithelial cancers) and has been particularly useful in studies of breast cancer, kidney cancer, colon and other gastrointestinal cancers, endometrial (uterine epithelium) cancer, and ovarian cancer. Adenocarcinomas that have a largely diploid pattern are said to be well differentiated and have a better prognosis than the same cancers with aneuploidy (nonintegral multiples of the haploid amount of DNA) and tetraploidy.

Enzyme Digestion

Enzyme digestion of a section adjacent to one stained for a specific component, such as glycogen, DNA, or RNA, can be used to confirm the identity of the stained material

Intracellular material that stains with the PAS reaction may be identified as glycogen by pretreatment of sections with diastase or amylase. Abolition of the staining after these treatments positively identifies the stained material as glycogen.

Similarly, pretreatment of tissue sections with deoxyribonuclease (DNAse) will abolish the Feulgen staining in those sections, and treatment of sections of protein secretory epithelia with ribonuclease (RNAse) will abolish the staining of the ergastoplasm with basic dyes.

Enzyme Histochemistry

Histochemical methods are also used to identify and localize enzymes in cells and tissues

To localize enzymes in tissue sections, special care must be taken in fixation to preserve the enzyme activity. Usually, mild aldehyde fixation is the preferred method.

In these procedures, the reaction product of the enzyme activity, rather than the enzyme itself, is visualized. In general, a ***capture reagent,*** either a dye or a heavy metal, is used to trap or bind the reaction product of the enzyme by precipitation at the site of reaction. In a typical reaction to display a hydrolytic enzyme, the tissue section is placed in a solution containing a substrate (AB) and a trapping agent (T) that precipitates one of the products as follows:

$$AB + T \xrightarrow{\text{enzyme}} AT + B$$

where AT is the trapped end product and B is the hydrolyzed substrate.

By using such methods, the lysosome (see page 32), first identified in differential centrifugation studies of cells, was equated with a vacuolar component seen in electron micrographs. In lightly fixed tissues, the acid hydrolases and esterases contained in lysosomes react with an appropriate substrate. The reaction mixture also contains lead ions to precipitate, e.g., lead phosphate derived from the action of acid phosphatase. The precipitated reaction product can then be observed with both light and electron microscopy.

Similar light and electron histochemical procedures have been developed to demonstrate alkaline phosphatase, adenosinetriphosphatases (ATPases) of many varieties (including the Na^+/K^+-ATPase that is the enzymatic basis of the sodium pump in cells and tissues), various esterases, and many respiratory enzymes (Fig. 1.3).

Immunocytochemistry

A foreign protein or other antigen injected into an animal results in production of antibodies

An antibody is a protein produced by certain white blood cells that binds to the foreign substance that stimulated its production. In the laboratory, antibodies can be purified and conjugated (i.e., chemically bound) to a fluorescent dye such as fluorescein. This reagent can then be applied to sections of lightly fixed or frozen tissue on glass slides to localize the antigen in cells and tissues. The reaction can then be examined and photographed with a fluorescence microscope.

The specificity of the reaction between antigen and antibody is the underlying basis of immunocytochemistry

In a typical procedure, a specific protein, such as actin, is isolated from the muscle cells of one species, such as a rat, and injected into the circulation of another species, such as a rabbit. The actin stimulates the formation of antiactin antibodies that circulate in the bloodstream of the rabbit. The antibodies are then removed from the blood of the rabbit, conjugated with a fluorescent dye, and used to stain tissues or cells of the rat suspected of containing actin, such as fibroblasts in connective tissue. If actin is present, the antibodies bind to it, and the reaction is visualized by virtue of

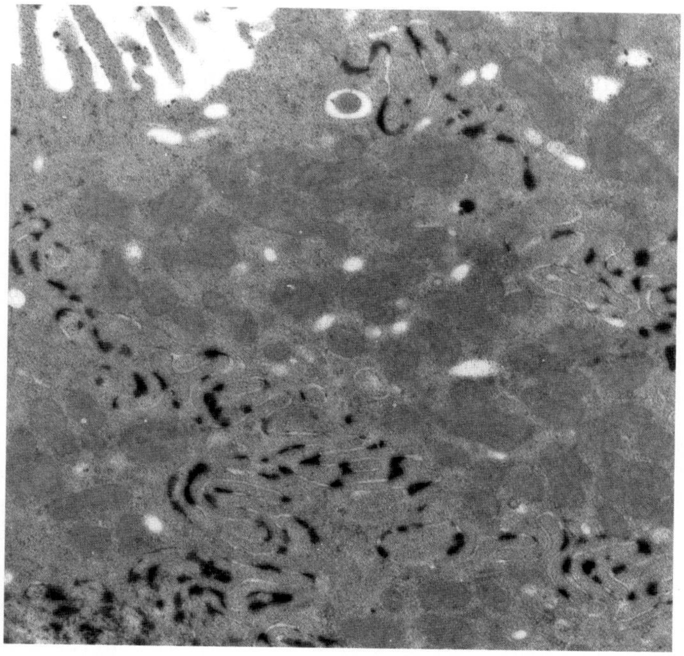

FIGURE 1.3
Electron histochemical procedure for localization of membrane ATPase in epithelial cells of rabbit gallbladder. *Dark areas* visible on the electron micrograph show the location of the enzyme ATPase. This enzyme is detected in the plasma membrane at lateral domains of epithelial cells, which corresponds to the location of sodium pumps. These epithelial cells are involved in active transport of molecules across the plasma membrane. ×26,000.

the fluorescent dye bound to the antibodies (Fig. 1.4). A fluorescence microscope is used to display the fluorescein now attached indirectly to the antigen. It is also possible to conjugate substances such as gold or ferritin (an iron-containing molecule) to the antibody molecule. These markers can be visualized directly with the EM.

Enzyme histochemical methods are combined with traditional immunocytochemical methods to amplify the localization reaction between an antigen and an antibody

In these methods, horseradish peroxidase enzyme is conjugated with a **primary antibody.** Following the antigen–antibody reaction, the histochemical procedure for demonstrating peroxidase activity is run to reveal the location of the antigen–antibody complex (direct reaction). A further refinement of this method attaches the peroxidase to an anti–γ-globulin ***(secondary antibody)*** that binds to the ***primary antibody,*** further amplifying the reaction (indirect reaction). Because the end product of the peroxidase reaction is also visible in the EM, this method is easily adapted to EM immunocytochemistry. Monoclonal antibodies conjugated with ferritin or gold particles may be used as primary antibody stains to achieve even more precise localization of antigens in tissue sections examined in the TEM than is possible with traditional polyclonal antibodies.

An additional advantage of the indirect labeling method is that a single secondary antibody can be used to localize the intracellular or tissue-specific binding of several different primary antibodies. For light microscopic studies, the secondary antibody can be conjugated with different fluorescent dyes so that multiple labels can be shown in the same tissue section (see page 49).

Autoradiography

Autoradiography makes use of a photographic emulsion placed over a tissue section to localize radioactive material within tissues

Many small molecular precursors of larger molecules, such as the amino acids that make up proteins and the nucleotides that make up nucleic acids, may be tagged by incorporation of a radioactive atom or atoms into their molecular structure. The radioactivity is then traced to localize the larger molecules in cells and tissues. Labeled precursor molecules can be injected into animals or introduced into

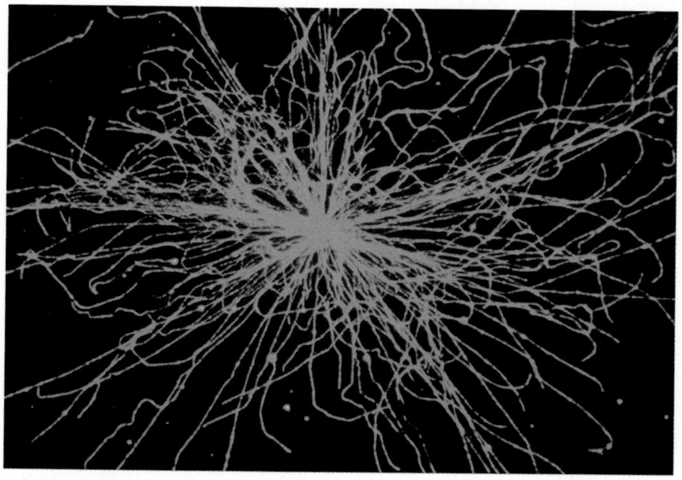

FIGURE 1.4
Microtubules visualized by immunocytochemical methods. The behavior of microtubules (elements of the cell cytoskeleton) obtained from human breast tumor cells can be studied in vitro by measuring their nucleation activity, which is initiated by the centrosome. This image was photographed in the fluorescence microscope. By use of indirect immunofluorescence techniques, microtubules were labeled with a mixture of anti–α-tubulin and anti–β-tubulin monoclonal antibodies (primary antibodies) and visualized by secondary antibodies conjugated with fluorescein dye (fluorescein isothiocyanate–goat antimouse immunoglobulin G). The antigen–antibody reaction, performed directly on the glass coverslip, resulted in visualization of tubulin molecules responsible for the formation of more than 120 microtubules visible on this image. They originate from the centriole and extend outward approximately 20 to 25 μm in a uniform radial array. ×1,400. (Photomicrograph courtesy of Dr. Wilma L. Lingle and Ms. Vivian A. Negron.)

cell or organ cultures. In this way, synthesis of DNA and subsequent cell division, synthesis and secretion of proteins by cells, and localization of synthetic products within cells and in the extracellular matrix have been studied.

Sections of specimens that have incorporated radioactive material are mounted on slides. In the dark, the slide is usually dipped in a melted photographic emulsion, thus producing a thin photographic film on the surface of the slide. After appropriate exposure in a light-tight box, usually for days to weeks, the exposed emulsion on the slide is developed by standard photographic techniques and permanently mounted with a coverslip. The slides may be stained either before or after exposure and development. The silver grains in the emulsion over the radioactively labeled molecules are exposed and developed by this procedure and appear as dark grains overlying the site of the radioactive emission when examined with the light microscope (Fig. 1.5a).

These grains may be used simply to indicate the location of a substance, or they may be counted to provide semiquantitative information about the amount of a given substance in a specific location. For instance, after injection of an animal with tritiated thymidine, cells that incorporated this nucleotide into their DNA prior to dividing but that have not yet divided will have approximately twice as many silver grains overlying their nuclei as will cells that have divided after incorporating the labeled nucleotide.

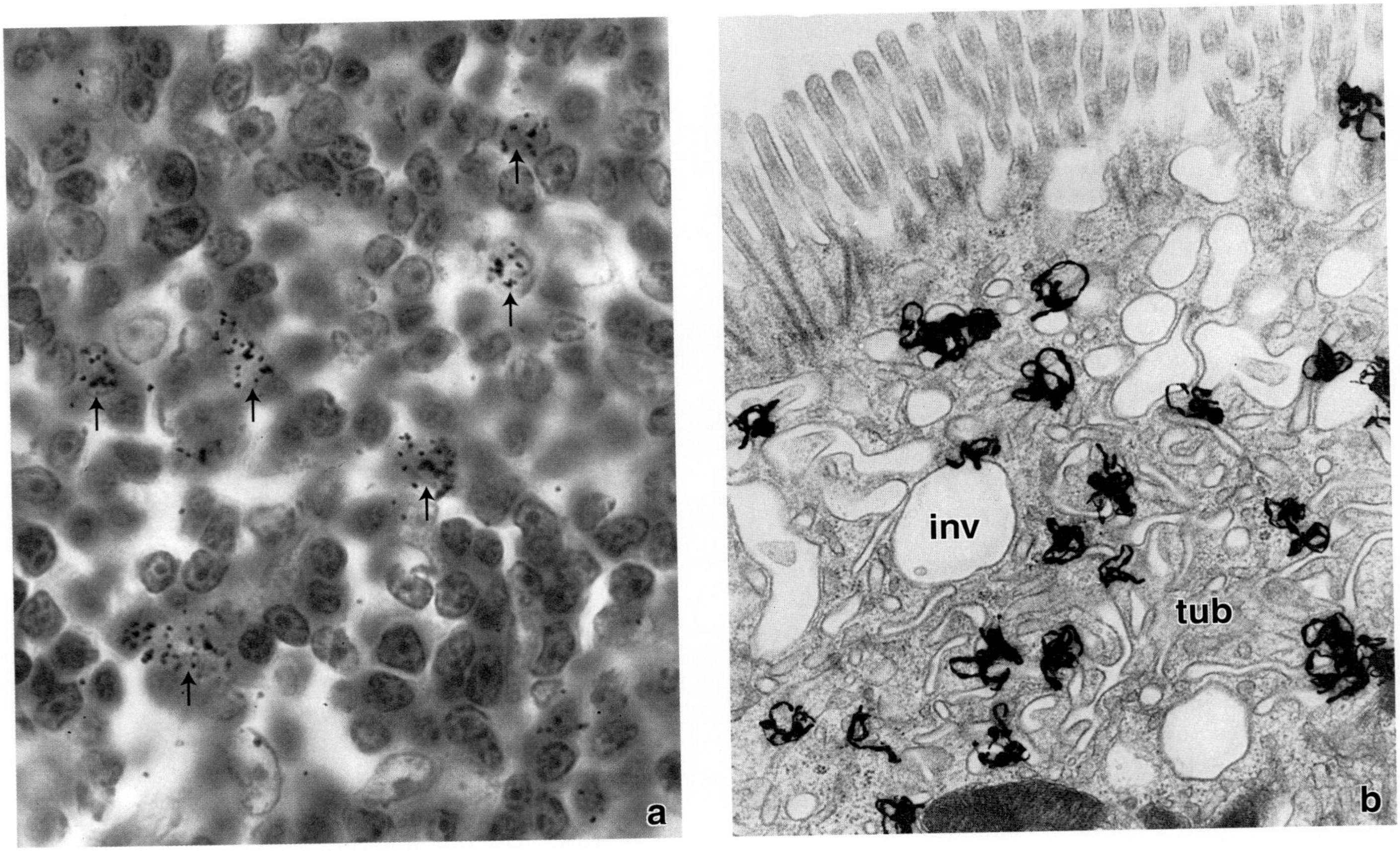

FIGURE 1.5
Examples of autoradiography used in light and electron microscopy. a. Photomicrograph of a lymph node section from an animal injected with tritiated (^{3}H) thymidine. Some of the cells exhibit aggregates of metallic silver grains, which appear as small black particles *(arrows)*. These cells synthesized DNA in preparation for cell division and have incorporated the [^{3}H]thymidine into newly formed DNA. Over time, the low-energy radioactive particles emitted from the [^{3}H]thymidine strike silver halide crystals in a photographic emulsion covering the specimen (exposure) and create a latent image (much like light striking photographic film in a camera). During photographic development of the slide with its covering emulsion, the latent image, actually the activated silver halide in the emulsion, is reduced to the metallic silver, which then appears as black grains in the microscope. ×1,200. (Original slide specimen courtesy of Dr. Ernst Kallenbach.) **b.** Electron microscopic autoradiograph of the apical region of an intestinal absorptive cell. In this specimen, ^{125}I bound to nerve growth factor (NGF) was injected into the animal, and the tissue was removed 1 hour later. The specimen was prepared in a manner similar to that for light microscopy. The relatively small size of the silver grains aids precise localization of the ^{125}I–NGF complexes. Note that the silver grains are concentrated over apical invaginations *(inv)* and early endosomal tubular profiles *(tub)*. ×32,000. (Electron micrograph courtesy of Dr. Marian R. Neutra.)

Autoradiography can also be carried out by using thin plastic sections for examination with the EM. Essentially the same procedures are used, but as with all TEM preparation techniques, the processes are much more delicate and difficult; however, they also yield much greater resolution and more precise localization (Fig. 1.5b).

Historadiography

Historadiography is the production of an x-ray photograph (microradiograph) of a specimen on a slide

A ***historadiograph*** displays mass just as a regular x-ray does. Although x-rays can be used to examine soft tissues, their greatest utility is in the examination of ground sections of bone or other mineralized tissue. In practice, the ground section of bone is placed in contact with a photographic emulsion on a glass slide and exposed to a beam of x-rays. The photographic emulsion is then developed and viewed with a microscope (Fig. 1.6). Standards of known mass can be added to the slide or to a similarly treated companion slide to provide semiquantitative information on the amount of bone mineral in different parts of the ground section.

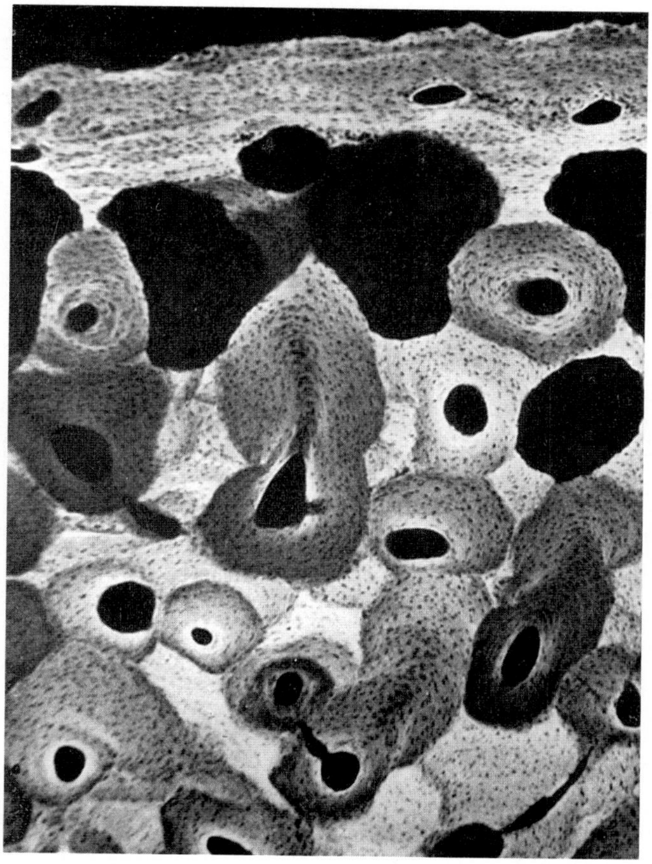

FIGURE 1.6
Microradiograph of a 200-μm-thick section of bone. *Black areas* are sites of soft tissue, *white areas* contain high concentrations of calcium salts, and *light gray to dark gray areas* reflect decreasing amounts of calcium salts. ×157. (Microradiograph courtesy of Dr. Jenifer Jowsey.)

▼ MICROSCOPY

Light Microscopy

A microscope, whether simple (one lens) or compound (multiple lenses), is an instrument that magnifies an image and allows visualization of greater detail than is possible with the unaided eye. The simplest microscope is a magnifying glass or a pair of reading glasses.

The resolving power of the human eye, i.e., the distance by which two objects must be separated to be seen as two objects (0.2 mm), is determined by the spacing of the photoreceptor cells in the retina. The role of a microscope is to magnify an image to a level at which the retina can resolve the information that would otherwise be below its limit of resolution. Table 1.4 compares the resolution of the eye with that of various instruments.

Resolving power is the ability of a microscope lens or optical system to produce separate images of closely positioned objects

Resolution depends not only on the optical system but also on the wavelength of the light source and other factors, such as specimen thickness, quality of fixation, and staining intensity. With light whose wavelength is 540 nm (see Table 1.1), a green-filtered light to which the eye is extremely sensitive, and with appropriate objective and condenser lenses, the greatest attainable resolving power of a bright-field microscope would be about 0.2 μm (see page 16 for method of calculation). This is the theoretical resolution and, as mentioned, depends on all conditions being optimal. *The ocular or eyepiece lens magnifies the image produced by the objective lens, but it cannot increase resolution.*

Various light microscopes are available for general and specialized use in modern biologic research. Their differences are based largely on such factors as the wavelength of specimen illumination, physical alteration of the light coming to or leaving the specimen, and specific analytic processes that can be applied to the final image. These instruments and their applications are described briefly in this section.

TABLE 1.4. **Eye Versus Instrument Resolution**

	Distance Between Resolvable Points
Human eye	0.2 mm
Bright-field microscope	0.2 μm
SEM	2.5 nm
TEM	
Theoretical	0.05 nm
Tissue section	1.0 nm

The microscope used by most students and researchers is the bright-field microscope

The bright-field microscope is the direct descendant of the microscopes that became widely available in the 1800s and opened the first major era of histologic research. The bright-field microscope (Fig. 1.7) essentially consists of

- ***Light source*** for illumination of the specimen, e.g., a substage lamp
- ***Condenser lens*** to focus the beam of light at the level of the specimen
- ***Stage*** on which the slide or other specimen is placed
- ***Objective lens*** to gather the light that has passed through the specimen
- ***Ocular lens*** (or a pair of ocular lenses in the more commonly used binocular microscopes) through which the image formed by the objective lens may be examined directly

A specimen to be examined with the bright-field microscope must be sufficiently thin for light to pass through it. Although some light is absorbed while passing through the specimen, the optical system of the bright-field microscope does not produce a useful level of contrast in the unstained specimen. For this reason, the various staining methods discussed earlier are used. Other optical systems, described below, may be used to enhance the contrast without staining.

The phase contrast microscope enables examination of unstained cells and tissues and is especially useful for living cells

The phase contrast microscope takes advantage of small differences in the refractive index in different parts of a cell or tissue sample. Light passing through areas of relatively high refractive index (denser areas) is deflected and becomes out of phase with the rest of the beam of light that has passed through the specimen. The phase contrast microscope adds other induced-out-of-phase wavelengths through a series of optical rings in the condenser and objective lenses, essentially abolishing the amplitude of the initially deflected portion of the beam and producing contrast in the image. Dark portions of the image correspond to dense portions of the specimen; light portions of the image correspond to less dense portions of the specimen. The phase contrast microscope is therefore used to examine living cells and tissues, such as cells in tissue culture, and is used extensively to examine unstained semithin (approximately 0.5-μm) sections of plastic-embedded tissue.

Two modifications of the phase contrast microscope are the ***interference microscope***, which also allows quantification of tissue mass, and the ***differential interference microscope*** (using Nomarski optics), which is especially useful for assessing surface properties of cells and other biologic objects.

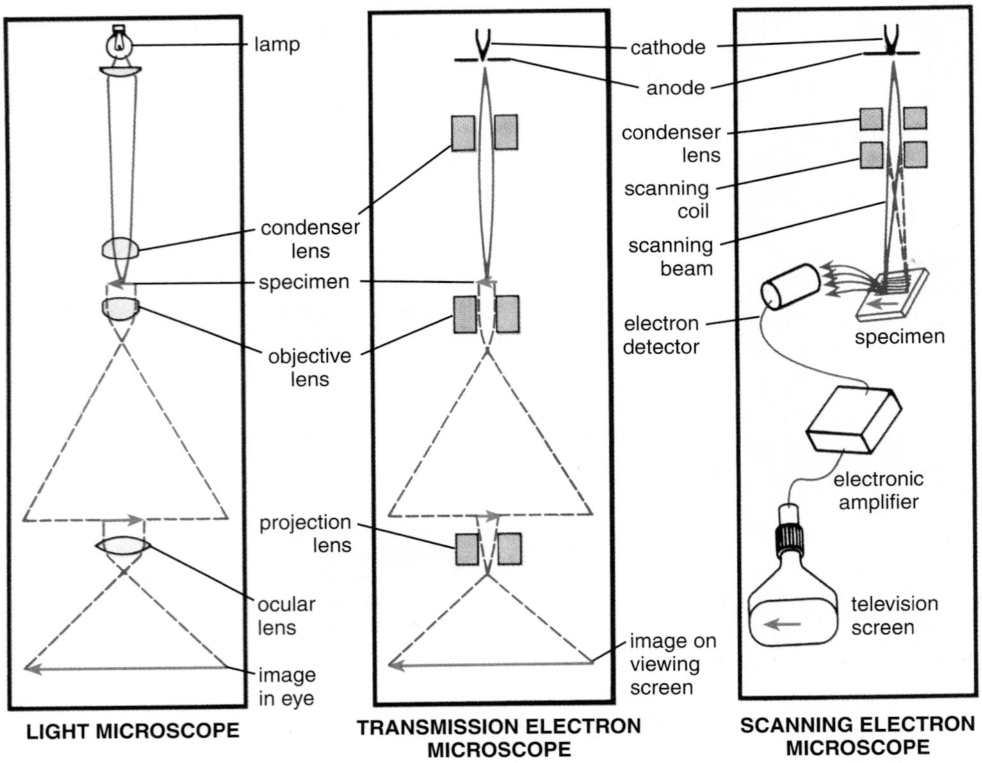

FIGURE 1.7
Diagram comparing the optical paths in different types of microscopes. The light microscope *(left)* is shown as if it were turned upside down; TEM *(middle)*; and SEM *(right)*. The specimen and the projected magnified image are depicted by *red arrows*.

In dark-field microscopy, no direct light from the light source is gathered by the objective lens

In *dark-field microscopy,* only light that has been scattered or diffracted by structures in the specimen reaches the objective. The dark-field microscope is equipped with a special condenser that illuminates the specimen with strong, oblique light. Thus, the field of view appears as a dark background on which small particles in the specimen that reflect some light into the objective appear bright.

The effect is similar to that of dust particles seen in the light beam emanating from a slide projector in a darkened room. The light reflected off the dust particles reaches the retina of the eye, thus making the particles visible.

The resolution of the dark-field microscope cannot be better than that of the bright-field microscope, using, as it does, the same wavelength source. Smaller individual particles can be detected in dark-field images, however, because of the enhanced contrast that is created.

The dark-field microscope is useful in examining autoradiographs, in which the developed silver grains appear white in a dark background. Clinically, it is useful in examining urine for crystals, such as those of uric acid and oxalate, and in demonstrating spirochetes, particularly *Treponema pallidum,* the organism that causes syphilis, a sexually transmitted disease.

The fluorescence microscope makes use of the ability of certain molecules to fluoresce under ultraviolet light

A molecule that fluoresces emits light of wavelengths in the visible range when exposed to an ultraviolet (UV) source. The *fluorescence microscope* is used to display naturally occurring fluorescent (autofluorescent) molecules, such as vitamin A and some neurotransmitters. Because autofluorescent molecules are not numerous, however, its most widespread application is the display of introduced fluorescence, as in the detection of antigens or antibodies in immunocytochemical staining procedures (see Fig. 1.4). Specific fluorescent molecules can also be injected into an animal or directly into cells and used as tracers. Such methods have been useful in studying intercellular (gap) junctions, in tracing the pathway of nerve fibers in neurobiology, and in detecting fluorescent growth markers of mineralized tissues.

Various filters are inserted between the UV light source and the specimen to produce monochromatic or near-monochromatic (single-wavelength or narrow-band-wavelength) light. A second set of filters inserted between the specimen and the objective allows only the narrow band of wavelength of the fluorescence to reach the eye or to reach a photographic emulsion or other analytic processor.

The confocal scanning microscope combines components of a light optical microscope with a scanning system to dissect a specimen optically

The *confocal scanning microscope* is a relatively new microscope system used to study the structure of biologic materials. The illuminating laser light system that it uses is strongly convergent and therefore produces a shallow scanning spot. The light emerging from the spot is directed to a photomultiplier tube, where it is analyzed. A mirror system is used to move the laser beam across the specimen, illuminating a single spot at a time (Fig. 1.8). The data from each point of the specimen scanned by this moving spot are recorded and stored in a computer. This information is then displayed on a high-resolution video monitor to create a visual image. The major advantage of this system is its ability to visualize a specimen in very thin optical sections (approximately 1 μm thick). The out-of-focus regions are subtracted from the image by the computer program, thus creating an extremely sharp image. In these aspects, confocal microscopy resembles the imaging process in computed axial tomography (x-ray) scanning (CAT scans). Ordinary or nonconfocal light imaging contains superimposed in-focus and out-of-focus specimen parts, thereby reducing image quality.

Furthermore, by using only the narrow depth of the in-focus image, it is possible to create multiple images at varying depths within the specimen. Thus, one can literally dissect layer by layer through the thickness of the specimen. It is also possible to use the computer to make three-dimensional reconstructions of a series of these images. Because each individual image located at a specific depth within the specimen is extremely sharp, the resulting assembled three-dimensional image is equally sharp.

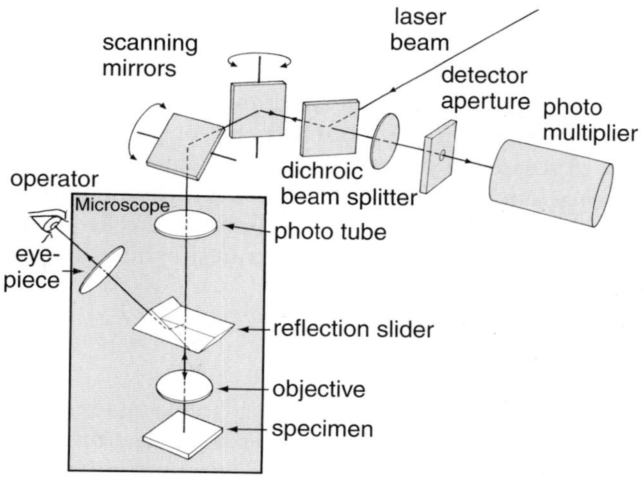

FIGURE 1.8
Diagram of the beam path in the confocal microscope. (Courtesy of Sarastro, Inc., Ypsilanti, MI.)

Moreover, once the computer has assembled each of the sectioned images, the reconstructed three-dimensional image can be rotated and viewed from any orientation desired.

The ultraviolet microscope uses quartz lenses with an ultraviolet light source

The image in the **ultraviolet (UV) microscope** depends on the absorption of UV light by molecules in the specimen. The UV source has a wavelength of approximately 200 nm. Thus, the UV microscope may achieve a resolution of 0.1 μm. In principle, UV microscopy resembles the workings of a spectrophotometer; the results are usually recorded photographically. The specimen cannot be inspected directly through an ocular because the UV light is not visible and is injurious to the eye.

The method is useful in detecting nucleic acids, specifically the purine and pyrimidine bases of the nucleotides. It is also useful for detecting proteins that contain certain amino acids. Using specific illuminating wavelengths, UV spectrophotometric measurements are commonly made through the UV microscope to determine quantitatively the amount of DNA and RNA in individual cells. As described on page 8, it is used clinically to evaluate the degree of ploidy (multiples of normal DNA quantity) in sections of tumors.

The polarizing microscope uses the fact that highly ordered molecules or arrays of molecules can rotate the angle of the plane of polarized light

The ***polarizing microscope*** is a simple modification of the light microscope, in which a polarizing filter, called the ***polarizer,*** is located between the light source and the specimen, and a second polarizer, called the ***analyzer,*** is located between the objective lens and the viewer.

Both the polarizer and the analyzer can be rotated; the difference between their angles of rotation is used to determine the degree by which a structure affects the beam of polarized light. The ability of a crystal or paracrystalline array to rotate the plane of polarized light is called ***birefringence*** (double refraction). Striated muscle and the crystalloid inclusions in the testicular interstitial cells (Leydig cells), among other common structures, exhibit birefringence.

Electron Microscopy

Two kinds of EMs can provide morphologic and analytic data on cells and tissues: the ***transmission electron microscope (TEM)*** and the ***scanning electron microscope (SEM).*** The primary improvement in the EM versus the light microscope is that the wavelength of the EM beam is approximately 1/2,000th that of the light microscope beam, thereby increasing resolution by a factor of 10^3.

The TEM uses the interaction of a beam of electrons with a specimen to produce an image

The "optics" of the TEM are, in principle, similar to those of the light microscope (see Fig. 1.7), except that the TEM uses a beam of electrons rather than a beam of light. The principle of the microscope is as follows:

- A ***source,*** such as a heated tungsten filament, emits electrons ***(cathode).***
- The electrons are attracted toward an ***anode.***
- An electrical difference between the cathode cover and the anode imparts an accelerating voltage of between 20,000 and 200,000 volts to the electrons, creating the beam.
- The beam then passes through a series of ***electromagnetic lenses*** that serve the same function as the glass lenses of a light microscope.

The ***condenser lens*** shapes and changes the diameter of the beam that reaches the specimen plane. The beam that has passed through the specimen is then focused and magnified by an ***objective lens*** and further magnified by one or more ***projector lenses.*** The final image is viewed on a phosphor-coated ***screen.*** Portions of the specimen through which electrons have passed appear bright; those portions of the specimen that have absorbed or scattered electrons because of their inherent density or because of heavy metals added during specimen preparation appear dark. A photographic plate or video detector can be placed above or below the viewing screen to record the image on the screen permanently.

Specimen preparation for transmission electron microscopy is similar to that for light microscopy except that it requires finer methods

The principles used in the preparation of sections for viewing with the TEM are essentially the same as those used in light microscopy, with the added constraint that at every step one must work with specimens 3 to 4 orders of magni-

BOX 1.2

Functional Considerations: Development of Electron Microscopy

The electronic principles of both the TEM and the SEM are similar to those of a cathode ray tube (CRT), such as those used in television sets. In fact, the first EMs, built in the early 1930s, were developed independently in several countries by scientists and engineers working on the development of television. Although some viruses and other dried paracrystalline materials were studied with the EM in the 1930s, it was not until adequate fixation, embedding, and sectioning methods were developed in the 1950s that the TEM could be applied as a routine tool in biologic research.

tude smaller or thinner than those used for light microscopy. The TEM, whose electron beam has a wavelength of approximately 0.1 nm, has a theoretical resolution of 0.05 nm.

Because of the exceptional resolution of the TEM, the quality of fixation, i.e., the degree of preservation of subcellular structure, must be the best achievable.

Routine preparation of specimens for transmission electron microscopy begins with glutaraldehyde fixation followed by a buffer rinse and fixation with osmium tetroxide

Glutaraldehyde, a dialdehyde, preserves protein constituents by cross-linking them; the osmium tetroxide reacts with lipids, particularly phospholipids. The osmium also imparts electron density to cell and tissue structures because it is a heavy metal, thus enhancing subsequent image formation in the TEM.

Ideally, tissues should be perfused with buffered glutaraldehyde before excision from the animal. More commonly, tissue pieces no more than 1 mm^3 are fixed for the TEM (compared with light microscope specimens, which may be measured in centimeters). The dehydration process is identical to that used in light microscopy, and the tissue is infiltrated with a monomeric resin, usually an epoxy resin, which is subsequently polymerized.

The plastic-embedded tissue is sectioned on specially designed microtomes using diamond knives

Because of the limited penetrating power of electrons, sections for routine transmission electron microscopy range from 50 nm to no more than 150 nm. Because abrasives used to sharpen steel knives leave unacceptable scratches on sections viewed in the TEM, diamond knives with nearly perfect sharpness are used. Sections cut by the diamond knife are much too thin to handle; they are floated away from the knife edge on the surface of a fluid-filled trough and picked up from the surface onto plastic-coated copper mesh grids. The grids have 50 to 400 holes/inch or special slots for viewing serial sections. The beam passes through the holes in the copper grid, then through the specimen, and the image is then focused on the viewing screen or photographic film.

Routine staining of transmission electron microscopy sections is necessary to increase the inherent contrast so that the details of cell structure are readily visible and photographable

In general, transmission electron microscopy sections are stained by adding materials of great density, such as ions of heavy metals, to the specimen. Heavy-metal ions may be bound to the tissues during fixation or dehydration or by soaking the sections in solutions of such ions after sectioning. Osmium tetroxide, routinely used in the fixative, binds to the phospholipid components of membranes, imparting additional density to the membranes.

Uranyl nitrate is often added to the alcohol solutions used in dehydration to increase the density of components of cell junctions and other sites. Sequential soaking in solutions of uranyl acetate and lead citrate is routinely used to stain sections before viewing with the TEM to provide high-resolution, high-contrast electron micrographs.

Freeze fracture is a special method of sample preparation for transmission electron microscopy, especially important in the study of membranes

The tissue to be examined may be fixed or unfixed; if it has been fixed, the fixative is washed out of the tissue before proceeding. A cryoprotectant, such as glycerol, is allowed to infiltrate the tissue, and the tissue is then rapidly frozen to about −160°C. Ice crystal formation is prevented by the use of cryoprotectants, rapid freezing, and extremely small tissue samples. The frozen tissue is then placed in a vacuum in the freeze fracture apparatus and struck with a knife edge or razor blade.

The fracture plane passes preferentially through the hydrophobic portion of the plasma membrane, exposing the interior of the plasma membrane

The resulting fracture of the plasma membrane produces two new surfaces. The surface of the membrane that is

BOX 1.3

Functional Considerations: Special Staining for Transmission Electron Microscopy

Many of the histochemical methods used in light microscopy have been adapted for electron microscopy. The use of low-molecular-weight dialdehydes, particularly glutaraldehyde, as primary fixatives has allowed application of many of the standard enzyme histochemical methods to tissue for TEM examination, often requiring only minor modifications of buffers and capture reagents. The phosphatase and esterase procedures have been well adapted for the TEM. The reactions are usually run on 50-μm tissue slices that are subsequently fixed in osmium tetroxide and embedded for TEM sectioning (see Fig. 1.3).

Substitution of a heavy metal–containing compound for the fluorescent dye usually conjugated with an antibody has allowed adaptation of immunocytochemical methods to transmission electron microscopy, as has the adaptation of the diaminobenzidine-based peroxidase reaction. Similarly, refinement of techniques has also allowed development of routine EM autoradiography as an investigative method (see Fig. 1.5b). These methods have been particularly useful in elucidating the cellular sources and intracellular pathways of certain secretory products, the location on the cell surface of specific receptors, and the intracellular location of ingested drugs and substrates.

BOX 1.4

Proper Use of the Light Microscope

This brief introduction to the proper use of the light microscope is directed to those students who will use the microscope for the routine examination of tissues. If the following comments appear elementary, it is only because most users of the microscope fail to use it to its fullest advantage. Despite the availability of today's fine equipment, relatively little formal instruction is given on the correct use of the light microscope.

Expensive and highly corrected optics perform optimally only when the illumination and observation beam paths are centered and properly adjusted. The use of proper settings and proper alignment of the optic pathway will contribute substantially to the recognition of minute details in the specimen and to the faithful display of color for the visual image and for photomicrography.

Köhler illumination is one key to good microscopy and is incorporated in the design of practically all modern laboratory and research microscopes. Figure 1.9 shows the two light paths and all the controls for alignment on a modern laboratory microscope; it should be referred to in following the instructions given below to provide appropriate illumination in your microscope.

The alignment steps necessary to achieve good Köhler illumination are few and simple:

- Focus the specimen.
- Close the field diaphragm.
- Focus the condenser by moving it up or down until the outline of its field diaphragm appears in sharp focus.
- Center the field diaphragm with the centering controls on the (condenser) substage. Then, open the field diaphragm until the light beam covers the full field observed.
- Remove the eyepiece (or use a centering telescope or a phase telescope accessory if available) and observe the exit pupil of the objective. You will see an illuminated circular field, whose radius is directly proportional to the numerical aperture of the objective. As you close the condenser diaphragm, its outline will appear in this circular field. For most stained materials, set the condenser diaphragm to cover approximately two thirds of the objective aperture. This setting results in the best compromise between resolution and contrast (contrast simply being the intensity difference between dark and light areas in the specimen).

Using only these five simple steps, the image obtained will be as good as the optics allow. Now let us find out why.

First, why do we adjust the field diaphragm to cover only the field observed? Illuminating a larger field than the optics can "see" only leads to internal reflections or stray light, resulting in more "noise" or a decrease in image contrast.

Second, why do we emphasize the setting of the condenser diaphragm, i.e., the illuminating aperture? This diaphragm greatly influences the resolution and the contrast with which specimen detail can be observed.

For most practical applications, the resolution is determined by the equation

$$d = \frac{\lambda}{NA_{objective} + NA_{condenser}}$$

where

d	=	point-to-point distance of resolved detail (in nm)
λ	=	wavelength of light used (green = 540 nm)
NA	=	numerical aperature or sine of half angle picked up by the objective or condenser of a central specimen point multiplied by the refractive index of the medium between objective or condenser and specimen

How do wavelength and numerical aperture directly influence resolution? Specimen structures diffract light. The diffraction angle is directly proportional to the wavelength and inversely proportional to the spacing of the structures. According to Ernst Abbé, a given structural spacing can be resolved only when the observing optical system (objective) can see some of the diffracted light produced by the spacing. The larger the objective's aperture, the more diffracted the light that participates in the image formation, resulting in resolution of smaller detail and sharper images.

Our simple formula, however, shows that the condenser aperture is just as important as the objective aperture. This point is only logical when you consider the diffraction angle for an oblique beam or one of higher aperture. This angle remains essentially constant but is presented to the objective in such a fashion that it can be picked up easily.

How does the aperture setting affect the contrast? Theoretically, the best contrast transfer from object to image would be obtained by the interaction (interference) between nondiffracted and all the diffracted wavefronts.

For the transfer of contrast between full transmission and complete absorption in a specimen, the intensity relationship between diffracted and nondiffracted light would have to be 1:1 to achieve full destructive interference (black) or full constructive interference (bright). When the condenser aperture matches the objective aperture, the nondiffracted light enters the objective with full intensity, but only part of the diffracted light can enter, resulting in decreased contrast. In other words, closing the aperture of the condenser to two thirds of the objective aperture brings the intensity relationship between diffracted and nondiffracted light close to 1:1 and thereby optimizes the contrast. Closing the condenser aperture (or lowering the condenser) beyond this equilibrium will produce interference phenomena or image artifacts such as diffraction rings or artificial lines around specimen structures. Most microscope techniques used for the enhancement of contrast, such as dark-field, oblique illumination, phase contrast, or modulation contrast, are based on the same principle; i.e., they suppress or reduce the intensity of the nondiffracted light to improve an inherently low specimen contrast.

By observing the steps outlined above and maintaining clean lenses, the quality and fidelity of visual images will vary only with the performance capability of the optical system.

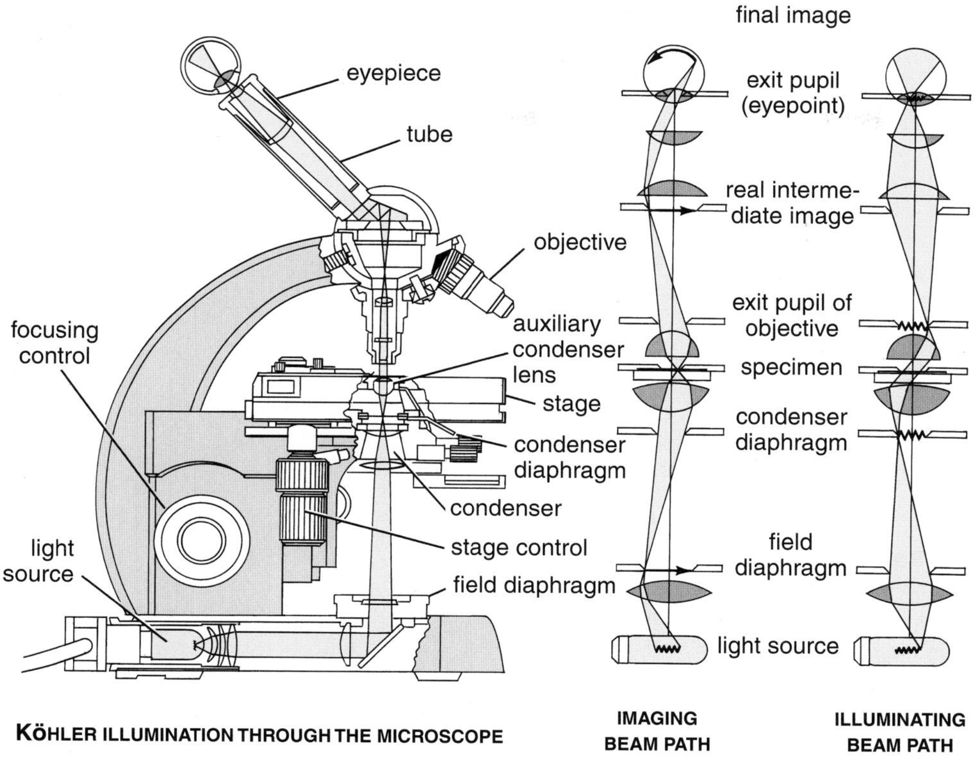

FIGURE 1.9
Diagram of a typical light microscope. This drawing shows a cross-sectional view of the microscope, its operating components, and light path. (Courtesy of Carl Zeiss, Inc., Thornwood, NY.)

backed by extracellular space is called the ***E-face***; the face backed by the protoplasm (cytoplasm) is called the ***P-face***. The specimen is then coated, typically with evaporated platinum, to create a replica of the fracture surface. The tissue is then dissolved, and the surface replica, not the tissue itself, is picked up on grids to be examined with the TEM. Such a replica displays details at the macromolecular level (see Fig. 2.5, page 23).

In scanning electron microscopy, the electron beam does not pass through the specimen but is scanned across its surface

In many ways, the SEM more closely resembles a television tube than the TEM. For examination of most tissues, the sample is fixed, dehydrated by critical point drying, coated with an evaporated gold–carbon film, mounted on an aluminum stub, and placed in the specimen chamber of the SEM. For mineralized tissues, it is possible to remove all the soft tissues with a bleach and then examine the structural features of the mineral.

Scanning is accomplished by the same type of raster that scans the electron beam across the face of a television tube. Electrons reflected from the surface ***(backscattered electrons)*** and electrons forced out of the surface ***(secondary electrons)*** are collected by one or more detectors and reprocessed to form a three-dimensional-like image on a high-resolution CRT.

Photographs may then be taken of the CRT to record data, or the image may be recorded on videotape. Other detectors can be used to measure x-rays emitted from the surface, cathodoluminescence of molecules in the tissue below the surface, and Auger electrons emitted at the surface.

The scanning-transmission electron microscope combines features of the TEM and SEM to allow electron probe x-ray microanalysis

The SEM configuration can be used to produce a transmission image by inserting a grid holder at the specimen level, collecting the transmitted electrons with a detector, and reconstructing the image on a CRT. This latter configuration of a SEM or scanning-transmission electron microscope (STEM) facilitates the use of the instrument for ***electron probe x-ray microanalysis.***

Detectors can be fitted to the microscope to collect the x-rays emitted as the beam bombards the section, and with appropriate analyzers, a map can be constructed that shows the distribution in the sections of elements with an atomic number above 12 and a concentration sufficient to produce enough x-rays to analyze. Semiquantitative data can also be derived for elements in sufficient concentration. Thus, both the TEM and the SEM can be converted into sophisticated analytical tools in addition to being used as "optical" instruments.

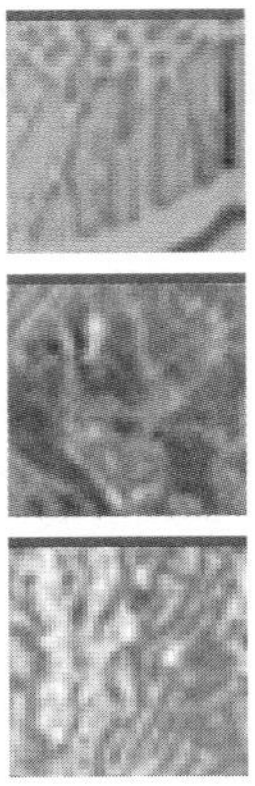

2

The Cell

OVERVIEW OF CELL STRUCTURE

Cells are the basic structural and functional units of all multicellular organisms

The processes we normally associate with the daily activities of organisms, such as protection, ingestion, digestion, absorption of metabolites, elimination of wastes, movement, reproduction, and even death, are all reflections of similar processes occurring within each of the billions of cells that constitute the human body. To a very large extent, similar mechanisms are used by cells of different types to synthesize protein, transform energy, and move essential substances into the cell; they use the same kinds of molecules to engage in contraction, and they duplicate their genetic material in the same manner.

Specific functions are identified with specific structural components and domains within the cell

Some cells develop one or more of these functions to such a degree of specialization that they are identified by the function and the cell structures associated with it. For example, although all cells contain contractile filamentous proteins, some cells, such as ***muscle cells,*** contain large amounts of these proteins in specific arrays. This allows them to carry out their specialized function of contraction at both the cellular and tissue level. The specialized activity or function of a cell may be reflected not only by the presence of a larger amount of the specific structural component performing the activity but also by the shape of the cell, its organization with respect to other similar cells, and its products (Fig. 2.1).

CYTOPLASM

Cells can be divided into two major compartments: the ***cytoplasm*** and the ***nucleus.*** The cytoplasm and the nucleus not only play distinct functional roles but also work in concert to maintain the cell's viability.

The cytoplasm contains organelles and inclusions in a cytoplasmic matrix

Organelles, or "little organs," include the membrane systems of the cell and the membrane-limited compartments that perform the metabolic, synthetic, energy-requiring, and energy-generating functions of the cell, as well as nonmembranous structural components.

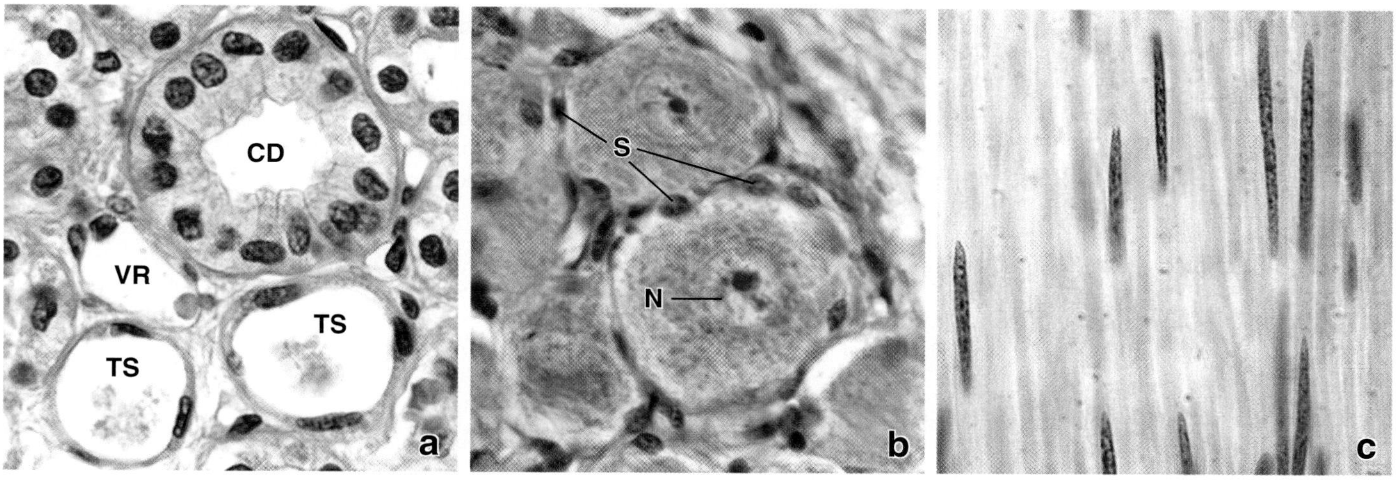

FIGURE 2.1
Different histologic features of different cell types. These three photomicrographs show different types of cells in three different organs of the body. The distinguishing features include size, shape, orientation, and cytoplasmic contents that can be related to each cell's specialized activity or function. **a.** Epithelial cells in the kidney. Note several shapes of epithelial cells: columnar cells with well-defined borders in collecting duct *(CD)*, squamous cells in the thin segment *(TS)* of nephron, and even more flattened cells lining blood vessels, the vasa recta in the kidney *(VR)*. ×380. **b.** Dorsal root ganglion cells. Note the large size of these nerve cell bodies and the large, pale (euchromatic) nuclei *(N)* with distinct nucleoli. Each ganglion cell is surrounded by flattened satellite cells *(S)*. The size of the ganglion cell and the presence of a euchromatic nucleus, prominent nucleolus, and Nissl bodies (rough-surfaced endoplasmic reticulum [rER] visible as darker granules within the cytoplasm) reflect the extensive synthetic activity required to maintain the exceedingly long processes (axons) of these cells. ×380. **c.** Smooth muscle cells of the small intestine. Note that these cells are typically elongated, fusiform-shaped, and organized in a parallel array. The nuclei are also elongated to conform to the general shape of the cell. ×380.

Inclusions are materials in the cytoplasm that may or may not be surrounded by a membrane. They comprise such diverse materials as secretory granules, pigment, neutral fat, glycogen, and stored waste products.

The cytoplasmic ground substance was called *cytosol* in older texts because it was believed to be an amorphous fluid. The term ***cytoplasmic matrix*** is now used to emphasize that it is a concentrated aqueous gel of different-size molecules and has an organized structure.

Intracellular membranes increase surface area and delimit compartments

Many organelles and inclusions are membrane-limited structures; i.e., they are surrounded by a membrane. The membranes form vesicular, tubular, and other structural patterns that may be convoluted (as in the case of the smooth-surfaced endoplasmic reticulum [sER]) or plicated (as in the case of the inner mitochondrial membrane). These membrane configurations greatly increase the surface area on which essential physiologic processes and biochemical reactions take place.

Moreover, the spaces enclosed by membranes constitute intracellular microcompartments in which substrates, products, or other substances are segregated or concentrated. For example, the enzymes of lysosomes are separated by a membrane from the cytoplasmic matrix because their hydrolytic activity would be detrimental to the cell.

Organelles are described as membranous (membrane-limited) or nonmembranous

All cells have the same basic set of intracellular organelles, which can be classified into one of two groups: (1) ***membranous organelles*** with plasma membranes that separate the internal environment of the organelle from the cytoplasm, and (2) ***nonmembranous organelles*** without plasma membranes.

The membranous organelles include

- ***Plasma*** (cell) ***membrane,*** a lipid bilayer that forms the cell boundary as well as the boundaries of many organelles within the cell.
- ***Rough-surfaced endoplasmic reticulum (rER),*** a region of endoplasmic reticulum associated with ribosomes. It is the site of protein synthesis and modification of newly synthesized proteins.
- ***Smooth-surfaced endoplasmic reticulum (sER),*** a region of endoplasmic reticulum involved in lipid and steroid synthesis. It is not associated with ribosomes.
- ***Golgi apparatus,*** a membranous organelle composed of multiple flattened cisternae responsible for modifying, sorting, and packaging proteins and lipids for intracellular or extracellular transport.
- ***Endosomes,*** membrane-bounded compartments interposed within endocytotic pathways. Their major function is sorting proteins delivered to them via endocytotic vesicles and redirecting them to different cellular compartments for their final destination.
- ***Lysosomes,*** small organelles containing digestive enzymes; their derivatives include ***phagosomes, phagolysosomes, autophagosomes,*** and ***autophagolysosomes.***
- ***Transport vesicles,*** which include ***pinocytotic vesicles, endocytotic vesicles,*** and ***coated vesicles.*** These vesicles are involved in both endocytosis and exocytosis and vary in shape and the material that they transport.
- ***Mitochondria,*** organelles that provide most of the energy to the cell by producing adenosine triphosphate (ATP) in the process of oxidative phosphorylation.
- ***Peroxisomes,*** small organelles involved in the production and degradation of H_2O_2 and degradation of fatty acids.

The nonmembranous organelles include

- ***Microtubules,*** which together with actin and intermediate filaments form elements of the ***cytoskeleton.*** Microtubules continuously elongate (by adding tubulin dimers) and shorten (by removing tubulin dimers), a property referred to as ***dynamic instability.***
- ***Filaments,*** which are also part of the cytoskeleton. In general, filaments can be classified into one of two groups: ***actin filaments,*** which are flexible chains of globular actin molecules, and ***intermediate filaments,*** which are rope-like fibers formed from a variety of proteins. Both provide tensile strength to withstand tension and confer resistance to shearing forces.
- ***Centrioles,*** short, paired cylindrical structures found in the center of the ***centrosome.*** Derivatives of centrioles give rise to basal bodies of cilia.
- ***Ribosomes,*** structures composed of ribosomal RNA (rRNA) and ribosomal proteins (including proteins attached to membranes of the rER and proteins free in the cytoplasm). Ribosomes are essential for protein synthesis.

An outline of the key features relating to the identification of cell organelles and inclusions is provided at the end of the chapter (see Table 2.3, page 76). The normal function and the related pathologies are also summarized (see Table 2.4, page 77).

▼ MEMBRANOUS ORGANELLES

Plasma Membrane

The plasma membrane is a lipid-bilayered structure visible with transmission electron microscopy

The ***plasma membrane (cell membrane)*** is a dynamic structure that actively participates in many physiologic and biochemical activities essential to cell function and survival.

When the plasma membrane is properly fixed, sectioned, stained, and viewed on edge with the transmission electron

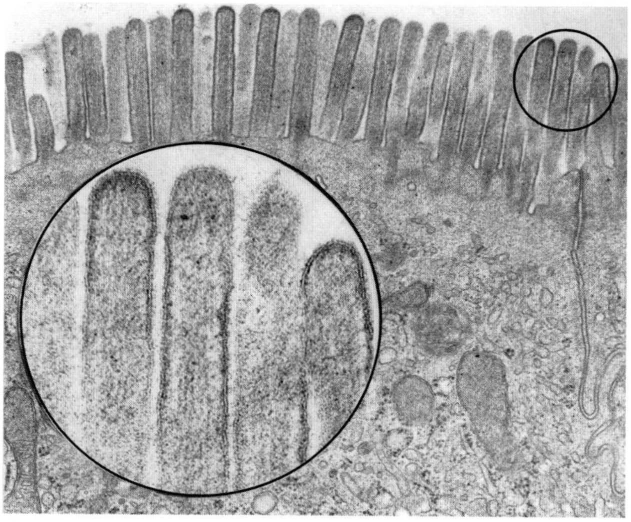

FIGURE 2.2
Absorptive cells of the small intestine. This electron micrograph shows the apical portion of absorptive cells with microvilli. ×29,000. **Inset.** Higher magnification of the area within the *circle.* Note that at this magnification the plasma membrane displays its characteristic appearance, showing two electron-dense lines separated by an electron-lucent intermediate layer. ×95,000.

microscope (TEM), it appears as two electron-dense layers separated by an intermediate, electron-lucent (nonstaining) layer (Fig. 2.2). The total thickness of the plasma membrane is about 8 to 10 nm.

The plasma membrane is composed of amphipathic lipids and two types of proteins

The current interpretation of the molecular organization of the plasma membrane is referred to as the ***modified fluid-mosaic model*** (Fig. 2.3). The membrane consists primarily of ***phospholipid, cholesterol,*** and ***protein*** molecules. The lipid molecules form a ***lipid bilayer*** with an amphipathic character (it is both hydrophobic and hydrophilic). The fatty acid chains of the lipid molecules face each other, making the inner portion of the membrane ***hydrophobic*** (i.e., having no affinity for water). The surfaces of the membrane are formed by the polar head groups of the lipid molecules, thereby making the surfaces ***hydrophilic*** (i.e., having an affinity for water).

In most plasma membranes, protein molecules constitute approximately half of the total membrane mass. Most

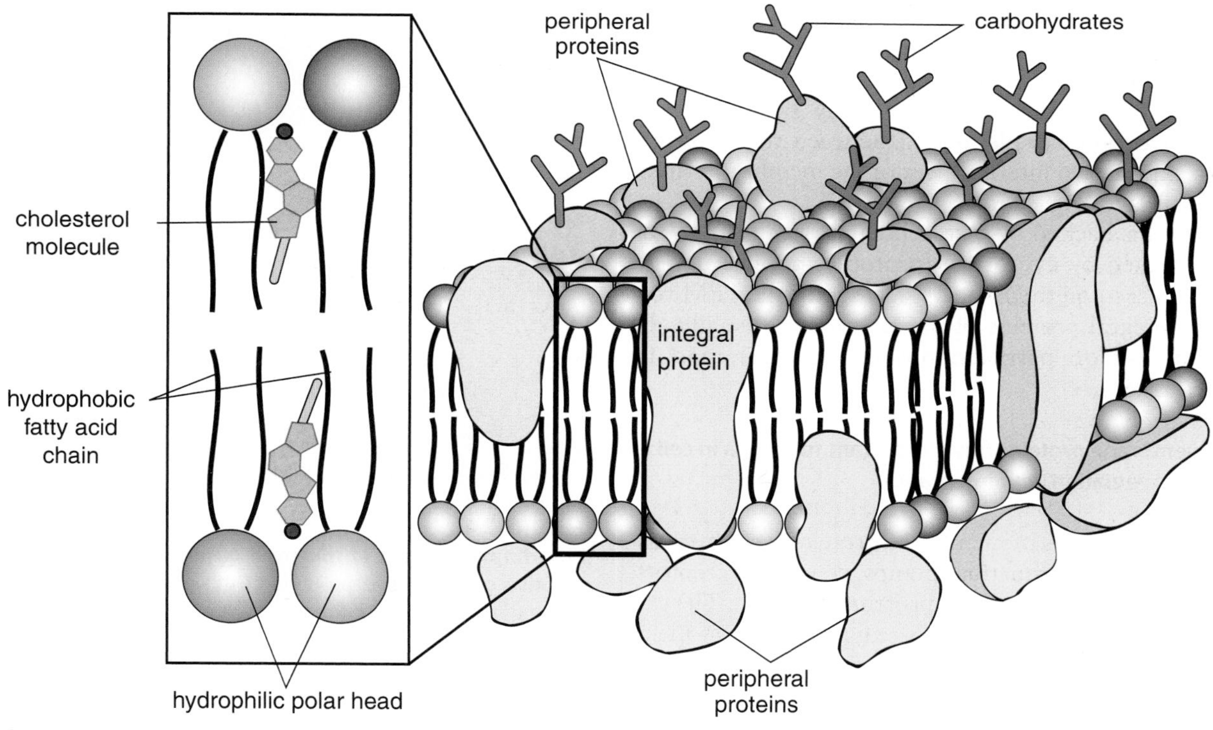

FIGURE 2.3
Diagram of a plasma membrane showing the modified fluid-mosaic model. The plasma membrane is a lipid bilayer consisting primarily of phospholipid molecules, cholesterol, and protein molecules. The hydrophobic fatty acid chains of phospholipids face each other to form the inner portion of the membrane, while the hydrophilic polar heads of the phospholipids form the extracellular and intracellular surfaces of the membrane. Cholesterol molecules are incorporated within the gaps between phospholipids equally on both sides of the membrane. Note the asymmetric distribution of specific phospholipids in the membrane bilayer *(indicated by the different colors of the phospholipid heads).* The diagram also shows integral membrane proteins and peripheral membrane proteins. Carbohydrate chains attach to both integral and peripheral membrane proteins, forming glycoproteins, and to polar phospholipid heads, forming glycolipids.

of the proteins are embedded within the lipid bilayer or pass through the lipid bilayer completely. These proteins are called ***integral membrane proteins.*** Integral membrane proteins can move within the plane of the membrane; this movement can be compared to the movement of icebergs floating in the ocean (see Fig. 2.3). The other types of protein, called ***peripheral membrane proteins,*** are not embedded within the lipid bilayer. They are associated with the plasma membrane by strong ionic interactions, mainly with integral proteins on both the extracellular and intracellular surfaces of the membrane (see Fig. 2.3). In addition, on the extracellular surface of the plasma membrane, carbohydrates may be attached to proteins, thereby forming ***glycoproteins,*** or to lipids of the bilayer, thereby forming ***glycolipids.*** These surface molecules constitute a layer at the surface of the cell, referred to as the ***cell coat*** or ***glycocalyx*** (Fig. 2.4). They help establish extracellular microenvironments at the membrane surface that have specific functions in metabolism, cell recognition and cell association, and serve as receptor sites for hormones.

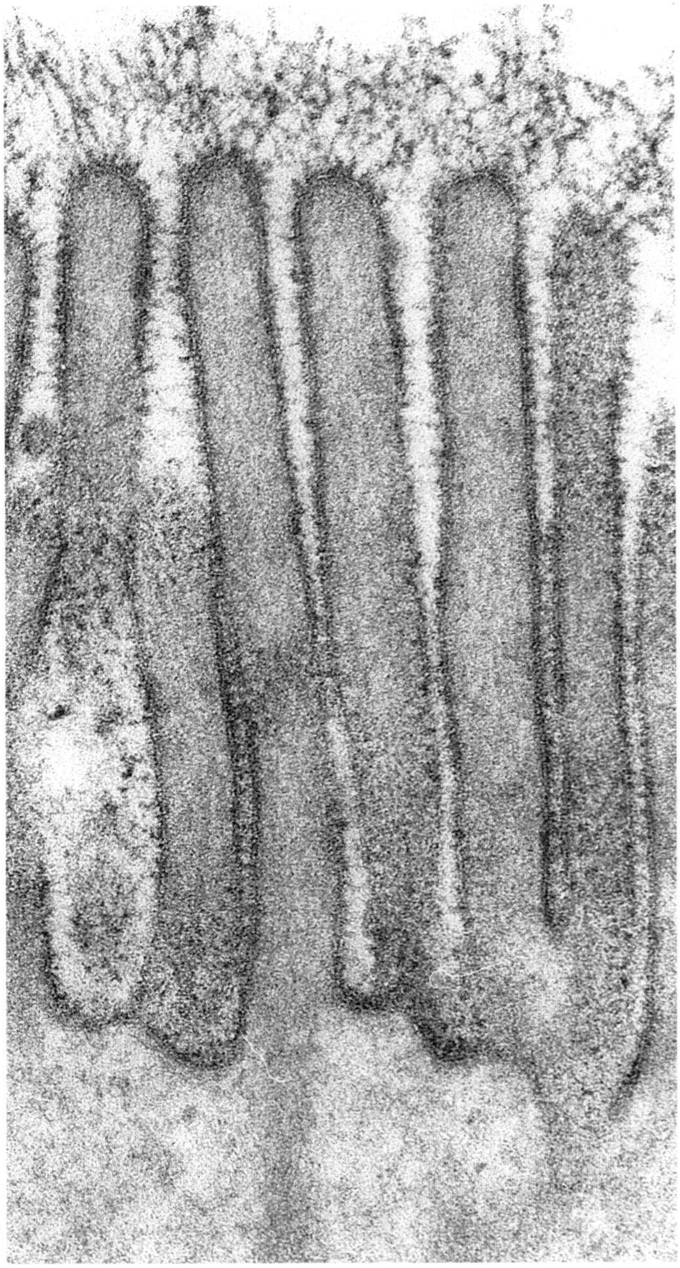

FIGURE 2.4
Electron micrograph of microvilli on the apical surface of an absorptive cell. The glycoproteins of the glycocalyx can be seen extending from the tips of the microvilli into the lumen. At this magnification, the relationship between the outer plasma membrane leaflet and the glycocalyx is particularly well demonstrated. Glycoproteins of the glycocalyx include terminal digestive enzymes such as dipeptidases and disaccharidases. ×100,000. (Courtesy of Dr. Ray C. Henrikson.)

Integral membrane proteins can be visualized with the special tissue preparation technique of freeze fracture

The existence of protein within the substance of the plasma membrane, i.e., integral proteins, was confirmed by a technique called ***freeze fracture.*** When tissue is prepared for electron microscopy by the freeze fracture process (Fig. 2.5a), membranes typically split or cleave along the hydrophobic plane (i.e., between the two lipid layers) to expose two interior faces of the membrane, an E-face and a P-face (Fig. 2.5b).

The ***E-face*** is backed by extracellular space, whereas the ***P-face*** is backed by cytoplasm (protoplasm). The numerous particles seen on the E- and P-faces with the TEM represent the integral proteins of the membrane. Usually, the P-face displays more particles, thus more protein, than the E-face (Fig. 2.5c).

Integral membrane proteins have important functions in cell metabolism, regulation, and integration

Six broad categories of membrane proteins have been defined in terms of their function: pumps, channels, receptors, linkers, enzymes, and structural proteins (Fig. 2.6). The categories are not mutually exclusive; e.g., a structural membrane protein may simultaneously serve as a receptor, an enzyme, a pump, or any combination of these functions.

- ***Pumps*** serve to transport certain ions, such as Na^+, actively across membranes. Pumps also transport metabolic precursors of macromolecules, such as amino acids and sugars, across membranes, either by themselves or linked to the Na^+ pump.
- ***Channels*** allow the passage of small ions and molecules across the plasma membrane in either direction, i.e.,

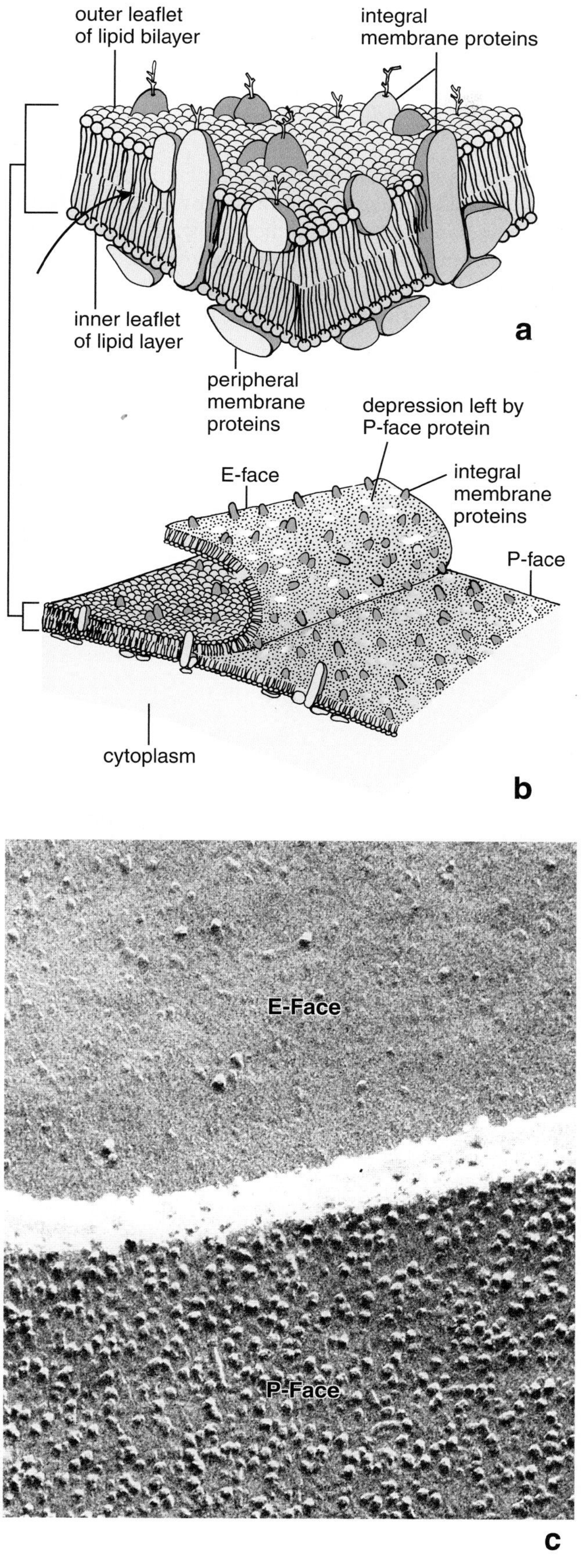

FIGURE 2.5
Freeze fracture examination of the plasma membrane. a. View of the plasma membrane seen on edge, with *arrow* indicating the preferential plane of splitting of the lipid bilayer through the hydrophobic portion of the membrane. When the membrane splits, some proteins are carried with the outer leaflet, though most are retained within the inner leaflet. **b.** View of the plasma membrane with the leaflets separating along the cleavage plane. The surfaces of the cleaved membrane are coated, forming replicas; the replicas are separated from the tissue and examined with the TEM. Proteins appear as bumps. The replica of the inner leaflet is called the P-face; it is backed by cytoplasm (protoplasm). A view of the outer leaflet is called the E-face; it is backed by extracellular space. **c.** Electron micrograph of a freeze fracture replica shows the E-face of the membrane of one epithelial cell and the P-face of the membrane of the adjoining cell. The cleavage plane has jumped from the membrane of one cell to the membrane of the other cell, as indicated by the clear space (intercellular space) across the middle of the figure. Note the paucity of particles in the E-face compared with the P-face, from which the majority of the integral membrane proteins project. (Courtesy of Dr. Giuseppina d'Elia Raviola.)

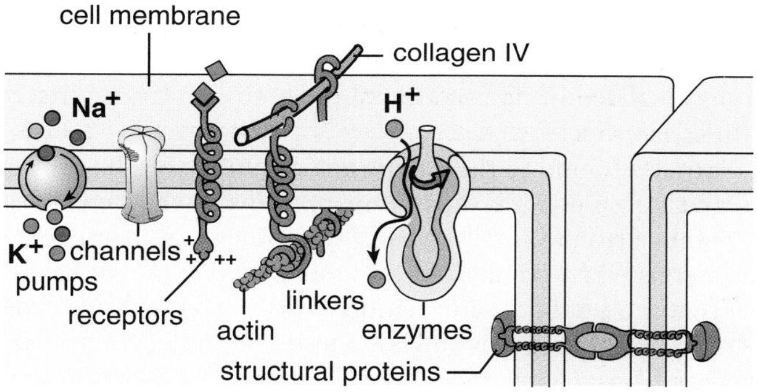

FIGURE 2.6
Different functions of integral membrane proteins. The six major categories of integral membrane proteins are shown in this diagram. These are pumps, channels, receptors, linkers, enzymes, and structural proteins. These categories are not mutually exclusive. A structural membrane protein involved in cell-to-cell junctions might simultaneously serve as receptor, enzyme, linker, or any combination of these functions.

passive diffusion. Gap junctions formed by aligned channels in the membranes of adjacent cells permit passage of ions and small molecules from the cytoplasm of one cell to the cytoplasm of the adjacent cells.

- ***Receptor proteins*** allow recognition and localized binding of ligands (molecules that bind to the extracellular surface of the plasma membrane) in processes such as hormonal stimulation, coated-vesicle endocytosis, and antibody reactions.

- ***Linker proteins*** anchor the intracellular cytoskeleton to the extracellular matrix. Examples of linker proteins include the family of integrins that link cytoplasmic actin filaments to an extracellular matrix protein (fibronectin).
- ***Enzymes*** have a variety of roles. Adenosine triphosphatases (ATPases) have specific roles in ion pumping: ATP synthase is the major protein of the inner mitochondrial membrane, and digestive enzymes such as disaccharidases and dipeptidases are integral membrane proteins.
- ***Structural proteins*** are visualized by the freeze fracture method, especially where they form junctions with neighboring cells. Often, certain proteins and lipids are concentrated in localized regions of the plasma membrane to carry out specific functions. Examples of such regions can be recognized in polarized cells, such as epithelial cells.

Integral membrane proteins move within the lipid bilayer of the membrane

The fluidity of the plasma membrane is not revealed in static electron micrographs. However, experiments show that the membrane behaves as though it were a two-dimensional lipid fluid. Proteins with their hydrophobic regions localized in the interior of the lipid bilayer are free to diffuse laterally.

Particles bound to the membrane can move on the surface of a cell; even integral membrane proteins, such as enzymes, may move from one cell surface to another, e.g., from apical to lateral, when barriers to flow, such as cell junctions, are disrupted. The fluidity of the membrane is a function of the types of phospholipids in the membrane and variations in their local concentration.

Integral membrane proteins may move to mediate a hormone response or to sort (or move) to a different region of the plasma membrane. The lateral diffusion of proteins is often limited by physical connections between membrane proteins and intracellular or extracellular structures. Such connections may exist

- Between proteins associated with cytoskeletal filaments and portions of the membrane proteins that extend into the adjacent cytoplasm
- Between the cytoplasmic domains of membrane proteins
- Between peripheral proteins associated with the extracellular matrix and the integral membrane proteins that extend from the cell surface, i.e., the extracellular domain

Through these connections, proteins can be localized or restricted to "specialized" regions of the plasma membrane or act as transmembrane linkers between intracellular and extracellular filaments (see below).

MEMBRANE TRANSPORT AND VESICULAR TRANSPORT

Substances that enter or leave the cell must traverse the plasma membrane

Some substances (fat-soluble and small, uncharged molecules) cross the plasma membrane by ***simple diffusion*** down their concentration gradient (Fig. 2.7a). All other molecules require ***membrane transport proteins*** to provide them with individual passage across the plasma membrane.

There are generally two classes of transport proteins:

- ***Carrier proteins*** transfer small, water-soluble molecules. They are highly selective, often transporting only one type of molecule. After binding to a molecule designated for transport, the carrier protein undergoes a series of conformational changes and releases the molecule on the other side of the membrane (Fig. 2.7b). Some carrier proteins, such as the Na^+/K^+ pump or H^+ pump, require

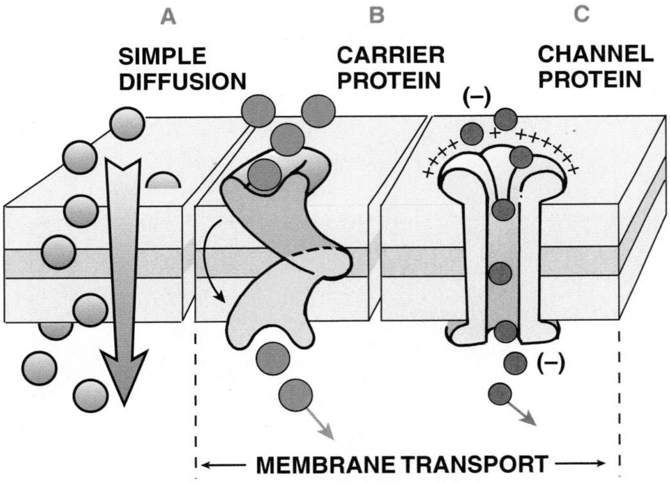

FIGURE 2.7
Movement of molecules through the plasma membrane. a. Fat-soluble and other small uncharged molecules (in *green*) cross the plasma membrane by simple diffusion down their concentration gradient. **b.** Other molecules require membrane transport proteins to provide them with individual passage across the plasma membrane. Small water-soluble molecules (in *blue*) require highly selective carrier proteins to transfer them across the plasma membrane. After binding with a molecule, the carrier protein undergoes a series of conformational changes and releases the molecule on the other side of the membrane. If the process requires energy, it is called active transport (e.g., transport of H^+ ions against their concentration gradient). The process is called passive transport when energy is not required (e.g., glucose transport). **c.** Ions and other small charged molecules (in *red*) are transported through the plasma membrane by ion-selective channel proteins. In neurons, for instance, ion transport is regulated by membrane potentials (voltage-gated ion channels); in skeletal muscle cells, neuromuscular junctions possess ligand-gated ion channels.

energy for ***active transport*** of molecules against their concentration gradient. Other carrier proteins, such as glucose carriers, do not require energy and participate in ***passive transport.***

- ***Channel proteins*** also transfer small, water-soluble molecules. Channel proteins create hydrophilic channels through the plasma membrane that regulate the transport of the molecule (Fig. 2.7c). They are ion selective and are regulated on the basis of the cell's needs. Channel protein transport can be regulated by membrane potentials (e.g., ***voltage-gated ion channels*** in neurons), neurotransmitters (e.g., ***ligand-gated ion channels*** such as acetylcholine receptors in muscle cells), or mechanical stress (e.g., ***stress-activated channels*** in the inner ear).

Vesicular transport maintains the integrity of the plasma membrane and also provides for the transfer of molecules between different cellular compartments

Some substances enter and leave cells by ***vesicular transport,*** a process that involves conformational changes in the plasma membrane at localized sites and subsequent formation of vesicles from the membrane or fusion of vesicles with the membrane (Fig. 2.8).

The major mechanism by which large molecules enter, leave, and move within the cell is called ***vesicle budding.*** Vesicles formed by budding from the plasma membrane of one compartment fuse with the plasma membrane of another compartment. Within the cell, this process ensures intercompartmental transfer of the vesicle contents.

Vesicular transport involving the cell membrane may also be described in more specific terms:

- ***Endocytosis*** is the general term for processes of vesicular transport in which substances enter the cell.
- ***Exocytosis*** is the general term for processes of vesicular transport in which substances leave the cell.

Both processes can be visualized with the electron microscope.

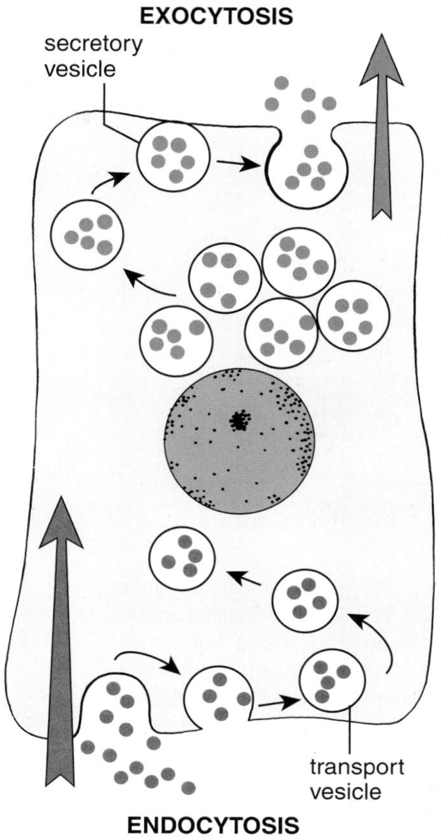

FIGURE 2.8
Endocytosis and exocytosis are two major forms of vesicular transport. Endocytosis brings molecules and other substances into the cell. In exocytosis, synthesized molecules and other substances leave the cell. Endocytosis is associated with the formation and budding of vesicles from the plasma membrane; exocytosis is associated with the fusion of vesicles originating from intracellular organelles with the plasma membrane and is a primary secretory modality.

ENDOCYTOSIS

Uptake of fluid and macromolecules during endocytosis depends on three different mechanisms

Some of the endocytotic mechanisms require special proteins during vesicle formation. The best known protein that interacts with the plasma membrane in vesicle formation is ***clathrin.*** Therefore, endocytosis can be also be classified as either clathrin dependent or clathrin independent. In general, three mechanisms of endocytosis are recognized in the cell:

- ***Pinocytosis*** *[Gr., cell drinking]* is the ingestion of fluid and small protein molecules via small vesicles, usually smaller than 150 nm in diameter. Pinocytosis is performed by virtually every cell in the organism, and it is ***constitutive;*** i.e., it involves a continuous dynamic formation of small vesicles at the cell surface (Fig. 2.9a). Recent studies indicate that mechanoenzymes such as GTPase (dynamin) are involved in pinocytotic vesicle scission (the process of pinching off from the plasma membrane). Pinocytotic vesicles are visible with the TEM, and they have a smooth surface. These smooth pinocytotic vesicles are especially numerous in the endothelium of blood vessels (Fig. 2.9b) and in smooth muscle cells. Pinocytosis does not require clathrin and therefore may be referred to as ***clathrin-independent endocytosis.***
- ***Receptor-mediated endocytosis*** allows entry of specific molecules into the cell. In this mechanism, receptors for specific molecules, called ***cargo receptors,*** accumulate in

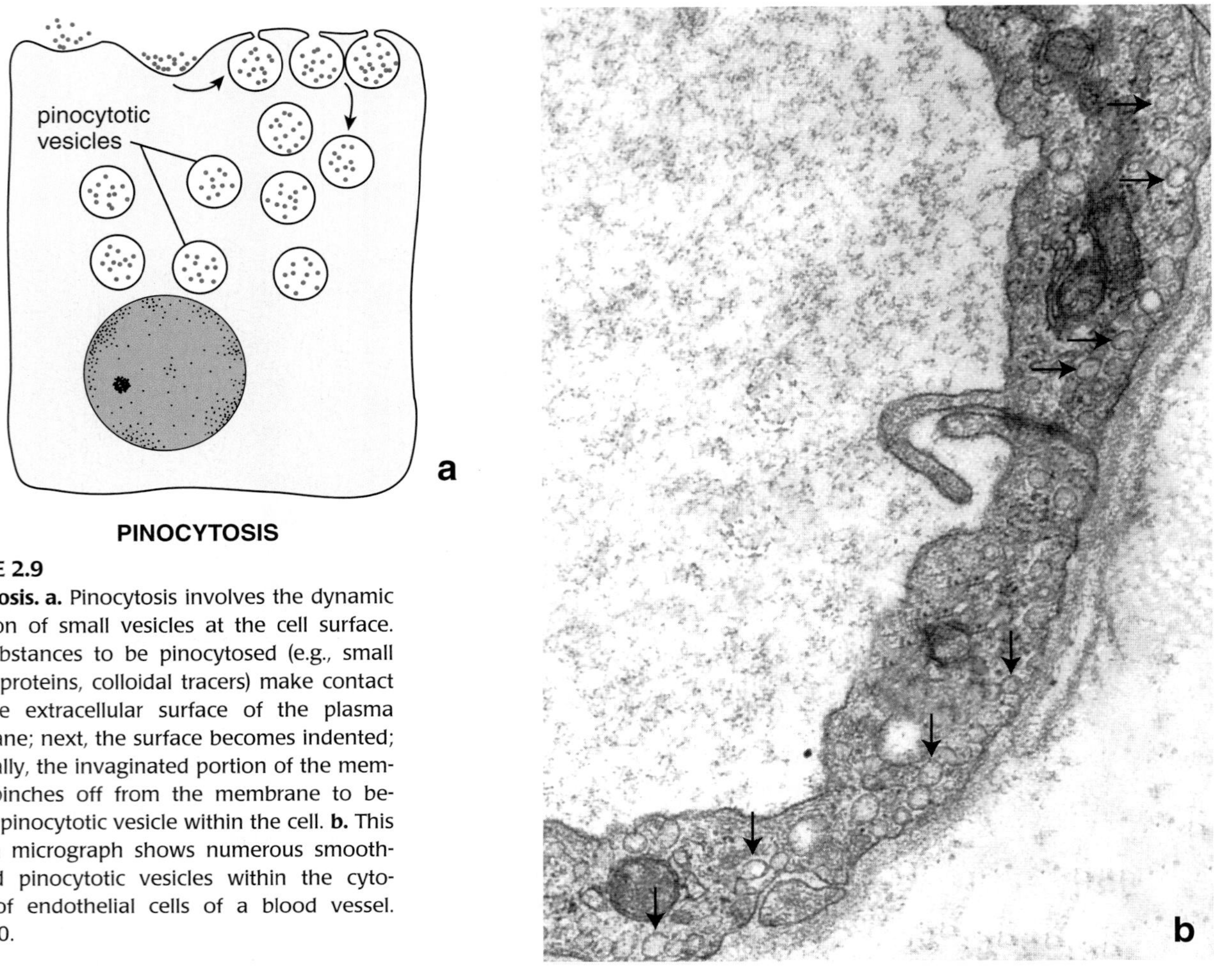

FIGURE 2.9
Pinocytosis. a. Pinocytosis involves the dynamic formation of small vesicles at the cell surface. First, substances to be pinocytosed (e.g., small soluble proteins, colloidal tracers) make contact with the extracellular surface of the plasma membrane; next, the surface becomes indented; and finally, the invaginated portion of the membrane pinches off from the membrane to become a pinocytotic vesicle within the cell. **b.** This electron micrograph shows numerous smooth-surfaced pinocytotic vesicles within the cytoplasm of endothelial cells of a blood vessel. ×60,000.

well-defined regions of the cell membrane. These regions eventually become ***coated pits*** (Fig. 2.10a). The name "coated pit" is derived from their appearance in the electron microscope as an accumulation of electron-dense material that represents aggregation of clathrin molecules on the cytoplasmic surface of the plasma membrane. Cargo receptors recognize and bind to specific molecules that come in contact with the plasma membrane. Clathrin molecules then assemble into a basket-like cage that helps change the shape of the plasma membrane at that site into a vesicle-like invagination (Fig. 2.10b). Clathrin interacts with the cargo receptor via another coating protein, ***adaptin,*** which is instrumental in selecting appropriate cargo molecules for transport into the cells. Thus, selected cargo proteins and their receptors are pulled from the extracellular space into the lumen of a forming vesicle. The large (100-kDa) mechanoenzyme (GTPase, also called ***dynamin***) mediates the liberation of forming clathrin-coated vesicles from the plasma membrane during receptor-mediated endocytosis. The type of vesicle formed as a result of receptor-mediated endocytosis is referred to as a ***coated vesicle,*** and the process itself is known as ***clathrin-dependent endocytosis.*** Clathrin-coated vesicles are also involved in the movement of the cargo material from the plasma membrane to endosomes and from the Golgi apparatus to the plasma membrane.

- ***Phagocytosis*** *[Gr., cell eating]* is the ingestion of large particles such as cell debris, bacteria, and other foreign materials. In this process, large vesicles (larger than approximately 250 nm in diameter) called phagosomes are produced. Phagocytosis is performed mainly by a specialized group of cells belonging to the mononuclear phagocytotic system (MPS). Phagocytosis is generally a receptor-mediated process in which receptors on the cell surface recognize non–antigen-binding domains (F_c fragments) of antibodies coating the surface of an invading microorganism or cell (Fig. 2.11a). However, nonbiologic materials such as inhaled carbon particles, inorganic dusts, and asbestos fibers, as well as biologic debris from inflammation, wound healing, and dead cells, are sequestered by cells

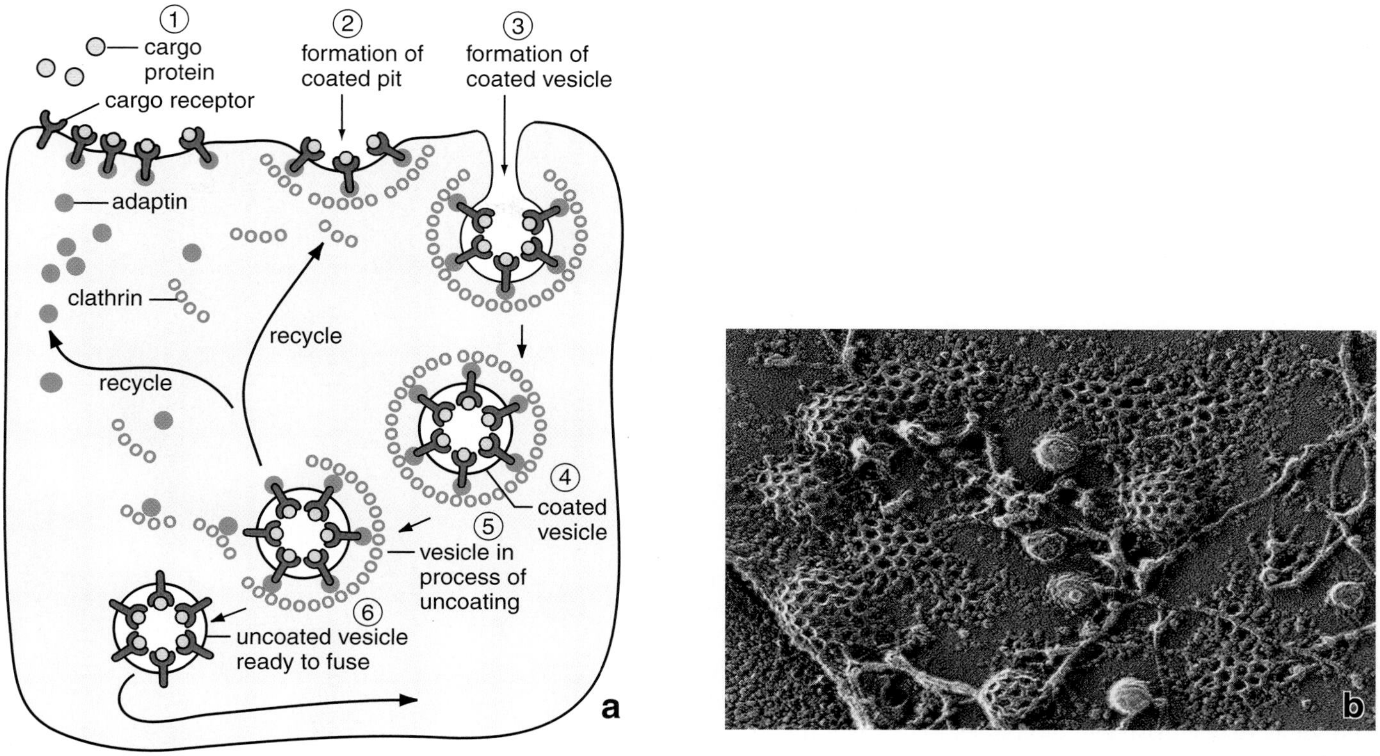

FIGURE 2.10

Receptor-mediated endocytosis. a. This diagram shows the steps in receptor-mediated endocytosis, a transport mechanism that allows selected molecules to enter the cell. ① Cargo receptors recognize and bind specific molecules that come in contact with the plasma membrane. Cargo receptor–molecule complexes are recognized by adaptin, a protein that helps select and gather appropriate complexes in specific areas of the plasma membrane for transport into cells. ② Clathrin molecules then bind to the adaptin–cargo receptor–molecule complex to assemble into a shallow basket-like cage, forming a coated pit. ③ Clathrin interactions then assist the plasma membrane to change shape to form a deep depression, a fully formed coated pit that then pinches off from the plasma membrane as a coated vesicle ④ (i.e., budding from the membrane). Selected cargo proteins and their receptors are thus pulled from the extracellular space into the lumen of a forming coated vesicle. After budding and internalization of the vesicle, the coat proteins are removed ⑤ and recycled for further use. ⑥ The uncoated vesicle travels to its destination to fuse with a cytoplasmic organelle. **b.** Electron micrograph of the cytoplasmic surface of the plasma membrane of A431 cells prepared by the quick-freeze deep-etch technique. This image shows coated pits and clathrin-coated vesicles in different stages of their formation. Note that the coated pits and clathrin-coated vesicles are formed in areas devoid of actin filaments. The small uniform pinocytotic vesicles do not have a clathrin coat and are located in close proximity to actin filaments. ×200,000. (Courtesy of Dr. John E. Heuser, Washington University School of Medicine.)

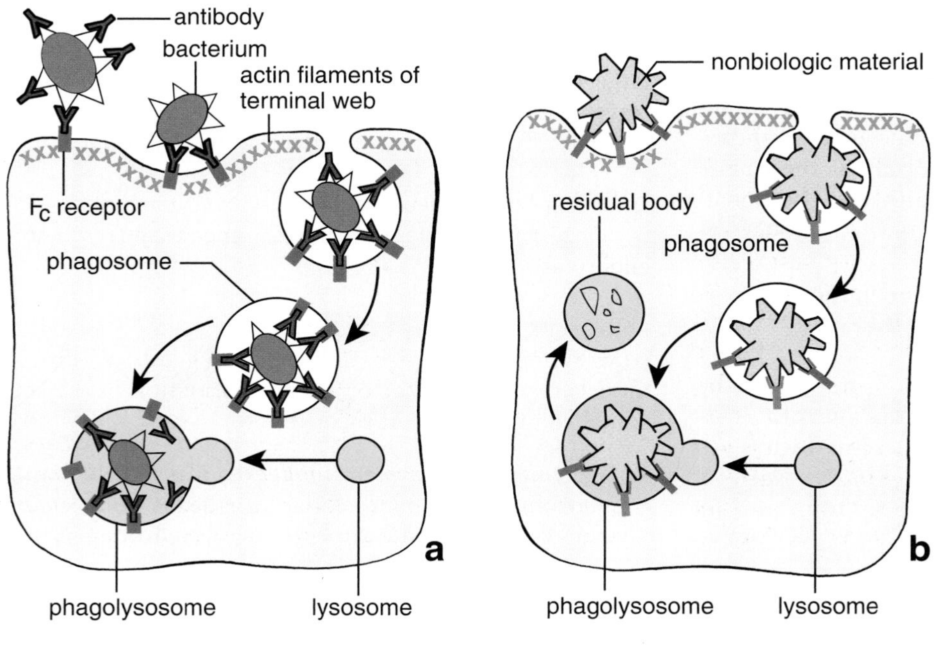

FIGURE 2.11

Phagocytosis. a. This drawing shows the steps in the phagocytosis of a large particle, such as a bacterium that has been killed as a result of an immune response. The bacterium is surrounded by antibodies attached to the bacterial surface antigens. F_c receptors on the surface of the plasma membrane of the phagocytotic cells recognize the F_c portion of the antibodies. This interaction triggers formation of phagosomes and intracellular destruction of the microorganism. Because of the large size of the phagosomes, the actin cytoskeleton is rearranged by depolymerization and repolymerization of actin filaments. **b.** Nonbiologic materials such as inhaled carbon particles, inorganic dusts, and asbestos fibers, as well as cellular debris resulting from inflammation, are internalized without involvement of antibodies and F_c receptors. These particles are bound to multiple receptors on the plasma membrane.

of the MPS without involvement of F_c receptors (Fig. 2.11b). This process does not require clathrin. However, because of the large size of the vesicle, the actin cytoskeleton must be rearranged in a process that requires depolymerization and repolymerization of the actin filaments. Thus phagocytosis is referred to as *clathrin-independent* and *actin-dependent endocytosis.*

EXOCYTOSIS

Exocytosis is the process by which a vesicle moves from the cytoplasm to the plasma membrane, where it discharges its contents to the extracellular space

A variety of molecules produced by the cell for export are initially delivered from the site of their formation to the Golgi apparatus. The next step involves sorting and packaging the secretory product into transport vesicles that are destined to fuse with the plasma membrane in a process known as *exocytosis.* The molecules that travel this route are often chemically modified (e.g., glycosylated, sulfated) as they pass through different cellular compartments. The membrane that is added to the plasma membrane by exocytosis is recovered into the cytoplasmic compartment by an endocytotic process. There are two general pathways of exocytosis:

- In the *constitutive pathway*, substances designated for export are continuously delivered in transport vesicles to the plasma membrane. Proteins that leave the cell by this process are secreted immediately after their synthesis and exit from the Golgi apparatus, as seen in the secretion of immunoglobulins by plasma cells and of tropocollagen by fibroblasts. This pathway is present to some degree in all cells. The TEM reveals that these cells lack secretory granules.
- In the *regulated secretory pathway,* specialized cells, such as endocrine and exocrine cells and neurons, concentrate secretory proteins and transiently store them in secretory vesicles within the cytoplasm (Fig. 2.12). In this case, a regulatory event (hormonal or neural stimulus) must be activated for secretion to occur, as in the release of zymogen granules by chief cells of the gastric mucosa and by acinar cells of the pancreas. The signaling stimulus causes a transient influx of Ca^{2+} into the cytoplasm, which in turn stimulates secretory vesicles to fuse with the plasma membrane and discharge their contents (Fig. 2.13).

In addition to excretory pathways, proteins can be transported between the Golgi apparatus and other organelles along endosomal pathways. These pathways are used for delivery of organelle-specific proteins, such as lysosomal structural proteins, into the appropriate organelles.

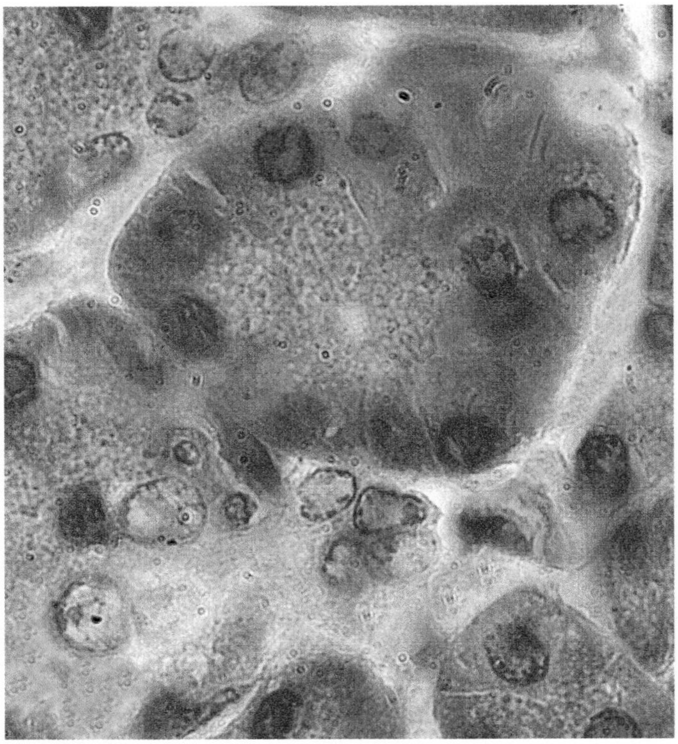

FIGURE 2.12
Photomicrograph of secretory cells of the pancreas. Note that secretory vesicles containing protein ready for secretion fill the apical portion of the cells. This process requires an external signaling mechanism for the cell to discharge the accumulated granules. ×860.

Endosomes

The TEM reveals the presence in the cytoplasm of membrane-enclosed compartments associated with all the endocytotic pathways described above (Fig. 2.14). These compartments, called *early endosomes,* are restricted to a portion of the cytoplasm near the cell membrane where vesicles originating from the cell membrane fuse. From here, many vesicles return to the plasma membrane. However, large numbers of vesicles originating in early endosomes travel to deeper structures in the cytoplasm, called *late endosomes.* The latter typically develop into *lysosomes.*

Endosomes can be viewed either as stable cytoplasmic organelles or as transient structures formed as the result of endocytosis

Recent experimental observations of endocytotic pathways conducted in vitro and in vivo suggest two different models that explain the origin and formation of the endosomal compartments in the cell:

- The *stable compartment model* describes early and late endosomes as stable cellular organelles connected by vesicular transport with the external environment of the

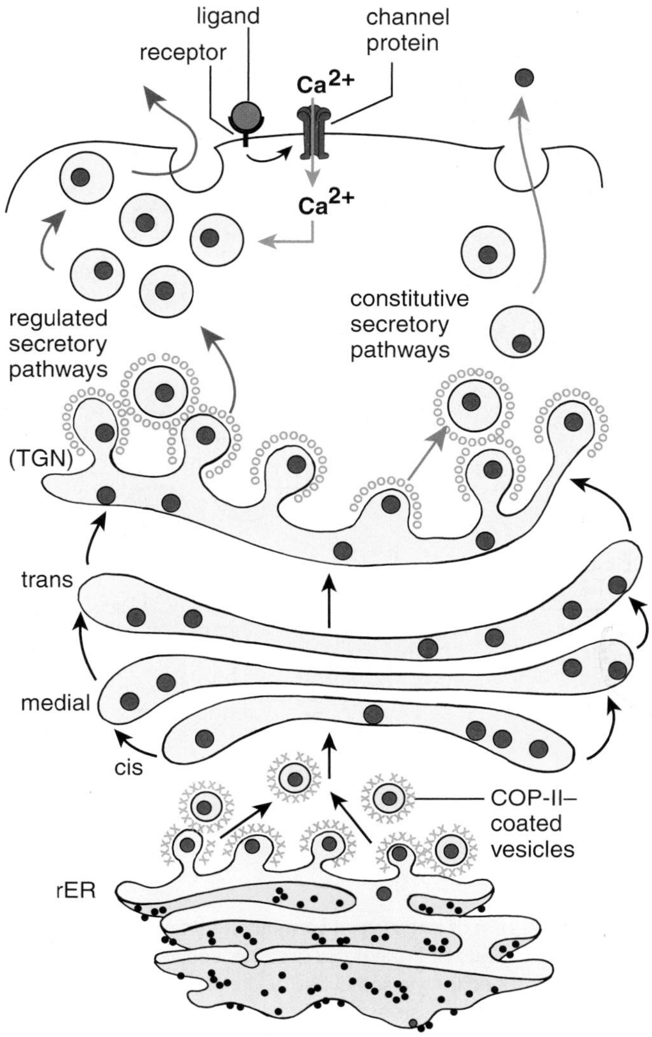

FIGURE 2.13
Diagram showing two pathways for exocytosis. Newly synthesized proteins are synthesized in the rER. After their initial posttranslational modification, they are delivered in COP-II–coated vesicles to the Golgi apparatus. After additional modification in the Golgi apparatus, sorting, and packaging, the final secretory product is transported to the plasma membrane in vesicles that form from the *trans*-Golgi network (TGN). Two distinct pathways are recognized. *Blue arrows* indicate the constitutive pathway in which proteins leave the cell immediately after their synthesis. In cells using this pathway, little secretory product accumulates, and thus few secretory vesicles are present in the cytoplasm. *Red arrows* indicate the regulated secretory pathway in which protein secretion is regulated by hormonal or neural stimuli. In cells using this pathway, such as the pancreatic acinar cells in Figure 2.12, secretory proteins are concentrated and transiently stored in secretory vesicles within the cytoplasm. After appropriate stimulation, the secretory vesicles fuse with the plasma membrane and discharge their contents.

cell and with the Golgi apparatus. Coated vesicles formed at the plasma membrane fuse only with early endosomes because of their expression of specific surface receptors. The receptor remains a resident component of the early endosomal membrane.

- In the ***maturation model***, early endosomes are formed de novo from endocytotic vesicles originating from the plasma membrane. Therefore, the composition of the early endosomal membrane changes progressively as some components are recycled between the cell surface and the Golgi apparatus. This maturation process leads to formation of late endosomes and then to lysosomes. Specific receptors present on early endosomes, e.g., for coated vesicles, are removed by recycling, degradation, or inactivation as this compartment matures.

Both models actually complement rather than contradict each other in describing, identifying, and studying the pathways of internalized molecules.

Endosomes destined to become lysosomes receive newly synthesized lysosomal enzymes that are targeted via the mannose-6-phosphate receptor

Some endosomes also communicate with the vesicular transport system of the rER. This pathway provides constant delivery of newly synthesized lysosomal enzymes, or hydrolases. Hydrolases are synthesized in the rER and are glycosylated. The protein then folds in a specific way so that a ***signal patch*** is formed and exposed on the surface of the molecule. This recognition signal is created when specific amino acids are brought into close proximity by the three-dimensional folding of the protein. The sig-

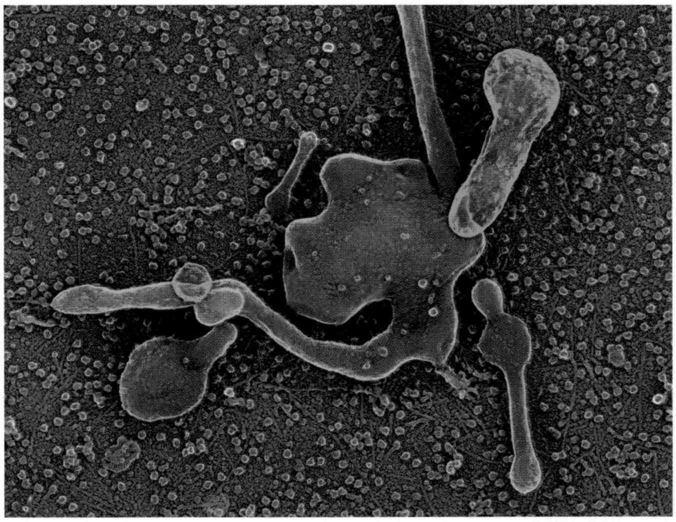

FIGURE 2.14
Electron micrograph of an early endosome. This deep-etch electron micrograph shows the structure of an early endosome in *Dictyostelium*. Early endosomes are located near the plasma membrane and have a typical tubulovesical structure. The lumen of the endosome is subdivided into multiple compartments or cisternae by the invagination of its membrane and undergoes frequent change in shape. ×15,000. (Courtesy of Dr. John E. Heuser, Washington University School of Medicine.)

nal patch on a protein destined for a lysosome is then modified by several enzymes that attach ***mannose-6-phosphate (M-6-P)*** to the enzyme surface. M-6-P acts as a target for specific proteins possessing a ***M-6-P receptor.*** M-6-P receptors are present in early and late endosomes, lysosomes, and the Golgi apparatus that is involved in sorting and retrieving secreted hydrolyses destined for transport to endosomes (Fig. 2.15).

Early and late endosomes differ in their cellular localization, morphology, and state of acidification and function

Early and late endosomes are localized in different areas of the cell. Early endosomes can be found in the more peripheral cytoplasm, whereas late endosomes are often positioned near the Golgi apparatus and the nucleus. Early endosomes have a tubulovesicular structure: The lumen is subdivided into cisternae that are separated by invagination of its membrane. They exhibit only a slightly more acidic environment (pH 6.2 to 6.5) than the cytoplasm of the cell. In contrast, late endosomes have a more complex structure and often exhibit onion-like internal membranes. Their pH is more acidic, averaging 5.5. TEM studies reveal specific vesicles that transport substances between early and late endosomes. These vesicles, called ***multivesicular bodies (MVB),*** are highly selective transporters. Within early endosomes, proteins destined to be transported to late endosomes are sorted and separated from proteins destined for recycling and packaging into MVBs (Fig. 2.16). In general, substances transported to late endosomes are eventually degraded in lysosomes in a default process that does not require any

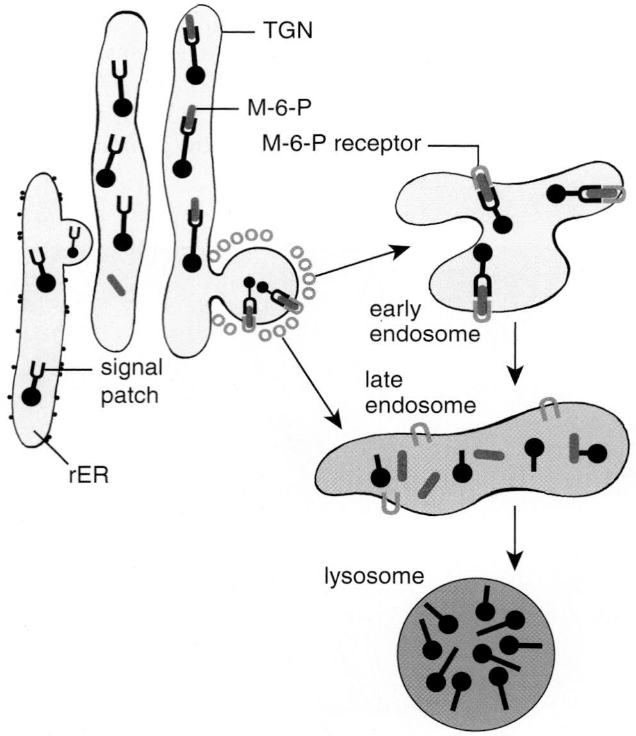

FIGURE 2.15
Pathways for delivery of newly synthesized lysosomal enzymes. Lysosomal enzymes (such as lysosomal hydrolases) are synthesized and glycosylated within the rER. The enzymes then fold in a specific way so that a signal patch is formed, which allows for further modification by the addition of mannose-6-phospate (M-6-P). M-6-P allows the enzyme to be targeted to specific proteins that possess M-6-P receptor activity. M-6-P receptors are present in the *trans*-Golgi network (TGN) of the Golgi apparatus, where the lysosomal enzymes are sorted and packaged into vesicles later transported to the early or late endosomes and lysosomes.

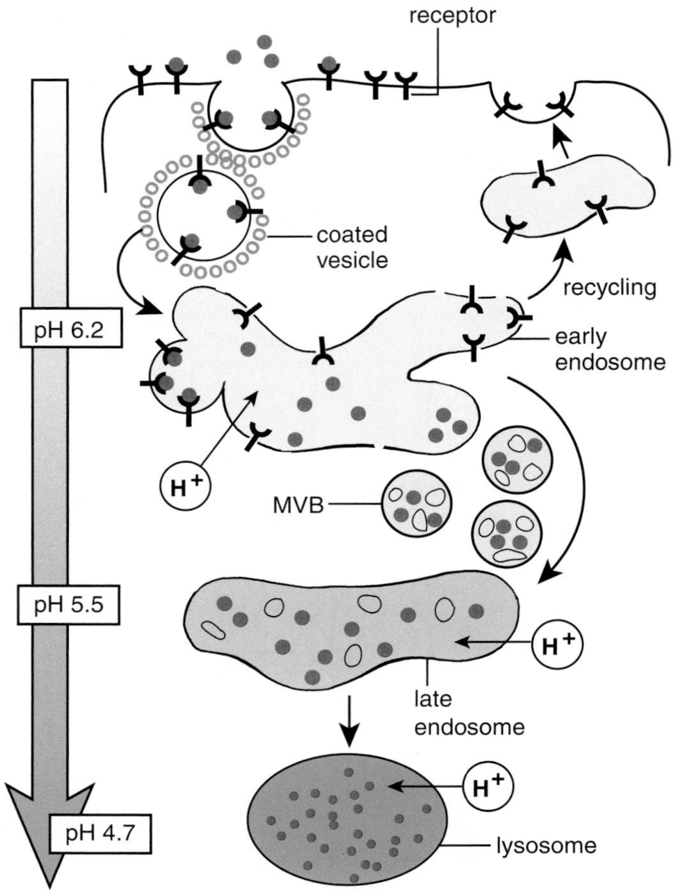

FIGURE 2.16
Schematic diagram of endosomal compartments of the cell. This diagram shows the fate of protein *(red circles)* endocytosed from the cell surface and destined for lysosomal destruction. Proteins are first found in endocytotic (coated) vesicles that deliver them to early endosomes, which are located in the peripheral part of cytoplasm. Because of the sorting capability of the early endosomes, receptors are usually recycled to the plasma membrane, and endocytosed proteins are transported via multivesicular bodies *(MVB)* to late endosomes positioned near the Golgi apparatus and the nucleus. The proteins transported to late endosomes eventually will be degraded in lysosomes. Note the acidification scale *(left)* that illustrates changes of pH from early endosomes to lysosomes. The acidification is accomplished by the active transport of protons into endosomal compartments.

additional signals. For that reason, late endosomes are also called prelysosomes.

The major function of early endosomes is to sort and recycle proteins internalized by endocytotic pathways

Early endosomes sort proteins that have been internalized by endocytotic processes. The morphologic shape and geometry of the tubules and vesicles emerging from the early endosome create an environment in which localized changes in pH constitute the basis of the sorting mechanism. This mechanism includes dissociation of ligands from their receptor protein; thus, in the past, early endosomes were referred to as *compartments of uncoupling receptors and ligands (CURLs)*. In addition, the narrow diameter of the tubules and vesicles may also aid in the sorting of large molecules, which can be mechanically prevented from entering specific sorting compartments. After sorting, most of the protein is rapidly recycled, and the excess membrane is returned to the plasma membrane.

The fate of the internalized ligand–receptor complex depends on the sorting and recycling ability of the early endosome

The following pathways for processing internalized ligand–receptor complexes are present in the cell:

- ***The receptor is recycled and the ligand is degraded.*** Surface receptors allow the cell to bring in substances selectively through the process of endocytosis. This pathway occurs most often in the cell; it is important because it allows surface receptors to be recycled. Most ligand–receptor complexes dissociate in the acidic pH of the early endosome. The receptor, most likely an integral membrane protein (see page 22), is recycled to the surface via vesicles that bud off the ends of narrow-diameter tubules of the early endosome. Ligands are usually sequestered in the spherical vacuolar part of the endosome that will later form MVBs, which will transport the ligand to late endosomes for further degradation in the lysosome (Fig. 2.17a). This pathway is described for the ***low-density lipoprotein (LDL)–receptor***

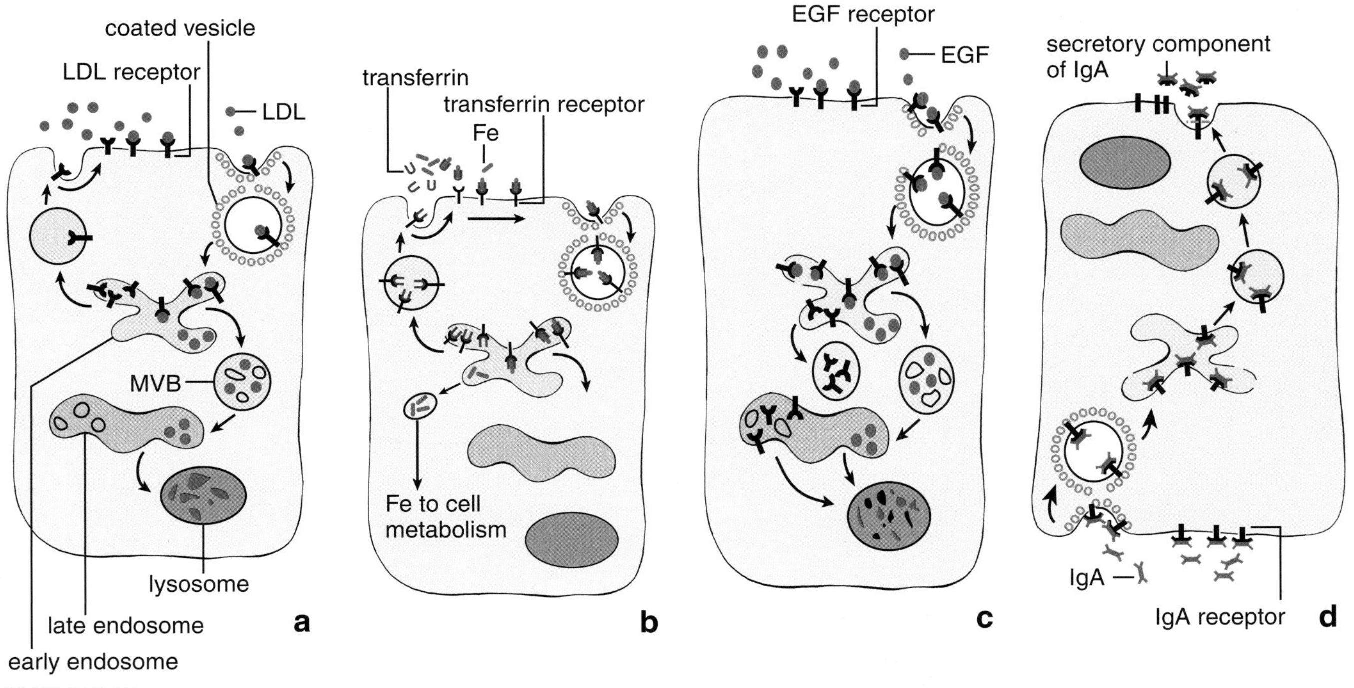

FIGURE 2.17
Fate of receptor and ligand in receptor-mediated endocytosis. This diagram shows four major pathways along which the fate of internalized ligand–receptor complexes is determined. **a.** The internalized ligand–receptor complex dissociates, the receptor is recycled to the cell surface, and the ligand is directed to late endosomes and eventually degraded within lysosomes. This processing pathway is used by the LDL/LDL–receptor complex, insulin–GLUT receptor complex, and a variety of peptide hormone–receptor complexes. **b.** Both internalized receptor and ligand are recycled. Ligand–receptor complex dissociation does not occur, and the entire complex is recycled to the surface. An example is the iron-transferrin/transferrin–receptor complex that uses this processing pathway. Once iron is released in the endosome, the transferrin–receptor complex returns to the cell surface, where transferrin is released. **c.** The internalized ligand–receptor complex dissociates in the early endosome. The free ligand and the receptor are directed to the late endosomal compartment for further degradation. This pathway is used by many growth factors (i.e., epidermal growth factor (EGF)/EGF–receptor.) **d.** The internalized ligand–receptor complex is transported through the cell. Dissociation does not occur, and the entire complex undergoes transcytosis and release at a different site of the cell surface. This pathway is used during secretion of immunoglobulins (secretory IgA) into saliva. The antibody IgA–receptor complex is internalized at the basal surface of the secretory cells in the salivary gland and released at the apical surface.

complex, insulin–glucose transporter (GLUT) receptor complex, and a variety of ***peptide hormones*** and their receptors.

- ***Both receptor and ligand are recycled.*** Ligand–receptor complex dissociation does not always accompany receptor recycling. For example, the low pH of the endosome dissociates iron from the iron-carrier protein transferrin, but transferrin remains associated with its receptor. Once the transferrin–receptor complex returns to the cell surface, however, transferrin is released. At neutral extracellular pH, transferrin must again bind iron to be recognized by and bound to its receptor. A similar pathway is recognized for ***major histocompatibility complex (MHC) I and II molecules,*** which are recycled to the cell surface with a foreign antigen protein attached to them (Fig. 2.17b).
- ***Both receptor and ligand are degraded.*** This pathway has been identified for epidermal growth factor (EGF) and its receptor. Like many other proteins, EGF binds to its receptor on the cell surface. The complex is internalized and carried to the early endosomes. Here, EGF dissociates from its receptor, and both are sorted, packaged in separate MVBs, and transferred to the late endosome. From there, both ligand and receptor are transferred to lysosomes, where they are degraded (Fig. 2.17c).
- ***Both receptor and ligand are transported through the cell.*** This pathway is used for secretion of immunoglobulins (secretory IgA) into saliva or secretion of maternal IgG into milk. During this process, commonly referred as ***transcytosis,*** substances can be altered as they are transported across the epithelial cell (Fig. 2.17d).

Lysosomes

Lysosomes are digestive organelles that were recognized only after histochemical procedures were used to demonstrate lysosomal enzymes

Lysosomes are organelles rich in hydrolytic enzymes such as proteases, nucleases, glycosidases, lipases, and phospholipases. They are responsible for degradation of macromolecules derived from endocytotic pathways as well as from the cell itself in a process known as ***autophagy*** (removal of cytoplasmic components, particularly membrane-bounded organelles, by digesting them within lysosomes).

The first hypothesis for lysosomal biogenesis, formulated almost a half century ago, postulated that lysosomes arise as complete and functional organelles budding from the Golgi apparatus. These newly formed lysosomes were termed ***primary lysosomes,*** in contrast to ***secondary lysosomes,*** which had already fused with incoming endosomes. However, the primary and secondary lysosome hypothesis has proved to have little validity as new research data allow a better understanding of the details of protein secretory pathways and the fate of endocytotic vesicles.

Lysosomes have a unique membrane that is resistant to the hydrolytic digestion occurring in their lumen

Lysosomes contain a collection of hydrolytic enzymes and are surrounded by a unique membrane that resists hydrolysis by their own enzymes (Fig. 2.18). Most of the structural lysosomal membrane proteins are classified into ***lysosome-associated membrane proteins (lamps),***

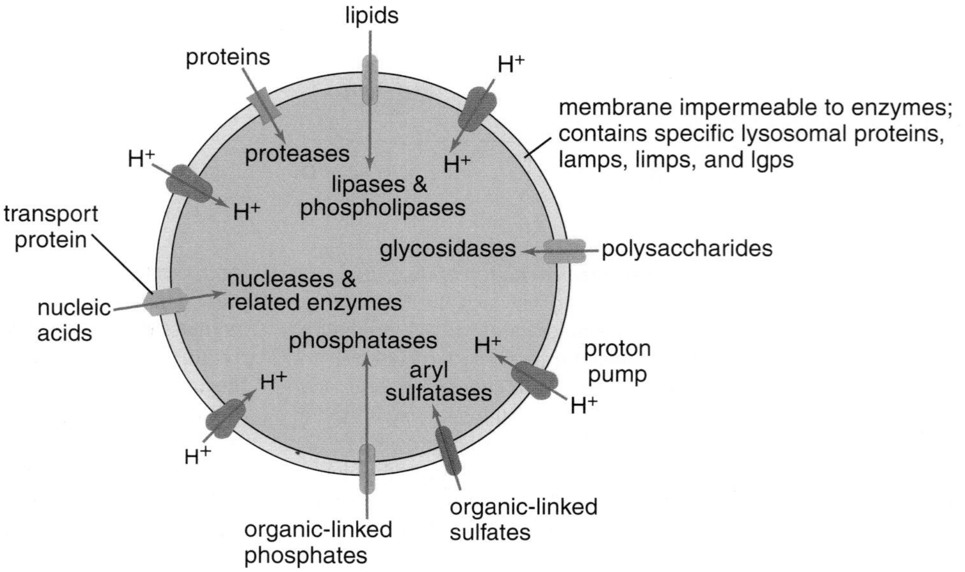

FIGURE 2.18
Schematic diagram of a lysosome. This diagram shows a few selected lysosomal enzymes residing inside the lysosome and their respective substrates. The major lysosomal membrane-specific proteins, as well as a few other proteins associated with membrane transport, are also shown.

lysosomal membrane glycoproteins (lgps), and ***lysosomal integral membrane proteins (limps).*** The lamps, lgps, and limps represent more than 50% of the total membrane proteins in lysosomes and are highly glycosylated on the luminal surface. Sugar molecules cover almost the entire luminal surface of these proteins, thus protecting them from digestion by hydrolytic enzymes. The same family of proteins is also detected in late endosomes. In addition, lysosomes and late endosomes contain ***proton (H^+) pumps*** that transport H^+ ions into the lysosomal lumen, maintaining a low pH (~4.7). The lysosomal membrane also contains ***transport proteins*** that transport the final products of digestion (amino acids, sugars, nucleotides) to the cytoplasm, where they are used in the synthetic processes of the cell or are exocytosed. All membrane proteins destined for lysosomes (and late endosomes) are synthesized in the rER, transported to the Golgi apparatus, and reach their destination by one of two pathways:

- In the ***constitutive secretory pathway,*** limps that exit the Golgi apparatus are delivered to the cell surface. From here, they are endocytosed and, via the early and late endosomal compartments, finally reach lysosomes (Fig. 2.19). This pathway does not require the M-6-P receptor targeting mechanism.
- In the ***Golgi-derived coated vesicle secretory pathway,*** limps, after sorting and packaging, exit the Golgi apparatus in clathrin-coated vesicles (see Fig. 2.19). These vesicles are delivered to the early and/or late endosome in a manner similar to that described for soluble lysosomal enzymes; thus, the M-6-P targeting mechanism is required for this pathway (see page 29).

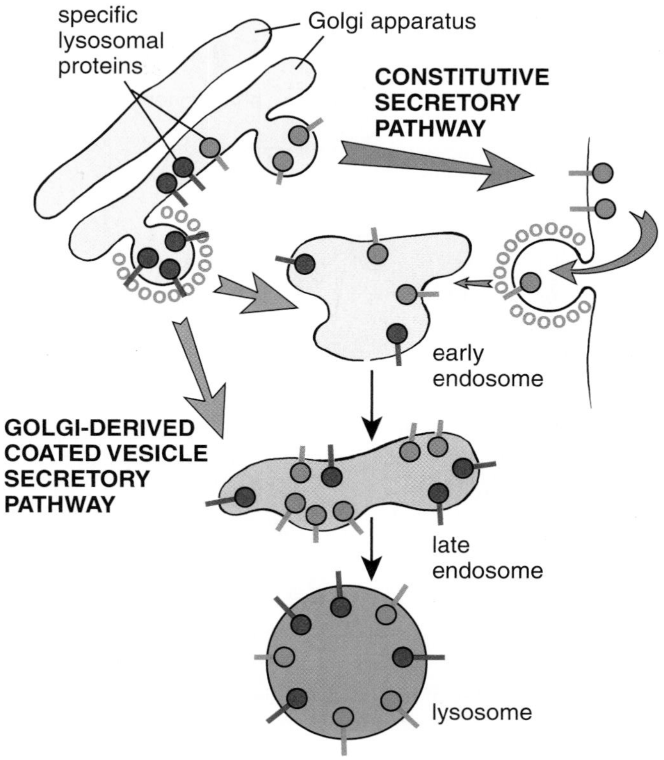

FIGURE 2.19
Lysosome biogenesis. This diagram shows regulated and constitutive pathways for delivery of lysosomal specific membrane proteins into early and late endosomes. The lysosomal membrane possesses highly glycosylated specific membrane proteins that protect the membrane from digestion by lysosomal enzymes. These lysosome-specific proteins are synthesized in the rER, transported to the Golgi apparatus, and reach their destination by two pathways. *Blue arrows* indicate the constitutive secretory pathway in which certain lysosomal membrane proteins exit the Golgi apparatus and are delivered to the cell surface. From there they are endocytosed and, via the early and late endosomal compartments, finally reach lysosomes. *Green arrows* indicate the endosomal Golgi-derived coated vesicle secretory pathway. Here, other lysosomal proteins, after sorting and packaging, exit the Golgi apparatus in clathrin-coated vesicles. These vesicles are delivered to the early and/or late endosome by use of the M-6-P targeting mechanism.

Three different pathways deliver material for intracellular digestion in lysosomes

Depending on the nature of the digested material, different pathways deliver material for digestion within the lysosomes (Fig. 2.20). In the digestion process, most of the digested material comes from endocytotic processes; however, the cell also uses lysosomes to digest its own obsolete parts, nonfunctional organelles, and unnecessary molecules. Three pathways for digestion exist:

- ***Extracellular large particles*** such as bacteria, cell debris, and other foreign materials are engulfed in the process of phagocytosis. A ***phagosome,*** formed as the material is internalized within the cytoplasm, subsequently fuses with a lysosome to create a ***phagolysosome.***
- ***Extracellular small particles*** such as extracellular proteins, plasma membrane proteins, and ligand–receptor complexes are internalized by endocytosis and receptor-mediated endocytosis. These particles follow the endocytotic pathway through early and late endosomal compartments and are finally delivered to lysosomes for degradation.
- ***Intracellular particles*** such as entire organelles, cytoplasmic proteins, and other cellular components are isolated from the cytoplasmic matrix by endoplasmic reticulum membranes, transported to lysosomes, and degraded in the process called ***autophagy*** (see below).

In addition, some cells (e.g., osteoclasts involved in bone resorption and neutrophils involved in acute inflammation) may release lysosomal enzymes directly into the extracellular space to digest components of the extracellular matrix.

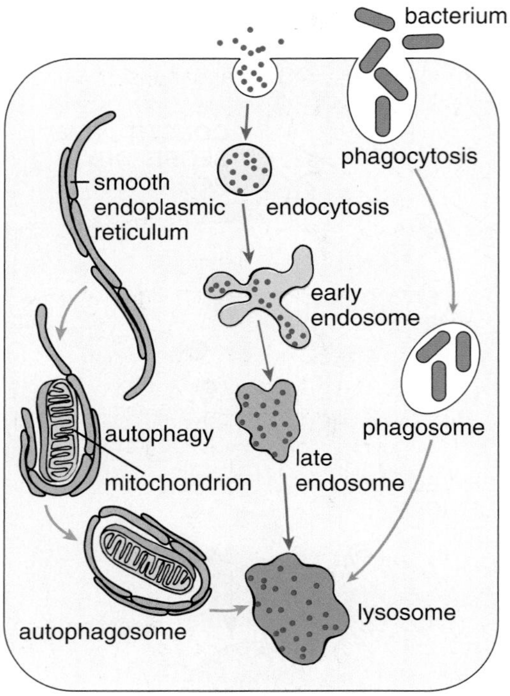

FIGURE 2.20
Pathways of delivery of materials for digestion in lysosomes. Most of the material to be digested comes from endocytotic pathways *(red arrows).* It consists of small extracellular particles that are internalized by both endocytosis and receptor-mediated endocytosis. Large extracellular particles such as bacteria and cellular debris are delivered to lysosomes via the phagocytotic pathway *(blue arrows).* The cell also uses lysosomes to digest its own proteins and other intracellular particles via the autophagic pathway *(green arrows).* Intracellular particles are isolated from the cytoplasmic matrix by the membranes of the endoplasmic reticulum, transported to lysosomes, and subsequently degraded.

Cytoplasmic proteins and organelles are also substrates for lysosomal degradation in the process of autophagy

A number of cytosolic proteins, organelles, and other cellular structures can be degraded in the lysosomes (Fig. 2.21). Generally, this process can be divided into three well-characterized pathways:

- ***Macroautophagy*** is a nonspecific process in which a portion of the cytoplasm or an entire organelle is surrounded by an intracellular membrane of endoplasmic reticulum to form a vacuole called an ***autophagosome.*** After fusion with a lysosome ***(autophagolysosome),*** the contents of the vacuole are degraded in a manner similar to that occurring within the phagolysosome. Macroautophagy occurs in the liver during the first stages of starvation (Fig. 2.22).
- ***Microautophagy*** is also a nonspecific process in which cytoplasmic proteins are degraded in a slow, continuous process under normal physiologic conditions. In microautophagy, small cytoplasmic soluble proteins are internalized into the lysosomes by invagination of the lysosomal membrane.
- ***Chaperone-mediated direct transport*** to lysosomes is the only selective process of protein degradation and requires assistance from a specific ***chaperone protein*** called ***hsc73.*** This process is activated during nutrient deprivation and requires the presence of targeting signals on the degraded proteins and a specific receptor on the lysosomal membrane. Chaperone-mediated direct transport resembles the process of protein import to various other cellular organelles: hsc73 binds to the protein

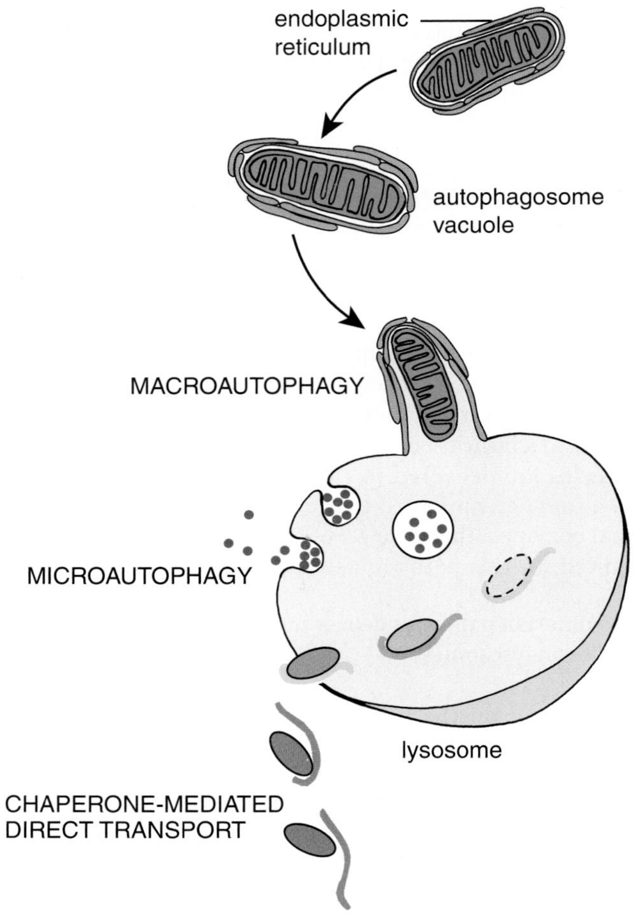

FIGURE 2.21
Three autophagic pathways for degradation of cytoplasmic constituents. In *macroautophagy,* a portion of the cytoplasm or an entire organelle is surrounded by an intracellular membrane of the endoplasmic reticulum to form an autophagosome vacuole. After fusion with a lysosome, the contents of the vacuole are degraded. In *microautophagy,* cytoplasmic proteins are internalized into lysosomes by invagination of the lysosomal membrane. *Chaperone-mediated direct transport* to lysosomes is the most selective process for degradation of specific cytoplasmic proteins. It requires assistance of proteins called chaperones. Chaperones bind to the protein and help transport it into the lysosomal lumen, where it is finally degraded.

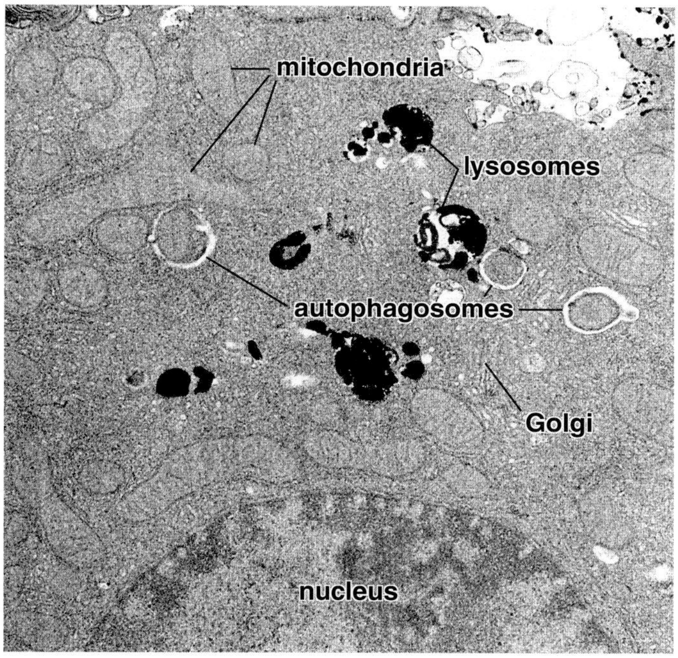

FIGURE 2.22
Electron micrograph of autophagosomes in an hepatocyte. This electron micrograph shows several autophagosomes containing degenerating mitochondria. Note the surrounding lysosomes that had been stained with acid phosphatase. ×12,600. (Courtesy of Dr. William A. Dunn, Jr.)

and assists in its transport through the lysosomal membrane into the lumen, where it is finally degraded.

Lysosomes in some cells are recognizable in the light microscope because of their number, size, or contents

The numerous azurophilic granules of ***neutrophils (polymorphonuclear neutrophilic leukocytes)*** are lysosomes and are recognized in aggregate by their specific staining. Lysosomes that contain phagocytized bacteria and fragments of damaged cells are often recognized in macrophages.

Hydrolytic breakdown of the contents of lysosomes often produces a debris-filled vacuole called a ***residual body,*** which may remain for the entire life of the cell. For example, in neurons, residual bodies are called "age pigment" or lipofuscin granules. Residual bodies are a normal feature of cell aging. The absence of certain lysosomal enzymes can cause the pathologic accumulation of undigested substrate in residual bodies. This can lead to several disorders collectively termed ***lysosomal storage diseases.*** In ***Tay-Sachs disease,*** for example, which was first described in 1881, the absence of a lysosomal galactosidase (β-hexosaminidase) in neurons produces concentric lamellated structures in residual bodies that accumulate in the cell and interfere with normal functions.

Rough-Surfaced Endoplasmic Reticulum

The protein synthetic system of the cell consists of the rough endoplasmic reticulum and ribosomes

The cytoplasm of a variety of cells engaged chiefly in protein synthesis stains intensely with basic dyes. The basophilic staining is due to the presence of RNA. That portion of the cytoplasm that stains with the basic dye is called ***ergastoplasm.*** The ergastoplasm in secretory cells, e.g., pancreatic acinar cells, is the light microscopic image of the organelle called the ***rough endoplasmic reticulum (rER).***

With the TEM, the rER appears as a series of interconnected, membrane-limited flattened sacs called ***cisternae,*** with particles studding the exterior surface of the membrane (Fig. 2.23). These particles, called ***ribosomes,*** are at-

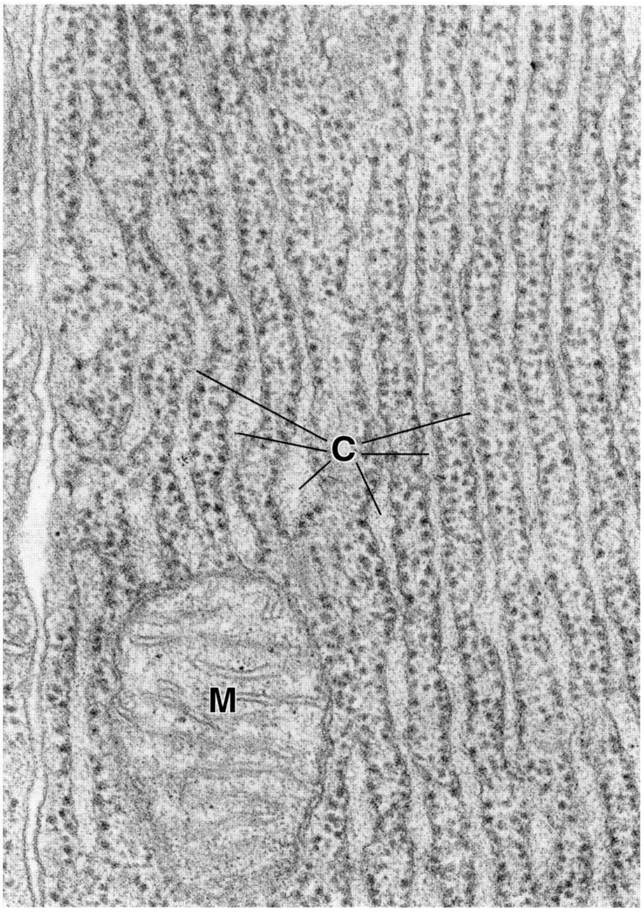

FIGURE 2.23
Electron micrograph of the rER. This image of rER in a chief cell of the stomach shows the membranous cisternae *(C)* closely packed in parallel arrays. Polyribosomes are present on the cytoplasmic surface of the membrane surrounding the cisternae. The image of ribosome-studded membrane is the origin of the term "rough endoplasmic reticulum." A few ribosomes are free in the cytoplasm. *M,* mitochondrion. ×50,000.

tached to the membrane of the rER by ribosomal docking proteins. Ribosomes measure 15 to 20 nm in diameter and contain RNA and protein. In many instances, the rER is continuous with the outer membrane of the nuclear envelope (see below). Groups of ribosomes form short spiral arrays called ***polyribosomes*** or ***polysomes*** (Fig. 2.24), in which many ribosomes are attached to a thread of ***messenger RNA (mRNA).***

Protein synthesis involves transcription and translation

The production of proteins by the cell begins with ***transcription,*** in which the genetic code for a protein is transcribed from DNA to mRNA. Transcription is followed by ***translation,*** in which the coded message contained in the mRNA is "read" to form a polypeptide. A typical single molecule of mRNA may bind to many ribosomes spaced as close as 80 nucleotides apart, thus forming a polyribosome complex, or ***polysome.*** A polysome can translate a single mRNA molecule and simultaneously produce many copies of a particular protein.

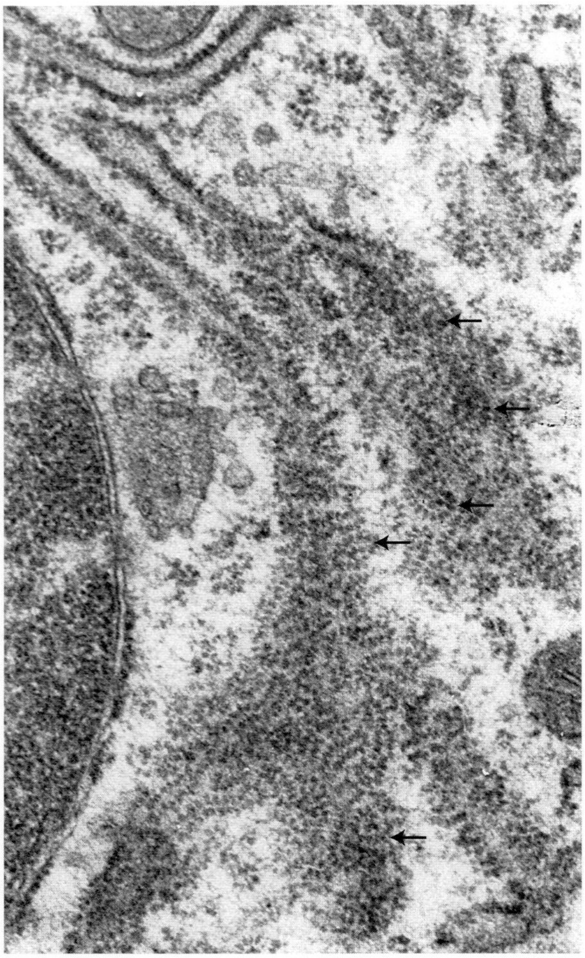

FIGURE 2.24
Electron micrograph of the rER and polyribosome complexes. This image shows a small section of the rER adjacent to the nucleus sectioned in two planes. The reticulum has turned within the section. Thus, in the upper right and left, the membranes of the reticulum have been cut at a right angle to their surface. In the center, the reticulum has twisted and is shown as in an aerial view (from above the membrane). The large spiral cytoplasmic assemblies *(arrows)* are chains of ribosomes that form polyribosomes that are actively engaged in translation of the mRNA molecule. ×38,000.

Polysomes of the rER synthesize proteins for export from the cell and integral proteins of the plasma membrane

As polypeptide chains are synthesized by the membrane-bound polysomes, the protein is injected into the lumen of the cisterna, where it may be further modified, concentrated, or carried to another part of the cell in the continuous channels of the rER. The rER is particularly well developed in those cells that synthesize protein destined to leave the cell (secretory cells) as well as in cells with large amounts of plasma membrane, such as neurons. Secretory cells include glandular cells, fibroblasts, plasma cells, odontoblasts, ameloblasts, and osteoblasts. The rER is not limited, however, to secretory cells and neurons. Virtually every cell of the body contains profiles of rER. However, they may be few in number, a reflection of the amount of protein secretion, and dispersed so that in the light microscope they are not evident as areas of basophilia.

In agreement with the observation that the rER is most highly developed in active secretory cells, secretory proteins are synthesized exclusively by the ribosomes of the rER. In all cells, however, the ribosomes of the rER synthesize proteins that are to become permanent components of the lysosome, Golgi apparatus, rER, or nuclear envelope (these structures are discussed below) or integral components of the plasma membrane.

Signal peptides are attached to secretory proteins and integral proteins of the plasma membrane

If the protein to be synthesized is destined for export or will become part of the plasma membrane, the first group of amino acids that are linked to one another form a hydrophobic ***signal peptide (signal sequence)*** that binds to a receptor on the membrane of the rER (Fig. 2.25). When the ribosome (polysome) binds to the rER membrane, the signal peptide or a subsequent sequence instructs the newly formed peptide to pass through the membrane into the lumen of the rER cisterna. For simple secretory proteins, the polypeptide continues to be inserted into the lumen as it is synthesized. For integral membrane proteins, sequences along the polypeptide may instruct the forming protein to pass back and forth through the membrane, creating the functional domains that the protein will exhibit at its final membrane location.

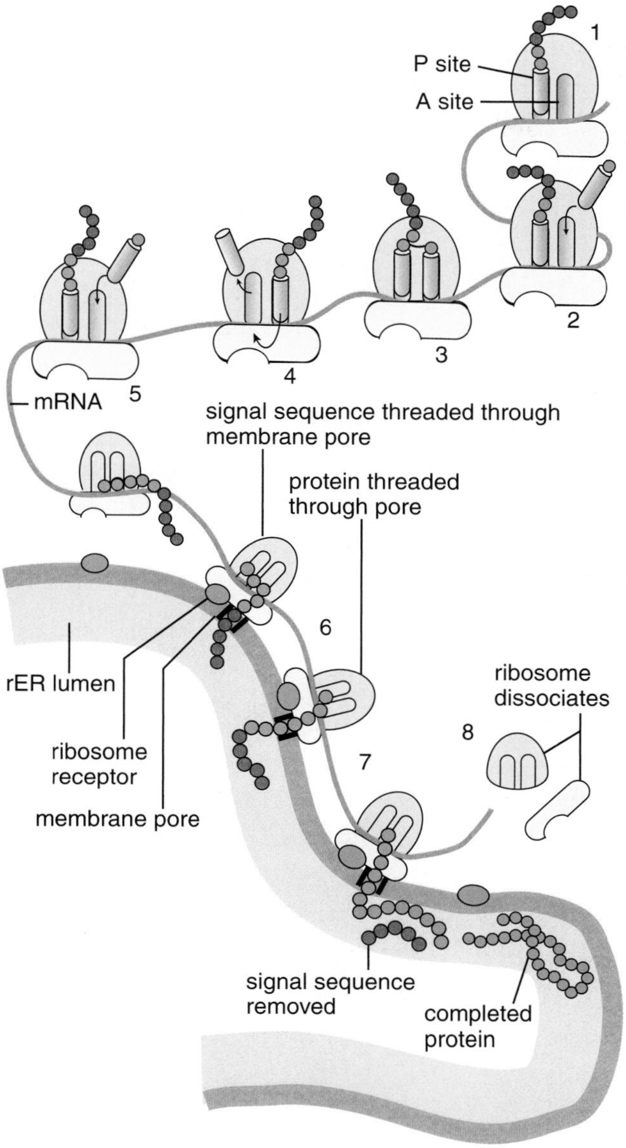

FIGURE 2.25
Summary of events during protein synthesis. Prior to the events depicted here, DNA has been "translated" into mRNA, and the large and small ribosomal subunits have assembled into a ribosome. Notice that the ribosome has two binding sites: the "P" site and the "A" site. **1.** Transfer RNA (tRNA) with a growing peptide chain is bound to the P site of the ribosome. The initial amino acids of the nascent protein constitute the signal sequence *(red)*. The nascent protein grows by adding amino acids at the end of the chain opposite to the signal sequence. **2.** An incoming tRNA with an amino acid attached binds to the A site. **3.** A peptide bond forms between the last amino acid of the growing peptide chain and the new amino acid brought to the ribosome by the incoming tRNA. **4.** The previous tRNA is released from the P site. **5.** The "new" tRNA with the growing peptide chain is translocated to the A site, and the ribosome moves along the mRNA. **6.** The ribosome is attached to the membrane of the rER, and after recognizing the membrane pore proteins, the signal sequence becomes translocated into the lumen of the rER. **7.** By enzymatic action of a signal peptidase, signal sequence is cleaved from the peptide. **8.** After the stop codon is recognized by the ribosome, the synthesis is terminated, and both of the ribosomal subunits dissociate from the mRNA and the surface of the rER.

Secretory proteins pass through the membrane of the rER to its lumen, where they are modified and stored

The hydrophobic signal domain of a forming secretory protein attaches to a receptor on the membrane of the rER; as synthesis proceeds, the protein is inserted into and through the membrane. This process is described as ***cotranslational*** insertion of protein into the rER. If the forming protein is not to be threaded in its entirety through the membrane, a new hydrophobic signal domain stops the threading process, permanently anchoring the protein in the membrane at this site.

On completion of protein synthesis, the ribosome detaches from the rER membrane and is again free in the cytoplasm. The region of the newly formed protein that extends into the lumen of the rER is modified by enzymes present there; these modifications include core glycosylation, disulfide and internal hydrogen bond formation, folding of the newly synthesized protein, and partial subunit assembly. The rER also serves as a quality checkpoint in the process of protein production. If the newly synthesized protein is not properly modified, it cannot exit the rER.

Except for the few proteins that remain permanent residents of the rER membranes and those proteins secreted by the constitutive pathway, the newly synthesized proteins are normally delivered to the Golgi apparatus within minutes. In cells in which the constitutive pathway is dominant, namely, plasma cells and developing fibroblasts, newly synthesized proteins may accumulate in the rER cisternae, causing their engorgement and distension.

Coatomers mediate bidirectional traffic between the rER and Golgi apparatus

Experimental data indicate that two classes of coated vesicles are involved in the transport of protein from and to the rER. A protein coat similar to clathrin surrounds vesicles transporting proteins between the rER and the Golgi apparatus (page 25). However, unlike clathrins, which mediate bidirectional transport from and to the plasma membrane, one class of proteins is involved only in ***anterograde transport*** from the rER to the *cis*-Golgi network (CGN), the Golgi cisternae closest to the rER. Another class of proteins mediates ***retrograde transport*** from the CGN back to the rER (Fig. 2.26). These two classes of proteins are called ***coatomers*** or ***COPs:***

- ***COP-I*** mediates transport vesicles originating in the CGN back to the rER (Fig. 2.27a). This retrograde transport mediates a salvage operation that returns rER proteins mistakenly transferred to the CGN during normal anterograde transport.

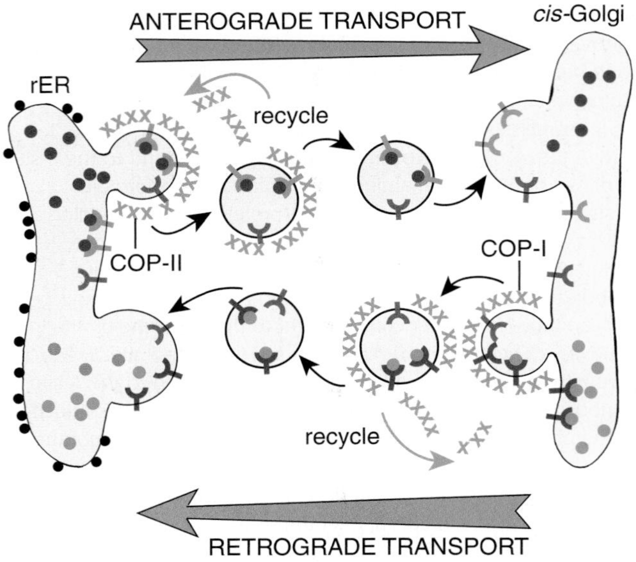

FIGURE 2.26
Anterograde and retrograde transport between the rER and *cis*-Golgi network. Two classes of coated vesicles are involved in protein transport to and from the rER. These vesicles are surrounded by COP-I and COP-II protein coat complex, respectively. COP-II is involved in anterograde transport from the rER to the *cis*-Golgi network (CGN), and COP-I is involved in retrograde transport from the CGN back to the rER. After a vesicle is formed, the coat components dissociate from the vesicle and are recycled to their site of origin.

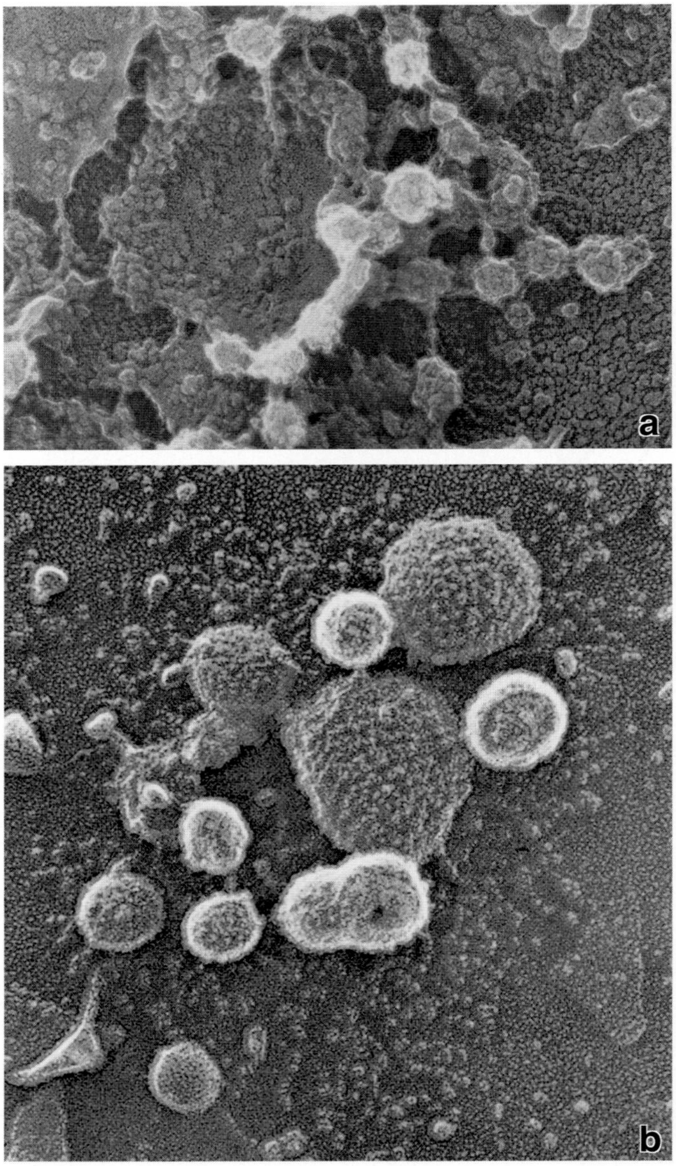

FIGURE 2.27
Electron micrograph of COP-I– and COP-II–coated vesicles. a. This image shows COP-I–coated vesicles that initiate retrograde transport from the *cis*-Golgi network to the rER. In this image, taken of a quick-freeze deep-etch preparations, note the structure of the *cis*-Golgi network and emerging vesicles. ×27,000. **b.** Image of COP-II–coated vesicles that are responsible for anterograde transport. Note that the surface coat of these vesicles is different from that of clathrin-coated vesicles. ×50,000. (Courtesy of Dr. John E. Heuser, Washington University School of Medicine.)

- *COP-II* is responsible for anterograde transport, forming rER transport vesicles destined for the CGN (Fig. 2.27b). COP-II assists in the physical deformation of rER membranes into sharply curved buds and further separation of vesicles from the rER membrane. Most proteins produced in the rER use COP-II–coated vesicles to reach the CGN.

Shortly after formation of COP-I– or COP-II–coated vesicles, the coats dissociate from the newly formed vesicles, allowing the vesicle to fuse with its target. The coat components then recycle to their site of origin.

"Free" ribosomes synthesize proteins that will remain in the cell as cytoplasmic structural or functional elements

Cytoplasmic basophilia is also associated with cells that produce large amounts of protein that will remain in the cell. Such cells and their products include developing red blood cells (hemoglobin), developing muscle cells (the contractile proteins actin and myosin), nerve cells (neurofilaments), and keratinocytes of the skin (keratin). In addition, most enzymes of the mitochondrion are synthesized by free polysomes and transferred into that organelle.

Basophilia in these cells was formerly called *ergastoplasm* and is due to the presence of large amounts of RNA. In this case, the ribosomes and polysomes are "free" in the cytoplasm; i.e., they are not attached to membranes of the endoplasmic reticulum. The large basophilic bodies of nerve cells, called Nissl bodies, consist of both rER and large numbers of free ribosomes (Fig. 2.28). All ribosomes

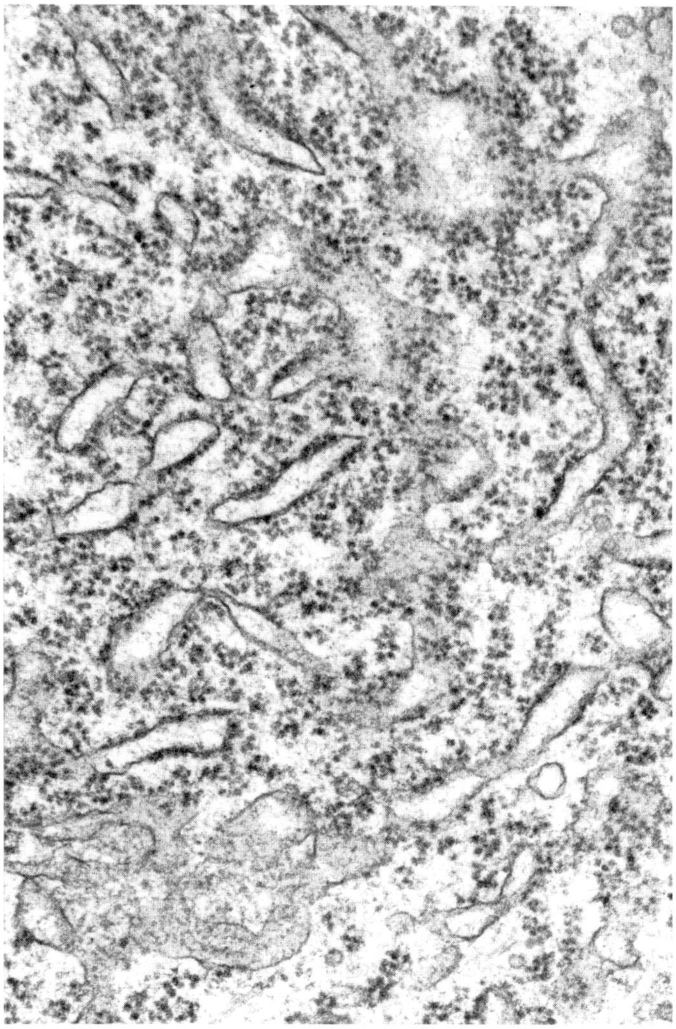

FIGURE 2.28
Electron micrograph of a nerve cell body. This image shows profiles of rER as well as numerous free ribosomes located between the membranes of the rER. Collectively, the free ribosomes and membrane-attached ribosomes are responsible for the characteristic cytoplasmic basophilia (Nissl bodies) observed in the light microscope in the perinuclear cytoplasm of neurons. ×45,000.

contain RNA; it is the phosphate groups of the RNA of the ribosomes, not the membranous component of the endoplasmic reticulum, that accounts for basophilic staining of the cytoplasm.

Smooth-Surfaced Endoplasmic Reticulum

sER consists of short anastomosing tubules that are not associated with ribosomes

Cells with large amounts of ***smooth endoplasmic reticulum (sER)*** may exhibit distinct cytoplasmic eosinophilia (acidophilia) when viewed in the light microscope. It is biochemically similar to the rER but lacks the ribosome-docking proteins. sER tends to be tubular rather than sheet-like, and it may be separate from the rER or an extension of it. The sER is abundant in cells that function in lipid metabolism, and it proliferates in hepatocytes when animals are challenged with lipophilic drugs. The sER is well developed in cells that synthesize and secrete steroids, such as adrenocortical cells and testicular Leydig (interstitial) cells (Fig. 2.29). In skeletal and cardiac muscle, the sER is also called the ***sarcoplasmic reticulum***. It sequesters Ca^{2+} that is essential for the contractile process and is closely apposed to the plasma membrane invaginations that conduct the contractile impulses to the interior of the cell.

sER is the principal organelle involved in detoxification and conjugation of noxious substances

The sER is particularly well developed in the liver and contains a variety of detoxifying enzymes related to cytochrome P450 that are anchored directly into sER plasma membranes. The degree to which the liver is involved in detoxification at any given time may be estimated by the amount of sER present in liver cells. The sER is also involved in

- Lipid and steroid metabolism
- Glycogen metabolism
- Membrane formation and recycling

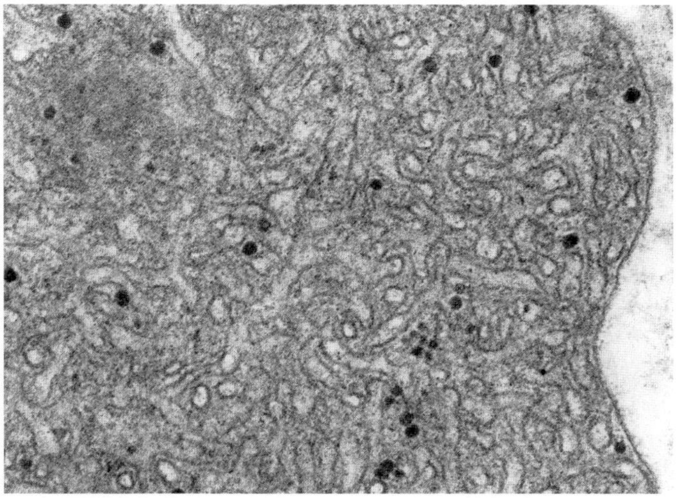

FIGURE 2.29
Electron micrograph of the sER. This image shows numerous profiles of sER in an interstitial (Leydig) cell of the testis, a cell that produces steroid hormones. The sER seen here is a complex system of anastomosing tubules. The small dense objects are glycogen particles. ×60,000.

Because of these widely disparate functions, numerous other enzymes, including hydrolases, methylases, glucose-6-phosphatase, ATPases, and lipid oxidases, are associated with the sER, depending on its functional role.

Golgi Apparatus

The Golgi apparatus is well developed in secretory cells and does not stain with hematoxylin or eosin

The *Golgi apparatus* was described more than 100 years ago by histologist Camillo Golgi. In studies of osmium-impregnated nerve cells, he discovered an organelle that formed networks around the nucleus. It was also described as well developed in secretory cells. Changes in the shape and location of the Golgi apparatus relative to its secretory state were described even before it was viewed with the electron microscope and its functional relationship to the rER was established. It is active both in cells that secrete protein by exocytosis and in cells that synthesize large amounts of membrane and membrane-associated proteins, such as nerve cells. In the light microscope, secretory cells that have a large Golgi apparatus, e.g., plasma cells, osteoblasts, and cells of the epididymis, typically exhibit a clear area partially surrounded by ergastoplasm (Fig. 2.30). In electron micrographs, the Golgi appears as a series of stacked, flattened, membrane-limited sacs or cisternae and tubular extensions embedded in a network of microtubules near the microtubule-organizing center (MTOC) (see page 53). Small vesicles involved in vesicular transport are seen in association with the cisternae. The Golgi apparatus is polarized both morphologically and functionally. The flattened cisternae located closest to the rER represent the forming face, or ***cis-Golgi network (CGN)***; the cisternae located away from the rER represent the maturing face, or ***trans-Golgi network (TGN)*** (Figs. 2.31 and 2.32). The cisternae located between the TGN and CGN are commonly referred as the medial Golgi.

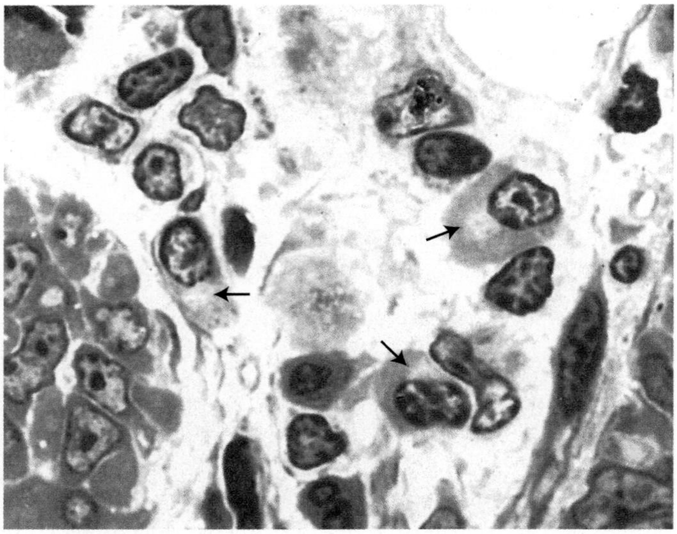

FIGURE 2.30
Photomicrograph of plasma cells. This photomicrograph of a plastic-embedded specimen showing the lamina propria of the small intestine is stained with toluidine blue. The plasma cells, where appropriately oriented, exhibit a clear area in the cytoplasm near the nucleus. These negatively stained regions *(arrows)* represent extensive accumulation of membranous cisternae that belong to the Golgi apparatus. The surrounding cytoplasm is deeply metachromatically stained because of the presence of ribosomes associated with the extensive rER. ×1,200.

The Golgi apparatus functions in the posttranslational modification, sorting, and packaging of proteins

Small vesicles called ***transport vesicles*** carry newly synthesized proteins (both secretory and membrane) from the rER to the CGN. From there, they travel within the transport vesicles from one cisterna to the next. The vesicles bud from one cisterna and fuse with the adjacent cisternae. As proteins and lipids travel through the Golgi stacks, they undergo a series of posttranslational modifications that involve remodeling of N-linked oligosaccharides previously added in the rER.

In general, glycoproteins and glycolipids have their oligosaccharides trimmed and translocated. Glycosylation of proteins and lipids uses several carbohydrate-processing enzymes that add, remove, and modify sugar moieties of oligosaccharide chains. M-6-P is added to those proteins destined to travel to late endosomes and lysosomes (page 28). In addition, glycoproteins are phosphorylated and sulfated. The proteolytic cleavage of certain proteins is also initiated within the cisternae (Fig. 2.33).

Four major pathways of protein secretion from the Golgi apparatus disperse proteins to various cell destinations

As noted, proteins exit the Golgi apparatus from the TGN. This network and the associated tubulovesicular array serve as the sorting station for shuttling vesicles that deliver proteins to various locations (Fig. 2.34). These locations are

- ***Basolateral plasma membrane.*** Proteins targeted to the basolateral domain have a specific sorting signal attached to them by the TGN. This constitutive pathway uses clathrin-coated vesicles with an epithelium-specific adaptor protein; the transported membrane proteins are continuously incorporated into the basolateral cell surface.
- ***Apical plasma membrane.*** Many extracellular and membrane proteins are delivered to this site. This pathway represents another example of constitutive secretion. Secretory proteins also use clathrin-coated vesicles for their transport to the apical surface, which is mediated by specific carbohydrate–lecithin interactions.

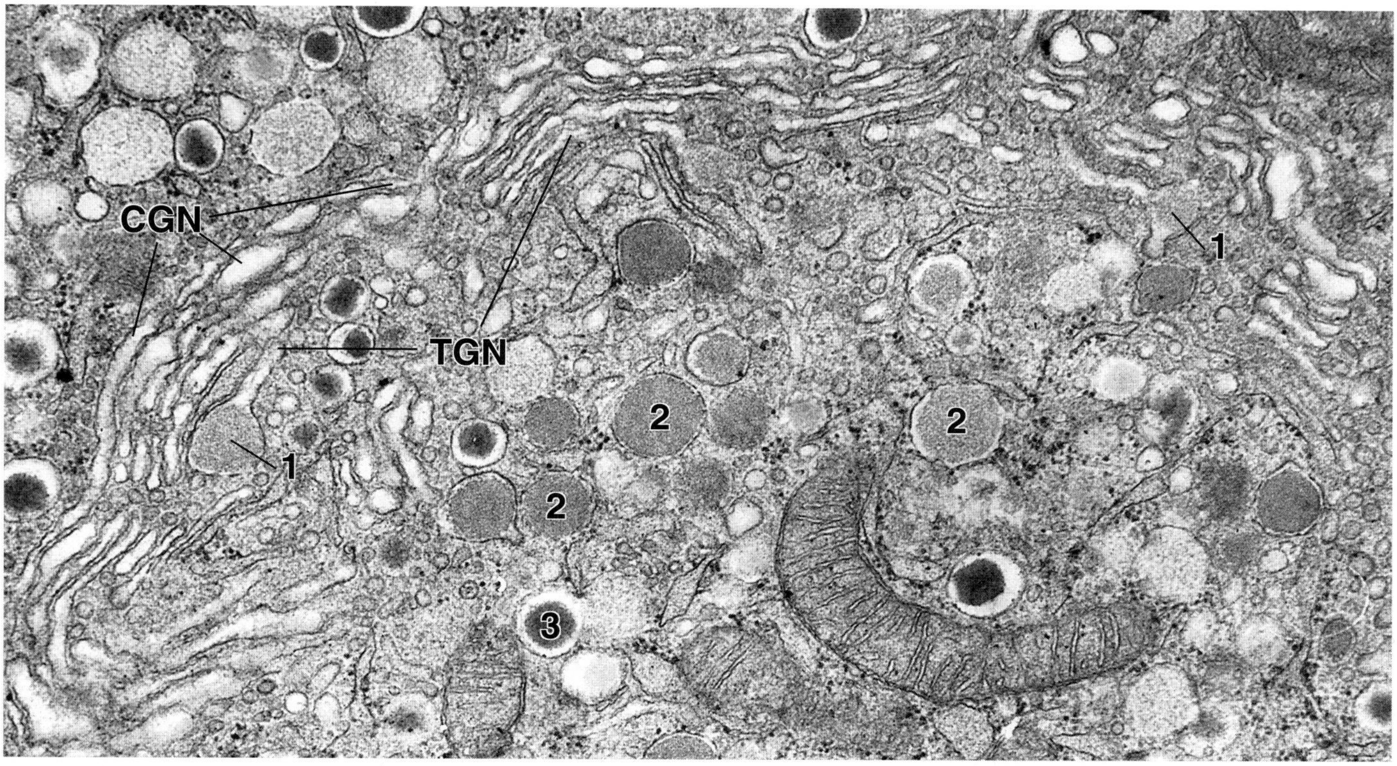

FIGURE 2.31
Electron micrograph of the Golgi apparatus. This electron micrograph shows the extensive Golgi apparatus in an islet cell of the pancreas. The flattened membrane sacs of the Golgi apparatus are arranged in layers. The *cis*-Golgi network *(CGN)* is represented by the flattened vesicles on the outer convex surface, whereas the flattened vesicles of the inner convex region constitute the *trans*-Golgi network *(TGN)*. Budding off the TGN are several vesicles *(1)*. These vesicles are released *(2)* and eventually become secretory vesicles *(3)*. ×55,000.

- ***Endosomes or lysosomes.*** Most of the proteins bearing M-6-P markers are destined for these sites (see page 28).
- ***Apical cytoplasm.*** Proteins that were aggregated or crystallized in the TGN because of changes in pH and Ca^{2+} concentration are stored in large secretory vesicles. These vesicles eventually fuse with the plasma membrane to release the secretory product by exocytosis. This type of secretion is characteristic of secretory cells found in exocrine glands.

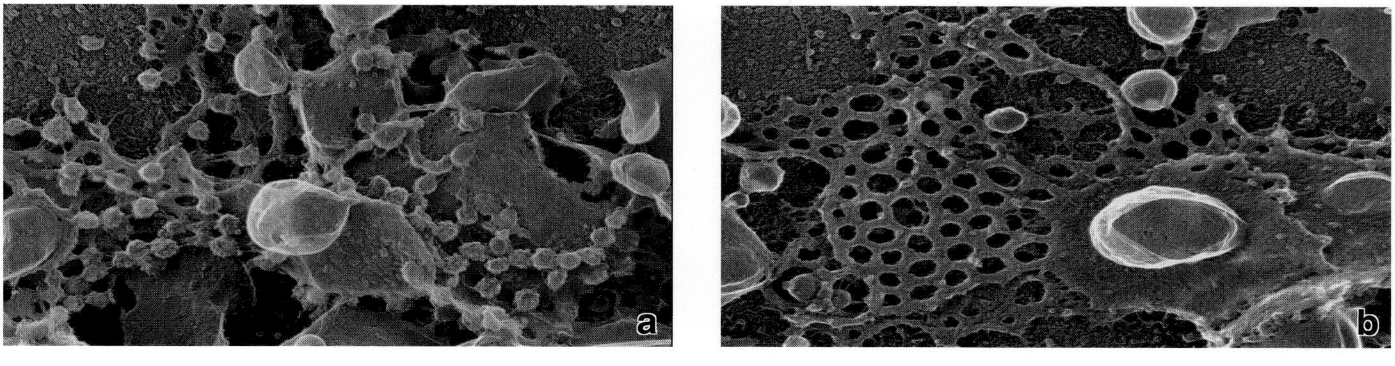

FIGURE 2.32
Electron micrograph of Golgi cisternae. a. This transmission electron micrograph shows a quick-frozen isolated Golgi apparatus replica from a cultured CHO cell line. The *trans*-Golgi cisternae are in the process of coated vesicle formation. **b.** Incubation of the *trans*-Golgi cisternae with the coatomer-depleted cytosol shows a decrease in vesicle formation activity. Note the lack of vesicles and the fenestrated shape of the *trans*-Golgi cisternae. ×85,000. (Courtesy of Dr. John E. Heuser, Washington University School of Medicine.)

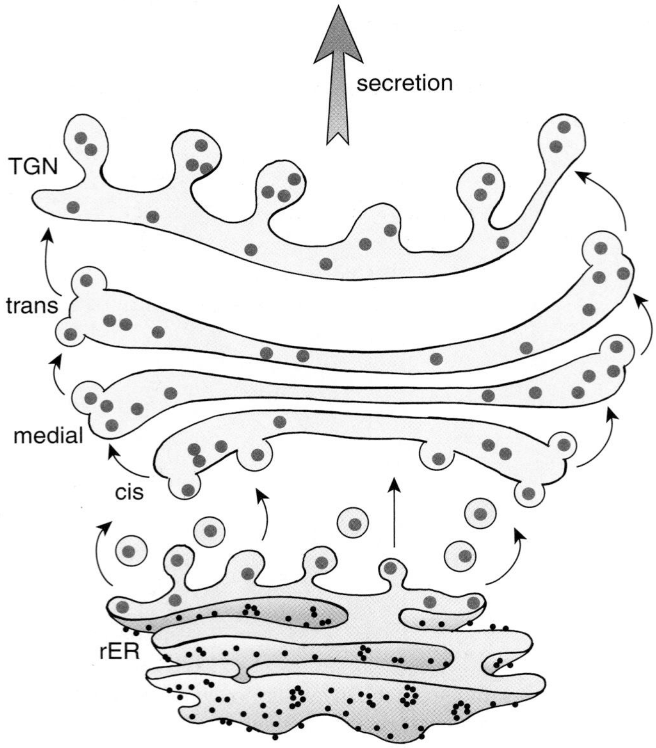

FIGURE 2.33
Structure and function of the Golgi apparatus. The Golgi apparatus contains several stacks of flattened cisternae with dilated edges. The Golgi cisternae form separate functional compartments. The closest compartment to the rER represents the *cis*-Golgi network (CGN), to which transport vesicles originating from the rER fuse and deliver newly synthesized proteins. The CGN represents the first compartment of the Golgi apparatus, where posttransitional modification of the proteins occurs (i.e., phosphorylation). Once proteins have been modified within the CGN, the transport vesicles bud off dilated ends of this compartment, and proteins are transferred into *medial* Golgi cisternae, where they are further modified (i.e., glycosylated). The process continues, and in the same fashion, proteins are translocated into the *trans*-Golgi cisternae and further into the *trans*-Golgi network (TGN), where they are sorted into different transport vesicles that deliver them to their final destinations.

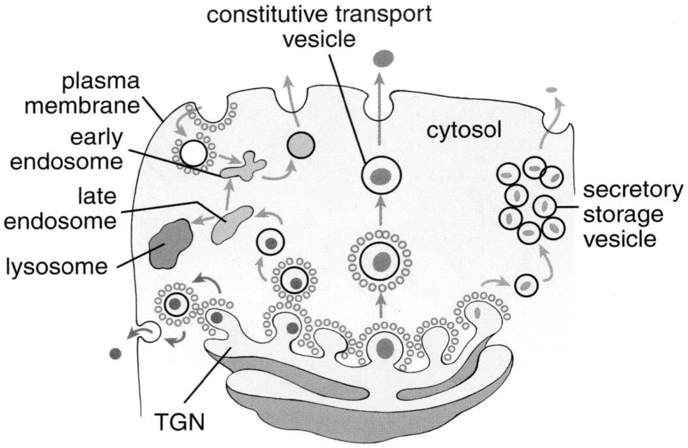

FIGURE 2.34
Summary of events in protein trafficking from the *trans*-Golgi network (TGN). The tubulovesicular array of the TGN serves as the sorting station for transporting vesicles that deliver proteins to four major locations in the cell. The constitutive secretory pathway to the basolateral plasma membrane *(red arrows)* uses clathrin-coated vesicles. The endosomal pathway *(green arrows)* is an organelle-specific protein delivery system. Another constitutive secretory pathway to the apical plasma membrane *(purple arrows)* also uses clathrin-coated vesicles. The regulated secretory pathway *(orange arrows)* directs protein to the apical region of the cell, where proteins are stored in large secretory vesicles. These vesicles eventually fuse with the plasma membrane and release the secretory product by exocytosis.

Mitochondria

Mitochondria are abundant in cells that generate and expend large amounts of energy

Mitochondria were also known to early cytologists who observed them in cells vitally stained with Janus green B. It is now evident that mitochondria increase in number by division throughout interphase, and their divisions are not synchronized with the cell cycle. Videomicroscopy confirms that mitochondria can both change their location and undergo transient changes in shape. They may therefore be compared to mobile power generators as they migrate from one area of the cell to another to supply needed energy.

Because mitochondria generate ATP, they are more numerous in cells that use large amounts of energy, such as striated muscle cells and cells engaged in fluid and electrolyte transport. Mitochondria also localize at sites in the cell where energy is needed, as in the middle piece of the sperm, the intermyofibrillar spaces in striated muscle cells, and adjacent to the basolateral plasma membrane infoldings in the cells of the proximal convoluted tubule of the kidney.

Mitochondria evolved from aerobic bacteria that were engulfed by eukaryotic cells

Mitochondria are believed to have evolved from an aerobic prokaryote (bacterium) that lived symbiotically within primitive eukaryotic cells. This hypothesis received support with the demonstration that mitochondria possess their own genome, increase their numbers by division, and synthesize some of their structural (constituent) proteins. Mitochondrial DNA is a closed circular molecule that encodes 13 enzymes involved in the oxidative phosphorylation pathway, 2 rRNAs, and 22 transfer RNAs (tRNAs)

used in the translation of the mitochondrial mRNA. Mitochondria possess a complete system for protein synthesis including the synthesis of their own ribosomes. The remainder of the mitochondrial proteins are encoded by nuclear DNA; new polypeptides are synthesized by free ribosomes in the cytoplasm and then imported into mitochondria with the help of protein chaperones.

Mitochondria are present in all cells except red blood cells and terminal keratinocytes

The number, shape, and internal structure of mitochondria are often characteristic for specific cell types. When present in large numbers, mitochondria contribute to the acidophilia of the cytoplasm because of the large amount of membrane they contain. Mitochondria may be stained specifically by histochemical procedures that demonstrate some of their constituent enzymes, such as those involved in ATP synthesis and electron transport.

Mitochondria possess two membranes that delineate distinct compartments

Mitochondria display a variety of shapes, including spheres, rods, elongated filaments, and even coiled structures. All mitochondria, unlike other organelles described above, possess two membranes (Fig. 2.35). The inner mitochondrial membrane surrounds a space called the *ma-*

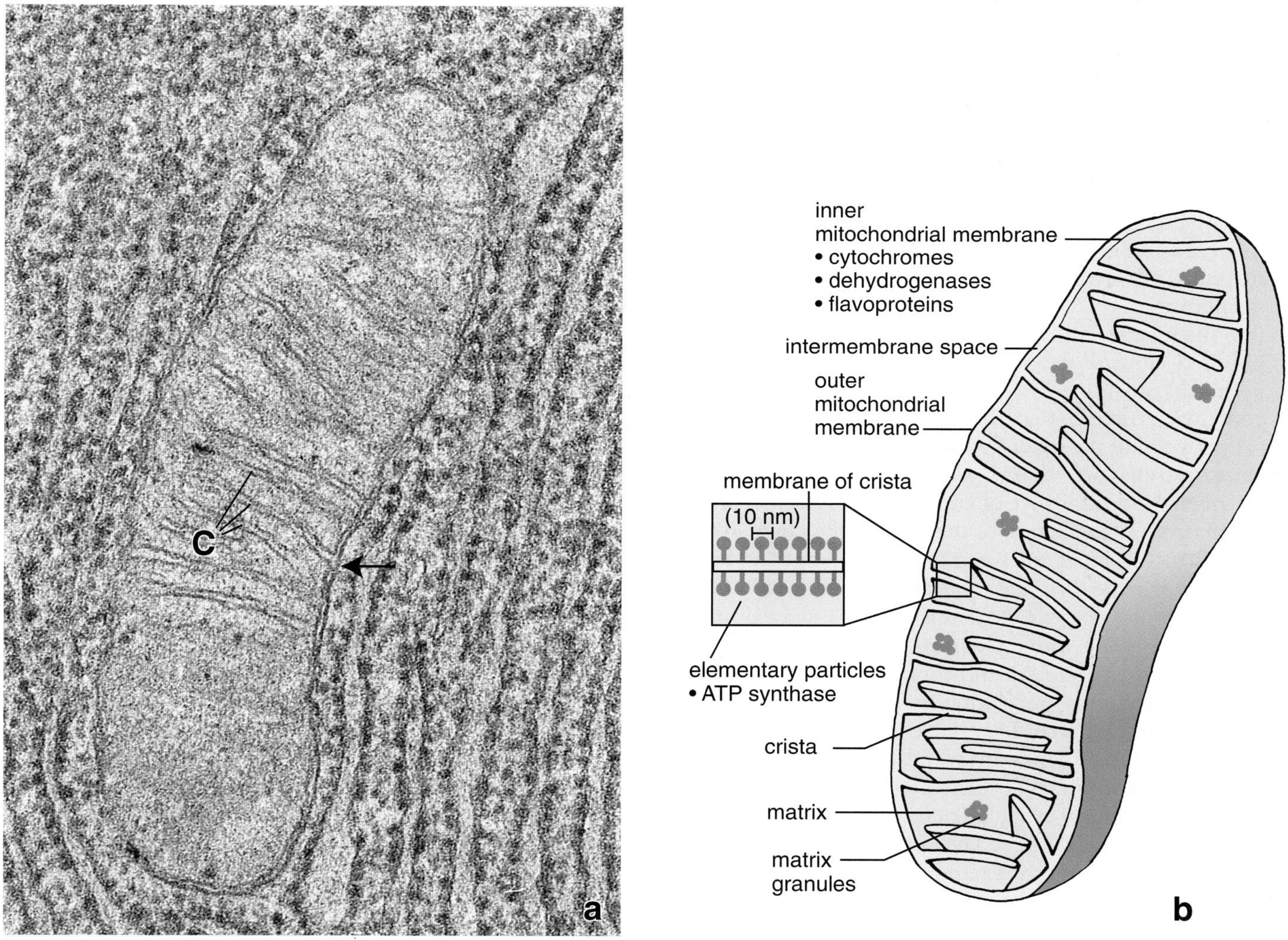

FIGURE 2.35
Structure of the mitochondrion. a. This electron micrograph shows a mitochondrion in a pancreatic acinar cell. Note that the inner mitochondrial membrane forms the cristae *(C)* through a series of infoldings, as is evident in the region of the *arrow.* The outer mitochondrial membrane is a smooth continuous envelope that is separate and distinct from the inner membrane. ×200,000. **b.** Schematic diagram showing the components of a mitochondrion. Note the location of the elementary particles **(inset),** the shape of which relates to the three-dimensional structure of ATP synthase.

trix. The outer mitochondrial membrane is in close contact with the cytoplasm. The space between the two membranes is called the ***intermembrane space.*** The structural components of mitochondria possess specific characteristics related to their function:

- ***Outer mitochondrial membrane.*** This 6- to 7-nm-thick smooth membrane contains many ***voltage-dependent anion channels*** (also called ***mitochondrial porins***). These large channels (approximately 3 nm in diameter) are permeable to uncharged molecules up to 5,000 Da. Thus small molecules, ions, and metabolites can enter the intermembrane space but cannot penetrate the inner membrane. The environment of the intermembrane space is therefore similar to that of cytoplasm with respect to ions and small molecules. The outer membrane possesses receptors for proteins and polypeptides that translocate into the intermembrane space. It also contains several enzymes, including phospholipase A_2, monoamine oxidase, and acetyl coenzyme A (CoA) synthase.
- ***Inner mitochondrial membrane.*** The TEM reveals that this membrane is thinner than the outer mitochondrial membrane. It is arranged into numerous folds *(cristae)* that significantly increase the inner membrane surface area (see Fig. 2.35). These folds project into the matrix that constitutes the inner compartment of the organelle. In some cells involved in steroid metabolism, the inner membrane may form tubular or vesicular projections into the matrix. The inner membrane is rich in the phospholipid ***cardiolipin,*** which makes the membrane impermeable to ions. The membrane forming the cristae contains proteins that have three major functions: (1) performing the oxidation reactions of the respiratory electron-transport chain, (2) synthesizing ATP, and (3) regulating transport of metabolites into and out of the matrix. The enzymes of the respiratory chain are attached to the inner membrane and project their heads into the matrix (Fig. 2.35, *rectangle*). With the TEM, these enzymes appear as tennis racquet–shaped structures called ***elementary particles.*** Their heads measure about 10 nm in diameter and contain enzymes that carry out oxidative phosphorylation, which generates ATP.
- ***Intermembrane space.*** This space is located between the inner and outer membranes and contains specific enzymes that use the ATP generated in the inner membrane. These enzymes include creatine kinase, adenylate kinase, and cytochrome *c*. The latter is an important factor in initiating apoptosis (see page 45).
- ***Matrix.*** The mitochondrial matrix is surrounded by the inner mitochondrial membrane and contains the soluble enzymes of the citric acid cycle (Krebs cycle) and the enzymes involved in fatty acid β-oxidation. The major products of the matrix are CO_2 and reduced NADH, which is the source of electrons for the electron transport chain. Mitochondria contain dense ***matrix granules*** that store Ca^{2+} and other divalent and trivalent cations. These granules increase in number and size when the concentration of divalent (and trivalent) cations increases in the cytoplasm. Mitochondria can accumulate cations against a concentration gradient. Thus, in addition to ATP production, mitochondria also regulate the concentration of certain ions of the cytoplasmic matrix, a role they share with the sER. The matrix also contains mitochondrial DNA, ribosomes, and tRNAs.

Mitochondria contain the enzyme system that generates ATP by means of the citric acid cycle and oxidative phosphorylation

Mitochondria generate ATP in a variety of metabolic pathways including oxidative phosphorylation, the citric acid cycle, and β-oxidation of fatty acids. The energy generated from these reactions, which take place in the mitochondrial matrix, is represented by hydrogen ions (H^+) derived from reduced NADH. These ions drive a series of ***proton pumps*** located within the inner mitochondrial membrane that transfer H^+ from the matrix to the intermembrane space (Fig. 2.36). These pumps constitute the

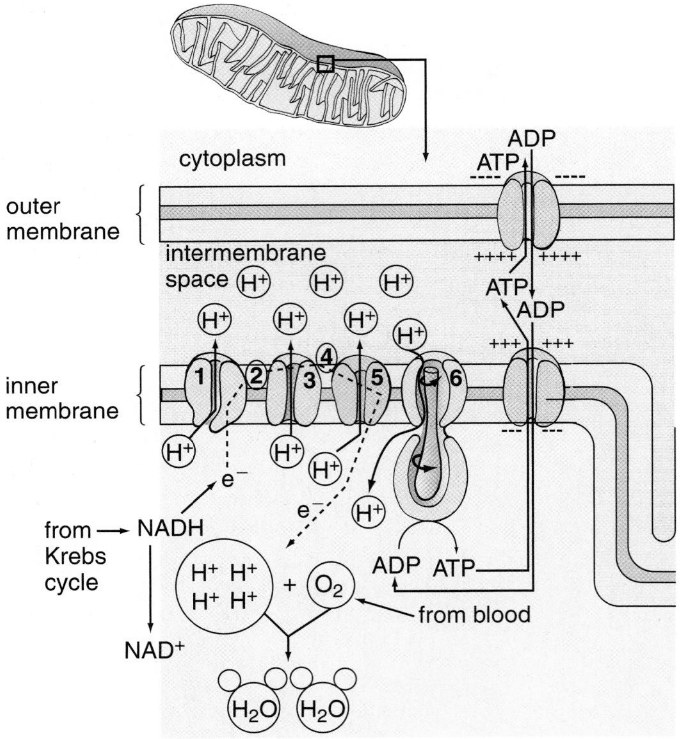

FIGURE 2.36
Schematic diagram illustrating how mitochondria generate energy. The diagram indicates the ATP synthase complex and the electron transport chain of proteins located in the inner mitochondrial membrane. The electron transport chain generates a proton gradient between the matrix and intermembrane space that is used to produce ATP. *Numbers* represent sequential proteins involved in the electron transport chain and ATP production: *1,* NADH dehydrogenase complex; *2,* ubiquinone; *3,* cytochrome *b-c₁* complex; *4,* cytochrome *c*; *5,* cytochrome oxidase complex; and *6,* ATP synthase complex.

electron-transport chain of respiratory enzymes (see Fig. 2.36). The transfer of H^+ across the inner mitochondrial membrane establishes an ***electrochemical proton gradient.*** This gradient creates a ***large proton motive force*** that causes the movement of H^+ down its electrochemical gradient through a large, membrane-bound enzyme called ***ATP synthase.*** ATP synthase provides a pathway across the inner mitochondrial membrane in which H^+ ions are used to drive the energetically unfavorable reactions leading to synthesis of ATP. This movement of protons back to the mitochondrial matrix is referred to as ***chemiosmotic coupling.*** The newly produced ATP is transported from the matrix to the intermembrane space by the voltage gradient–driven ***ATP/ADP exchange protein*** located in the inner mitochondrial membrane. From here, ATP leaves the mitochondria via voltage-dependent anion channels in the outer membrane to enter the cytoplasm. At the same time, ADP produced in the cytoplasm rapidly enters the mitochondria for recharging.

Mitochondria undergo morphologic changes related to their functional state

TEM studies show mitochondria in two distinct configurations. In the ***orthodox configuration,*** the cristae are prominent and the matrix compartment occupies a large part of the total mitochondrial volume. This configuration corresponds to a ***low level*** of oxidative phosphorylation. In the ***condensed configuration,*** cristae are not easily recognized, the matrix is concentrated and reduced in volume, and the intermembrane space increases to as much as 50% of the total volume. This configuration corresponds to a ***high level*** of oxidative phosphorylation.

Mitochondria decide if the cell lives or dies

Recent experimental studies indicate that mitochondria sense cellular stress and are capable of deciding whether the cell lives or dies by initiating ***apoptosis*** (programmed cell death). The major cell death event generated by the mitochondria is the release of cytochrome *c* from the mitochondrial intermembranous space into the cell cytoplasm. This event, regulated by the ***Bcl-2 protein family*** (see page 74), initiates the cascade of proteolytic enzymatic reactions that leads to apoptosis.

Peroxisomes (Microbodies)

Peroxisomes are single membrane-bounded organelles containing oxidative enzymes

Peroxisomes (microbodies) are small (0.5 μm diameter), membrane-limited spherical organelles that contain oxidative enzymes, particularly catalase and other peroxidases. Virtually all oxidative enzymes produce ***hydrogen peroxide (H_2O_2)*** as a product of the oxidation reaction. Hydrogen peroxide is a toxic substance. The catalase universally present in peroxisomes carefully regulates the cellular hydrogen peroxide content by breaking down hydrogen peroxide, thus protecting the cell. In addition, peroxisomes contain D-amino acid oxidases, β-oxidation enzymes, and numerous other enzymes.

Oxidative enzymes are particularly important in liver cells (hepatocytes), where they perform a variety of detoxification processes. Peroxisomes in hepatocytes are responsible for detoxification of ingested alcohol by converting it to acetaldehyde. β-Oxidation of fatty acids is also a major function of peroxisomes. In some cells, peroxisomal fatty acid oxidation may equal that of mitochondria. The proteins contained in the peroxisome lumen and membrane are synthesized on cytoplasmic ribosomes and imported into the peroxisome. A protein destined for peroxisomes must have a ***peroxisomal targeting signal*** attached to its C-terminus.

Although abundant in liver and kidney cells, peroxisomes are found in most other cells. The number of peroxisomes present in a cell increases in response to diet, drugs, and hormonal stimulation. In most animals, but not humans, peroxisomes also contain urate oxidase (uricase), which often appears as a characteristic ***crystalloid inclusion (nucleoid).***

Various human metabolic disorders are caused by the inability to import peroxisomal proteins into the organelle because of faulty peroxisomal targeting signal. Several severe disorders are associated with nonfunctional peroxisomes. In the most common inherited disease related to nonfunctional peroxisomes, ***Zellweger syndrome,*** which leads to early death, peroxisomes lose their ability to function because of lack of necessary enzymes. Therapies for peroxisomal disorders have been unsatisfactory to date.

▼ NONMEMBRANOUS ORGANELLES

Microtubules

Microtubules are nonbranching and rigid hollow tubes of protein that can rapidly disassemble in one location and reassemble in another. In general, they grow from the ***microtubule-organizing center (MTOC)*** located near the nucleus (page 53) and extend toward the cell periphery. Microtubules create a system of connections within the cell, frequently compared to railroad tracks, along which vesicular movement occurs.

Microtubules are elongated polymeric structures composed of equal parts of α-tubulin and β-tubulin

Microtubules measure 20 to 25 nm in diameter (Fig. 2.37). The wall of the microtubule is approximately 5 nm thick and consists of 13 circularly arrayed globular ***dimeric tubulin molecules.*** The tubulin dimer has a molecular weight of 110 kDa and is formed from an α-tubulin and a β-tubulin molecule, each with a molecular weight of 55 kDa. (Fig.

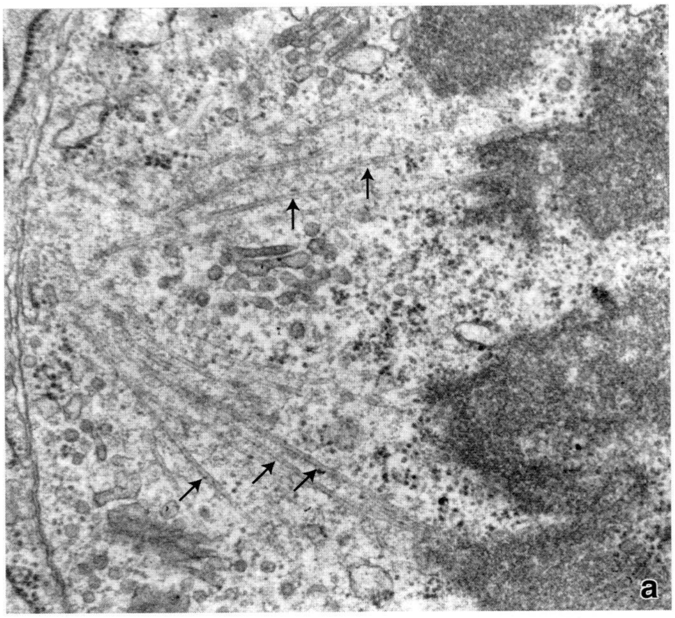

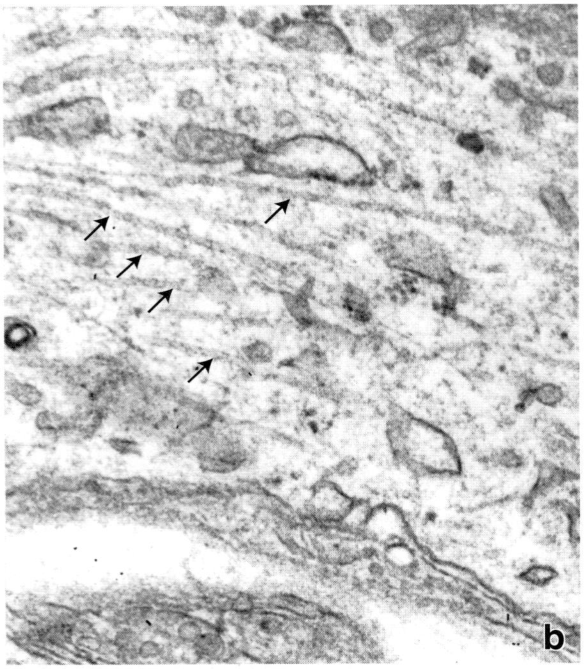

FIGURE 2.37

Electron micrographs of microtubules. a. Micrograph showing microtubules *(arrows)* of the mitotic spindle in a dividing cell. On the right, the microtubules are attached to chromosomes. ×30,000. **b.** Micrograph of microtubules *(arrows)* in the axon of a nerve cell. In both cells, the microtubules are seen in longitudinal profile. ×30,000.

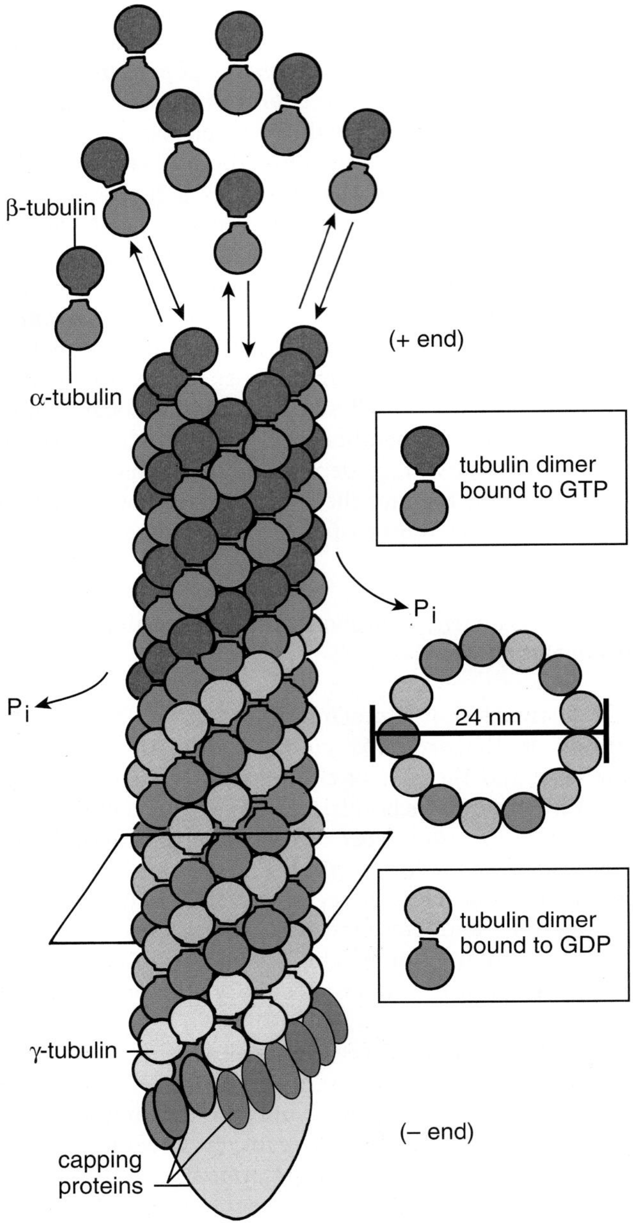

FIGURE 2.38

Diagram of a microtubule in a longitudinal and cross-sectional profile. At the left, the diagram depicts the process of polymerization and depolymerization of tubulin dimers during the process of microtubule assembly. Each tubulin dimer consists of an α-tubulin and a β-tubulin subunit. On the right, each microtubule contains 13 tubulin dimers within its cross section. The minus (−) end of the microtubule contains a ring of γ-tubulin, which is necessary for microtubule nucleation. This end is usually embedded within the MTOC and possesses numerous capping proteins. The plus (+) end of the microtubule is the growing end to which tubulin dimers bound to GTP molecules are incorporated. Incorporated tubulin dimers hydrolyze GTP, which releases the phosphate groups to form polymers with GDP–tubulin molecules.

2.38). The dimers polymerize in an end-to-end fashion, head to tail, with the α molecule of one dimer bound to the β molecule of the next dimer in a repeating pattern. The polymer thus formed is called a protofilament. Axial periodicity seen along the 5-nm-diameter dimers corresponds to the length of the protein molecules. A small, 1-μm segment of microtubule contains approximately 16,000 tubulin dimers.

Microtubules grow from γ-tubulin rings within the MTOC that serve as nucleation sites for each microtubule

Microtubule formation can be traced to hundreds of γ-tubulin rings that form an integral part of the MTOC (Fig. 2.39). The α- and β-tubulin dimers are added to a γ-tubulin ring in an end-to-end fashion (see Fig. 2.38). Polymerization of tubulin dimers requires the presence of guanosine triphosphate (GTP) and Mg^{2+}. Each tubulin molecule binds GTP before it is incorporated into the forming microtubule.

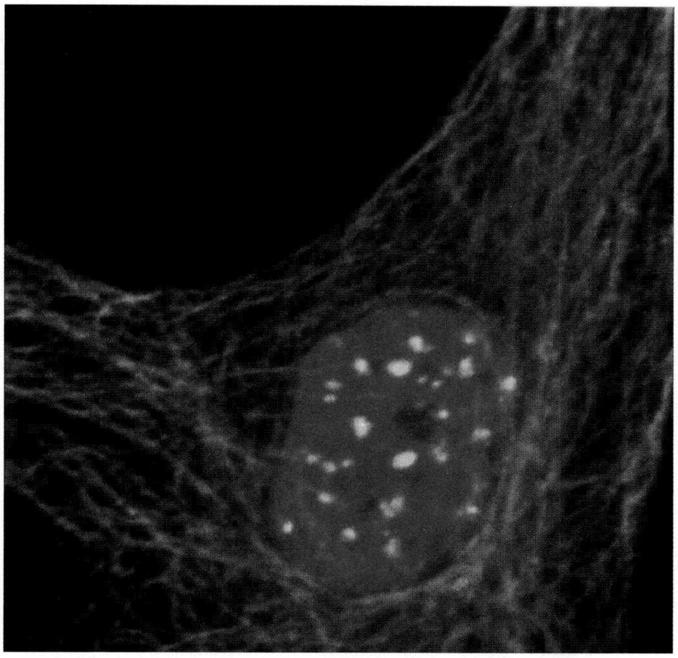

FIGURE 2.39
Staining of microtubules with fluorescent dye. This confocal immunofluorescent image shows the organization of the microtubules within an epithelial cell in tissue culture. In this example, the specimen was immunostained with three primary antibodies against tubulin *(green)*, centrin *(red)*, and kinetochores *(light blue)* and then incubated in a mixture of three different fluorescently tagged secondary antibodies that recognized the primary antibodies. Nuclei were stained *(dark blue)* with a fluorescent molecule that intercalates into the DNA double helix. Note that the microtubules are focused at the MTOC or centrosome *(red)* located adjacent to the nucleus. The cell is in the S phase of the cell cycle, as indicated by the presence of both large unduplicated kinetochores and smaller pairs of duplicated kinetochores. ×3,000. (Courtesy of Dr. Wilma L. Lingle and Ms. Vivian A. Negron.)

The GTP–tubulin complex is then polymerized, and at some point GTP is hydrolyzed to guanosine diphosphate (GDP). As a result of this polymerization pattern, each microtubule possesses a ***minus*** (nongrowing) ***end*** embedded in the MTOC and a ***plus*** (growing) ***end*** elongating toward the cell periphery. Tubulin dimers dissociate from microtubules in the steady state, which adds a pool of free tubulin dimers to the cytoplasm. This pool is in equilibrium with the polymerized tubulin in the microtubules; therefore, polymerization and depolymerization are in equilibrium. The equilibrium can be shifted in the direction of depolymerization by exposing the cell or isolated microtubules to low temperatures or high pressure. Repeated exposure to alternating low and high temperature is the basis of the purification technique for tubulin and microtubules. The speed of polymerization or depolymerization can also be modified by interaction with specific ***microtubule-associated proteins (MAPs)***. These proteins, such as MAP-1, 2, 3, and 4, MAP-t, and TOGp, regulate microtubule assembly and anchor the microtubules to specific organelles. MAPs are also responsible for the existence of stable populations of nondepolymerizing microtubes in the cell, such as those found in cilia and flagella.

The length of microtubules changes dynamically as tubulin dimers are added or removed in a process of dynamic instability

Microtubules observed in cultured cells with real-time video microscopy appear to be constantly growing toward the cell periphery (by addition of tubulin dimers) and then suddenly shrinking in the direction of the MTOC (by removal of tubulin dimers). This constant remodeling process, known as ***dynamic instability***, is linked to a pattern of GTP hydrolysis during the microtubule assembly and disassembly process. The MTOC can be compared to a feeding chameleon, which fires its long, projectile tongue to make contact with potential food. The chameleon then retracts its tongue back into its mouth and repeats this process until it is successful in obtaining food. The same strategy of "firing" microtubules from the MTOC toward the cell periphery and subsequently retracting them enables the cell to establish an organized system of microtubules linking peripheral structures and organelles with the MTOC. As mentioned above, association of a microtubule with MAPs, such as occurs within the axoneme of a cilium or flagellum, effectively blocks this dynamic instability and stabilizes the microtubules.

The structure and function of microtubules in mitosis and in cilia and flagella are discussed later in this chapter and in Chapter 4.

Microtubules can be visualized in the light microscope and are involved in intracellular transport and cell motility

Microtubules may be seen in the light microscope by using special stains, polarization, or phase contrast optics.

Because of the limited resolution of the light microscope, in the past microtubules were erroneously called fibers, such as the "fibers" of the mitotic spindle. Microtubules may now be distinguished from filamentous and fibrillar cytoplasmic components even at the light microscopic level by using antibodies to tubulin, the primary protein component of microtubules, conjugated with fluorescent dyes (Fig. 2.39).

In general, microtubules are found in the cytoplasm, where they originate from the MTOC; in cilia and flagella, where they form the axoneme and its anchoring basal body; in centrioles and the mitotic spindle; and in elongating processes of the cell, such as those in growing axons.

Microtubules are involved in numerous essential cellular functions:

- Intracellular vesicular transport (e.g., movement of secretory vesicles, endosomes, lysosomes)
- Movement of cilia and flagella
- Attachment of chromosomes to the mitotic spindle and their movement during mitosis and meiosis
- Cell elongation and movement (migration)
- Maintenance of cell shape, particularly its asymmetry

Movement of intracellular organelles is generated by molecular motor proteins associated with microtubules

In cellular activities that involve movement of organelles and other cytoplasmic structures, such as transport vesicles, mitochondria, and lysosomes, microtubules serve as guides to the appropriate destinations. ***Molecular motor proteins*** attach to these organelles or structures and ratchet along the microtubule track (Fig. 2.40). The energy required for the ratcheting movement is derived from ATP hydrolysis. Two families of molecular motors have been identified that allow for unidirectional movement:

- ***Dyneins*** constitute one family of molecular motors. They move along the microtubules toward the minus end of the tubule. Therefore, ***cytoplasmic dyneins*** are capable of transporting organelles from the cell periphery toward the MTOC. One member of the dynein family, ***axonemal dynein,*** is present in cilia and flagella. It is responsible for the sliding of one microtubule against an adjacent microtubule of the axoneme that effects their movement.
- ***Kinesins,*** members of the other family, move along the microtubules toward the plus end; therefore, they are capable of moving organelles from the cell center toward the cell periphery.

Both dyneins and kinesins are involved in mitosis and meiosis. In these activities, dyneins move the chromosomes along the kinetochore microtubules toward the spindle pole. Kinesins are simultaneously involved in movement of polar microtubules. These microtubules extend from one spindle pole past the metaphase plate and overlap with microtubules extending from the opposite spindle pole. Kinesins located between these microtubules generate a sliding movement that reduces the overlap, thereby pushing the two spindle poles apart to each daughter cell (Fig. 2.41).

Actin Filaments

Actin filaments are present in virtually all cell types

Actin molecules (42 kDa) are abundant and may constitute up to 20% of the total protein of some nonmuscle cells (Fig. 2.42). Similar to the tubulin in microtubules, actin molecules also assemble spontaneously by polymerization into a linear helical array to form filaments 6 to 8 nm in diameter. They are thinner, shorter, and more flexible than microtubules. Free actin molecules in the cytoplasm are referred to as ***G-actin (globular actin)*** in contrast to the polymerized actin of the filament, called ***F-actin (filamentous actin).*** Actin filaments are polarized structures; their fast-growing end is referred to as the ***plus*** or ***barbed end,*** and their slow-growing end is referred to as the ***minus*** or ***pointed end.*** The dynamic process of actin polymerization requires the presence of K^+, Mg^{2+}, and ATP, which is hydrolyzed to ADP after each G-actin molecule is incorporated into the filament (Fig. 2.43). The control and regulation of the polymerization process depends on the local concentration of G-actin and the interaction of ***actin-binding proteins (ABPs),*** which can prevent or enhance polymerization.

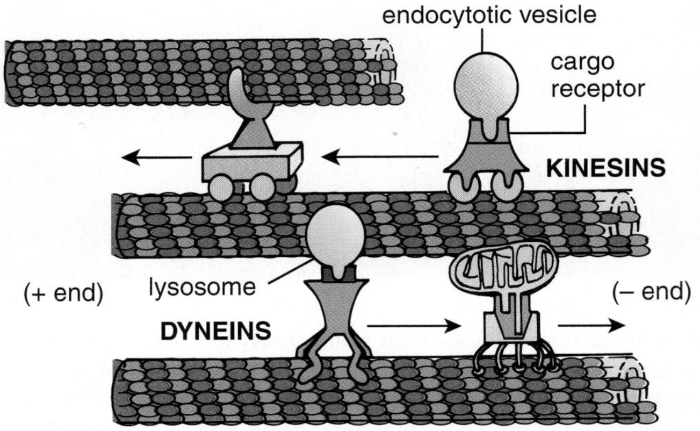

FIGURE 2.40
The molecular motor proteins associated with microtubules. Microtubules serve as guides for molecular motor proteins. These ATP-driven microtubule-associated motor proteins are attached to moving structures (such as organelles) and ratchet them along a tubular track. Two types of molecular motors have been identified: dyneins that move along microtubules toward their minus (–) end (i.e., toward the center of the cell) and kinesins that move toward their plus (+) end (i.e., toward the cell periphery).

In addition to controlling the rate of polymerization of actin filaments, ABPs are responsible for their organization. For example, a number of proteins can modify or act on actin filaments to give them various specific characteristics:

- ***Actin-bundling proteins*** cross-link actin filaments into parallel arrays, creating actin filament bundles. An example of this modification occurs inside the microvillus, where actin filaments are cross-linked by the actin-bundling proteins ***fascin*** and ***fimbrin*** (see Fig. 4.3, page 92). This cross-linkage provides support and imparts rigidity to the microvilli.
- ***Actin filament–severing proteins*** sever long actin filaments into short fragments. An example of such proteins is ***gelsolin,*** a 90-kDa ABP that normally initiates actin polymerization but at high Ca^{2+} concentrations causes severing of the actin filaments, converting an actin gel into a fluid state.

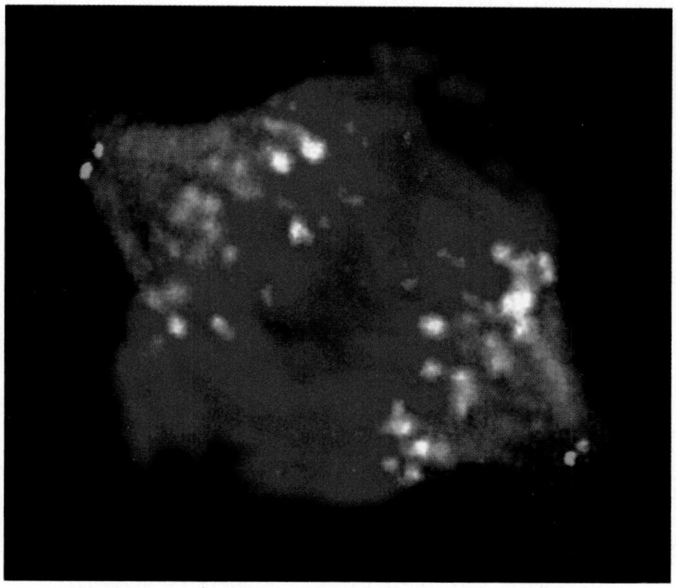

FIGURE 2.41
Distribution of kinesin-like motor protein within the mitotic spindle. This confocal immunofluorescent image shows a mammary gland epithelial cell in anaphase of mitosis, Each mitotic spindle pole contains two centrioles *(green).* A mitosis-specific kinesin-like molecule called Eg5 *(red)* is associated with the subset of the mitotic spindle microtubules that connect the kinetochores *(white)* to the spindle poles. The motor action of Eg5 is required to separate the sister chromatids *(blue)* into the daughter cells. This cell was first immunostained with three primary antibodies against Eg5 *(red),* centrin *(green),* and kinetochores *(white)* and then incubated in three different fluorescently tagged secondary antibodies that recognize the primary antibodies. Chromosomes were stained with a fluorescent molecule that intercalates into the DNA double helix. ×3,500. (Courtesy of Dr. Wilma L. Lingle and Ms. Vivian A. Negron.)

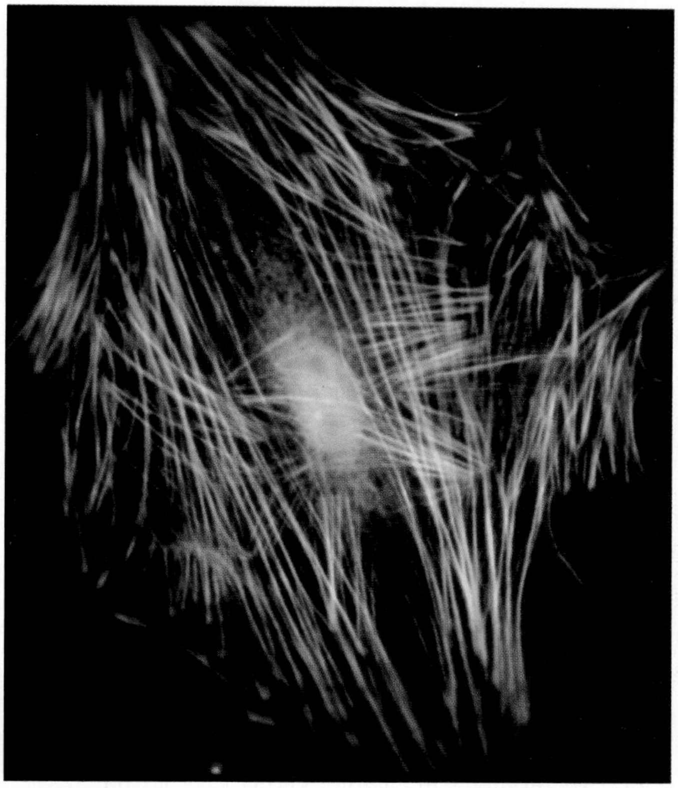

FIGURE 2.42
Distribution of actin filaments in a human fibroblast in culture. The cell was stained with an actin-specific antibody conjugated with the dye fluorescein. The antigen–antibody reaction, performed directly in the culture, results in localization of the actin. The actin filaments organized in linear bundles fluoresce and thus show their distribution in this nonmigrating cell. (Courtesy of Dr. Elias Lazarides.)

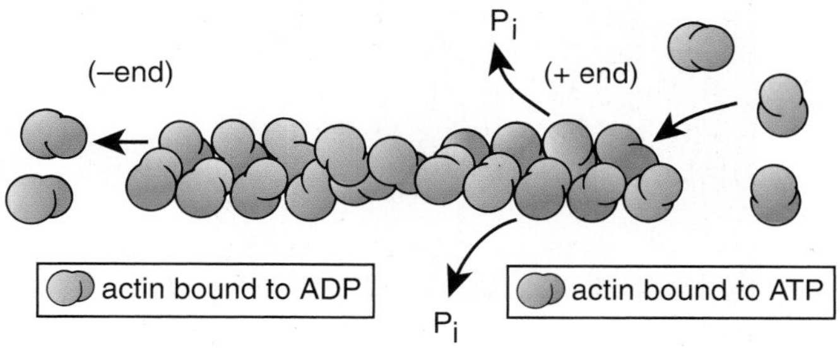

FIGURE 2.43
Polymerization of actin filaments. Actin filaments are polarized structures. Their fast-growing end is referred to as the plus (+) or barbed end; the slow-growing end is referred to as the minus (–) or pointed end. The dynamic process of actin polymerization requires energy in the form of an ATP molecule that is hydrolyzed to ADP after a G-actin molecule is incorporated into the filament.

- ***Actin-capping proteins*** block further addition of actin molecules by binding to the free end of an actin filament. An example is ***tropomodulin,*** which can be isolated from skeletal and cardiac muscle cells. Tropomodulin binds to the free end of actin myofilaments, regulating the length of the filaments in a sarcomere.
- ***Actin cross-linking proteins*** are responsible for cross-linking actin filaments with each other. An example of such proteins can be found in the cytoskeleton of erythrocytes. Several proteins, such as spectrin, adductin, protein 4.1, or protein 4.9, are involved in cross-linking actin filaments (see Fig. 9.4, page 219).
- ***Actin motor proteins*** belong to the myosin family, which hydrolyzes ATP to provide the energy for movement along the actin filament from the minus end to the plus end. Some cells, such as muscle cells, are characterized by the size, amount, and nature of the filaments and actin-motor proteins they contain. There are two types of filaments ***(myofilaments)*** present in muscle cells: 6- to 8-nm actin filaments (called ***thin filaments***) (Fig. 2.44) and 15-nm filaments (called ***thick filaments***) of myosin II, which is the predominant protein in muscle cells. Myosin II is a double-headed molecule with an elongated rod-like tail. The specific structural and functional relationships among actin, myosin, and other ABPs in muscle contraction are discussed in Chapter 10 (Muscle Tissue).

In addition to myosin II, nonmuscle cells contain ***myosin I,*** a protein with a single globular domain and short tail that attaches to other molecules or organelles. Extensive studies have revealed the presence of a variety of other nonmuscle myosin isoforms that are responsible for motor functions in many specialized cells, such as melanocytes, kidney and intestinal absorptive cells, nerve growth cones, and inner ear hair cells.

Actin filaments participate in a variety of cell functions

Actin filaments are often grouped in bundles close to the plasma membrane. Functions of these membrane-associated actin filaments include

- ***Anchorage and movement of membrane protein.*** Actin filaments are distributed in three-dimensional networks throughout the cell and are used as anchors within specialized cell junctions such as focal adhesions.
- ***Formation of the structural core of microvilli*** on absorptive epithelial cells. Actin filaments may also help maintain the shape of the apical cell surface, e.g., the apical terminal web of actin filaments serves as tension cables under the cell surface.
- ***Locomotion of cells.*** Locomotion is achieved by the force exerted by actin filaments by polymerization at their growing ends. This mechanism is used in many migrating cells, in particular on transformed cells of invasive tumors. As a result of actin polymerization at their leading edge, cells extend processes from their surface by pushing the plasma membrane ahead of the growing actin filaments. The leading-edge extensions of a crawling cell are called ***lamellipodia;*** they contain elongating organized bundles of actin filaments with their plus ends directed toward the plasma membrane.
- ***Extension of cell processes.*** These processes can be observed in many other cells that exhibit small protrusions

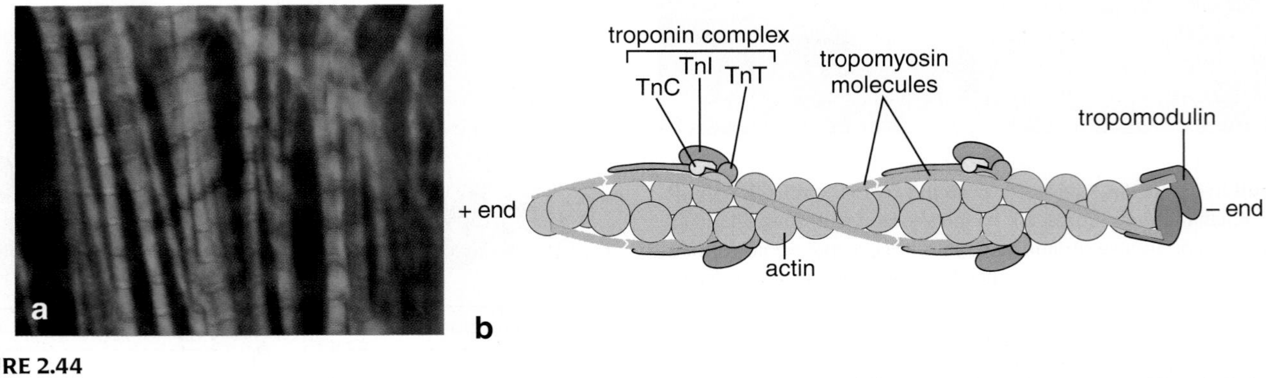

FIGURE 2.44
Thin filament organization and structure in cardiac cells. a. Immunofluorescence micrograph of a chick cardiac myocyte stained for actin *(green)* to show the thin filaments and for tropomodulin *(red)* to show the location of the slow-growing (–) ends of the thin filaments. Tropomodulin appears as regular striations because of the uniform lengths and alignments of the thin filaments in sarcomeres. **b.** Diagram of a thin filament. The polarity of the thin filament is indicated by the fast-growing (+) end and the slow-growing (–) end. Only a portion of the entire thin filament is shown for clarity. Tropomodulin is bound to actin and tropomyosin at the slow-growing (–) end. The troponin complex binds to each tropomyosin molecule every seven actin monomers along the length of the thin filament. (Courtesy of Drs. Velia F. Fowler and Ryan Littlefield.)

called *filopodia,* located around their surface. As in lamellipodia, these protrusions contain loose aggregations of 10 to 20 actin filaments organized in the same direction, again with their plus ends directed toward the plasma membrane. Actin filaments are also essential in cytoplasmic streaming, i.e., the stream-like movement of cytoplasm that can be observed in cultured cells.

Intermediate Filaments

Intermediate filaments play a supporting or general structural role. These rope-like filaments are called "intermediate" because their diameter of 8 to 10 nm is "intermediate" between that of actin filaments and microtubules. Nearly all intermediate filaments consist of subunits with a molecular weight of about 50 kDa. Some evidence suggests that many of the stable structural proteins in intermediate filaments evolved from highly conserved enzymes, with only minor genetic modification.

Intermediate filaments are formed from nonpolar and highly variable intermediate filament subunits

Unlike those of microfilaments and microtubules, the protein subunits of intermediate filaments show considerable diversity and tissue specificity. In addition, they do not posses enzymatic activity and form nonpolar filaments. Intermediate filaments also do not typically disappear and re-form in the continuous manner characteristic of most microtubules and actin filaments. For these reasons, intermediate filaments are believed to play a primarily structural role within the cell and to compose the cytoplasmic link of a tissue-wide continuum of cytoplasmic, nuclear, and extracellular filaments (Fig. 2.45).

Intermediate filament proteins are characterized by a highly variable central ***rod-shaped domain*** with strictly conserved globular domains at either end (Fig. 2.46). Although the various classes of intermediate filaments differ in the amino acid sequence of the rod-shaped domain and show some variation in molecular weight, they all share a homologous region that is important in filament self-assembly. Intermediate filaments are assembled from a pair of helical monomers that twist around each other to form ***coiled-coil dimers.*** Then, two coiled-coil dimers twist around each other in antiparallel fashion (parallel but pointing in opposite directions) to generate a ***staggered tetramer*** of two coiled-coil dimers, thus forming the nonpolarized unit of the intermediate filaments (see Fig. 2.46). Each tetramer, acting as an individual unit, is aligned along the axis of the filament. The ends of the tetramers are bound together to form the free ends of the filament. This assembly process provides a stable, staggered, helical array in which filaments are packed together and additionally stabilized by lateral binding interactions between adjacent tetramers.

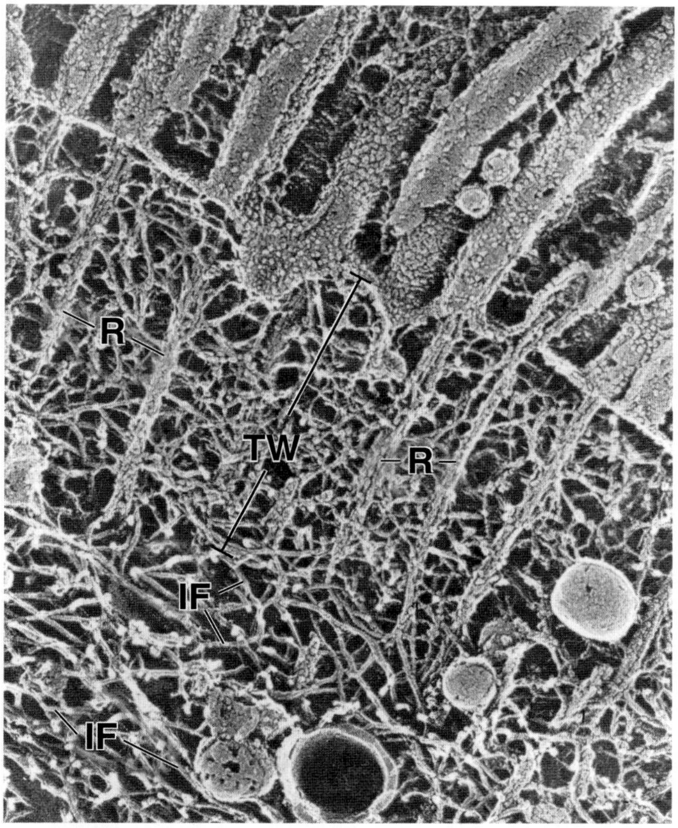

FIGURE 2.45
Electron micrograph of the apical part of an epithelial cell. This electron micrograph, obtained using the quick-freeze deep-etch technique, shows the terminal web *(TW)* of an epithelial cell and underlying intermediate filaments *(IF)*. The long straight actin filament cores or rootlets *(R)* extending from the microvilli are cross-linked by a dense network of actin filaments containing numerous actin-binding proteins. The network of intermediate filaments can be seen beneath the terminal web anchoring the actin filaments of the microvilli. × 47,000. (From Hirokawa N, et al. *J Cell Biol* 1983;96:1325.)

Intermediate filaments are a heterogeneous group of cytoskeletal elements found in various cell types

Intermediate filaments are organized into four major classes on the basis of protein composition and cellular distribution (Table 2.1):

- ***Keratins (cytokeratins),*** the most diverse group of intermediate filaments, contain more than 50 different isoforms. Keratin filaments are formed from a variety of different keratin subunits and are found in different cells of epithelial origin. Specialized keratins called ***hard keratins*** are found in skin appendages such as hair and nails. Keratin filaments span the cytoplasm of epithelial cells and, via desmosomes, connect with keratin filaments in neighboring cells. Keratin subunits do not coassemble with

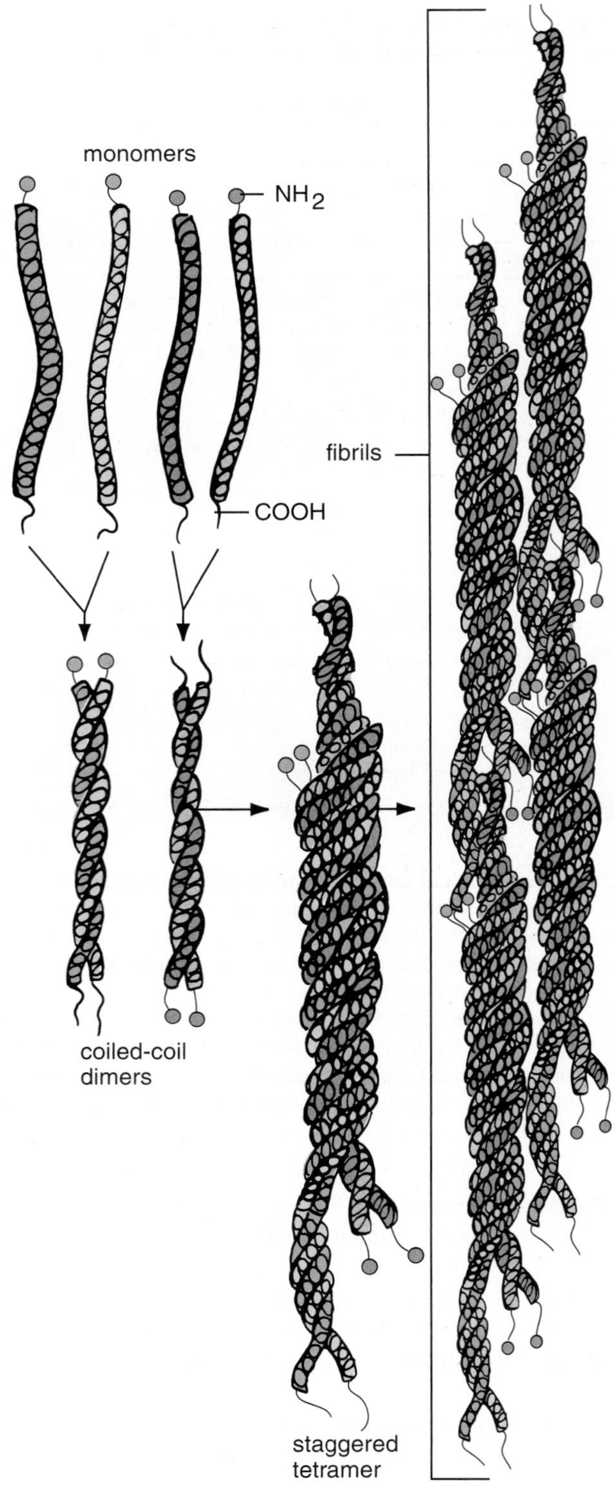

FIGURE 2.46
Polymerization and structure of intermediate filaments. Intermediate filaments are self-assembled from a pair of monomers that twist around each other in parallel fashion to form a stable dimer. Two coiled-coil dimers then twist around each other in antiparallel fashion to generate a staggered tetramer of two coiled-coil dimers. This tetramer forms the nonpolarized unit of the intermediate filaments. Each tetramer, acting as an individual unit, aligns along the axis of the filament and binds to the free end of the elongating structure. This staggered helical array is additionally stabilized by lateral binding interactions between adjacent tetramers.

other types of intermediate filaments; therefore, they form a distinct cell-specific and tissue-specific system.

- ***Vimentin and vimentin-like filaments*** represent a diverse family of cytoplasmic filaments found in many cell types. In contrast to keratins, they form homopolymeric filaments containing only one type of intermediate protein. ***Vimentin*** is the most abundant intermediate filament found in all mesoderm-derived cells. Vimentin-like filaments include ***desmin,*** characteristic of muscle cells; ***glial fibrillary acidic protein (GFAP),*** found in glial cells and astrocytes; ***peripherin,*** found in many neurons; and ***synemin*** and ***paranemin,*** found also in muscle cells.
- ***Neurofilaments*** are formed from the group of neurofilament-triplet (NF) proteins that contain three proteins of different molecular weights: *NF-L* (low-weight protein), *NF-M* (a medium-weight protein) and *NF-H* (a high-weight protein). All three proteins form neurofilaments that extend from the cell body into the ends of axons and dendrites, providing structural support.
- ***Lamins,*** specifically nuclear lamins, are associated with the nuclear envelope and are formed by two types of proteins, lamin A and lamin B. In contrast to other types of intermediate filaments found in the cytoplasm, lamins are located within the nucleoplasm of almost all differentiated cells in the body. A description of their structure and function can be found on page 64.

Intermediate filament–associated proteins are essential for the integrity of cell-to-cell and cell-to-extracellular matrix junctions

A variety of intermediate filament–associated proteins function within the cytoskeleton as integral parts of the molecular architecture of cells. Some proteins, such as those of the ***plectin family,*** possess binding sites for actin filaments, microtubules, and intermediate filaments and are thus important in the proper assembly of the cytoskeleton. Another important family of intermediate filament–associated proteins consists of ***desmoplakins, desmoplakin-like proteins,*** and ***plakoglobins.*** These pro-

TABLE 2.1. **Classes of Intermediate Filaments Based on Their Molecular Structure and Assembly**

Type of Protein	Molecular Weight (kDa)	Cellular Distribution	Where Found
		Class I: Keratins	
Acid cytokeratins	40–64	Cytoplasm	All epithelial cells
Basic cytokeratins	52–68	Cytoplasm	All epithelial cells
		Class 2: Vimentin and Vimentin-like	
Vimentin	55	Cytoplasm	Cells of mesenchymal origin (including endothelial cells, myofibroblasts, some smooth muscle cells) and some cells of neuroectodermal origin
Desmin	53	Cytoplasm	Muscle cells
Glial fibrillary acidic protein (GFAP)	50–52	Cytoplasm	Neuroglial cells (including oligodendroglia, astrocytes, microglia), Schwann cells, ependymal cells, and pituicytes
Peripherin	54	Cytoplasm	Neurons
Synemin	182	Cytoplasm	Muscle cells
Paranemin	178	Cytoplasm	Muscle cells
Nestin	240	Cytoplasm	Muscle cells, some cells of neuroectodermal origin
		Class 3: Neurofilaments	
Neurofilament L (NF-L)	68	Cytoplasm	Neurons
Neurofilament M (NF-M)	110	Cytoplasm	Neurons
Neurofilament H (NF-H)	130	Cytoplasm	Neurons
		Class 4: Lamins	
Lamin A/C[A]	62–72	Nucleus	Most differentiated cells
Lamin B	65–68	Nucleus	All nucleated cells

[A]Lamin C is a splice product of lamin A.

teins form the attachment plaques for intermediate filaments, an essential part of desmosomes and hemidesmosomes. The interaction of intermediate filaments with cell-to-cell and cell-to-extracellular matrix junctions provides mechanical strength and resistance to extracellular forces. Table 2.2 summarizes the characteristics of the three types of cytoskeletal filaments.

Centrioles and Microtubule-Organizing Centers

Centrioles represent the focal point around which the MTOC assembles

Centrioles, visible in the light microscope, are paired, short, rod-like cytoplasmic cylinders built from nine microtubule triplets. In resting cells, centrioles have an orthogonal orientation: one centriole in the pair is arrayed at right angles to the other. Centrioles are usually found in close proximity to the nucleus, often partially surrounded by the Golgi apparatus, and associated with a zone of amorphous, dense pericentriolar material. The region of the cell containing the centrioles and pericentriolar material is called the ***MTOC*** or ***centrosome*** (Fig. 2.48). The MTOC is the region where most microtubules are formed and from which they are then directed to specific destinations within the cell. Therefore, the MTOC controls the number, polarity, direction, orientation, and organization of microtubules formed during interphase of the cell cycle. Development of the MTOC itself depends solely on the presence of centrioles. When centrioles are missing, the MTOCs disappear, and formation of microtubules is severely impaired.

The MTOC contains centrioles and numerous ring-shaped structures that initiate microtubule formation

The MTOC contains an amorphous matrix of more than 200 proteins, including γ-tubulins that are organized in ring-shaped structures. Each γ-tubulin ring serves as the starting point (nucleation site) for the growth of one microtubule that is assembled from tubulin dimers; α- and β-tubulin dimers are added with specific orientation to the γ-tubulin ring. The minus end of the microtubule remains attached to the MTOC, and the plus end represents the growing end directed toward the plasma membrane (see Fig. 2.48).

TABLE 2.2. **Summary Characteristics of Three Types of Cytoskeletal Elements**

	Actin Filaments (Microfilaments)	Intermediate Filaments	Microtubules
	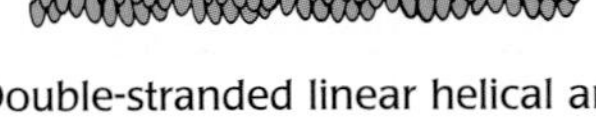	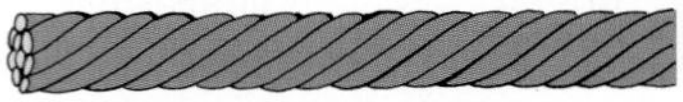	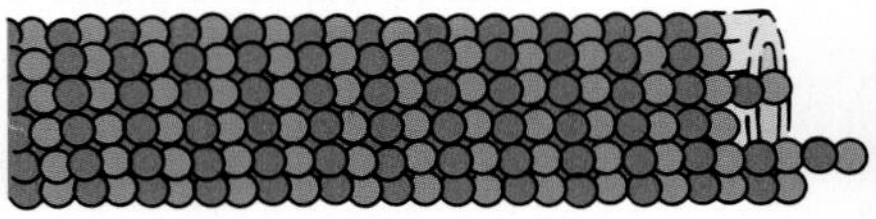
Shape	Double-stranded linear helical array	Rope-like fibers	Nonbranching long hollow cylinders
Diameter (nm)	6–8	8–10	20–25
Basic protein subunit	Monomer of G-actin (MW 42 kDa)	Various intermediate filament proteins (MW about 50 kDa)	Dimers of α- and β-tubulin (MW 54 kDa); γ-tubulin found in MTOC is necessary for nucleation of microtubules
Enzymatic activity	ATP hydrolytic activity	None	GTP hydrolytic activity
Polarity	Yes; minus (–) or pointed end is slow-growing end; plus (+) or barbed end is faster-growing end	Nonpolar structures	Yes; minus (–) end is nongrowing end embedded in MTOC; plus (+) end is the growing end
Assembly process	Monomers of G-actin are added to growing filament; polymerization requires the presence of K^+, Mg^{2+}, and ATP, which is hydrolyzed to ADP after each G-actin molecule is incorporated into the filament	Two pairs of monomers form two coiled-coil dimers; then, two coiled-coil dimers twist around each other to generate a staggered tetramer, which aligns along the axis of the filament and binds to the free end of the elongating structure	At the nucleation site, α- and β-tubulin dimers are added to γ-tubulin ring in an end-to-end fashion; each tubulin dimer molecule binds GTP before it becomes incorporated into the microtubule; polymerization also requires the presence of Mg^{2+}; GTP–tubulin complex is polymerized, and after incorporation, GTP is hydrolyzed to GDP
Source of energy required for assembly	ATP	N/A	GTP
Characteristics	Thin, flexible filaments	Strong, stable structures	Exhibit dynamic instability
Associated proteins	Variety of actin-binding proteins (ABPs) with different functions: fascin–bundling; gelsolin–filament severing; CP protein–capping; spectrin–cross-linking; myosin I and II–motor functions	Intermediate filament–associated proteins: plectins–bind microtubules, actin, and intermediate filaments; desmoplakins and plakoglobins–attach intermediate filaments to desmosomes and hemidesmosomes	Microtubule-associated proteins: MAP-1, 2, 3, and 4, MAP-τ, and TOGρ regulate assembly, stabilize and anchor microtubules to specific organelles; motor proteins–dyneins and kinesins–required for organelle movement
Location in cell	Core of microvilli; terminal web; concentrated beneath the plasma membrane; contractile elements of muscles; contractile ring in dividing cells	Extend across cytoplasm connecting desmosomes and hemidesmosomes; in the nucleus just beneath inner nuclear membrane	Core of cilia; emerge from MTOC and spread into periphery of the cell; mitotic spindle, centrosome
Major functions	Provide essential components to contractile elements of muscle cells (sarcomeres)	Provide mechanical strength and resistance to shearing forces	Provide network "railroad tracks" for movement of organelles within the cell; provide movement for cilia and for chromosomes during cell division

BOX 2.1

Clinical Correlations: Abnormalities in Microtubules and Filaments

Abnormalities related to the organization and structure of microtubules, actin, and intermediate filaments underlie a variety of pathologic disorders. These abnormalities lead to defects in the cytoskeleton and can produce a variety of defects related to intracellular vesicular transport, intracellular accumulations of pathologic proteins, and impairment of cell mobility.

MICROTUBULES

Defects in the organization of microtubules and microtubule-associated proteins can immobilize the cilia of respiratory epithelium, interfering with the ability of the respiratory system to clear accumulated secretions. This syndrome, known as ***Kartagener's syndrome*** (see page 95), also causes dysfunction of microtubules that affects sperm motility, leading to male sterility. It may also cause infertility in females because of impaired ciliary transport of the ovum through the oviduct.

Microtubules are essential for vesicular transport (endocytosis and exocytosis) as well as cell motility. Certain drugs, such as ***colchicine,*** bind to tubulin molecules and prevent their polymerization; this drug is useful in the treatment of acute attacks of gout, to prevent neutrophil migration and to lower their ability to respond to urate crystal deposits in the tissues. ***Vinblastine*** and ***vincristine*** represent another family of drugs that bind to microtubules and inhibit the formation of the mitotic spindle essential for cell division. These drugs are used as antimitotic and antiproliferative agents in cancer therapy. Another drug, ***Taxol,*** is used in chemotherapy for breast cancer. It stabilizes microtubules, preventing them from depolymerizing (an action opposite to that of colchicine), thus arresting cancer cells in various stages of cell division.

ACTIN FILAMENTS

Actin filaments are essential for various stages of leukocyte migration as well as for the phagocytotic functions of various cells (see page 28). Some drugs, such as ***cytochalasin B*** and ***cytochalasin D,*** prevent actin polymerization by binding to the plus end of the actin filament inhibiting lymphocyte migration and phagocytosis. Several toxins of poisonous mushrooms, such as ***phalloidin,*** also bind to actin filaments, preventing their depolymerization. Prolonged exposure of the cell to these substances can disrupt the dynamic equilibrium between F-actin and G-actin, causing cell death.

INTERMEDIATE FILAMENTS

As noted, the molecular structure of intermediate filaments is tissue specific and consists of many different types of proteins. Several diseases are caused by defects in the proper assembly of intermediate filaments. These defects have also been induced experimentally by mutations in intermediate filament genes in laboratory animals. Changes in neurofilaments within brain tissue are characteristic of ***Alzheimer's disease,*** which produces ***neurofibrillary tangles*** containing neurofilaments and other microtubule-associated proteins. A prominent feature of ***alcoholic liver cirrhosis*** is the presence of eosinophilic intracytoplasmic inclusions composed predominantly of keratin intermediate filaments. These inclusions, called ***Mallory bodies,*** are visible in light microscopy within the hepatocyte cytoplasm (Fig. 2.47).

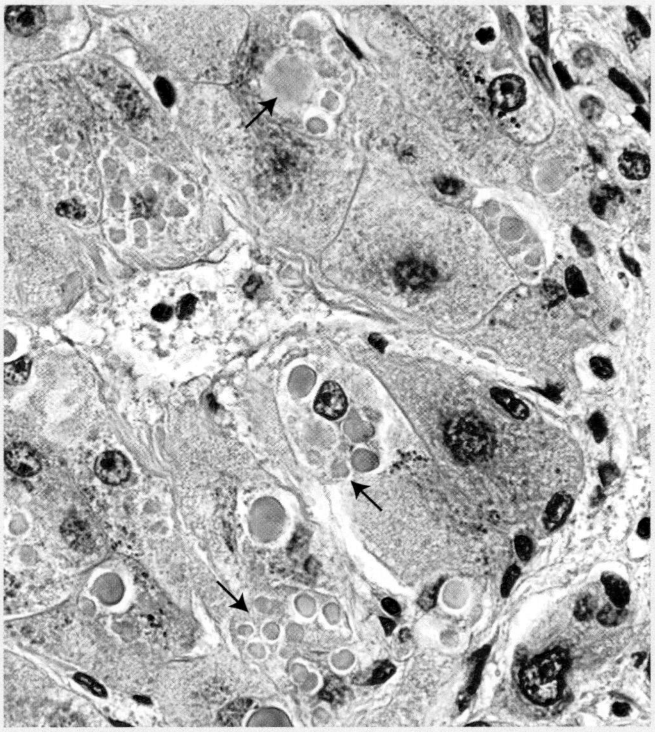

FIGURE 2.47
Photomicrograph of Mallory bodies. Accumulation of keratin intermediate filaments forming intercellular inclusions is frequently associated with specific cell injuries. In alcoholic liver cirrhosis, hepatocytes exhibit such inclusions *(arrows),* known as a Mallory bodies. Note that lymphocytes and macrophages responsible for an intense inflammatory reaction surround cells containing Mallory bodies. ×900.

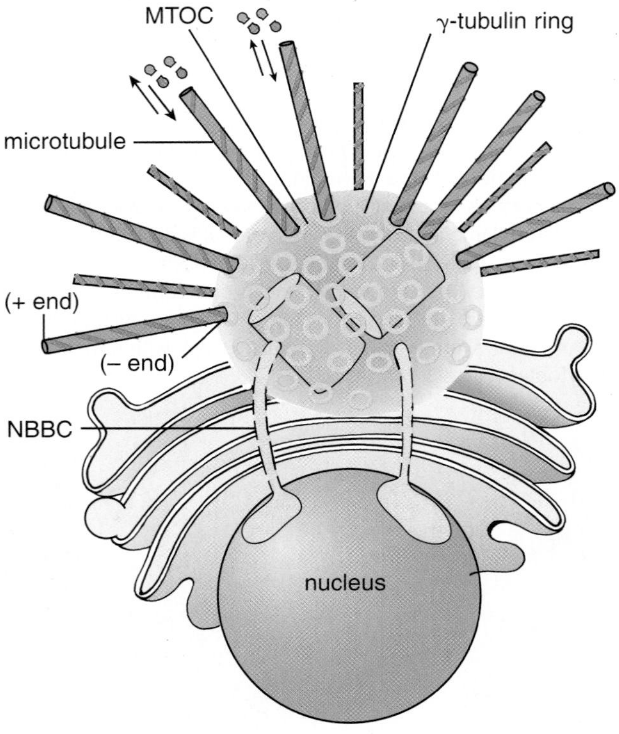

FIGURE 2.48
Structure of the microtubule-organizing center (MTOC). This diagram shows the location of the MTOC in relation to the nucleus and the Golgi apparatus. In some species, the MTOC is tethered to the nuclear envelope by a contractile protein, the nucleus–basal body connector *(NBBC)*. The MTOC contains the centrioles and an amorphous protein matrix with an abundance of γ-tubulin rings. Each γ-tubulin ring serves as the nucleation site for the growth of a single microtubule. Note that the minus (–) end of the microtubule remains attached to the MTOC and the plus (+) end represents the growing end directed toward the plasma membrane.

Centrioles provide basal bodies for cilia and flagella and align the mitotic spindle during cell division

Although centrioles were discovered over a century ago, their precise functions, replication, and assembly remain largely unclear. The functions of centrioles can be organized into two categories:

- ***Basal body formation.*** One of the important functions of the centriole is to provide basal bodies, which are necessary for the assembly of cilia and flagella (Fig. 2.49). Basal bodies are formed by replication of centrioles that give rise to multiple ***procentrioles.*** Each procentriole migrates to the appropriate site on the surface of the cell, where it becomes a basal body. The basal body acts as the organizing center for a cilium. Microtubules grow upward from the basal body, pushing the cell membrane outward, and elongate to form the mature cilium. The process of ciliary formation is described on page 95.
- ***Mitotic spindle formation.*** During mitosis, centrioles are necessary for the formation of the MTOC and ***astral microtubules.*** Astral microtubules are formed around each individual centriole in a star-like fashion. They are crucial in establishing the axis of the developing mitotic spindle. In some animal cells, the mitotic spindle itself (mainly kinetochore microtubules) is formed by MTOC-independent mechanisms and consists of microtubules that originate from the chromosomes. Recent experimental data indicate that in the absence of centrioles, astral microtubules fail to develop, causing errors in mitotic spindle orientation (Fig. 2.50). Thus, the primary role of centrioles in mitosis is to position the mitotic spindle properly by recruit-

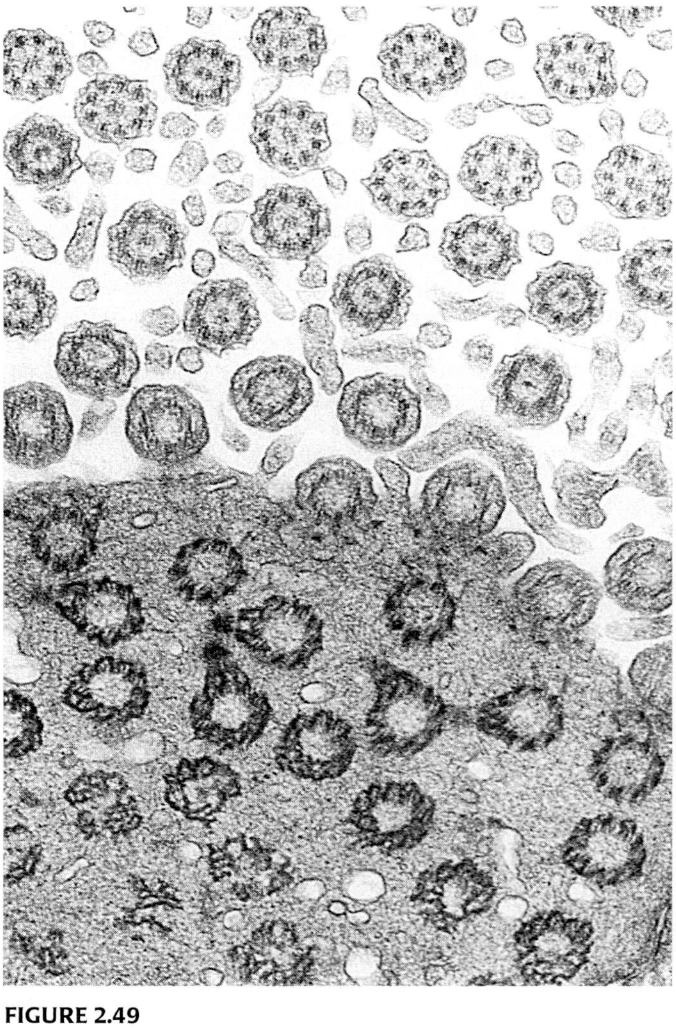

FIGURE 2.49
Basal bodies and cilia. This electron micrograph shows the basal bodies and cilia in cross-sectional profile as seen in an oblique section through the apical part of a ciliated cell in the respiratory tract. Note the 9 + 2 microtubule arrangement of the cilia. The basal bodies lack the central tubule pair. The triplet microtubule configuration in the basal body appears as a more dense structure than the doublet microtubule configuration in the cilia. × 28,000. (Courtesy of Patrice C. Abell-Aleff.)

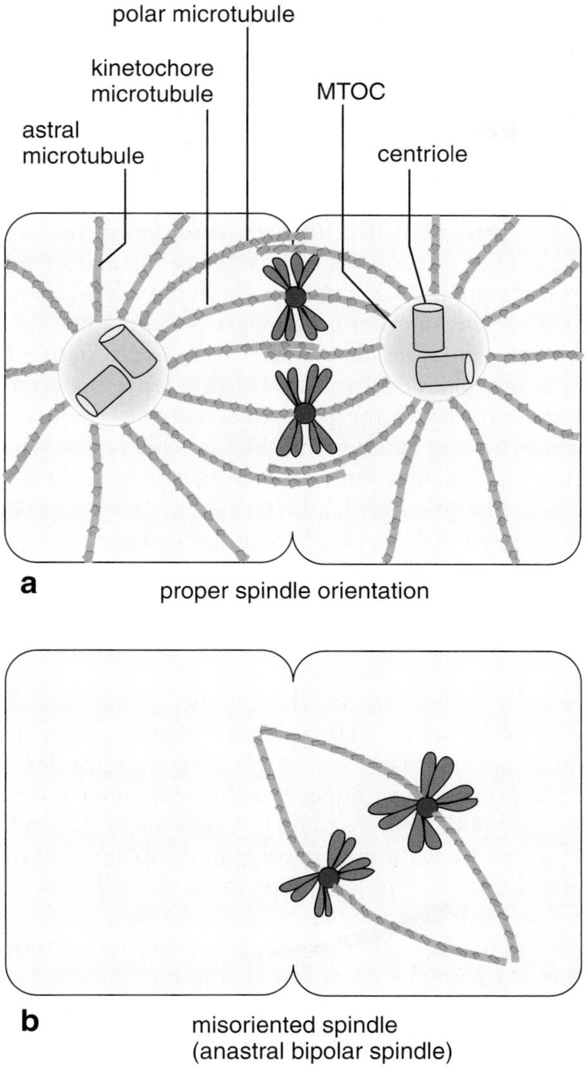

FIGURE 2.50
Mitotic spindle during normal cell division and in cells lacking centrioles. a. This schematic drawing shows the orientation of the astral bipolar spindle in a normal cell undergoing mitosis. Note the positions of the centrioles and the distribution of the spindle microtubules. **b.** In a cell that lacks centrioles, mitosis occurs and a mitotic spindle containing only kinetochore microtubules is formed. However, both poles of the mitotic spindle lack astral microtubules, which position the spindle in proper plane during the mitosis. Such a misoriented spindle is referred to as an anastral bipolar spindle. (Based on Marshall WF, Rosenbaum JL. *Curr Opin Cell Biol* 2000;112:119–125.)

ing the MTOC from which astral microtubules can grow and establish the axis for the developing spindle.

The dominant feature of centrioles is the cylindrical array of triplet microtubules with associated proteins

The TEM reveals that each rod-shaped centriole is about 0.2 μm long and consists of nine triplets of microtubules that are oriented parallel to the long axis of the organelle and run in slightly twisted bundles (Fig. 2.51). The three microtubules of the triplet are fused, with adjacent microtubules sharing a common wall. The innermost or ***A microtubule*** is a complete ring of 13 α- and β-tubulin dimers; the middle and outer microtubules, ***B*** and ***C***, respectively, appear C-shaped because they share tubulin dimers with each other and with the ***A*** microtubule. The microtubules of the triplets are not equal in length. The C microtubule of the triplet is usually shorter than A and B.

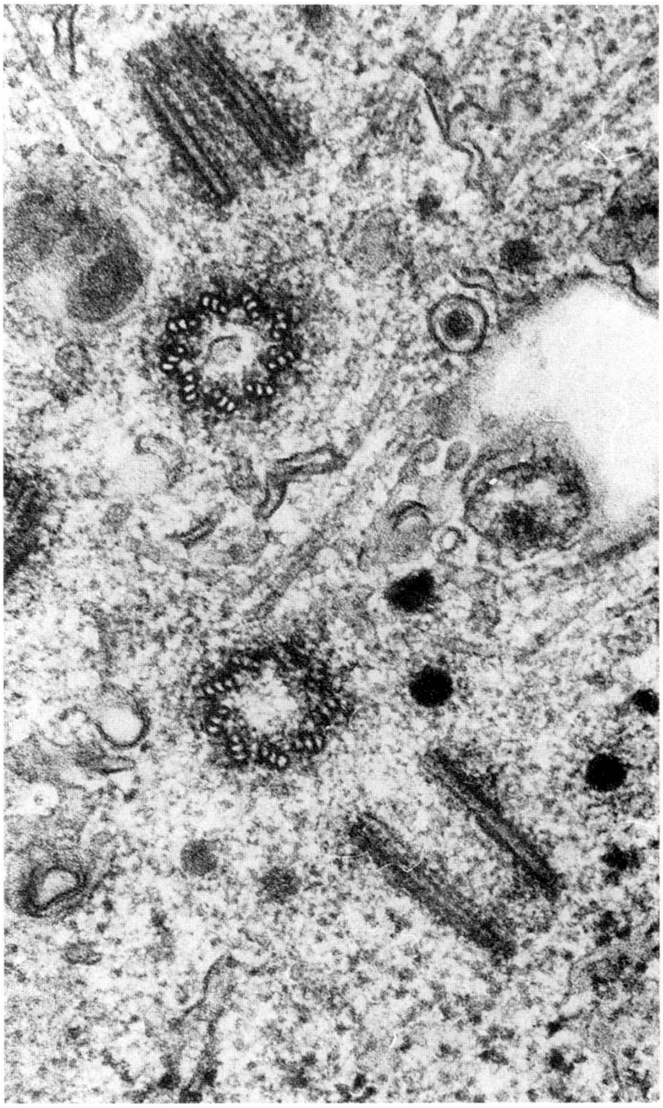

FIGURE 2.51
Electron micrograph showing parent and daughter centrioles in a fibroblast. Note that the transverse-sectioned centriole in each of the pairs reveals the triplet configuration of microtubules. The lower right centriole represents a midlongitudinal section, whereas the upper left centriole has also been longitudinally sectioned, but along the plane of its wall. ×90,000. (Courtesy of Drs. Manley McGill, D. P. Highfield, T. M. Monahan, and Bill R. Brinkley.)

The microtubule triplets of the centriole surround an internal lumen. The distal part of the lumen (away from the nucleus) contains a 20-kDa Ca^{2+}-binding protein, ***centrin*** (Fig. 2.52). The proximal part of the lumen (close to the nucleus) is lined by ***γ-tubulin,*** which provides the template for the arrangement of the triplet microtubules. A group of proteins generally known as ***pericentrins*** has also been associated with the centrioles. Newly identified ***protein p210*** forms a ring of molecules that appears to link the distal end of the centriole to the plasma membrane. Filamentous connections between the centriole pair have been identified in human lymphocytes. In other organisms, two protein bridges, the ***proximal*** and ***distal connecting fibers,*** connect each centriole in a pair (see Fig. 2.52). In dividing cells, these connections participate in segregating the centrioles to each daughter cell. In some organisms, the proximal end of each centriole is attached to the nuclear envelope by contractile proteins called ***nucleus–basal body connectors (NBBCs).*** Their function is to link the centriole to the mitotic spindle poles during mitosis. In human cells, the centrosome–nucleus connection appears to be maintained by filamentous structures of cytoskeleton. A distinctive feature of mammalian centrioles is the difference between individual centrioles in the pair. One centriole (termed the ***mature centriole***) contains stalk-like satellite processes and sheet-like appendages whose function is not known (see Fig. 2.52). The other centriole (termed the ***immature centriole***) does not possess satellites or appendages.

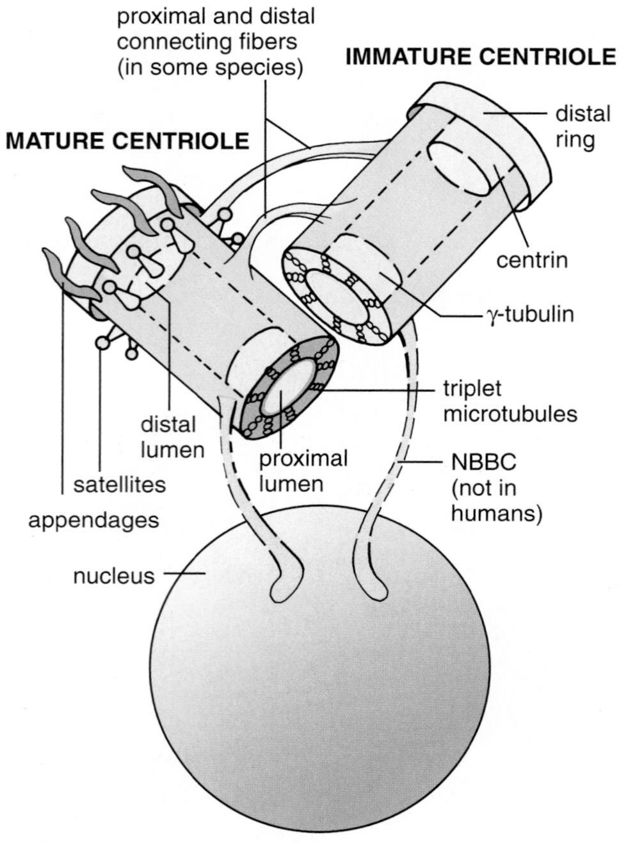

FIGURE 2.52
Schematic structure of centrioles. In nondividing cells, centrioles are arranged in pairs in which one centriole is aligned at a right angle to the other. One centriole is also more mature (generated at least two cell cycles ago) than the other centriole, which was generated in the previous cell cycle. Centrioles are located in close proximity to the nucleus. The basic building components of each centrosome are microtubule triplets that form the cylindrical structure surrounding an internal lumen. The proximal part of the lumen is lined by γ-tubulin, which provides the template for nucleation and arrangement of the microtubule triplets. The distal part of each lumen contains the protein centrin. In some species, two protein bridges, the proximal and distal connecting fibers, connect each centriole in a pair. In some species, but not in humans, the proximal end of each centriole is attached to the nuclear envelope by a contractile protein known as nucleus–basal body connector *(NBBC).*

Prior to cell division, a single new centriole is formed at a right angle and adjacent to each preexisting centriole

Prior to cell division, when DNA is being replicated during the S phase of the cell cycle (see page 68), centrioles also duplicate. A small mass of granular and fibrillar material, the ***procentriole,*** appears at the side of each centriole and gradually enlarges to form a right-angle appendage to the parent. Microtubules develop in the mass as it grows (usually during the S to late G^2 phase of the cell cycle), appearing first as single tubules, then as doublets, and finally as triplets. Thus, a single new immature centriole is formed adjacent to each existing centriole, and its duplication occurs at a precise right angle to the preexisting centriole. Centrioles are the only organelles besides the cell nucleus that undergo such exact duplication. After duplication, the parent–daughter pairs separate and produce astral microtubules. In doing so, they define the poles between which the mitotic spindle develops.

However, during certain processes (e.g., development of ciliated epithelium), large clusters of centrioles may assemble de novo, independent of preexisting centrioles. The phenomenon of de novo centriole formation can be explained by simple maturation of invisible procentrioles already existing in the cytoplasm of the cell.

Basal Bodies

Development of cilia on the cell surface requires the presence of basal bodies, structures derived from centrioles

Each cilium requires a *basal body.* Repeated replications of centrioles and the migration of the newly replicated centrioles to the apical surface of the cell are responsible for the production of basal bodies. Each

centriole-derived basal body then serves as the organizing center for the assembly of the microtubules of the cilium. The core structure (axoneme) of a cilium is composed of a complex set of microtubules consisting of two central microtubules surrounded by nine microtubule doublets (see Fig. 4.6, page 94). The organizing role of the basal body differs from that of the MTOC. The axonemal microtubule doublets are continuous with the A and B microtubules of the basal body from which they develop by addition of α- and β-tubulin dimers at the growing plus end.

Inclusions

Inclusions consist largely of secretory vesicles, pigment granules, neutral fat, other lipid droplets, and glycogen

Inclusions are cytoplasmic or nuclear structures with characteristic staining properties. They are considered "nonliving" components of the cell. Some of them, such as secretory vesicles and pigment granules, are surrounded by a plasma membrane; others, e.g., lipid droplets and glycogen, are not and reside within the cytoplasmic or nuclear matrix.

Secretory vesicles and ***neutral fat*** often constitute most of the cytoplasmic volume, compressing the other formed organelles into a thin rim at the margin of the cell. This structure is typical of the intestinal goblet cell (see Fig. 16.23, page 497) and the adipose cell of connective tissue (see Fig. 6.2, page 159). Cells with ***regulated secretory pathways*** store proteins within large vesicles in their cytoplasm for hours or even days. These vesicles do not fuse with the plasma membrane until the cell is activated for exocytosis by an external signaling mechanism (see page 28).

Glycogen may be seen in the light microscope only after special fixation and staining procedures. It is usually lost during routine processing of tissue for light microscopy. Liver and striated muscle cells, which usually contain large amounts of glycogen, may display empty regions where the glycogen was localized. Glycogen appears in electron micrographs as granules 25 to 30 nm in diameter or as clusters of such granules that often occupy significant portions of the cytoplasm (Fig. 2.53).

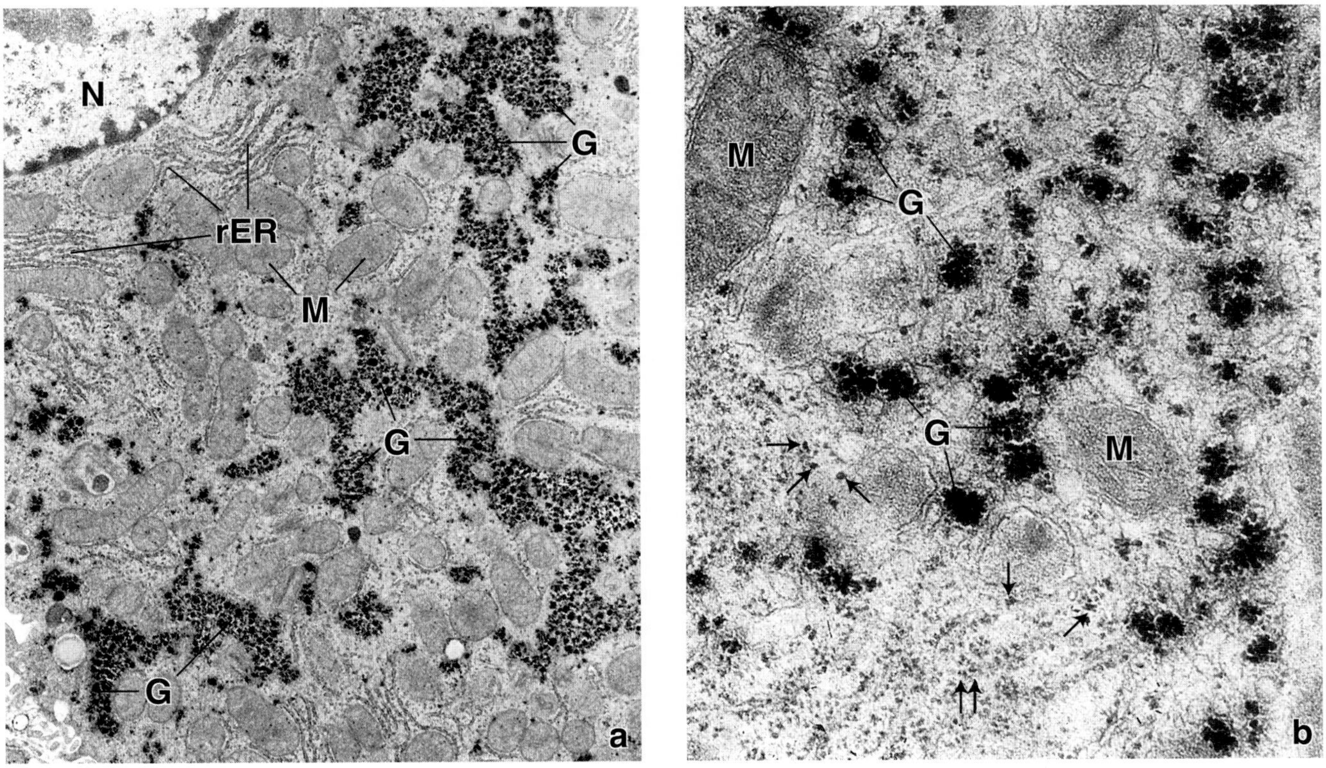

FIGURE 2.53
Electron micrographs of a liver cell with glycogen inclusions. a. Low-magnification electron micrograph showing a portion of an hepatocyte with part of the nucleus *(N, upper left).* Glycogen *(G)* appears as irregular electron-dense masses. Profiles of rough endoplasmic reticulum *(rER)* and mitochondria *(M)* are also evident. ×10,000. **b.** This higher-magnification electron micrograph reveals glycogen *(G)* as aggregates of small particles. Even the smallest aggregates *(arrows)* appear to be composed of several smaller glycogen particles. The density of the glycogen is considerably greater than that of the ribosomes *(lower left).* ×52,000.

Lipid inclusions (fat droplets) are also usually extracted by the organic solvents used to prepare tissues for both light and electron microscopy. What is seen as a "fat droplet" in light microscopy is actually a hole in the cytoplasm that represents the site from which the lipid was extracted.

Crystalline inclusions contained in certain cells are recognized in the light microscope. In humans, such inclusions are found in the Sertoli (sustentacular) and Leydig (interstitial) cells of the testis. With the TEM, crystalline inclusions have been found in many cell types and in virtually all parts of the cell, including the nucleus and most cytoplasmic organelles. Although some of these inclusions contain storage material or remnants of cellular structures, the significance of others is not clear.

Cytoplasmic Matrix

The cytoplasmic matrix is a concentrated aqueous gel consisting of molecules of different sizes and shapes

The ***cytoplasmic matrix*** (ground substance, or ***cytosol***) shows little specific structure by light microscopy or conventional TEM and has traditionally been described as a concentrated aqueous solution containing molecules of different size and shape (e.g., electrolytes, metabolites, RNA, and synthesized proteins). In most cells, it is the largest single compartment. The cytoplasmic matrix is the site of physiologic processes that are fundamental to the cell's existence (protein synthesis, breakdown of nutrients). Studies with high-voltage electron microscopy (HVEM) of 0.25- to 0.5-μm sections reveal a complex three-dimensional structural network of thin ***microtrabecular strands*** and ***cross-linkers.*** This network provides a structural substratum on which cytoplasmic reactions occur, such as those involving free ribosomes, and along which regulated and directed cytoplasmic transport and movement of organelles occur.

▼ NUCLEUS

The nucleus is a membrane-limited compartment that contains the genome (genetic information) in eukaryotic cells

The nucleus of a nondividing cell, also called an ***interphase cell,*** consists of the following components:

- ***Chromatin,*** nuclear material organized as euchromatin and heterochromatin. It contains DNA, histones, and various nuclear proteins that are necessary for DNA to function.
- ***Nucleolus*** (pl., ***nucleoli***), a small dense area within the nucleus that contains RNA and proteins. The nucleolus is the site of rRNA synthesis.
- ***Nuclear envelope,*** the membrane system that surrounds the nucleus of the cell. It consists of inner and outer membranes separated by a perinuclear cisternal space and perforated by nuclear pores. The outer membrane of the nuclear envelope is continuous with that of the rER and is often studded with ribosomes.
- ***Nucleoplasm,*** the nuclear contents other than the chromatin and nucleolus.

Chromatin

Chromatin, a complex of DNA and proteins, is responsible for the characteristic basophilia of the nucleus

In most cells, chromatin does not have a homogeneous appearance; rather, clumps of densely staining chromatin are embedded in a more lightly staining background. The densely staining material is highly condensed chromatin called ***heterochromatin,*** and the lightly staining material is a dispersed form called ***euchromatin.*** It is the phosphate groups of the DNA of the chromatin that are responsible for the characteristic basophilia of chromatin (page 7). The proteins of chromatin include five basic proteins called ***histones*** and other ***nonhistone proteins.*** Heterochromatin is disposed in three locations (Fig. 2.54):

- ***Marginal chromatin*** is found at the perimeter of the nucleus (the structure light microscopists formerly referred to as the nuclear membrane actually consists largely of marginal chromatin).
- ***Karyosomes*** are discrete bodies of irregular size and shape, found throughout the nucleus.
- ***Nucleolar associated chromatin*** is chromatin found in association with the nucleolus.

Heterochromatin stains with hematoxylin and basic dyes; it is also readily displayed with the Feulgen procedure (a specific histochemical reaction for the deoxyribose of DNA, page 7) and fluorescent vital dyes such as Hoechst dyes and propidium iodide. It is the heterochromatin that accounts for the conspicuous staining of the nucleus in hematoxylin and eosin (H&E) preparations.

Euchromatin indicates active chromatin, i.e., chromatin that is stretched out so that the genetic information in the DNA can be read and transcribed. It is prominent in metabolically active cells such as neurons and liver cells. Heterochromatin predominates in metabolically inactive cells such as small circulating lymphocytes and sperm or in cells that produce one major product, such as plasma cells.

Euchromatin is not evident in the light microscope. It is present within the nucleoplasm in the "clear" areas between the heterochromatin. In routine electron micrographs, there is no sharp delineation between euchromatin and heterochromatin; both have a granular, filamentous appearance, but the euchromatin is less tightly packed.

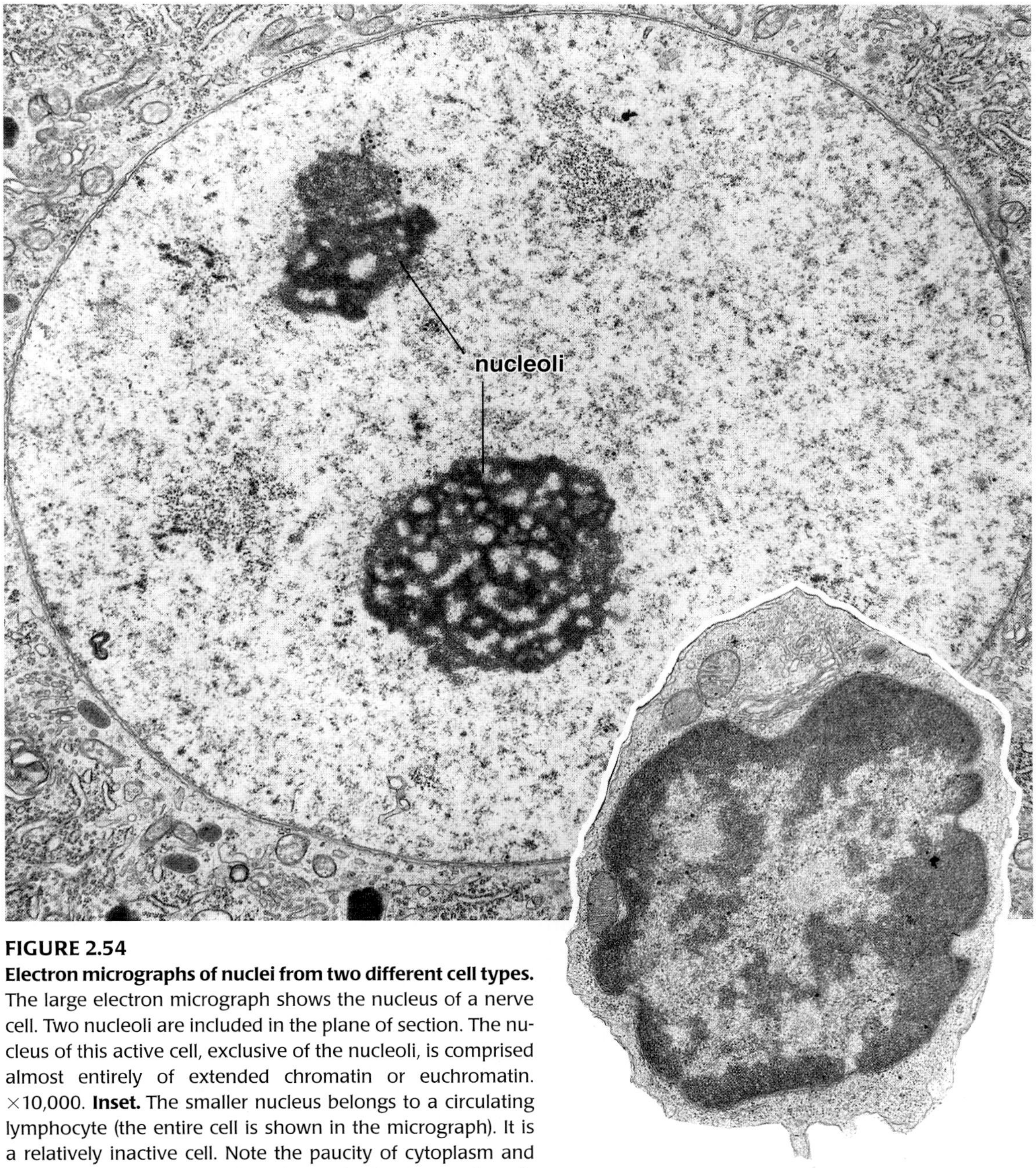

FIGURE 2.54
Electron micrographs of nuclei from two different cell types. The large electron micrograph shows the nucleus of a nerve cell. Two nucleoli are included in the plane of section. The nucleus of this active cell, exclusive of the nucleoli, is comprised almost entirely of extended chromatin or euchromatin. ×10,000. **Inset.** The smaller nucleus belongs to a circulating lymphocyte (the entire cell is shown in the micrograph). It is a relatively inactive cell. Note the paucity of cytoplasm and cytoplasmic organelles. The chromatin in the nucleus is largely condensed (heterochromatin). The lighter areas represent euchromatin. ×13,000.

The smallest units of chromatin structure are macromolecular complexes of DNA and histones, called nucleosomes

Nucleosomes are found in both euchromatin and heterochromatin and in chromosomes (see below). A nucleosome is a 10-nm-diameter particle that consists of a core of eight histone molecules. Approximately two loops of DNA (about 146 nucleotide pairs) are wrapped around the core octamer. The DNA extends between each particle as a 1.5-nm filament that joins adjacent nucleosomes. The nucleosomal substructure of chromatin is often described as "***beads on a string.***"

A long strand of nucleosomes is coiled to produce a unit ***chromatin fibril*** that is about 25 to 30 nm in diameter. Six

nucleosomes form one turn in the coil of the chromatin fibril. Both interphase chromatin and chromosomes are formed from the 25- to 30-nm unit fibril. In heterochromatin, the unit chromatin fibrils are tightly packed and folded on each other; in euchromatin, the unit fibrils are more loosely arranged. This loose arrangement allows DNA polymerases access to the DNA in euchromatin.

In dividing cells, chromatin is condensed and organized into discrete bodies called chromosomes

Chromosomes *[Gr., colored bodies]* are formed during mitosis by condensation of the euchromatin and combination with heterochromatin. Each chromosome is formed by two ***chromatids*** that are joined together at a point called the ***centromere.*** The double nature of the chromosome is produced in the preceding synthetic (S) phase of the cell cycle (see page 69), during which DNA is replicated in anticipation of the next mitotic division.

The area located at each end of the chromosome is called the telomere. Telomeres shorten with each cell division. Recent studies indicate that telomere length is an important indicator of the lifespan of the cell. To survive indefinitely (become "immortalized"), cells must activate a mechanism that maintains telomere length. For example, in cells that have been transformed into malignant cells, an enzyme called telomerase is present that adds repeated nucleotide sequences to the telomere ends. Recently, expression of this enzyme has been shown to extend the life span of cells.

With the exception of the mature gametes, the egg and sperm, human cells contain ***46 chromosomes*** organized as ***23 homologous pairs*** (each chromosome in the pair has the same shape and size). Twenty-two pairs have identical chromosomes, i.e., each chromosome of the pair contains the same portion of the genome, and are called ***autosomes.*** The twenty-third pair of chromosomes are the ***sex chromosomes,*** designated X and Y. Females contain two X chromosomes; males contain one X and one Y chromosome. The chromosomal number, 46, is found in most of the somatic cells of the body and is called the diploid (2n) number. Diploid chromosomes have the 2n amount of DNA immediately after cell division but have twice that amount, i.e., the 4n amount of DNA, after the S phase (see page 69).

As a result of ***meiosis*** (see below), eggs and sperm have only 23 chromosomes, the haploid ($1n$) number, as well as the haploid ($1n$) amount of DNA. The somatic chromosome number and the diploid ($2n$) amount of DNA are reestablished at ***fertilization*** by the fusion of the sperm nucleus with the egg nucleus.

In a karyotype, chromosome pairs are sorted according to their size and shape

A preparation of chromosomes derived from mechanically ruptured, dividing cells that are then fixed, plated on a microscope slide, and stained with Giemsa stain is called a metaphase spread (Fig. 2.55a). Such spreads are then photographed. The chromosome pairs are cut from the photograph and sorted according to their morphology to form a ***karyotype*** (Fig. 2.55b). Karyotypes are used to detect chromosome abnormalities such as deletions, nondisjunctions, and additions; for determination of sex in fetuses; and for prenatal diagnosis of certain genetic disorders. Special stains and molecular probes allow study of localized regions of specific chromosomes to determine duplications or deletions of specific gene sites (loci).

The Barr body can be used to identify the sex of a fetus

Some chromosomes are repressed in the interphase nucleus and exist only in the tightly packed heterochromatic form. One X chromosome of the female is an example of such a chromosome. This fact can be used to identify the sex of a fetus. This chromosome was discovered in 1949 by Barr and Bartram in nerve cells of female cats, where it appears as a well-stained round body, now called the ***Barr body,*** adjacent to the nucleolus.

Although the Barr body was originally found in sectioned tissue, it was subsequently shown that any relatively large number of cells prepared as a smear (e.g., scrapings of the oral mucous membrane from the inside of the cheeks or neutrophils from a blood smear) can be used to search for the Barr body. In cells of the oral mucous membrane, the Barr body is located adjacent to the nuclear envelope. In neutrophils, the Barr body forms a drumstick appendage on one of the nuclear lobes (Fig. 2.56). In both sections and smears, many cells must be examined to find those whose orientation is suitable for the display of the Barr body.

Nucleolus

The nucleolus is the site of rRNA synthesis and initial ribosomal assembly

The nucleolus is a nonmembranous, intranuclear structure formed by ***fibrillar material (pars fibrosa)*** and ***granular material (pars granulosa)*** (Fig. 2.57). It varies in size but is particularly well developed in cells active in protein synthesis. Some cells contain more than one nucleolus. The nucleolus consists largely of DNA loops of different chromosomes containing genes for rRNA clustered together, large amounts of rRNA, and proteins.

rRNA is present in both granular and fibrillar material and is organized, respectively, as both granules and extremely fine filaments packed tightly together. The network formed by the granular and the fibrillar materials is called the ***nucleolonema.*** DNA containing genes for the ri-

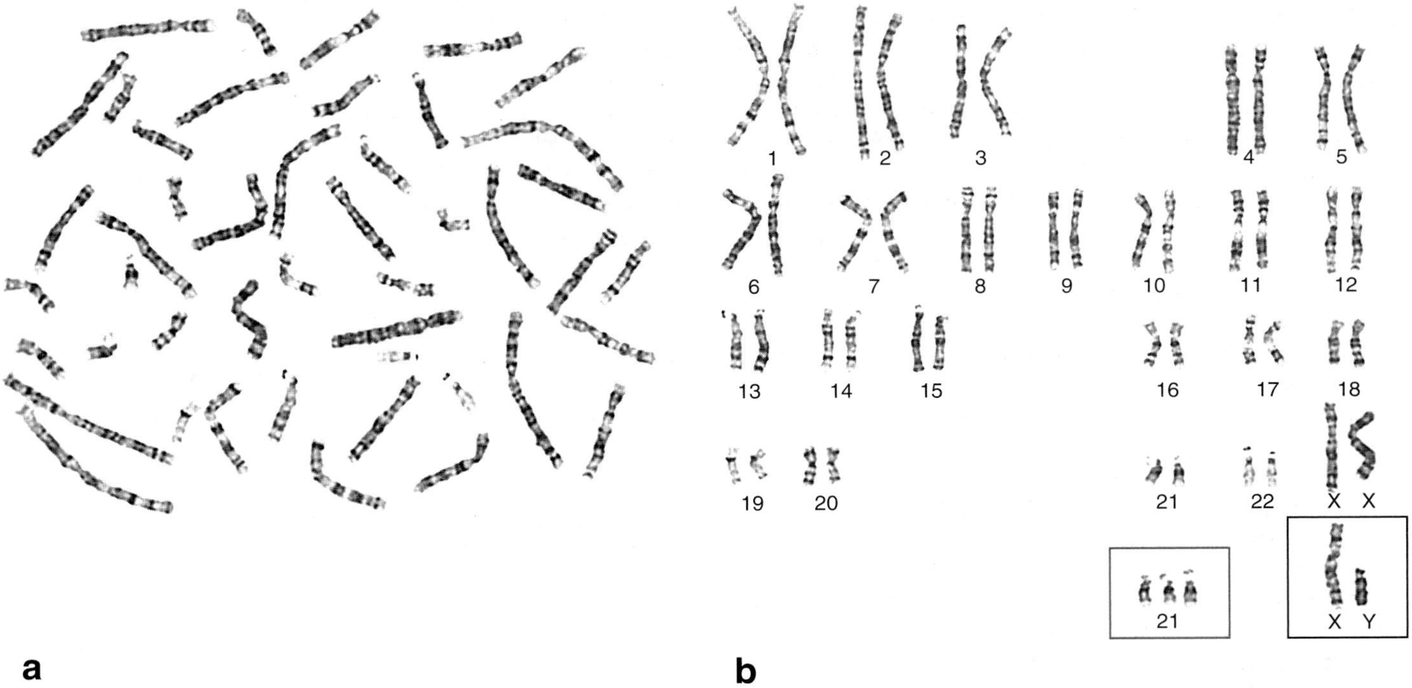

FIGURE 2.55
Examination of chromosomes. a. Metaphase spread. **b.** Karyotype of a normal female. The paired chromosomes are numbered in the karyotype, and the female sex chromosomes are indicated by X and X. The *black box insert* below the XX chromosomes shows the XY chromosome pair in the male. Note in the *red box insert* below the chromosome 21 pair is an example of trisomy 21, an error in chromosome number that causes Down's syndrome. (Courtesy of the University of Florida Cytogenetics Laboratory.)

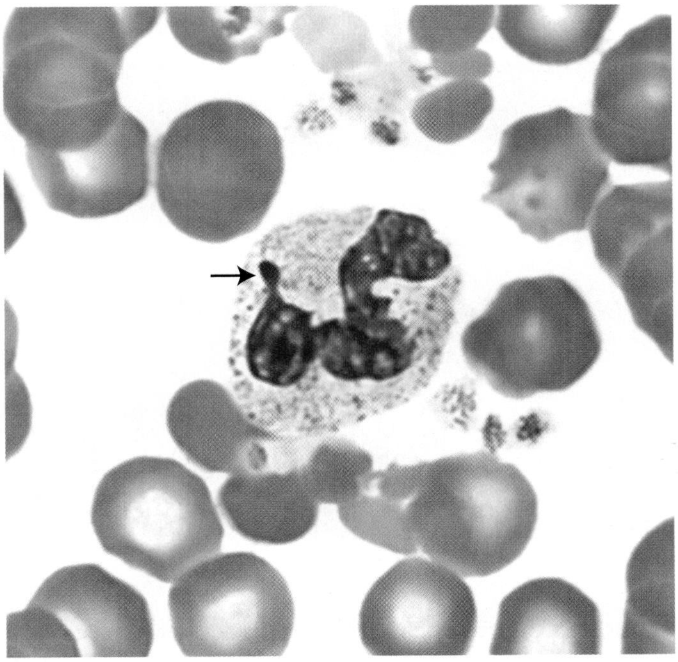

FIGURE 2.56
Photomicrograph of a neutrophil from a female blood smear. The second X chromosome of the female is repressed in the interphase nucleus and can be demonstrated in the neutrophil as a drumstick-appearing appendage *(arrow)* on a nuclear lobe. ×250.

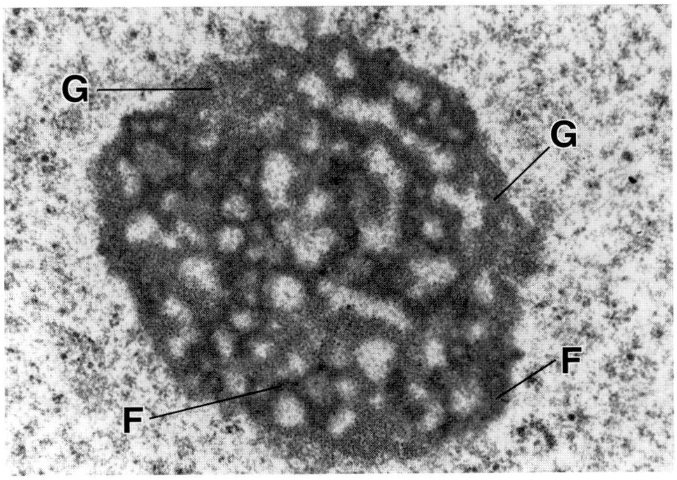

FIGURE 2.57
Electron micrograph of the nucleolus. This nucleolus from a nerve cell shows the fibrillar *(F)* and granular *(G)* materials. Such a network of both materials is referred to as the nucleolonema. The rRNA, DNA-containing genes for the rRNA, and specific proteins are localized in the interstices of the nucleolonema. ×15,000.

bosomal subunits is localized in the interstices of this network.

rRNA genes are transcribed by RNA polymerase I, and subunits of rRNA are assembled using ribosomal proteins imported from the cytoplasm. The partially assembled ribosomal subunits leave the nucleus via nuclear pores (see below), to be fully assembled into ribosomes in the cytoplasm.

The nucleolus stains intensely with hematoxylin and basic dyes and metachromatically with thionine dyes

That the basophilia and metachromasia of the nucleolus are due to the phosphate groups of the nucleolar RNA is confirmed by predigestion of specimens with ribonuclease (RNAse), which abolishes the staining. DNA is present in the nucleolus but in such small amounts that it appears Feulgen negative when examined in the light microscope. However, Feulgen-positive material, nucleolus-associated chromatin, often rims the nucleolus.

Nuclear Envelope

The nuclear envelope, formed by two membranes with a perinuclear cisternal space between them, separates the nucleoplasm from the cytoplasm

The *nuclear envelope* is assembled from two (outer and inner) nuclear membranes containing a *perinuclear cisternal space* between them. The nuclear envelope encloses the chromatin, defines the nuclear compartment, and serves as a membranous boundary between the nucleoplasm and the cytoplasm. The perinuclear clear cisternal space is continuous with the cisternal space of the rER (Fig. 2.58). The two membranes of the envelope are perforated at intervals by *nuclear pores* that mediate the active transport of proteins, ribonucleoproteins, and RNAs between the nucleus and cytoplasm. The membranes of the nuclear envelope differ in structure and functions:

- The outer nuclear membrane closely resembles the membrane of the endoplasmic reticulum and in fact is contin-

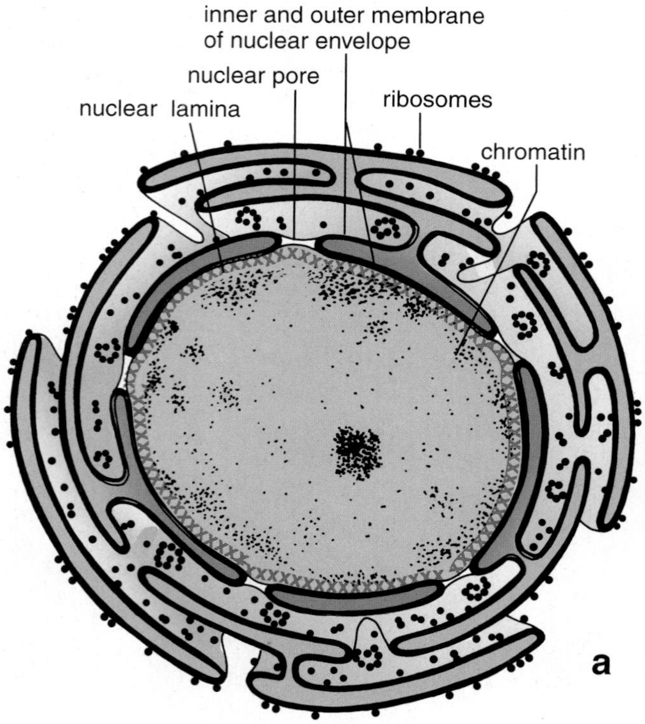

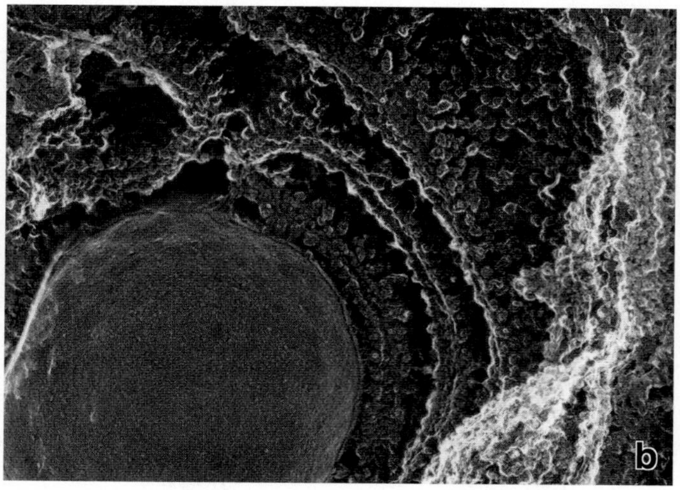

FIGURE 2.58
Structure of the nuclear envelope and its relationship to the rER. a. This schematic drawing shows the organization of the nuclear wall. A double membrane envelope surrounds the nucleus. The outer membrane is continuous with the membranes of rER; thus, the perinuclear space communicates with the rER lumen. The inner membrane is adjacent to nuclear intermediate filaments that form the nuclear lamina.

b. This electron micrograph, prepared by the quick-freeze deep-etch technique, shows the nucleus, the large spherical object, surrounded by the nuclear envelope. Note that the outer membrane possesses ribosomes and is continuous with the rER. ×12,000. (Courtesy of Dr. John E. Heuser, Washington University School of Medicine.)

uous with rER membrane (see Fig 2.58). Polyribosomes are often attached to ribosomal docking proteins present on the cytoplasmic side of the outer nuclear membrane.

- The inner nuclear membrane is supported by a rigid network of protein filaments attached to its inner surface, called the ***nuclear lamina.*** In addition, the inner nuclear membrane contains specific lamin receptors and several lamina-associated protein receptors that bind to chromosomes and secure the attachment of the nuclear lamina.

The nuclear lamina lies adjacent to the inner surface of the nuclear envelope, between the membrane and the marginal heterochromatin

The ***nuclear (fibrous) lamina,*** a thin, electron-dense protein layer, has a supporting or "nucleoskeletal" function. If the membranous component of the nuclear envelope is disrupted by exposure to detergent, the fibrous lamina remains, and the nucleus retains its shape.

The major components of the lamina, as determined by biochemical isolation, are ***nuclear lamins,*** a specialized type of nuclear intermediate filament (see page 53), and ***lamina-associated proteins*** (Fig. 2.59). Unlike other cytoplasmic intermediate filaments, lamins disassemble during mitosis and reassemble when mitosis ends. The nuclear lamina appears to serve as a scaffolding for chromatin, chromatin-associated proteins, nuclear pores, and the membranes of the nuclear envelope. In addition, it is involved in nuclear organization, cell cycle regulation, and differentiation. Impairment in nuclear lamina architecture or function is associated with certain genetic diseases and apoptosis.

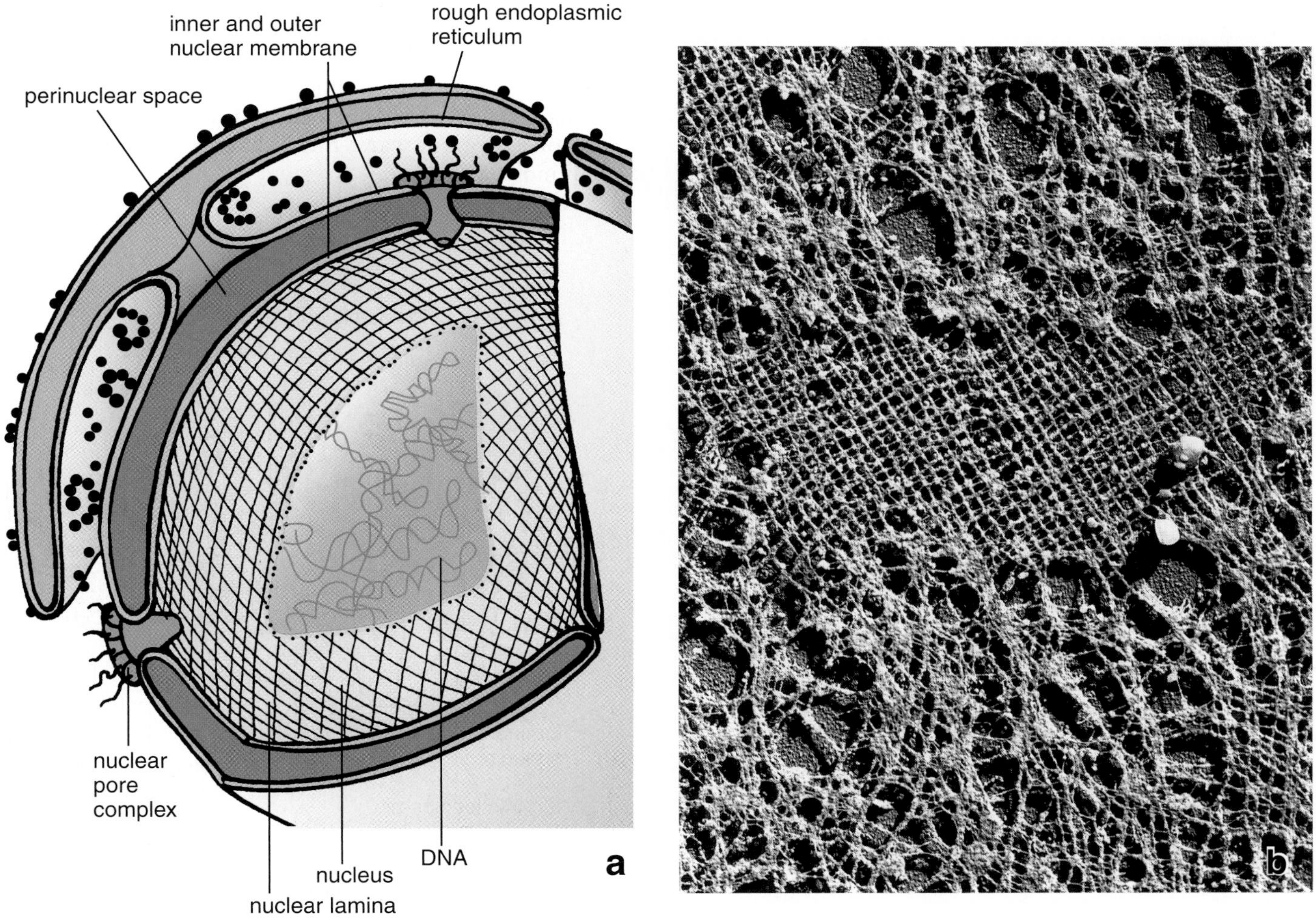

FIGURE 2.59
Structure of the nuclear lamina. a. This schematic drawing shows the structure of the nuclear lamina adjacent to the inner nuclear membrane. The cut window in the nuclear lamina shows the DNA within the nucleus. Note that the nuclear envelope is pierced by nuclear pore complexes, which allow for selective bidirectional transport of molecules between nucleus and cytoplasm. **b.** Electron micrograph of a portion of the nuclear lamina from a *Xenopus* oocyte. It is formed by intermediate filaments (lamins) that are arranged in a square lattice. ×43,000. (Adapted from Aebi U, et al. *Nature* 1986;323: 560–564.)

The nuclear envelope possesses an array of openings called nuclear pores

At numerous sites, the paired membranes of the nuclear envelope are punctuated by 70- to 80-nm "openings" through the envelope. These openings, or ***nuclear pores,*** are formed from the fusion of the inner and outer membranes of the nuclear envelope. With an ordinary TEM, a diaphragm-like structure appears to cross the pore opening (Fig. 2.60). Often, a small dense body is observed in the center of the opening. Such profiles are thought to represent either ribosomes or other protein complexes (transporters) captured during their passage through the pore at the time of fixation.

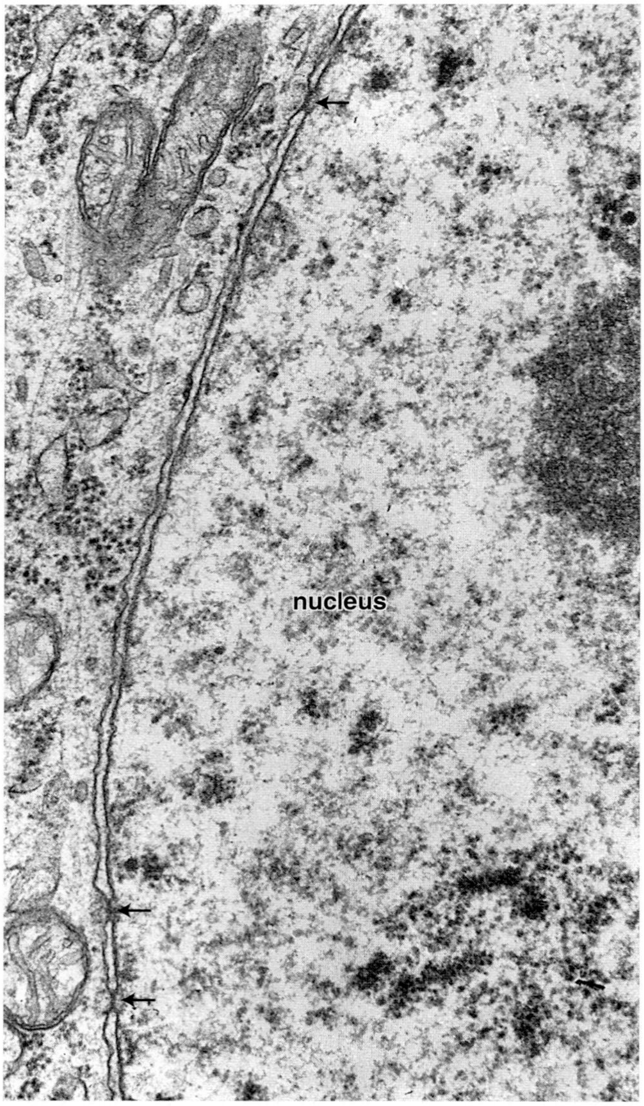

FIGURE 2.60
Electron micrograph of the nuclear envelope. Note the visible nuclear pore complexes *(arrows)* and the two membranes that constitute the nuclear envelope. At the periphery of each pore, the outer and inner membranes of the nuclear envelope appear continuous. $\times$30,000.

With special techniques, such as negative staining and high-voltage transmission electron microscopy, the nuclear pore exhibits additional structural detail. Eight multidomain protein subunits arranged in an octagonal ***central framework*** at the periphery of each pore form a cylinder-like structure known as the ***nuclear pore complex (NPC).*** The NPC, whose total mass is estimated at 125×10^6 Da, is composed of about 50 different nuclear pore complex proteins collectively referred to as ***nucleoporins (Nup proteins).*** This central framework is inserted between two ***cytoplasmic*** and ***nuclear rings*** (Fig. 2.61). From the cytoplasmic ring, eight short ***protein fibrils*** protrude into the cytoplasm. The nucleoplasmic ring complex anchors a ***basket*** (or ***nuclear "cage,"*** which resembles a fish trap) assembled from eight thin 50-nm-long filaments joined distally by a 30- to 50-nm-diameter ring. The cylinder-shaped central framework encircles the ***central pore*** of the NPC, which acts as a close-fitting diaphragm or gated channel. In addition, each NPC contains one or more water-filled channels for transport of small molecules.

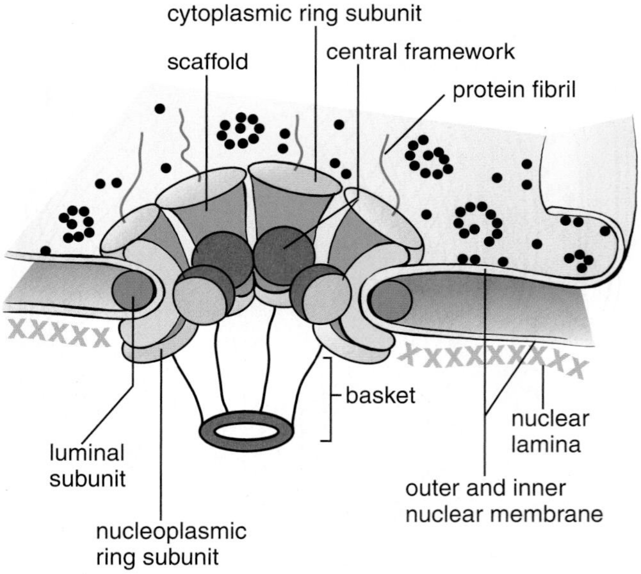

FIGURE 2.61
Schematic drawing of the structure of the nuclear pore complex. Each pore contains eight protein subunits arranged in an octagonal central framework at the periphery of the pore. These subunits form a nuclear pore complex that is inserted between two cytoplasmic and nuclear rings. Eight short protein fibrils protrude from the cytoplasmic ring into the cytoplasm. The nuclear ring anchors a basket assembled from eight thin filaments joined distally by a protein ring. The cylindrical central framework encircles the central pore, which acts as a close-fitting diaphragm.

The NPC mediates bidirectional nucleocytoplasmic transport

Various experiments have shown that the nuclear pore complex regulates the passage of proteins between the nucleus and the cytoplasm (Fig. 2.62). The significance of the NPC can be readily appreciated, as the nucleus does not carry out protein synthesis. Ribosomal proteins are partially assembled into ribosomal subunits in the nucleolus and are transported through nuclear pores to the cytoplasm. Conversely, nuclear proteins, such as histones and lamins, are produced in the cytoplasm and are transported through nuclear pores into the nucleus. Transport through the NPC largely depends on the size of the molecules:

- **Large molecules** (such as RNAs, large proteins, and macromolecular complexes) depend for passage on the presence of an attached signal sequence called the ***nuclear localization signal.*** Labeled proteins destined for the nucleus then bind to a soluble cytosolic receptor called a ***nuclear import receptor*** that directs them from the cytoplasm to an appropriate NPC. They are then actively transported through the pore by a GTP energy-dependent mechanism. The NPC transports proteins as well as ribosomal subunits in their fully folded configuration.
- ***Ions*** and ***smaller water-soluble molecule***s (less than 9 Da) may cross the ***water-filled channels*** of the NPC by simple diffusion. This process is nonspecific and does not require nuclear signal proteins. The effective size of the pore is about 9 nm for substances that diffuse, rather than the 70- to 80-nm measurement of the pore boundary. However, even the smaller nuclear proteins that are capable of diffusion are selectively transported, presumably because the rate is faster than by simple diffusion.

During cell division, the nuclear envelope is disassembled to allow chromosome separation and is later reassembled as the daughter cells form

In early prophase of cell division, enzymes (kinases) are activated that cause phosphorylation of the nuclear lamins and other lamina-associated proteins of the nuclear envelope. After phosphorylation, the proteins become soluble, and the nuclear envelope disassembles. The lipid component of the nuclear membranes then disassociates from the proteins and is retained in small cytoplasmic vesicles. The replicated chromosomes then attach to the microtubules of the mitotic spindle and undergo active movement.

Reassembly of the nuclear envelope begins in late anaphase, when phosphatases are activated to remove the phosphate residues from the nuclear lamins. During telophase, the nuclear lamins begin to repolymerize and form the nuclear lamina material around each set of daughter chromosomes. At the same time, vesicles containing the lipid components of the nuclear membranes and structural membrane protein components fuse, and an envelope is formed on the surface of the already-reassembled nuclear lamina. By the end of telophase, formation of a nuclear envelope in each daughter cell is complete.

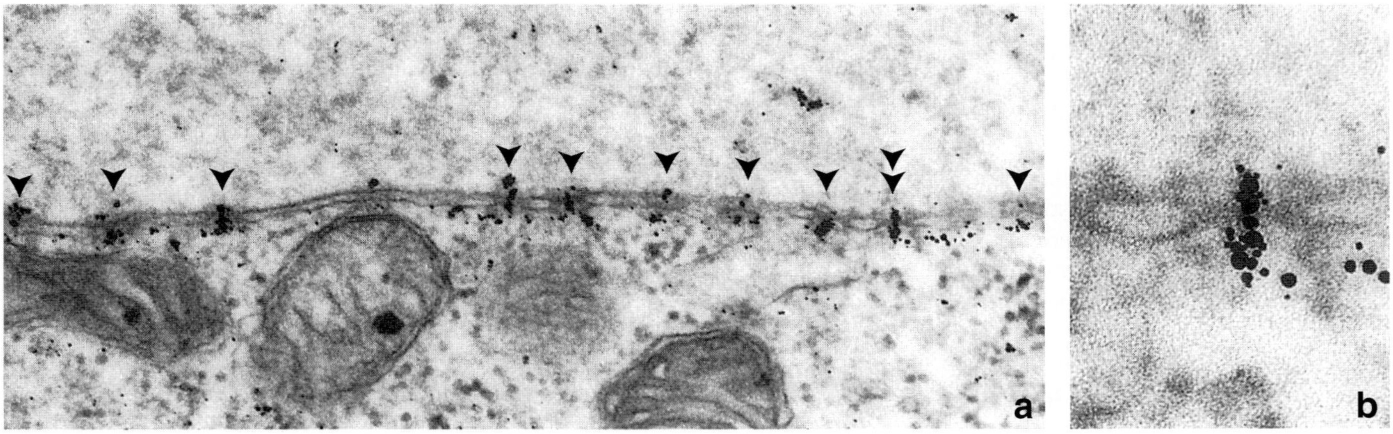

FIGURE 2.62
Electron micrographs showing protein-coated gold particles passing through nuclear pore complexes. a. Protein coated with gold particles was injected into the cytoplasm of an oocyte. Within 15 minutes of injection, the coated gold particles are largely concentrated in the region of the nuclear pore complexes of the nuclear envelope *(arrowheads).* ×60,000. **b.** A higher magnification of the area marked by the *double arrowhead* in *a* shows an elongate cluster of gold particles at the site of the nuclear pore complex. The particles are in a linear array and appear to be in transit through the nuclear pore complex from the cytoplasm to the nucleoplasm. The path of the particles illustrates the pathway taken by proteins synthesized in the cytoplasm as they are transported into the nucleus. ×200,000. (Courtesy of Dr. Carl M. Feldherr.)

Nucleoplasm

Nucleoplasm is the material enclosed by the nuclear envelope exclusive of the chromatin and the nucleolus

Although crystalline, viral, and other inclusions are sometimes found in the ***nucleoplasm,*** until recently, morphologic techniques showed it to be amorphous. It must be assumed, however, that many proteins and other metabolites reside in or pass through the nucleus in relation to the synthetic and metabolic activity of the chromatin and nucleolus. New structures have recently been identified within the nucleoplasm, including intranuclear lamin-based arrays, the protein filaments emanating inward from the nuclear pore complexes, as well as the active gene-tethered RNA transcription and processing machinery itself. It is likely that improved TEM and immunocytochemical methods will further elucidate the nature of the nucleoplasm, but the possibility remains that chromatin is the main constituent of the nuclear structure.

▽ CELL RENEWAL

Somatic cells in the adult organism may be classified according to their mitotic activity

The level of mitotic activity in a cell can be assessed by the number of mitotic metaphases visible in a single high-magnification light microscopic field or by autoradiographic studies of the incorporation of tritiated thymidine into the newly synthesized DNA prior to mitosis. Using these methods, cell populations may be classified either static, stable, or renewing:

- ***Static cell populations*** consist of cells that no longer divide (postmitotic cells), such as cells of the central nervous system, or cells that divide only rarely, such as skeletal and cardiac muscle cells.
- ***Stable cell populations*** consist of cells that divide episodically and slowly to maintain normal tissue or organ structure. These cells may be stimulated by injury to become more mitotically active. Periosteal and perichondrial cells, smooth muscle cells and endothelial cells of blood vessels, and fibroblasts of the connective tissue may be included in this category.
- ***Renewing cell populations*** may be slowly or rapidly renewing but display ***regular mitotic activity.*** Division of such cells usually results in two daughter cells that differentiate both morphologically and functionally or two cells that remain as stem cells. Daughter cells may divide one or more times before their mature state is reached. The differentiated cell may ultimately be lost from the body.

Slowly renewing populations include smooth muscle cells of most hollow organs, fibroblasts of the uterine wall, and epithelial cells of the lens of the eye. Slowly renewing populations may actually slowly increase in size during life, as do the smooth muscle cells of the gastrointestinal tract and the epithelial cells of the lens.

Rapidly renewing populations include blood cells, epithelial cells and dermal fibroblasts of the skin, and the epithelial cells and subepithelial fibroblasts of the mucosal lining of the alimentary tract.

▽ CELL CYCLE

Somatic cell division is a cyclic process divided into two phases: mitosis and interphase

For renewing cell populations and growing cell populations, including embryonic cells, cells in tissue culture, and even tumor cells, the ***cell cycle*** has two principal phases: ***mitosis (M phase)*** and ***interphase.*** Three other phases, ***gap*** $_1$ (G_1), ***synthesis phase (S),*** and ***gap*** $_2$ (G_2), further subdivide interphase (Fig. 2.63). Mitosis nearly always includes both ***karyokinesis*** (division of the nucleus into two daughter nuclei) and ***cytokinesis*** (division of the cell into two daughter cells) and lasts about 1 hour. It is usually followed by G_1, a period in which no DNA synthesis occurs. G_1 is usually a period of ***cell growth*** and may last only a few hours in a rapidly dividing cell or may last a lifetime in a nondividing cell. A cell that leaves the cycle in G_1 to begin "terminal" differentiation enters the ***G_O phase,*** "O" for "outside" the cycle.

The ***S*** or ***DNA synthesis phase*** follows G_1 and usually lasts about 7 hours. The DNA of the cell is doubled during the S phase, and new chromatids are formed that will become obvious at prophase or metaphase (see Figs. 2.64 and 2.65) of the next M phase. The brevity of the S phase allows the use of tritiated thymidine to label only those cells engaged in DNA synthesis at the time the radioactively labeled nucleotide is present.

The S phase is also followed by a period in which no DNA synthesis occurs, a second gap or G_2 phase. G_2 may be as short as 1 hour in rapidly dividing cells or of nearly indefinite duration in some polyploid cells and in cells, such as the primary oocyte, that are arrested in G_2 for extended periods.

Cells identified as ***reserve stem cells*** may be thought of as G_O cells that may be induced to reenter the cell cycle in response to injury of the cell populations within the tissues of the body. Activation of these cells may occur in normal wound healing and in the repopulation of the seminiferous epithelium after intense acute exposure of the testis to x-irradiation or during regeneration of an organ, such as the liver, after removal of a major portion. If the damage to the tissues is too severe, even the reserve stem cells die, and there is no potential for regeneration.

Mitosis

Cell division is a crucial process that increases the number of cells, permits renewal of cell populations, and allows wound repair.

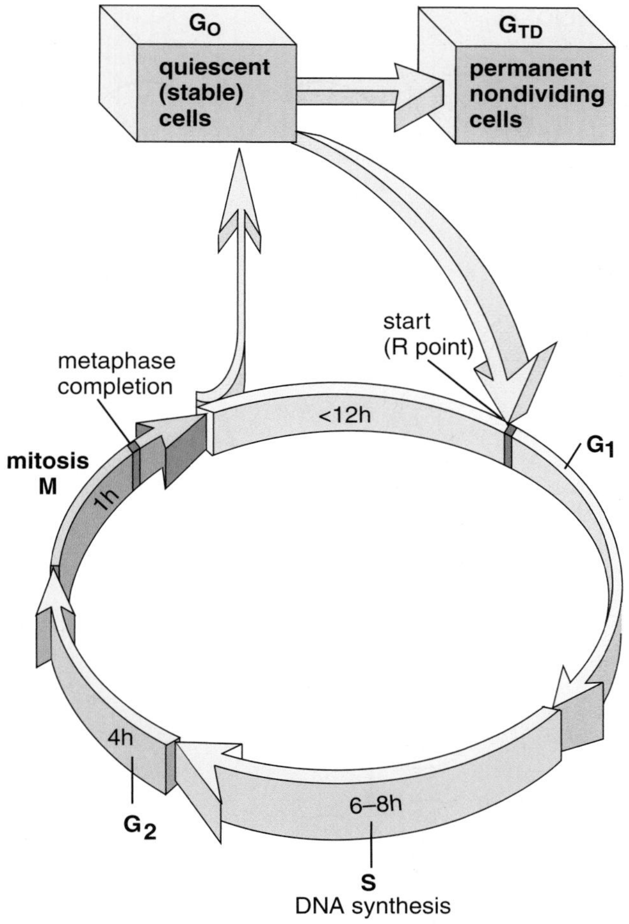

FIGURE 2.63
Cell cycle. This diagram illustrates the cell cycle of rapidly dividing cells in relation to DNA synthesis. After mitosis, the cell is in interphase. G_1 represents the period during which a gap occurs in DNA synthesis. S represents the period during which DNA synthesis occurs. During this phase, tritiated thymidine can be incorporated into the DNA to serve as an experimental tracer. G_2 represents a second gap in DNA synthesis. G_O represents the path of a cell that has stopped dividing; however, such a cell may reenter the cell cycle at the R point after an appropriate stimulus. The cell residing in G_O may undergo terminal differentiation, G_{TD}, and produce a population of permanent nondividing cells (e.g., adult neurons). The average timing of each phase of the cell cycle is indicated on the diagram.

Mitosis is a cell division process that produces two daughter cells with the same chromosome number and DNA content as the parent cell

The process of cell division usually includes division of both the nucleus *(karyokinesis)* and the cytoplasm *(cytokinesis)*. In the strictest sense, the terms mitosis and meiosis are used to describe the duplication and distribution of the chromosomes. If cytokinesis does not follow karyokinesis, a binucleate cell is formed.

Cells that are not in the process of dividing are called *resting or interphase cells*. Prior to entering mitosis (or the first meiotic division; see page 70), cells duplicate their DNA. This phase of the cell cycle is called the ***S*** or ***synthesis phase***. At the beginning of this phase, the chromosome number is $2n$, and the DNA content is $2n$; at the end, the chromosome number is $4n$, and the DNA content is $4n$ (see page 70).

Mitosis follows the S phase and is described in four phases

Mitosis consists of four phases:

- ***Prophase*** begins as the chromosomes condense and become visible. As the chromosomes continue to condense, each of the four chromosomes derived from each homologous pair can be seen to consist of two ***chromatids***. The chromatids are held together by the ***centromere*** or ***kinetochore***. Other changes at this time include disappearance of the nucleolus, replication of the centrioles, and disintegration of the nuclear envelope.
- ***Metaphase*** (Fig. 2.66) begins as the mitotic spindle, consisting of three types of microtubules, becomes organized around the MTOCs located at opposite poles of the cell. The first type of ***astral microtubules*** are nucleated from the γ-tubulin rings in a star-like fashion around each MTOC. The second type of ***polar microtubules*** also originates from the MTOC; however, these microtubules extend away from the MTOC. The third type of ***kinetochore microtubules*** is formed by MTOC-independent mechanisms that involve kinetochores. These microtubules and their associated microtubule motor proteins direct the movements of the chromosomes to the plane in the middle of the cell, the ***equatorial*** or ***metaphase plate***.
- ***Anaphase*** (Fig. 2.66) begins as the chromatids separate and are pulled to opposite poles of the cell by the molecular motors (dyneins) sliding along kinetochore microtubules toward the MTOC.
- ***Telophase*** (Fig. 2.67) is marked by the reconstitution of a nuclear envelope around the chromosomes at each pole. The chromosomes uncoil and become indistinct except at regions that remain condensed in the interphase nucleus. The nucleoli reappear, and the cytoplasm divides to form two daughter cells. Because the chromosomes in the daughter cells contain identical copies of the duplicated DNA, the daughter cells are genetically identical and contain the same kind and number of chromosomes. The daughter cells are $2n$ in DNA content and chromosome number.

Meiosis

Meiosis is a process consisting of two sequential cell divisions that produces gametes containing half the number of chromosomes and half the DNA found in somatic cells

The zygote and all the somatic cells derived from it are *diploid (2n)* in chromosome number; the ***gametes***, having

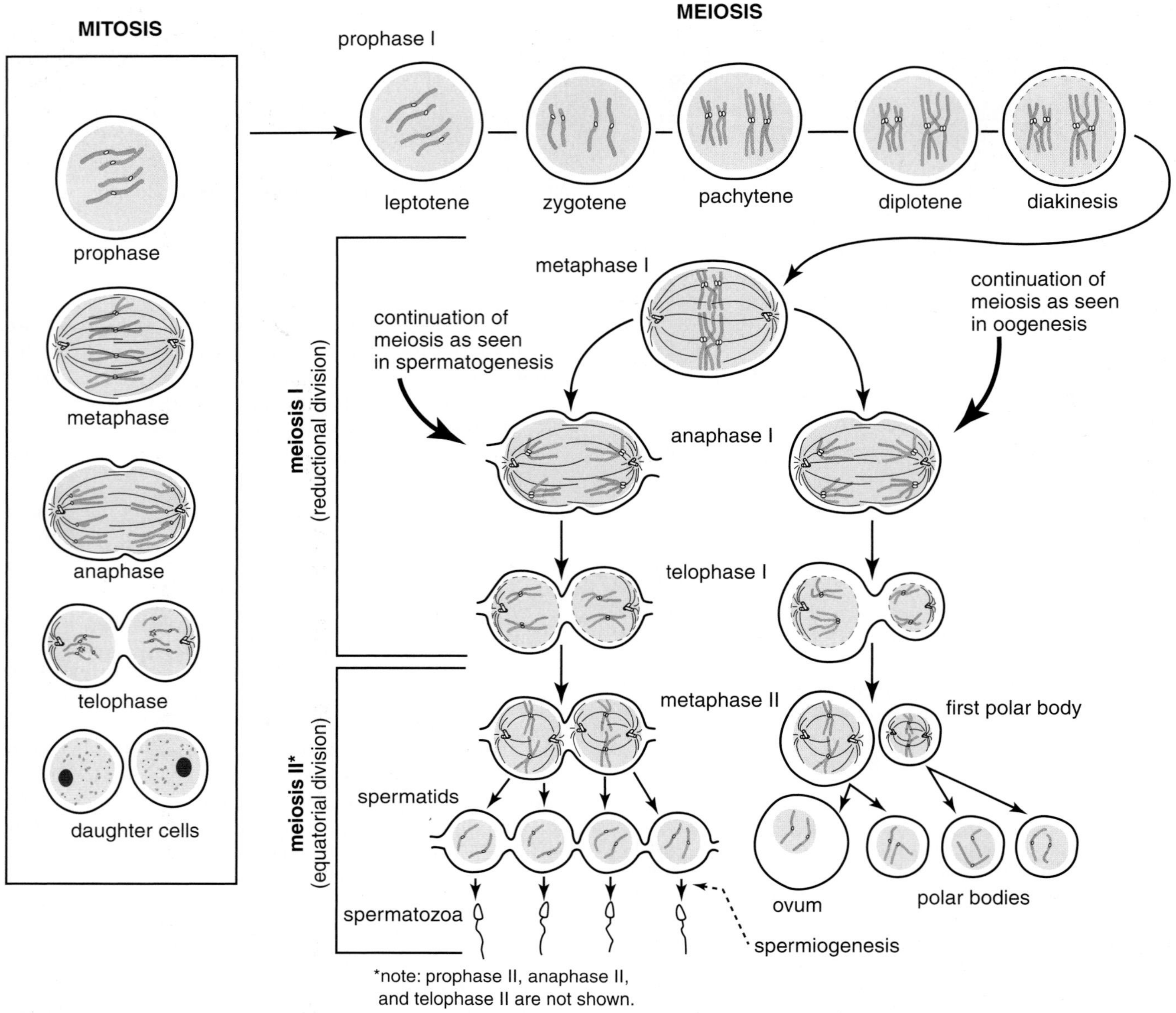

FIGURE 2.64

Comparison of mitosis and meiosis in an idealized cell with two pairs of chromosomes (2*n*). The chromosomes of maternal and paternal origin are depicted in *red* and *blue,* respectively. The mitotic division produces daughter cells that are genetically identical to the parental cell (2*n*). The meiotic division, which has two components, a reductional division and an equatorial division, produces a cell that has only two chromosomes (*n*). In addition, during the chromosome pairing in prophase I of meiosis, chromosome segments are exchanged, leading to further genetic diversity. It should be noted that in humans the first polar body does not divide. Division of the first polar body does occur in some species.

only one member of each chromosome pair, are described as ***haploid (1n).*** During gametogenesis, reduction in chromosome number to the haploid state (23 chromosomes in humans) occurs through ***meiosis,*** a process that involves two successive cell divisions, the second of which is not preceded by an S phase. This reduction is necessary to maintain a constant number of chromosomes in the species. Reduction in chromosome number in the first meiotic division is followed by reduction in DNA content to the haploid (1*n*) amount in the second meiotic division.

During meiosis, the chromosomes pair and may exchange chromosome segments, thus altering the genetic composition of the chromosomes. This genetic exchange, called ***crossing-over,*** and the random assortment of each member of the chromosome pairs into haploid gametes give rise to infinite genetic diversity.

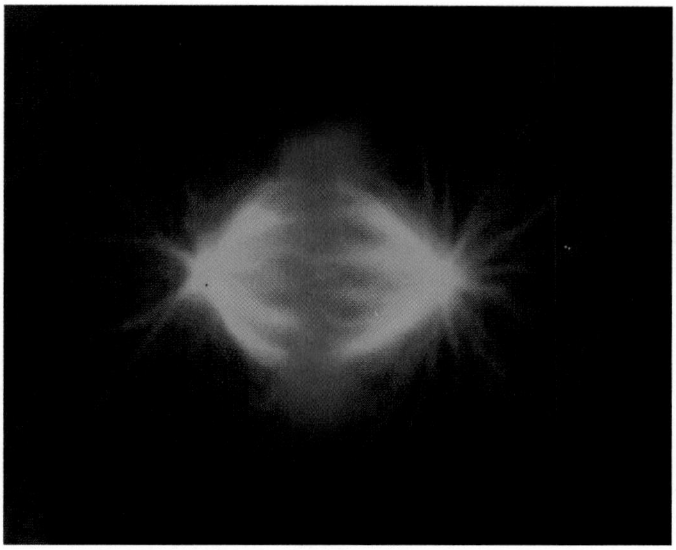

FIGURE 2.65
Mitotic spindle in metaphase. Using indirect immunofluorescence techniques, the mitotic spindle in a *Xenopus* XL-177 cell was labeled with an antibody against α-tubulin conjugated with fluorescein *(green).* DNA was stained *blue* with fluorescent DAPI stain. In metaphase, the nuclear membrane disassembles, DNA is condensed into chromosomes, and microtubules form a mitotic spindle. The action of microtubule-associated motor proteins on the microtubules of the mitotic spindle creates the metaphase plate along which the chromosomes align in the center of the cell. ×1,400. (Courtesy of Dr. Thomas U. Mayer.)

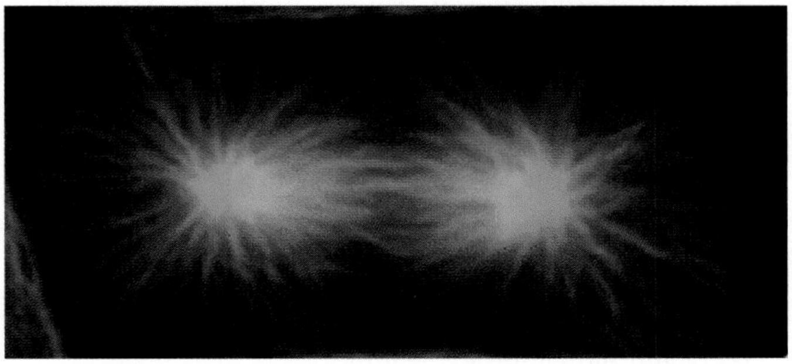

FIGURE 2.66
Mitotic spindle in anaphase. This immunofluorescent image comes from the same cell type and identical preparation as in Figure 2.65. Connections that hold the sister chromatids together break at this stage. The chromatids are then moved to opposite poles of the cell by microtubule-associated molecular motors (dyneins and kinesins) that slide along the kinetochore microtubules toward the centriole and are also pushed by the polar microtubules (visible between the separated chromosomes) away from each other, thus moving opposite poles of the mitotic spindle into the separate cells. ×1,400. (Courtesy of Dr. Thomas U. Mayer.)

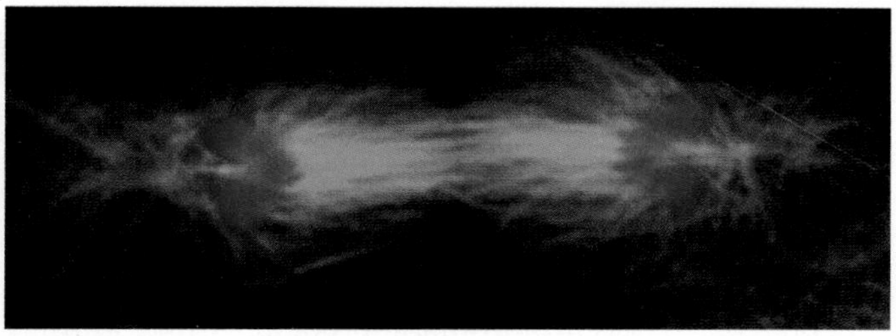

FIGURE 2.67
Mitotic spindle in telophase. In this phase, DNA is segregated and a nuclear envelope is reconstituted around the chromosomes at each pole of the mitotic spindle. The cell divides into two during cytokinesis. In the middle of the cell, actin, septins, myosins, microtubules, and other proteins gather as the cell establishes a ring of proteins that will constrict, forming a bridge between the two sides of what was once one cell. The chromosomes uncoil and become indistinct except at regions that remain condensed in interphase. The cell types and preparation are the same as those in Figures 2.65 and 2.66. ×1,400. (Courtesy of Dr. Thomas U. Mayer.)

The cytoplasmic events associated with meiosis differ in the male and female

The nuclear events of meiosis are the same in males and females, but the cytoplasmic events are markedly different. Figure 2.64 illustrates the key nuclear and cytoplasmic events of meiosis as they occur in spermatogenesis and oogenesis. The events of meiosis through metaphase I are the same in both sexes. Therefore, the figure illustrates the differences in the process as they diverge after metaphase I.

In males, the two meiotic divisions of a primary spermatocyte yield four structurally identical, although genetically unique, haploid spermatids. Each spermatid has the capacity to differentiate into a spermatozoon. In contrast, in females, the two meiotic divisions of a primary oocyte yield one haploid ovum and three haploid polar bodies. The ovum receives most of the cytoplasm and becomes the functional gamete. The polar bodies receive very little cytoplasm and degenerate.

The nuclear events of meiosis are similar in males and females

During the ***S phase*** that precedes meiosis, chromosomes are replicated. The DNA content becomes ***4n,*** and the chromosome number becomes ***4n.*** The cells then undergo a ***reductional division (meiosis I)*** and an ***equatorial division (meiosis II).*** During meiosis I, the maternal and paternal chromosomes pair and exchange segments. They then separate from one another. At the end of meiosis I, each daughter cell contains one member of each pair of chromosomes (the diploid or *2n* amount), and the amount of DNA is reduced to ***2n.*** In meiosis II, the chromatids separate from one another, establishing the haploid number ***(n)*** of chromosomes and reducing the DNA content to the haploid amount ***(n).***

Phases in the process of meiosis are similar to the phases of mitosis

PROPHASE I

The prophase of meiosis I is an extended phase that is subdivided into five stages (see Fig. 2.64):

- ***Leptotene.*** The chromosomes become visible as thin strands.
- ***Zygotene.*** Homologous chromosomes of maternal and paternal origin pair. This pairing involves the formation of a synaptonemal complex, a tripartite structure that brings the chromosomes into physical association so that crossing-over may occur.
- ***Pachytene.*** As the chromosomes condense, the individual chromatids become visible. Crossing-over occurs early in this phase.
- ***Diplotene.*** The chromosomes condense further, and ***chiasmata*** or contacts between the chromatids appear. The chiasmata indicate crossing-over may have occurred.
- ***Diakinesis.*** The chromosomes reach their maximum thickness, the nucleolus disappears, and the nuclear envelope disintegrates.

METAPHASE I

Metaphase I is similar to the metaphase of mitosis except that the paired chromosomes are aligned at the equatorial plate with one member on either side. ***Anaphase I*** and ***telophase I*** are similar to the same phases in mitosis except that the centromeres do not split and the paired chromatids, held by the centromere, remain together. A maternal or paternal member of each homologous pair, now containing exchanged segments, moves to each pole. ***Segregation*** or ***random assortment*** occurs because the maternal and paternal chromosomes of each pair are randomly aligned on one side or the other of the metaphase plate, thus contributing to genetic diversity. At the completion of meiosis I, or the reductional division, the cytoplasm divides. Each resulting daughter cell (a secondary ***spermatocyte*** or ***oocyte***) is haploid in chromosome number ($1n$), containing one member of each chromosome pair, but is still diploid in DNA content ($2n$).

MEIOSIS II

After meiosis I, without passing through an S phase, the cells quickly enter meiosis II, the equatorial division, which is more like mitosis because the centromeres divide. The chromatids then separate at ***anaphase II*** and move to opposite poles of the cell. During meiosis II, the cells pass through prophase II, metaphase II, anaphase II, and telophase II. These stages are essentially the same as those in mitosis except that they involve a haploid set of chromosomes and produce daughter cells that have only the haploid DNA content ($1n$). Unlike the cells produced by mitosis, which are genetically identical to the parent cell, the cells produced by meiosis are genetically unique.

▼ CELL DEATH

In humans, as in all other multicellular organisms, the rates of cell proliferation and cell death determine the net cell production. An abnormality in any of these rates can cause ***disorders of cell accumulation*** (e.g., hyperplasia, cancer, autoimmune diseases) or ***disorders of cell loss*** (atrophy, degenerative diseases, AIDS, ischemic injury). Therefore, the balance (homeostasis) between cell production and cell death must be carefully maintained (Fig. 2.68).

Cell death may occur as a result of acute cell injury or an internally encoded suicide program

Cell death may result from accidental cell injury or mechanisms that cause cells to self-destruct. The two different mechanisms of cell death are

- ***Necrosis,*** or accidental cell death. Necrosis is a pathologic process. It occurs when cells are exposed to an unfavorable physical or chemical environment (e.g., hypothermia, hypoxia, radiation, low pH, cell trauma) that causes acute cellular injury and damage to the plasma membrane. Under physiologic conditions, damage to the plasma membrane may also be initiated by viruses, substances such as complement, or proteins called perforins. Rapid cell swelling and lysis are two characteristic features of this process.
- ***Apoptosis*** *[Gr., falling off, as petals from flowers],* also referred to as ***programmed cell death.*** Apoptosis represents a physiologic process. During apoptosis, cells that are no longer needed are eliminated from the organism. This process may occur during normal embryologic development or other normal physiologic processes, such as follicular atresia in the ovaries. Cells can initiate their own death through activation of an internally encoded suicide program. Apoptosis is characterized by controlled autodigeston, which maintains cell membrane integrity; thus, the cell "dies with dignity" without spilling its contents and damaging its neighbors.

In addition, certain cells or their secretions found in the immune system are toxic to other cells (e.g., cytotoxic $CD8^+$ T lymphocytes, NK cells); they initiate processes that destroy designated cells (e.g., cancer-transformed or virus-infected cells). In contrast to necrosis and apoptosis, cytotoxic death does not involve one specific mechanism. For example, cell death mediated by cytotoxic $CD8^+$ T lymphocytes combines some aspects of both necrosis and apoptosis.

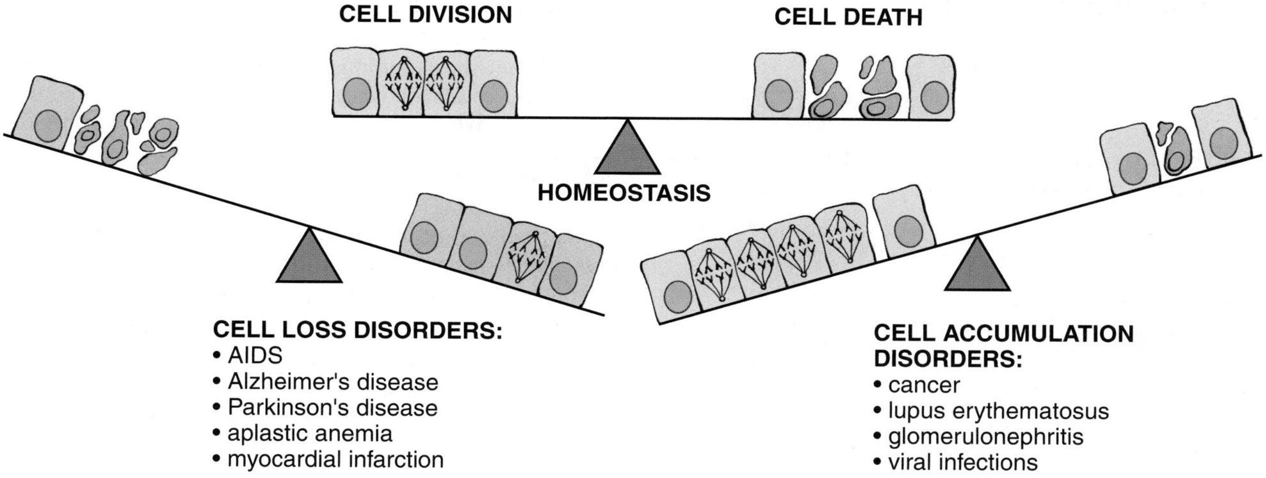

FIGURE 2.68
Schematic diagram showing the relationship between cell death and cell division. Under normal physiologic conditions (homeostasis), the rate of cell division and the rate of cell death are similar. If the rate of cell death is higher than that of cell divisions, a net loss of cell number will occur. Such conditions are categorized as cell loss disorders. When the situation is reversed and the rate of cell division is higher than the rate of cell death, the net gain in cell number will be prominent, leading to a variety of disorders of cell accumulation.

Necrosis begins with impairment of the cell's ability to maintain homeostasis

As a result of cell injury, damage to the cell membrane leads to an influx of water and extracellular ions. Intracellular organelles, such as the mitochondria, rER, and nucleus, undergo irreversible changes that are caused by cell swelling and cell membrane rupture (cell lysis). As a result of the ultimate breakdown of the plasma membrane, the cytoplasmic contents, including lysosomal enzymes, are released into the extracellular space. Therefore, necrotic cell death is often associated with extensive surrounding tissue damage and an ***intense inflammatory response*** (Fig. 2.69).

Apoptosis is a mode of cell death that occurs under normal physiologic conditions

In apoptosis, the cell is an active participant in its own demise ("cellular suicide"). This process is activated by a variety of extrinsic and intrinsic signals. Cells undergoing apoptosis show characteristic morphologic and biochemical features (see Fig. 2.69):

- ***DNA fragmentation*** occurs in the nucleus and is an irreversible event that commits the cell to die. DNA fragmentation is a result of Ca^{2+}-dependent and Mg^{2+}-dependent activation of nuclear endonucleases. These enzymes selectively cleave DNA, generating small oligonucleosomal fragments. Nuclear chromatin then aggregates, and the nucleus may divide into several discrete fragments bounded by the nuclear envelope.
- ***Decrease in cell volume*** is achieved by shrinking of the cytoplasm. The cytoskeletal elements become reorganized in bundles parallel to the cell surface. Ribosomes become clumped within the cytoplasm, the rER forms a series of concentric whorls, and most of the endocytotic vesicles fuse with the plasma membrane.
- ***Loss of mitochondrial function*** is caused by changes in the permeability of the mitochondrial membrane channels. The integrity of the mitochondrion is breached, the mitochondrial transmembrane potential drops, and the electron transport chain is disrupted. Proteins from the mitochondrial intermembrane space, such as ***cytochrome c,*** are released into the cytoplasm to activate a cascade of proteolytic enzymes called caspases that are responsible for dismantling the cell. The regulated release of cytochrome *c* suggests that mitochondria, under the influence of Bcl-2 proteins (see page 74), are the decision makers for initiating apoptosis. Thus many researchers view mitochondria either as the "headquarters for the leader of a crack suicide squad" or as a "high security prison for the leaders of a military coup."
- ***Membrane blebbing*** results from cell membrane alterations. One alteration is related to translocation of certain molecules (e.g., phosphatidylserine) from the cytoplasmic surface to the outer surface of the plasma membrane. These changes cause the plasma membrane

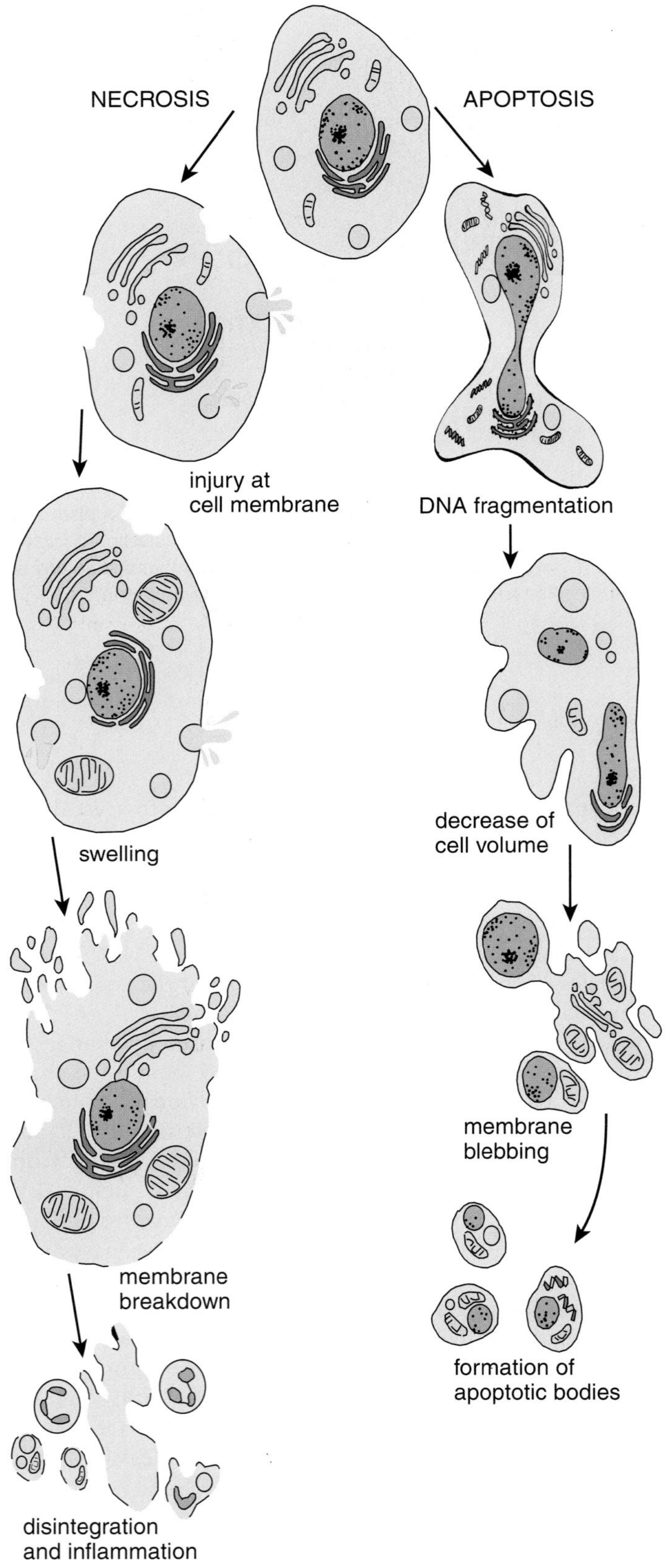

FIGURE 2.69
Schematic diagram of changes occurring in necrosis and apoptosis. This diagram shows the major steps in necrosis and apoptosis. In necrosis *(left column)*, breakdown of the cell membrane results in an influx of water and extracellular ions, causing the organelles to undergo irreversible changes. Lysosomal enzymes are released into the extracellular space, causing damage to neighboring tissue and an intense inflammatory response. In apoptosis *(right column)*, the cell shows characteristic morphologic and biochemical features such as DNA fragmentation, decrease in cell volume, membrane blebbing without loss of membrane integrity, and formation of apoptotic bodies, causing cell breakage. Apoptotic bodies are later removed by phagocytotic cells without inflammatory reactions.

to change its physical and chemical properties and lead to blebbing without loss of membrane integrity (see Fig. 2.69).

- ***Formation of apoptotic bodies,*** the final step of apoptosis, results in cell breakage (Fig. 2.70). These membrane-bounded vesicles originate from the cytoplasmic bleb containing organelles and nuclear material. They are rapidly removed by phagocytotic cells. The removal of apoptotic bodies is so efficient that ***no inflammatory response is elicited.***

Apoptosis is regulated by external and internal stimuli

Apoptotic processes can be activated by a variety of external and internal stimuli. Some factors, such as ***tumor necrosis factor (TNF),*** acting on cell membrane receptors, trigger apoptosis by recruiting and activating the caspase cascade. Consequently, the TNF receptor is known as the ***"death receptor."*** Other external activators of apoptosis include transforming growth factor β (TGF-β), certain neurotransmitters, free radicals, oxidants, and UV and ioning radiation. Internal activators of apoptosis include oncogenes (e.g., *myc* and *rel*), tumor suppressors such as p53, and nutrient deprivation antimetabolites (Fig. 2.71).

Apoptosis can also be inhibited by signals from other cells and the surrounding environment via so-called ***survival factors.*** These include growth factors, hormones such as estrogen and androgens, neutral amino acids, zinc, and interactions with extracellular matrix proteins. However, the most important regulatory function in apoptosis is ascribed to internal signals from the ***Bcl-2 family*** of proteins. Members of this family consist of antiapoptotic and proapoptotic members that determine the life or death of a cell. These proteins interact with each other to suppress or propagate their own activity by acting on downstream activation of various executional steps of apoptosis. They also act independently on mitochondria to regulate the release of cytochrome *c*, the most potent apoptosis-inducing agent.

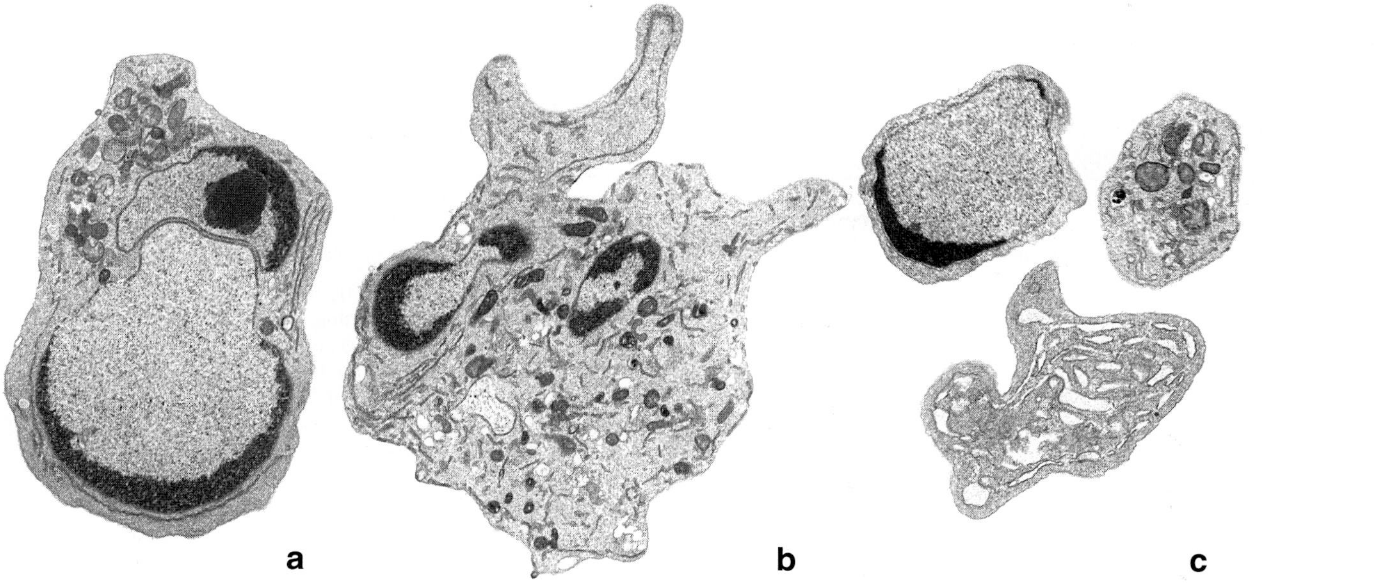

FIGURE 2.70

Electron micrograph of apoptotic cells. a. This electron micrograph shows an early stage of apoptosis in a lymphocyte. The nucleus is already fragmented, and the irreversible process of DNA fragmentation is turned on. Note the regions containing condensed heterochromatin adjacent to the nuclear envelope. ×5,200. **b.** Further fragmentation of DNA. The heterochromatin in one of the nuclear fragments *(left)* begins to bud outward through the envelope, initiating a new round of nuclear fragmentation. Note the reorganization of the cytoplasm and budding of the cytoplasm to produce apoptotic bodies. ×5,200. **c.** Apoptotic bodies containing fragments of the nucleus, organelles, and cytoplasm. These bodies will eventually be phagocytosed by cells from the mononuclear phagocytotic system. ×5,200. (Courtesy of Dr. Scott H. Kaufmann, Mayo Clinic.)

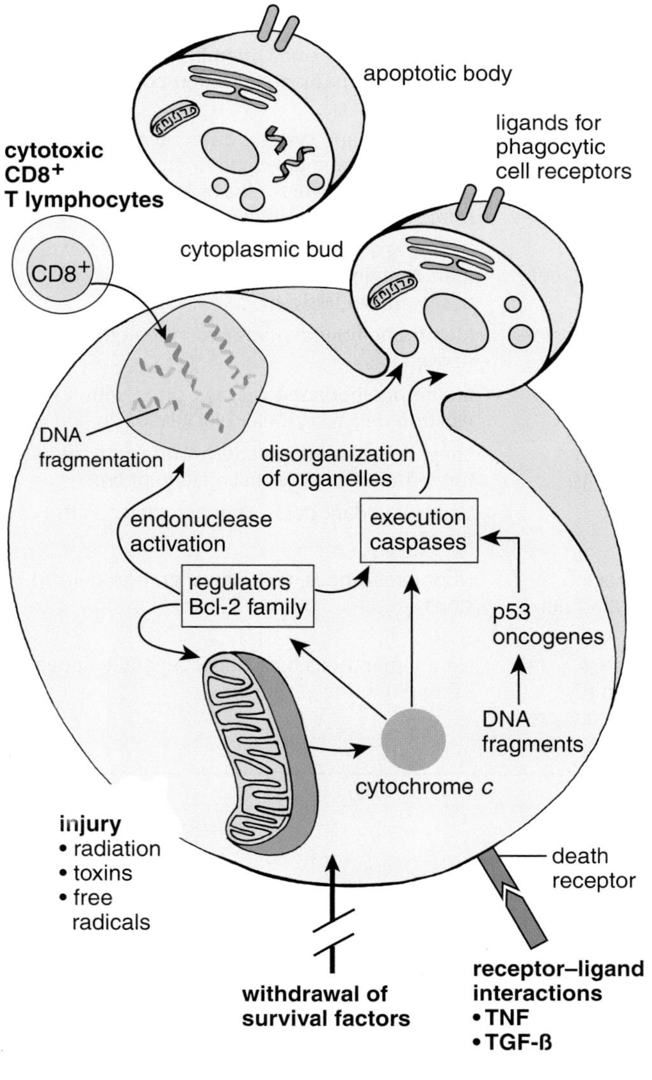

FIGURE 2.71

Schematic drawing of mechanisms leading to apoptosis. Both external and internal stimuli can trigger apoptosis by activating the enzymatic caspase cascade. Many external activators act on the cell to initiate signals leading to apoptosis; note that TNF and TGF-β act through a "death receptor." Controlled release of cytochrome *c* from mitochondria is an important internal step in the activation of apoptosis.

TABLE 2.3. **Review of Organelles and Cytoplasmic Inclusions: A Key to Light Microscopic and Electron Microscopic Identification**

Organelle or Inclusion	Size (μm)	Light Microscopic Features	Electron Microscopic Features
Nucleus	3–10	Largest organelle within the cell with distinct boundary; often visible nucleoli and chromatin pattern regions	Surrounded by two membranes (nuclear envelope) containing nuclear pore complexes and perinuclear cisternal space; regions with condensed and diffuse chromatin pattern (heterochromatin and euchromatin)
Nucleolus	1–2	Roughly circular, basophilic region within the nucleus; visible in living cells throughout interphase with interference microscopy	Dense, nonmembranous structure containing fibrillar and granular material
Plasma membrane	0.008–0.01	Not visible	The external membrane and membranes surrounding membranous organelles of the cell; two inner and outer electron-dense layers separated by an intermediate electron-lucent layer
rER	Area ~5–10	Often observed as a basophilic region of cytoplasm referred as "ergastoplasm"	Flattened sheets, sacs, and tubes of membranes with attached ribosomes
sER	Throughout cytoplasm	Not visible; cytoplasm in region of sER may exhibit distinct eosinophilia	Flattened sheets, sacs, and tubes of membranes *without* attached ribosomes
Golgi apparatus	Area ~5–10	Sometimes observed as "negative-staining" region; appears as network in heavy-metal–stained preparations; visible in living cells with interference microscopy	Stack of flattened membrane sheets, often adjacent to one side of the nucleus
Secretory vesicles	0.050–1.0	Observed only when vesicles are very large (e.g., zymogen granules in pancreas)	Many relatively small, membrane-bounded vesicles of uniform diameter; often polarized on one side of cell
Mitochondria	0.2–2 × 2–7	Sometimes observed in favorable situations (e.g., liver or nerve cells) as very small, dark dots; visible in living cells stained with vital dyes, e.g., Janus green	Two-membrane system: outer membrane and inner membrane arranged in numerous folds (cristae); in steroid-producing cells inner membrane arranged in tubular cristae
Endosomes	0.02–0.5	Not visible	Tubolovesicular structures with subdivided lumen containing electron-lucent material or other smaller vesicles
Lysosomes	0.2–0.5	Visible only after special enzyme histochemical staining	Membrane-bounded vesicles, often electron dense
Peroxisomes	0.2–0.5	Visible only after special enzyme histochemical staining	Membrane-bounded vesicles, often with electron-dense crystalloid inclusions
Cytoskeletal elements	0.006–0.025	Only observed when organized into large structures (e.g., muscle fibrils)	Long, linear staining pattern with width and features characteristic of each filament type
Ribosomes	0.025	Not visible	Very small dark dots, often associated with the rER
Glycogen	0.010–0.040	Observed as a "purple haze" region of cytoplasm (metachromasia) with toluidine blue–stained specimen	Nonmembranous, very dense grape-like inclusions
Lipid droplets	0.2–5, up to 80	Readily visible when very large (e.g., in adipocytes); appear as large empty holes in section (lipid itself is usually removed by embedding solvents)	Nonmembranous inclusions; generally appear as a void in the section

TABLE 2.4. **Organelles and Cytoplasmic Inclusions: Functions and Pathologies**

Organelle or Inclusion	Function	Examples of Associated Pathologies
Nucleus	Storage and use of genome	Inherited genetic diseases; environmentally induced mutations
Nucleolus	Synthesis of rRNA and partial assembly of ribosomal subunits	?
Plasma membrane	Ion and nutrient transport; recognition of environmental signals; cell-to-cell and cell-to-extracellular matrix adhesions	Cystic fibrosis Intestinal malabsorption syndromes Lactose intolerance
rER	Binds ribosomes engaged in translating mRNA for proteins destined for secretion or for membrane insertion; also involved in chemical modifications of proteins and membrane lipid synthesis	Pseudoachondroplasia Calcium phosphate dihydrate crystal deposition disease
sER	Similar to the rER but lacks the ribosome-binding function; involved in lipid and steroid metabolism	Hepatic endoplasmic reticular storage disease
Golgi apparatus	Chemical modification of proteins: sorting and packaging of molecules for secretion or transport to other organelles	I-cell disease Polycystic kidney disease
Secretory vesicles	Transport and storage of secreted proteins to plasma membrane	Lewy bodies of Parkinson's disease Proinsulin diabetes
Mitochondria	Aerobic energy supply (oxidative phosphorylation, ATP); initiation of apoptosis	Mitochondrial myopathies such as MERRF,[A] MELAS,[B] Kearns-Sayre syndromes, and Laber's hereditary optic atrophy
Endosomes	Transport of endocytosed material; biogenesis of lysosomes	M-6-P receptor deficiency
Lysosomes	Digestion of macromolecules	Glycogen storage disease type II Tay-Sachs disease Metachromatic leukodystrophy
Peroxisomes	Oxidative digestion, e.g., fatty acids	Zellweger's syndrome
Cytoskeletal element	Various functions including cell motility, intracellular and extracellular transport; maintenance of cellular skeleton	Immotile cilia syndrome, Alzheimer's disease, epidermolysis bullosa
Ribosomes	Synthesize protein by translating protein-coding sequence from mRNA	Many antibiotics act selectively on bacterial ribosomes, e.g., tetracyclines, aminoglycosides (gentamicin, streptomycin)
Glycogen	Short-term storage of glucose in the form of branched polymer; found in liver, skeletal muscle, and adipose tissue	There are several known glycogen storage diseases, including major groups of hepatic–hypoglycemic and muscle-energy pathophysiologies
Lipid droplets	Storage of esterified forms of fatty acids as high-energy storage molecules	Lipid storage diseases such as Gaucher's and Niemann-Pick disease, liver cirrhosis

[A]Myoclonic epilepsy and ragged red fibers syndrome.
[B]Mitochondrial myopathy, encephalopathy, lactic acidosis, and stroke-like episodes syndrome.

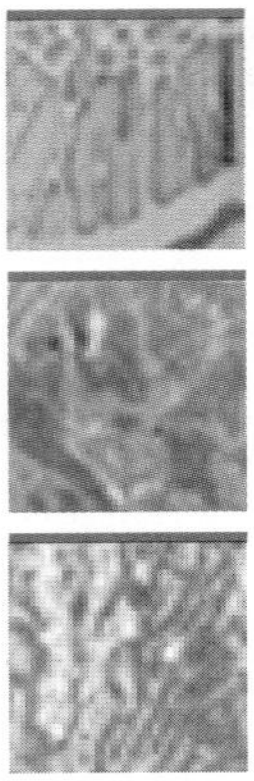

3

Tissues: Concept and Classification

OVERVIEW OF TISSUES

Tissues are aggregates or groups of cells organized to perform one or more specific functions

At the light microscope level, the cells and extracellular components of the various organs of the body exhibit a recognizable and often distinctive pattern of organization. This organized arrangement reflects the cooperative effort of cells performing a particular function. Therefore, an organized aggregation of cells that function in a collective manner is called a **tissue** *[Fr. tissu, woven; L. texo, to weave]*.

Although it is frequently said that the cell is the basic functional unit of the body, it is really the tissues, through the collaborative efforts of their individual cells, that are responsible for maintaining body functions. Cells within tissues communicate through specialized intercellular junctions (gap junctions, page 101), thus facilitating this collaborative effort and allowing the cells to operate as a functional unit. Other mechanisms that permit the cells of a given tissue to function in a unified manner include specific membrane receptors and anchoring junctions between cells.

Despite their disparate structure and physiologic properties, all organs are made up of only four basic tissue types

The tissue concept provides a basis for understanding and recognizing the many cell types within the body and how they interrelate. Despite the variations in general appearance, structural organization, and physiologic properties of the various body organs, the tissues that compose them are classified into four basic tissues:

- ***Epithelium (epithelial tissue),*** which covers body surfaces, lines body cavities, and forms glands
- ***Connective tissue,*** which underlies or supports the other three basic tissues, both structurally and functionally

- *Muscle tissue,* which is made up of contractile cells and is responsible for movement
- *Nerve tissue,* which receives, transmits, and integrates information from outside and inside the body to control the activities of the body

Each of these basic tissues is defined by a set of general morphologic characteristics or functional properties. Each type may be further subdivided according to specific characteristics of their various cell populations and any special extracellular substances that may be present.

In classifying the basic tissues, two different definitional parameters are used. The basis for definition of epithelium and connective tissue is primarily morphologic, whereas for muscle and nerve tissue, it is primarily functional. Moreover, the same parameters exist in designating the tissue subclasses. For example, while muscle tissue itself is defined by its function, it is subclassified into smooth and striated categories, a purely morphologic distinction, not a functional one. Another kind of contractile tissue, myoepithelium, functions as muscle tissue but is typically designated epithelium because of its location.

For these reasons, tissue classification cannot be reduced to a simple formula. Rather, students are advised to learn the features or characteristics of the different cell aggregations that define the four basic tissues and their subclasses.

▼ EPITHELIUM

Epithelium is characterized by close cell apposition and presence at a free surface

Epithelial cells, whether arranged in a single layer or in multiple layers, are always contiguous with one another. In addition, they are usually joined by specialized cell-to-cell junctions, which create a barrier between the free surface and the adjacent connective tissue. The intercellular space between epithelial cells is minimal and is devoid of any structure except where junctional attachments are present.

Free surfaces are characteristic of the exterior of the body, the outer surface of many internal organs, and the lining of the body cavities, tubes, and ducts, both those that ultimately communicate with the exterior of the body and those that are enclosed. The enclosed body cavities and tubes include the pleural, pericardial, and peritoneal cavities as well as the cardiovascular system. All of these are lined by epithelium.

Subclassifications of epithelium are usually based on the shape of the cells and the number of cell layers rather than on function. Cell shapes include squamous (flattened), cuboidal, and columnar. Layers are described as simple (single layer) or stratified (multiple layers). Figure 3.1

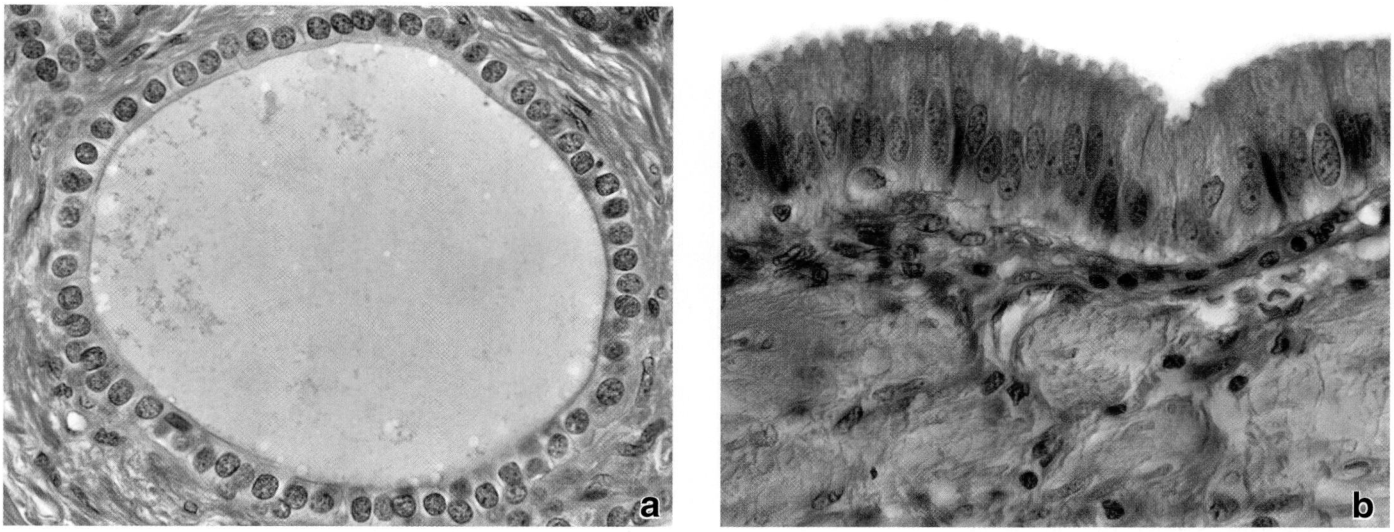

FIGURE 3.1
Simple epithelia. a. A H&E–stained section showing a pancreatic duct lined by a single layer of contiguous cuboidal epithelial cells. The free surface of the cells faces the lumen; the basal surface is in apposition to the connective tissue. ×540. **b.** A H&E–stained section showing a single layer of tall columnar epithelial cells lining the gallbladder. Note that the cells are much taller than the lining cells of the pancreatic duct. The free surface of the epithelial cells is exposed to the lumen of the gallbladder, and the basal surface is in apposition to the adjacent connective tissue. ×540.

shows epithelia from two sites. Both are simple epithelia, i.e., one cell layer thick. The major distinction between the two examples is the shape of the cells, cuboidal versus columnar. In both epithelia, however, the cells occupy a surface position.

CONNECTIVE TISSUE

Connective tissue is characterized on the basis of its extracellular matrix

Unlike epithelial cells, connective tissue cells are conspicuously separated from one another. The intervening spaces are occupied by material produced by the cells. This extracellular material is called the ***extracellular matrix.*** The nature of the cells and matrix varies according to the function of the tissue. Thus, subclassification of connective tissue takes into account not only the cells but also the composition and organization of the extracellular matrix.

A type of connective tissue found in close association with most epithelia is ***loose connective tissue*** (Fig. 3.2a). In fact, it is the connective tissue that most epithelia rest upon. The extracellular matrix of loose connective tissue contains loosely arranged collagen fibers and numerous cells. Some of these cells, the fibroblasts, form and maintain the extracellular matrix. However, most of the cells are migrants from the vascular system and have roles associated with the immune system.

In contrast, where only strength is required, collagen fibers are more numerous and densely packed. Also, the cells are relatively sparse and limited to the fiber-forming cell, the fibroblast (Fig. 3.2b). This type of connective tissue is described as ***dense connective tissue.***

Bone and cartilage are two other types of connective tissue characterized by the material associated with collagen, i.e., calcium (bones) and hyaluronic acid (cartilage). Again, in both of these tissues, it is the extracellular material that characterizes the tissue, not the cells.

MUSCLE TISSUE

Muscle tissue is categorized on the basis of a functional property, the ability of its cells to contract

Muscle cells are characterized by large amounts of the contractile proteins actin and myosin in their cytoplasm and by their particular cellular arrangement in the tissue. To function efficiently to effect movement, most muscle cells are aggregated into distinct bundles that are easily distinguished from the surrounding tissue. Muscle cells are typically elongated and oriented with their long axes in the same direction (Fig. 3.3). The arrangement of nuclei is also consistent with the parallel orientation of muscle cells.

Although the shape and arrangement of cells in specific muscle types, e.g., smooth muscle, skeletal muscle, and cardiac muscle, are quite different, all muscle types share

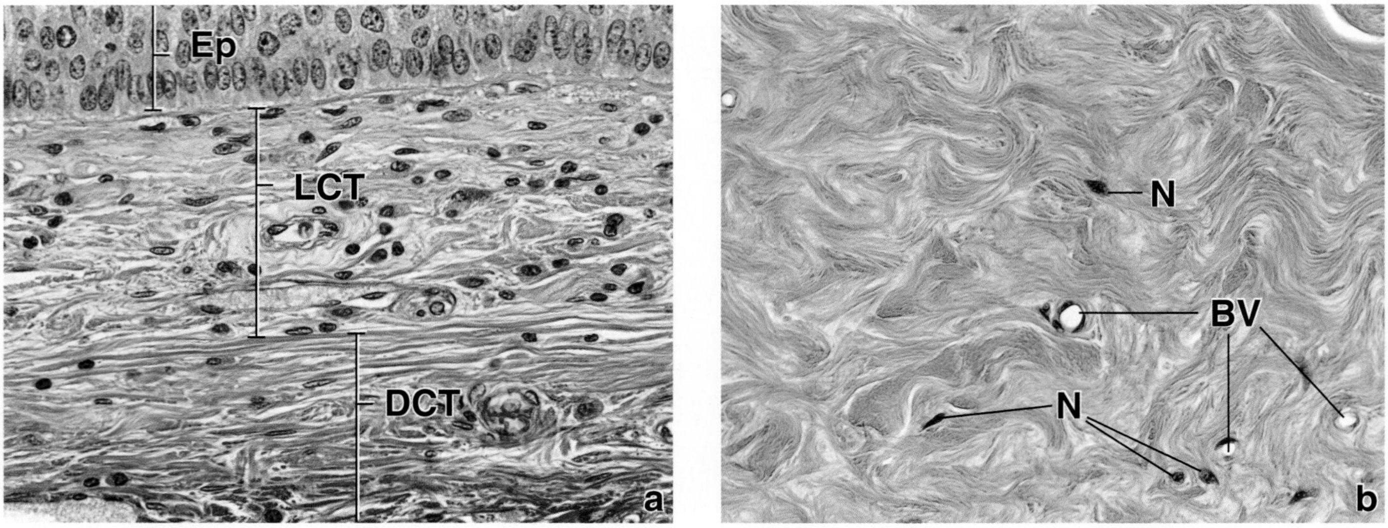

FIGURE 3.2
Loose and dense connective tissue. a. Mallory-Azan–stained specimen of a section through the epiglottis, showing the lower part of its stratified epithelium *(Ep)*, subjacent loose connective tissue *(LCT)*, and dense connective tissue *(DCT)* below. Loose connective tissue typically contains many cells of several types. Their nuclei vary in size and shape. The elongate nuclei most likely belong to fibroblasts. Because dense connective tissue contains thick collagen bundles, it stains more intensely with the blue dye. Also, note the relatively fewer nuclei. ×540. **b.** A Mallory-stained specimen of dense connective tissue, showing a region composed of numerous, densely packed collagen fibers. The few nuclei *(N)* that are present belong to fibroblasts. The combination of densely packed fibers and the paucity of cells characterizes dense connective tissue. Relatively few small blood vessels *(BV)* are shown on this section. ×540.

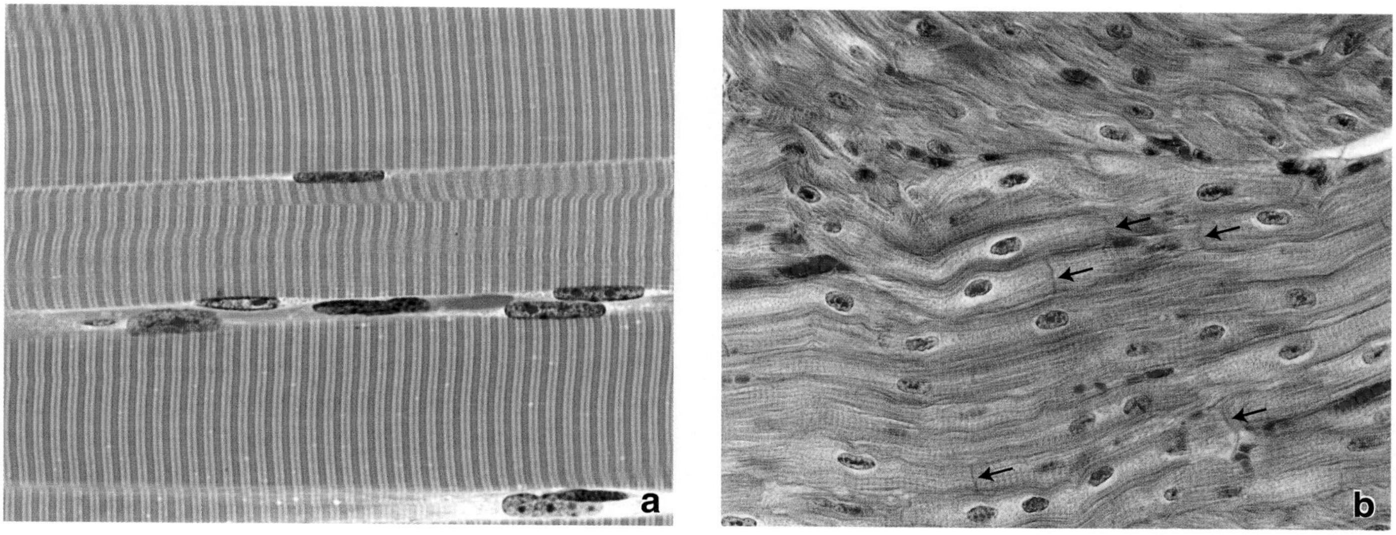

FIGURE 3.3
Muscle tissue. a. A H&E–stained specimen showing a portion of three longitudinally sectioned skeletal muscle fibers (cells). Two striking features of these large, long cells are their characteristic cross-striations and the many nuclei located along the periphery of the cell. ×420. **b.** A Mallory-stained specimen showing cardiac muscle fibers that also exhibit striations. These fibers are composed of individual cells that are much smaller than those of skeletal muscle and are arranged end to end to form long fibers. Most of the fibers are seen in longitudinal array. The organized aggregation, i.e., the parallel array of the fibers in the case of muscle tissue, allows for collective effort in performing their function. Intercalated disks *(arrows)* mark the junction of adjoining cells. ×420.

a common characteristic: The bulk of the cytoplasm consists of the contractile proteins actin and myosin. Although these proteins are ubiquitous in all cells, only in muscle cells are they present in such large amounts and organized in such highly ordered arrays that their contractile activity can produce movement in an entire organ or organism.

▽ NERVE TISSUE

Nerve tissue consists of nerve cells (neurons) and associated supporting cells of several types

Although all cells exhibit electrical properties, nerve cells or ***neurons*** are highly specialized to transmit electrical impulses from one site in the body to another; they are also specialized to integrate those impulses. Nerve cells receive and process information from the external and internal environment and may have specific sensory receptors and sensory organs to accomplish this function. Neurons are characterized by two different types of processes through which they interact with other nerve cells and with cells of epithelia and muscle. A single, long ***axon*** (sometimes longer than a meter) carries impulses away from the ***cell body,*** which contains the neuron's nucleus. Multiple **dendrites** receive impulses and carry them toward the cell body. (In histologic sections, it is usually impossible to differentiate axons and dendrites because they have the same structural appearance.) The axon terminates at a neuronal junction called a ***synapse,*** where electrical impulses are transferred from one cell to the next by secretion of ***neuromediators.*** These chemical substances are released at synapses to generate electric impulses in the adjacent communicating neuron.

In the central nervous system (CNS), i.e., the brain and spinal cord, the supporting cells are called ***neuroglial cells.*** In the peripheral nervous system (PNS), i.e., the nerves in all other parts of the body, the supporting cells are called ***Schwann (neurilemmal) cells*** and ***satellite cells.*** Supporting cells are responsible for several important functions. They separate neurons from one another, produce the myelin sheath that insulates and speeds conduction in certain types of neurons, provide active phagocytosis to remove cellular debris, and contribute to the blood–brain barrier in the CNS.

In an ordinary hematoxylin and eosin (H&E)–stained section, nerve tissue may be observed in the form of a nerve, which consists of varying numbers of neuronal processes along with their supporting cells (Fig. 3.4a). Nerves are most commonly seen in longitudinal or cross sections in loose connective tissue. Nerve cell bodies in the PNS, including the autonomic nervous system (ANS), are seen in aggregations called ganglia, where they are surrounded by satellite cells (Fig. 3.4b).

Neurons and supporting cells are derived from neuroectoderm, which forms the neural tube in the embryo. Neuroectoderm originates by invagination of an epithelial

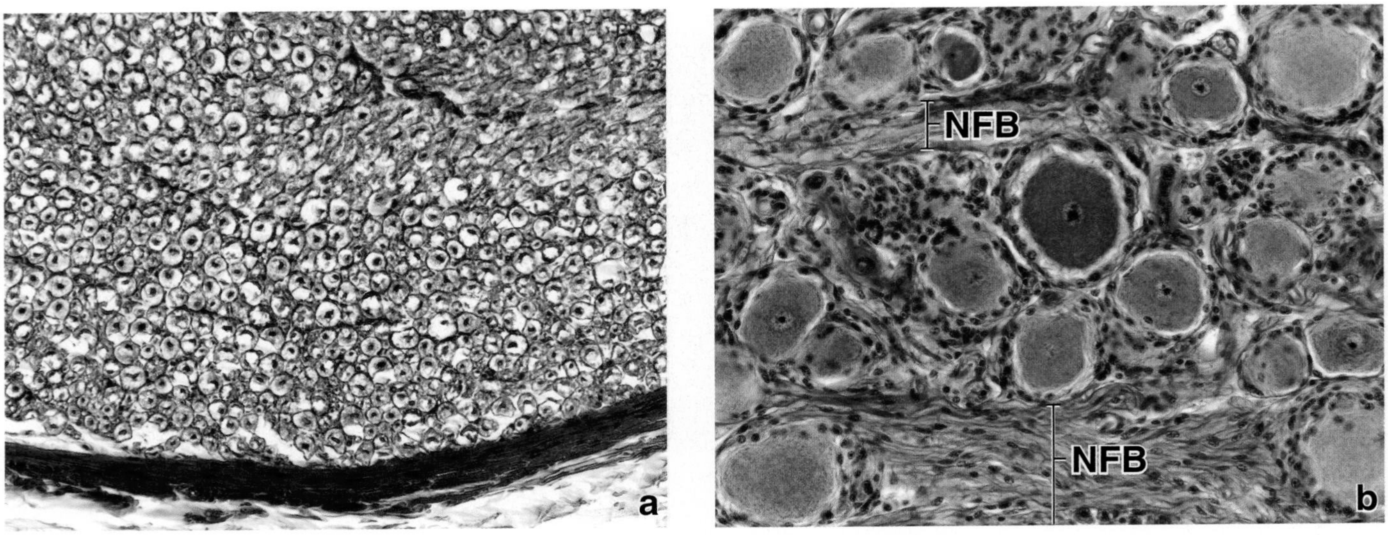

FIGURE 3.4

Nerve tissue. a. A Mallory-stained section of a peripheral nerve. Nerve tissue consists of a vast number of thread-like myelinated axons held together by connective tissue. The axons have been cross-sectioned and appear as small, red, dot-like structures. The clear space surrounding the axons previously contained myelin that was dissolved and lost during preparation of the specimen. The connective tissue is stained blue. It forms a delicate network around the myelinated axons and ensheathes the bundle, thus forming a structural unit, the nerve. ×270. **b.** An Azan-stained section of a nerve ganglion, showing the large, spherical nerve cell bodies and the nuclei of the small satellite cells that surround the nerve cell bodies. The axons associated with the nerve cell bodies are unmyelinated. They are seen as nerve fiber bundles *(NFB)* between clusters of the cell bodies. ×270.

BOX 3.1

Clinical Correlations: Ovarian Teratomas

It is of clinical interest that, under certain conditions, abnormal differentiation may occur. The result is formation of a tumor mass that contains a variety of mature tissues arranged in an unorganized fashion. Such masses are referred to as ***teratomas.*** Teratomas almost always occur in the gonads. In the ovary, these tumors usually develop into solid masses that contain characteristics of the mature basic tissues. Although the tissues fail to form functional structures, frequently organ-like structures may be seen, i.e., teeth, hair, epidermis, bowel segments, etc. These tissues are thought to arise through parthenogenic oocyte development. Teratomas may also develop in the testis, but they are rare. Moreover, ovarian teratomas are usually benign, whereas teratomas in the testis are composed of less differentiated tissues that usually lead to malignancy. An example of a solid-mass ovarian teratoma containing fully differentiated tissue is shown in the center micrograph of Figure 3.5. The low power reveals the lack of organized structures but does not allow identification of the specific tissues present. However, with higher magnification, as shown in the *insets* (a–f), mature differentiated tissues are evident.

The example given in Figure 3.5 shows that one can readily identify tissue characteristics, even in an unorganized structure. Again, the important point is the ability to recognize aggregates of cells and to determine the special characteristics that they exhibit.

FIGURE 3.5

Ovarian teratoma. In the center is a H&E–stained section of an ovarian teratoma seen at low magnification. This mass is composed of various basic tissues that are well differentiated and easy to identify at higher magnification. The abnormal feature is the lack of organization of the tissues to form functional organs. The tissues within the *boxed areas* are seen at higher magnification in micrographs *a–f.* ×10. The higher magnification allows identification of some of the basic tissues that are present within this tumor. **a.** Simple columnar epithelium lining a cavity of a small cyst. ×170. **Inset.** Higher magnification of the epithelium and the underlying connective tissue. ×320. **b.** Dense regular connective tissue forming a tendon-like structure. ×170. **c.** Area showing hyaline cartilage *(C)* and developing bone spicules *(B).* ×170. **d.** Brain tissue with glial cells. ×170. **e.** Cardiac muscle fibers. ×220. **Inset.** Higher magnification showing intercalated disks *(arrows).* ×320. **f.** Skeletal muscle fibers cut in cross section. ×220.

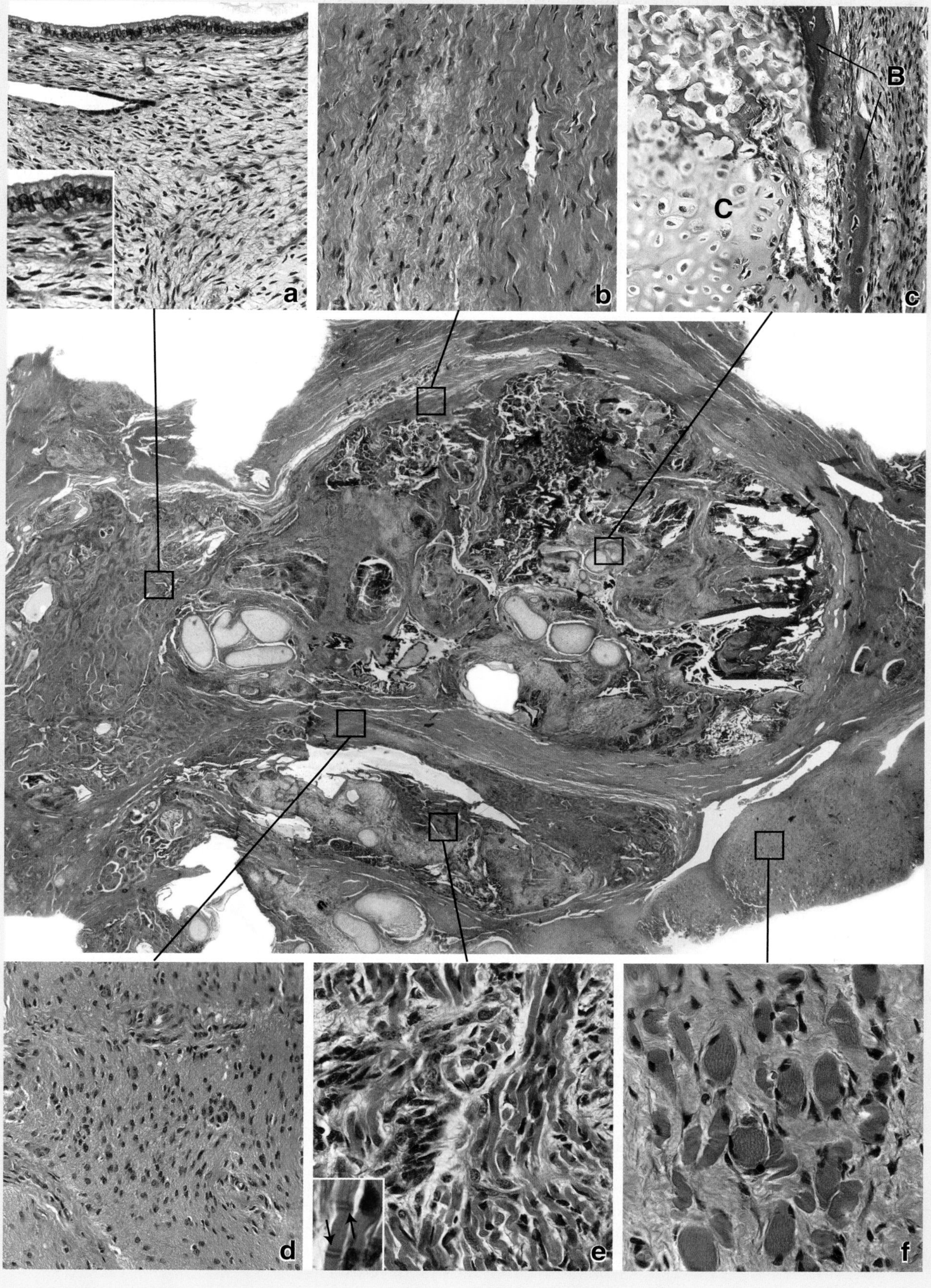
B
C
a
b
c
d
e
f

layer, the dorsal ectoderm of the embryo. Some nervous system cells, such as ***ependymal cells*** and cells of the choroid plexus in the CNS, retain the absorptive and secretary functions characteristic of epithelial cells.

▼ IDENTIFYING TISSUES

Recognition of tissues is based on the presence of specific components within cells and on specific cellular relationships

Keeping these few basic facts and concepts about the fundamental four tissues in mind can facilitate the task of examining and interpreting histologic slide material. The first goal is to recognize aggregates of cells as tissues and determine the special characteristics that they present. Are the cells present at a surface? Are they in contact with their neighbors, or are they separated by definable intervening material? Do they belong to a group with special properties, such as muscle or nerve?

The structure and the function of each fundamental tissue are examined in subsequent chapters. In focusing on a single specific tissue we are, in a sense, artificially separating the constituent tissues of organs. However, this separation is necessary to understand and appreciate the histology of the various organs of the body and the means by which they operate as functional units and integrated systems.

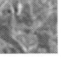

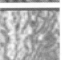
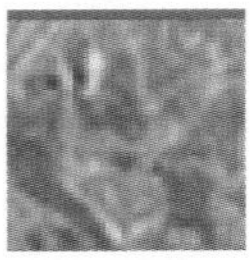
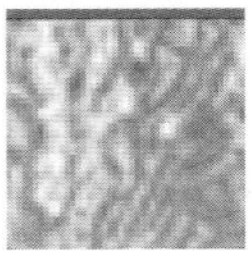

4

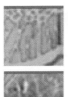

Epithelial Tissue

BOXES

OVERVIEW OF EPITHELIAL STRUCTURE AND FUNCTION

Epithelium covers body surfaces, lines body cavities, and constitutes glands

Epithelium is an avascular tissue composed of cells that cover the exterior body surfaces and line internal closed cavities (including the vascular system) and body tubes that communicate with the exterior (the alimentary, respiratory, and genitourinary tracts). Epithelium also forms the secretory portion (parenchyma) of glands and their ducts. In addition, specialized epithelial cells function as receptors for the special senses (smell, taste, hearing, and vision).

The cells that make up epithelium have three principal characteristics:

- They are closely apposed and adhere to one another by means of specific cell-to-cell adhesion molecules that form specialized ***cell junctions*** (Fig. 4.1).
- They exhibit functional as well morphologic polarity; i.e., different functions are associated with three distinct morphologic surface domains: a ***free surface*** or ***apical domain***, a ***lateral domain***, and a ***basal domain***. (The properties of each domain are determined by specific membrane proteins.)
- Their basal surface is attached to an underlying ***basement membrane***, a noncellular, protein–polysaccharide-rich layer demonstrable at the light microscopic level by histochemical methods (see Fig. 1.2, page 7).

In special situations, epithelial cells lack a free surface (epithelioid tissues)

In some locations, cells are closely apposed to one another but lack a free surface. Although the close apposition of these cells and the presence of a basement membrane would classify them as epithelium, the absence of a free surface more appropriately classifies such cell aggregates as ***epithelioid tissues***. Epithelioid organization is typical of most endocrine glands; examples of such tissue

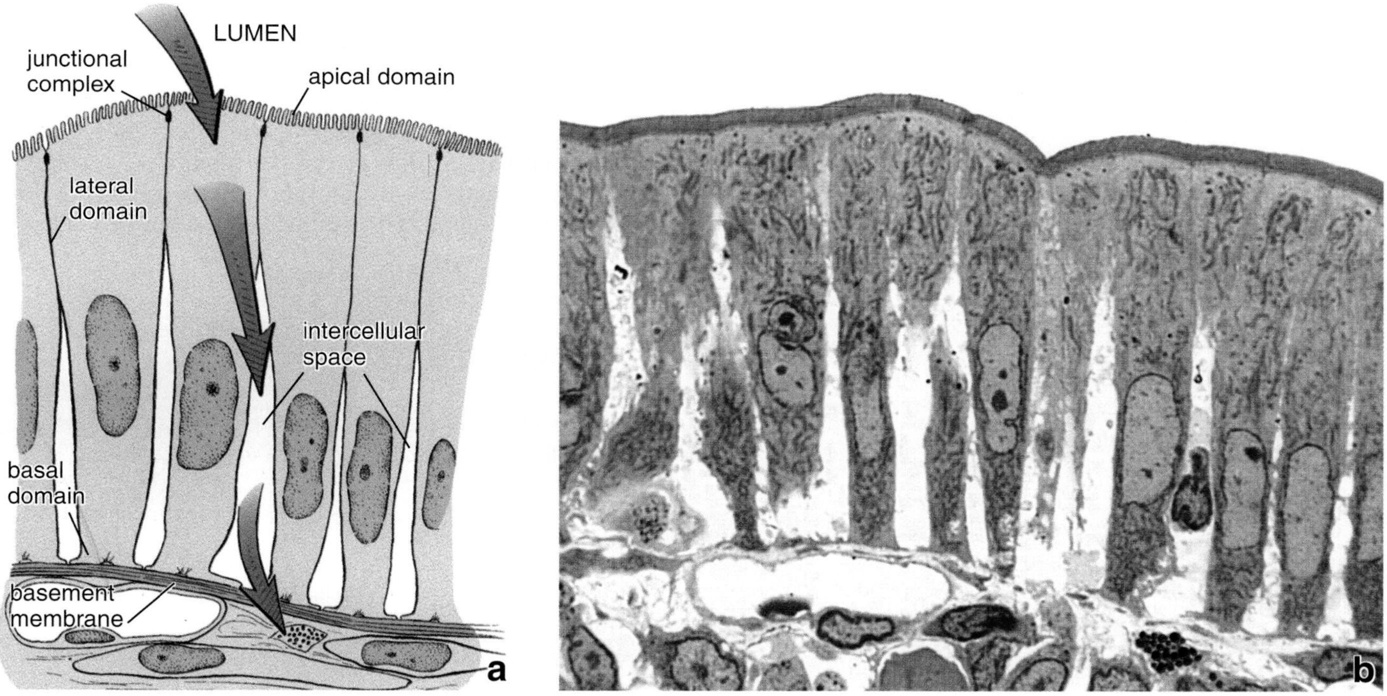

FIGURE 4.1
Diagram of small intestine absorptive epithelial cells. a. All three cellular domains of a typical epithelial cell are indicated on the diagram. The junctional complex provides adhesion between adjoining cells and separates the luminal space from the intercellular space, limiting the movement of fluid between the lumen and the underlying connective tissue. The pathway of fluid movement during absorption *(arrows)* is from the intestinal lumen into the cell, then across the lateral cell membrane into the intercellular space, and, finally, across the basement membrane to the connective tissue. **b.** This photomicrograph of a plastic-embedded, thin section of intestinal epithelium, stained with toluidine blue, shows cells actively engaged in fluid transport. Like the adjacent diagram, the intercellular spaces are prominent, reflecting fluid passing into this space before entering the underlying connective tissue. ×1,250.

include the interstitial cells of Leydig in the testis, the lutein cells of the ovary, the islets of Langerhans in the pancreas, the parenchyma of the adrenal gland, and the anterior lobe of the pituitary gland. Epithelioreticular cells of the thymus also may be included in this category. Epithelioid patterns are also formed by accumulations of connective tissue macrophages in response to certain types of injury and infections, as well as by many tumors derived from epithelium.

Epithelium creates a selective barrier between the external environment and the underlying connective tissue

Covering and lining epithelium forms a sheet-like cellular investment that separates underlying or adjacent connective tissue from the external environment, internal cavities, or fluid connective tissue such as the blood and lymph. Among other roles, this epithelial investment functions as a selective barrier that facilitates or inhibits the passage of specific substances between the exterior (including the body cavities) environment and the underlying connective tissue compartment.

CLASSIFICATION OF EPITHELIUM

The traditional classification of epithelium is descriptive and based on two factors: the number of cell layers and the shape of the surface cells. The terminology, therefore, reflects only structure, not function. Thus, epithelium is described as

- ***Simple,*** when it is one cell layer thick
- ***Stratified,*** when it has two or more cell layers

The individual cells that compose an epithelium are described as

- ***Squamous,*** when the width of the cell is greater than its height
- ***Cuboidal,*** when the width, depth, and height are approximately the same
- ***Columnar,*** when the height of the cell appreciably exceeds the width (the term ***low columnar*** is often used when a cell's height only slightly exceeds its other dimensions)

Thus, by describing the number of cell layers (i.e., simple or stratified) and the surface cell shape, the various configurations of epithelia are easily classified. The cells in some exocrine glands are more or less ***pyramidal,*** with their apices directed toward a lumen. However, these cells are still classified as either cuboidal or columnar, depending on their height relative to their width at the base of the cell.

In a stratified epithelium, the shape and height of the cells usually vary from layer to layer, but *only the shape of the cells that form the surface layer is used in classifying the epithelium.* For example, stratified squamous epithelium consists of more than one layer of cells, and the surface layer consists of flat or squamous cells.

In some instances, a third factor—specialization of the apical cell surface domain—can be added to this classification system. For example, some simple columnar epithelia are classified as simple columnar ciliated when the apical surface domain possesses cilia. The same principle applies to stratified squamous epithelium, in which the surface cells may be keratinized or nonkeratinized. Thus, epidermis would be designated as stratified squamous keratinized epithelium because of the keratinized cells at the surface.

Pseudostratified epithelium and transitional epithelium are special classifications of epithelium

Two special categories of epithelium are pseudostratified and transitional.

- ***Pseudostratified epithelium*** appears stratified, although some of the cells do not reach the free surface; all rest on the basement membrane. Thus, it is actually a simple epithelium. The distribution of pseudostratified epithelium is limited in the body. Also, it is often difficult to discern whether all of the cells contact the basement membrane. For these reasons, identification of pseudostratified epithelium usually depends on knowing where it is normally found.
- ***Transitional epithelium (urothelium)*** is a term applied to the epithelium lining the lower urinary tract, extending from the minor calyces of the kidney down to the proximal part of the urethra. Urothelium is a stratified epithelium with specific morphologic characteristics that allow it to distend. This epithelium is described in Chapter 19.

The cellular configurations of the various types of epithelia and their appropriate nomenclature are illustrated in Table 4.1.

Endothelium and mesothelium are the simple squamous epithelia lining the vascular system and body cavities

Specific names are given to epithelium in certain locations:

- ***Endothelium*** is the epithelial lining of the vascular system.
- ***Mesothelium*** is the epithelium that lines the walls and covers the contents of the closed cavities of the body, i.e., the abdominal, pericardial, and pleural cavities.

Both endothelium and mesothelium are almost always simple squamous epithelia. An exception is found in postcapillary venules of certain lymphatic tissues, where the endothelium is cuboidal. These venules are called high endothelial venules (HEV). Another exception is found in the spleen, in which endothelial cells of the venous si-

TABLE 4.1. **Types of Epithelium**

	Classification	Some Typical Locations	Major Function
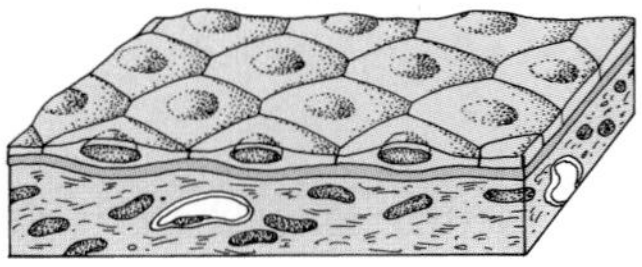	Simple squamous	Vascular system (endothelium) Body cavities (mesothelium) Bowman's capsule (kidney) Respiratory spaces in lung	Exchange, barrier in central nervous system Exchange and lubrication Barrier Exchange
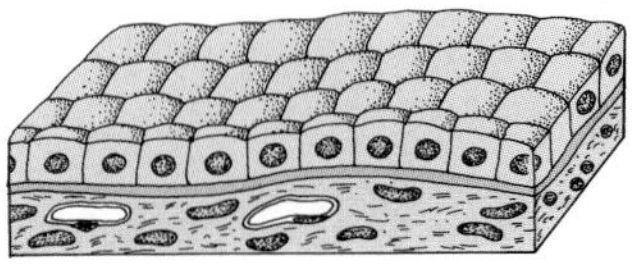	Simple cuboidal	Small ducts of exocrine glands Surface of ovary (germinal epithelium) Kidney tubules	Absorption, conduit Barrier Absorption and secretion
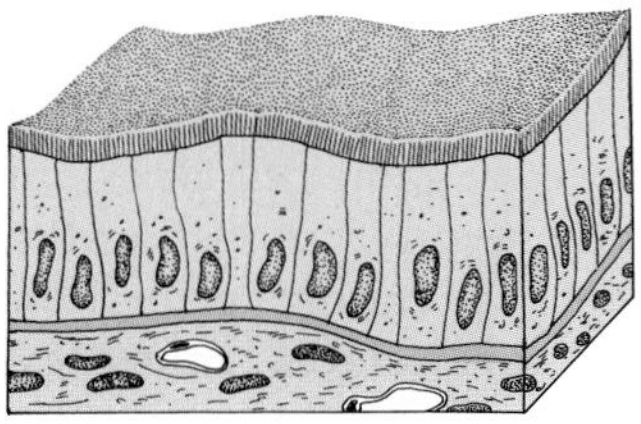	Simple columnar	Small intestine and colon Stomach lining and gastric glands Gallbladder	Absorption and secretion Secretion Absorption
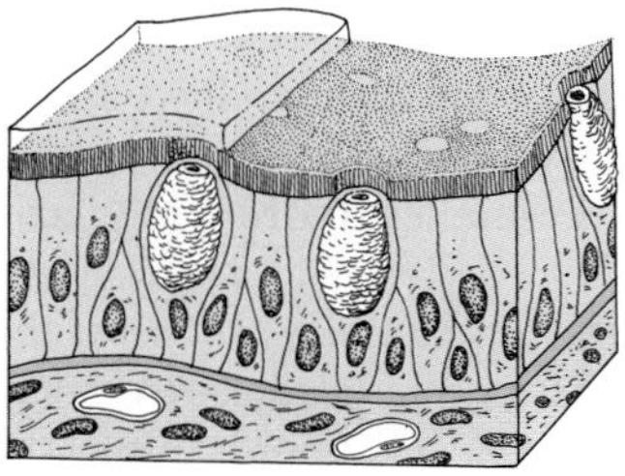	Pseudostratified	Trachea and bronchial tree Ductus deferens Efferent ductules of epididymis	} Secretion, conduit Absorption, conduit
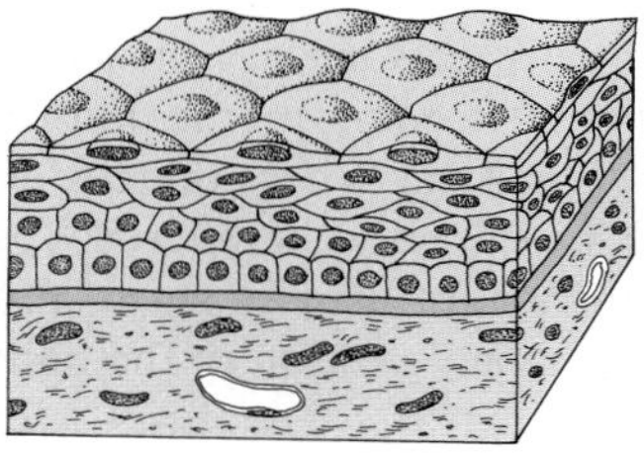	Stratified squamous	Epidermis Oral cavity and esophagus Vagina	} Barrier, protection
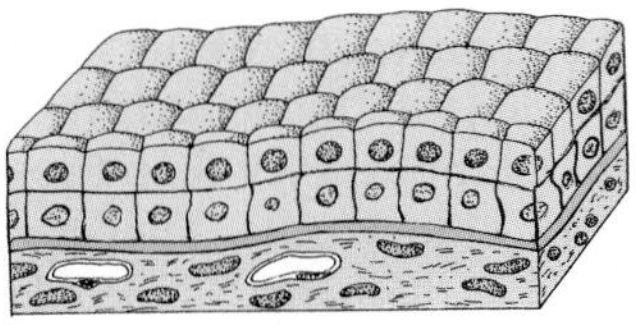	Stratified cuboidal	Sweat gland ducts Large ducts of exocrine glands Anorectal junction	} Barrier, conduit
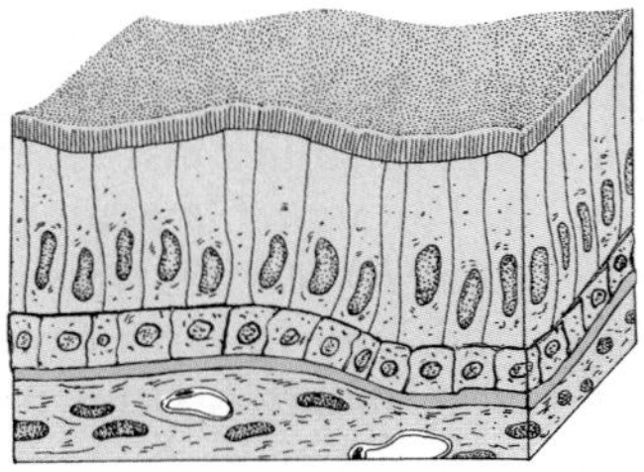	Stratified columnar	Largest ducts of exocrine glands Anorectal junction	} Barrier, conduit
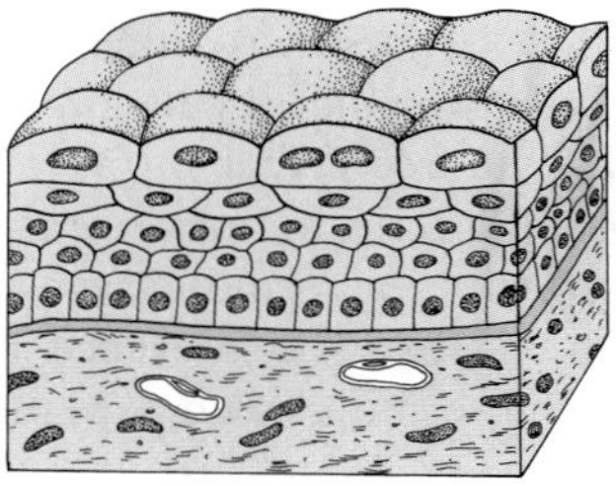	Transitional (urothelium)	Renal calyces Ureters Bladder Urethra	} Barrier, distensible property

nuses are rod-shaped and arranged like the staves of a barrel.

Diverse epithelial functions can be found in different organs of the body

A given epithelium may serve one or more functions, depending on the activity of the cell types that are present:

- ***Secretion,*** as in the columnar epithelium of the stomach and the gastric glands
- ***Absorption,*** as in the columnar epithelium of the intestines and proximal convoluted tubules in the kidney
- ***Transport,*** as in transport of materials or cells along the surface of an epithelium by motile cilia or in transport of materials across an epithelium to and from the connective tissue
- ***Protection,*** as in the stratified squamous epithelium of the skin (epidermis) and the transitional epithelium of the urinary bladder
- ***Receptor function,*** to receive and transduce external stimuli, as in the taste buds of the tongue, olfactory epithelium of the nasal mucosa, and the retina of the eye

Epithelia involved in secretion or absorption are typically simple or, in a few cases, pseudostratified. The height of the cells often reflects the level of secretory or absorptive activity. Simple squamous epithelia are compatible with a high rate of transepithelial transport. Stratification of the epithelium usually correlates with transepithelial impermeability. Finally, in some pseudostratified epithelia, basal cells are the stem cells that give rise to the mature functional cells of the epithelium, thus balancing cell turnover.

▽ CELL POLARITY

Epithelial cells exhibit distinct ***polarity.*** They have an **apical domain,** a **lateral domain,** and a **basal domain.** Specific biochemical characteristics are associated with each cell surface. These characteristics and the geometric arrangements of the cells in the epithelium determine the functional polarity of all three cell domains.

The free or apical domain is always directed toward the exterior surface or the lumen of an enclosed cavity or tube. The lateral domain communicates with adjacent cells and is characterized by specialized attachment areas. The basal domain rests on the basal lamina anchoring the cell to underlying connective tissue.

▽ THE APICAL DOMAIN AND ITS MODIFICATIONS

In many epithelial cells, the apical domain exhibits special structural surface modifications to carry out specific functions. In addition, the apical domain may contain specific enzymes (e.g., hydrolases), ion channels, and carrier proteins (e.g., glucose transporters). The structural surface modifications include

- ***Microvilli,*** cytoplasmic processes that extend from the cell surface
- ***Stereocilia (stereovilli),*** microvilli of unusual length
- ***Cilia,*** motile cytoplasmic processes

Microvilli are finger-like cytoplasmic projections on the apical surface of most epithelial cells

As observed with the electron microscope (EM), microvilli vary widely in appearance. In some cell types, microvilli are short, irregular, bleb-like projections. In other cell types, they are tall, closely packed, uniform projections that greatly increase the free cell surface area. In general, the number and shape of the microvilli of a given cell type correlate with its absorptive capacity. Thus, cells that principally transport fluid and absorb metabolites have many closely packed, tall microvilli. Cells in which transepithelial transport is less active have smaller, more irregularly shaped microvilli.

Among the fluid-transporting epithelia, e.g., those of the intestine and kidney tubule, a distinctive border of vertical striations at the apical surface of the cell, representing the close packed microvilli, is easily seen in the light microscope. In intestinal absorptive cells, this surface structure was originally called the ***striated border;*** in the kidney tubule cells, it is called the ***brush border.*** Where there is no apparent surface modification based on light microscope observations, microvilli, if present, are usually short and not numerous; thus, they may escape detection in the light microscope.

The variations seen in microvilli of various types of epithelia are shown in Figure 4.2. The microvilli of the intestinal epithelium (striated border) are the most highly ordered and are even more uniform in appearance than those that constitute the brush border of kidney cells. They also contain a conspicuous core of actin filaments (microfilaments). Actin filaments are anchored to ***villin*** located in the tip of the microvillus and extend down into the apical cytoplasm. Here, they interact with a horizontal network of actin filaments, the ***terminal web,*** which lies just below the base of the microvilli (Fig. 4.3a). The actin filaments inside the microvillus are cross-linked at 10-nm intervals by the actin-bundling proteins ***fascin*** and ***fimbrin.*** This cross-linkage provides support and gives rigidity to the microvilli. In addition, the core of actin filaments is associated with ***myosin I,*** a molecule that binds the actin filaments to the plasma membrane of the microvillus. The addition of villin to epithelial cells growing in cultures induces formation of microvilli on the free apical surface.

The terminal web is composed of actin filaments stabilized by ***spectrin,*** which also anchors the terminal web to the apical cell membrane (Fig. 4.3b). The presence of ***myosin II*** and ***tropomyosin*** in the terminal web explains

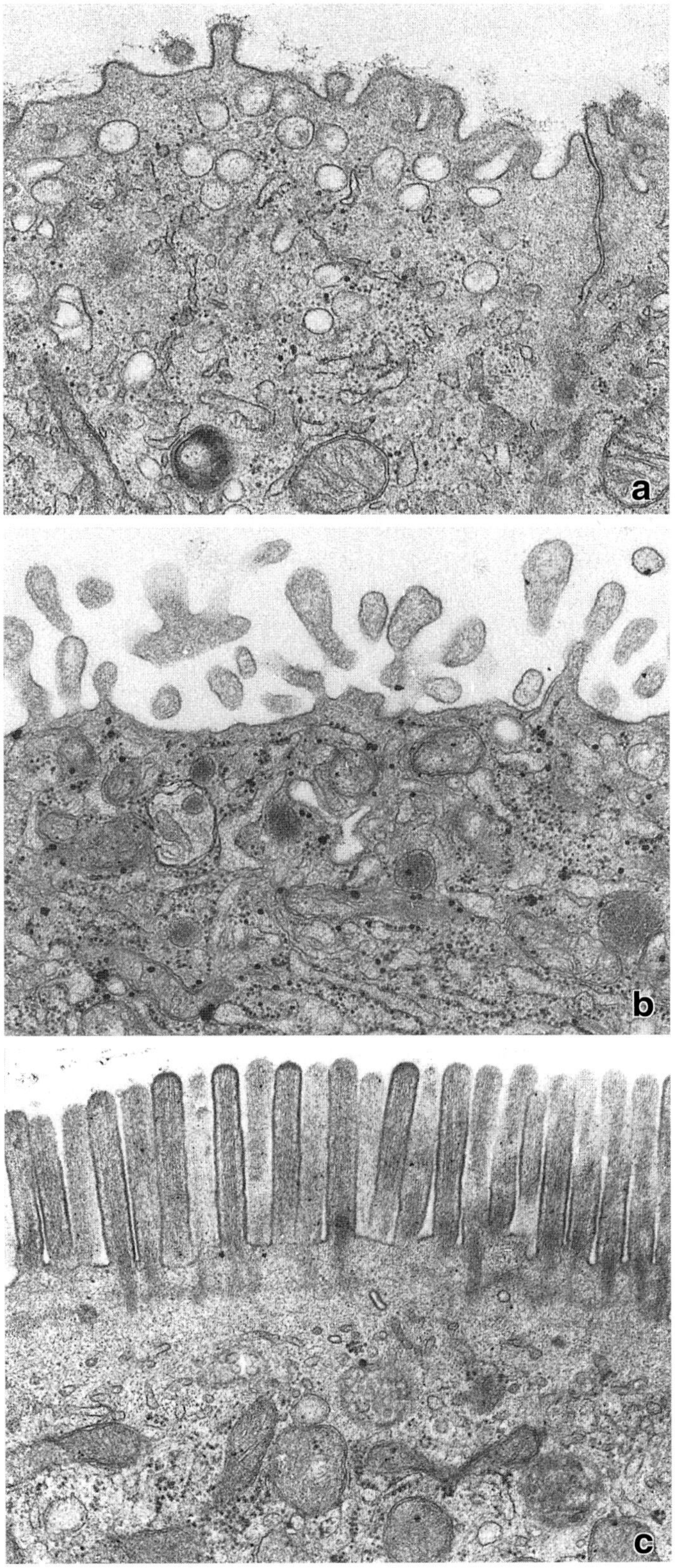

FIGURE 4.2
Electron micrographs showing variation in microvilli of different cell types. a. Epithelial cell of uterine gland; small projections. **b.** Syncytiotrophoblast of placenta; irregular, branching microvilli. **c.** Intestinal absorptive cell; uniform, numerous, and regularly arranged microvilli. All figures ×20,000.

its contractile ability, which could have the effect of decreasing the diameter of the apex of the cell, causing the microvilli, whose stiff actin cores are anchored into the terminal web, to spread apart and increase the intermicrovillous space.

Stereocilia are unusually long, immotile microvilli

Stereocilia are not widely distributed among epithelia. They are, in fact, limited to the epididymis, to the proximal part of the ductus deferens of the male reproductive system, and to the sensory (hair) cells of the ear. They are included in this section because this unusual surface modification is traditionally treated as a separate structural entity.

Stereocilia of the genital ducts are extremely long processes that extend from the apical surface of the cell and facilitate absorption. Unique features include an apical cell protrusion from which they arise and thick stem portions that are interconnected by cytoplasmic bridges. Because electron microscopy reveals their internal structure to be that of unusually long microvilli, some histologists now use the term *stereovilli* (Fig. 4.4a). Seen in the light microscope, these processes frequently resemble the hairs of a paint brush because of the way they aggregate into pointed bundles.

Like microvilli, stereocilia are supported by internal actin filament bundles that are cross-linked by fimbrin. Unlike microvilli, a plasma membrane–associated molecule, ***erzin,*** anchors the actin filaments to the plasma membrane of stereocilia. The stem portion of the stereocilium and the apical cell protrusion contain the cross-bridge–forming molecule ***α-actinin*** (Fig. 4.4b). A striking difference between microvilli and stereocilia, other than size and the presence of erzin, is the absence of villin from the tip of the stereocilium.

Stereocilia of the sensory epithelium of the ear are uniform in diameter and possess an internal structure similar to that of genital duct stereocilia. However, they lack both erzin and α-actinin. These stereocilia serve as sensory receptors rather than absorptive structures.

Cilia are motile cytoplasmic structures capable of moving fluid and particles along epithelial surfaces

Cilia possess an internal structure that provides for their movement. In most ciliated epithelia, such as the trachea, bronchi, or oviducts, cells may have as many as several hundred cilia, all arranged in orderly rows. In the tracheobronchial tree, the cilia sweep mucus and trapped particulate material toward the oropharynx where it is swallowed with saliva and thus eliminated from the body. In the oviducts, cilia help transport ova and fluid toward the uterus.

In some epithelia, only a single cilium per cell may be present, e.g., the epithelial cells of the rete testis in the male reproductive tract and the vestibular hair cells of the ear. In these instances, the single cilium is thought to have a sensory role.

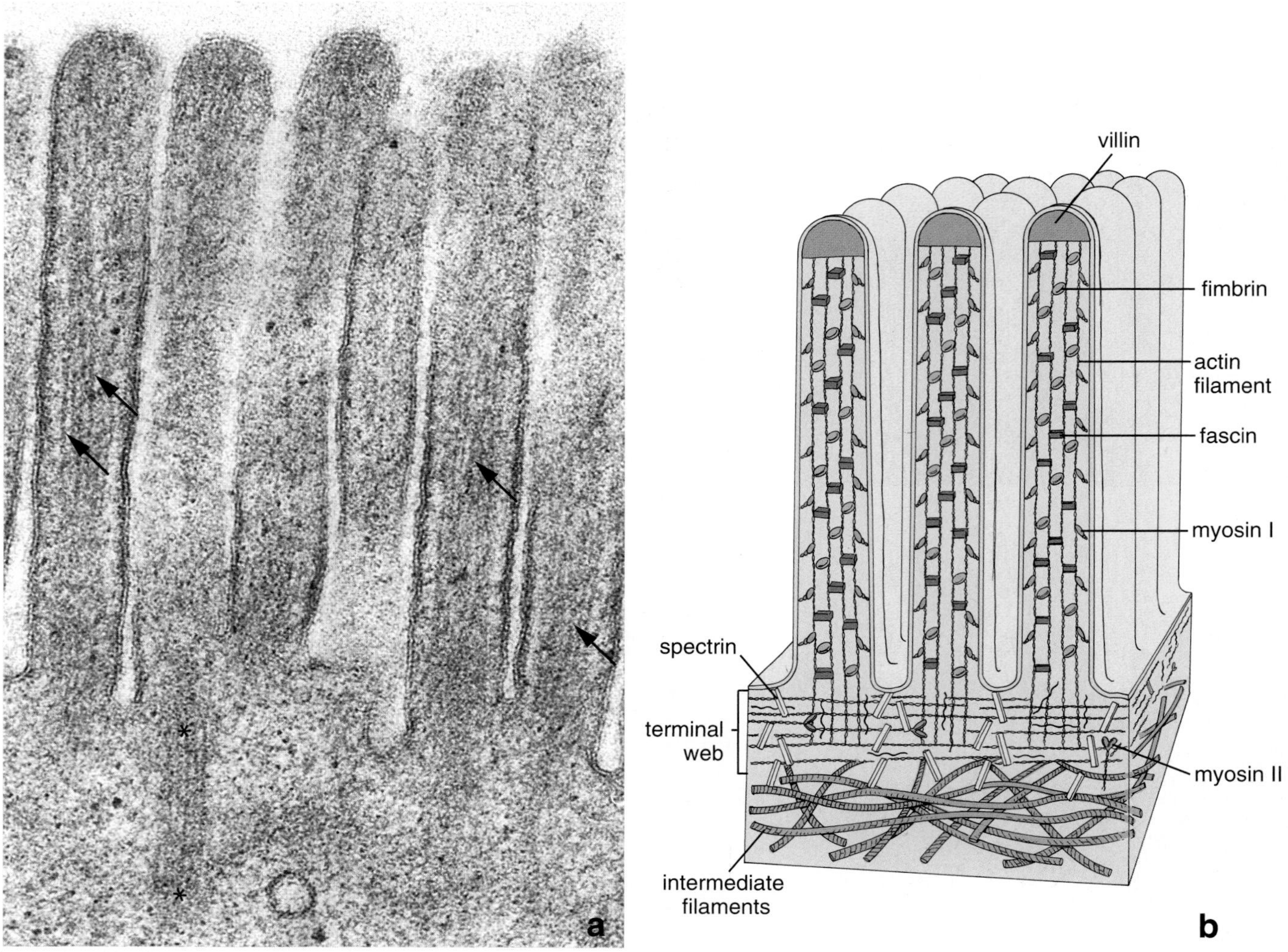

FIGURE 4.3
Molecular structure of microvilli. a. High magnification of microvilli from Figure 4.2c. Note the presence of the actin filaments in the microvilli *(arrows),* which extend into the apical cytoplasm. ×80,000. **b.** Schematic diagram showing molecular structure of microvilli and the location of specific actin filament–bundling proteins. Note the distribution of myosin I within the microvilli and myosin II within the terminal web. The spectrin molecules stabilize the actin filaments within the terminal web and anchor them into the apical plasma membrane.

Cilia give a "crew-cut" appearance to the epithelial surface

In the light microscope, cilia appear as short, fine, hairlike structures emanating from the free surface of the cell (Fig. 4.5). A thin, dark-staining band is usually seen extending across the cell at the base of the cilia. This dark-staining band represents structures known as ***basal bodies.*** These structures take up stain and appear as a continuous band when viewed in the light microscope. When viewed with the EM, however, the basal body of each cilium appears as a distinct individual structure.

Cilia contain an organized core of microtubules arranged in a 9 + 2 pattern

Electron microscopy of a cilium in longitudinal profile reveals an internal core of microtubules (Fig. 4.6a). A cross-sectional view reveals a characteristic configuration of nine pairs or doublets of circularly arranged microtubules surrounding two central microtubules (Fig. 4.6b).

The microtubules composing each doublet are constructed so that the wall of one microtubule, designated the ***B microtubule,*** is actually incomplete; it shares a portion of the wall of the other microtubule of the doublet, the ***A microtubule.*** The A microtubule is composed of 13 tubulin dimers, arranged in side-by-side configuration, whereas the B microtubule is composed of 10 tubulin dimers. When seen in cross section at high resolution, each doublet exhibits a pair of "arms" that contain ***ciliary dynein,*** a microtubule-associated motor protein. This motor protein uses the energy of adenosine triphosphate (ATP) hydrolysis to move along the surface of the adjacent microtubule (see Fig. 4.6b). The dynein arms occur at 24-nm intervals along the length of the A microtubule and extend out to form temporary

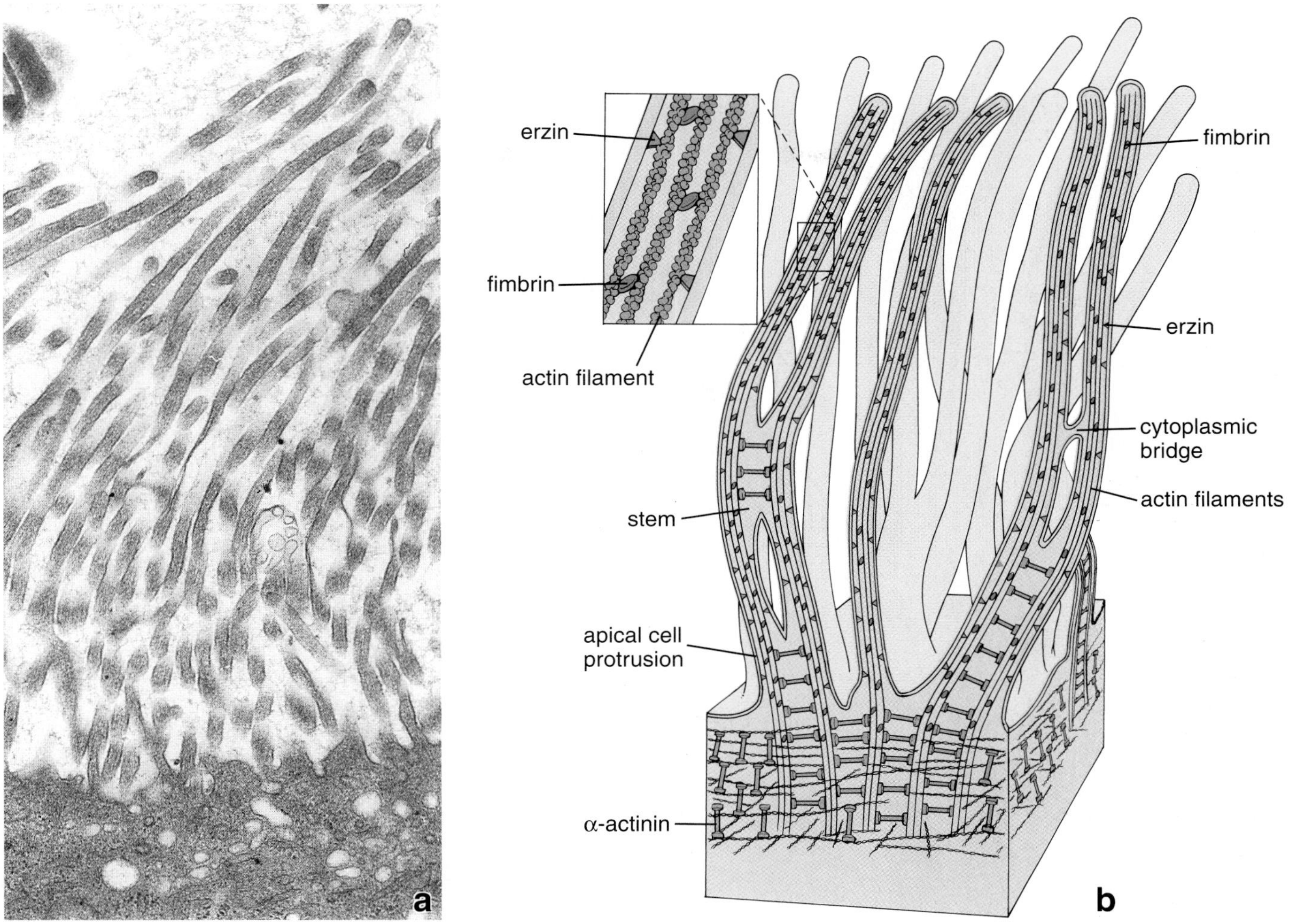

FIGURE 4.4

Molecular structure of stereocilia. a. Electron micrograph of stereocilia from the epididymis. The cytoplasmic projections are similar to microvilli, but they are extremely long. ×20,000. **b.** Schematic diagram showing the molecular structure of stereocilia. They arise from the apical cell protrusions, having thick stem portions that are interconnected by cytoplasmic bridges. Note the distribution of actin filaments within the core of the stereocilium and the actin-associated proteins: fimbrin and erzin in the elongated portion *(enlarged box)*, and α-actinin in the terminal web and apical cell protrusion.

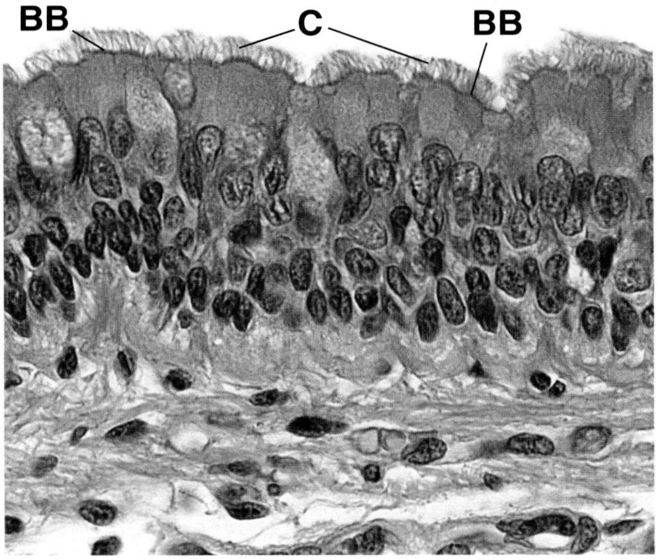

FIGURE 4.5

Ciliated epithelium. Photomicrograph of a H&E–stained specimen of tracheal pseudostratified ciliated epithelium. The cilia *(C)* appear as hair-like processes extending from the apical surface of the cells. The dark line immediately below the ciliary processes is produced by the basal bodies *(BB)* associated with the cilia. ×750.

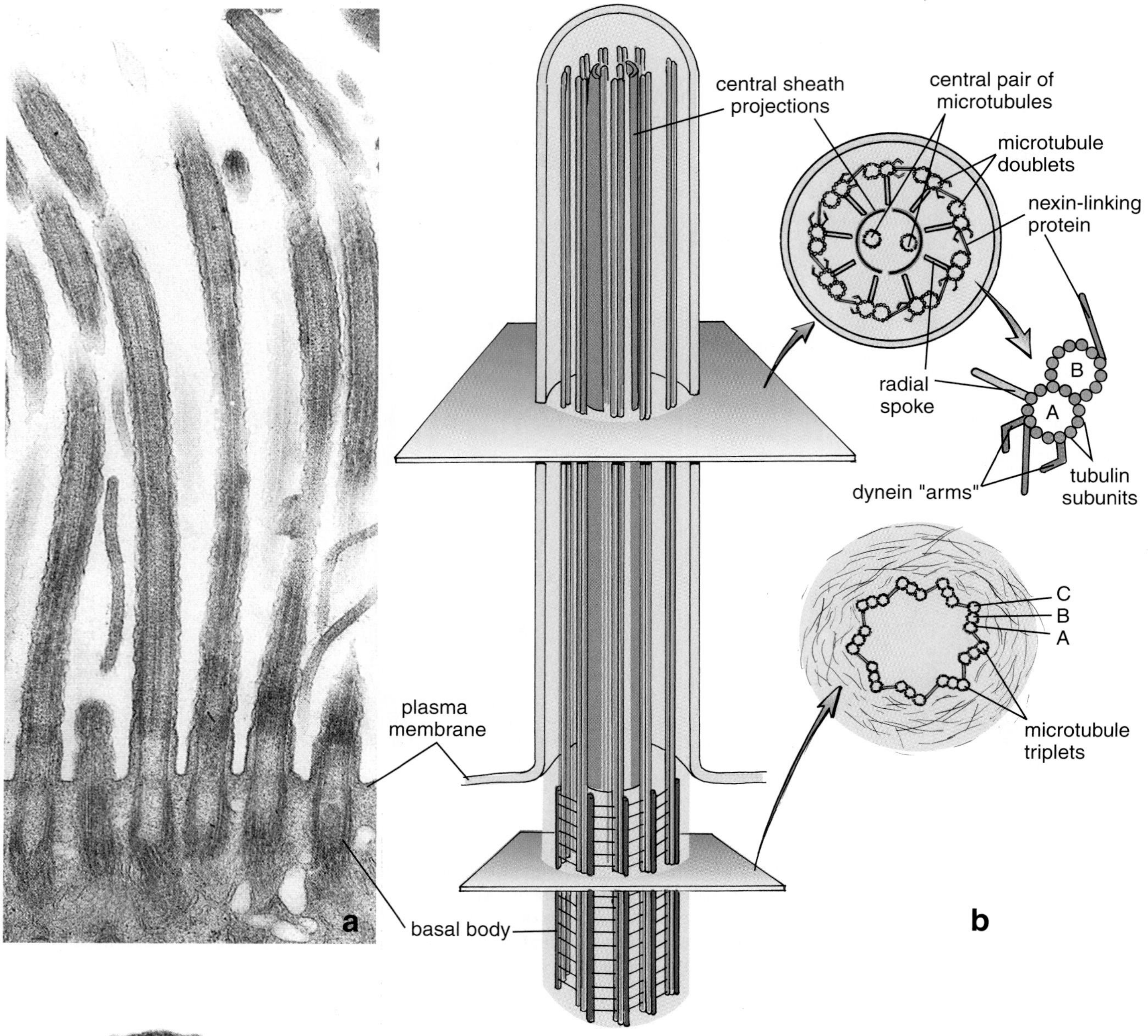

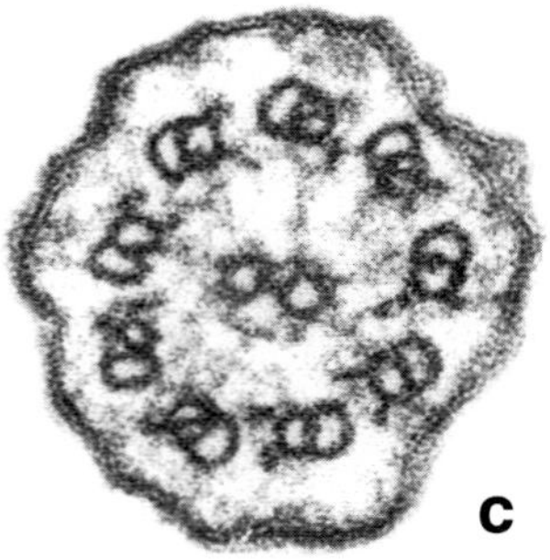

FIGURE 4.6

Molecular structure of cilia. a. Electron micrograph of longitudinally sectioned cilia from the oviduct. The internal structures within the ciliary process are microtubules. Most of the basal bodies appear "empty" because of the absence of the central pair of microtubules in this portion of the cilium. One basal body *(second from left)* has been sectioned peripherally through the outer microtubule triplet. ×20,000. **b.** Schematic diagram of cilium, showing its cross section *(upper plane)* with the pair of central microtubules and the nine surrounding microtubule doublets. The dynein arms extend from the A microtubule and make temporary cross-bridges with the B microtubule of the adjacent doublet. **Inset.** Compare the diagram with the cross section in the electron micrograph *(**c**)* and identify corresponding structures. ×180,000. The molecular structure of the microtubule doublet is shown adjacent to the cross section. Note that the A microtubule of the doublet is composed of 13 tubulin dimers arranged in a side-by-side configuration, whereas the B microtubule is composed of 10 tubulin dimers and shares the remaining dimers with those of the A microtubule. The cross section of the basal body *(lower plane)* shows the arrangement of nine microtubule triplets. These structures form a ring structure. Each microtubule doublet of the cilium is an extension of two inner microtubules of the corresponding triplet.

cross-bridges with the B microtubule of the adjacent doublet. A passive elastic component formed by **nexin** permanently links the A microtubule with the B microtubule of adjacent doublets at 86-nm intervals. The two central microtubules are separate but are partially enclosed by a central sheath projection at 14-nm intervals along the length of the cilium. Radial spokes extend from each of the nine doublets toward the two central microtubules at 29-nm intervals. The proteins forming the radial spokes and the nexin connections between the outer doublets make large-amplitude oscillations of the cilia possible.

The 9 + 2 microtubule array courses from the tip of the cilium to its base, where the outer paired microtubules join the basal body. The basal body is a modified centriole consisting of nine short microtubule triplets arranged in a ring. Each of the paired microtubules of the cilium is continuous with two of the triplet microtubules of the basal body. The two central microtubules of the cilium end at the level of the top of the basal body. Therefore, a cross section of the basal body would reveal nine circularly arranged microtubule triplets but not the two central single microtubules of the cilium.

Cilia develop from procentrioles

The process of ciliary formation in differentiating cells involves the replication of the centriole to give rise to multiple ***procentrioles,*** one for each cilium. The procentrioles grow and migrate to the apical surface of the cell, where each becomes a basal body. From each of the nine triplets that make up the basal body, a microtubule doublet grows upward, creating a projection of the apical membrane containing the nine doublets found in the mature cilium. Simultaneously, the two single central microtubules form within the ring of doublet microtubules, thus yielding the characteristic 9 + 2 arrangement.

Cilia beat in a synchronous pattern

Cilia display a regular and synchronous undulating movement. A cilium remains rigid as it exhibits a rapid forward movement called the ***effective stroke;*** it becomes flexible and bends on the slower return movement, the ***recovery stroke.*** The plane of movement of a cilium is perpendicular to a line joining the central pair of microtubules. Cilia in successive rows start their beat so that each row is slightly more advanced in its cycle than the following row, thus creating a wave that sweeps across the epithelium. This ***metachronal rhythm*** is responsible for moving mucus over epithelial surfaces or facilitating the flow of fluid and other substances through tubular organs and ducts.

Ciliary activity is based on the movement of the doublet microtubules in relation to one another. Ciliary movement is initiated by the dynein arms (see Fig. 4.6b). The ciliary dynein located in the arms of the A microtubule forms temporary cross-bridges with the B microtubule of the adjacent doublet. Hydrolysis of ATP produces a sliding movement of the bridge along the B microtubule. The dynein molecules produce a continuous

BOX 4.1

Clinical Correlations: Immotile Cilia Syndrome

Cilia play a significant role in the human body. The mucociliary transport that occurs in the respiratory epithelium is one of the important mechanisms protecting the body against invading bacteria and other pathogens. Failure of the mucociliary transport system is caused by several hereditary disorders grouped under the general name of immotile cilia syndrome. ***Kartagener's syndrome,*** for instance, is caused by a structural abnormality involving absence of dynein arms (see electron micrograph at right). ***Young's syndrome*** is characterized by malformation of the radial spokes and the dynein arms. The most prominent symptom of immotile cilia syndrome is chronic respiratory difficulty (including bronchitis and sinusitis), although ***situs inversus*** of the viscera is also common. Respiratory problems are caused by severely impaired or absent ciliary motility that results in reduced or absent mucociliary transport in the tracheobronchial tree. The transposition of the viscera may be related to the lack of ciliary activity during the developmental process. Another possibility is that microtubules that designate a form of polarity within cells may also indirectly influence the polarity of organ systems. It may also result from abnormal microtubular structure. Males with Kartagener's syndrome are sterile. The flagellum of the sperm, which is similar in structure to the cilium, is immotile. In contrast, some females with the syndrome may be fertile. In such individuals, the ciliary movement may be sufficient, though impaired, to permit transport of the ovum through the oviduct. (Photomicrograph courtesy of Patrice Abell-Aleff. ×180,000.)

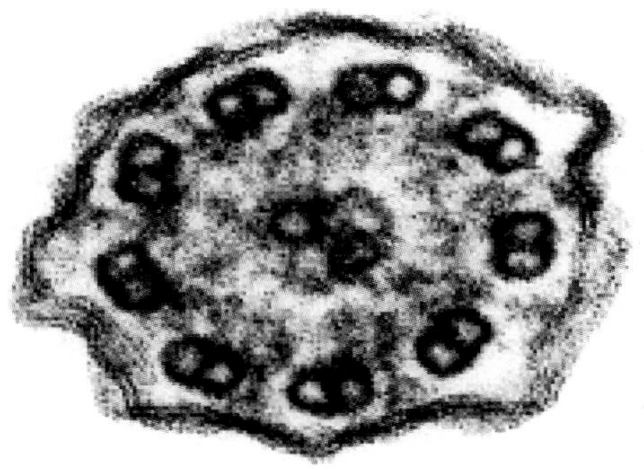

shear force during this interdoublet sliding directed toward the ciliary tip. As a result of this ATP-dependent phase of the effective stroke, the cilium bends. At the same time, the passive elastic connections provided by nexin and the radial spokes accumulate the energy necessary to bring the cilium back to the straight position, thus producing the recovery stroke.

However, if all dynein arms along the length of the A microtubules in all nine doublets attempted to form temporary cross-bridges simultaneously, no effective stroke of the cilium would result. Thus, regulation of the active shear force is required. Current evidence suggests that the central pair of microtubules undergo rotation with respect to the nine outer doublets. This rotation may be driven by another motor protein, kinesin, which is associated with the central pair of microtubules. The central microtubule pair can act as a "distributor" that regulates the sequence of interactions of the dynein arms in a progressive manner to produce the effective stroke.

THE LATERAL DOMAIN AND ITS SPECIALIZATIONS IN CELL-TO-CELL ADHESION

The lateral domain of epithelial cells is in close contact with the opposed lateral domains of neighboring cells. Like the other domains, the lateral domain is characterized by the presence of unique proteins, in this case the adhesion molecules that are part of junctional specializations. The molecular composition of the lipids and proteins that form the lateral cell membrane differ significantly from the composition of those that form the apical cell membrane. In addition, the lateral cell surface membrane in some epithelia may form folds and processes, invaginations and evaginations that create interdigitating and interleaving tongue-and-groove margins between neighboring cells.

Terminal bars represent epithelial cell attachment sites

Before the advent of electron microscopy, the close apposition of epithelial cells was attributed to the presence of a viscous adhesive substance referred to as "intercellular cement." This cement stained deeply at the apicolateral margin of most cuboidal and columnar epithelial cells. When viewed in a plane perpendicular to the epithelial surface, the stained material appears as a dot-like structure. When the plane of section passes parallel to and includes the epithelial surface, however, the dot-like component is seen as a dense bar or line between the apposing cells (Fig. 4.7). The bars, in fact, form a polygonal structure (or band) at the periphery of each cell.

Because of its location in the terminal or apical portion of the cell and its bar-like configuration, the stainable material visible in light microscopy was called the ***terminal bar.*** It is now evident that intercellular cement as such does not exist. The terminal bar, however, does represent a significant structural complex. Electron microscopy has shown it includes a specialized site that joins epithelial cells (Fig. 4.8a). It is also the site of a barrier to the passage (diffusion) of substances across the epithelium. The specific structural components that make up the barrier and the attachment device are readily identified with the EM and are collectively referred to as a ***junctional complex*** (see Table 4.4). These complexes are responsible for joining individual cells together and contain three types of junctions (Fig. 4.8b):

- ***Occluding junctions,*** as a result of their impermeable nature, allow epithelial cells to function as a barrier. Also called ***tight junctions,*** occluding junctions form the intercellular diffusion barrier between adjacent cells; by limiting the movement of water and other molecules through the intercellular space, they maintain physicochemical separation of tissue compartments. Because they are located at the most apical point between adjoining epithelial cells, occluding junctions prevent the migration of specialized membrane proteins between the apical and lateral surfaces, thus maintaining the integrity of these two domains.
- ***Anchoring junctions*** provide mechanical stability to epithelial cells by linking the cytoskeleton of one cell to the cytoskeleton of an adjacent cell. These junctions are important in creating and maintaining the structural unity of the epithelium. Anchoring junctions interact with both actin and intermediate filaments and can be found not only on the lateral cell surface but also on the basal domain of the epithelial cell.
- ***Communicating junctions*** allow direct communication between adjacent cells by diffusion of small (<1000 Da)

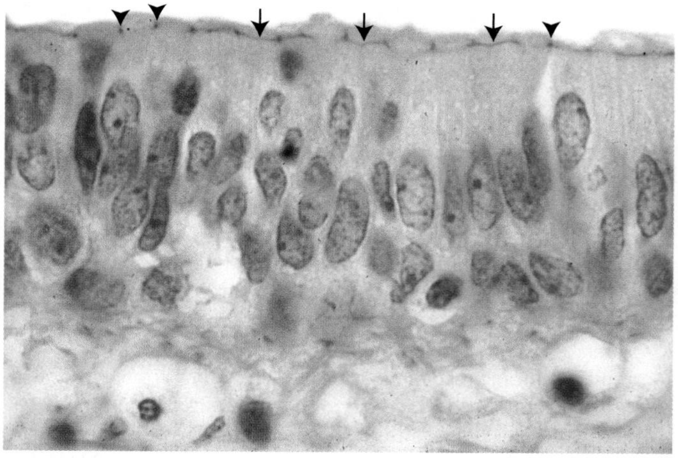

FIGURE 4.7
Terminal bars in pseudostratified epithelium. Photomicrograph of a H&E–stained specimen, showing the terminal bars in a pseudostratified epithelium. The bar appears as a dot *(arrowheads)* when seen on its cut edge. When the bar is coursing parallel to the cut surface and lying within the thickness of the section, it is seen as a linear or bar-like profile *(arrows).* ×550.

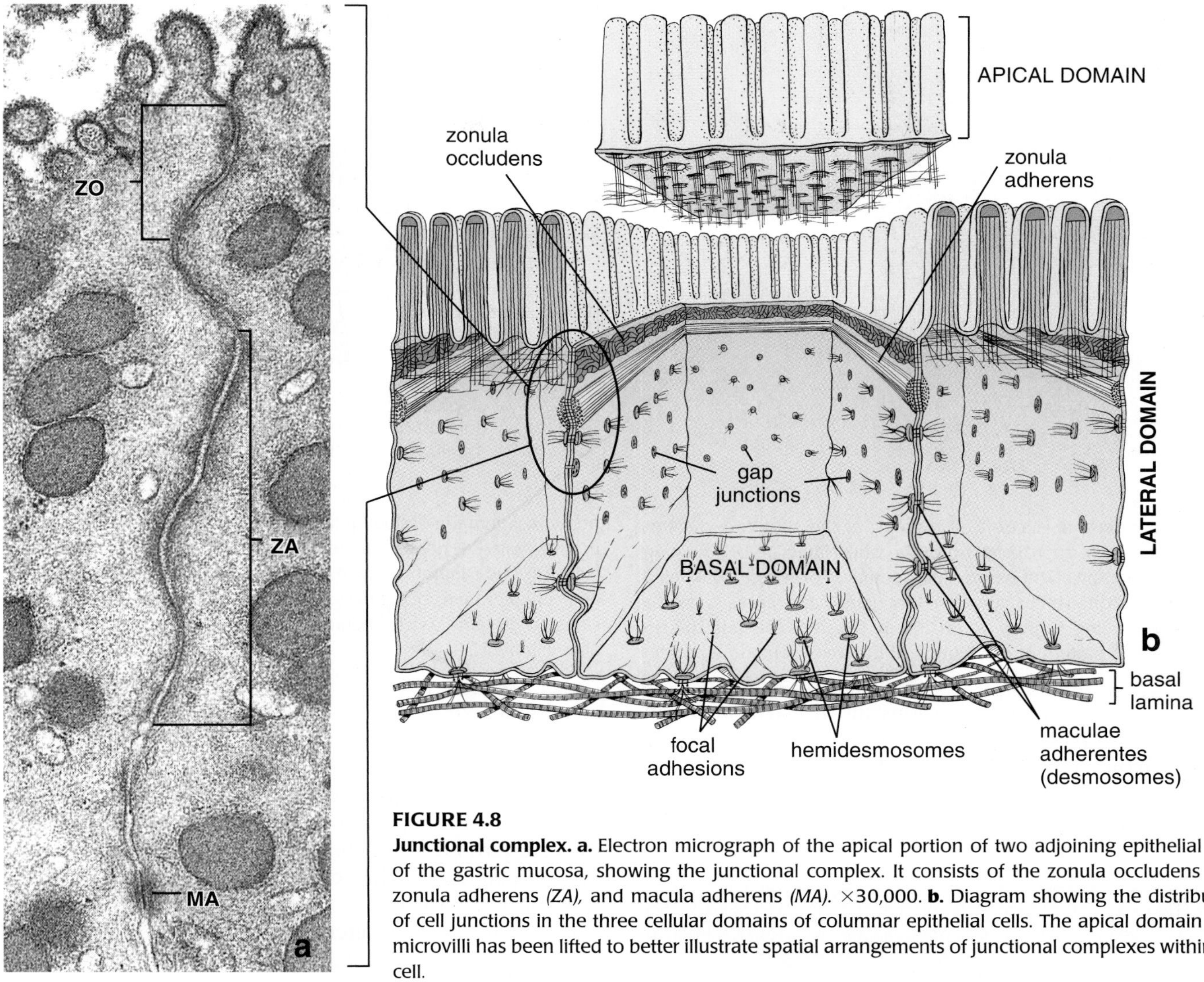

FIGURE 4.8
Junctional complex. a. Electron micrograph of the apical portion of two adjoining epithelial cells of the gastric mucosa, showing the junctional complex. It consists of the zonula occludens *(ZO)*, zonula adherens *(ZA)*, and macula adherens *(MA)*. ×30,000. **b.** Diagram showing the distribution of cell junctions in the three cellular domains of columnar epithelial cells. The apical domain with microvilli has been lifted to better illustrate spatial arrangements of junctional complexes within the cell.

molecules (e.g., ions, amino acids, second messengers, metabolites). This type of intercellular communication permits the coordinated cellular activity that is important for maintaining organ homeostasis.

Occluding Junctions

The ***zonula occludens*** (pl., ***zonulae occludentes***) represents the most apical component in the junctional complex between epithelial cells.

The zonula occludens is created by localized sealing of adjacent plasma membranes

Examination of the zonula occludens or tight junction with the transmission electron microscope (TEM) reveals a narrow region in which the plasma membranes of adjoining cells come in close contact to seal off the intercellular space (Fig. 4.9a). The high-resolution TEM similarly reveals that the zonula occludens is not a continuous seal but rather a series of focal fusions between the cells. These focal fusions are created by specific transmembrane proteins of adjoining cells that traverse the cell membrane and join in the intercellular space. The transmembrane protein **occludin** has been identified as the sealing protein. The cytoplasmic portion of occludin is associated with the ***zonula occludens proteins ZO-1, ZO-2,*** and ***ZO-3*** (Fig. 4.9b,c). Occludin interacts with the actin cytoskeleton through ZO-1. Regulatory functions during the formation of the zonula occludens have been suggested for all ZO proteins. In addition, ZO-1 is a tumor suppressor, and ZO-2 is required in the epidermal growth factor–receptor signaling mechanism. The ZO-3 protein interacts with ZO-1 and the cytoplasmic domain of occludin. Many pathogenic agents, such as cytomegalovirus (CMV) and cholera toxins, act on ZO-1 and ZO-2, causing the junction to become permeable.

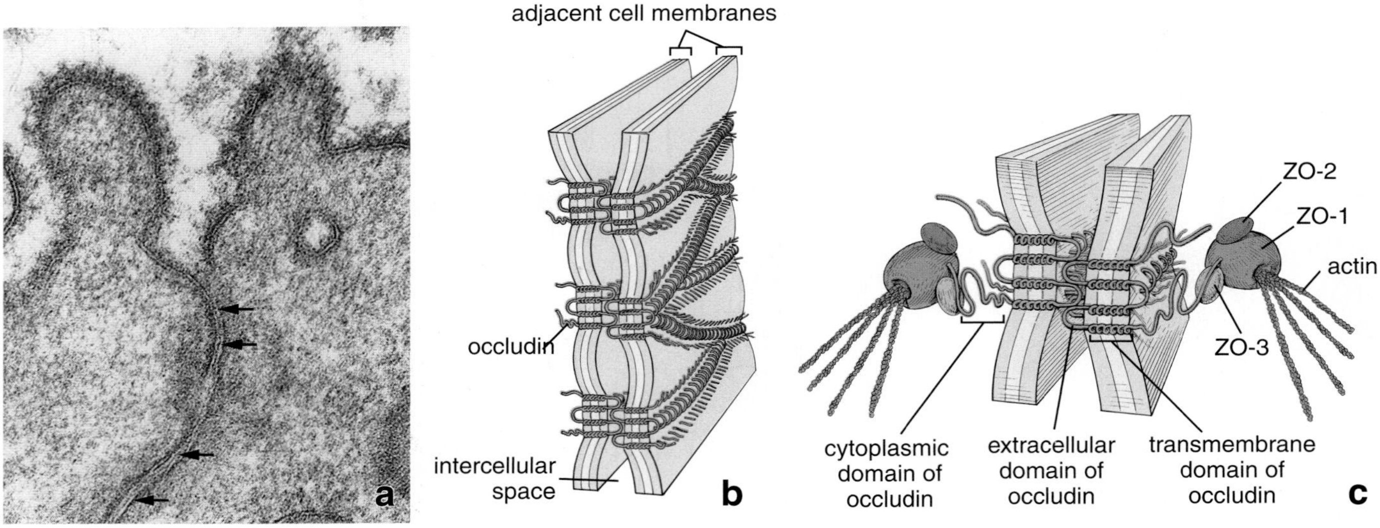

FIGURE 4.9
Zonula occludens. a. Electron micrograph of the zonula occludens, showing the close approximation of the outer lamellae of adjoining plasma membranes. The extracellular domains of proteins involved in the formation of this junction (occludins) appear as a single electron-dense line *(arrows)*. ×100,000. **b.** Diagram showing the organization and pattern of distribution of the transmembrane protein occludin within the occluding junction. Compare the linear pattern of grooves with the ridges detected in the freeze-fracture preparation in Figure 4.10. **c.** Diagram showing the occludin molecule and the major associated proteins of the occluding junction. Note that one of the associated proteins, ZO-1, interacts with the cell cytoskeleton binding actin filaments.

The arrangement of the various junctional proteins in forming the zona occludens seal is best visualized by the freeze fracture technique (Fig. 4.10). When the plasma membrane is fractured at the site of the zonula occludens, the junctional proteins are observed on the P-face of the membrane, where they appear as ridge-like structures. The opposing surface of the fractured membrane, the E-face, reveals complementary grooves that result from detachment of the protein particles from the opposing surface. The ridges and grooves are arranged as a network of anastomosing strands, thus creating a functional seal within the intercellular space. They correspond to the location of the rows of transmembrane proteins.

Observations of different kinds of epithelia reveal that the complexity and number of strands forming the zonulae occludentes varies. In epithelia in which anastomosing strands or fusion sites are sparse, such as certain kidney tubules, the intercellular pathway is partially permeable to water and solutes. In contrast, in epithelia in which the strands are numerous and extensively intertwined, e.g., in-

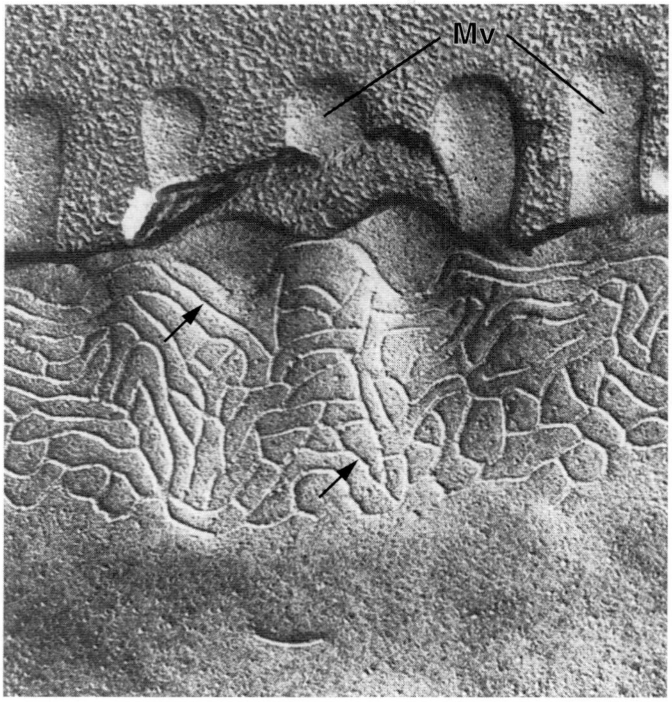

FIGURE 4.10
Freeze fracture preparation of zonula occludens. The fracture membrane surface shown here reveals an anastomosing network of ridges *(arrows)* located near the apical surface of the cell (note microvilli *(Mv)* present at the cell surface). This is the P-face of the membrane. (The E-face of the fractured membrane would show a complementary pattern of grooves.) The ridges represent linear arrays of transmembrane proteins (most likely occludins) involved in the formation of the zonula occludens. The membrane of the opposing cell contains a similar network of proteins, which is in register with the first cell. The actual sites of protein interaction between the cells form the anastomosing network. ×100,000. (From Hull BE, Staehelin LA. *J Cell Biol* 1976; 68:688–704.)

testinal and urinary bladder epithelia, the intercellular region is highly impermeable.

The zonula occludens separates the luminal space from the intercellular space and connective tissue compartment

It is now evident that the zonula occludens plays an essential role in the selective passage of substances from one side of an epithelium to the other. Because the diffusion of water and solutes between cells is restricted by the zonula occludens, transport must occur by active means. Active transport requires specialized membrane transport proteins that move selected substances across the apical plasma membrane into the cytoplasm and then across the lateral membrane below the level of the junction.

The zonula occludens establishes functional domains in the plasma membrane

As a junction, the zonula occludens restricts not only the passage of water, electrolytes, and other small molecules across the epithelial layer but also the diffusion of molecules within the plasma membrane itself. Thus, the cell is able to segregate certain internal membrane proteins on the apical (free) surface and restrict others to the lateral or basal surfaces. In the intestine, for instance, the enzymes for terminal digestion of peptides and saccharides (dipeptidases and disaccharidases) are localized in the membrane of the microvilli of the apical surface. The Na^+/K^+-ATPase that drives salt and water transport, as well as amino acid and sugar transport, is restricted to the lateral plasma membrane below the zonula occludens.

Anchoring Junctions

Anchoring junctions provide lateral adhesions between epithelial cells, using proteins that link into the cytoskeleton of the adjacent cells. Two types of anchoring cell-to-cell junctions can be identified on the lateral cell surface:

- ***Zonula adherens*** (pl., ***zonulae adherentes***), which interacts with the network of actin filaments inside the cell
- ***Macula adherens*** (pl., ***maculae adherentes***) or ***desmosome,*** which interacts with intermediate filaments

In addition, two other types of anchoring junctions can be found where epithelial cells rest on the connective tissue matrix. These ***focal adhesions*** (focal contacts) and ***hemidesmosomes*** are discussed in the section on the basal domain (see pages 109 to 111).

The zonula adherens provides lateral adhesion between epithelial cells

The integrity of epithelial surfaces depends in large part on the lateral adhesion of the cells with one another and their ability to resist separation. Although the zonula occludens involves a fusion of adjoining cell membranes, their resistance to mechanical stress is limited. Reinforcement of this region depends on a strong bonding site below the zonula occludens. Like the zonula occludens, this lateral adhesion device occurs in a continuous band or belt-like configuration around the cell; thus, the adhering junction is referred to as a **zonula adherens.** The zonula adherens is composed of the transmembrane adhesion molecule ***E-cadherin.*** On the cytoplasmic side, the tail of E-cadherin is bound to ***catenin*** (Fig. 4.11a). The resulting ***cadherin–catenin complex*** binds to ***vinculin*** and α-actinin and is required for the interaction of cadherins with the actin filaments of cytoskeleton. The extracellular components of the E-cadherin molecules from adjacent cells are linked by Ca^{2+} ions or an additional extracellular link protein. Therefore, the morphologic and functional integrity of the zonula adherens is calcium dependent. Removal of Ca^{2+} leads to dissociation of E-cadherin molecules and disruption of the junction.

When examined with the TEM, the zonula adherens is characterized by a uniform 15- to 20-nm space between the opposing cell membranes (Fig. 4.11b). The intercellular space is of low electron density, appearing almost clear, but it is evidently occupied by extracellular components of adjacent E-cadherin molecules and Ca^{2+} ions. Within the confines of the zonula adherens, a moderately electron-dense material called ***fuzzy plaque*** is found along the cytoplasmic side of the membrane of each cell. This material corresponds to the location of the cytoplasmic component of the E-cadherin–catenin complex and the associated proteins (α-actinin and vinculin) into which actin filaments attach. Evidence also suggests that the fuzzy plaque represents the stainable substance in light microscopy, the terminal bar. Associated with the electron-dense material is an array of 6-nm actin filaments that stretch across the apical cytoplasm of the epithelial cell, the terminal web.

The fascia adherens is a sheet-like junction that stabilizes nonepithelial tissues

Physical attachments that occur between cells in tissues other than epithelia are usually not prominent, but there is at least one notable exception. Cardiac muscle cells are arranged end to end, forming thread-like contractile units. The cells are attached to each other by a combination of typical desmosomes, or maculae adherentes, and broad adhesion plates that morphologically resemble the zonula adherens of epithelial cells. Because the attachment is not ring-like but rather has a broad face, it is called the ***fascia adherens*** (Fig. 4.12). At the molecular level, the structure of the fascia adherens is similar to that of the zonula adherens; it also contains the zonula occludens ZO-1 protein found in the tight junctions of epithelial cells.

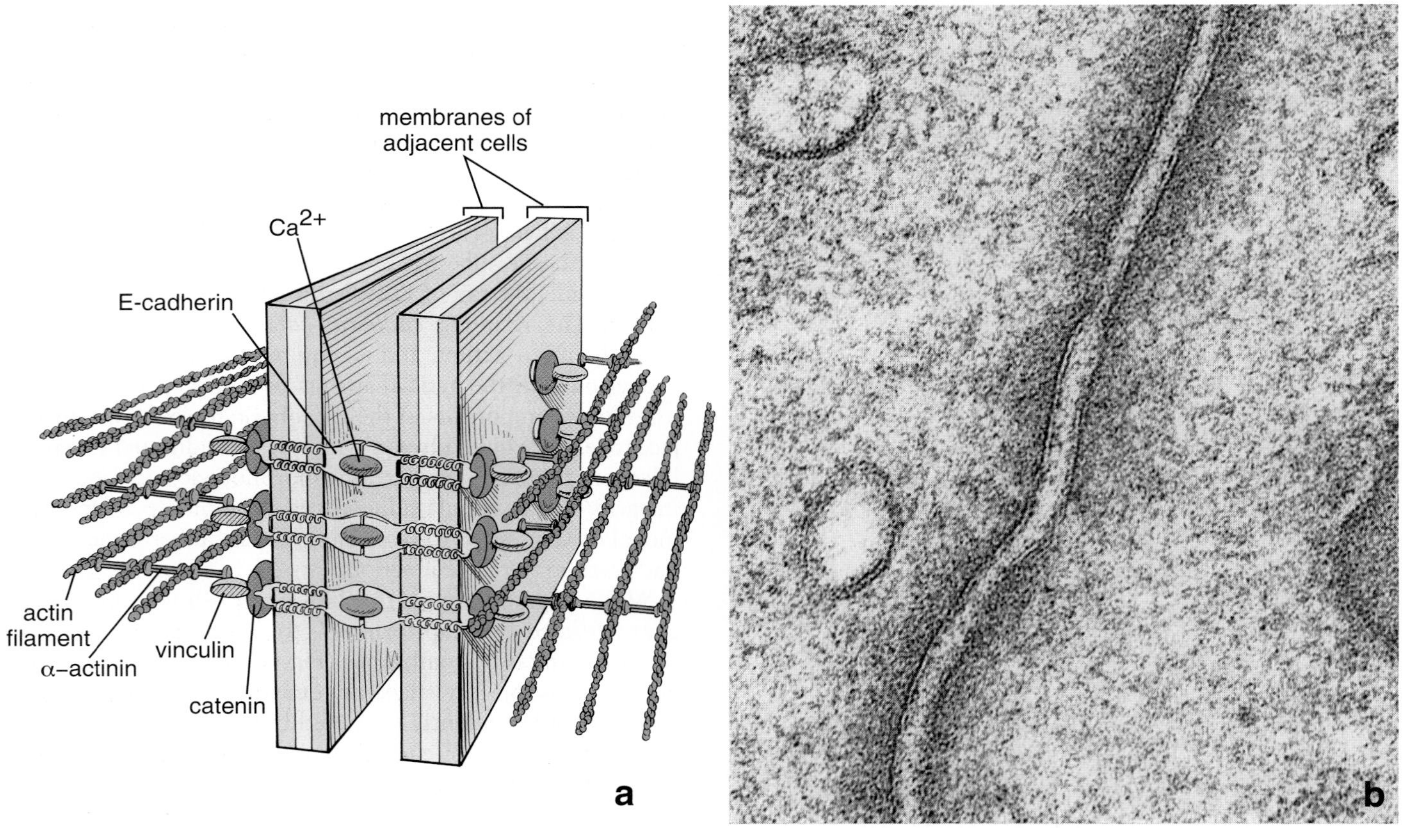

FIGURE 4.11
Zonula adherens. a. Diagram showing molecular organization of zonula adherens. Actin filaments of adjacent cells are attached to the E-cadherin–catenin complex by α-actinin and vinculin. The E cadherin–catenin complex interacts with identical molecules embedded in the plasma membrane of the adjacent cell. Interactions between transmembrane proteins are mediated by calcium ions. **b.** Electron micrograph of the zonula adherens from Figure 4.8a at higher magnification. The plasma membranes are separated here by a relatively uniform intercellular space. This space appears clear, showing only a sparse amount of diffuse electron-dense substance, which represents extracellular domains of E-cadherin. The cytoplasmic side of the plasma membrane exhibits a moderately electron-dense material containing actin filaments. ×100,000.

The macula adherens (desmosome) provides localized spot-like adhesion between epithelial cells

The ***macula adherens*** is an anchoring cell-to-cell junction that provides a particularly strong attachment, as shown by microdissection studies. These junctions are localized on the lateral domain of the cell, much like a series of spot welds (see Fig. 4.8a). The macula adherens was originally described in epidermal cells and called a ***desmosome*** *[Gr. desmo, bond + soma, body]*. The name is often used interchangeably with macula adherens *[L. macula, spot]*. In epidermal cells, the macula adherens is the only attachment device present. In other epithelia, particularly those with cuboidal or columnar cells, the macula adherens is found in conjunction with a zonula adherens. The macula adherens occupies small, localized sites on the lateral cell surface, however; it is not a continuous structure around the cell, as is the zonula adherens. Thus, a section perpendicular to the surface of a cell that cuts through the entire lateral surface will often not include a macula adherens. The section will always, however, include the zonula adherens.

Electron microscopy reveals that the macula adherens has a complex structure. On the cytoplasmic side of the plasma membrane of each of the adjoining cells is a disk-shaped structure consisting of very dense material called the desmosomal ***attachment plaque.*** This structure measures about 400 × 250 × 10 nm and anchors intermediate filaments (Fig. 4.13a). The filaments appear to loop through the attachment plaques and extend back out into the cytoplasm. They are thought to play a role in dissipating physical forces throughout the cell from the attachment site. At the molecular level, each attachment plaque is composed of several constitutive proteins, mainly ***desmoplakins*** and ***plakoglobins,*** which are capable of anchoring the intermediate filaments (Fig. 4.13b).

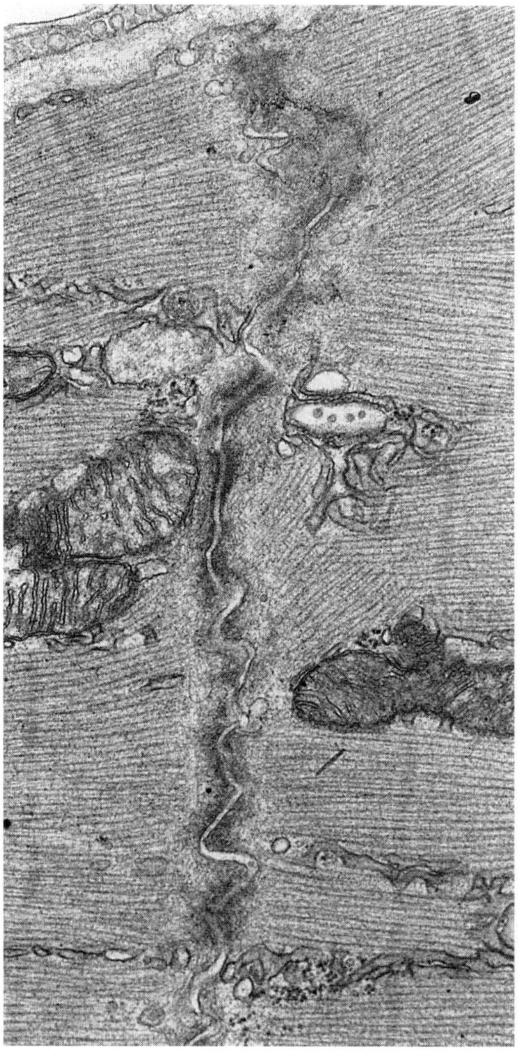

FIGURE 4.12
Fascia adherens. Electron micrograph showing the end-to-end apposition of two cardiac muscle cells. The intercellular space appears as a clear undulating area. On the cytoplasmic side of the plasma membrane of each cell, there is a dense material similar to that seen in a zonula adherens containing actin filaments. Because the attachment site here involves a portion of the end face of the two cells, it is called a fascia adherens. ×38,000.

The intercellular space of the macula adherens is conspicuously wider (up to 30 nm) than that of the zonula adherens and is occupied by a dense medial band, the ***intermediate line.*** This line represents extracellular portions of transmembrane glycoproteins, the ***desmogleins*** and ***desmocollins,*** which are members of the cadherin family of Ca^{2+}-dependent cell adhesion molecules. In the presence of Ca^{2+}, extracellular portions of desmogleins and desmocollins bind adjacent identical molecules of neighboring cells. X-ray crystallographic studies suggest that the extracellular binding domain of proteins from one cell interacts with two adjacent cadherin domains in an antiparallel orientation, thus forming a continuous ***cadherin zipper*** in the area of the desmosome (see Fig. 4.13b). The cytoplasmic portions of desmogleins and desmocollins are integral components of the desmosomal attachment plaque. They interact with the placoglobins and desmoplakins that are involved in desmosome assembly and the anchoring of intermediate filaments.

The cells of different epithelia require different types of attachments

In epithelia that serve as physiologic barriers, the junctional complex is particularly significant because it serves to create a long-term barrier, allowing the cells to compartmentalize and restrict the free passage of substances across the epithelium. Although it is the zonula occludens of the junctional complex that principally effects this function, it is the adhesive properties of the zonulae and maculae adherens that guard against physical disruption of the barrier. In other epithelia, there is need for substantially stronger attachment between cells in several planes. In the stratified epithelial cells of the epidermis, for example, numerous maculae adherentes maintain adhesion between adjacent cells. In cardiac muscle, where there is a similar need for strong adhesion, a combination of the macula adherens and the fascia adherens serves this function.

Communicating Junctions

Communicating junctions, also called ***gap junctions*** or ***nexus,*** are present in a wide variety of tissues, including epithelia, smooth and cardiac muscle, and nerves. They are important in tissues in which activity of adjacent cells must be coordinated, such as epithelia engaged in fluid and electrolyte transport, vascular and intestinal smooth muscle, and heart muscle. A gap junction consists of an accumulation of transmembrane channels or pores in a tightly packed array. The pores in one cell membrane are precisely aligned with corresponding pores on the membrane of an adjacent cell, thus, as the name implies, allowing communication between the cells. The gap junctions allow cells to exchange ions, regulatory molecules, and small metabolites through the pores. The number of pores in a gap junction can vary widely, as can the number of gap junctions between adjacent cells.

Organized concentrations of integral membrane proteins form the gap junctions

Various procedures have been used to study gap junctions, including the injection of dyes, radiolabeled compounds, or electric current into cells and the measurement of these probes in adjacent cells. In dye studies, a

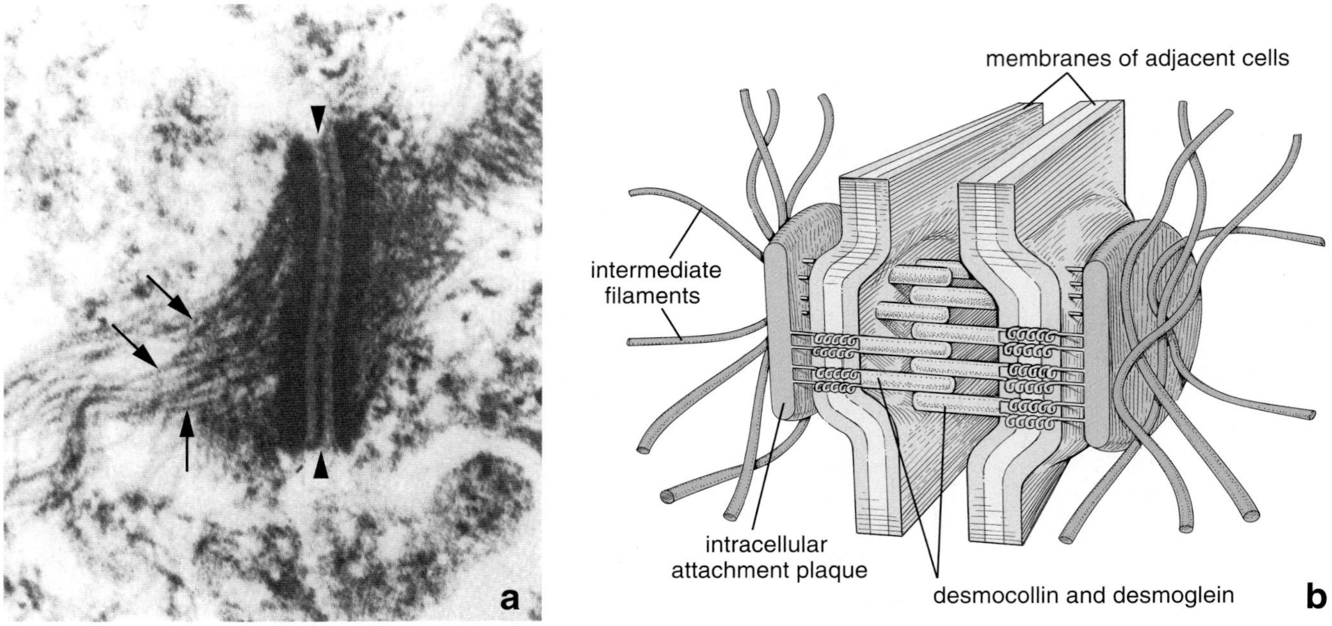

FIGURE 4.13
Molecular structure of the macula adherens (desmosome). a. Electron micrograph of a macula adherens, showing the intermediate filaments *(arrows)* attaching into a dense intracellular attachment plaque located on the cytoplasmic side of the plasma membrane. The intercellular space is also occupied by electron-dense material *(arrowheads)* containing desmocollins and desmogleins. The intercellular space above and below the macula adherens is not well defined because of extraction of the plasma membrane to show components of this structure. ×40,000. (Courtesy of Dr. Ernst Kallenbach.) **b.** Schematic diagram showing the structure of a macula adherens. Note the intracellular attachment plaque with anchored intermediate filaments. The extracellular portions of desmocollins and desmogleins from opposing cells interact with each other in the localized area of the desmosome, forming the cadherin "zipper."

fluorescent dye is injected with a micropipette into one cell of an epithelial sheet. The readily visualized dye can be seen to pass to the immediately adjacent cells. These experiments confirm that adjacent cells share communicating channels that allow small molecules and ions to pass directly between cells without entering the extracellular space.

Gap junctions reduce resistance to passage of electric current between adjacent cells

Electrical conductance studies of gap junctions involve the introduction of microelectrodes into neighboring cells and the establishment of a voltage difference between the electrodes. Current flow between the cells is then measured. If no gap junctions are present between the neighboring cells, the current flow is low, primarily because of the high electrical resistance of the plasma membranes. In contrast, if neighboring cells are joined by gap junctions, there is little electrical resistance between them, and current flow is high. The low resistance reflects the direct cytoplasmic continuity between the two cells, resulting from the presence of the gap junctions. Therefore, gap junctions are also called ***low-resistance junctions.***

Gap junctions can be visualized in TEM sections and freeze fracture preparations

When viewed with the TEM, the gap junction appears as an area of contact between the plasma membranes of adjacent cells (Fig. 4.14a). When uranyl acetate is applied as a "stain" before embedding the tissue (en bloc staining), a gap junction appears as two parallel, closely apposed plasma membranes separated by a gap of 2 nm.

Freeze fracture images of gap junctions reveal groups of channels formed by the apposition of identical structures in the facing membranes. Known as ***connexons,*** these structures consist of six integral membrane proteins called ***connexins,*** configured in a circular arrangement (Fig. 4.14b). Each channel is composed of two connexons, one belonging to the plasma membrane of each cell. Channels in gap junctions can fluctuate rapidly between an open 2-nm-diameter channel and a closed state through reversible changes in the confirmation of the individual connexins (Fig. 4.14c). The molecular mechanism of channel regulation is not yet fully understood. Like many other cellular organelles whose electron microscopic appearance suggests a static structure, gap junctions are actually dynamic.

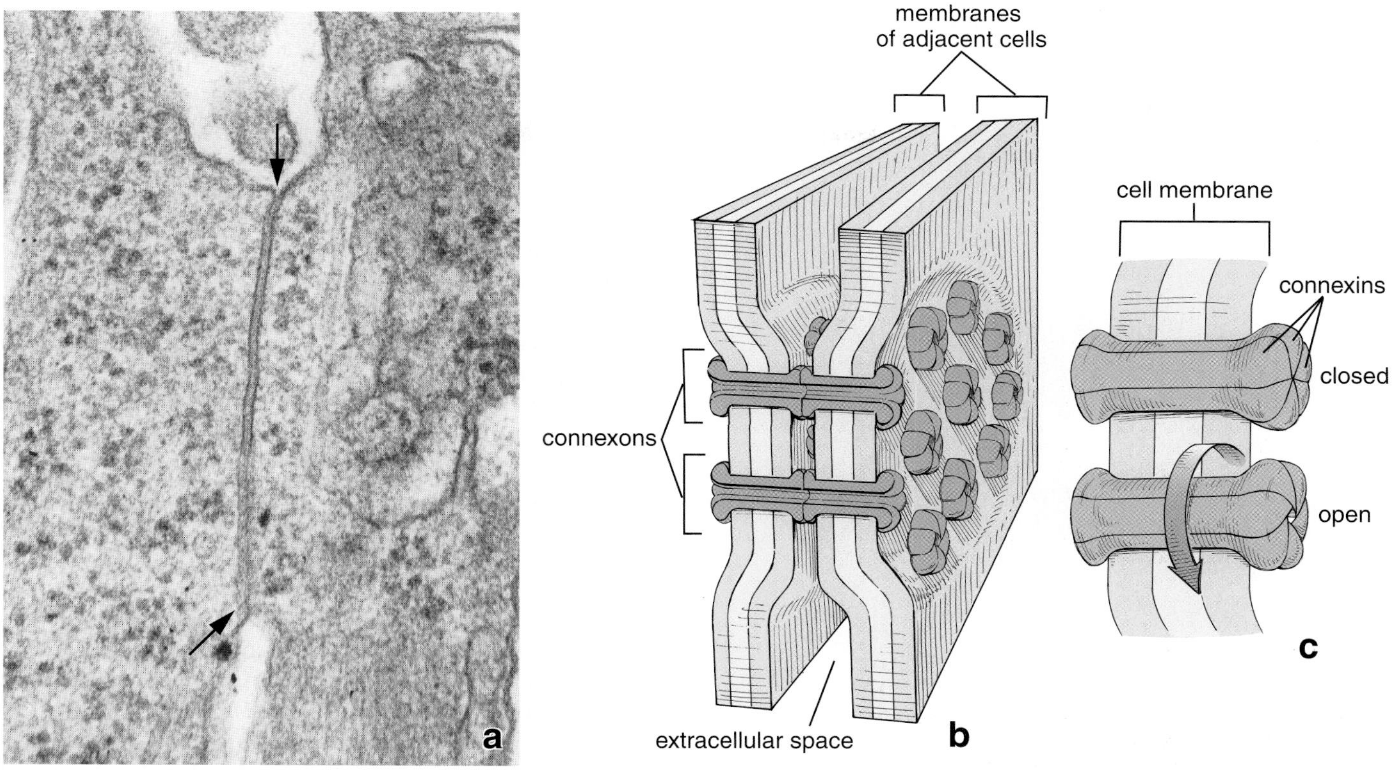

FIGURE 4.14
Structure of a gap junction. a. Electron micrograph showing the plasma membranes of two adjoining cells forming a gap junction. The unit membranes *(arrows)* approach one another, narrowing the intercellular space to produce a 2-nm-wide gap. ×76,000. **b.** Drawing of a gap junction, showing the membranes of adjoining cells and the structural components of the membrane that form channels or passageways between the two cells. Each passageway is formed by a circular array of six subunits, dumbbell-shaped transmembrane proteins that span the plasma membrane of each cell. These complexes, called connexons, have a central opening of about 2-nm in diameter. The channels formed by the registration of the adjacent complementary pairs of connexons permit the flow of small molecules through the channel but not into the intercellular space. Conversely, substances in the intercellular space can permeate the area of a gap junction by flowing around the connexon complexes, but they cannot enter the channels. **c.** The diameter of the channel in an individual connexon is regulated by reversible changes in the confirmation of the individual connexins.

Morphologic Specializations of the Lateral Cell Surface

Lateral cell surface folds (plicae) create interdigitating cytoplasmic processes of adjoining cells

The lateral surfaces of certain epithelial cells show a tortuous boundary due to infoldings or ***plicae*** along the border of each cell with its neighbor (Fig. 4.15). These infoldings increase the lateral surface area of the cell and are particularly prominent in epithelia that are engaged in fluid and electrolyte transport, such as the intestinal and gallbladder epithelium. In active fluid transport, sodium ions are pumped out of the cytoplasm at the lateral plasma membrane by Na^+/K^+-ATPase localized in that membrane. Anions then diffuse across the membrane to maintain electrical neutrality, and water diffuses from the cytoplasm into the intercellular space, driven by the osmotic gradient between the salt concentration in the intercellular space and the concentration in the cytoplasm. The intercellular space distends because of the accumulating fluid moving across the epithelium, but it can distend only to a limited degree because of junctional attachments in the apical and basal portions of the cell. Hydrostatic pressure gradually builds up in the intercellular space and drives an essentially isotonic fluid from the space into the underlying connective tissue. The occluding junction at the apical end of the intercellular space prevents fluid from moving in the opposite direction. As the action of the sodium pump depletes the cytoplasm of salt and water, these are replaced by diffusion across the apical plasma membrane, whose surface area is greatly increased by the presence of microvilli, thus allowing the continuous movement of fluid from the lumen to the connective tissue as long as the Na^+/K^+-ATPase is active.

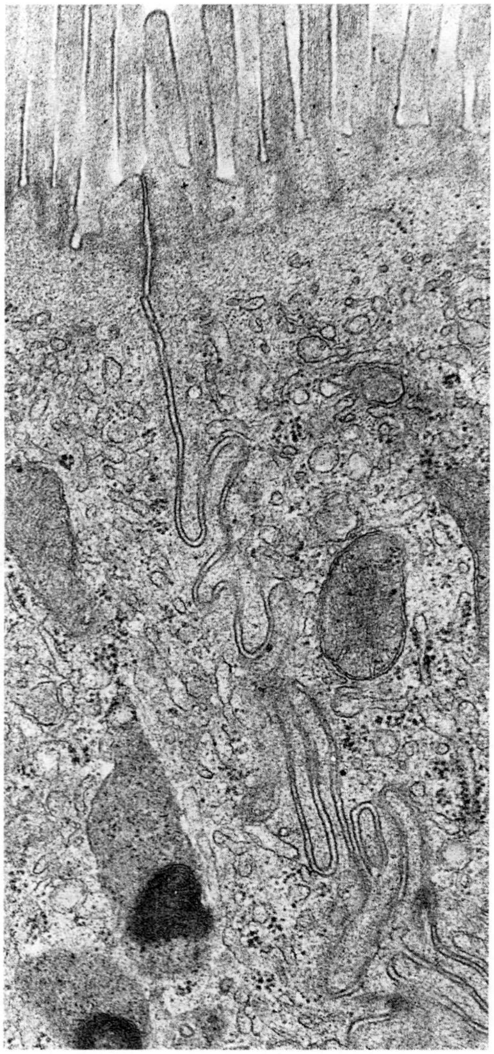

FIGURE 4.15
Lateral interdigitations. Electron micrograph showing infoldings or interdigitations at the lateral surfaces of two adjoining intestinal absorptive cells. ×25,000.

▽ THE BASAL DOMAIN AND ITS SPECIALIZATIONS IN CELL-TO-EXTRACELLULAR MATRIX ADHESION

The basal domain of epithelial cells is characterized by several features:

- *Basement membrane,* which is located next to the basal surface of epithelial cells
- *Cell-to-extracellular matrix junctions,* which anchor the cell to the extracellular matrix
- *Plasma membrane* **infoldings,** which increase surface area and facilitate morphologic interactions between adjacent cells

Basement Membrane Structure and Function

The term *basement membrane* was originally given to a layer of variable thickness at the basal surfaces of epithelia. Although a prominent structure referred to as basement membrane is observed with hematoxylin and eosin (H&E) stain in a few locations, such as the trachea (Fig. 4.16) and, occasionally, the urinary bladder and ureters, basement membrane requires special staining to be seen in the light microscope. This requirement is due, in part, to its thinness and to the effect of the eosin stain, which makes it indistinguishable from the immediately adjacent connective tissue. In the trachea, the structure that is often described as basement membrane includes not only the true basement membrane but an additional layer of closely spaced and aligned collagen fibrils that belong to the connective tissue.

In contrast to H&E (Fig. 4.17a), the periodic acid–Schiff (PAS) staining technique (Fig. 4.17b) results in a positive reaction at the site of the basement membrane. It appears as a thin, well-defined magenta layer between the epithelium and the connective tissue. The stain reacts with the sugar moieties of proteoglycans, accumulating in sufficient amounts and density to make the basement membrane visible in the light microscope. Techniques involving the reduction of silver salts by the sugars blacken the basement membrane and are also used to demonstrate this structure. Although the basement membrane is classically described as exclusively associated with epithelia, similar PAS-positive and silver-reactive sites can be demonstrated surrounding peripheral nerve supporting cells, adipocytes, and mus-

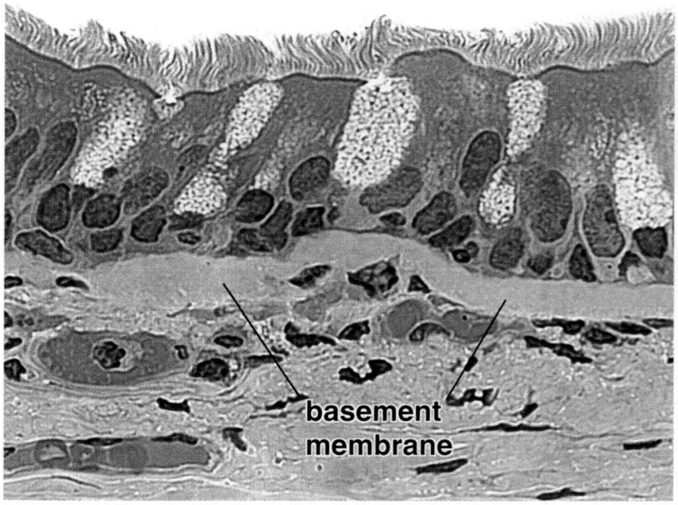

FIGURE 4.16
Tracheal basement membrane. Photomicrograph of a H&E–stained section of the pseudostratified ciliated epithelium of the trachea. The basement membrane appears as a thick homogeneous layer immediately below the epithelium. It is actually a part of the connective tissue and is composed largely of densely packed collagen fibrils. ×450.

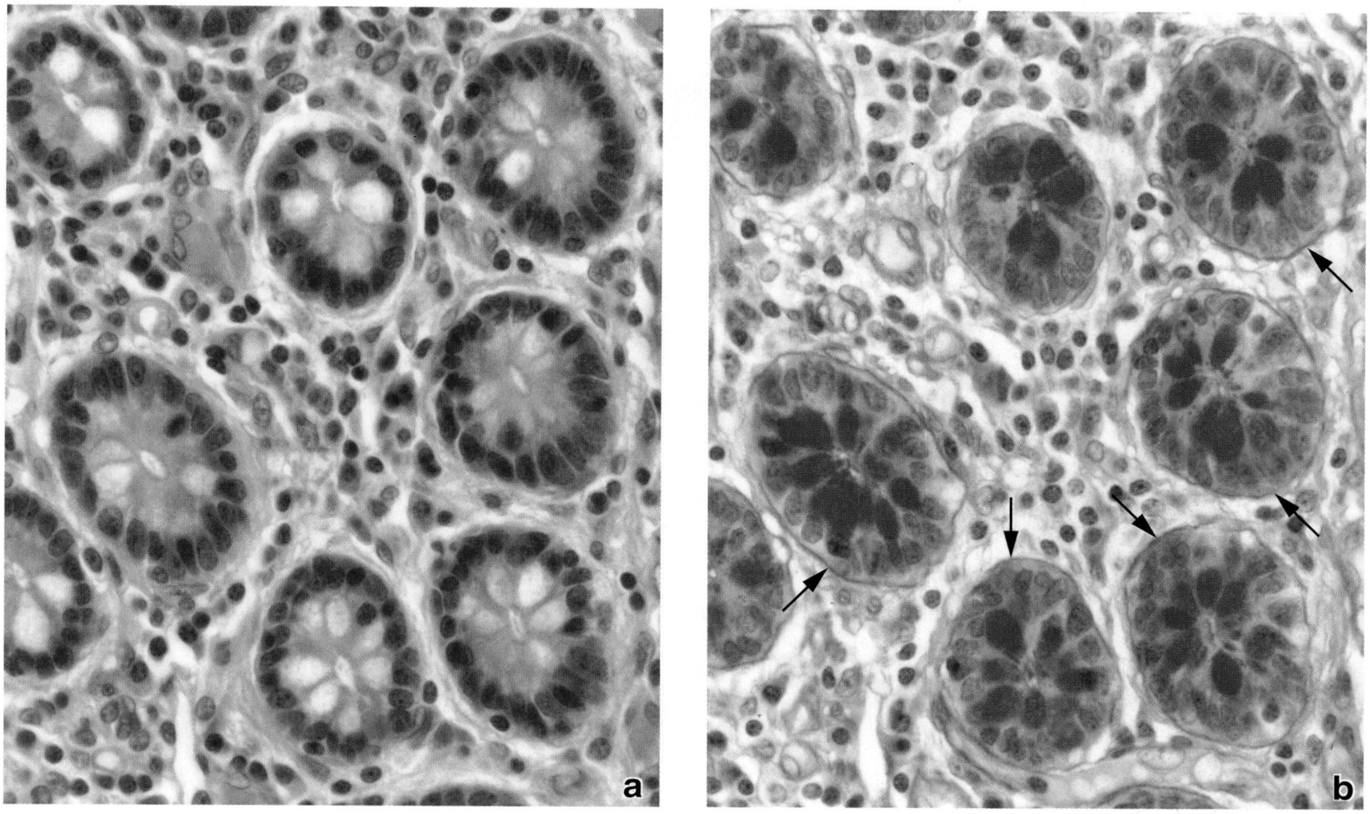

FIGURE 4.17
Photomicrographs showing serial sections of intestinal glands of the colon. The glands in this specimen have been cross-sectioned and appear as round profiles. **a.** This specimen was stained with H&E. Note that neither the basement membrane nor the mucin that is located within the goblet cells is stained. ×550. **b.** This section was stained by the PAS method. It reveals the basement membrane as a thin, magenta layer *(arrows)* between the base of the epithelial cells of the glands and the adjacent connective tissue. The mucin within the goblet cells is also PAS-positive. ×550.

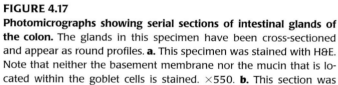

cle cells (Fig. 4.18); this helps to delineate them from the surrounding connective tissue in histologic sections. Connective tissue cells other than adipocytes do not show a similar PAS-positive or silver reaction. That most connective tissue cells are not surrounded by basement membrane material is consistent with their lack of adhesion to the connective tissue fibers. In fact, they must migrate within the tissue under appropriate stimuli to function.

The basal lamina is the structural attachment site for overlying cells and underlying connective tissue

Examination of the site of epithelial basement membranes with the EM reveals a discrete layer of electron-dense matrix material 40- to 60-nm thick between the ep-

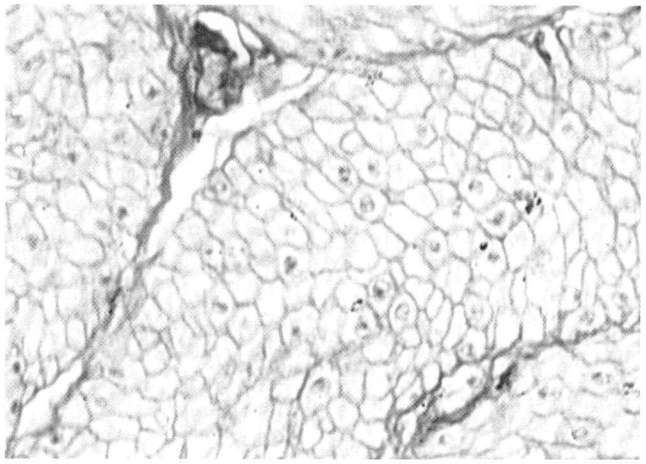

FIGURE 4.18
Photomicrograph of smooth muscle cells stained by the PAS method. This photomicrograph is stained by the PAS method and counterstained with hematoxylin (pale nuclei). The muscle cells have been cut in cross section and appear as polygonal profiles because of the presence of PAS-positive basement membrane material surrounding each cell. As the plane of section passes through each smooth muscle cell, it may or may not pass through the portion of the cell that includes the nucleus. Therefore, in some of the polygonal profiles, nuclei can be seen; in other profiles, no nuclei are seen. The cytoplasm is not stained. ×850.

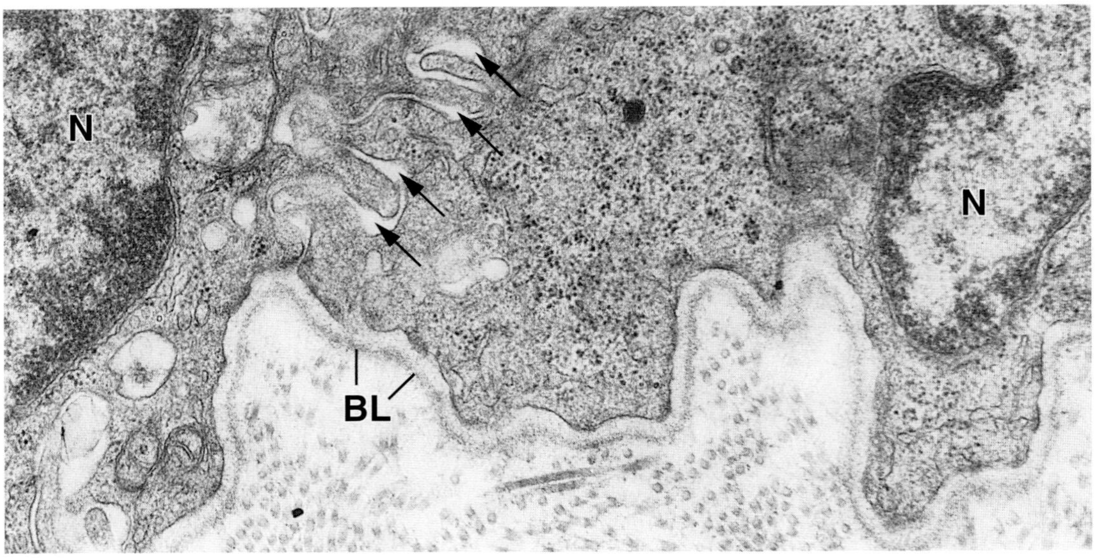

FIGURE 4.19
Electron micrograph of two adjoining epithelial cells with their basal lamina. The micrograph shows only the basal portions of the two cells and parts of their nuclei *(N)*. The intercellular space is partially obscured by lateral interdigitations between the two cells *(arrows)*. The basal lamina *(BL)* appears as a thin layer that follows the contours of the basal domain of the overlying cell. Below the basal lamina are numerous cross-sectioned collagen (reticular) fibrils. ×30,000.

ithelium and the adjacent connective tissue (Fig. 4.19) called the ***basal lamina*** or, sometimes, ***lamina densa***. This layer exhibits a network of fine, 3- to 4-nm filaments when observed at high resolution. Between the basal lamina and the cell is a relatively clear or electron-lucent area, the **lamina lucida** (also about 40 nm wide). This area contains extracellular portions of cell adhesion molecules, mainly ***fibronectin receptors***. These receptors are members of the large family of transmembrane proteins called ***integrins***. Integrins are linked to the cytoskeleton intracellularly and have extracellular portions that bind to the principal glycoproteins of the extracellular matrix (collagen, laminin, fibronectin).

The basal lamina includes at least four groups of molecules

Analyses of basal laminae derived from epithelia in many locations (kidney glomeruli, lung, cornea, lens of the eye) indicate that it consists of collagens, proteoglycans, laminin, and the glycoproteins entactin and fibronectin.

- ***Collagen.*** Several collagen species are present in the basal lamina. The major component, ***type IV collagen***, represents one of approximately 19 types of collagen currently characterized in the body (see Table 5.2). Unlike most of the other collagens in the body, which are products of fibroblasts and related cells, type IV collagen and the other collagens of the basal lamina are products of the epithelial cells and other cell types that possess a basal or external lamina. Type IV collagen consists of short filaments that are thought to provide structural integrity to the basal lamina. It has more hydroxyproline and hydroxylysine than other collagens as well as a larger number of carbohydrate side chains. ***Type VII collagen*** forms anchoring fibrils that link the basal lamina to the underlying reticular lamina (described below). These molecular associations are reinforced by fibronectin and additional glycoproteins. Still incompletely characterized, these glycoproteins (some of which may be additional minor collagen types) interconnect or cross-link the other molecules to impart even greater stability in the interactions between the basal lamina and its associated cells and structures.
- ***Proteoglycans.*** Much of the volume of the basal lamina is probably due to the proteoglycans (heparan sulfate and chondroitin sulfate proteoglycans). Owing to their highly anionic character, these molecules are extensively hydrated. Because of their high negative charge density, sulfated proteoglycans are believed to play an important role in the regulation of the passage of ions across the basal lamina.
- ***Laminin.*** This cross-shaped glycoprotein molecule bridges the lamina lucida to link the basal lamina to the integrins of the basal domain of the overlying epithelial cells (Fig. 4.20). Laminin, heparan sulfate, and chondroitin sulfate proteoglycans are products of these cells; when secreted along with type IV collagen, they self-assemble into basal lamina sheets.
- ***Entactin and fibronectin.*** The remaining two substances are less well characterized. Entactin is a small, sulfated glycoprotein whose specific location and function within the basal lamina are not yet elucidated. It has binding sites for collagen type IV. It also binds to laminin, forming a stable entactin–laminin complex. Fibronectin, an-

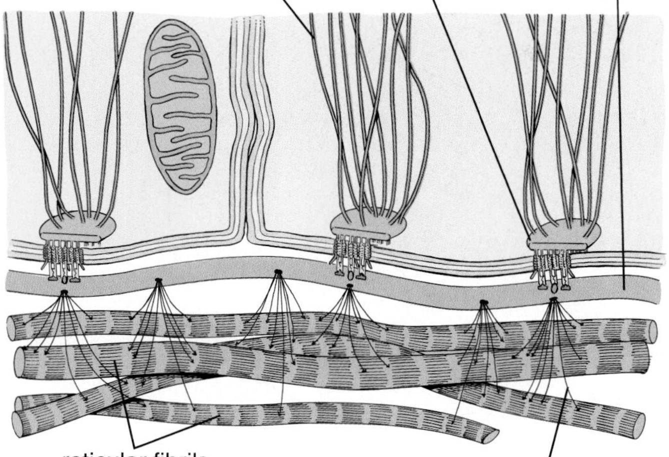

FIGURE 4.20
Schematic diagram of the basal portions of two epithelial cells. This diagram shows the cellular and extracellular components that provide attachment between epithelial cells and the underlying connective tissue. On the connective tissue side of the basal lamina, anchoring fibrils extend from the basal lamina to the collagen (reticular) fibrils of the connective tissue, providing structural attachment at this site. On the epithelial side, laminin *(green)*, collagen XVII *(red)*, and integrins *(yellow)* are present in the lamina rara and lamina densa and provide adhesion between the basal lamina and the intracellular attachment plaques of hemidesmosomes.

other glycoprotein, has binding sites for all of the basal lamina components and probably serves to bind it to the subjacent connective tissue.

A layer of reticular fibers underlies the basal lamina

There is still lack of agreement as to the extent to which the basal lamina seen with the EM corresponds to the structure described as the basement membrane in the light microscope. Some investigators contend that the basement membrane includes not only the basal lamina but also a secondary layer of small-unit fibrils of ***type III collagen*** (reticular fibers) that forms the reticular lamina. The reticular lamina, as such, belongs to the connective tissue and is not a product of the epithelium. The reticular lamina was once regarded as the component that reacted with silver, whereas the polysaccharides of the basal lamina and the ground substance associated with the reticular fibers were thought to be the components stained with the PAS reaction. However, convincing arguments can be made for the basal lamina reacting with both PAS and silver in several sites. In normal kidney glomeruli, for example, no collagen (reticular) fibers are associated with the basal lamina of the epithelial cells (Fig. 4.21), although a positive reaction occurs with both PAS staining and silver impregnation. Also, in the spleen, where the basal lamina of the venous sinuses forms a unique pattern of ring-like bands rather than a thin, sheath-like layer around the vessel, exactly corresponding images are seen with the PAS and silver techniques as well as with the EM (Fig. 4.22).

Several structures are responsible for attachment of the basal lamina to the underlying connective tissue

On the opposite side of the basal lamina, the connective tissue side, several mechanisms provide attachment of the basal lamina to the underlying connective tissue:

- ***Anchoring fibrils*** *(type VII collagen)* (see Table 5.2) are usually found in close association with hemidesmosomes. They extend from the basal lamina matrix and appear to attach to connective tissue reticular fibrils (see Fig. 4.20).
- ***Fibrillin microfibrils*** are 10 to 12 nm in diameter and attach the lamina densa to elastic fibers. Fibrillin microfibrils are known to have elastic properties. A mutation in the fibrillin gene *(FBN1)* causes Marfan's syndrome and other related connective tissue disorders.
- ***Discrete projections of the lamina densa*** on its connective tissue side interact directly with the reticular lamina to form an additional binding site with type III collagen.

The multiple roles of the basal lamina and basement membrane are not yet fully elucidated. It is generally accepted that they facilitate attachment of epithelia to underlying connective tissue and that they influence the differentiation and proliferation of the epithelial cells that contact them.

Muscle cells, adipocytes, and peripheral nerve supporting cells exhibit an extracellular electron-dense material that resembles the basal lamina of epithelium. This mate-

BOX 4.2

Functional Considerations: Basement Membrane and Basal Lamina Terminology

The terms ***basement membrane*** and ***basal lamina*** are used inconsistently in the literature. Some authors use *basement membrane* when referring to both light and electron microscopic images. Others dispense with the term *basement membrane* altogether and use *basal lamina* in both light and electron microscopy. Because the term *basement membrane* originated with light microscopy, it is used in this book only in the context of light microscopic descriptions and only in relation to epithelia. The electron microscopic term *basal lamina* is reserved for the ultrastructural content to denote the layer present at the interface of connective tissue with epithelial cells. The term ***external lamina*** is used to identify this same layer when it forms a peripheral cellular investment, as in muscle cells and peripheral nerve supporting cells.

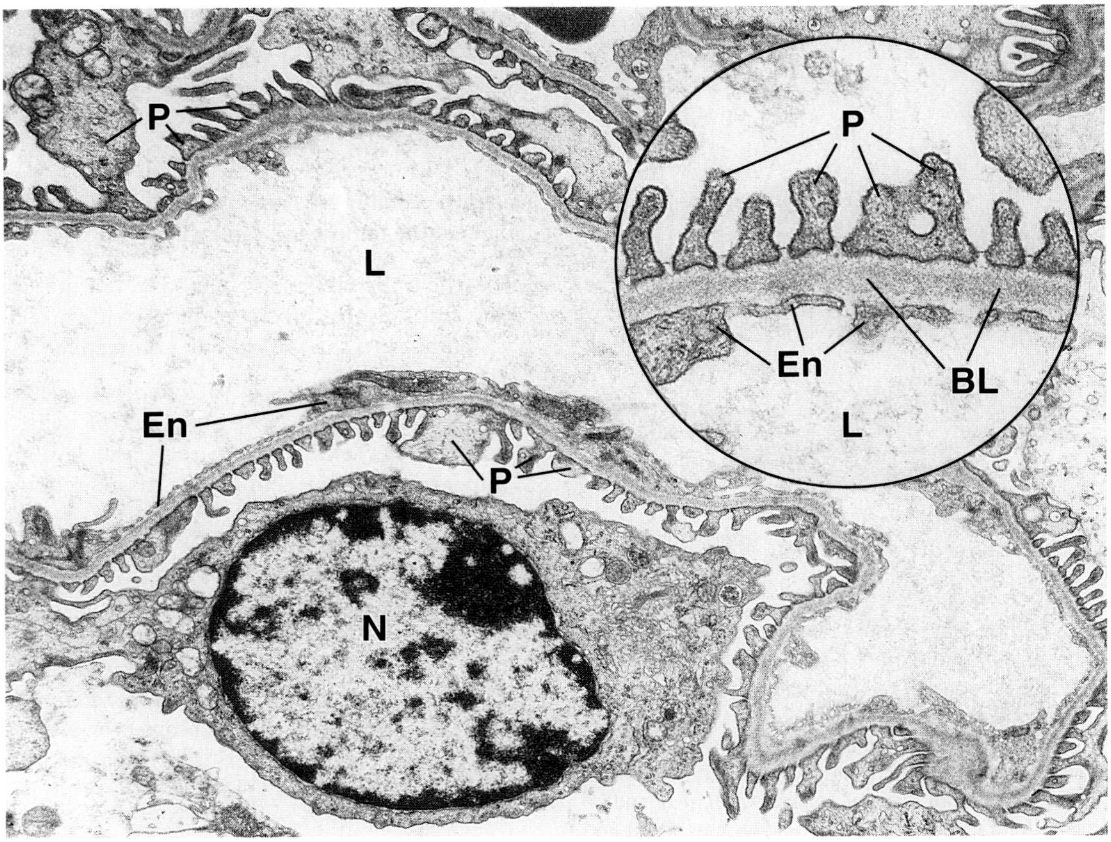

FIGURE 4.21
Basal lamina in the kidney glomerulus. Electron micrograph of a kidney glomerular capillary, showing the basal lamina *(BL)* interposed between the capillary endothelial cell *(En)* and the cytoplasmic processes *(P)* of epithelial cells (podocytes). The epithelial cell is located on the outer (abluminal) surface of the endothelial cell. ×12,000. **Inset.** Relationship at higher magnification. Note that the endothelial cells and epithelial cells are separated by the shared basal lamina and that no collagen fibrils are present. *N*, nucleus of epithelial cell; *L*, lumen of capillary. ×40,000.

rial also corresponds to a PAS-positive staining reaction, as described above (see Fig. 4.18). Although the term "basement membrane" is not ordinarily applied to the extracellular stainable material of these nonepithelial cells in light microscopy, the terms "basal lamina" or "external lamina" are typically used at the EM level.

Basal laminae have multiple functions

Various functions are now attributed to the basal lamina:

- ***Structural attachment.*** As noted, the basal lamina serves as an intermediary structure in the attachment of cells to the adjacent connective tissue.
- ***Compartmentalization.*** Structurally, basal and external laminae separate or isolate the connective tissue from epithelia, nerve, and muscle tissues. Connective tissue—including all of its specialized tissues, such as bone and cartilage (with the exception of adipose tissue, in that its cells possess an external lamina)—can be viewed as a single, continuous compartment. In contrast, epithelia, muscles, and nerves are separated from adjacent connective tissue by intervening basal or external laminae. For any substance to move from one tissue to another (e.g., from one compartment to another), it must cross such a lamina.
- ***Filtration.*** The movement of substances to and from the connective tissue is regulated in part by the basal lamina, largely through ionic charges and integral spaces. Filtration is well characterized in the kidney, where the plasma filtrate must cross the compound basal laminae of capillaries and adjacent epithelial cells to reach the urinary space within a renal corpuscle.
- ***Polarity induction.*** Epithelial cells exhibit functionally different membrane properties as a result of surface exposure. Specific properties attributable to the basal membrane surface, as opposed to the apical and lateral membrane surfaces, are induced by the presence of the basal lamina. For example, epithelial cells grown in ordinary tissue culture flatten as they proliferate and grow in the culture. When grown on the surface of an artificial basal lamina in the culture medium, the same cells display their characteristic shape as well as normal polarity and function.
- ***Tissue scaffolding.*** The basal lamina serves as a guide or scaffold during regeneration. Newly formed cells or

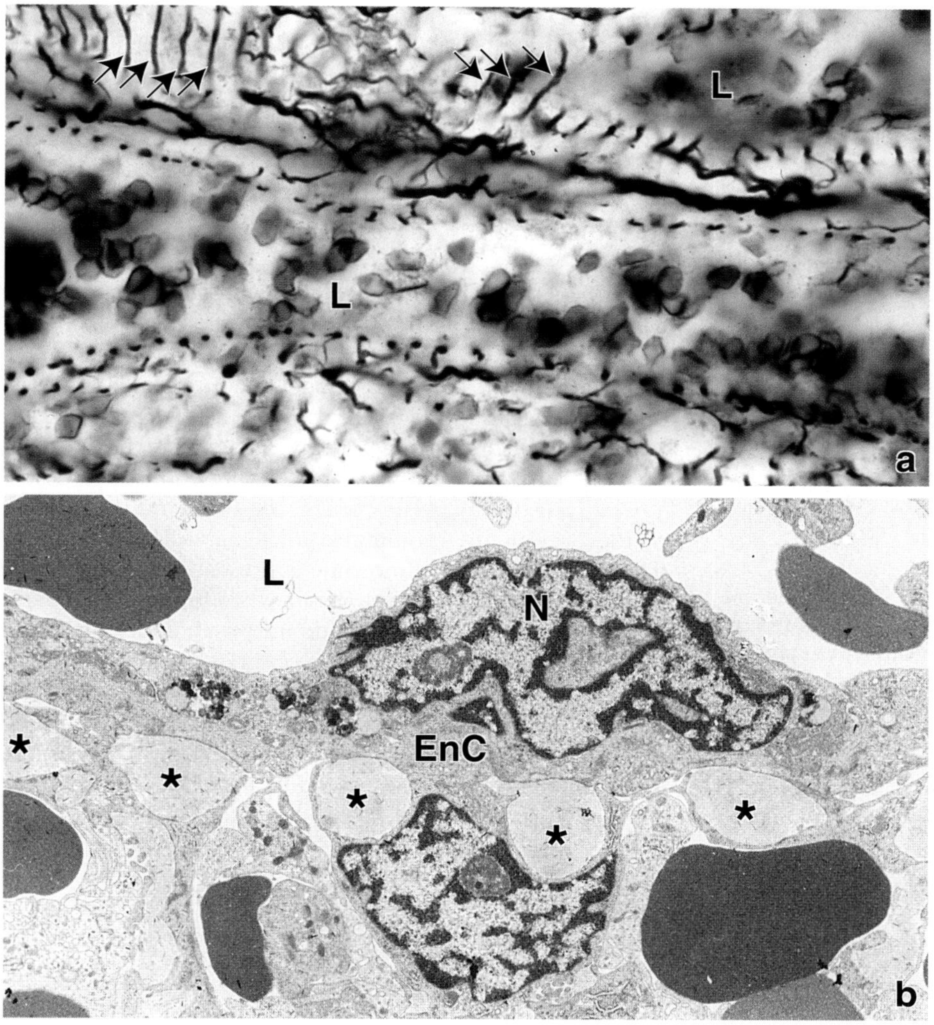

FIGURE 4.22
Demonstration of basement membrane material in splenic vessels. a. Photomicrograph of a silver preparation revealing two longitudinally sectioned venous sinuses in the spleen. These blood vessels are surrounded by a modified basement membrane, which takes the form of a ring-like structure, much like the hoops of a barrel, rather than a continuous layer or lamina. The rings are blackened by the silver and appear as bands where the walls of the vessel have been tangentially sectioned *(arrows)*. To the right, the cut has penetrated deeper into the vessel and shows the lumen *(L)*. Here, the cut edges of the rings are seen on both sides of the vessel. In the lower vessel, the cut rings have been sectioned in a virtually perpendicular plane, and the rings appear as a series of dots. ×400. **b.** Electron micrograph of the wall of a venous sinus, showing a longitudinally sectioned endothelial cell *(EnC)*. The nucleus *(N)* of the cell is protruding into the lumen. The basal lamina material *(asterisks)* has the same homogeneous appearance as seen by electron microscopy in other sites except that it is aggregated into ring-like structures rather than into a flat layer or lamina. Moreover, its location and plane of section correspond to the silver-reactive, dot-like material in the panel above. ×25,000.

growing processes of a cell use the basal lamina that remains after cell loss, thus helping to maintain the original tissue architecture. For example, when nerves are damaged, new neuromuscular junctions from a growing axon will be established only if the external lamina remains intact after injury.

Cell-to-Extracellular Matrix Junctions

The organization of cells in epithelium depends on the support provided by the extracellular matrix, on which the basal surface of each cell rests. ***Anchoring junctions*** maintain the morphologic integrity of the epithelium–connective tissue interface. The two major anchoring junctions are

- ***Focal adhesions,*** which anchor actin filaments of the cytoskeleton into the basement membrane
- ***Hemidesmosomes,*** which anchor the intermediate filaments of cytoskeleton into the basement membrane

In addition, transmembrane proteins located in the basal cell domain (mainly related to the integrin family of adhesion molecules) interact with the basal lamina.

Focal adhesions create a dynamic link between the actin cytoskeleton and extracellular matrix proteins

Focal adhesions are responsible for attaching long bundles of actin filaments (stress fibers) into the basal lamina. They play a prominent role during dynamic changes that occur in epithelial cells, e.g., migration of epithelial cells in wound repair. These focal adhesions form dynamic attachments to the underlying connective tissue by linking actin filaments to extracellular matrix proteins (Fig. 4.23).

In general, focal adhesions consist of a cytoplasmic face to which actin filaments are bound, a transmembrane connecting region, and an extracellular face that binds to the proteins of the extracellular matrix. The main family of transmembrane proteins involved in focal adhesions are integrins, which are concentrated in clusters within the areas

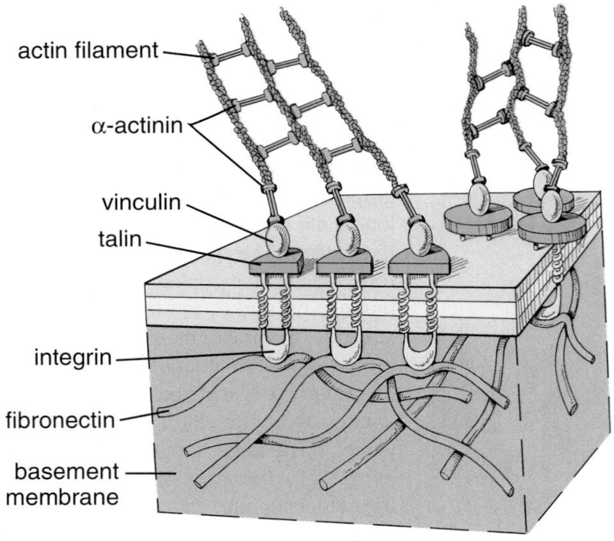

FIGURE 4.23
Molecular structure of focal adhesions. Diagram showing the molecular organization of focal adhesions. On the cytoplasmic side, note the arrangement of different actin-binding proteins. These proteins interact with integrins, the transmembrane proteins, the extracellular domains of which bind to fibronectin.

where the junctions can be detected. Integrins are capable of transducing signals to the interior of the cell, where they affect cell migration, differentiation, and growth. On the cytoplasmic face, integrins interact with actin-binding proteins (α-actinin, vinculin, ***talin, paxillin***) as well as many regulatory proteins, such as ***focal adhesion kinase*** or ***tyrosine kinase.*** On the extracellular side, integrins bind to extracellular matrix glycoproteins, usually laminin and fibronectin.

Hemidesmosomes occur in epithelia that require strong, stable adhesion to the connective tissue

A variant of the anchoring junction similar to the desmosome is found in certain epithelia subject to abrasion and mechanical shearing forces that would tend to separate the epithelium from the underlying connective tissue. Typically, it occurs in the cornea, the skin, and the mucosa of the oral cavity, esophagus, and vagina. In these locations, only half the desmosome is present, hence the name ***hemidesmosome.*** Hemidesmosomes are found on the basal cell surface, where they provide increased adhesion to the basal lamina (Fig. 4.24a). When observed with the EM, the hemidesmosome exhibits an ***attachment plaque*** on the cytoplasmic side of the basal plasma membrane. The protein composition of this structure is similar to that of the desmosomal plaque, as it contains *desmoplakin-like* pro-

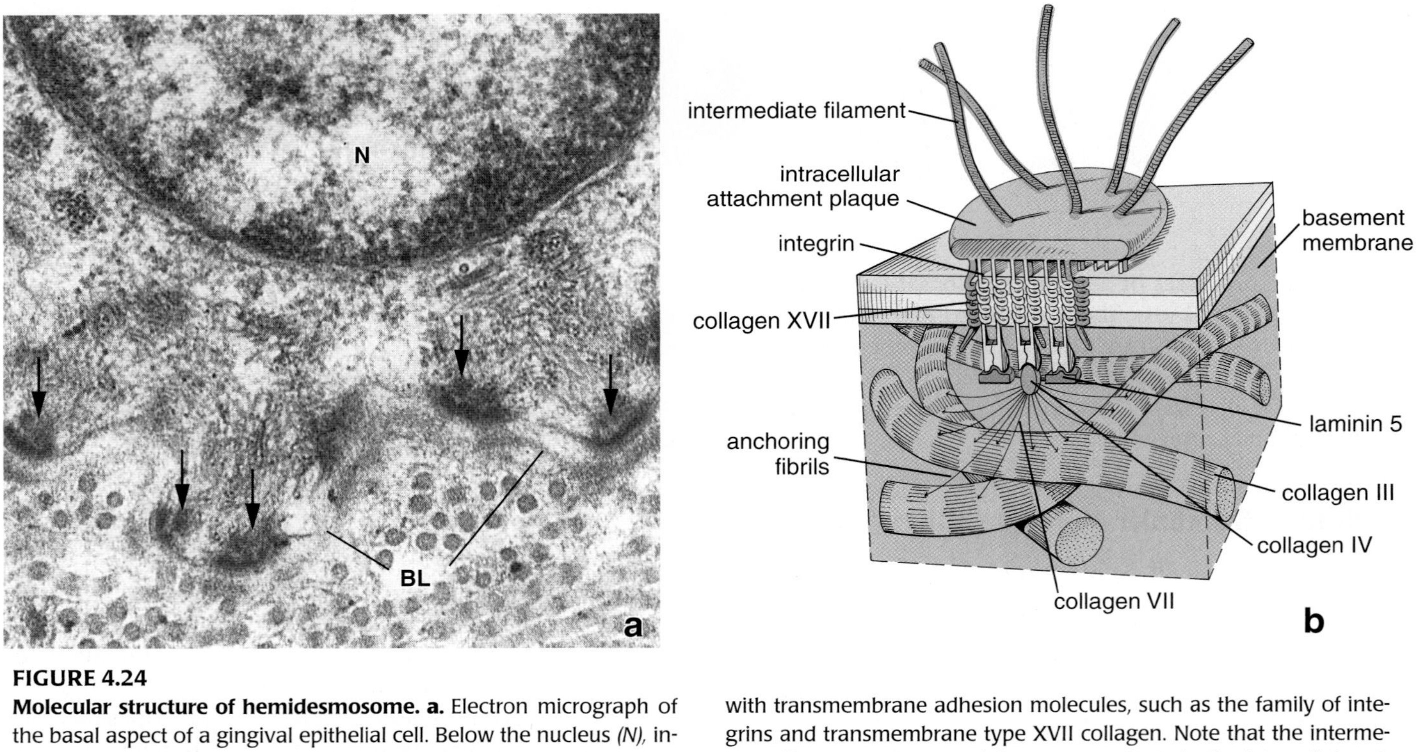

FIGURE 4.24
Molecular structure of hemidesmosome. a. Electron micrograph of the basal aspect of a gingival epithelial cell. Below the nucleus *(N)*, intermediate filaments are seen converging on the intracellular attachment plaques *(arrows)* of the hemidesmosome. Below the plasma membrane are the basal lamina *(BL)* and collagen (reticular) fibrils (most of which are cut in cross section) of the connective tissue. ×40,000. **b.** Diagram showing the molecular organization of a hemidesmosome. The intracellular attachment plaque is associated with transmembrane adhesion molecules, such as the family of integrins and transmembrane type XVII collagen. Note that the intermediate filaments seem to originate or terminate in the intracellular attachment plaque. Extracellular portions of integrins bind to laminin 5 and type IV collagen. With the help of anchoring fibrils (type VII collagen) laminin and integrin, the attachment plaque is secured to the reticular fibers (type III collagen) of extracellular matrix.

teins capable of anchoring intermediate filaments of the cytoskeleton. In contrast to the desmosome, whose transmembrane proteins belong to the cadherin family of calcium-dependent molecules, the transmembrane proteins found in the hemidesmosome include the integrin class of cell matrix receptors. The extracellular portions of these integrins enter the basal lamina and interact with its proteins, including laminin and type IV collagen. In addition, ***type XVII collagen,*** a transmembrane molecule, can be detected within the hemidesmosome (Fig. 4.24b). In certain skin diseases characterized clinically by blister formation, such as bullous pemphigoid, high levels of antibodies directed against components of the hemidesmosome, including antibodies against type XVII collagen, can be detected.

Morphologic Modifications of the Basal Cell Surface

Many cells that transport fluid have infoldings at the basal cell surface. These basal surface modifications are prominent in proximal and distal tubules of the kidney (Fig. 4.25) and in certain ducts of the salivary glands. Mitochondria are typically concentrated at this basal site to provide the energy requirements for active transport. The mitochondria are usually oriented vertically within the folds. The orientation of the mitochondria, combined with the basal membrane infoldings, results in a striated appearance along the basal aspect of the cell when observed in the light microscope. Because of this phenomenon, the salivary gland ducts that possess these cells are referred to as ***striated ducts.***

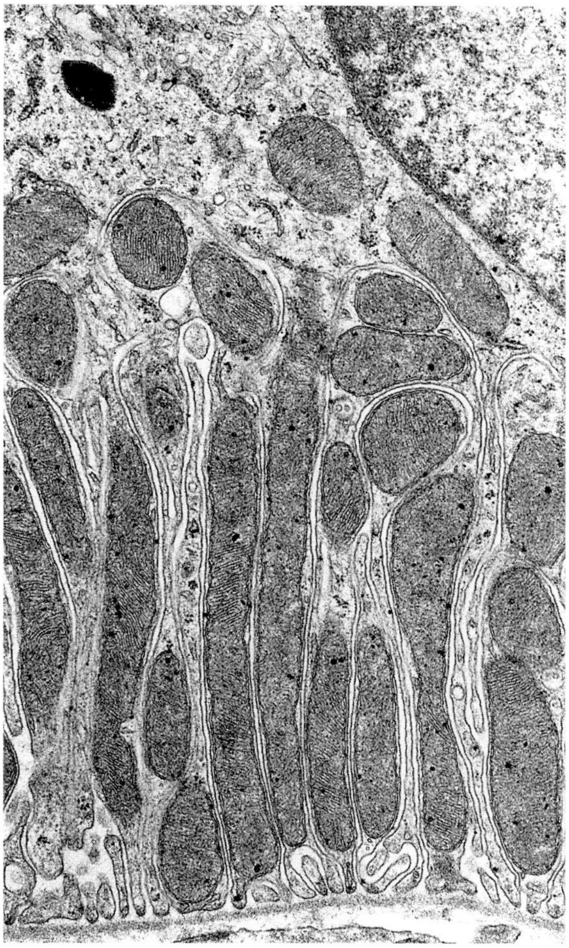

FIGURE 4.25
Basal infoldings. Electron micrograph of the basal portion of a kidney tubule cell, showing the infolding of the plasma membrane. Note the aligned mitochondria. The infoldings of adjoining cells result in the interdigitations of cytoplasm between the two cells. ×25,000.

GLANDS

Typically, glands are classified into two major groups according to how their products are released (Table 4.2):

- ***Exocrine glands*** secrete their products onto a surface directly or through epithelial ducts or tubes that are connected to a surface. Ducts may convey the secreted material in an unaltered form or may modify the secretion by concentrating it or adding or reabsorbing constituent substances.
- ***Endocrine glands*** lack a duct system. They secrete their products into the connective tissue, where they enter the bloodstream to reach their target cells. The products of endocrine glands are called ***hormones.***

In some epithelia, individual cells secrete a substance that does not reach the bloodstream but rather affects other cells within the same epithelium. Such secretory activity is referred to as ***paracrine.*** The secretory material reaches the target cells by diffusion through the extracellular space or immediately subjacent connective tissue.

Cells of exocrine glands exhibit different mechanisms of secretion

The cells of exocrine glands have three basic release mechanisms for secretory products (see Table 4.2):

- ***Merocrine secretion.*** The secretory product is delivered in membrane-bounded vesicles to the apical surface of the cell. Here, vesicles fuse with the plasma membrane and extrude their contents by exocytosis. This is the most common mechanism of secretion and is found, for example, in pancreatic acinar cells.
- ***Apocrine secretion.*** The secretory product is released in the apical portion of the cell, surrounded by a thin layer of cytoplasm within an envelope of plasma membrane. This mechanism of secretion is found in the lactating mammary gland, where it is responsible for releasing large lipid droplets into the milk. It also occurs in the apocrine glands of skin, ciliary (Moll's) glands of the eyelid, and the ceruminous glands of the external auditory meatus.
- ***Holocrine secretion.*** The secretory product accumulates within the maturing cell, which simultaneously undergoes programmed cell death. Both secretory products

TABLE 4.2. Types of Glands

Exocrine Glands			Endocrine Glands	Paracrine Glands
Merocine	Apocrine	Holocrine		

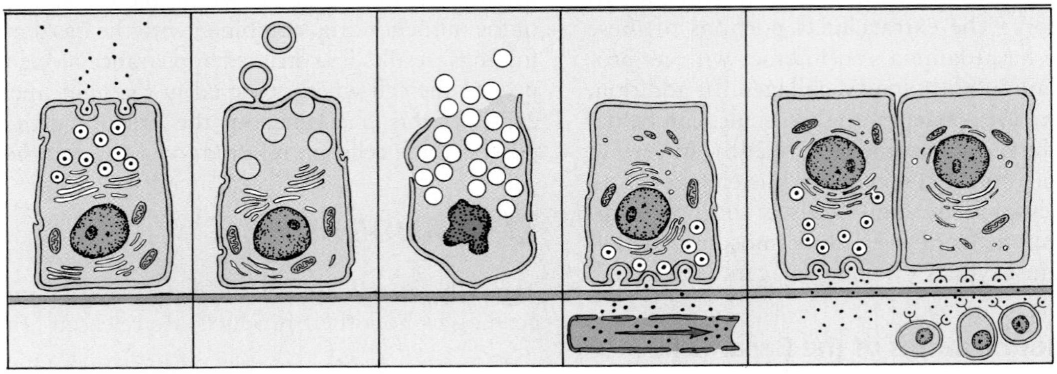

and cell debris are discharged into the lumen of the gland. This mechanism is found in sebaceous glands of skin and the tarsal (Meibomian) glands of the eyelid.

Exocrine glands are classified as either unicellular or multicellular

Unicellular glands are the simplest in structure. In unicellular exocrine glands, the secretory component consists of single cells distributed among other nonsecretory cells. A typical example is the goblet cell, a mucus-secreting cell positioned among other columnar cells (Fig. 4.26). Goblet cells are located in the surface lining and glands of the intestines and in certain passages of the respiratory tract.

Multicellular glands are composed of more than one cell. They exhibit varying degrees of complexity. Their structural organization allows subclassification according to the arrangement of the secretory cells (parenchyma) and the presence or absence of branching of the duct elements.

The simplest arrangement of a multicellular gland is a cellular sheet in which each surface cell is a secretory cell. For example, the lining of the stomach and its gastric pits is a sheet of mucus-secreting cells (Fig. 4.27).

Other multicellular glands typically form tubular invaginations from the surface. The end pieces of the gland contain the secretory cells; the portion of the gland connecting the secretory cells to the surface serves as a duct. If the duct is unbranched, the gland is called ***simple;*** if the duct is branched, it is called ***compound.*** If the secretory portion is shaped like a tube, the gland is ***tubular;*** if it is shaped like a flask, the gland is ***alveolar*** or ***acinar;*** if the tube ends in a sac-like dilation, the gland is ***tubuloalveolar.*** Tubular secretory portions may be straight, branched, or coiled; alveolar portions may be single or branched. Various combinations of duct and secretory portion shapes are found in the body. Classification and description of exocrine glands may be found in Table 4.3.

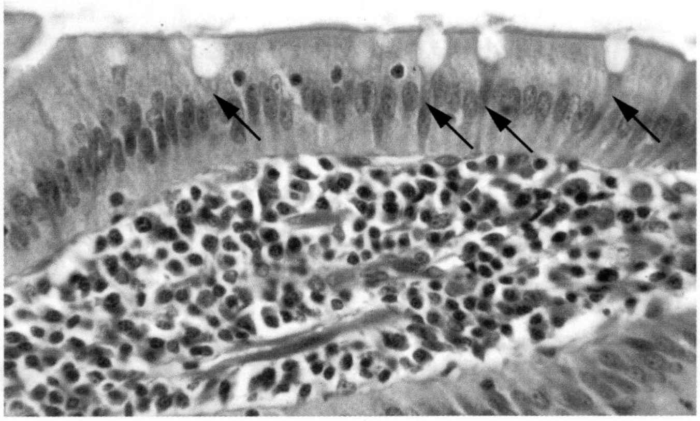

FIGURE 4.26
Unicellular glands. Photomicrograph of intestinal epithelium, showing single goblet cells *(arrows)* dispersed among absorptive cells. Each goblet cell may be regarded as a unicellular gland—the simplest exocrine type gland. ×350.

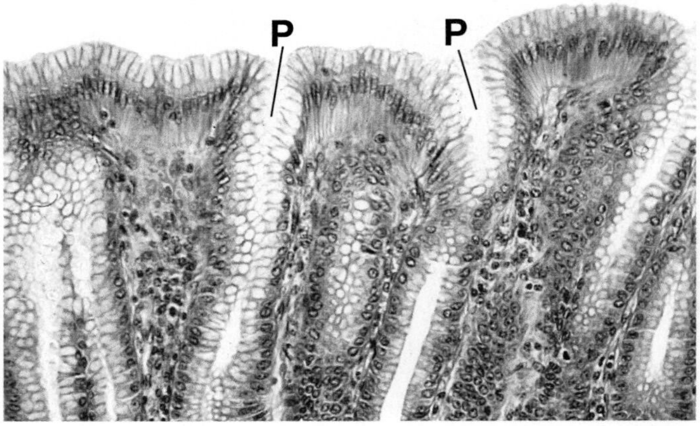

FIGURE 4.27
Mucus surface cells of stomach. Photomicrograph of stomach surface. The epithelial cells lining the surface are all mucus-secreting cells, as are the cells lining the gastric pits *(P)*. The cells of the gastric pit form simple tubular glands. ×260.

TABLE 4.3. **Classification of Multicellular Glands**

	Classification		Typical location	Features
Simple Glands	Simple tubular	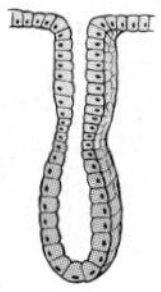	Large intestine: intestinal glands of the colon	Secretory portion of the gland is a straight tube formed by the secretory cells (goblet cells)
	Simple coiled tubular	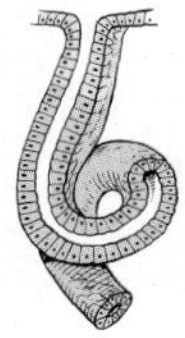	Skin: eccrine sweat gland	Coiled tubular structure is composed of the secretory portion located deep in the dermis
	Simple branched tubular	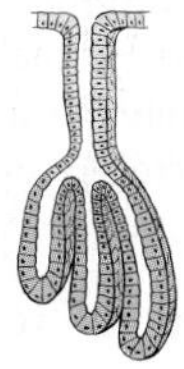	Stomach: mucus-secreting glands of the pylorus	Branched tubular glands with wide secretory portions are formed by the secretory cells and produce a viscous mucous secretion
	Simple acinar	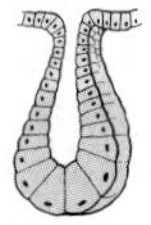	Urethra: paraurethral and periurethral glands	Simple acinar glands develop as an outpouching of the transitional epithelium and are formed by a single layer of secretory cells
	Branched acinar	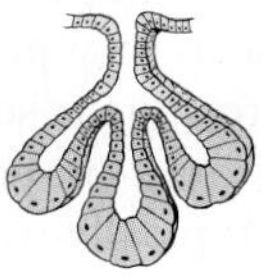	Stomach: mucus-secreting glands of cardia	Branched acinar glands with secretory portions are formed by mucus-secreting cells; the short, single-duct portion opens directly into the lumen
Compound Glands	Compound tubular	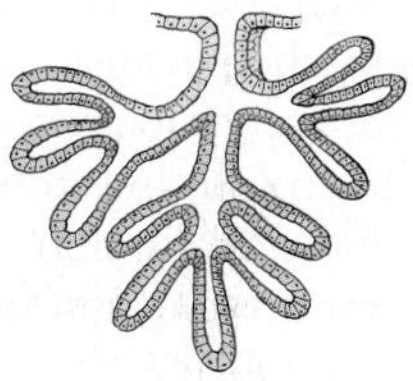	Duodenum: submucosal glands of Brunner	Compound tubular glands with coiled secretory portions are located deep in the submucosa of the duodenum
	Compound acinar	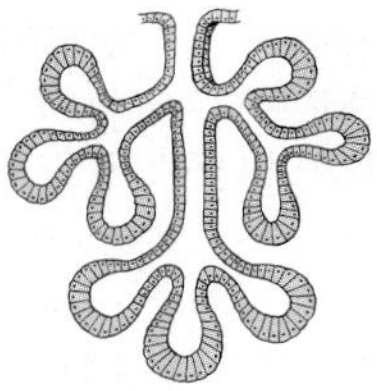	Pancreas: excretory portion	Compound acinar glands with alveolar-shaped secretory units are formed by pyramid-shaped serous-secreting cells
	Compound tubuloacinar	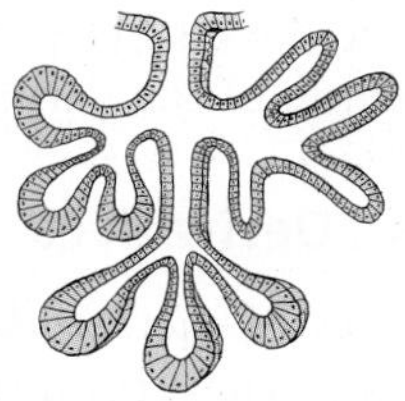	Submandibular salivary gland	Compound tubuloacinar glands can have both mucous branched tubular and serous branched acinar secretory units; they have serous end-caps (demilunes)

Mucous and serous glands are so named because of the type of secretion produced

The secretory cells of exocrine glands associated with the various body tubes, e.g., the alimentary canal, respiratory passages, and urogenital system, are often described as being ***mucous, serous,*** or both.

Mucous secretions are viscous and slimy, whereas serous secretions are watery. Goblet cells, secretory cells of the sublingual salivary glands, and surface cells of the stomach are examples of mucus-secreting cells. The mucous nature of the secretion results from extensive glycosylation of the constituent proteins with anionic oligosaccharides. The mucinogen granules, the secretory product within the cell, are therefore PAS positive (see Fig. 4.17a). However, they are water soluble and lost during routine tissue preparation. For this reason, the cytoplasm of mucous cells appears to be empty in H&E–stained paraffin sections. Another characteristic feature of a mucous cell is that its nucleus is usually flattened against the base of the cell by accumulated secretory product (Fig. 4.28).

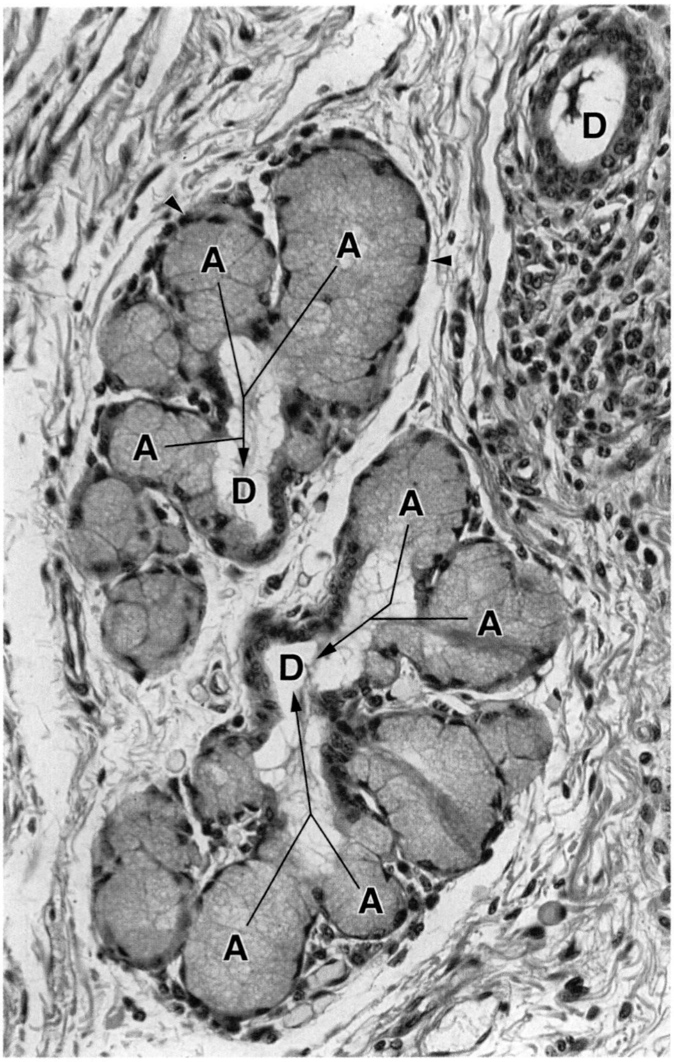

FIGURE 4.28
Mucus-secreting compound gland. Photomicrograph showing two small lobes of a mucus-secreting gland associated with the larynx. Each displays the beginning of a duct *(D)* into which mucin is secreted *(arrows).* The individual secretory cells that form the acinus *(A)* are difficult to define. Their nuclei *(arrowheads)* are flattened and located in the very basal portion of the cell, a feature typical of mucus-secreting glands. The cytoplasm is filled with mucin that has been retained during preparation of the tissue and appears stained. ×350.

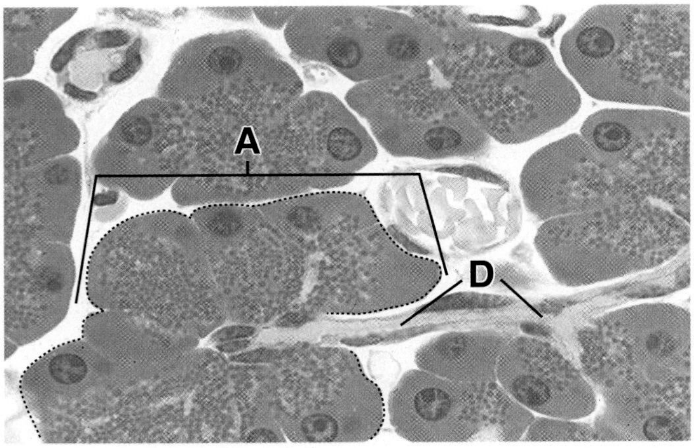

FIGURE 4.29
Serous-secreting compound gland. Photomicrograph of pancreatic acinus *(A)* (outlined by the *dotted line)* with its duct *(D).* The small round objects within the acinar cells represent the zymogen granules, the stored secretory precursor material. ×320.

In contrast to mucus-secreting cells, serous cells produce poorly glycosylated or nonglycosylated protein secretions. The nucleus is typically round or oval (Fig. 4.29). The apical cytoplasm is often intensely stained with eosin if its secretory granules are well preserved. The perinuclear cytoplasm often appears basophilic because of an extensive rough endoplasmic reticulum, a characteristic of protein-synthesizing cells.

Serous cell–containing ***acini*** (sing., ***acinus***) are found in the parotid gland and pancreas. Acini of some glands, such as the submandibular gland, contain both mucous and serous cells. In routine tissue preparation, the serous cells are more removed from the lumen of the acinus and are shaped as crescents or ***demilunes*** ("half-moons") (see page 455 for an explanation of demilune formation) at the periphery of the mucous acinus.

▼ HISTOGENESIS OF EPITHELIUM

The three germ layers in the developing embryo contribute to the formation of the various epithelia.

Ectodermal Derivatives

The derivatives of the ***ectoderm*** may be divided into two major classes: surface ectoderm and neuroectoderm.

Surface ectoderm gives rise to

- ***Epidermis*** and its derivatives (hair, nails, sweat glands, sebaceous glands, and the parenchyma and ducts of the mammary glands)
- ***Cornea*** and ***lens epithelia*** of the eye
- ***Enamel organ*** and ***enamel*** of the teeth
- ***Components of the inner ear***
- ***Adenohypophysis*** (anterior lobe of pituitary gland)

Neuroectoderm gives rise to

- ***Neural tube*** and its derivatives (the central nervous system, including ependyma, pineal body, and neurohy-

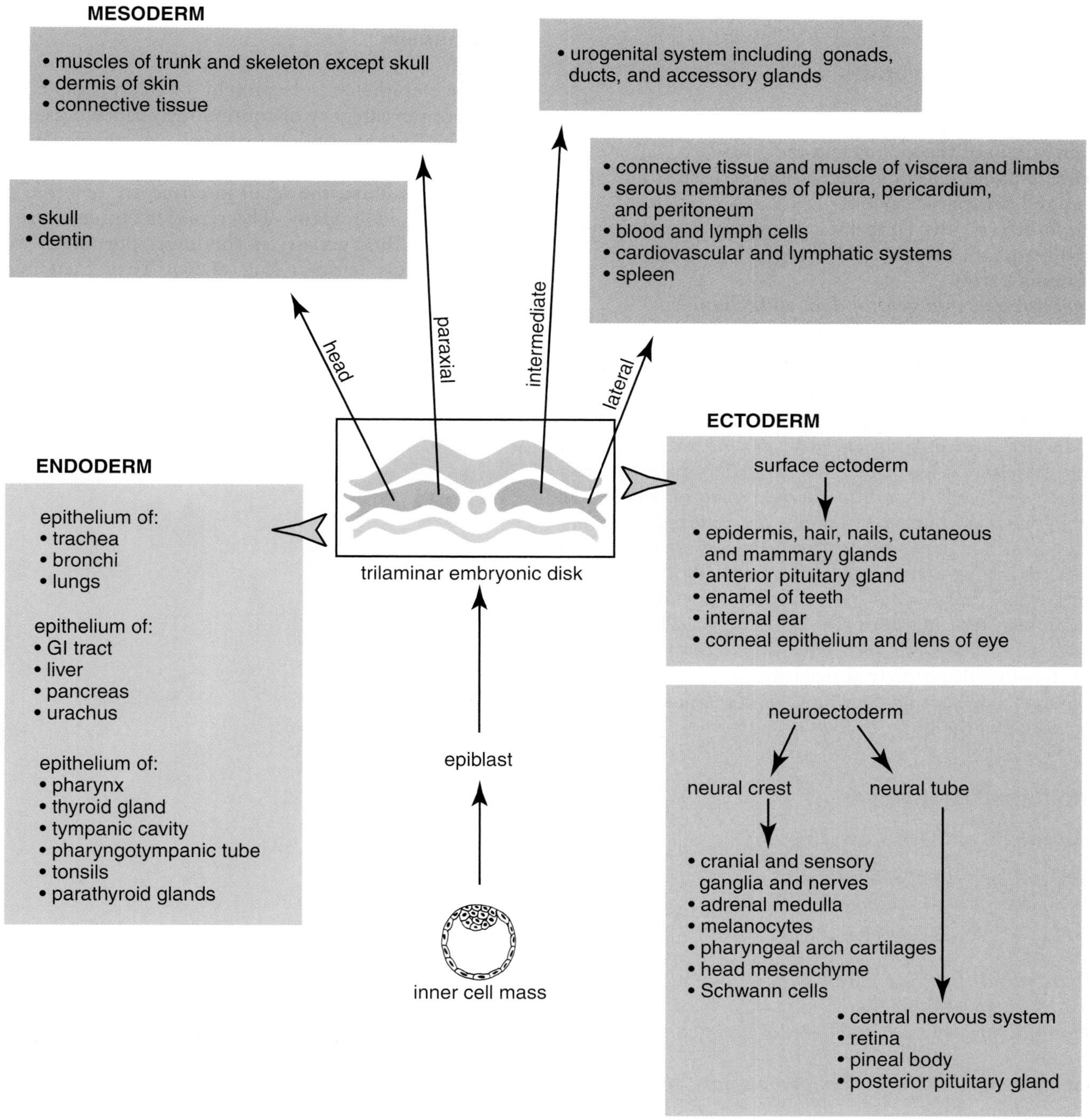

FIGURE 4.30
Derivatives of the three germ layers. Schematic drawing illustrating the derivatives of the three germ layers: ectoderm, endoderm, and mesoderm. (Based on Moore KL, Persaud TVN. *The Developing Human, Clinically Oriented Embryology*. Philadelphia: WB Saunders, 1998.)

pophysis, and the sensory epithelium of the eye, ear, and nose)

- *Neural crest* and its derivatives (components of the peripheral nervous system, including ganglia, nerves, and glial cells; medullary cells of the adrenal gland; the ***amine precursor uptake and decarboxylation (APUD)*** cells of the diffuse neuroendocrine system; melanoblasts, the precursors of melanocytes; and the mesenchyme of the head and its epithelial derivatives, such as corneal endothelium and vascular endothelium)

Mesodermal Derivatives

Mesoderm gives rise to

- *Epithelium* of the kidney and the gonads
- *Mesothelium,* the epithelium lining the pericardial, pleural, and peritoneal cavities
- *Endothelium,* the epithelium lining the cardiovascular and lymphatic vessels
- *Adrenal cortex*
- *Seminiferous and genital duct epithelium*

Many of the more atypical epithelia arise from mesoderm. For example, the adrenocortical cells of the adrenal gland, the Leydig cells of the testis, and the lutein cells of the ovary, all of which are endocrine components, lack a free surface, which is not characteristic of most epithelia. These secretory cells, which are derived from progenitor mesenchymal cells (nondifferentiated cells of embryonic origin found in connective tissue), are referred to as epithelioid. Although the progenitor cells of these epithelioid tissues may have arisen from a free surface or the immature cells may have had a free surface at some time during development, the mature cells lack a surface location or surface connection. Endothelium and mesothelium also differ from epithelia derived from the other two germ layers, in that they have no continuity or communication with the exterior of the body.

Endodermal Derivatives

Endoderm (or entoderm) gives rise to

- *Respiratory system epithelium*
- *Alimentary canal epithelium* (excluding the epithelium of the oral cavity and anal region, which are of ectodermal origin)
- *Extramural digestive gland epithelium,* e.g., the liver, pancreas, and gallbladder
- *Thyroid, parathyroid,* and *thymus gland* epithelial components
- Lining *epithelium of the tympanic cavity* and *auditory (Eustachian) tubes*

Thyroid and parathyroid glands develop as epithelial outgrowths from the floor and walls of the pharynx; they then lose their attachments from these sites of original outgrowth. As an epithelial outgrowth of the pharyngeal wall, the thymus grows into the mediastinum and also loses its original connection. Figure 4.30 (see page 115) summarizes the derivatives of the three germ layers.

▼ EPITHELIAL CELL RENEWAL

Most epithelial cells have a finite life span less than that of the whole organism

Surface epithelia and epithelia of many simple glands belong to the category of continuously renewing cell populations. The rate of cell turnover, i.e., the replacement rate, is characteristic of a specific epithelium. For example, the cells lining the small intestine are renewed every 4 to 6 days in humans. The replacement cells are produced by mitotic activity in the lower portion of the intestinal glands (crypts) (Fig. 4.31). They then migrate

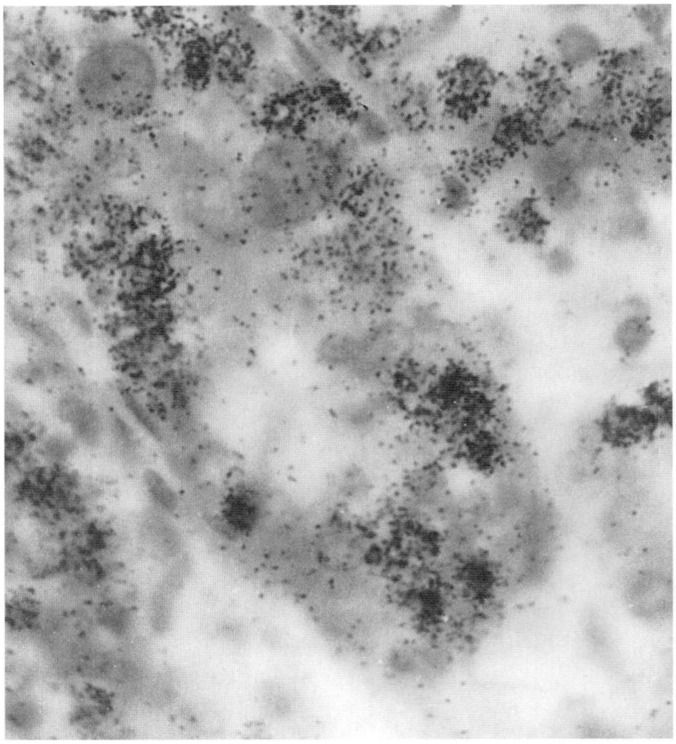

FIGURE 4.31
Autoradiograph of intestinal gland (crypt). Autoradiograph of crypts in the jejunum of a rabbit that had been injected with tritiated thymidine 8 hours prior to death and fixation. Nearly all of the epithelial cells in this replicative zone of the intestinal mucosa are labeled, indicating that they were synthesizing DNA at the time the animal was injected. ×600. (From Parker FG, Barnes EN, Kaye GI. *Gastroenterology* 1974;67:607–621.)

along the villi to the surface of the intestinal lumen. The migration of these new cells continues until they reach the tips of the villi, where they undergo apoptosis and slough off into the lumen.

Similarly, the stratified squamous epithelium of skin is replaced in most sites over a period of approximately 28 days. Cells in the basal layer of the epidermis, appropriately named the ***stratum basale (germinativum),*** undergo mitosis to provide for cell renewal. As these cells differentiate, they are pushed toward the surface by new cells in the basal layer. Ultimately, the cells become keratinized and slough off. In both of the above examples, a steady state is maintained within the epithelium, with new cells normally replacing exfoliated cells at the same rate.

In other epithelia, particularly in more complex glands, individual cells may live for a long time, and cell division is rare after the mature state is reached. These epithelial cells are characteristic of stable cell populations in which relatively little mitotic activity occurs, such as in liver. However, loss of significant amounts of liver tissue through physical trauma or acute toxic destruction is accommodated by active proliferation of undamaged liver cells. The liver tissue is essentially restored by the stimulated mitotic activity of healthy liver tissue.

BOX 4.3

Functional Considerations: Mucous and Serous Membranes

In two general locations, surface epithelium and its underlying connective tissue are regarded as a functional unit called a ***membrane.*** The two types of membrane are mucous membrane and serous membrane. The term "membrane" as used here should not be confused with the biologic membranes of cells, nor should the designations "mucous" and "serous" be confused with the nature of the gland secretion as discussed above.

Mucous membrane, also called **mucosa,** lines those cavities that connect with the outside of the body, namely, the alimentary canal, the respiratory tract, and the genitourinary tract. It consists of surface epithelium (with or without glands), a supporting connective tissue called the ***lamina propria,*** a basement membrane separating the epithelium from the lamina propria, and sometimes a layer of smooth muscle called the ***muscularis mucosae*** as the deepest layer.

Serous membrane, also called ***serosa,*** lines the peritoneal, pericardial, and pleural cavities. These cavities are usually described as closed cavities of the body, although in the female the peritoneal cavity communicates with the exterior via the genital tract. Structurally, the serosa consists of a lining epithelium, the ***mesothelium,*** a supporting connective tissue, and a basement membrane between the two. Serous membranes do not contain glands, but the fluid on their surface is watery.

TABLE 4.4. **Summary of Junctional Features**

Type	Classification	Major Link Proteins	Extracellular Ligands	Cytoskeleton Components	Associated Intracellular Attachment Proteins	Functions
Occluding Junction *(cell-to-cell)*	Zonula occludens (tight junction) 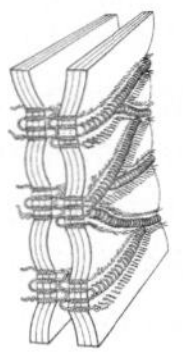	Occludins	Occludins in adjacent cell	Actin filaments	ZO-1, ZO-2, ZO-3	Seals adjacent cells together to inhibit passage of molecules between them (control of permeability)
Anchoring Junctions *(cell-to-cell)*	Zonula adherens 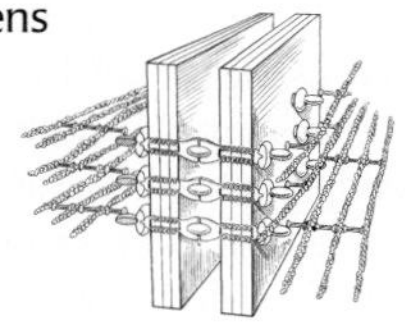	E-cadherin–catenin complex	E-cadherin–catenin complex in adjacent cell	Actin filaments	α-Actinin, vinculin	Couples the actin cytoskeleton to the plasma membrane at regions of cell-cell adhesion
	Macula adherens (desmosome) 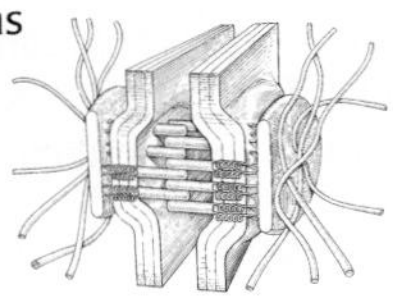	Cadherins (e.g., desmogleins, desmocollins)	Desmogleins, desmocollins in adjacent cell	Intermediate filaments	Desmoplakins, plakoglobins	Couples the intermediate filaments to the plasma membrane at regions of cell-cell adhesion
Anchoring Junctions *(cell-to-extracellular matrix)*	Focal adhesion 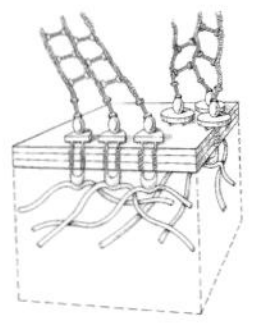	Integrins	Extracellular matrix proteins (e.g., fibronectin)	Actin filaments	Vinculin, talin, α-actinin	Anchors the actin cytoskeleton to the extracellular matrix
	Hemidesmosome 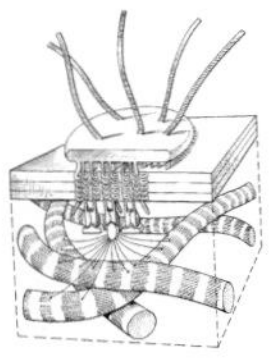	Integrins	Extracellular matrix protein (e.g., laminin 5, collagen IV)	Intermediate filaments	Desmoplakin-like proteins, collagen XVII	Anchors the intermediate filaments to the extracellular matrix
Communicating Junction *(cell-to-cell)*	Gap junction (nexus) 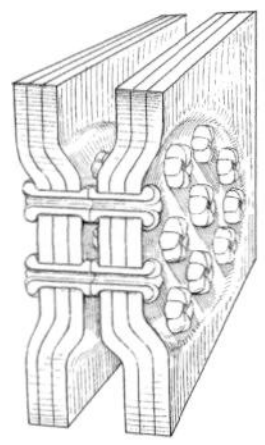	Connexin	Connexin in adjacent cell	None	Not known	Creates a conduit between two adjacent cells for passage of small ions and informational micromolecules

PLATE 1. SIMPLE SQUAMOUS AND CUBOIDAL EPITHELIA

Selected examples of epithelia characteristic of different organs are presented here and on the next several pages. For each example, note the shape and arrangement of the epithelial cells, the number of layers of cells, the location of their free surfaces, the shape of the cells at the free surface, and the location of the underlying or adjacent connective tissue. Remember that the morphologic characteristics of an epithelium are directly related to its functions in protection, secretion, absorption, or transport.

Figure 1, intestine, monkey, H&E ×640.

This shows the ***simple squamous epithelium*** (mesothelium) covering the outer surface of the intestine. The epithelium overlies a well-defined layer of connective tissue *(CT)* containing several small blood vessels *(BV);* deeper is a layer of smooth muscle *(SM).* The epithelial cells are very flat, as judged by the shape of their nuclei *(N).* Note that cell boundaries are not evident and the nuclei are unevenly spaced. The uneven spacing is because the sectioning knife passes through some cells without including the nucleus. This phenomenon can be understood better and visualized more easily in a nonsectioned (whole mount), silver-impregnated preparation of a piece of a very thin mesentery (the structure that holds the intestines in place), as in Figure 2.

Figure 2, mesentery, monkey, silver ×640.

The mesentery is lying on the slide, and the microscope is focused on its upper surface to reveal the surface epithelial cells. Cell boundaries are revealed by a deposition of reduced silver along the intercellular spaces. The nuclei *(N)* appear oval or round when viewed from the surface, as opposed to flat or elongate when seen on edge, as in a section. If one were to draw a line representing a knife cut across the cells as revealed in this figure, it would be possible to envision why the epithelial nuclei are unevenly spaced in sectioned material; the knife would pass through the cytoplasm of each cell but would not necessarily cut across the nucleus of each cell. Some of the more ovoid nuclei in the preparation belong to fibroblasts *(F)* in the underlying connective tissue. Because of the thinness of the mesentery, they are in the same focal plane as the epithelial cells and are thus superimposed.

Figure 3, kidney, human, H&E ×640.

This micrograph, another example of a ***simple squamous epithelium,*** reveals a sectioned renal corpuscle and adjacent kidney tubules. The renal corpuscle consists of a special capillary bed, the glomerulus, that is enclosed by Bowman's capsule, part of which (the visceral layer) is directly adjacent to the capillaries and part of which (the parietal layer) forms a thin-walled spherical structure composed of simple squamous epithelium. The nuclei *(N)* of the cells forming the parietal layer appear as flattened bodies that show the same uneven spacing as in Figure 1. The free surface of the epithelium faces Bowman's space *(B).* The cross sections of tubules, marked with *asterisks* (lower left), provide a good example of a ***simple cuboidal epithelium.*** Although the cell boundaries are not evident, one can judge that the height of each cell approximates its width by the spacing of the nuclei. Thus, it is a cuboidal epithelium.

Figure 4, ovary, monkey, H&E ×640.

This example of a ***simple cuboidal epithelium*** *(Ep)* shows the cells that cover the surface of the ovary. The epithelium rests on a highly cellular connective tissue *(CT).* The surface epithelial cells are approximately square or cuboidal in three dimensions. The free surfaces of these cells face the abdominal cavity and are a modification of the simple squamous epithelium or mesothelium shown in Figures 1 and 2.

Figure 5, liver, human, H&E ×400.

These cells also approximate a cube, but they are arranged in sheets separated by blood vessels *(BV)* called sinusoids. The epithelium is unusual, in that several surfaces of the cell possess a groove that represents the free surface. Where a grooved surface is present on one cell, the adjoining cell possesses a mirror-imaged grooved surface. The opposing grooves form a small lumen or *canaliculus* through which the bile produced by the cells reaches a bile duct. The canaliculi are not visible at this magnification but are located at the points of the *arrows* (see bile canaliculus, Plate 62).

KEY

AV, arteriole, vessel supplying glomerulus
B, Bowman's space
BV, blood vessel
CT, connective tissue
Ep, epithelium
F, fibroblast nucleus
N, nucleus
SM, smooth muscle
arrows, site of bile canaliculus
asterisk, tubule possessing simple cuboidal epithelium

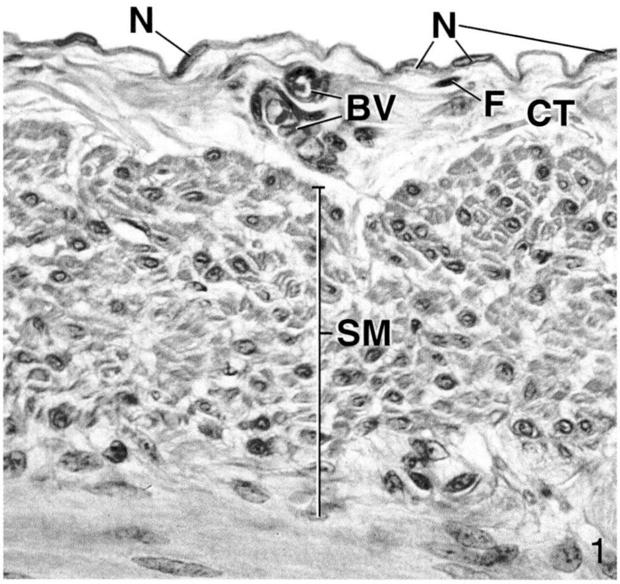
N
N
BV
F
CT
SM
1

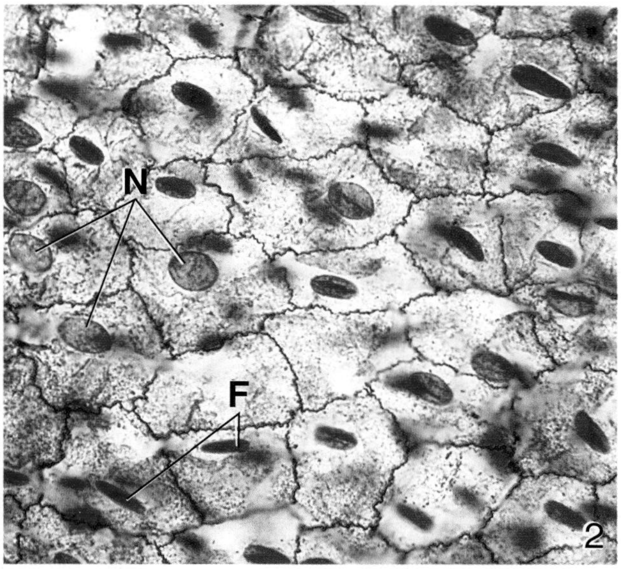
N
F
2

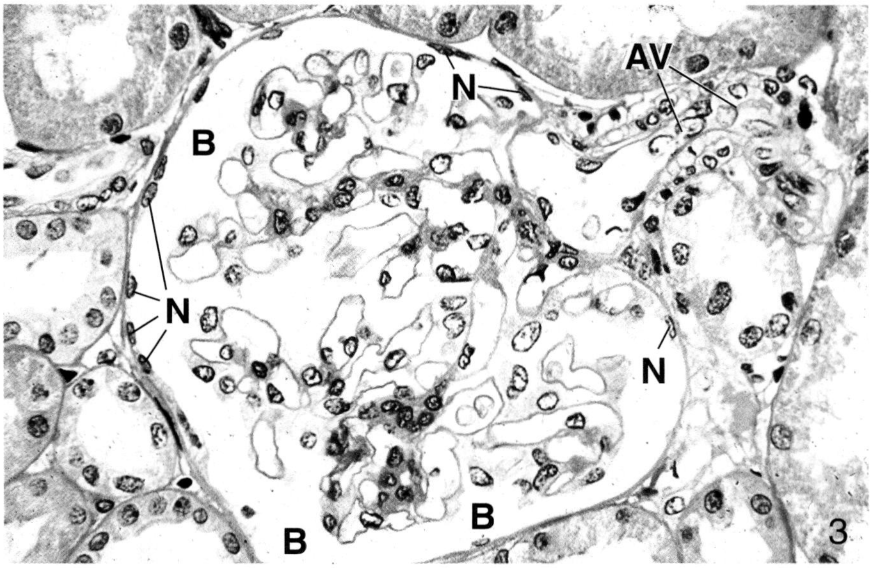
AV
N
B
N
N
B
B
3

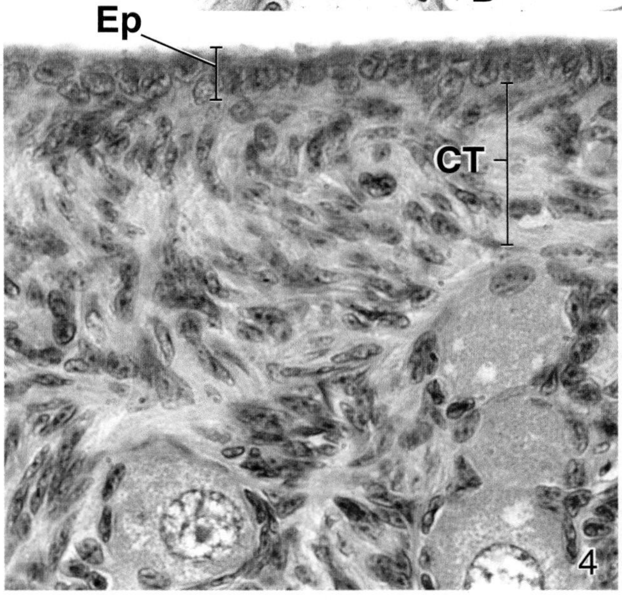
Ep
CT
4

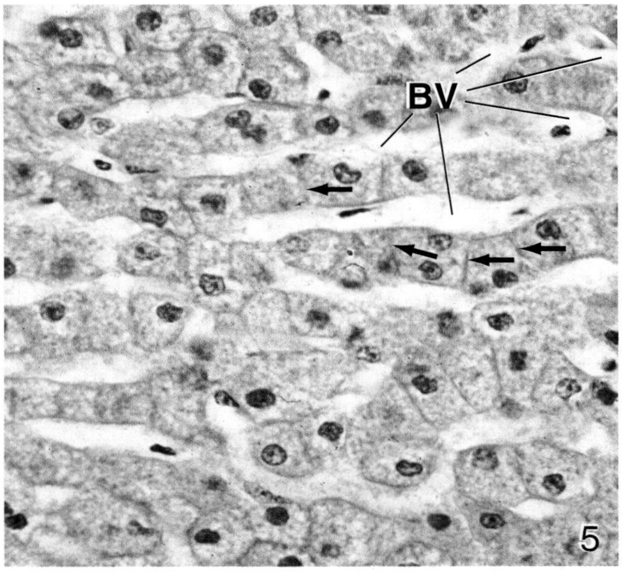
BV
5

PLATE 2. SIMPLE AND STRATIFIED EPITHELIA

Simple epithelia are only one cell layer thick. They are characteristic of organs and organ systems primarily concerned with transport, absorption, and secretion, such as the intestine, the vascular system, the digestive glands and other exocrine glands, and the kidney. Stratified epithelia have more than one layer and are typical of surfaces that are subject to frictional stress, such as skin, oral mucosa and esophagus, and vagina.

Figure 1, exocrine pancreas, monkey, H&E ×450.
This shows three epithelial forms. In the *circle* is a well-oriented acinus, a functional group of secretory cells, each of which is pyramidal in shape. The secretory cells form a spherical or tubular structure. The free surface of the cells and the lumen are located in the center of the *circle.* The lumen is not evident here but is evident in a similar cell arrangement in Figure 4 (see *circle).* Because the height of the cells (the distance from the edge of the *circle* to the lumen) is greater than the width, the epithelium is ***simple columnar.*** The second epithelial type is represented by a small, longitudinally sectioned duct *(arrows)* extending across the field. It is composed of flattened cells (note the nuclear shape), and on this basis, the epithelium is ***simple squamous.*** Finally, there is a larger cross-sectioned duct *(asterisk)* into which the smaller duct enters. The nuclei of this larger duct tend to be round, and the cells tend to be square in profile. Thus, these duct cells are a ***simple cuboidal epithelium.***

Figure 2, kidney, human, H&E ×450.
This section shows cross-sectioned tubules of several types. Those that are labeled with the *arrows* provide another example of a simple cuboidal epithelium. The *arrows* point to the lateral cell boundaries; note that cell width approximates cell height. The cross-sectioned structures marked with *asterisks* are another type of tubule; they are smaller in diameter but are also composed of a simple cuboidal epithelium.

Figure 3, colon, human, H&E ×350.
The simple columnar lining epithelium of the colon shown here consists of a single layer of absorptive cells and mucus-secreting cells (goblet cells). The latter can be recognized by the light staining "goblet" *(arrows)* that contains the cell's secretory product. The epithelium lines the lumen of the colon and extends down into the connective tissue to form the intestinal glands *(GL).* Both cell types are tall with their nuclei located at the base of the cell. The connective tissue *(CT)* contains numerous cells, many of which are lymphocytes and plasma cells.

Figure 4, trachea, monkey, H&E ×450.
In addition to the tall columnar cells *(CC)* in this columnar epithelium, there is a definite layer of basal cells *(BC).* The columnar cells, which contain elongate nuclei and possess cilia *(C),* extend from the surface to the basement membrane (clearly visible in the trachea as a thick, acellular, homogeneous region that is part of the connective tissue *(CT)*). The basal cells are interspersed between the columnar cells. Because all of the cells rest on the basement membrane, they are regarded as a single layer, as opposed to two discrete layers, one over the other. Because the epithelium appears to be stratified but is not, it is called ***pseudostratified columnar epithelium.*** The *circle* in the micrograph delineates a tracheal gland similar to the acinus in Figure 1 *(circle).* Note that the lumen of the gland is clearly visible and the cell boundaries are also evident. The gland epithelium is simple columnar.

Figure 5, epididymis, human, H&E ×450.
This is another example of pseudostratified columnar epithelium. Again, two layers of nuclei are evident, those of basal cells *(BC)* and those of columnar cells *(CC).* As in the previous example, however, although not evident, the columnar cells rest on the basement membrane; thus, the epithelium is pseudostratified. Note that where the epithelium is vertically oriented, on the right of the micrograph, there appear to be more nuclei, and the epithelium is thicker. This is a result of a tangential plane of section. As a rule, always examine the thinnest area of an epithelium to visualize its true organization.

Figure 6, vagina, human, H&E ×225.
This is the ***stratified squamous epithelium*** of the vaginal wall. The deeper cells, particularly those of the basal layer, are small, with little cytoplasm, and thus the nuclei appear closely packed. As the cells become larger, they tend to flatten out, forming disk-like squames. Because the surface cells retain this shape, the epithelium is called stratified squamous.

KEY

BC, basal cell
C, cilia
CC, columnar cell
CT, connective tissue
GL, intestinal gland
arrows: Fig. 1, tubule composed of simple squamous epithelium; Fig. 2, lateral boundaries of cuboidal tubule cells; Fig. 3, mucus cups of goblet cells
asterisk, duct or tubule of simple cuboidal epithelium

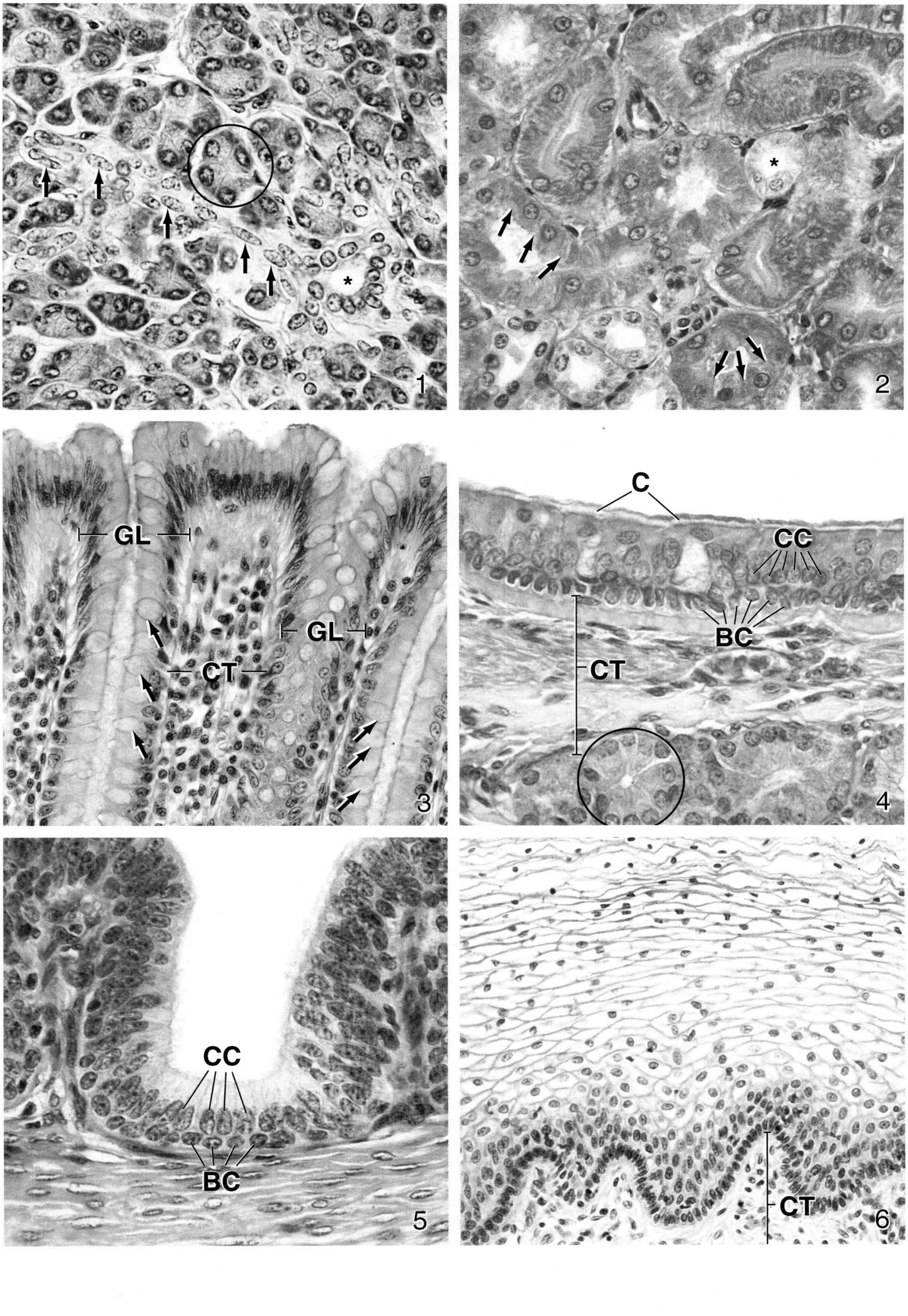
1
2
GL
GL
CT
3
C
CC
BC
CT
4
CC
BC
5
CT
6

PLATE 3. STRATIFIED EPITHELIA AND EPITHELIOID TISSUES

Tissues that resemble epithelia but lack the characteristic free surface are designated epithelioid tissues. This is the characteristic structure of the endocrine organs, which develop from typical epithelia but lose their connection to a surface during development.

Figure 1, esophagus, monkey, H&E ×250.
This part of the wall of the esophagus reveals two different epithelia. On the left is the lining epithelium of the esophagus. It is multilayered with squamous surface cells; therefore, it is a ***stratified squamous epithelium*** *(SS)*. On the right is the duct of an esophageal gland cut in several planes. By examining a region where the plane of section is at a right angle to the surface, the true character of the epithelium becomes apparent. In this case, the epithelium consists of two cell layers with cuboidal surface cells; thus, it is ***stratified cuboidal epithelium*** *(SC)*.

Figure 2, skin, human, H&E ×450.
This shows a portion of the duct of a sweat gland just before the duct enters the stratified squamous epithelium *(SS)* of the skin. The *dashed line* traces the duct within the epidermis. This duct also consists of a stratified cuboidal epithelium *(SC)* in two layers; the cells of the inner layer (the surface cells) appear more or less square. Because the epidermal surface cells are not included in the field, the designation stratified squamous cannot be derived from the information offered by the micrograph.

Figure 3, anorectal junction, human, H&E ×300.
The area shown here is the terminal part of the intestine. The luminal epithelium on the left is typical simple columnar *(SCol)* epithelium of the colon. This epithelium undergoes an abrupt transition *(arrowhead)* to a stratified cuboidal epithelium *(StCu)* at the anal canal. Note the general cuboidal shape of most of the surface cells *(arrows)* and the underlying layers of cells. The simple columnar epithelium on the left is part of an intestinal gland that is continuous with the simple columnar epithelium at the intestinal luminal surface. The connective tissue *(CT)* at this site is heavily infiltrated with lymphocytes, giving it an appearance unlike the connective tissue of other specimens on this page.

Figure 4, urinary bladder, monkey, H&E ×400.
The epithelium of the urinary bladder is called ***transitional epithelium,*** a stratified epithelium that changes in appearance according to the degree of distension of the bladder. In the nondistended state, as here, it is about four or five cells deep. The surface cells are large and dome shaped *(asterisks)*. The cells immediately under the surface cells are pear shaped and slightly smaller. The deepest cells are the smallest, and their nuclei appear more crowded. When the bladder is distended, the superficial cells are stretched into squamous cells, and the epithelium is reduced in thickness to about three cells deep. The bladder wall usually contracts when it is removed, unless special steps are taken to preserve it in a distended state. Thus, its appearance is usually like that in Figure 4.

Figure 5, testis, monkey, H&E ×350.
This shows the interstitial (Leydig) cells of the testis. These cells possess certain epithelial characteristics. They do not possess a free surface, however, nor do they develop from a surface; instead, they develop from mesenchymal cells. They are referred to as ***epithelioid cells*** because they contact similar neighboring cells much the same as epithelial cells contact each other. Leydig cells are endocrine in nature.

Figure 6, endocrine pancreas, human, H&E ×450.
Cells of the endocrine islet (of Langerhans) *(En)* of the pancreas also have an epithelioid arrangement. The cells are in contact but lack a free surface, although they have developed from an epithelial surface by invagination. In contrast, the surrounding alveoli of the exocrine pancreas *(Ex),* which developed from the same epithelial surface, are made up of cells with a free surface onto which the secretory product is discharged. Capillaries *(C)* are prominent in endocrine tissues. Similar examples of epithelioid tissue are seen in the adrenal and the parathyroid and pituitary glands, all of which are endocrine glands.

KEY

C, capillary
CT, connective tissue
En, endocrine cells
Ex, exocrine cells
IC, interstitial (Leydig) cells
SC, stratified cuboidal epithelium
SCol, stratified columnar epithelium
SS, stratified squamous epithelium
StCu, stratified cuboidal epithelium
arrowhead, transition site of simple stratified epithelium to stratified cuboidal
arrows, surface cuboidal cells
asterisks, dome-shaped cells

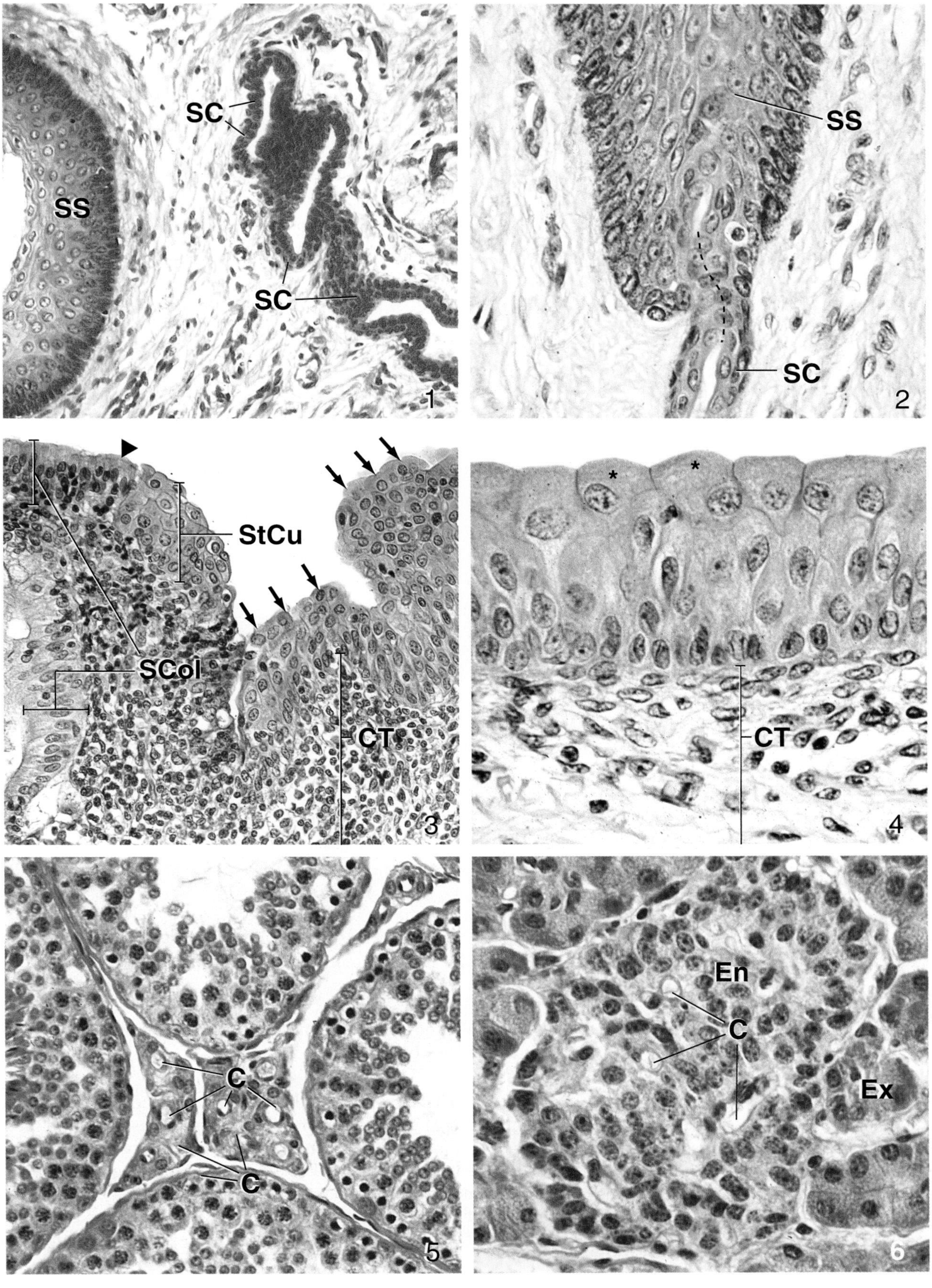
SC
SS
SC
1
SS
SC
2
StCu
SCol
CT
3
*
*
CT
4
C
C
5
En
C
Ex
6

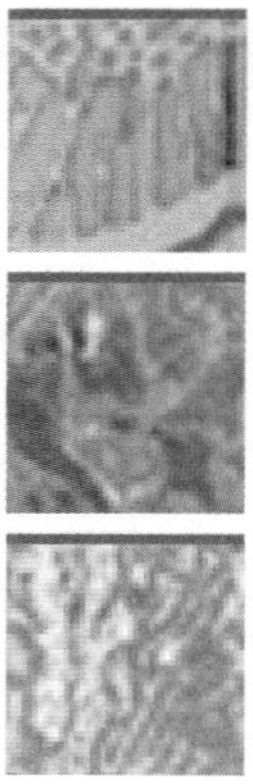

5

Connective Tissue

GENERAL STRUCTURE AND FUNCTION OF CONNECTIVE TISSUE

Connective tissue comprises a diverse group of cells embedded in a tissue-specific extracellular matrix

In general, ***connective tissue*** consists of cells and an ***extracellular matrix*** that includes fibers, ground substance, and tissue fluid. It forms a vast and continuous compartment throughout the body, bounded by basal laminae of the various epithelia and by the basal or external lamina of muscle cells and nerve supporting cells.

Different types of connective tissue are responsible for a variety of functions

The functions of the various connective tissues are reflected in the types of cells and fibers present within the tissue and the character of the ground substance in the extracellular matrix. For example, in loose connective tissue, many different cell types are present (Fig. 5.1). One type, the fibroblast, produces the extracellular fibers that serve a structural role in the tissue. They also produce and maintain the ground substance. Other cell types, such as lym-

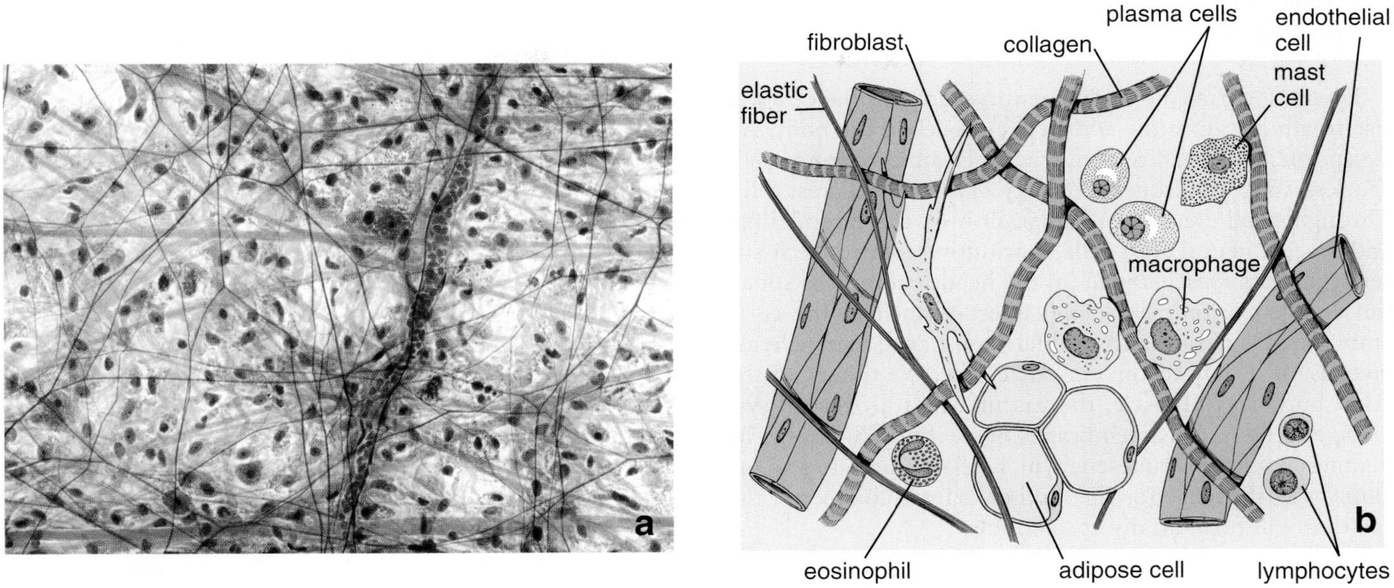

FIGURE 5.1
Loose connective tissue. a. Photomicrograph of a mesentery spread stained with Verhoeff's hematoxylin to show nuclei and elastic fibers, counterstained with safranin for identification of mast cell granules and with orange G for identification of other proteins (mainly collagen fibers). The elastic fibers appear as blue-black, thin, long, and branching threads without discernable beginnings or endings. Collagen fibers appear as orange-stained, long, straight profiles and are considerably thicker than the elastic fibers. Most of the visible nuclei are presumed to be those of fibroblasts. Nuclei of other cell types, i.e., lymphocytes, plasma cells, and macrophages, are also present but are not identifiable. Mast cells are identified by the bright reddish granules within their cytoplasm. Note the presence of the small blood vessel filled with red blood cells. ×150. **b.** Schematic diagram illustrating the components of loose connective tissue. Note the association of different cell types with the surrounding extracellular matrix, which contains blood vessels and different types of fibers.

phocytes, plasma cells, macrophages, and eosinophils, are associated with the body's defense system; they function within the ground substance of the tissue. In contrast, bone tissue, another form of connective tissue, contains only a single cell type, the osteocyte. This cell produces the fibers that make up the bulk of bone tissue. A unique feature of bone is that its fibers are organized in a specific pattern and become calcified to create the hardness associated with this tissue. Similarly, in tendons and ligaments, fibers are the prominent feature of the tissue. These fibers are arranged in parallel array and are densely packed to impart maximum strength.

Classification of connective tissue is based on the composition and organization of its cellular and extracellular components and on its functions

The term ***connective tissue*** includes a variety of tissues with differing functional properties but with certain common characteristics that allow them to be grouped together. For convenience they are classified in a manner that reflects these features. Table 5.1 provides a classification including subtypes of the principal connective tissues.

TABLE 5.1. **Classification of Connective Tissue**

Embryonic connective tissue
Mesenchyme
Mucous connective tissue

Connective tissue proper
Loose connective tissue
Dense connective tissue
  Irregular
  Regular

Specialized connective tissue[A]
Adipose tissue (Chapter 6)
Blood (Chapter 9)
Bone (Chapter 8)
Cartilage (Chapter 7)
Hemopoietic tissue (Chapter 9)
Lymphatic tissue (Chapter 13)

[A]In the past, the designations elastic tissue and reticular tissue have been listed as separate categories of specialized connective tissue. The tissues usually cited as examples of elastic tissue are certain ligaments associated with the spinal column and the tunica media of elastic arteries. The identifying feature of reticular tissue is the presence of reticular fibers and reticular cells together forming a three-dimensional stroma. Reticular tissue serves as the stroma for hemopoietic tissue (specifically the red bone marrow) and lymphatic tissue organs (lymph nodes and spleen, but not the thymus).

EMBRYONIC CONNECTIVE TISSUE

Embryonic mesenchyme gives rise to the various connective tissues of the body

The mesoderm, the middle embryonic germ layer, gives rise to almost all of the connective tissues of the body. An exception is the head region, where certain progenitor cells are derived from ectoderm by way of the neural crest cells. Through proliferation and migration of the mesodermal and specific neural crest cells, a primitive connective tissue referred to as ***mesenchyme*** (in the head region, it is sometimes called ***ectomesenchyme***) is established in the early embryo. Maturation and proliferation of the mesenchyme give rise not only to the various connective tissues of the adult but also to muscle, the vascular and urogenital systems, and the serous membranes of the body cavities. The manner in which the mesenchymal cells proliferate and organize sets the stage for the kind of mature connective tissue that will form at any specific site.

Embryonic connective tissue is present in the embryo and within the umbilical cord

Embryonic connective tissue is classified into two subtypes:

- ***Mesenchyme*** is primarily found in the embryo. It contains small, spindle-shaped cells of relatively uniform appearance (Fig. 5.2a). Processes extend from these cells and contact similar processes of neighboring cells, forming a three-dimensional cellular network. Gap junctions are present where the processes make contact. The extracellular space is occupied by a viscous ground substance. Collagen (reticular) fibers are present; they are very fine and relatively sparse. The paucity of collagen fibers is consistent with the limited physical stress on the growing fetus.
- ***Mucous connective tissue*** is present in the umbilical cord. It consists of a specialized, almost gelatin-like extracellular matrix whose ground substance is frequently referred to as ***Wharton's jelly.*** It occupies large intercellular spaces located between thin, wispy collagen fibers (Fig. 5.2b). The spindle-shaped cells contained in the matrix are widely separated and appear much like fibroblasts in the near-term umbilical cord, e.g., the cytoplasmic processes are thin and difficult to visualize in routine hematoxylin and eosin (H&E) preparations.

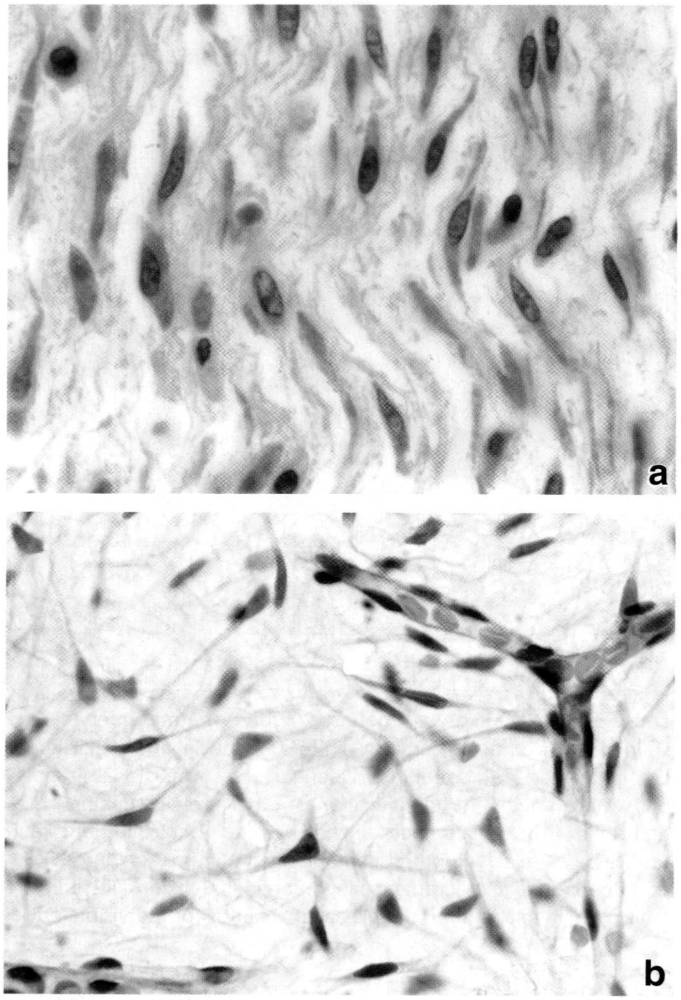

FIGURE 5.2
Embryonic connective tissue. a. Photomicrograph of mesenchymal tissue from a developing fetus stained with H&E. Although morphologically the mesenchymal cells appear as a homogeneous population, they will give rise to cells that differentiate into various cell types. Their cytoplasmic processes often give the cell a tapering or spindle appearance. The extracellular component of the tissue contains a sparse arrangement of reticular fibers and abundant ground substance. ×480. **b.** Photomicrograph of Wharton's jelly from the umbilical cord stained with H&E. Wharton's jelly consists of a specialized, almost gelatin-like ground substance that occupies large intercellular spaces located between the spindle-shaped mesenchymal cells. ×480.

CONNECTIVE TISSUE PROPER

Connective tissues that belong to this category are divided into two general subtypes:

- ***Loose connective tissue,*** also sometimes called ***areolar tissue***
- ***Dense connective tissue,*** which can be further subcategorized into two basic types based on the organization of its collagen fibers: ***dense irregular connective tissue*** and ***dense regular connective tissue***

Loose connective tissue is characterized by loosely arranged fibers and abundant cells

Loose connective tissue is a cellular connective tissue with thin and relatively sparse collagen fibers (Fig. 5.3).

The ground substance, however, is abundant; in fact, it occupies more volume than the fibers do. It has a viscous to gel-like consistency and plays an important role in the diffusion of oxygen and nutrients from the small vessels that course through this connective tissue as well as in the diffusion of carbon dioxide and metabolic wastes back to the vessels.

Loose connective tissue is primarily located beneath those epithelia that cover the body surfaces and line the internal surfaces of the body. It is also associated with the epithelium of glands and surrounds the smallest blood vessels. This tissue is thus the initial site where pathogenic agents, such as bacteria, that have breached an epithelial surface can be challenged and destroyed by cells of the immune system. Most cell types in loose connective tissue are transient wandering cells that migrate from local blood vessels in response to specific stimuli. This tissue is, therefore, the site of inflammatory and immune reactions. During these reactions, loose connective tissue can undergo considerable swelling. In areas of the body where foreign substances are continually present, large populations of defending cells are maintained. For example, the ***lamina propria,*** the loose connective tissue of mucous membranes, such as those of the respiratory and alimentary systems, contains large numbers of these cells.

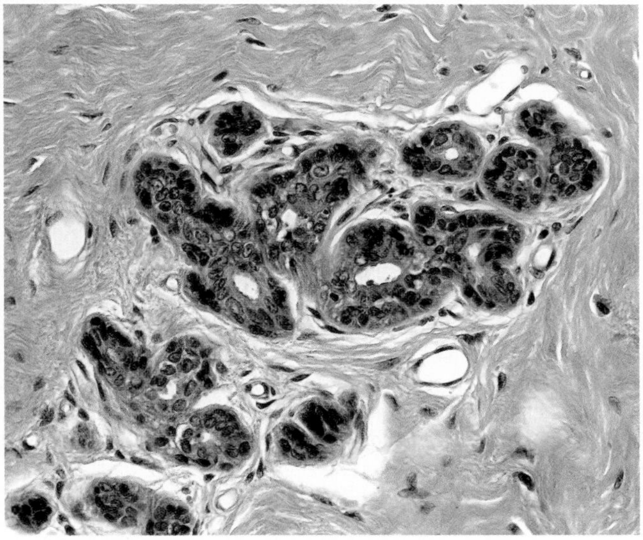

FIGURE 5.3
Loose and dense irregular connective tissue. Photomicrograph comparing loose and dense irregular connective tissue from the mammary gland stained with Masson's trichrome. In the center, loose connective tissue surrounds the glandular epithelium. The loose connective tissue is composed of a wispy arrangement of collagen fibers with many cells. Note the large number of nuclei visible at this low magnification. On the upper left and lower right of the figure is dense irregular connective tissue. In contrast, few nuclei are revealed in the dense connective tissue. However, collagen is considerably more abundant and is composed of very thick fibers. ×100.

Dense irregular connective tissue is characterized by abundant fibers and few cells

Dense irregular connective tissue contains mostly collagen fibers. Cells are sparse and are typically of a single type, the fibroblast. This tissue also contains relatively little ground substance. Because of its high proportion of collagen fibers, dense irregular connective tissue provides significant strength. Typically, the fibers are arranged in bundles oriented in various directions (thus the term "irregular") that can withstand stresses on organs or structures. Hollow organs (e.g., the intestinal tract) possess a distinct layer of dense irregular connective tissue, called the ***submucosa,*** in which the fiber bundles course in varying planes. This arrangement allows the organ to resist excessive stretching and distension. Similarly, skin contains a relatively thick layer of dense irregular connective tissue in the dermis, called the ***reticular*** or ***deep layer*** of the dermis. It provides resistance to tearing as a consequence of stretching forces from different directions.

Dense regular connective tissue is characterized by ordered and densely packed arrays of fibers and cells

Dense regular connective tissue is the main functional component of ***tendons, ligaments,*** and ***aponeuroses.*** As in dense irregular connective tissue, the fibers of dense regular connective tissue are the prominent feature, and there is little ground substance. However, in dense regular connective tissue, the fibers are arranged in parallel array and are densely packed to provide maximum strength. The cells that produce and maintain the fibers are packed and aligned between fiber bundles.

- ***Tendons*** are cord-like structures that attach muscle to bone. They consist of parallel bundles of collagen fibers. Situated between these bundles are rows of fibroblasts called ***tendinocytes*** (Fig. 5.4). In H&E–stained cross sections of tendon, the tendinocytes appear stellate. In transmission electron micrograph sections parallel to the long axis of tendons, the cytoplasmic projections of the cell are seen to lie between the fibers and appear as thin cytoplasmic sheets. In most H&E–stained longitudinal sections, however, tendinocytes appear only as rows of typically flattened basophilic nuclei. The cytoplasmic sheets that extend from the body of the tendinocytes are not usually evident in longitudinal H&E–stained sections because they blend in with the collagen fibers.
- The substance of the tendon is surrounded by a thin connective tissue capsule, the ***epitendineum,*** in which the collagen fibers are not nearly as orderly. Typically, the tendon is subdivided into fascicles by ***endotendineum,*** a connective tissue extension of the epi-

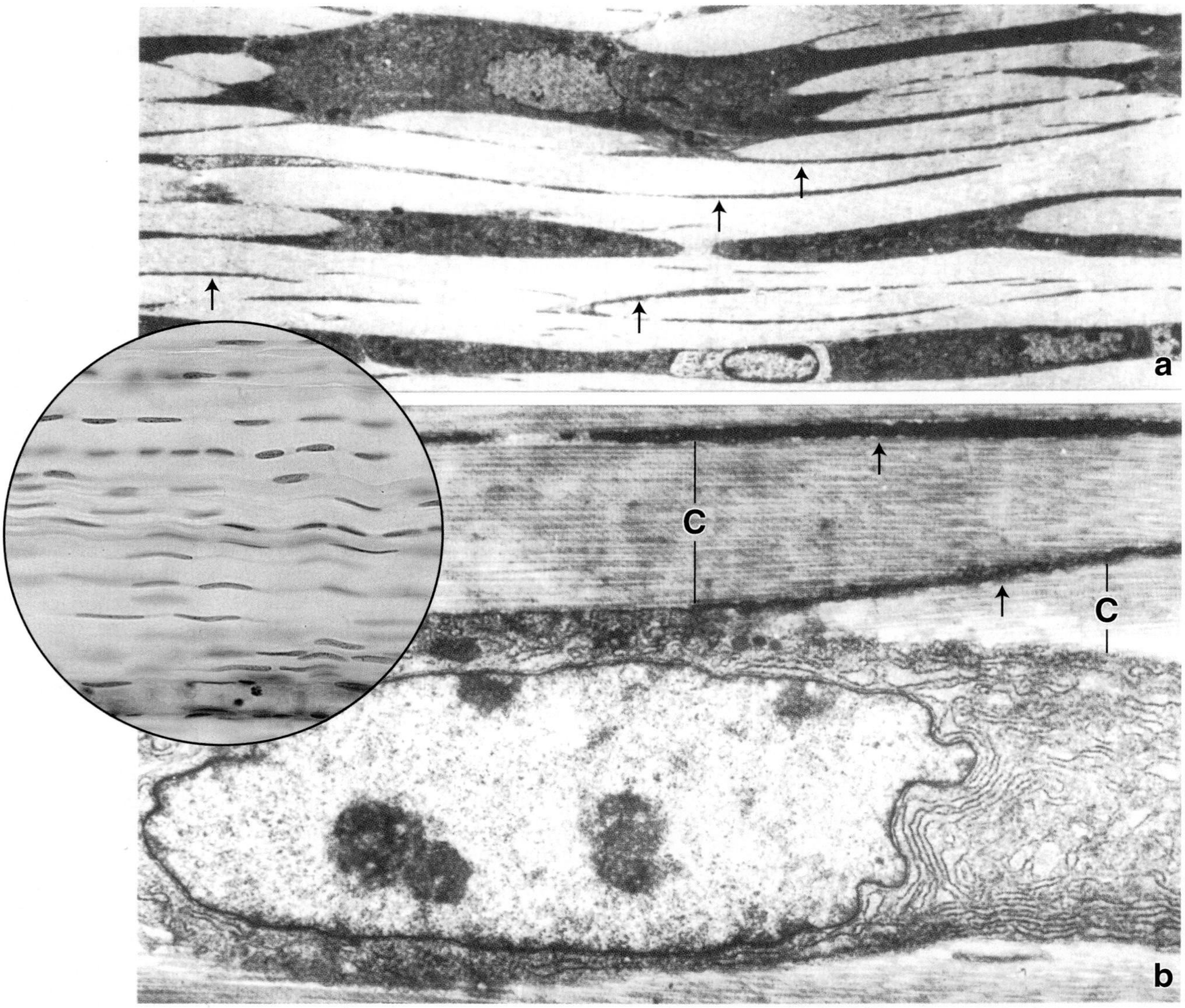

FIGURE 5.4

Dense regular connective tissue—tendon. a. Electron micrograph of a tendon at low magnification, showing tendinocytes (fibroblasts) and their thin processes (*arrows*) lying between the collagen bundles. ×1,600. **b.** A tendinocyte with prominent profiles of rough endoplasmic reticulum (rER) is shown at higher magnification. The collagen fibers (*C*) can be resolved as consisting of very tightly packed collagen fibrils. The *arrows* indicate processes of tendinocytes. ×9,500. **Inset.** Photomicrograph of a tendon. Note the orderly and regular alignment of the bundles of collagen fibers. Tendinocytes are aligned in rows between the collagen fibers. ×200. (Electron micrographs modified from Rhodin J. *Histology.* New York: Oxford University Press, 1974.)

tendineum. It contains the small blood vessels and nerves of the tendon.

- ***Ligaments,*** like tendons, consist of fibers and fibroblasts arranged in parallel. The fibers of ligaments, however, are less regularly arranged than those of tendons. Ligaments join bone to bone, which in some locations, such as in the spinal column, requires some elasticity. Although collagen is the major extracellular fiber of most ligaments, some of the ligaments associated with the spinal column (e.g., ligamenta flava) contain many elastic fibers and fewer collagen fibers. These ligaments are called ***elastic ligaments.***
- ***Aponeuroses*** resemble broad, flattened tendons. Instead of fibers lying in parallel arrays, the fibers of aponeuroses are arranged in multiple layers. The bundles of collagen fibers in one layer tend to be arranged at a 90° angle to those in the neighboring layers. The fibers within each of the layers are arranged in regular arrays; thus it is a dense regular connective tissue. This ***orthogonal ar-***

ray is also found in the cornea of the eye and is believed to be responsible for its transparency.

▼ CONNECTIVE TISSUE FIBERS

Connective tissue fibers are of three principal types

Connective tissue fibers are present in varying amounts, depending on the structural needs or function of the connective tissue. Each type of fiber is produced by fibroblasts and is composed of protein consisting of long peptide chains. The types of connective tissue fibers are

- *Collagen fibers*
- *Reticular fibers*
- *Elastic fibers*

Collagen Fibers and Fibrils

Collagen fibers are the most abundant type of connective tissue fiber

Collagen fibers are flexible and have a remarkably high tensile strength. In the light microscope, collagen fibers typically appear as wavy structures of variable width and indeterminate length. They stain readily with eosin and other acidic dyes. They can also be colored with the dye aniline blue, used in Mallory's connective tissue stain, or with the dye light green, used in Masson's stain.

When examined with the transmission electron microscope (TEM), collagen fibers appear as bundles of fine, thread-like subunits. These subunits are ***collagen fibrils*** (Fig. 5.5). Within an individual fiber, the collagen fibrils are relatively uniform in diameter. In different locations and at different stages of development, however, the fibrils differ in size. In developing or immature tissues, the fibrils may be as small as 15 or 20 nm in diameter. In dense regular connective tissue of tendons or other tissues that are subject to considerable stress, they may measure up to 300 nm in diameter.

Collagen fibrils have a 68-nm banding pattern

When collagen fibrils stained with osmium or other heavy metals are examined with the TEM, they exhibit a sequence of closely spaced transverse bands that repeat every 68 nm along the length of the fibril (Fig. 5.5, *inset*). This banding pattern reflects the fibril's subunit structure,

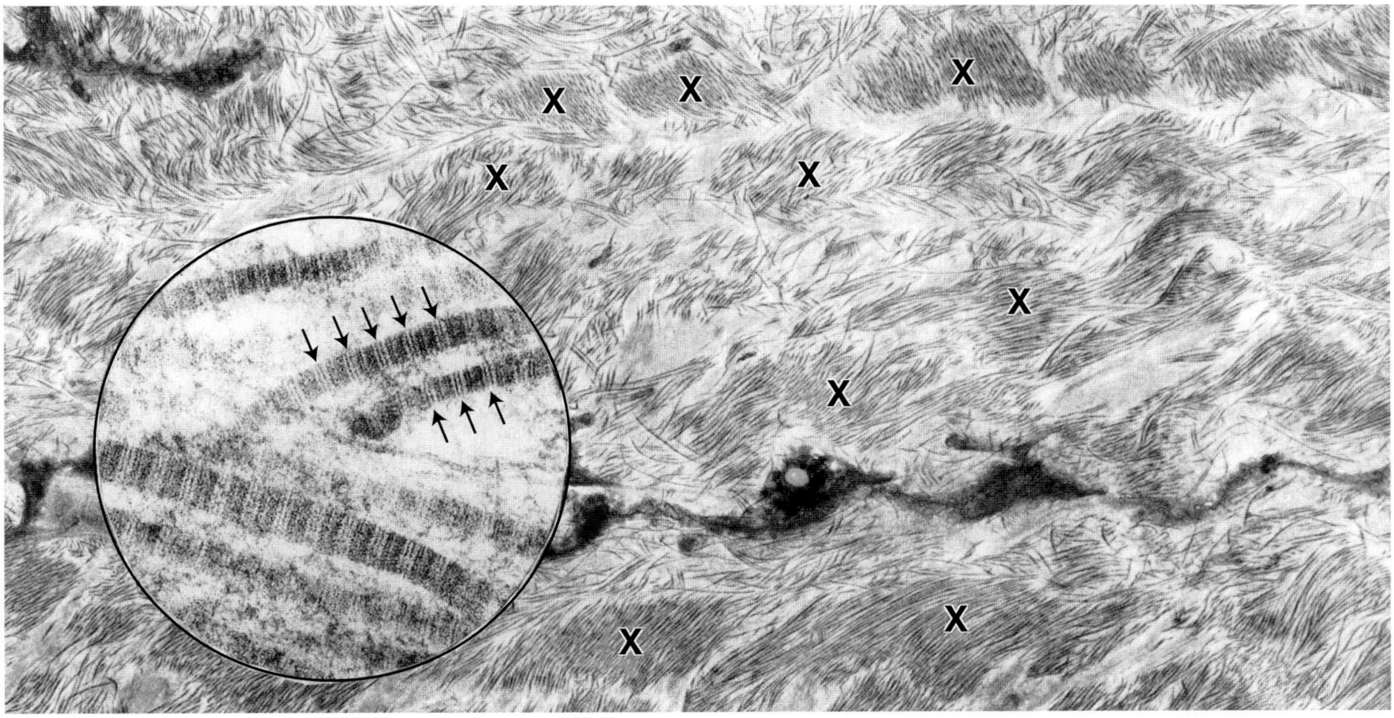

FIGURE 5.5
Collagen fibrils in dense irregular connective tissue. Electron micrograph of dense irregular connective tissue from the capsule of the testis of a young male. The thread-like collagen fibrils are aggregated in some areas (*X*) to form relatively thick bundles; in other areas, the fibrils are more dispersed. ×9,500. **Inset.** A longitudinal array of collagen fibrils from the same specimen seen at higher magnification. Note the banding pattern. The spacing of the *arrows* indicates the 68-nm repeat pattern. ×75,000.

specifically, the size and shape of the collagen molecule and the arrangement of the molecules that form the fibril (Fig. 5.6). The collagen molecule, also called ***tropocollagen,*** measures about 300 nm long by 1.5 nm thick, with a head and a tail. In forming a fibril, the collagen molecules align head to tail in overlapping rows with a gap between the molecules within each row and a one-quarter-molecule stagger between adjacent rows. The strength of the fibril is due to covalent bonds between the collagen molecules of adjacent rows, not to the head-to-tail attachment of the molecules in a row. The banding pattern observed with the TEM is caused largely by osmium deposition in the space between the heads and tails of the molecules in each row.

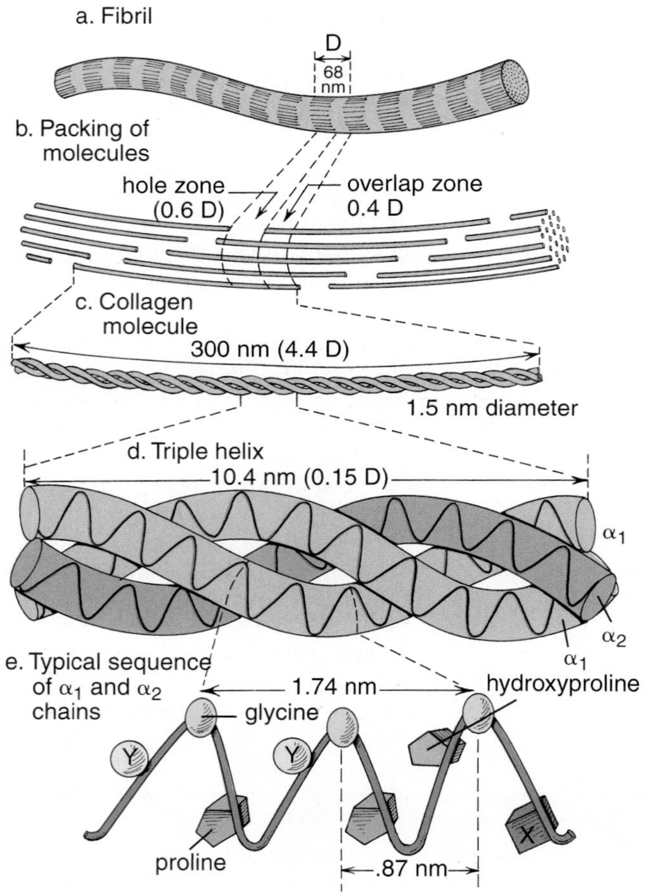

FIGURE 5.6
Diagram showing the molecular character of a type 1 collagen fibril in increasing order of structure. a. A collagen fibril displays periodic banding with a distance (D) of 68 nm between repeating bands. **b.** Each fibril is composed of staggered collagen molecules. **c.** Each molecule is about 300 nm long and 1.5 nm in diameter. **d.** The collagen molecule is a triple helix. **e.** The triple helix consists of three α chains. Every third amino acid of the α chain is a glycine. The X position following glycine is frequently a proline, and the Y position preceding the glycine is frequently a hydroxyproline.

Each collagen molecule is a triple helix composed of three intertwined polypeptide chains

A single collagen molecule consists of three polypeptides known as α ***chains.*** The α chains intertwine, forming a right-handed triple helix (Fig. 5.6d). Every third amino acid in the chain is a glycine molecule, except at the ends of the α chains. A hydroxyproline or hydroxylysine frequently precedes each glycine in the chain, and a proline frequently follows each glycine in the chain. Along with proline and hydroxyproline, the glycine is essential for the triple-helix conformation (Fig. 5.6e). Associated with the helix are sugar groups that are joined to hydroxylysyl residues. Because of these sugar groups, collagen is properly described as a ***glycoprotein.***

The α chains that constitute the helix are not all alike. They vary in size from 600 to 3,000 amino acids. To date, at least 27 types of α chains encoded by different genes have been identified. As many as 19 different types of collagens have been categorized on the basis of the combinations of α chains they contain. These various collagens are classified by Roman numerals I to XIX according to the chronology of their discovery.

For example, ***type I collagen*** is found in loose and dense connective tissue. Two of the α chains (α1) are identical, and one (α2) is different and identified as an α2 chain. Thus, in collagen nomenclature it is designated $[\alpha1(I)]_2\alpha2(I)$ (Table 5.2). ***Type II collagen*** is present in hyaline and elastic cartilage, where it occurs as very fine fibrils. The collagen molecules of type II collagen are composed of three identical α chains. Because these α chains differ from those of other collagens, type II collagen is designated $[\alpha1(II)]_3$.

Not only do the polypeptides of the various collagens differ, but the organization and arrangement of the molecules within the fibrils also differ. For example, the molecules of collagen types I, II, III, V, and XI aggregate to form 68-nm-banded fibrils (as diagramed in Fig. 5.6a). In contrast, ***type IV collagen*** forms a nonfibrillar network that provides structural cohesion to the basal lamina. Similarly, another nonfibrillar collagen, ***type IX collagen,*** binds and interacts with type II collagen of cartilage at the intersections of the fibrils. It serves to stabilize this tissue. Table 5.2 lists the collagens that have been characterized to date, including their structural variations and some of the roles presently ascribed to them.

Collagen fiber formation involves events that occur both within and outside the fibroblast

The production of fibrillar collagen (I, II, III, V, and XI) involves a series of events within the fibroblast that leads to production of ***procollagen,*** the precursor of the collagen molecule. These events take place in membrane-bounded organelles within the cell. Production of the actual fibril occurs outside the cell and involves enzymatic activity at the

TABLE 5.2. **Types of Collagen, Composition, Location, and Function**[A]

Type	Composition[B]	Location	Functions
I	$[\alpha1(I)]_2\alpha2(I)$	Connective tissue of skin, bone, tendon, ligaments, dentin, sclera, fascia, and organ capsules (accounts for 90% of body collagen)	Provides resistance to force, tension, and stretch
II	$[\alpha1(II)]_3$	Cartilage (hyaline and elastic), notochord, and intervertebral disc	Provides resistance to intermittent pressure
III	$[\alpha1(III)]_3$	Connective tissue of organs (uterus, liver, spleen, kidney, lung, etc.); smooth muscle; endoneurium; blood vessels; and fetal skin	Provides structural support and elasticity
IV	$[\alpha1(IV)]_2\alpha2(IV)$	Basal laminae of epithelia, kidney glomeruli, and lens capsule	Provides support and filtration barrier
V	$[\alpha1(V)]_2\alpha2(V)$ or $\alpha1(V)\alpha2(V)\alpha3(V)$	Distributed uniformly throughout connective tissue stroma; may be related to reticular network	Localized at the surface of type I collagen fibrils along with type XII and XIV collagen to modulate biomechanical properties of the fibril
VI	$[\alpha1(VI)]_2\alpha2(VI)$	Forms part of the cartilage matrix immediately surrounding the chondrocytes	Attaches the chondrocyte to the matrix
VII	$[\alpha1(VII)]_3$	Present in anchoring fibrils	Secures basal lamina to connective tissue fibers
VIII	$[\alpha1(VIII)]_2\alpha2(VIII)$	Product of endothelial cells	Facilitates movement of endothelial cells during angiogenesis
IX	$\alpha1(IX)\alpha2(IX)\alpha3(IX)$	Found in cartilage associated with type II collagen fibrils	Stabilizes network of cartilage type II collagen fibers by interaction with proteoglycan molecules at their intersections
X	$[\alpha1(X)]_3$	Produced by chondrocytes in the zone of hypertrophy of normal growth plate	Contributes to the bone mineralization process by forming hexagonal lattices necessary to arrange types II, IX, and XI collagen within cartilage.
XI	$[\alpha1(XI)]_2\alpha2(XI)$	Produced by chondrocytes; associated with type II collagen fibrils	Regulates size of type II collagen fibrils; it is essential for cohesive properties of cartilage matrix
XII	$[\alpha1(XII)]_3$	Isolated from skin and placenta; abundant in tissues where mechanical strain is high	Localized at the surface of type I collagen fibrils along with type V and XIV collagen to modulate biomechanical properties of the fibril
XIII	$[\alpha1(XIII)]_3$	An unusual transmembrane collagen detected in bone, cartilage, intestine, skin, placenta, and striated muscles	Associated with the basal lamina along with type VII collagen
XIV	$[\alpha1(XIV)]_3$	Isolated from placenta; also detected in the bone marrow	Localized at the surface of type I collagen fibrils along with type V and XII collagen to modulate biomechanical properties of the fibril; has a strong cell-cell binding property
XV	$[\alpha1(XV)]_3$	Present in tissues derived from mesenchyme	Involved in adhesion of basal lamina to the underlying connective tissue
XVI	$[\alpha1(XVI)]_3$	Localized in close association with fibroblasts and arterial smooth muscle cells, but not associated with type I collagen fibrils	Contributes to structural integrity of connective tissue
XVII	$[\alpha1(XVII)]_3$	Another unusual transmembrane collagen found in epithelial cell membranes	Interacts with integrins to stabilize hemidesmosome structure
XVIII	$[\alpha1(XVIII)]_3$	Found in epithelial and vascular basement membrane	Represents a basement membrane heparan sulfate proteoglycan thought to inhibit endothelial cell proliferation and angiogenesis
XIX	$[\alpha1(XIX)]_3$	Discovered from the sequence of rhabdomyosarcoma cDNA	The pronounced vascular and stromal interaction suggests involvement in angiogenesis

[A]Fibrillar collagens are indicated by blue type. Nonfibrillar collagens are indicated by black type.

[B]Each collagen molecule is composed of three polypeptide α chains intertwined in a helical configuration. The Roman numerals in the parentheses in the Composition column indicate that the α chains have a distinctive structure that differs from the chains with different numerals. Thus, collagen type I has two identical $\alpha1$ chains and one $\alpha2$ chain; collagen type II has three identical $\alpha1$ chains.

plasma membrane to produce the collagen molecule, followed by assembly of the molecules into fibrils in the extracellular matrix under guidance by the cell (Fig. 5.7).

Collagen synthesis involves a number of intracellular events

- *Polypeptide chains are produced by polyribosomes of the rough endoplasmic reticulum (rER).* This synthesis (translation) is directed by information provided by messenger RNA (mRNA), and newly synthesized polypeptides are simultaneously discharged into the cisternae of the rER.
- *Within the cisternae of the rER and the Golgi apparatus, a number of posttranslational modifications of the polypeptide chains occur.* These include

  1. Cleavage of the signal peptide
  2. Hydroxylation of proline and lysine residues while the polypeptides are still in the nonhelical conformation
  3. Addition of O-linked sugar groups to some hydroxylysine residues (glycosylation) and N-linked sugars to the two terminal positions
  4. Formation of a triple helix by three polypeptide chains, except at the terminals where the polypeptide chains remain uncoiled
  5. Formation of intrachain and interchain hydrogen bonds that influence the shape of the molecule and stabilize the interactions of the polypeptides.

  The resultant molecule is procollagen. Note that ascorbate (vitamin C) is required for the function of prolylhydroxylase and lysylhydroxylase; without posttranslational hydroxylation of proline and lysine, the hydrogen bonds essential to the final structure of the collagen molecule cannot form. This explains why wounds fail to heal and bone formation is impaired in vitamin C deficiency (scurvy).
- *The procollagen moves to the exterior of the cell by means of exocytosis of secretory vesicles.* Microtubules are involved in the movement of the secretory vesicles from the region of the Golgi apparatus to the cell surface. If the microtubules are disrupted with agents such as colchicine or vinblastine, the secretory vesicles accumulate in the Golgi region.

Collagen synthesis also involves extracellular events

- *As procollagen is secreted from the cell, it is converted to a collagen molecule by procollagen peptidase associated with the cell membrane, which cleaves the uncoiled ends of the molecule* (Fig. 5.8).
- *The aggregated collagen molecules then align to form the final collagen fibrils.* The cell controls the orderly array of the newly formed fibrils by directing the secretory vesicles to a localized surface site for discharge. The cell simultaneously creates a "cove" or indentation at its surface to allow molecules to concentrate where assembly will occur (see Fig. 5.7). Within the cove, the collagen fibril self-assembles: The collagen molecules align in rows and then cross-link by covalent bonds that form between the lysine and hydroxylysine aldehyde groups.

Reticular Fibers

Reticular fibers provide a supporting framework for the cellular constituents of various tissues and organs

Reticular fibers and collagen fibers share a prominent feature: They both consist of collagen fibrils. Unlike collagen fibers, however, reticular fibers are composed of type III collagen. The individual fibrils that constitute the reticular fiber exhibit a 68-nm banding pattern (the same as the fibrils of type I collagen). The fibrils have a narrow diameter (about 20 nm) and typically do not bundle to form thick fibers.

In routinely stained H&E preparations, reticular fibers cannot be identified positively. When visualized in the light microscope with special techniques, the reticular fibers have a thread-like appearance. Because they contain a greater relative content of sugar groups than collagen fibers, reticular fibers are readily displayed by means of the periodic acid–Schiff (PAS) reaction. They are also revealed with special silver-staining procedures, such as the Gomori and Wilder methods. After silver treatment, the fibers appear black; thus, they are said to be ***argyrophilic*** (Fig. 5.9). The thicker collagen fibers in such preparations are colored brown.

Reticular fibers are named for their arrangement in a mesh-like pattern or network

In loose connective tissue, networks of reticular fibers are found at the boundary of connective tissue and epithelium, as well as surrounding adipocytes, small blood vessels, nerves, and muscle cells. Reticular fibers also function as a supporting stroma in hemopoietic and lymphatic tissues (but not in the thymus). In these tissues, the collagen of the reticular fiber is produced by a special cell type, the ***reticular cell.*** This cell maintains a unique relationship to the fiber; it surrounds the fiber with its cytoplasm, thus isolating the fiber from other tissue components.

In most other locations, the reticular fiber is produced by fibroblasts. Important exceptions to this general rule include the endoneurium of peripheral nerves, where Schwann cells secrete reticular fibers, and the reticular and other collagen fibers secreted by smooth muscle cells of the tunica media of blood vessels and the muscularis of the alimentary canal.

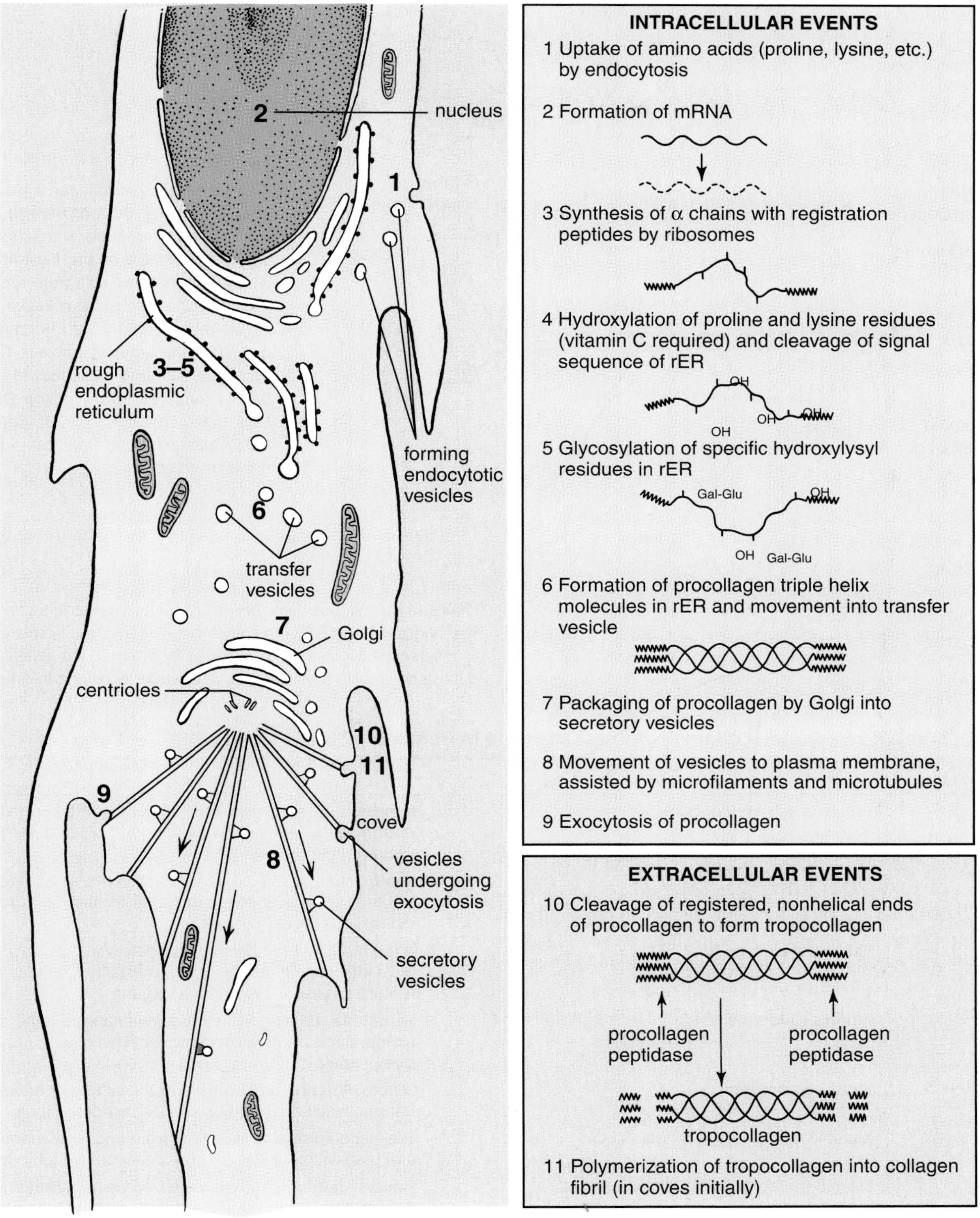

FIGURE 5.7

Collagen synthesis. Schematic representation of the biosynthetic events and organelles participating in collagen synthesis. *Bold numbers* within the cell diagram correspond to the events numbered in collagen production listed on the right.

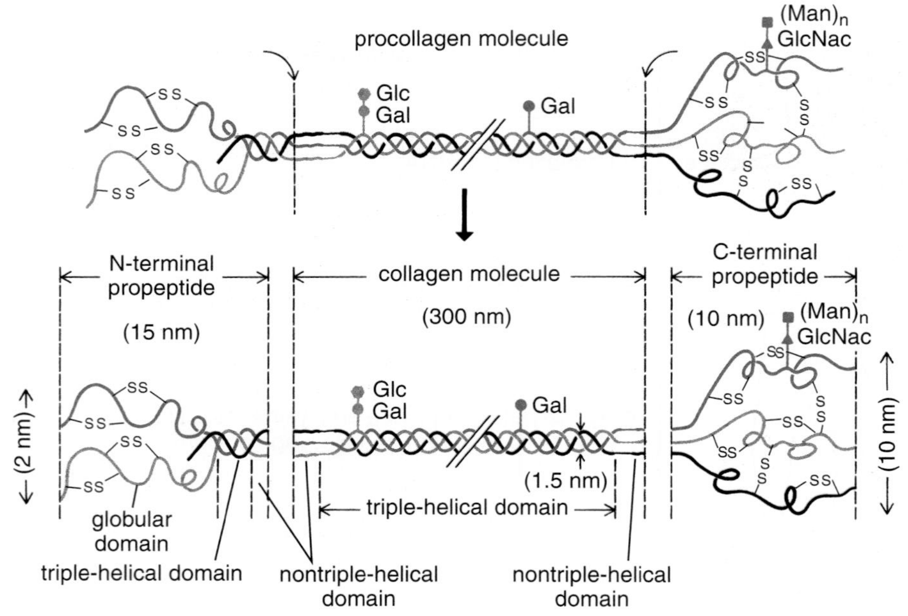

FIGURE 5.8
Cleavage of the procollagen molecule. Illustration showing the procollagen molecule with N- and C-terminals. *Small curved arrows* in the upper part of the illustration show where terminals are split from the procollagen molecule to form the collagen (tropocollagen) molecule. On the C-terminal of the molecule, the sugar subunit is GlcNac (*N*-acetylglucosamine) attached to mannose $(Man)_n$. (Adapted from Prockop DJ, et al. *N Engl J Med* 1979;301:13–23. Copyright © 1979 Massachusetts Medical Society. All rights reserved.)

BOX 5.1

Clinical Correlations: Collagenopathies

The important role of collagens in the body can be illustrated by collagenopathies (collagen diseases), which are caused by a deficit or abnormality in the production of specific collagens. Most collagenopathies are attributed to mutations in genes encoding the α chains in the various collagens. In the future, gene therapy could potentially be used either to control deposition of faulty collagen or to reverse the disease process caused by the mutated genes. Table 5.3 lists the most common collagenopathies occurring in humans.

TABLE 5.3. **The Most Common Collagenopathies Occurring in Humans**

Type of Collagen	Disease	Symptoms
I	Osteogenesis imperfecta	Repeated fractures after minor trauma, brittle bones, abnormal teeth, thin skin, weak tendons, blue sclerae, progressive hearing loss
II	Kniest dysplasia	Short stature, restricted joint mobility, ocular changes leading to blindness, wide metaphyses and joint abnormality seen in radiographs
III	Ehlers-Danlos type IV	Hypermobility of joints of digits, pale thin skin, severe bruisability, early morbidity and mortality resulting from rupture of vessels and internal organs
IV	Alport's syndrome	Hematuria resulting from structural changes in the glomerular basement membrane of the kidney, progressive hearing loss, and ocular lesions
VII	Kindler's syndrome	Severe blistering and scarring of the skin after minor trauma, resulting from absence of anchoring fibrils
IX	Multiple epiphyseal dysplasia (MED)	Skeletal deformations resulting from impaired endochondral ossification and premature degenerative joint disease
X	Schmid metaphyseal chondrodysplasia	Skeletal deformations characterized by modifications of the vertebral bodies and metaphyses of the long bone
XI	Stickler's syndrome type II	Craniofacial and skeletal deformations, severe myopia, retinal detachment, progressive hearing loss
XVII	Generalized atrophic benign epidermolysis bullosa (GABEB)	Blistering skin disease with mechanically induced dermal-epidermal separation, resulting from faulty hemidesmosomes, skin atrophy, nail dystrophy, and alopecia

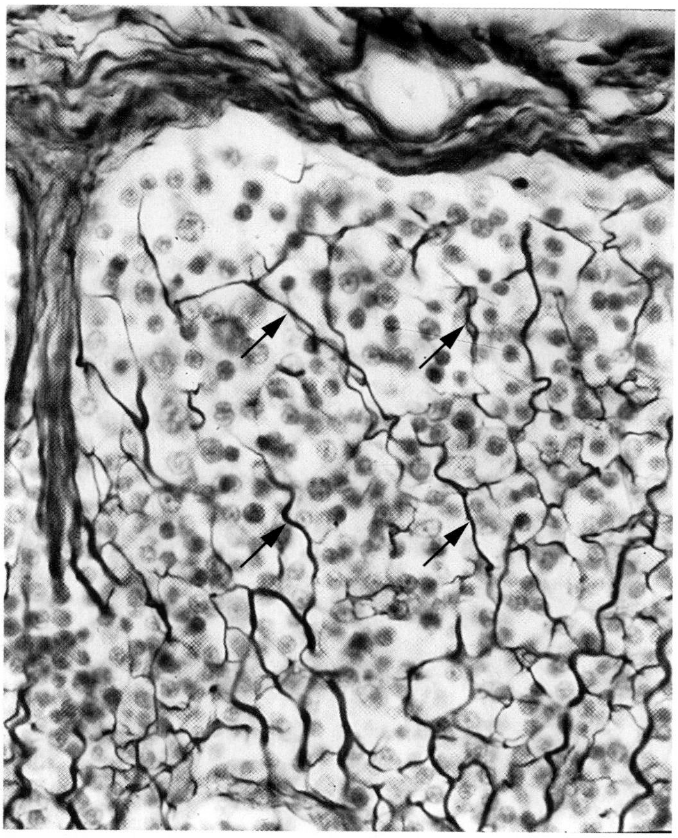

FIGURE 5.9
Reticular fibers in the lymph node. Photomicrograph of a lymph node silver preparation showing the connective tissue capsule at the top and a trabecula extending from it at the left. The reticular fibers (*arrows*) form an irregular anastomosing network. ×650.

Elastic Fibers

Elastic fibers allow tissues to respond to stretch and distension

Elastic fibers are typically thinner than collagen fibers and are arranged in a branching pattern to form a three-dimensional network. The fibers are interwoven with collagen fibers to limit the distensibility of the tissue and to prevent tearing from excessive stretching.

Elastic fibers stain with eosin, but not well; therefore, they cannot always be distinguished from collagen fibers in routine H&E preparations. Because elastic fibers become somewhat refractile with certain fixatives, they may be distinguished from collagen fibers in specimens stained with H&E when they display this characteristic. Elastic fibers can also be selectively stained with special dyes such as orcein or resorcin-fuchsin, as shown in Figure 5.10.

Elastic fibers are produced by most of the same cells that produce collagen and reticular fibers, particularly fibroblasts and smooth muscle cells. In contrast to collagen fibers, however, elastic fibers are composed of two structural components: a central core of elastin and surrounding fibrillin microfibrils.

- ***Elastin*** is a protein that, like collagen, is rich in proline and glycine. Unlike collagen, it is poor in hydroxyproline and completely lacks hydroxylysine. Elastin forms fibers of variable thickness or lamellar layers (as in elastic arteries).
- ***Fibrillin*** is a glycoprotein that forms fine microfibrils measuring 10 to 12 nm in diameter. During the early stages of elastogenesis, these microfibrils are formed first; elastin material is then deposited on the surface of the microfibrils. Elastin-associated ***fibrillin microfibrils*** play a major role in organizing elastin into fibers. The absence of fibrillin microfibrils during elastogenesis results in the formation of elastin sheets or lamellae, as found in blood vessels.

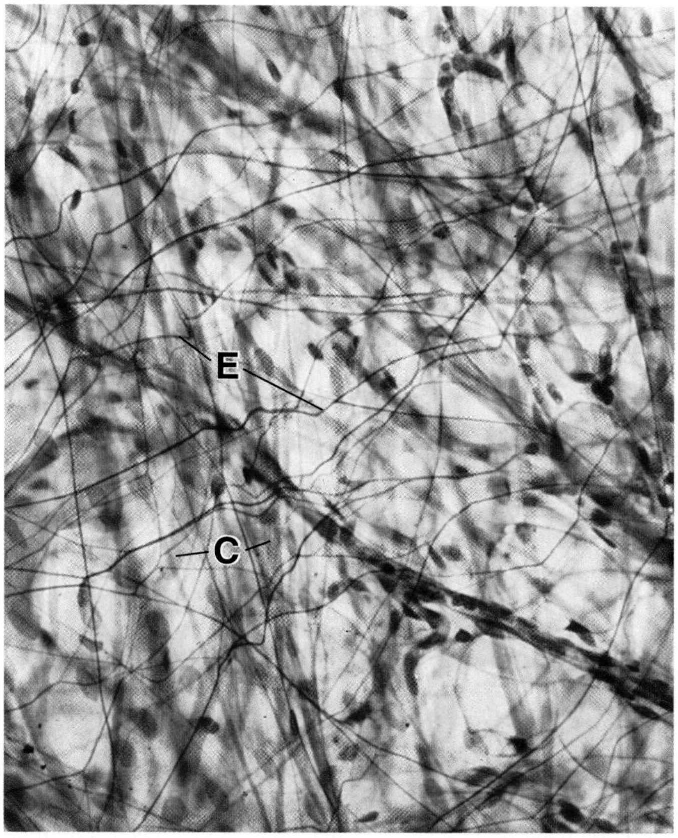

FIGURE 5.10
Collagen and elastic fibers. Photomicrograph of a mesentery spread stained with resorcin-fuchsin. The mesentery is very thin, and the microscope can be focused through the entire thickness of the tissue. The delicate thread-like branching strands are the elastic fibers (*E*). Collagen fibers (*C*) are also evident. They are much thicker, and although they cross one another, they do not branch. ×200.

The elastic property of the elastin molecule is due to its unusual polypeptide backbone that causes random coiling

The random coiling of the elastin molecule allows the elastic fiber to be stretched and then to recoil to its original state. Elastin also contains desmosine and isodesmosine, two large amino acids that are responsible for the covalent bonding of the elastin molecules to one another (Fig. 5.11). With the TEM, elastin appears as an amorphous structure of low electron density. In contrast, the fibrillin microfibrils are electron dense and are readily apparent even within the elastin matrix (Fig. 5.12). In mature fibers, the fibrillin microfibrils are located within the elastic fiber and at its periphery. The presence of microfibrils within the fiber is associated with the growth process; thus, as the fiber is formed and thickens, the microfibrils become entrapped within the newly deposited elastin.

In Marfan's syndrome, a complex, autosomal dominant, connective tissue disorder, expression of the fibrillin gene *(FBN1)* is abnormal. Immunofluorescence of a skin biopsy specimen from a person with Marfan's syndrome will show an absence of elastin-associated fibrillin microfibrils. One of the consequences of the disease is abnormal elastic tissue.

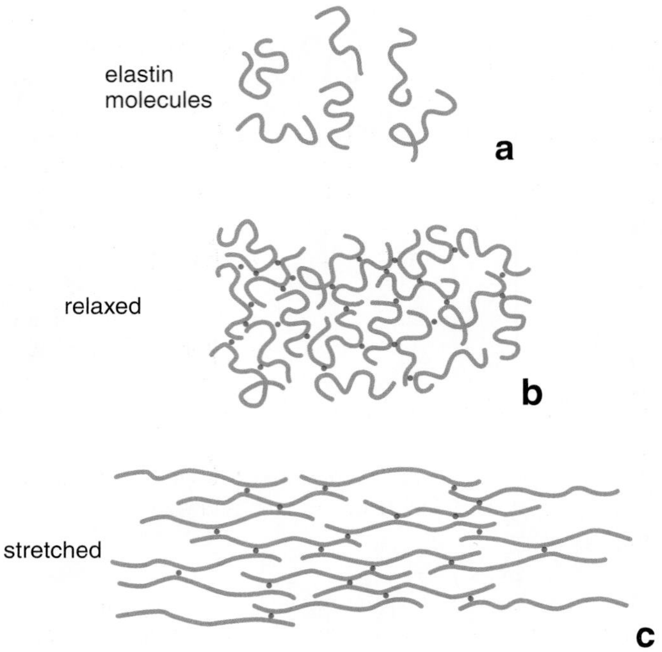

FIGURE 5.11
Diagram of elastin molecules and their interaction. a. Elastin molecules are depicted in their individual and random-coiled conformation. The configuration of the individual molecules continuously changes, oscillating from one form to another. **b.** Elastin molecules are shown joined by covalent bonding *(red)* to form a cross-linked network. **c.** The effect of stretching is shown. When the force is withdrawn, the network reverts to the relaxed state as in *panel b.* (Copyright 1997 from *Essential Cell Biology* by Bruce Alberts, et al, p. 153. Modified with permission of Routledge, Inc., part of The Taylor & Francis Group.)

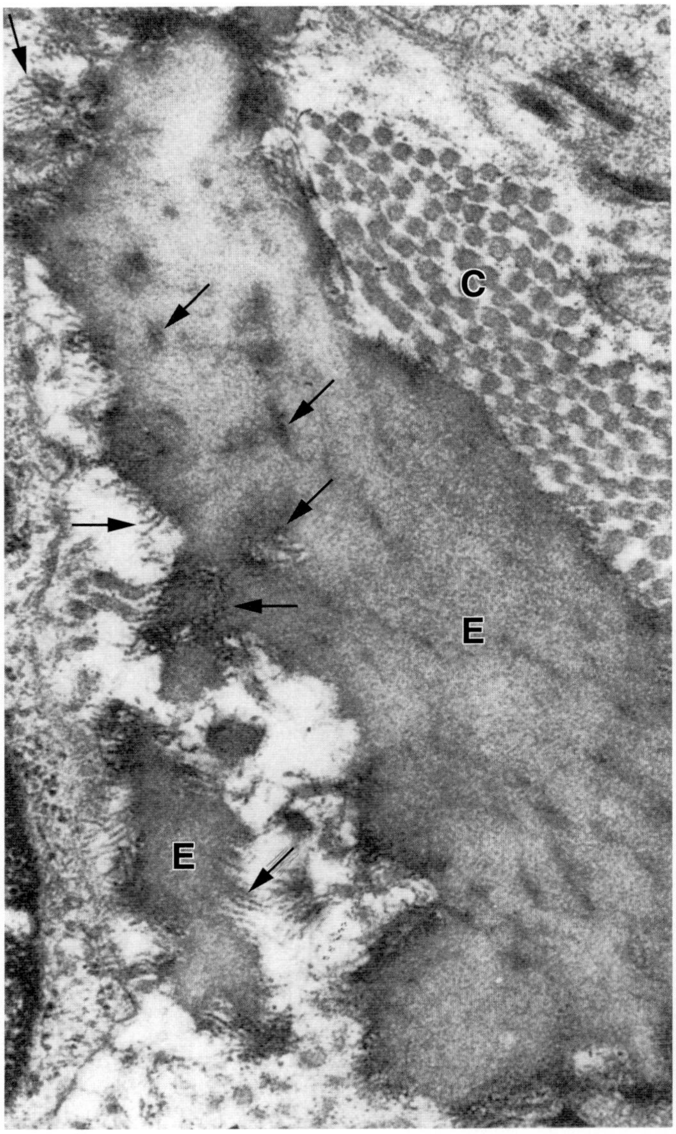

FIGURE 5.12
Electron micrograph of an elastic fiber. The elastin (*E*) of the fiber has a relatively amorphous appearance. The fibrillin microfibrils (*arrows*) are present at the periphery and within the substance of the fiber. A number of collagen fibrils (*C*) is also present in this electron micrograph. ×40,000.

Elastic material is a major extracellular substance in vertebral ligaments, larynx, and elastic arteries

In elastic ligaments, the elastic material consists of thick fibers interspersed with collagen fibers. Examples of this material are found in the ligamenta flava of the vertebral column and the ligamentum nuchae of the neck. Finer fibers are present in elastic ligaments of the vocal folds of the larynx.

In elastic arteries, the elastic material is in the form of fenestrated lamellae, sheets of elastin with gaps or openings. The lamellae are arranged in concentric layers

between layers of smooth muscle cells. Like the collagen fibers in the tunica media of blood vessel walls, the elastic material of arteries is produced by smooth muscle cells, not by fibroblasts. In contrast to elastic fibers, microfibrils are not found in the lamellae. Only the amorphous elastin component is seen in electron micrographs.

Elastin is synthesized by the same pathway as collagen

As noted, elastic fibers are produced by fibroblasts. Elastin synthesis parallels collagen production; in fact, both processes can occur simultaneously in a cell. The orderly modification and assembly of procollagen and proelastin, as well as the synthesis of other connective tissue components, are controlled by signal peptides that are built into the beginning of the polypeptide chains of each of the molecules.

Signal peptides can be compared to the airline tags on luggage. Just as the tags ensure that baggage moves correctly from one aircraft to another at airports, so signal peptides ensure that the components of procollagen and proelastin remain separate and properly identified as they pass through the organelles of the cell. During this transit, a series of synthetic events and posttranslational modifications occur before the polypeptides ultimately arrive at their proper destination.

▼ GROUND SUBSTANCE

Ground substance occupies the space between the cells and fibers

Ground substance is a viscous, clear substance with a slippery feel. It has a high water content and has little morphologic structure. In the light microscope, ground substance appears amorphous in sections of tissue preserved by freeze drying or in frozen sections stained with basic dyes or by the PAS method. In routine H&E preparations, ground substance is always lost because of its extraction during fixation and dehydration of the tissue. The result is an empty background; only cells and fibers are evident. Thus, in most histologic preparations, the appearance of ground substance—or its lack of appearance—belies its functional importance. Ground substance permits diffusion of oxygen and nutrients between the microvasculature and cellular components of the tissue.

Ground substance consists largely of proteoglycans and hyaluronic acid

Ground substance consists predominately of ***proteoglycans***, very large macromolecules composed of a core protein to which glycosaminoglycan molecules are covalently bound. *Glycosaminoglycans (GAGs)* are long-chain polysaccharides composed of repeating disaccharide units. They are named for glucosamine, a hexosamine sugar that is present in each disaccharide.

Proteoglycans and GAGs are responsible for the physical properties of ground substance

GAGs are highly negatively charged because of the sulfate and carboxyl groups located on many of the sugars, hence their propensity for staining with basic dyes. The high density of negative charges also attracts water, forming a hydrated gel. The gel-like composition of the ground substance permits rapid diffusion of water-soluble molecules but inhibits movement of large molecules and bacteria. In addition, proteoglycans contain binding sites for many growth factors, such as transforming growth factor β (TGF-β). The binding of growth factors to proteoglycans may cause either their local aggregation or dispersion, which in turn either inhibits or enhances the movement of migrating macromolecules, microorganisms, or metastatic cancer cells in the extracellular environment.

Based on differences in specific sugar residues, the nature of their linkages, and the degree of sulfation, a family of seven distinct GAGs is recognized. They are listed and partially characterized in Table 5.4. Several of these proteoglycans are modified by connective tissue cells after their synthesis. For example, heparin is formed by enzymatic cleavage of heparan sulfate; dermatan sulfate is similarly modified from chondroitin sulfate.

The GAG ***hyaluronic acid (HA)*** deserves special note because it differs from the other GAGs in several respects. It is an exceedingly long, rigid molecule composed of a carbohydrate chain of thousands of sugars, rather than the several hundred or fewer sugars found in other GAGs. Also, HA is not covalently bound to protein to form a proteoglycan. By means of special ***link proteins***, however, proteoglycans indirectly bind to HA, forming giant macromolecules, as in the ground substance of cartilage (Fig. 5.13). The swelling pressure, or turgor, that occurs in these giant hydrophilic macromolecules accounts for the ability of cartilage to resist compression without inhibiting flexibility.

▼ EXTRACELLULAR MATRIX

The extracellular matrix is a complex structural network that includes fibrous proteins, proteoglycans, and several glycoproteins

The current view of the extracellular components of connective tissue and their functional role reveals a dynamic system in which fibers, proteoglycans—some belonging to the ground substance and others associated with surfaces—and specific glycoproteins such as ***fibronectin*** and ***laminin*** interact with the other components. These structures compose the ***extracellular matrix***.

The attachment of the fibroblast to the extracellular matrix has functional implications

Tissue culture studies reveal that fibroblasts are anchored tightly to matrix elements and that these attach-

TABLE 5.4. **Glycosaminoglycans**

Name	Approximate Molecular Weight (Da)	Disaccharide Composition
Hyaluronic acid	1,000,000	D-Glucuronic acid + *N*-acetylglucosamine
Chondroitin 4-sulfate	25,000	D-Glucuronic acid + *N*-acetylgalactosamine 4-sulfate
Chondroitin 6-sulfate	25,000	D-Glucuronic acid + *N*-acetylgalactosamine 6-sulfate
Dermatan sulfate	35,000	L-Iduronic acid + *N*-acetylgalactosamine 4-sulfate
Keratan sulfate	10,000	Galactose or galactose 6-sulfate + *N*-acetylglucosamine 6-sulfate
Heparan sulfate	15,000	Glucuronic acid or L-iduronic acid 2-sulfate + *N*-sulfamylglucosamine or *N*-acetylglucosamine
Heparin	40,000	Glucuronic acid or L-iduronic acid 2-sulfate + *N*-sulfamylglucosamine or *N*-acetylglucosamine 6-sulfate

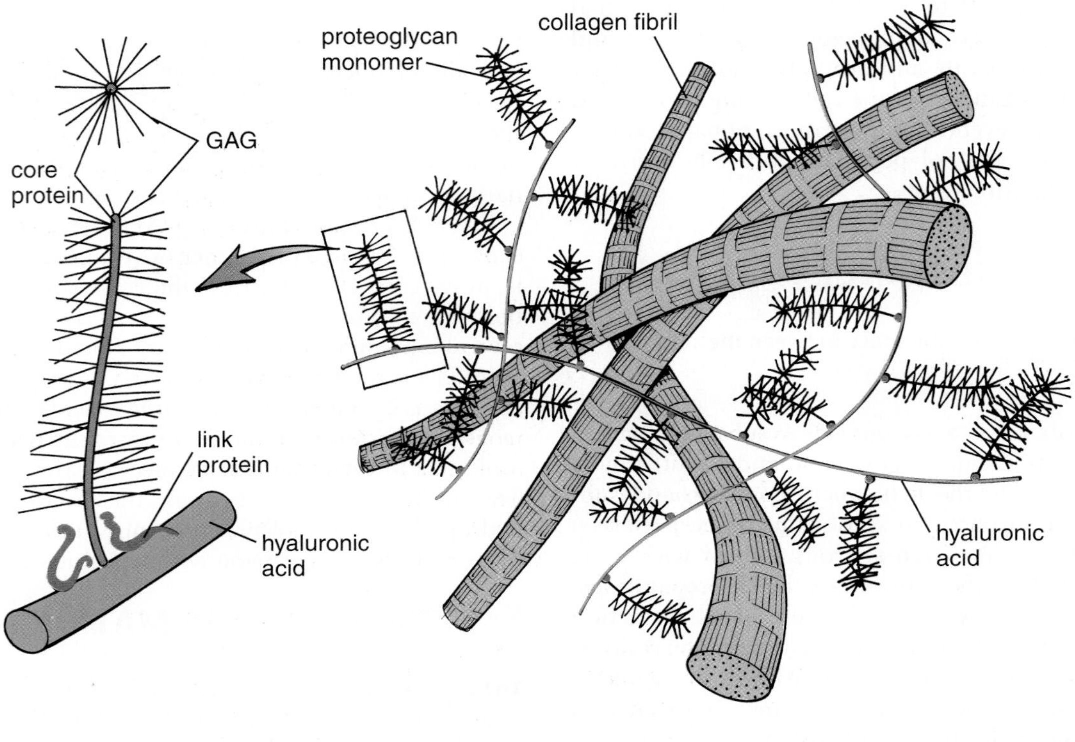

FIGURE 5.13
Proteoglycan structure. This schematic drawing shows, on the left, a proteoglycan monomer and its relationship to the hyaluronic acid (HA) molecule as represented in the ground substance of cartilage. The proteoglycan monomer is composed of a core protein to which glycosaminoglycans (GAGs) are covalently bound. The proteoglycan monomer consists of approximately 100 GAG units joined to the core protein. The end of the core protein contains a HA-binding region; interaction with the HA is strengthened by a link protein. On the right, HA molecules forming linear aggregates, each with many proteoglycan monomers, are interwoven with a network of collagen fibrils.

ments function in cellular movement. The attachments made by the fibroblasts involve several mechanisms that may be divided into two classes. The first class of mechanisms requires cell membrane receptors for fibril proteins, such as collagen, and for glycoproteins, such as fibronectin, which are attached to the fibrils. A second class appears to involve the covalent association of GAGs with specific integral plasma membrane proteins. The attachments established between fibroblasts and the matrix involve proteins that are distinct from the proteins that mediate cell-to-cell contacts. The functions of these proteins are similar to those involved in attachments of epithelial cells to the basal lamina. Small variations in the structure of the proteins involved in these contacts confer an individuality on the cell and matrix types with which they are associated. These variations may establish molecular speci-

ficity and, presumably, assist in specialization of function found at different tissue sites.

▼ CONNECTIVE TISSUE CELLS

Connective tissue cells can be resident or wandering

The cells that make up the ***resident cell population*** are relatively stable; they typically exhibit little movement and can be regarded as ***permanent residents*** of the tissue. These resident cells include

- ***Fibroblasts*** and a closely related cell type, the ***myofibroblast***
- ***Macrophages***
- ***Adipose cells***
- ***Mast cells***
- ***Undifferentiated mesenchymal cells***

The ***wandering or transient cell population*** consists primarily of cells that have migrated into the tissue from the blood in response to specific stimuli. These include

- ***Lymphocytes***
- ***Plasma cells***
- ***Neutrophils***
- ***Eosinophils***
- ***Basophils***
- ***Monocytes***

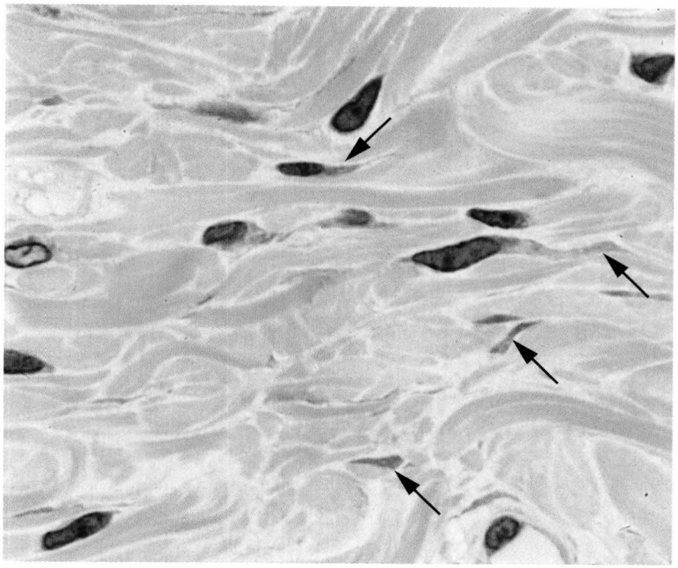

FIGURE 5.14
Fibroblasts in connective tissue. Photomicrograph of a connective tissue specimen fixed with glutaraldehyde, embedded in plastic, and stained with H&E. Thin strands of fibroblast cytoplasm (*arrows*) belonging to a few preferentially oriented cells can just barely be recognized between collagen fibers. In routine H&E–stained, paraffin-embedded preparations, it is usually impossible to distinguish the attenuated and poorly preserved fibroblast cytoplasm from the collagen fibers. Typically, only the nuclei of these cells are evident. ×600.

Fibroblasts and Myofibroblasts

The fibroblast is the principal cell of connective tissue

Fibroblasts are responsible for the synthesis of collagen, elastic and reticular fibers, and the complex carbohydrates of the ground substance. Research suggests that a single fibroblast is capable of producing all of the extracellular matrix components.

Fibroblasts reside in close proximity to collagen fibers. In routine H&E preparations, however, often only the nucleus is visible. It appears as an elongated or disk-like structure, sometimes with a nucleolus evident. The thin, pale-staining, flattened processes that form the bulk of the cytoplasm are usually not visible, largely because they blend with the collagen fibers. In some specially prepared specimens, it is possible to distinguish the cytoplasm of the cell from the fibrous components (Fig. 5.14). When examined with the TEM, the fibroblast cytoplasm exhibits profiles of rER and a prominent Golgi apparatus (Fig. 5.15). When extracellular matrix material is produced during active growth or in wound repair, the cytoplasm of the fibroblast is more extensive and may display basophilia as a result of increased amounts of rER associated with protein synthesis.

Fibroblasts in some locations (e.g., those immediately beneath the epithelium of the intestine, under the epidermis, and around tubular and glandular epithelia) constitute a ***replicating population*** of cells that have a particularly close physical relationship with the overlying epithelium. They are believed to interact with the epithelium in normal renewal and differentiation in the adult organism (epithelial–mesenchymal interaction).

The myofibroblast displays properties of both fibroblasts and smooth muscle cells

The ***myofibroblast*** is an elongate, spindly connective tissue cell not readily identifiable in routine H&E preparations. With the TEM, the myofibroblast displays typical cytologic characteristics of the fibroblast along with characteristics of smooth muscle cells. In addition to rER and Golgi profiles, the myofibroblast contains bundles of longitudinally disposed actin filaments and dense bodies similar to those observed in smooth muscle cells (Fig. 5.16). As in the smooth muscle cell, the nucleus often shows an undulating surface profile, a phenomenon associated with cell contraction. The myofibroblast differs from the smooth muscle cell in that it lacks a surrounding basal lamina (smooth muscle cells are surrounded by a basal or external lamina). Also, it usually exists as an isolated cell, although its processes may contact the processes of other myofibroblasts. Such points of contact exhibit gap junctions, indicating intercellular communication.

The myofibroblast is implicated in wound contraction, a natural process that results in closure of a wound in which

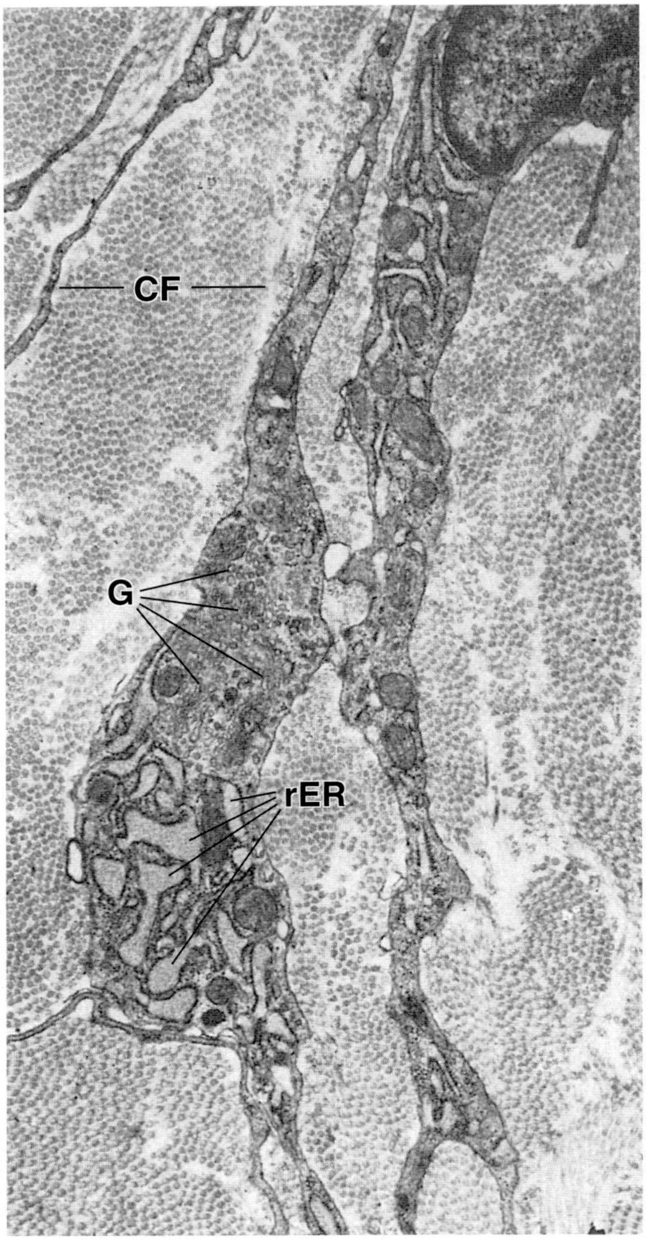

FIGURE 5.15
Electron micrograph of fibroblasts. The processes of several fibroblasts are shown. The nucleus of one fibroblast is in the upper right of the micrograph. The cytoplasm contains conspicuous profiles of rER. The cisternae of the reticulum are distended, indicating active synthesis. The membranes of the Golgi apparatus (*G*) are seen in proximity to the rER. Surrounding the cells are collagen fibrils (*CF*), almost all of which have been cut in cross section and thus appear as small dots at this magnification. ×11,000.

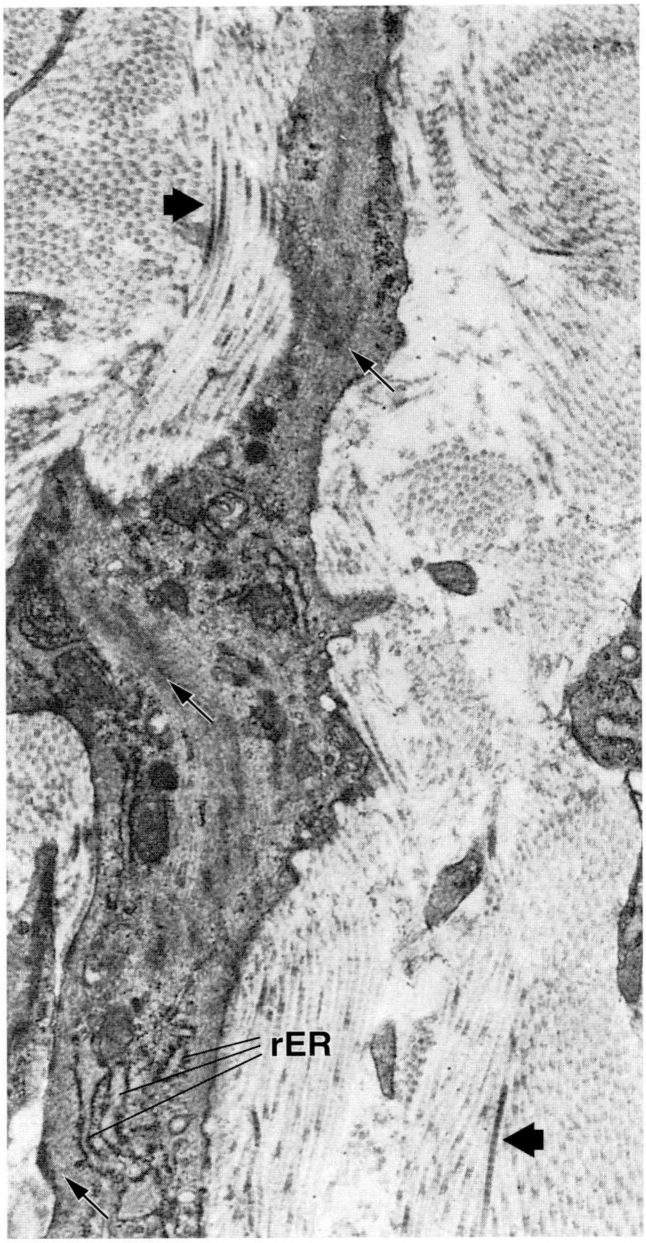

FIGURE 5.16
Electron micrograph of a myofibroblast. The cell exhibits some features of a fibroblast, such as areas with a moderate amount of rER. Compare with Figure 5.15. Other areas, however, contain aggregates of thin filaments and cytoplasmic densities (*arrows*), features characteristic of smooth muscle cells. The *arrowheads* indicate longitudinal profiles of collagen fibrils. ×11,000.

loss of tissue has occurred. TEM studies reveal numerous myofibroblasts in such wound sites, particularly in the granulation tissue of these wounds. Research suggests that these cells may represent modified fibroblasts that have responded to stimuli associated with tissue damage and repair.

Macrophages

Macrophages are phagocytotic cells derived from monocytes

Connective tissue ***macrophages,*** also known as tissue ***histiocytes,*** are derived from blood cells called mono-

cytes. Monocytes migrate from the bloodstream into the connective tissue, where they differentiate into macrophages.

In the light microscope and with conventional stains, tissue macrophages are difficult to identify unless they display obvious evidence of phagocytotic activity, i.e., visible ingested material within their cytoplasm. Another feature that assists in identifying macrophages is an indented or kidney-shaped nucleus. Lysosomes are abundant in the cytoplasm and can be revealed by staining for acid phosphatase activity (both in the light microscope and with the TEM); a positive reaction is a further aid in identification of the macrophage. With the TEM, the surface of the macrophage exhibits numerous folds and finger-like projections (Fig. 5.17a). The surface folds engulf the substances to be phagocytosed.

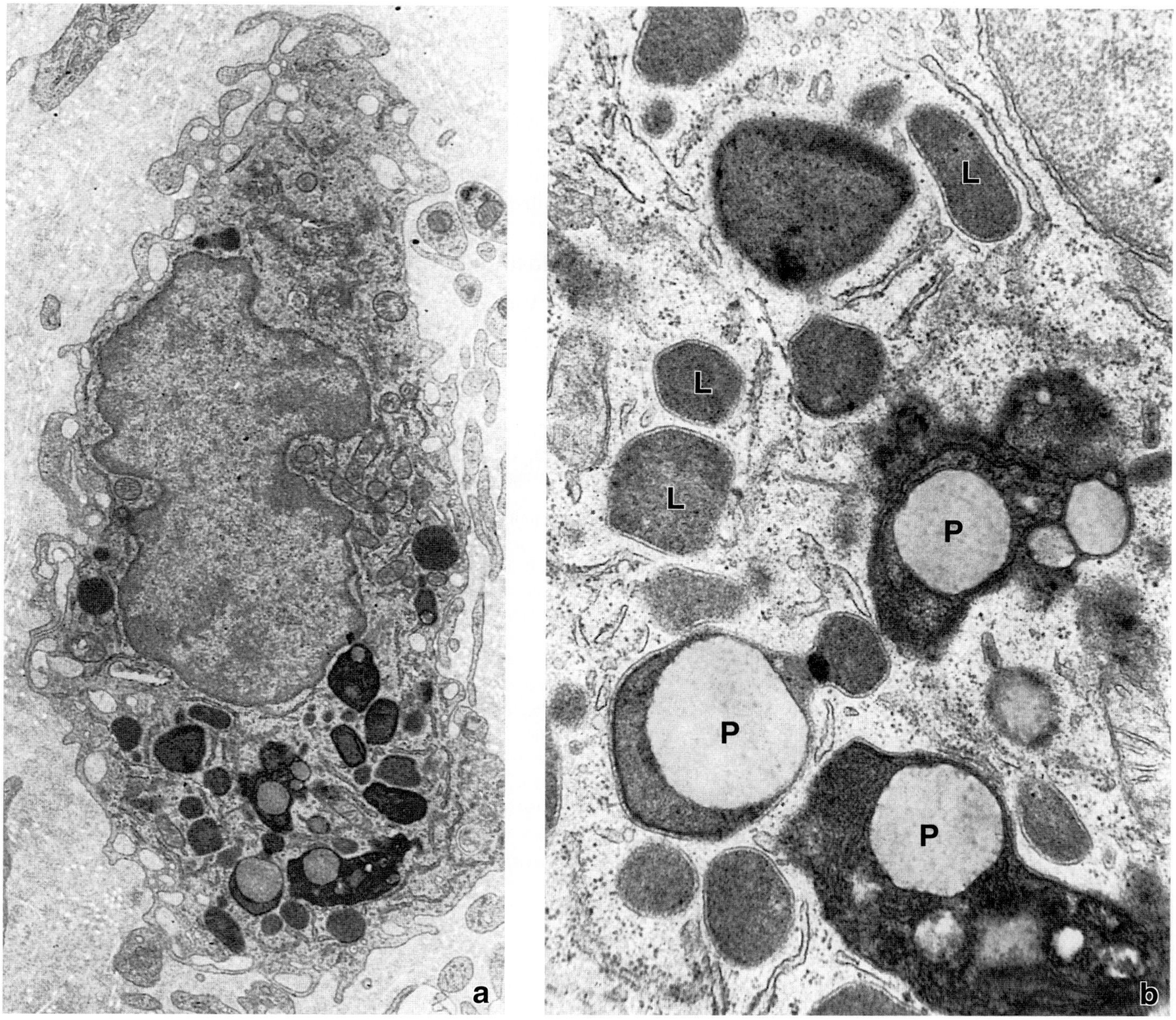

FIGURE 5.17

Electron micrograph of a macrophage. a. The most distinctive feature of the macrophage is its population of endocytotic vesicles, early and late endosomes, lysosomes, and phagolysosomes. The surface of the cell reveals a number of finger-like projections, some of which may be sections of surface folds. ×10,000. **b.** Higher magnification of the lysosomes and phagolysosomes from figure *a*. Most lysosomes possess an electron-dense homogeneous matrix (*L*). Many of the phagolysosomes (*P*) contain an electron-lucent phagocytosed material. ×45,000.

The macrophage contains a large Golgi apparatus, rER and sER, mitochondria, secretory vesicles, and lysosomes

The lysosomes of the macrophage, along with the surface cytoplasmic projections, are the structures most indicative of the specialized phagocytotic capability of the cell (Fig. 5.17b). The macrophage may also contain endocytotic vesicles, phagolysosomes, and other evidence of phagocytosis (i.e., residual bodies). The rER and Golgi apparatus support the synthesis of proteins involved in the phagocytotic and digestive functions, as well as in the cell's secretory functions. The secretory products leave the cell by both the constitutive and regulated exocytotic pathways. Regulated secretion can be activated by phagocytosis, immune complexes, complement, and signals from lymphocytes (including the release of ***lymphokines,*** biologically active molecules that influence the activity of other cells). The secretory products released by the macrophage include a wide variety of substances related to the immune response, anaphylaxis, and inflammation. The release of neutral proteases and GAGases (enzymes that break down GAGs) facilitates the migration of the macrophages through the connective tissue.

Although the main function of the macrophage is phagocytosis, either as a defense activity (e.g., phagocytosis of bacteria) or as a cleanup operation (e.g., phagocytosis of cell debris), it also plays an important role in immune response reactions. Macrophages have specific proteins on their surface known as ***major histocompatibility complex II (MHC II)*** molecules that allow them to interact with ***helper CD4⁺ T lymphocytes.*** When macrophages engulf a foreign cell, antigens—short polypeptides, 7 to 10 amino acids long, from the foreign cell—are displayed on the surface of MHC II molecules. If a $CD4^+$ T lymphocyte recognizes the displayed antigen, it becomes activated, triggering an immune response (see Chapter 13). Because macrophages "present" antigen to helper $CD4^+$ T lymphocytes, they are called ***antigen-presenting cells (APCs).***

When macrophages encounter large foreign bodies, they may fuse to form a large cell with up to 100 nuclei that engulfs the foreign body. These multinucleated cells are called ***foreign body giant cells*** (Langhans cells).

Mast Cells and Basophils

Mast cells are large, ovoid, connective tissue cells (20 to 30 μm in diameter) with a spherical nucleus and cytoplasm

BOX 5.2

Functional Considerations: The Mononuclear Phagocytotic System

The cells that are included in the ***mononuclear phagocytotic system (MPS)*** are derived from monocytes and denote a population of antigen-presenting cells involved in the processing of foreign substances. These cells are able to phagocytose avidly vital dyes such as trypan blue and India ink, which makes them visible and easy to identify in the light microscope. The common origin of MPS cells from monocytes serves as the major distinguishing feature of the system as it is currently perceived and is the basis for the system's name. In addition, cells of the MPS display receptors for complement and F_c fragments of immunoglobulins. The various cells of the MPS are listed in Table 5.5.

Most cells of the MPS become fixed in specific tissues and may adopt a variety of morphologic appearances as they differentiate. The main functions of MPS cells are phagocytosis, secretion (lymphokines), antigen processing, and antigen presentation to other cells of the immune system. Some functionally important phagocytotic cells are not derived from monocytes. For example, microglia are small, stellate cells located primarily along capillaries of the central nervous system, which function as phagocytotic cells. They are generally thought to arise from the mesectoderm of the neural crest and not from monocytes; nevertheless, they are included in the MPS. Similarly, fibroblasts of the subepithelial sheath of the lamina propria of the intestine and uterine endometrium have been shown to differentiate into cells with morphologic, enzymatic, and functional characteristics of connective tissue macrophages.

TABLE 5.5. **Cells of the Mononuclear Phagocytotic System**

Name of Cell	Location
Macrophage (histiocyte)	Connective tissue
Perisinusoidal macrophage (Kupffer cell)	Liver
Alveolar macrophage	Lungs
Macrophage	Spleen, lymph nodes, bone marrow, and thymus
Pleural and peritoneal macrophage	Serous cavities
Osteoclast	Bone
Microglia	Central nervous system
Langerhans' cell	Epidermis
Fibroblast-derived macrophage	Lamina propria of intestine, endometrium of uterus

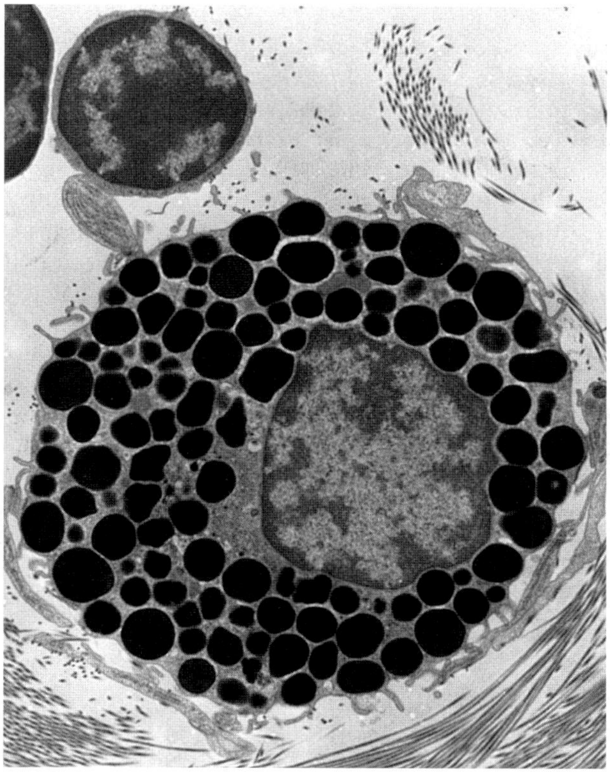

FIGURE 5.18
Electron micrograph of a mast cell. The cytoplasm is virtually filled with granules. Note a small lymphocyte present in the upper left of the figure. ×6,000.

filled with large, intensely basophilic granules (Fig. 5.18). The mast cell is related to, but not identical with, the basophil, a blood cell that contains similar granules (Table 5.6). The cell surface exhibits numerous microvilli and folds. The cytoplasm displays small amounts of rER, mitochondria, and a Golgi apparatus.

Mast cells are not easily identified in human tissue sections unless special fixatives are used to preserve the granules. After glutaraldehyde fixation, mast cell granules can be displayed with basic dyes, such as toluidine blue. It stains the granules intensely and metachromatically because they contain ***heparin,*** a highly sulfated proteoglycan (Fig. 5.19).

Several vasoactive and immunoreactive substances are contained in mast cell granules

Mast cells release their granules when appropriately stimulated, as when an individual is exposed to an antigen to which he or she has already been sensitized. Sensitization develops after the initial encounter with an antigen. During this first encounter, the immune system recognizes the antigen as "nonself." Immune system cells that express antibody molecules on their surface specific for the antigen ***(cognate antibodies)*** proliferate and differentiate into specialized antibody-secreting cells, plasma cells. These cells then produce antibodies against the antigen. Several major classes of antibodies, called ***immunoglobulins,*** are produced. Immunoglobulins of the IgE class are released by the plasma cells and bind to F_c receptors located on the plasma membrane of the mast cells. On subsequent exposure to the same antigen, an antigen–antibody reaction occurs at the mast cell surface that causes the discharge of mast cell granules.

The secretions of mast cell granules can result in immediate hypersensitivity reactions, allergy, and anaphylaxis

Several primary substances found inside mast cell granules are

- ***Histamine*** and ***slow-reacting substance of anaphylaxis (SRS-A),*** which increase the permeability of small blood vessels, causing edema in the surrounding tissue. In addition, both substances increase mucus production in the bronchial tree and trigger contraction of smooth muscles in the pulmonary airways, causing bronchospasm.
- ***Eosinophil chemotactic factor (ECF)*** and ***neutrophil chemotactic factor (NCF),*** which attract eosinophils and neutrophils to the site of inflammation. The secretions of eosinophils counteract the effects of the histamine and SRS-A.
- ***Heparin,*** a sulfated glycosaminoglycan, which is an anticoagulant. When it unites with antithrombin III, it can

TABLE 5.6. **Comparison of Features Characteristic of Mast Cells and Basophils**

Characteristic Features	Mast Cells	Basophils
Origin	Hemopoietic stem cell	Hemopoietic stem cell
Site of differentiation	Connective tissue	Bone marrow
Cell divisions	Yes (occasionally)	No
Life span	Weeks to months	Days
Size	20–30 μm	7–10 μm
Shape of nucleus	Round	Segmented (usually bilobar)
Granules	Many, large, metachromatic	Few, small, basophilic
Surface F_c receptors for IgE antibodies	Present	Present

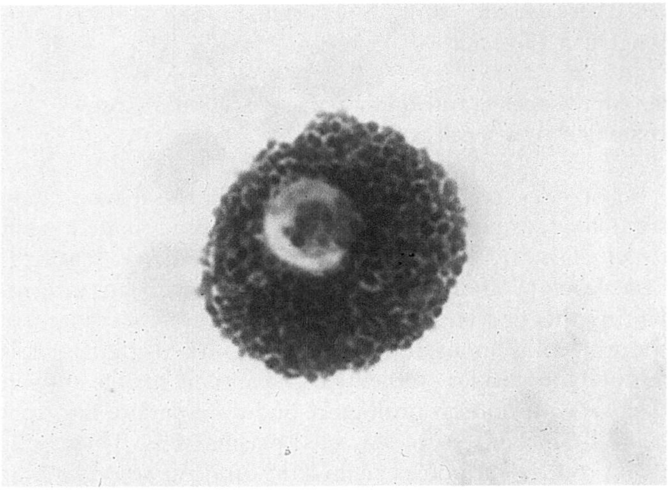

FIGURE 5.19
Photomicrograph of a mast cell stained with H&E. The granules stain intensely and, because of their numbers, tend to appear as a solid mass in some areas. The nucleus of the cell is represented by the pale-staining area. ×1,250.

block numerous coagulation factors. Based on its anticoagulant properties, heparin is useful for treatment of thrombosis.

In addition, several secondary mediators, namely, ***leukotrienes*** and ***prostaglandin D,*** are released during mast cell activation. These mediators are not stored in granules but are synthesized by the cell and released immediately into the extracellular matrix.

Mast cells are especially numerous in connective tissues of skin and mucous membranes but are not present in the brain and spinal cord

Mast cells are distributed chiefly in the vicinity of small blood vessels, a target of histamine and SRS-A. Mast cells are also present in the capsules of organs and the connective tissue that surrounds the blood vessels of organs. A notable exception is the central nervous system. Although the meninges (sheets of connective tissue that surround the brain and spinal cord) contain mast cells, the connective tissue around the small blood vessels within the brain and spinal cord is devoid of mast cells. The absence of mast cells protects the brain and spinal cord from the potentially disrupting effects of the edema characteristic of allergic reactions. Mast cells are also numerous in the thymus and, to a lesser degree, in other lymphatic organs, but they are not present in the spleen.

In certain immune reactions, basophils leave the circulation and function in the connective tissue

Basophils are also characterized by the presence of intensely basophilic secretory granules in the cytoplasm. Like that of mast cells, the basophil cell membrane exhibits specific receptors for the F_c fragment of IgE immunoglobulin, which is produced in response to allergens. In allergic reactions, IgE immunoglobulins become bound to the surface F_c receptor of the basophil. This binding triggers the rapid exocytosis of the basophil secretory granules. The release of histamine, heparan sulfate, ECF, NCF, and peroxidase contained in the granules enhances the vascular response in dermal hypersensitivity reactions, such as those that follow insect bites and stings. In highly sensitive individuals, the antigen injected by an insect can trigger a massive discharge of basophil granules. This often-explosive, life-threatening reaction, known as ***anaphylactic shock,*** is characterized by a decreased volume of circulating blood (leaky vessels) and constriction of smooth muscle cells in blood vessels and in the bronchial tree. The individual has difficulty breathing and may exhibit a rash as well as nausea and vomiting. Symptoms of anaphylactic shock usually develop within 1 to 3 minutes, and they require immediate treatment with vasoconstrictors such as epinephrine.

Adipose Cells

The adipose cell is a connective tissue cell specialized to store neutral fat

Adipose cells differentiate from undifferentiated mesenchymal cells and gradually accumulate fat in their cytoplasm. They are located throughout loose connective tissue as individual cells and groups of cells. When they accumulate in large numbers, they are called adipose tissue. This specialized connective tissue is discussed in Chapter 6.

Undifferentiated Mesenchymal Cells and Pericytes

Many researchers have postulated the existence of cells in loose connective tissue of the adult that retain the multiple potentials of embryonic mesenchymal cells. These cells, called ***undifferentiated mesenchymal cells,*** are thought to give rise to differentiated cells that function in repair and formation of new tissue, as in wound healing, and development of new blood vessels (neovascularization).

The pericyte may serve as one type of undifferentiated mesenchymal cell

Pericytes, also called ***adventitial cells*** or ***perivascular cells,*** are found around capillaries and venules (Fig. 5.20). They are surrounded by basal lamina material that is continuous with the basal lamina of the capillary endothelium; thus, they are not truly located in the connective tissue compartment. The pericyte is typically wrapped, at least partially, around the capillary, and its nucleus takes on a shape similar to that of endothelial cells, i.e., flattened but curved to conform to the tubular shape of the vessel.

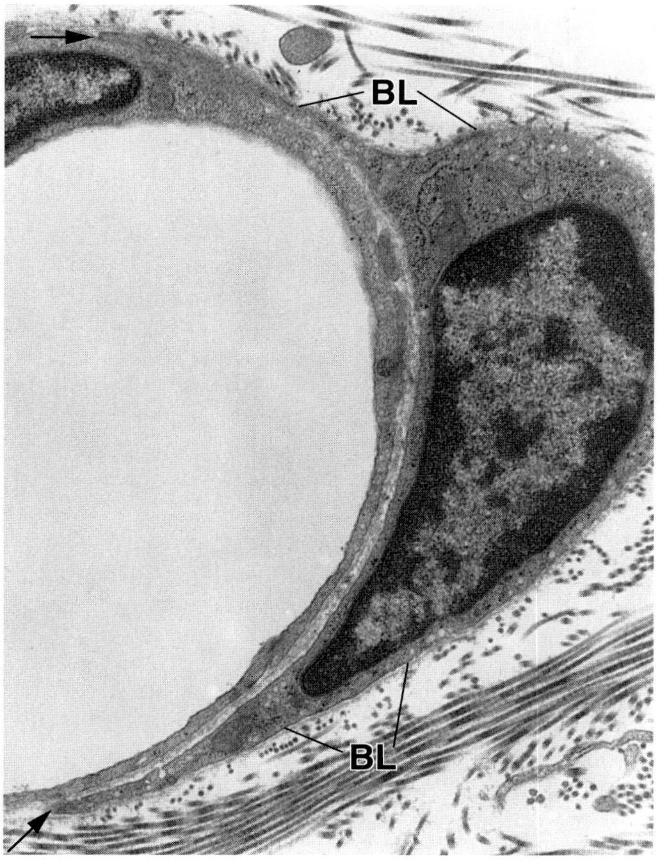

FIGURE 5.20
Electron micrograph of a small blood vessel. The nucleus at the upper left belongs to the endothelial cell that forms the wall of the vessel. At the right is another cell, a pericyte, that is in intimate relation to the endothelium. Note that the basal lamina (*BL*) covering the endothelial cell divides (*arrows*) to surround the pericyte. ×11,000.

TEM studies have shown that pericytes surrounding the smallest venules have cytoplasmic characteristics almost identical with those of the endothelial cells of the same vessel. Pericytes associated with larger venules have characteristics of smooth muscle cells of the tunica media of small veins. In fortuitous sections cut parallel to the long axis of venules, the distal portions and proximal portions of the same pericyte have characteristics of endothelial cells and smooth muscle cells, respectively. These studies suggest that during the development of new vessels, cells with characteristics of pericytes may differentiate into the smooth muscle of the vessel wall.

The fibroblasts and blood vessels within healing wounds develop from undifferentiated mesenchymal cells associated with the tunica adventitia of venules

Autoradiographic studies of wound healing using parabiotic (crossed-circulation) pairs of animals have established that undifferentiated mesenchymal cells located in the tunica adventitia of venules and small veins are the primary source of new cells in healing wounds. In addition, fibroblasts, pericytes, and endothelial cells in portions of the connective tissue adjacent to the wound divide and give rise to additional cells that form new connective tissue and blood vessels.

Lymphocytes, Plasma Cells, and Other Cells of the Immune System

Lymphocytes are principally involved in immune responses

Connective tissue lymphocytes are the smallest of the free cells in the connective tissue (see Fig. 5.18). They have a thin rim of cytoplasm surrounding a deeply staining, heterochromatic nucleus. Often, the cytoplasm of connective tissue lymphocytes may not be visible. Normally, small numbers of lymphocytes are found in the connective tissue throughout the body. The number increases dramatically, however, at sites of tissue inflammation caused by pathogenic agents. Lymphocytes are most numerous in the lamina propria of the respiratory and gastrointestinal tracts, where they are involved in immunosurveillance against pathogens and foreign substances that enter the body by crossing the epithelial lining of these systems.

Lymphocytes are a heterogeneous population of at least three functional cell types: T cells, B cells, and NK cells

At the molecular level, lymphocytes are characterized by the expression of specific molecules on the plasma membrane known as ***cluster of differentiation (CD) proteins.*** CD proteins recognize specific ligands on target cells. Because some CD proteins are present only on specific types of lymphocytes, they are considered specific marker proteins. On the basis of these specific markers, lymphocytes can be classified into three functional cell types:

- *T lymphocytes* are characterized by the presence of the *CD2, CD3*, and *CD7* marker proteins and the ***T cell receptors (TCRs).*** These cells have a long life span and are effectors in ***cell-mediated immunity.***
- *B lymphocytes* are characterized by the presence of *CD9, CD19, CD20*, and *CD24* proteins and attached immunoglobulins IgM and IgD. These cells recognize antigen, have a variable life span, and are effectors in ***antibody-mediated (humoral) immunity.***
- *Natural killer (NK) lymphocytes* are non-T, non-B lymphocytes that express the *CD16, CD56*, and *CD94* proteins, not found on other lymphocytes. These cells do not produce immunoglobulins, nor do they express TCR on their surface. Thus, NK lymphocytes are not antigen specific. Similar in action to T lymphocytes, however, they destroy virus-infected cells and some tumor cells by a cytotoxic mechanism.

In response to the presence of antigens, lymphocytes become activated and may divide several times, producing clones of themselves. In addition, clones of B lymphocytes mature into plasma cells. A description of B and T lymphocytes and their functions during immune response reactions is presented in Chapter 13.

Plasma cells are antibody-producing cells derived from B lymphocytes

Plasma cells are a prominent constituent of loose connective tissue where antigens tend to enter the body, e.g., the gastrointestinal and respiratory tracts. They are also a normal component of salivary glands, lymph nodes, and hemopoietic tissue. Once derived from its precursor, the B lymphocyte, a plasma cell has only limited migratory ability and a somewhat short life span of 10 to 30 days.

The plasma cell is a relatively large, ovoid cell (20 μm) with a considerable amount of cytoplasm. The cytoplasm displays strong basophilia because of an extensive rER (Fig. 5.21). The Golgi apparatus is usually prominent because of its relatively large size and lack of staining. It appears in light microscope preparations as a clear area, in contrast to the basophilic cytoplasm.

The nucleus is spherical and typically offset or eccentrically positioned. It is small, not much larger than the nucleus of the lymphocyte. It exhibits large clumps of peripheral heterochromatin alternating with clear areas of euchromatin. This arrangement has traditionally been described as resembling a cartwheel or analog clock face, with the heterochromatin resembling the spokes of the wheel or the numbers on a clock. The heterochromatic nucleus of the plasma cell is somewhat surprising, given the cell's function in synthesizing large amounts of protein. However, because the cells produce large amounts of *only one type of protein*—a specific antibody—only a small segment of the genome is exposed for transcription.

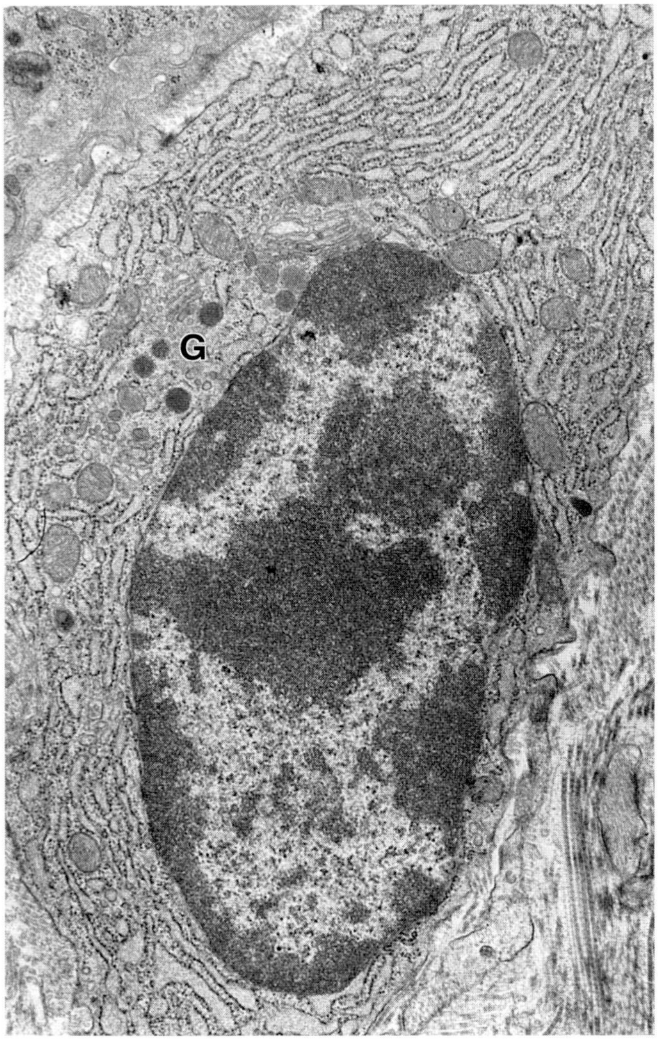

FIGURE 5.21
Electron micrograph of a plasma cell. An extensive rER occupies most of the cytoplasm. The Golgi apparatus (*G*) is also relatively large, a further reflection of the cell's secretory activity. ×15,000.

Eosinophils, monocytes, and neutrophils are also observed in connective tissue

As a result of immune responses and tissue injury, certain cells rapidly migrate from the blood to enter the connective tissue, particularly neutrophils and monocytes. Their presence generally indicates an acute inflammatory reaction. In these reactions, neutrophils migrate into the connective tissue in substantial numbers, followed by large numbers of monocytes. As noted, the monocytes then differentiate into macrophages. A description of these cells and their role is found in Chapter 9. The eosinophil, which functions in allergic reactions and parasitic infections, is also presented in that chapter. Eosinophils may be observed in normal connective tissue, particularly the lamina propria of the intestine, as a result of chronic immunologic responses that occur in these tissues.

PLATE 4. LOOSE AND DENSE CONNECTIVE TISSUE

A classification of connective tissue is presented in Table 1. The light microscopic appearance of loose connective tissue includes many cells, usually of various types, including fibroblasts, macrophages, leukocytes, and cells of the immune system, particularly lymphocytes and plasma cells; the cells are not organized in any special pattern. The collagen fibers are fine and wispy, and most of the ground substance is lost during fixation. Thus, the tissue usually stains lightly with eosin. In contrast, dense connective tissue is composed of thick collagen bundles that stain deeply with eosin. It has relatively few cells, most of which are fibroblasts. Both connective tissues contain elastic fibers that are visible only with special staining methods (see Plate 6).

TABLE 1. **Classification of Connective Tissue**

Connective tissue proper	Cartilage (Plates 7–10)
Loose connective tissue	Hemopoietic tissue (Plates 16–17)
Dense connective tissue	Lymphatic tissue (Plates 32–37)
Irregular	
Regular	
Specialized connective tissue	Embryonic connective tissue
Adipose tissue	Mesenchyme
Blood (Plates 16–17)	Mucous connective tissue
Bone (Plates 11–15)	

Figure 1, mammary gland, human, H&E ×160.
This micrograph shows, at low magnification, loose connective tissue (*LCT*) immediately surrounding the gland epithelium (*Ep*). It is relatively less strained with eosin, compared with the dense connective tissue (*DCT*) that occupies much of the field. The dense connective tissue, with its numerous thick fibers, is in contrast to the loose connective tissue that has a relative paucity of fibers. The typical wispy nature of the collagen fibers found in loose connective tissue is seen more clearly in Figure 2, which shows one of the lobules at higher magnification.

Figure 2, mammary gland, human, H&E ×250.
Although the magnification of this figure is not sufficiently high to explore cytologic detail, two general cell types are recognized in the loose connective tissue, based on nuclear shape. One population of cells contains elongate nuclei (*arrows*); these most likely belong to fibroblasts. The other population contains round nuclei; most of these nuclei represent lymphocytes (*L*), although some are of plasma cells. The significant feature, however, is that the loose connective tissue is highly cellular, considerably more so than the surrounding dense connective tissue. Typically, the cells of dense connective tissue are fibroblasts.

Figure 3, vagina, human, H&E ×250.
This example of loose connective tissue is from the wall of the vagina just below the epithelial surface. Again, note the myriad nuclear profiles. The area immediately to the right of the upper marked blood vessel (*BV*) is shown at high magnification in Figure 4.

Figure 4, vagina, human, H&E ×480.
Here the wispy nature of the fine collagen fibers is evident, and the variation of nuclear profiles is even more apparent. Identification of the cell type represented by each nucleus is not possible; however, certain cells of the total population can be identified with assurance. Thus, the small, dense, round nuclei without visible surrounding cytoplasm belong to lymphocytes (*L*). Some of the round nuclei exhibit a surrounding but eccentric mass of cytoplasm. These are plasma cells (*PC*). The cytoplasm of some cells is obscured partially by the nucleus, making identity less certain *(?)*. The size, density, chromatin pattern, and typically elongated nucleus make those cells more readily identifiable as fibroblasts. Two fibroblast nuclei *(F)* are indicated in the micrograph; both are elongate, but one appears quite narrow. It is being viewed on edge, whereas the broader nucleus profile represents an en face view of a fibroblast. This nucleus also shows prominent nucleoli, typical of active fibroblasts. Usually, the thin cytoplasmic processes of the fibroblasts are obscured by blending in with the collagen. Some of the nuclei seen here may represent macrophages or mast cells, but these cells cannot be definitively identified.

KEY

AT, adipose tissue
BV, blood vessel
DCT, dense connective tissue
Ep, epithelium
F, fibroblast nucleus
L, lymphocyte
LCT, loose connective tissue
PC, plasma cell
arrow, elongate nucleus

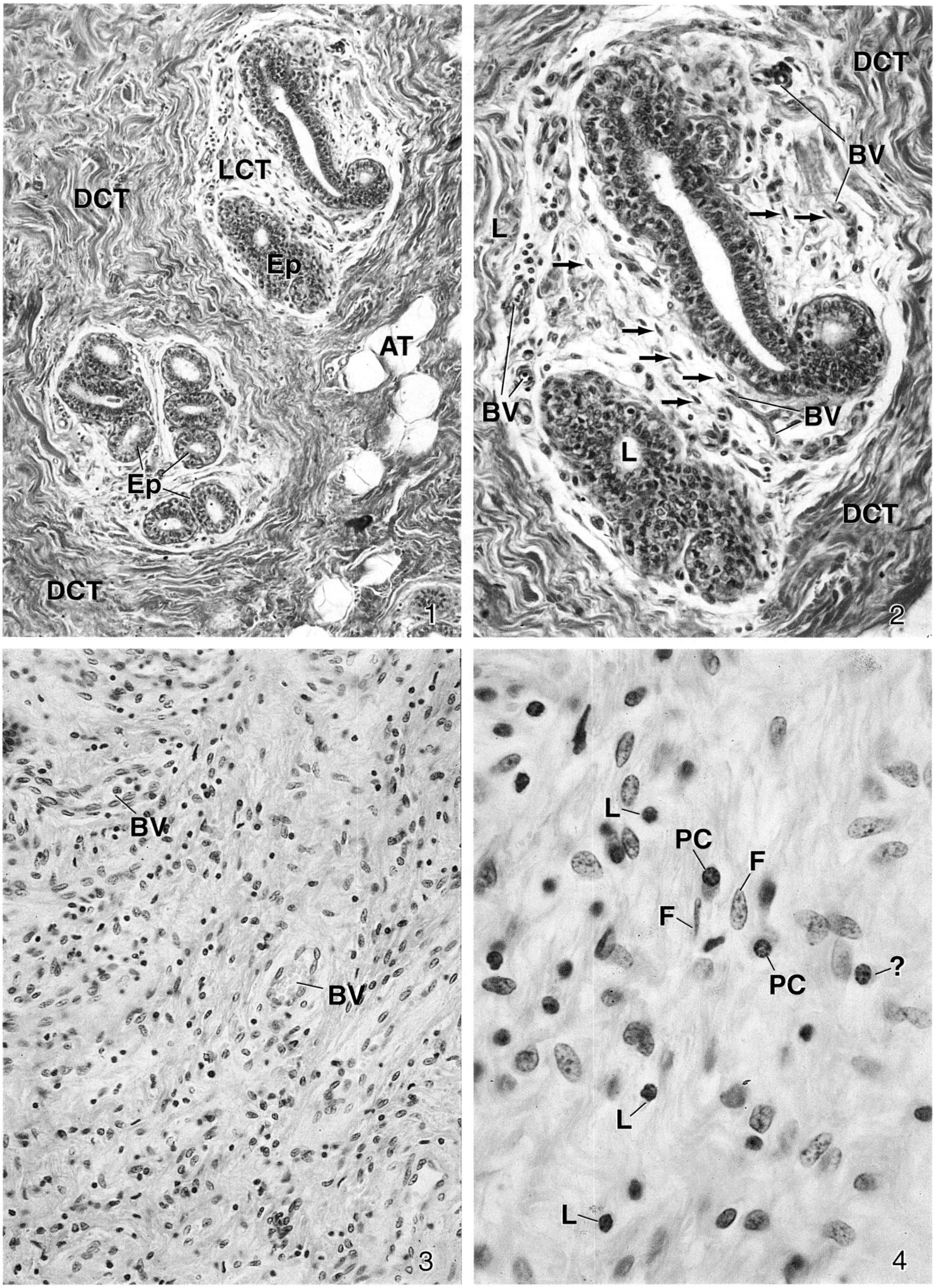
LCT
DCT
Ep
AT
Ep
DCT
1
DCT
BV
L
BV
BV
L
DCT
2
BV
BV
3
L
PC
F
F
PC
?
L
L
4

PLATE 5. DENSE REGULAR CONNECTIVE TISSUE, TENDONS, AND LIGAMENTS

Dense *regular connective tissue* is distinctive in that its fibers are very densely packed and are organized in parallel array into fascicles. The collagen fibrils that make up the fibers are also arranged in an ordered parallel array. *Tendons,* which attach muscle to bone, and *ligaments,* which attach bone to bone, are examples of this type of tissue. Ligaments are similar to tendons in most respects, but their fibers and the organization of the fascicles tend to be less ordered.

In tendons as well as ligaments, the fascicles are separated from one another by dense irregular connective tissue, the *endotendineum,* through which travel vessels and nerves. Also, a fascicle may be partially divided by connective tissue septa that extend from the endotendineum and contain the smallest vessels and nerves. Some of the fascicles may be grouped into larger functional units by a thicker, surrounding connective tissue, the *peritendineum.* Finally, the fascicles and groups of fascicles are surrounded by dense irregular connective tissue, the *epitendineum.*

The fibroblasts, also called tendon cells in tendons, are elongated cells that possess exceedingly thin, sheet-like cytoplasmic processes that reside between and embrace adjacent fibers. The margins of the cytoplasmic processes contact those of neighboring tendon cells, thus forming a syncytium-like cytoplasmic network.

The most regular dense connective tissue is that of the stroma of the cornea of the eye (see Plate 103). In this tissue, the collagen fibrils are arranged in parallel in lamellae that are separated by large, flattened fibroblasts. Adjacent lamellae are arranged at approximately right angles to one another, thus forming an *orthogonal array.* The extreme regularity of fibril size and fibril spacing in each lamella, in conjunction with the orthogonal array of the lamellae, is believed to be the basis of corneal transparency.

Figure 1, tendon, longitudinal section, human, H&E ×100.

This specimen includes the surrounding dense irregular connective tissue of the tendon, the epitendineum (*Ept*). The tendon fascicles (*TF*) that make up the tendon are surrounded by a less dense connective tissue than that associated with the epitendineum. In longitudinal sections such as this, the connective tissue that surrounds the individual fascicles, the endotendineum (*Ent*), seems to disappear at certain points, with the result that one fascicle appears to merge with a neighboring fascicle. This is due to an obliqueness in the plane of section rather than an actual merging of fascicles. The collagen that makes up the bulk of the tendon fascicle has a homogeneous appearance as a result of the orderly packing of the individual collagen fibrils. The nuclei of the tendon cells appear as elongate profiles arranged in linear rows. The cytoplasm of these cells blends in with the collagen, leaving only the nuclei as the representative feature of the cell.

Figure 2, tendon, longitudinal section, human, H&E ×400.

This higher magnification micrograph shows the ordered single-file array of the tendon cell nuclei (*TC*) along with the intervening collagen. The latter has a homogeneous appearance. The cytoplasm of the cells is indistinguishable from the collagen, as is typical in H&E paraffin specimens. The variation in nuclear appearance is due to the plane of section and the position of the nuclei within the thickness of the section. A small blood vessel (*BV*) coursing within the endotendineum is also present in the specimen.

Figure 3, tendon, cross section, human, H&E ×400.

This specimen is well preserved, and the densely packed collagenous fibers appear as a homogeneous field, even though the fibers are viewed on their cut ends. The nuclei appear irregularly scattered, as opposed to their more uniform pattern in the longitudinal plane. This is explained by examining the *dashed line* in Figure 2, which is meant to represent an arbitrary cross-sectional cut of the tendon. Note the irregular spacing of the nuclei that are in the plane of the cut. Lastly, several small blood vessels (*BV*) are present within the endotendineum (*Ent*) within a fascicle.

KEY

BV, blood vessel
Ent, endotendineum
Ept, epitendineum
TC, tendon cell nuclei
TF, fascicle of tendon
dashed line, arbitrary cross-sectional cut of tendon

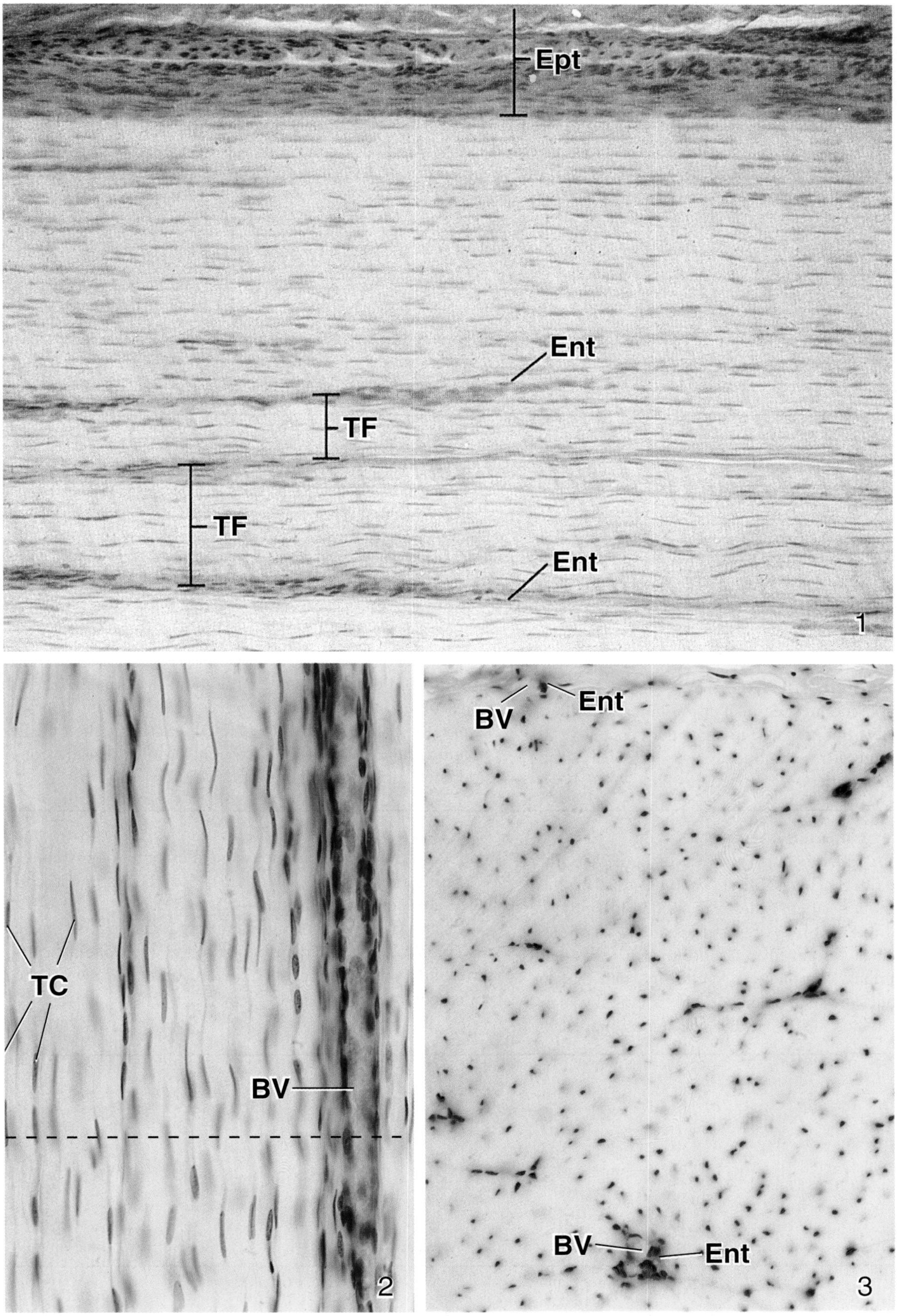
Ept
Ent
TF
TF
Ent
1
TC
BV
2
BV
Ent
BV
Ent
3

PLATE 6. ELASTIC FIBERS AND ELASTIC LAMELLAE

Elastic fibers are present in loose and dense connective tissue throughout the body, but in lesser amounts than collagenous fibers. Elastic fibers are not conspicuous in routine H&E sections but are visualized readily with special staining methods. (The following selectively color elastic material: Weigert's elastic tissue stain, purple-violet; Gomori's aldehyde fuchsin stain, blue-black; Verhoeff's hematoxylin elastic tissue stain, black; and modified Taenzer-Unna orcein stain, red-brown.) By using a combination of the special elastic stains and counterstains, such as H&E, not only the elastic fibers but also the other tissue components may be revealed, thus allowing study of the relationships between the elastic material and other connective tissue components.

Elastic material occurs in both fibrous and lamellar forms. In loose and dense connective tissue and in elastic cartilage (see Plate 9), the elastic material is in fibrous form. Similarly, the elastic ligaments that connect the cervical vertebrae and that are particularly prominent in grazing animals have a mixture of elastic and collagenous fibers in a tightly packed array. In the major, largest diameter arteries (e.g., aorta, pulmonary, common carotid, and other primary branches of the aorta), the *tunica media* consists of fenestrated layers of elastic tissue alternating with layers containing smooth muscle cells and collagenous tissue. This allows stretching and elastic rebound to assist in the propulsion of the blood. All arteries and most large arterioles have an *internal elastic lamina* that supports the delicate endothelium and its immediately subjacent connective tissue. It should be noted that both the collagen and elastic components of the tunica media are produced by the smooth muscle cells of this layer.

Figure 1, dermis, monkey, Weigert's ×160.

This shows the connective tissue of the skin, referred to as the dermis, stained to show the nature and distribution of the elastic fibers (*E*), which appear purple. The collagen fibers (*C*) have been stained by eosin, and the two fiber types are easily differentiated. The connective tissue at the top of the figure, close to the epithelium (the papillary layer of the dermis), contains thin elastic fibers (see upper left of figure) as well as less coarse collagen fibers. The lower portion of the figure shows considerably heavier elastic and collagen fibers. Also note that many of the elastic fibers appear as short rectangular profiles. These profiles simply represent fibers traveling through the thickness of the section at an oblique angle to the path of the knife. Careful examination will also reveal a few fibers that appear as dot-like profiles. They represent cross-sectioned elastic fibers. Overall, the elastic fibers of the dermis have a three-dimensional interlacing configuration, thus the variety of forms.

Figure 2, mesentery, rat, Weigert's ×160.

This is a whole mount specimen of mesentery, similar to Figure 2 in Plate 1 but prepared to show the connective tissue elements and differentially stained to reveal elastic fibers. The elastic fibers (*E*) appear as thin, long, criss-crossing and branching threads without discernable beginnings or endings and with a somewhat irregular course. Again, the collagen fibers (*C*) are contrasted by their eosin staining and appear as long, straight profiles that are considerably thicker than the elastic fibers.

Figure 3, artery, monkey, Weigert's ×80.

Elastic material also occurs in sheets or lamellae rather than string-like fibers. This figure shows the wall of an elastic artery (pulmonary artery) that was stained to show the elastic material. Each of the wavy lines is a lamella of elastic material that is organized in the form of a fenestrated sheet or membrane. The plane of section is such that the elastic membranes are seen on edge. This specimen was not subsequently stained with H&E. The empty-appearing spaces between elastic layers contain collagen fibers and smooth muscle cells, but they remain essentially unstained. In the muscular layer of blood vessel, both elastin and collagen are secreted by the smooth muscle cells.

Tissues of the body containing large amounts of elastic material are limited in distribution to the walls of elastic arteries and some ligaments that are associated with the spinal column.

KEY

BV, blood vessel
C, collagen fibers
D, duct of sweat gland
E, elastic fibers

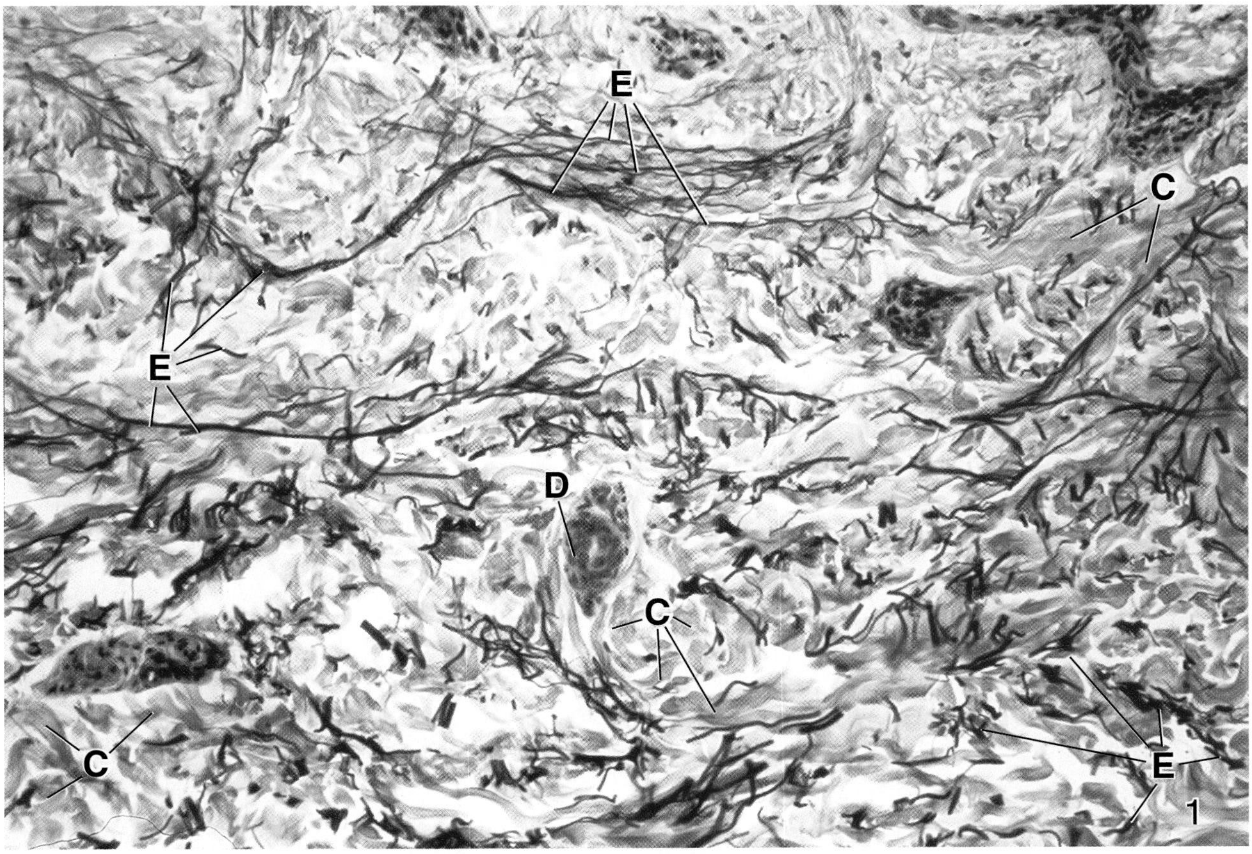
E
C
E
D
C
C
E
1

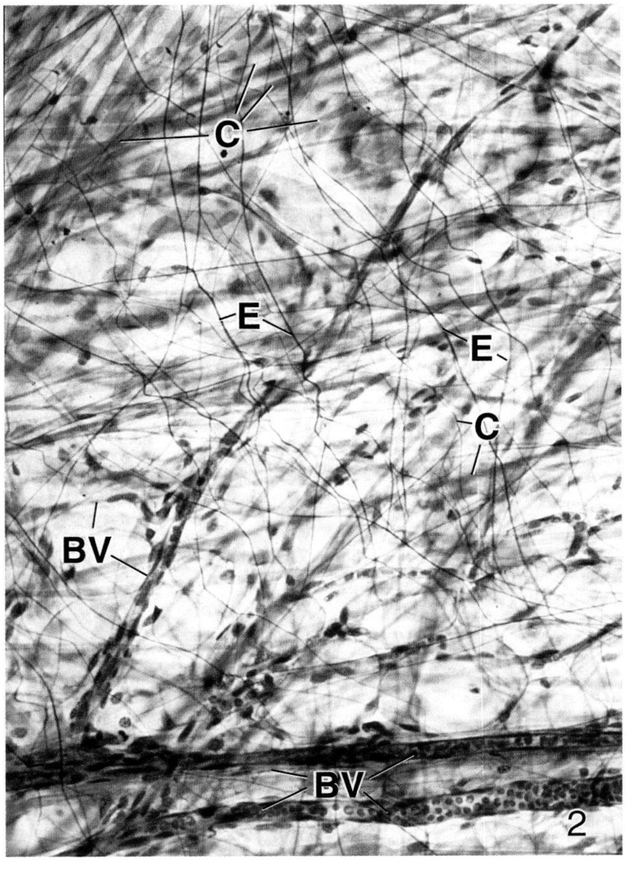
C
E
E
C
BV
BV
2

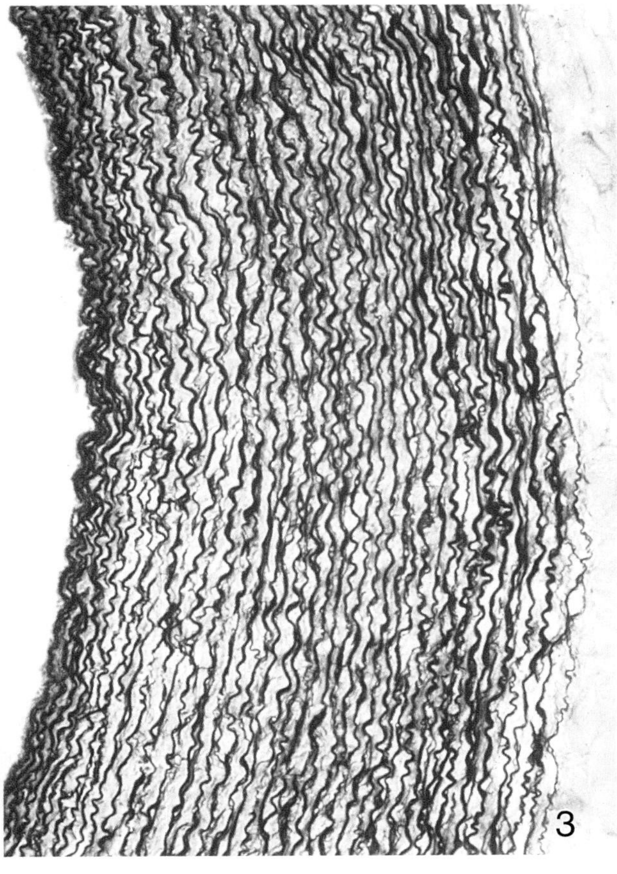
3

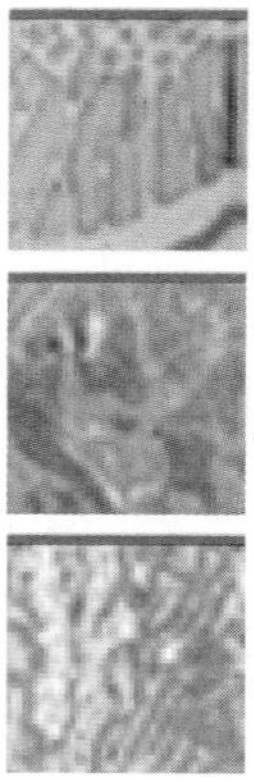

6

Adipose Tissue

OVERVIEW OF ADIPOSE TISSUE

Adipose tissue is a specialized connective tissue consisting of fat-storing cells (adipocytes) associated with a rich blood supply

Individual fat-storing cells, or ***adipocytes,*** and groups of adipocytes are found throughout loose connective tissue. Tissues in which adipocytes are the primary cell type are designated ***adipose tissue.*** Adipocytes function as fat-storage containers. The body has a limited capacity to store carbohydrate and protein; therefore, the fat contained within adipocytes represents the storage of excess nutritional calories that are not immediately used in metabolism or other activity. Fat is an efficient form of calorie storage because it has about twice the calorie density of carbohydrate and protein. The metabolism of fat can also be an essential source of water and energy for the body in the event of food deprivation. For example, the hump of a camel consists largely of fat and is a source of both energy and water for this desert animal.

There are two types of adipose tissue: white (unilocular) and brown (multilocular)

The two types of adipose tissue, ***white adipose tissue*** and ***brown adipose tissue,*** are so named because of their color in the living state.

- White adipose tissue is the predominant type in adult humans.
- Brown adipose tissue is present in humans during fetal life but diminishes during the first decade after birth.

WHITE ADIPOSE TISSUE

Function of White Adipose Tissue

Functions of white adipose tissue include energy storage, insulation, and cushioning of vital organs

Unilocular adipose tissue forms a layer called the ***panniculus adiposus*** or ***hypodermis*** in the connective tissue under the skin. This subcutaneous layer of connective tissue has a significant insulating function. Concentrations of adipose tissue are found in the connective tissue under the skin of the abdomen, buttocks, axilla, and thigh. Sex differences in the thickness of this fatty layer in the skin of

different parts of the body account, in part, for the differences in body contour between females and males. In both sexes, the breast is a preferential site for accumulation of adipose tissue; the nonlactating female breast is composed primarily of this tissue.

Internally, adipose tissue is preferentially located in the greater omentum, mesentery, and retroperitoneal space and is usually abundant around the kidneys. It is also found in bone marrow and between other tissues, where it fills in spaces. In the palms of the hands and the soles of the feet, beneath the visceral pericardium (around the outside of the heart), and in the orbits around the eyeballs, adipose tissue functions as a cushion. It retains this structural function even during reduced caloric intake; when adipose tissue elsewhere becomes depleted of lipid, this structural adipose tissue remains undiminished.

White adipose tissue produces the hormone leptin

Adipose tissue is exclusively responsible for the synthesis and secretion of ***leptin*** *[Gr. leptos, thin]*, a 16-kDa peptide hormone involved in the regulation of energy homeostasis. Generally accepted biologic effects of leptin are inhibition of food intake, loss of body weight, and stimulation of the metabolic rate. Thus, leptin fulfills the criteria for a ***circulating satiety factor*** that controls food intake when the body's store of energy is sufficient. Leptin most likely participates in an endocrine signaling pathway that communicates the energy state of adipose tissue to centers that regulate energy uptake. It acts on the central nervous system by binding to specific receptors, mainly in the hypothalamus. In addition, leptin communicates the fuel state of adipocytes from fat storage sites to other metabolically active tissues (i.e., from adipose tissue to muscle at a different site).

Histogenesis of Fat Cells

Early histologists debated whether adipose tissue was a specific tissue, distinct from connective tissue, or whether it was ordinary connective tissue in which fibroblasts stored fat globules. The current consensus is that adipocytes are a specific cell type and that they are derived from undifferentiated mesenchymal cells associated with the adventitia of small venules (Fig. 6.1). Therefore, adipocytes originate from the same stem cell population as fibroblasts and myofibroblasts in healing wounds. Even with the transmission electron microscope (TEM), it is still nearly impossible to distinguish ***early lipoblasts*** or ***preadipocytes*** from fibroblasts. Thus, many investigators describe the early lipoblast as a cell that is committed to differentiate into an adipocyte but is morphologically indistinguishable from a fibroblast.

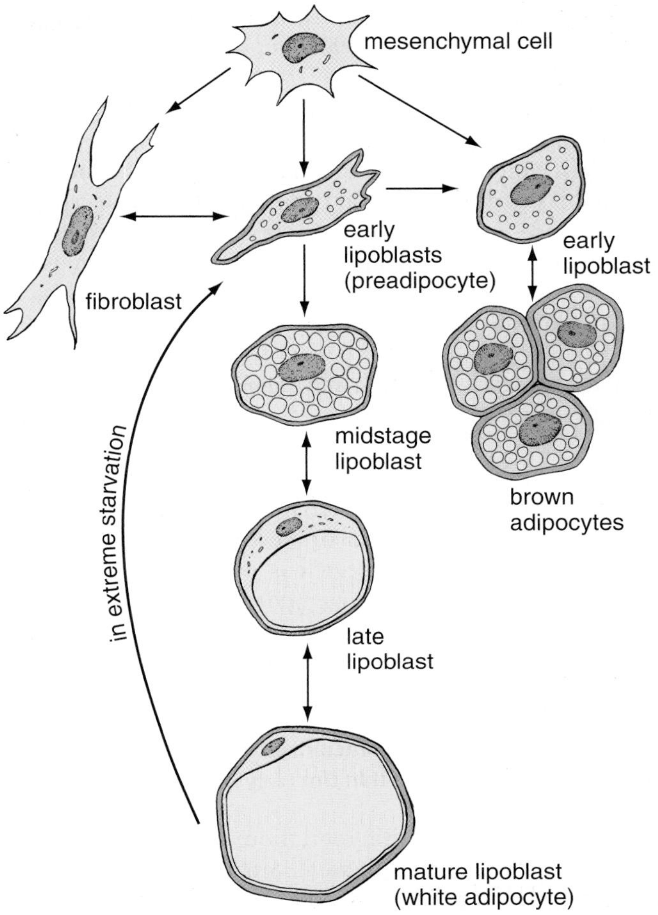

FIGURE 6.1
Diagram of the development of adipose tissue cells. Like all connective tissue cells, adipocytes are derived from mesenchymal cells (either mesodermally derived mesenchyme or ectomesenchyme derived from the neural crest). Mesenchymal cells give rise to fibroblasts and fibroblast-like cells that are committed to becoming lipoblasts (preadipocytes). Lipoblasts develop an external (basal) lamina and begin to accumulate numerous lipid droplets in their cytoplasm. In white adipose tissue, these droplets fuse to form a single large lipid droplet that ultimately fills the mature cell, compressing the nucleus, cytoplasm, and cytoplasmic organelles into a thin rim around the droplet. In brown adipose tissue, the individual lipid droplets remain separate. (Modified from Henrikson RC, Kaye GI, Mazurkiewicz JE. *NMS Histology.* Baltimore: Williams & Wilkins, 1997.)

White adipose tissue begins to form midway through fetal development

The lipoblasts that initially develop along the small blood vessels in the fetus are free of fat. Nevertheless, these cells are committed to becoming fat cells at this early stage; collections of such cells are sometimes called ***primitive fat organs.***

They are characterized by proliferating early lipoblasts and proliferating capillaries. Lipid accumulation in lipoblasts produces the typical morphology of the adipocytes.

Early lipoblasts look like fibroblasts but develop small lipid inclusions and a thin external lamina

TEM studies reveal that early lipoblasts have an elongated configuration, multiple cytoplasmic processes, and abundant endoplasmic reticulum and Golgi membranes. As lipoblastic differentiation begins, smooth-surfaced vesicles increase in number, with a corresponding decrease in rough endoplasmic reticulum (rER). Small lipid inclusions appear at one pole of the cytoplasm. Pinocytotic vesicles and an external lamina also appear.

Midstage lipoblasts become ovoid as lipid accumulation changes the cell dimensions

With further development, the cells assume an oval configuration. The most characteristic feature at this stage is the extensive concentration of smooth vesicles and small lipid droplets around the nucleus and extending toward both poles of the cell. Glycogen particles appear at the periphery of the lipid droplets, and pinocytotic vesicles and basal lamina become more apparent. These cells are designated ***midstage lipoblasts.***

The mature adipocyte is characterized by a single, large lipid inclusion surrounded by a thin rim of cytoplasm

In the late stage of differentiation, the cells increase in size and become more spherical. Small lipid droplets coalesce to form large lipid vacuoles that occupy the central portion of the cytoplasm. Smooth endoplasmic reticulum (sER) is abundant, whereas rER is less prominent. These cells are designated ***late lipoblasts.*** Eventually, the lipid mass compresses the nucleus to an eccentric position, producing a *signet-ring* appearance in hematoxylin and eosin (H&E) preparations. These cells are designated ***adipocytes*** or ***mature lipocytes.***

Structure of Adipocytes and Adipose Tissue

Unilocular adipocytes are large cells, sometimes 100 μm or more in diameter

When isolated, adipocytes are spherical, but they may appear polyhedral or oval when crowded together in adipose tissue. Their large size is due to the accumulated lipid in the cell. The nucleus is flattened and displaced to one side of the lipid mass; the cytoplasm forms a thin rim around the lipid. In routine histologic sections, the lipid is lost through extraction by organic solvents such as xylene; consequently, adipose tissue appears as a delicate meshwork of polygonal profiles (Fig. 6.2). The thin strand of meshwork that separates adjacent adipocytes represents the cytoplasm of both cells and the extracellular matrix. The strand is usually so thin, however, that it is not possible to resolve its component parts in the light microscope.

Adipose tissue is richly supplied with blood vessels, and capillaries are found at the angles of the meshwork where adjacent adipocytes meet. Silver stains show that adipocytes are surrounded by reticular fibers (type III collagen), which are secreted by the adipocytes. Special stains also reveal the presence of unmyelinated nerve fibers and numerous mast cells.

The lipid mass in the adipocyte is not membrane bounded

Transmission electron microscopy reveals that the interface between the contained lipid and surrounding cytoplasm of the adipocyte is composed of a 5-nm-thick condensed layer of lipid reinforced by parallel vimentin filaments measuring 5 to 10 nm in diameter. This layer separates the hydrophobic contents of the lipid droplet from the hydrophilic cytoplasmic matrix.

The perinuclear cytoplasm of the adipocyte contains a small Golgi apparatus, free ribosomes, short profiles of rER, microfilaments, and intermediate filaments. Filamentous mitochondria and multiple profiles of sER are also found in the thin rim of cytoplasm surrounding the lipid droplet (Fig. 6.3).

Regulation of Adipose Tissue

The amount of adipose tissue in an individual is determined by expression of the leptin (ob) gene

The recent discovery of the leptin *(ob)* gene, which encodes a fat-specific mRNA and *leptin,* has given some insight into the mechanism of energy homeostasis. Human leptin gene expression occurs in mature adipocytes and is highly regulated. Studies of obese individuals show that levels of leptin mRNA in adipose tissue as well as serum levels of leptin are elevated in all types of obesity, regardless of whether it is caused by genetic factors, hypothalamic lesions, or increased efficiency of food utilization. Studies of individuals who have lost weight and those with ***anorexia nervosa*** show that leptin mRNA levels in their adipose tissue and serum levels of leptin are significantly reduced. In experimental animal models, the addition of recombinant leptin to obese, leptin-deficient *ob/ob* mice causes them to reduce their food intake and lose about 30% of their total body weight after 2 weeks of treatment.

Genetic obesity is most likely related to the expression of defective leptin *(ob)* or leptin receptor genes. This may explain why identical twins usually have the same or close to the same amount of body fat. Even when the amount of body fat in identical twins varies, however, the patterns of distribution are always the same.

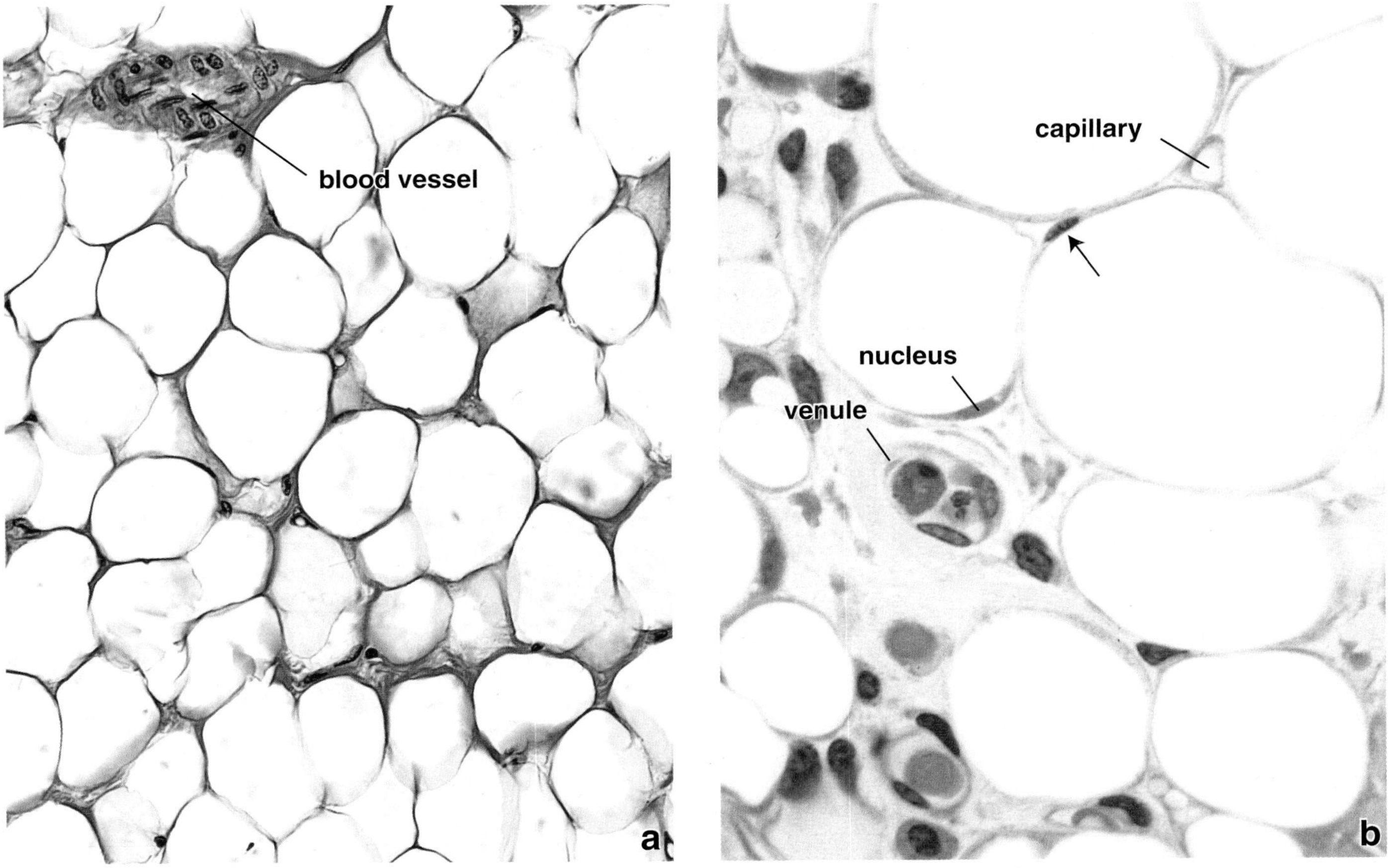

FIGURE 6.2
White adipose tissue. a. Photomicrograph of white adipose tissue, showing its characteristic meshwork in a H&E–stained paraffin preparation. Each space represents a single large drop of lipid before its dissolution from the cell during tissue preparation. The surrounding eosin-stained material represents the cytoplasm of the adjoining cells and some intervening connective tissue. ×320. **b.** High-power photomicrograph of a glutaraldehyde-preserved, plastic-embedded specimen of white adipose tissue. The cytoplasm of the individual adipose cells is recognizable in some areas, and part of the nucleus of one of the cells is included in the plane of section. A second nucleus *(arrow)*, which appears intimately related to one of the adipose cells, may actually belong to a fibroblast; it is difficult to tell with assurance. Because of the large size of adipose cells, the nucleus is infrequently observed in a given cell. A capillary and a small venule are also evident in the photomicrograph. ×950.

Deposition and mobilization of lipid are influenced by neural and hormonal factors

One of the major metabolic functions of adipose tissue involves the uptake of fatty acids from the blood and their conversion to triglyceride within the adipocyte. Triglyceride is then stored within the cell's lipid droplet. When adipose tissue is stimulated by neural or hormonal mechanisms, triglycerides are broken down into glycerol and fatty acids, a process called mobilization. The fatty acids pass through the adipocyte cell membrane to enter a capillary. Here, they are bound to the carrier protein albumin and transported to other cells, which use fatty acids as metabolic fuel.

Neural mobilization is particularly important during periods of fasting and exposure to severe cold. During early stages of experimental starvation in rodents, adipose cells in a denervated fat pad continue to deposit fat. Adipose cells in the intact contralateral fat pad mobilize fat. It is now known that norepinephrine (which is liberated by the endings of nerve cells of the sympathetic nervous system) initiates a series of metabolic steps that lead to the activation of lipase. This enzyme splits triglycerides (neutral fats), which constitute over 90% of the lipid in the fat of the adipocyte. The enzymatic activity is an early step in the mobilization of the lipid.

An unusual form of obesity is due to injury of the hypothalamus, the portion of the base of the brain where neurosecretions that control pituitary function are synthesized. Although the clinical manifestation of ***hypothalamic obesity*** is associated with increased food consumption, experiments with laboratory animals with hypothalamic injury show that caloric intake is not the only factor leading

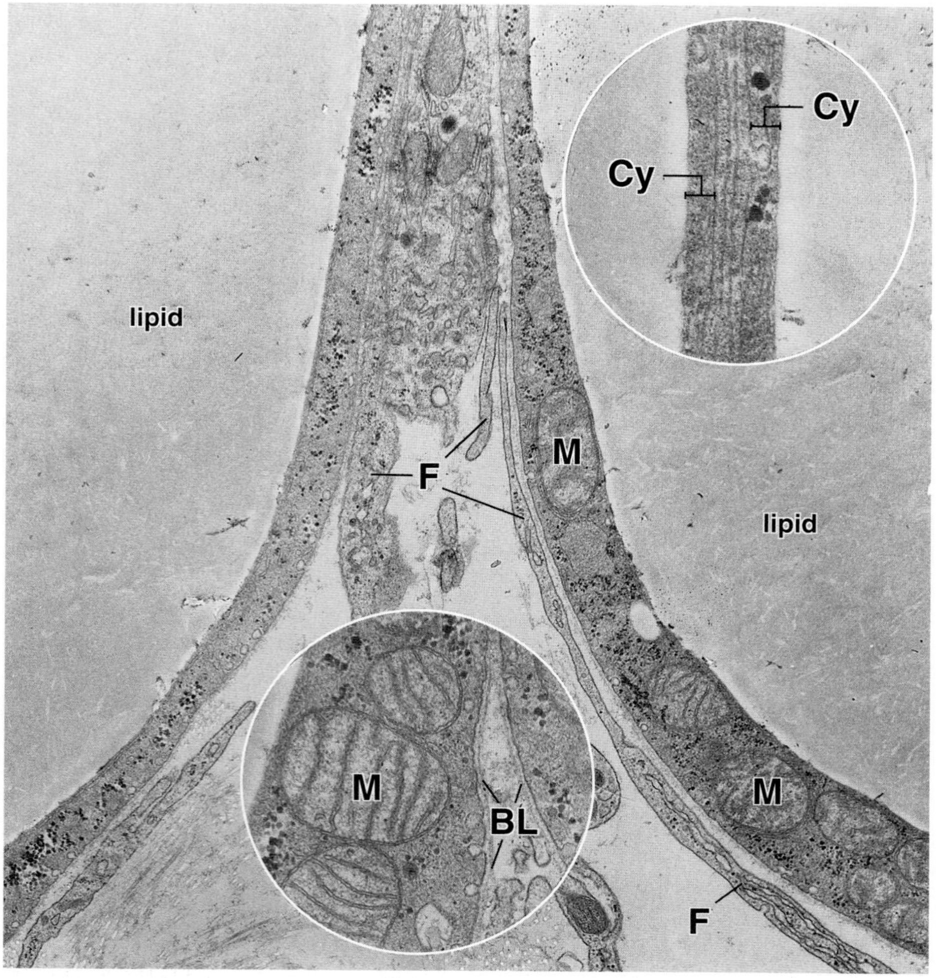

FIGURE 6.3
Electron micrograph showing portions of two adjacent adipose cells. The cytoplasm of the adipose cells reveals mitochondria *(M)* and glycogen (the latter appears as the very dark particles). ×15,000. **Upper inset.** Attenuated cytoplasm *(Cy)* of two adjoining adipose cells. Each cell is separated by a narrow space containing external (basal) lamina and an extremely attenuated process of a fibroblast. ×65,000. **Lower inset.** The external (basal) lamina *(BL)* of the adipose cells appears as a discrete layer where the cells are adequately separated from one another. *F,* fibroblast processes. ×30,000.

to obesity. Lesioned rats deposit more body fat than control animals fed the same amounts of food.

Hormonal mobilization involves insulin, a hormone that inhibits the action of hormone-sensitive lipase and thus blocks the release of fatty acids. It also enhances the conversion of glucose into the triglycerides of the lipid droplet by the adipocyte. In addition, other hormones modify various steps in the metabolism of adipose tissue, including thyroid hormone, glucocorticoids, prostaglandins, and hormones of the pituitary gland.

▼ BROWN ADIPOSE TISSUE

Adipocytes of brown, multilocular adipose tissue contain numerous fat droplets

The cells of brown adipose tissue are smaller than those of white adipose tissue. The nucleus of a mature multilocular adipocyte is typically in an eccentric position within the cell, but it is not flattened, as is the nucleus of a unilocular adipocyte.

In routine H&E–stained sections, the cytoplasm of the multilocular adipocyte consists largely of empty vacuoles because the lipid that ordinarily occupies the vacuolated spaces is lost during preparation (Fig. 6.4). Multilocular adipocytes depleted of their lipid bear a closer resemblance to epithelial cells than to connective tissue cells. The multilocular adipocyte contains numerous mitochondria, a small Golgi apparatus, and only small amounts of rER and sER. The mitochondria contain large amounts of cytochrome oxidase, which imparts the brown color to the cells.

Brown adipose tissue is subdivided into lobules by partitions of connective tissue, but the connective tissue stroma between individual cells within the lobules is sparse. The tissue has a rich supply of capillaries that enhance its color. Numerous unmyelinated nerve fibers are present among the fat cells.

Metabolism of lipid in brown adipose tissue generates heat

Hibernating animals have large amounts of brown adipose tissue. The tissue serves as a ready source of lipid.

When oxidized, it produces heat to warm the blood flowing through the brown fat on arousal from hibernation. This type of heat production is known as *nonshivering thermogenesis*.

Brown adipose tissue is also present in nonhibernating animals and again serves as a source of heat. In humans, multilocular adipose tissue is present in large amounts in the newborn, which helps offset the extensive heat loss that results from the newborn's high surface-to-mass ratio. The amount of brown adipose tissue gradually decreases as the body grows, but it remains widely distributed throughout the first decade of life. It then disappears from most sites except for regions around the kidney, adrenal glands, aorta, and regions in the neck and mediastinum. As in the mobilization of lipid in white adipose tissue, lipid is mobilized and heat is generated by multilocular adipocytes when they are stimulated by the sympathetic nervous system.

Thermogenic activity of brown adipose tissue is regulated by the unique uncoupling protein found in mitochondria

The mitochondria found in the cytoplasm of brown adipose tissue cells contain a unique ***uncoupling protein (UCP-1)***, which uncouples the oxidation of fatty acids from the production of ATP. At the molecular level, UCP-1 facilitates proton transport across the inner mitochondrial membrane. The movement of protons from the inner mitochondrial compartment dissipates the mitochondrial proton gradient, thus uncoupling respiration from ATP synthesis. The energy produced by the mitochondria is then used as heat. In experimental animals, UCP-1 activity has been shown to increase during cold stress.

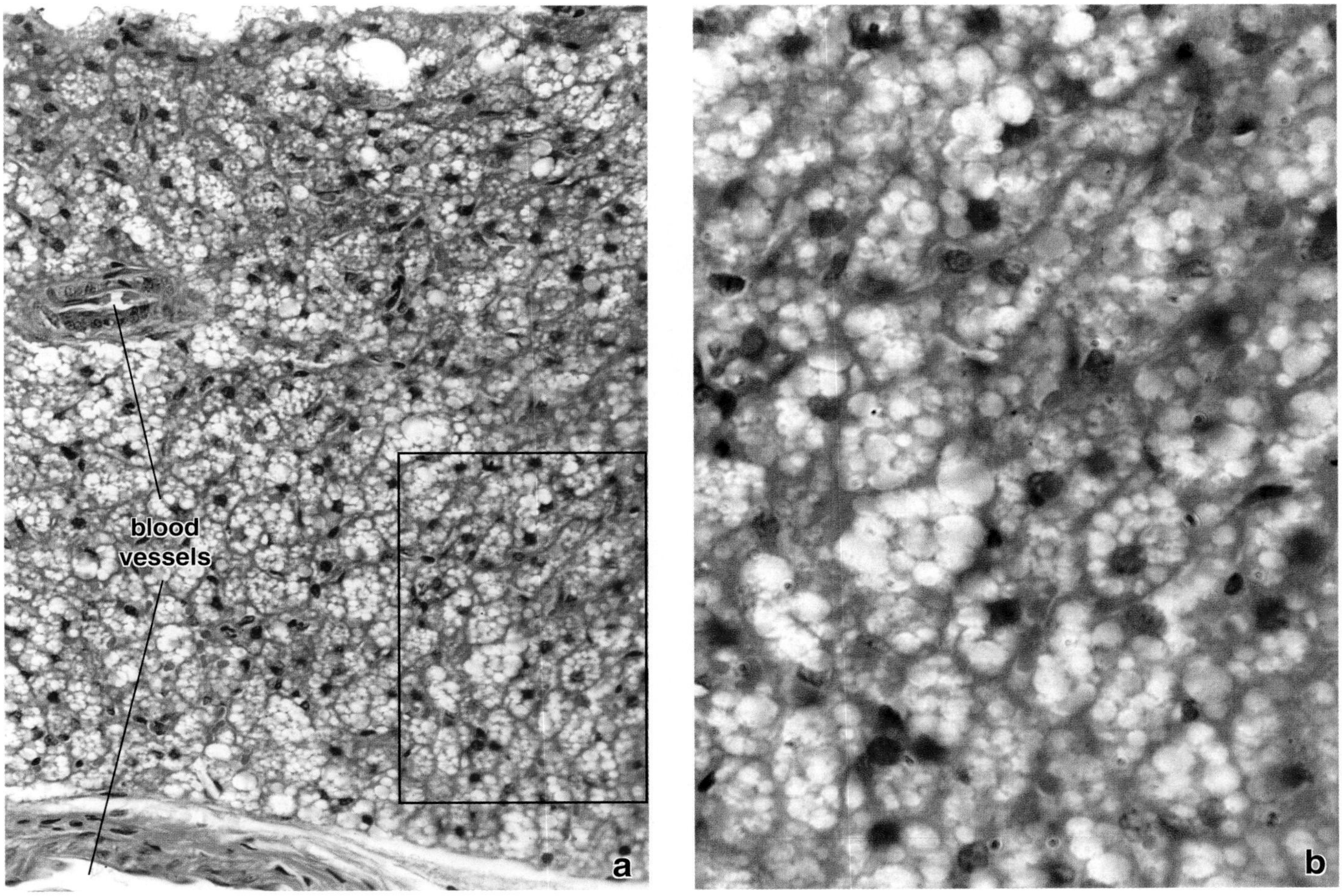

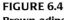

FIGURE 6.4
Brown adipose tissue. a. Photomicrograph of brown adipose tissue from a newborn in a H&E–stained paraffin preparation. The cells contain fat droplets of varying size. Note the large blood vessels within the tissue. ×150. **b.** This photomicrograph obtained at a higher magnification shows the brown adipose cells with round and often centrally located nuclei. Most of the cells are polygonal and are closely packed, with numerous lipid droplets. In some cells, large lipid droplets displace nuclei toward the cell periphery. A network of collagen fibers and capillaries surrounds the brown adipose cells. ×320.

BOX 6.1

Clinical Correlations: Adipose Tissue Tumors

The study of the numerous varieties of benign and malignant adipose tissue tumors provides further insight into, and confirmation of, the sequence of adipose tissue differentiation described above. Adipose tissue tumors are classified by the morphology of the predominant cell in the tumor (Fig. 6.5). As with epithelial tumors and tumors of fibroblast origin, the variety of adipose tissue tumors reflects the normal pattern of adipose tissue differentiation. That is, discrete tumor types can be described that consist primarily of cells resembling a given stage in adipose tissue differentiation. The most common adipose tissue tumor is the ***lipoma.*** It is more common than all other soft tissue tumors combined. Lipomas are usually found in subcutaneous tissues in middle-aged and elderly individuals. Although Figure 6.5 relates primarily to white adipose tissue tumors, tumors of brown adipose tissue are also found. Not surprisingly, these are called ***hibernomas.***

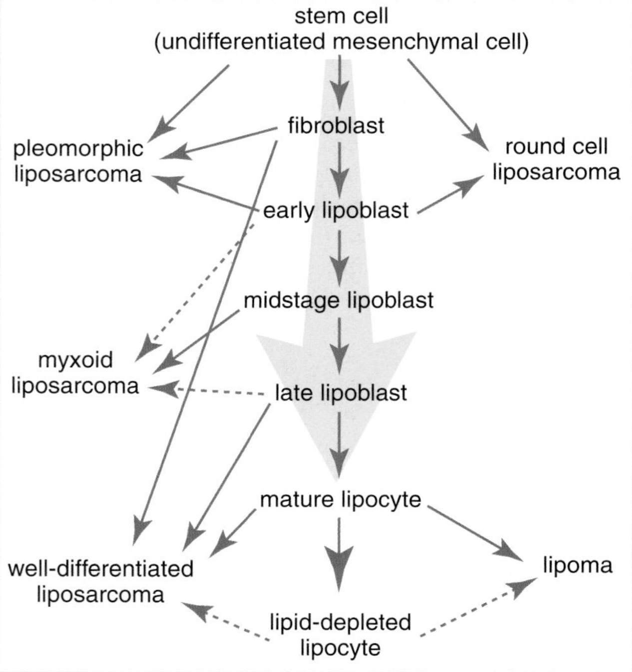

FIGURE 6.5
Adipocyte differentiation in relation to tumor cell development. Diagram summarizing the relationships between differentiation of normal adipose cells *(midcolumn)* and several types of adipose tissue tumors *(lateral columns).* Each type of adipose tissue tumor exhibits a predominant cell type that resembles one of the stages of differentiation of normal adipose cells. *Solid-line arrows* indicate the most frequently occurring cell type in each kind of tumor. *Dotted-line arrows* indicate the less frequently occurring cell type in that tumor. (Modified from Fu YS, et al. *Pathol Annu* 1980;15(Part 1):85, with permission of the McGraw-Hill Companies.)

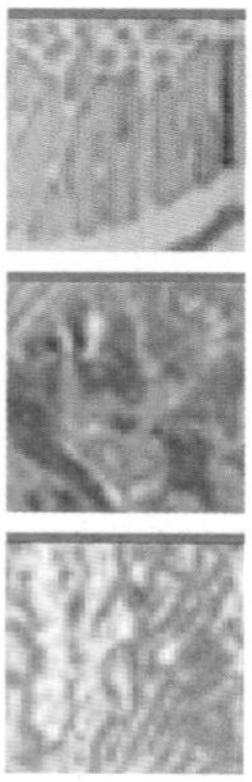

7

Cartilage

▽ OVERVIEW OF CARTILAGE

Cartilage is a form of connective tissue composed of cells called chondrocytes and a highly specialized extracellular matrix

Cartilage is an avascular tissue that consists of ***chondrocytes*** and an extensive extracellular matrix. Produced and maintained by chondrocytes, the cartilage matrix is solid and firm but also somewhat pliable, which accounts for its resilience. The large ratio of glycosaminoglycans to type II collagen in the cartilage matrix permits diffusion of substances between blood vessels in the surrounding connective tissue and the chondrocytes, thereby maintaining the viability of the tissue. Also, the presence of large amounts of hyaluronic acid in cartilage matrix makes it well adapted to bear weight, especially at points of movement, as in synovial joints. Because it maintains this property even while growing, cartilage is a key tissue in most growing bones.

Three different kinds of cartilage are distinguished on the basis of characteristics of the matrix:

- ***Hyaline cartilage,*** characterized by matrix containing type II collagen fibers, proteoglycans, and hyaluronic acid
- ***Elastic cartilage,*** characterized by elastic fibers and elastic lamellae in addition to the matrix material of hyaline cartilage
- ***Fibrocartilage,*** characterized by abundant type I collagen fibers in addition to the matrix material of hyaline cartilage

▽ HYALINE CARTILAGE

Hyaline cartilage is distinguished by a homogeneous, amorphous matrix

The matrix of ***hyaline cartilage*** appears glassy in the living state, hence the name hyaline *[Gr. hyalos, glassy]*. Throughout the cartilage matrix are spaces called ***lacunae.*** Located within these lacunae are the ***chondrocytes.*** Hyaline cartilage is not a simple, inert, homogeneous substance, but a complex living tissue. It provides a low friction surface, participates in lubrication in synovial joints, and distributes applied forces to the underlying bone. Although its capacity for repair is limited, under normal circumstances it shows no evidence of abrasive wear over a lifetime. The macromolecules of hyaline ***cartilage matrix*** consist of collagen (predominantly type II fibrils), proteoglycans, noncollagenous proteins, and glycoproteins that give it its mechanical and biologic properties.

Hyaline cartilage matrix is produced by chondrocytes and contains three major classes of molecules

Three classes of molecules are present in hyaline cartilage matrix:

- ***Collagen molecules.*** Collagen is the major matrix protein. Four collagen types participate in the formation of relatively thin (20-nm-diameter), short matrix fibrils.

Type II collagen constitutes the bulk of the fibril; ***type XI collagen*** regulates the fibril size; and ***type IX collagen*** facilitates fibril interaction with the matrix proteoglycan molecules. ***Type X collagen*** organizes the collagen fibrils into a three-dimensional hexagonal lattice. Because types II, IX, X, and XI are found in significant amounts only in the cartilage matrix, they are referred to as ***cartilage-specific collagen molecules.*** In addition, ***type VI collagen*** is also found in the matrix, mainly at the periphery of the chondrocytes, where it helps to attach these cells to the matrix framework. See Table 5.2 to review the different types of collagen.

- ***Proteoglycans.*** The ground substance of hyaline cartilage contains three kinds of glycosaminoglycans: ***hyaluronic acid, chondroitin sulfate,*** and ***keratan sulfate.*** As in loose connective tissue matrix, the chondroitin and keratan sulfates of cartilage matrix are joined to a ***core protein*** to form a ***proteoglycan monomer*** (Fig. 7.1). Each linear hyaluronic acid molecule is associated with approximately 80 proteoglycan monomers, which are bound to the hyaluronic acid by link proteins to form large ***hyaluronate proteoglycan aggregates.*** These aggregates are bound to the thin collagen matrix fibrils by electrostatic interactions and cross-linking glycoproteins.
- ***Noncollagenous proteins.*** The cartilage matrix also contains other proteoglycans that do not form aggregates, as well as noncollagenous and nonproteoglycan-linked glycoproteins. These small regulatory and structural proteins influence interactions between the chondrocytes and the matrix and have clinical value as markers of cartilage turnover and degeneration. Examples of such proteins are ***anchorin CII, tenascin,*** and ***fibronectin,*** which help anchor chondrocytes to the matrix.

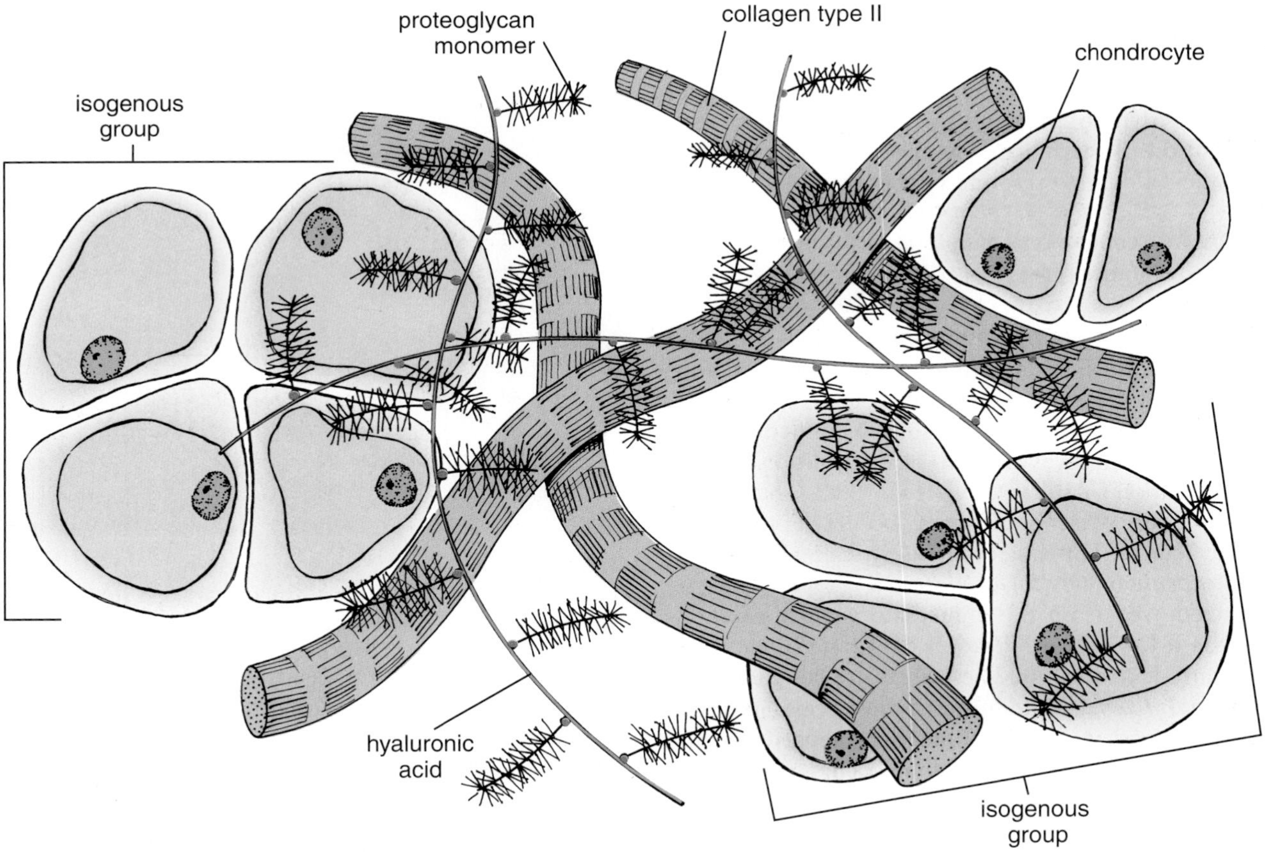

FIGURE 7.1
Molecular structure of the ground substance of hyaline cartilage. This schematic diagram shows the relationship of hyaluronate proteoglycan aggregates to type II collagen fibrils and chondrocytes in the ground substance of hyaline cartilage. A hyaluronic acid molecule forming a linear aggregate with many proteoglycan monomers is interwoven with a network of collagen fibrils. Proteoglycan monomers are linked electrostatically to the collagen fibrils as well as by cross-linking glycoproteins. Chondrocytes, the principal cells of hyaline cartilage, appear in isogenous groups.

Hyaline cartilage matrix is highly hydrated to permit diffusion of small metabolites and resilience

Like other connective tissue matrices, cartilage matrix is highly hydrated. Sixty to eighty percent of the net weight of hyaline cartilage is water. Much of this water is bound tightly to the hyaluronate proteoglycan aggregates, which imparts resilience to the cartilage. Some of the water is bound loosely enough, however, to allow diffusion of small metabolites to and from the chondrocytes.

In articular cartilage, both transient and regional changes occur in water content during joint movement and when the joint is subjected to pressure. The high degree of hydration and the movement of water in the matrix allow the cartilage matrix to respond to varying pressure loads and contribute to cartilage's weight-bearing capacity. Throughout life, cartilage undergoes continuous internal remodeling as the cells replace matrix molecules lost through degradation. New evidence indicates that normal matrix turnover depends on the ability of the chondrocytes to detect changes in matrix composition. The chondrocyte then responds by synthesizing appropriate types of new molecules. In addition, the matrix acts as a signal transducer for the embedded chondrocytes. Thus, pressure loads applied to the cartilage, as in synovial joints, create mechanical, electrical, and chemical signals that help direct the synthetic activity of the chondrocyte. As the body ages, the composition of the matrix changes, and the chondrocytes lose their ability to respond to these stimuli.

Ground substance components of hyaline cartilage matrix are not distributed uniformly

Because the proteoglycans of hyaline cartilage contain a high concentration of bound sulfate groups, ground substance stains with basic dyes and with hematoxylin. Thus, the basophilia and metachromasia seen in stained sections of cartilage provide information on the distribution and relative concentration of sulfated proteoglycans. The highest concentration of these substances occurs immediately around the lacunae. This ring of intensely staining matrix is called the ***capsule*** or ***territorial matrix*** (Fig. 7.2). The matrix more removed from the immediate vicinity of chondrocytes has a lower concentration of sulfated proteoglycans and stains less intensely. These areas are designated the ***interterritorial matrix.*** In addition to these regional differences in the concentration of sulfated proteoglycans, the decrease in proteoglycan content that occurs as cartilage ages is also reflected by staining differences.

Chondrocytes are specialized cells that produce and maintain the extracellular matrix

In hyaline cartilage, chondrocytes are distributed either singly or in clusters called ***isogenous groups.*** When the chondrocytes are present in isogenous groups, they represent cells that have recently divided. As the newly divided chondrocytes produce matrix material, which surrounds them, they become dispersed.

The cytoplasm of chondrocytes varies in appearance relative to their activity. Chondrocytes that are active in matrix production display areas of cytoplasmic basophilia, indicating protein synthesis, and clear areas, reflecting the large Golgi apparatus (Fig. 7.3). Chondrocytes secrete not only the collagen present in the matrix but also all of the gly-

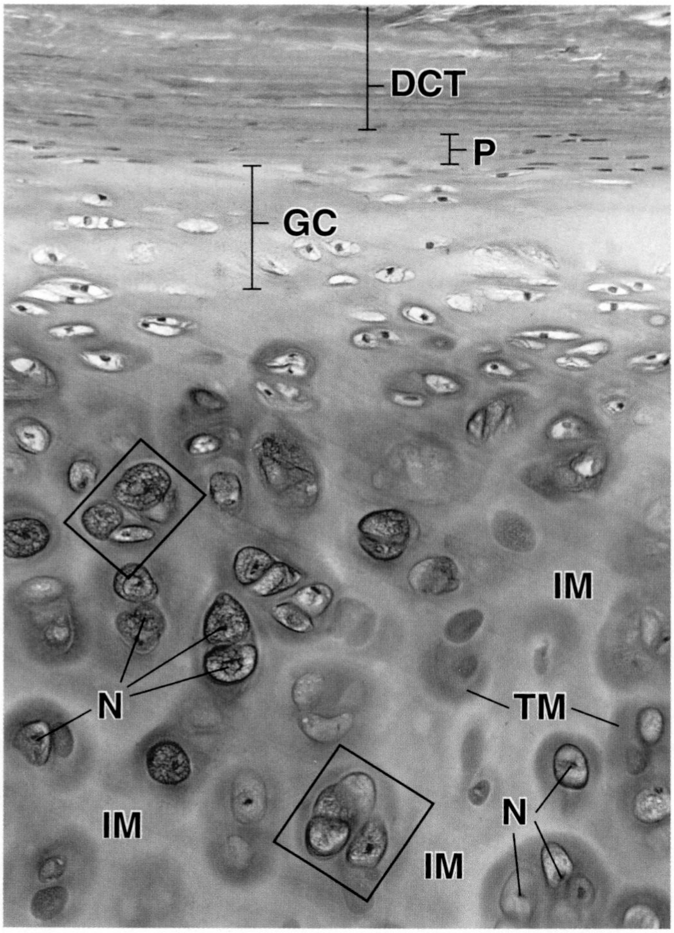

FIGURE 7.2
Photomicrograph of a typical hyaline cartilage specimen stained with H&E. The upper portion of the micrograph shows the dense connective tissue *(DCT)* overlying the perichondrium *(P),* from which new cartilage cells are derived. A slightly basophilic layer of growing cartilage *(GC)* underlying the perichondrium contains chondroblasts and immature chondrocytes that display little more than the nucleus residing in an empty-appearing lacuna. This layer represents deposition of new cartilage (appositional growth) on the surface of the existing hyaline cartilage below. Mature chondrocytes with clearly visible nuclei *(N)* reside in the lacunae and are well preserved in this specimen. They produce the cartilage matrix that shows the dark-staining capsule or territorial matrix *(TM)* immediately surrounding the lacunae. The interterritorial matrix *(IM)* is more removed from the immediate vicinity of chondrocytes and is less intensely stained. Growth from within the cartilage (interstitial growth) is reflected by the chondrocyte pairs and clusters that are responsible for the formation of isogenous groups *(rectangles).* ×480.

cosaminoglycans and proteoglycans. In older, less active cells, the Golgi apparatus is smaller; clear areas of cytoplasm, when evident, usually indicate sites of extracted lipid droplets and glycogen stores. In such specimens, chondrocytes also display considerable distortion because of shrinkage after the glycogen and lipid are lost during the preparation of the tissue. With the transmission electron microscope (TEM), the active chondrocyte displays numerous profiles of rough endoplasmic reticulum (rER), a large Golgi apparatus, secretory granules, vesicles, intermediate filaments, microtubules, and actin microfilaments (Fig. 7.4). In old cartilage cells, intermediate filaments are numerous.

Hyaline cartilage provides a model for the developing skeleton of the fetus

In early fetal development, hyaline cartilage is the precursor of bones that develop by the process of ***endochondral ossification*** (Fig. 7.5). Initially, most long bones are represented by cartilage models that resemble the shape of the adult bone. During the developmental process when much of the cartilage is replaced by bone, the remaining cartilage serves as a growth site called the ***epiphyseal growth plate (epiphyseal disc).*** This cartilage remains functional as long as the bone grows in length (Fig. 7.6). In the adult, the cartilage that remains from the developing skeleton is found on the articular surfaces of joints (articular cartilage), as seen in Figure 7.7, and within the rib cage (costal cartilages). Hyaline cartilage is also present in the adult as the skeletal unit in the trachea, bronchi, larynx, and nose.

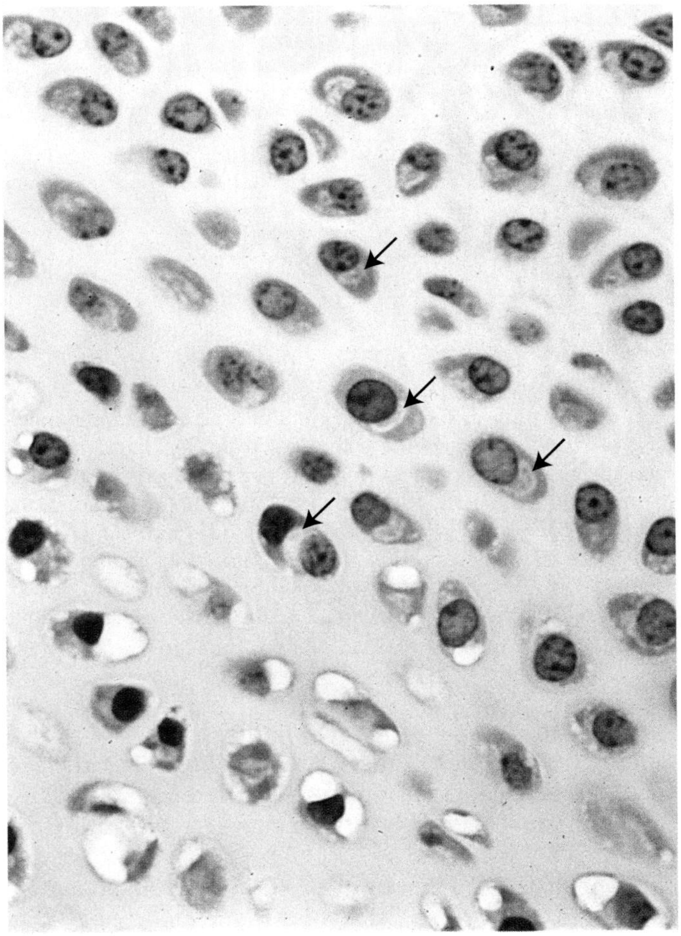

FIGURE 7.3
Photomicrograph of young, growing cartilage. This specimen was preserved in glutaraldehyde, embedded in plastic, and stained with H&E. The chondrocytes, especially those in the upper part of the photomicrograph, are well preserved. The cytoplasm is deeply stained, exhibiting a distinct and relatively homogeneous basophilia. The clear areas *(arrows)* represent sites of the Golgi apparatus. ×520.

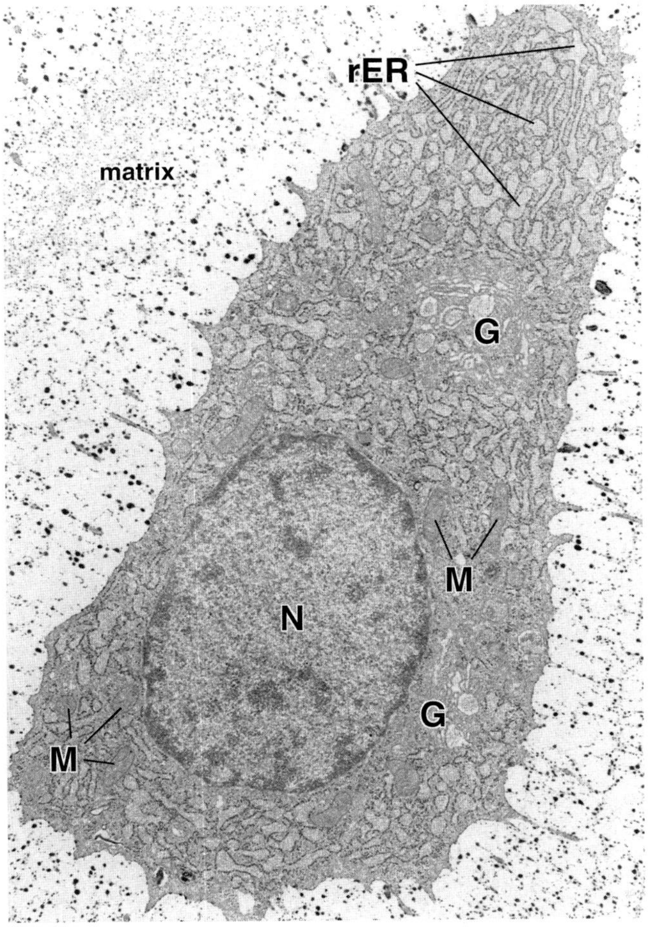

FIGURE 7.4
Electron micrograph of a young, active chondrocyte and surrounding matrix. The nucleus *(N)* of the chondrocyte is eccentrically located, like those in Figure 7.3, and the cytoplasm displays numerous and somewhat dilated profiles of rER, Golgi apparatus *(G)*, and mitochondria *(M)*. The large amount of rER and the extensive Golgi apparatus indicate that the cell is actively engaged in the production of cartilage matrix. The numerous dark particles in the matrix contain proteoglycans. The particularly large particles adjacent to the cell are located in the region of the matrix that is identified as the capsule or territorial matrix. ×15,000. (Courtesy of Dr. H. Clarke Anderson.)

A firmly attached connective tissue, the perichondrium, surrounds hyaline cartilage

The ***perichondrium*** is a dense connective tissue composed of cells that are indistinguishable from fibroblasts. In many respects, the perichondrium resembles the capsule that surrounds glands and many organs. It also serves as the source of new cartilage cells. When actively growing, the perichondrium appears divided into an ***inner cellular layer,*** which gives rise to new cartilage cells, and an ***outer fibrous layer.*** This division is not always evident, especially in perichondrium that is not actively producing new cartilage or in very slow growing cartilage. The changes that occur during the differentiation of new chondrocytes in growing cartilage are illustrated in Figure 7.3.

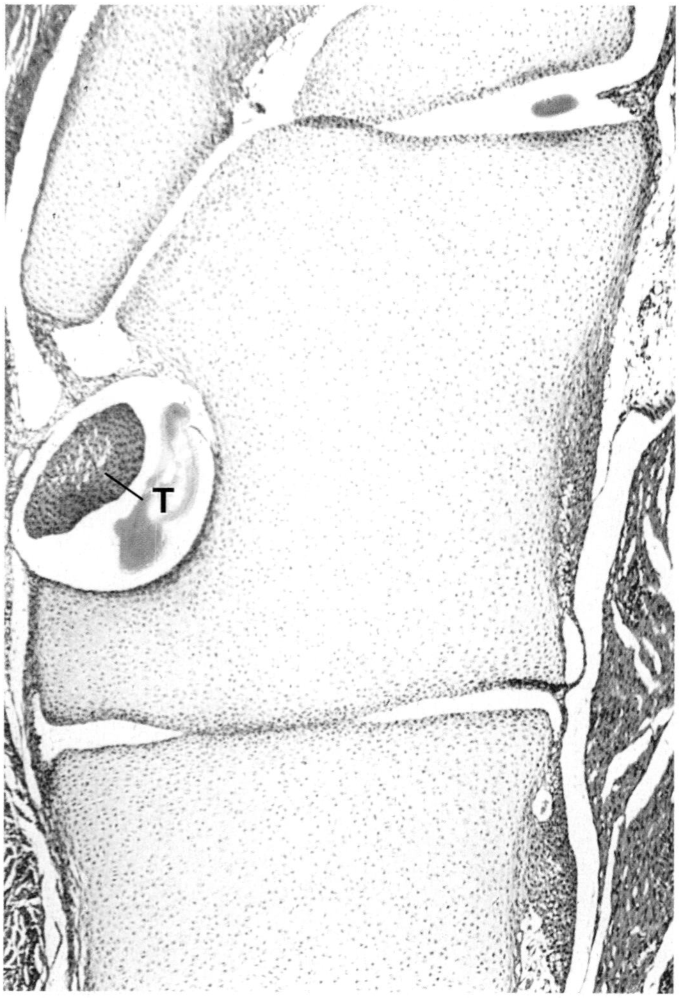

FIGURE 7.5
Photomicrograph of several cartilages that form the initial skeleton of the foot. The hyaline cartilage of developing tarsal bones will be replaced by bone as endochondral ossification proceeds. In this early stage of development, synovial joints are being formed between developing tarsal bones. Note that nonarticulating surfaces of the hyaline cartilage models of tarsal bones are covered by the perichondrium, which also contributes to the development of joint capsules. Also, a developing tendon *(T)* is evident in the indentation of the cartilage seen on the left side of the micrograph. ×85.

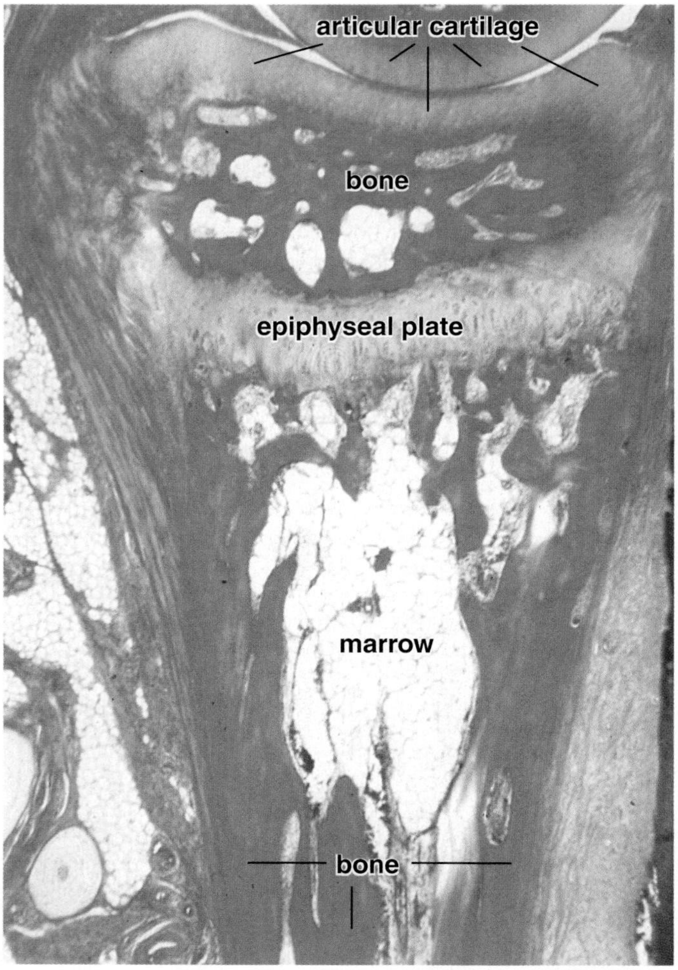

FIGURE 7.6
Photomicrograph of the proximal end of a growing long bone. A disc of hyaline cartilage—the epiphyseal plate—separates the more proximally located epiphysis from the funnel-shaped diaphysis located distal to the plate. The articular cartilage on the surface of the epiphysis contributes to the synovial joint and is also composed of hyaline cartilage. Whereas the cartilage of the epiphyseal plate disappears when lengthwise growth of the bone is completed, the articular cartilage remains throughout life. The spaces within the bone are occupied by marrow. ×85.

There are some exceptions to the general rule that hyaline cartilage is surrounded by a perichondrium. These include areas where cartilage forms a free surface, as in the articular surfaces in joints, and areas where cartilage makes direct contact with bone, as in the nasal and costal cartilages and sites of bone formation. In these areas, proliferation of chondrocytes within the cartilage lacunae provides the new cells for ***interstitial growth.***

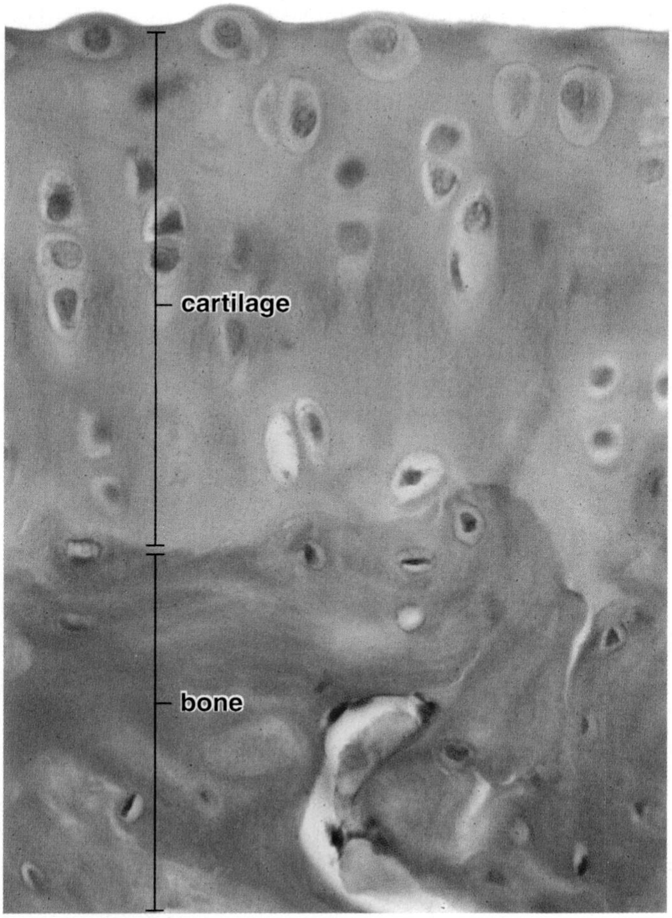

FIGURE 7.7
Photomicrograph of the epiphysis of a long bone. The smooth articular surface is composed of hyaline cartilage and does not possess a perichondrium. The irregularly shaped boundary between the articular cartilage and the underlying bone is clearly visible. ×480.

▼ ELASTIC CARTILAGE

Elastic cartilage is distinguished by the presence of elastin in the cartilage matrix

In addition to the normal components of hyaline cartilage matrix, elastic cartilage matrix also contains elastic fibers and interconnecting sheets of elastic material (Fig. 7.8). These fibers and lamellae are best demonstrated in paraffin sections with special stains such as resorcin-fuchsin and orcein. The elastic material gives the cartilage elastic properties in addition to the resilience and pliability that are characteristic of hyaline cartilage.

Elastic cartilage is found in the external ear, the walls of the external acoustic meatus, the auditory (Eustachian) tube, and the epiglottis of the larynx. The cartilage in all of these locations is surrounded by a perichondrium, similar to that found around most hyaline cartilage. Unlike hyaline cartilage, which calcifies with aging, the matrix of elastic cartilage does not calcify during the aging process.

▼ FIBROCARTILAGE

Fibrocartilage consists of chondrocytes and their matrix material in combination within dense connective tissue

Fibrocartilage is a combination of dense regular connective tissue and hyaline cartilage. The chondrocytes are dispersed among the collagen fibers, singly, in rows, and in isogenous groups (Fig. 7.9). They are similar in appearance to the chondrocytes of hyaline cartilage, but there is considerably less matrix material associated with them, and there is no surrounding perichondrium as in hyaline and elastic cartilage. In a section containing fibrocartilage, a population of cells with rounded nuclei and a small amount of surrounding amorphous matrix material is typically seen. These nuclei belong to the chondrocytes. Within the fibrous areas are nuclei that are flattened or elongated. These are fibroblast nuclei.

Fibrocartilage is typically present in intervertebral discs, the symphysis pubis, articular discs of the sternoclavicular and temporomandibular joints, menisci of the knee joint,

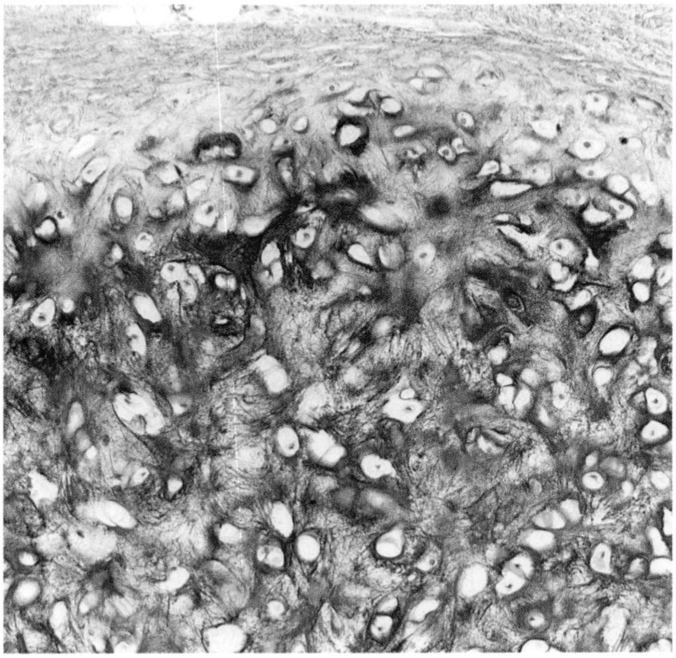

FIGURE 7.8
Photomicrograph of elastic cartilage from the epiglottis. This specimen was stained with orcein and reveals the elastic fibers, stained brown, within the cartilage matrix. The elastic fibers are of various sizes and constitute a significant part of the cartilage. Chondrocyte nuclei are evident in many of the lacunae. The perichondrium is visible at the top of the photomicrograph. ×180.

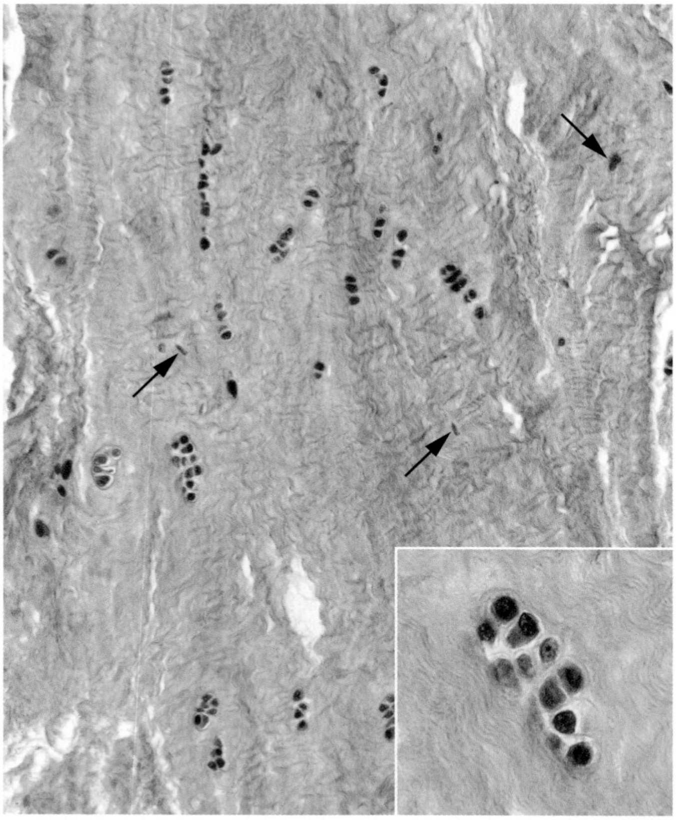

FIGURE 7.9
Photomicrograph of fibrocartilage from an intervertebral disc. The collagen fibers are stained green in this Gomori trichrome preparation. The tissue has a fibrous appearance and contains a relatively small number of fibroblasts with elongated nuclei *(arrows)* as well as more numerous chondrocytes with dark round nuclei. The chondrocytes exhibit close spatial groupings and are arranged either in rows among the collagen fibers or in isogenous groups. ×160. **Inset.** High magnification of an isogenous group. Chondrocytes are contained within lacunae. Typically, there is little cartilage matrix surrounding the chondrocytes. ×700.

and certain places where tendons attach to bones. The presence of fibrocartilage in these sites indicates that resistance to both compression and shearing forces is required of the tissue. The cartilage acts much like a shock absorber. The degree to which such forces occur is reflected in the amount of cartilage matrix material present.

HISTOGENESIS, GROWTH, AND REPAIR OF HYALINE CARTILAGE

Most cartilage arises from mesenchyme

The process of cartilage development begins when mesenchymal cells aggregate and form a mass of rounded, closely apposed cells. In the head, most of the cartilage arises from aggregates of ectomesenchyme derived from neural crest cells. Known as a ***blastema*** of precartilage ***(protochondral tissue)***, an aggregate of mesenchymal or ectomesenchymal cells marks the site of hyaline cartilage formation. The blastema cells begin to secrete cartilage matrix and at this point are called ***chondroblasts.*** They progressively move apart as they deposit matrix. When they are completely surrounded by matrix material, the cells are called chondrocytes. The mesenchymal tissue immediately surrounding the chondrogenic blastema gives rise to the perichondrium.

Cartilage is capable of two kinds of growth, appositional and interstitial

With the onset of matrix secretion, cartilage growth continues by a combination of two processes:

- ***Appositional growth,*** the process that forms new cartilage at the surface of an existing cartilage
- ***Interstitial growth,*** the process that forms new cartilage within an existing cartilage

New cartilage cells produced during ***appositional growth*** are derived from the inner portion of the surrounding perichondrium. The cells resemble fibroblasts in form and function, producing the collagen component of the perichondrium (type I collagen). When cartilage growth is initiated, however, the cells undergo a change: the cytoplasmic processes disappear, the nucleus becomes rounded, and the cytoplasm increases in amount and becomes more prominent. These changes result in the cell becoming a chondroblast. Chondroblasts function in cartilage matrix production including secretion of type II collagen. The new matrix increases the cartilage mass; at the same time, new fibroblasts are produced to maintain the cell population of the perichondrium.

New cartilage cells produced during ***interstitial growth*** arise from the division of chondrocytes within their lacunae (see Fig. 7.2). This is possible only because the chondrocytes retain the ability to divide and the surrounding matrix is distensible, thus permitting further secretory activity. Initially, the daughter cells of the dividing chondrocytes occupy the same lacuna. As new matrix is secreted, a partition is formed between the daughter cells; at this point each cell occupies its own lacuna. With continued secretion of matrix, the cells move even further apart. The overall growth of cartilage thus results from both the interstitial secretion of new matrix material by chondrocytes and the appositional secretion of matrix material by newly differentiated chondroblasts.

Cartilage has limited ability for repair

Cartilage can tolerate considerable amounts of intense and repetitive stress. However, when damaged, cartilage manifests a striking inability to heal, even in the most mi-

nor injuries. This lack of response to injury is due to cartilage's avascularity, the immobility of the chondrocytes, and the limited ability of mature chondrocytes to proliferate. Some repair can occur, but only if the defect involves the perichondrium. In these injuries, repair results from activity of the pluripotential progenitor cells located in the perichondrium. Even in this case, however, few cartilage cells, if any, are produced. Repair mostly involves the production of dense connective tissue.

At the molecular level, cartilage repair is a tentative balance between deposition of type I collagen in the form of scar tissue and repair by expression of the cartilage-specific collagens. However, in adults, new blood vessels commonly develop at the site of the healing wound, which stimulate the growth of bone rather than actual cartilage repair. The limited ability of cartilage to repair itself can cause significant problems in cardiothoracic surgery, such as coronary artery bypass surgery, when costal cartilage must be cut to enter the chest cavity. A variety of treatments may improve the healing of articular cartilage, including perichondral grafts, cell transplantation, insertion of artificial matrices, and application of growth factors.

When hyaline cartilage calcifies, it is replaced by bone

Hyaline cartilage is prone to calcification, a process in which calcium phosphate crystals become embedded in the cartilage matrix. The matrix of hyaline cartilage undergoes calcification as a regular occurrence in three well-defined situations:

- The portion of articular cartilage that is in contact with bone tissue in growing and adult bones, but not the surface portion, is calcified.
- Calcification always occurs in cartilage that is about to be replaced by bone (endochondral ossification) during the growth period of an individual.
- Hyaline cartilage in the adult calcifies with time as part of the aging process.

In most of these situations, given sufficient time, cartilage that calcifies will be replaced by bone. For example, in older individuals, it is not uncommon to find portions of the cartilage rings in the trachea replaced by bone tissue (Fig. 7.10). Chondrocytes normally derive all of their nutrients and dispose of wastes by diffusion of materials through the matrix. When the matrix becomes heavily calcified, diffusion is impeded and the chondrocytes swell and die. The ultimate consequence of this event is removal of the calcified matrix and its replacement by bone.

Some investigators have described a cell type, the ***chondroclast***, that resembles an osteoclast (page 190) in both morphology and function. This cell is thought to play a role in the digestion of calcified cartilage that is to be replaced by bone. These cells appear to enter the cartilage along with newly sprouting blood vessels and may, in fact, be derived from perivascular or bone marrow stem cells. Prechondroclasts resemble fibroblasts when seen with the TEM. Most studies of chondroclast structure and function have been carried out on the developing mandible, in which true endochondral ossification does not take place. It is still unclear whether chondroclasts are cells found where bone is replacing cartilage or whether they are limited to cartilages and bones that are derived from the ectomesenchyme that originates from neural crest cells.

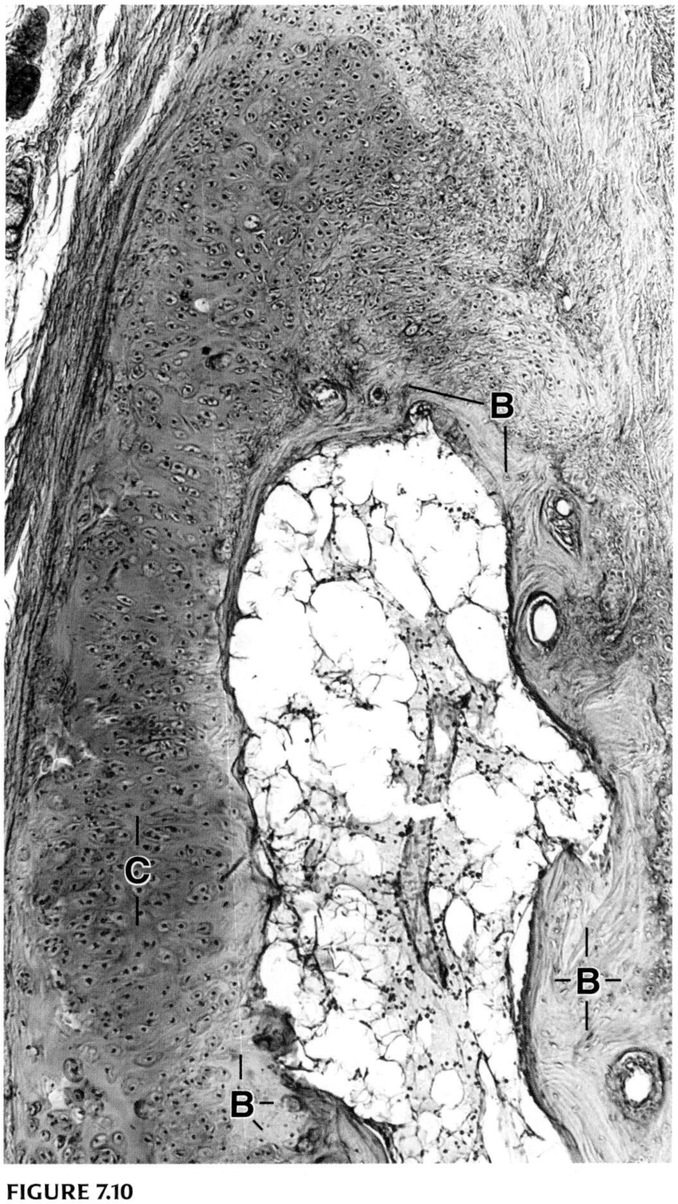

FIGURE 7.10
Photomicrograph of a tracheal ring from an elderly individual, stained with H&E. The darker, somewhat basophilic areas on the left side of the micrograph represent normal cartilage matrix *(C)*. The lighter and more eosinophilic areas represent bone tissue *(B)* that has replaced the original cartilage matrix. A large marrow cavity has formed within the cartilage structure and is visible in the center of the micrograph. ×75.

PLATE 7. HYALINE CARTILAGE

Cartilage is an avascular form of connective tissue composed of cells called *chondrocytes* and a highly specialized extracellular matrix. Three kinds of cartilage are described on the basis of characteristics of the matrix: *hyaline cartilage* (described here), *elastic cartilage* (described in Plate 9), and *fibrocartilage* (described in Plate 10). Hyaline cartilage has a homogeneous appearing amorphous matrix. It contains type II collagen. Type II collagen appears with the transmission electron microscope (TEM) as thin fibrils, ~20 nm in diameter, in which the characteristic 68-nm banding may not be obvious. The fibrils are arranged in a three-dimensional felt-like pattern. The matrix also contains large amounts of *glycosaminoglycans,* most of which form *proteoglycans* and *proteoglycan aggregates.*

Hyaline cartilage is found in the adult as the structural framework for the larynx, trachea, and bronchi; it is found on the articular ends of the ribs and on the surfaces of synovial joints. In addition, hyaline cartilage constitutes much of the fetal skeleton and plays an important role in the growth of most bones. Hyaline cartilage displays both *appositional growth,* the addition of new cartilage at its surface, and *interstitial growth,* the division and differentiation of chondrocytes within its substance.

Figure 1, cartilage, human, H&E ×450.

This micrograph reveals hyaline cartilage from the trachea as seen in a routinely prepared specimen. The cartilage appears as an avascular expanse of matrix material and a population of cells called chondrocytes *(Ch).* The chondrocytes produce the matrix; the space each chondrocyte occupies is called a lacuna *(L).* Surrounding the cartilage and in immediate apposition to it is a cover of connective tissue, the perichondrium *(P).* The perichondrium serves as a source of new chondrocytes during ***appositional growth*** of the cartilage. Often, the perichondrium reveals two distinctive layers: an outer, more fibrous layer and an inner, more cellular layer. The inner, more cellular layer is chondrogenic and provides for external growth.

Cartilage matrix contains collagenous fibrils masked by ground substance in which they are embedded; thus, the fibrils are not evident. The matrix also contains, among other components, sulfated glycosaminoglycans that exhibit basophilia with hematoxylin or other basic dyes. Also, the matrix material immediately surrounding a lacuna tends to stain more intensely with basic dyes. This region is referred to as a capsule *(Cap).* Not uncommonly, the matrix may appear to stain more intensely in localized areas *(asterisks)* that look much like the capsule matrix. This results from inclusion of a capsule within the thickness of the section, but not the lacuna it surrounds.

Frequently, two or more chondrocytes are located extremely close to one another, separated by only a thin partition of matrix. These are isogenous cell clusters that arise from a single predecessor cell. The proliferation of new chondrocytes by this means with the consequent addition of matrix results in ***interstitial growth*** of the cartilage.

Figure 2, hyaline cartilage, human, H&E ×160.

The hyaline cartilage in this micrograph is from a specimen obtained shortly after death and kept cool during fixation. The procedure reduces the loss of its negatively charged sulfate groups; thus, the matrix is stained more heavily with hematoxylin. Also, note the very distinct and deeply stained capsules *(arrows)* surrounding the chondrocytes. The capsule represents the site where the sulfated glycosaminoglycans are most concentrated. In contrast to the basophilia of the cartilage matrix, the perichondrium *(P)* is stained with eosin. The lightly stained region between the perichondrium and the deeply stained matrix is matrix that has not yet matured. It has fewer sulfate groups.

Figure 3, hyaline cartilage, human, H&E ×850.

This higher magnification micrograph reveals the area within the *rectangle* in Figure 2. The chondrocytes *(Ch)* in the upper part of the micrograph represent an isogenous group and are producing matrix material for interstitial growth. A prominent capsule is not yet evident. The lightly stained basophilic area reveals immature chondrocytes *(arrows)* within the perichondrium *(P).* Closest to the cartilage matrix, within the perichondrium *(P),* are several chondrocytes that exhibit just barely detectable cytoplasm and elongate nuclei *(FCh).* These cells are formative chondrocytes that are just beginning to, or will shortly, produce matrix material. In contrast, the nuclei near the bottom edge of the micrograph are fibroblast nuclei *(Fib);* they belong to the outer layer of the perichondrium. Note how attenuated their nuclei are compared with the formative chondroblast nuclei of the inner perichondrial layer.

KEY

Cap, capsule
Ch, chondrocytes
FCh, formative chondrocytes
Fib, fibroblasts
L, lacuna
P, perichondrium
arrows, immature chondrocytes
asterisk, capsule of a lacuna, but with lacuna and contained chondrocyte not included within the thickness of the section

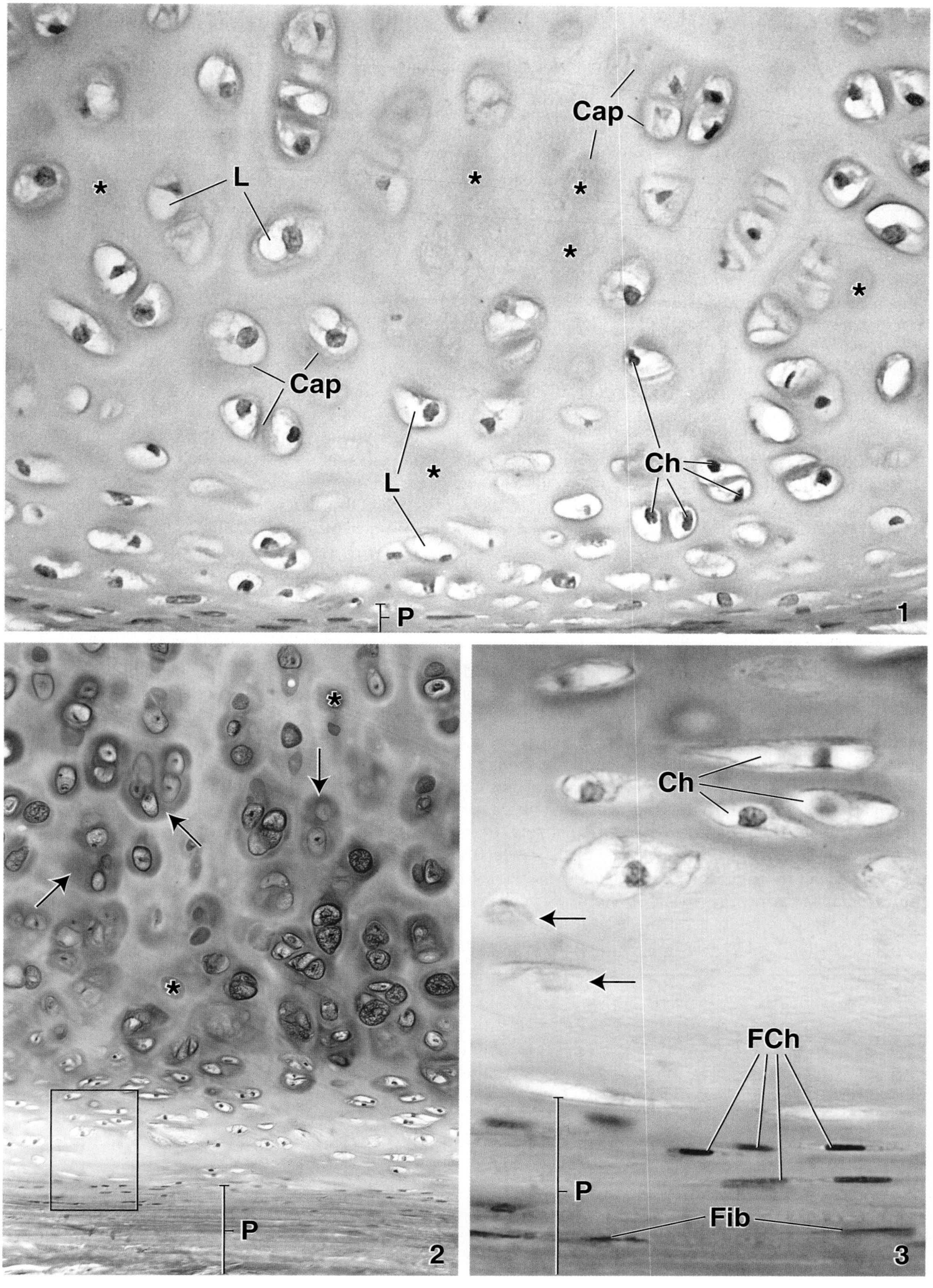
Cap
L
Cap
Ch
L
P
1
Ch
FCh
P
Fib
P
2
3

PLATE 8. CARTILAGE AND THE DEVELOPING SKELETON

Hyaline cartilage is present as a precursor to bones in the fetus. This cartilage is replaced by bone tissue except where one bone contacts another, as in a movable joint. In these locations, cartilage persists and covers the end of each bone as articular cartilage, providing a smooth, well-lubricated surface against which the end of one bone moves on the other in the joint. In addition, cartilage, being capable of interstitial growth, persists in weight-supporting bones and other long bones as a growth plate as long as growth in length occurs. The role of hyaline cartilage in bone growth is considered briefly below and in more detail in Plates 13 and 14.

Figure 1, fetal foot, rat, H&E ×85.

This section shows the cartilages that will ultimately become the bones of the foot. In several places, developing ligaments *(L)* can be seen where they join the cartilages. The nuclei of the fibroblasts within the ligaments are just barely perceptible. They are aligned in rows and are separated from other rows of fibroblasts by collagenous material. The hue and intensity of color of the cartilage matrix, except at the periphery, are due to the combined uptake of the H&E. The collagen of the matrix stains with eosin; however, the presence of sulfated glycosaminoglycans results in staining by hematoxylin. The matrix of cartilage that is about to be replaced by bone, such as that shown here, becomes impregnated with calcium salts, and the calcium is also receptive to staining with hematoxylin. The many enlarged lacunae (seen as light spaces within the matrix where the chondrocytes have fallen out of the lacunae) are due to hypertrophy of the chondrocytes, an event associated with calcification of the matrix. Thus, where these large lacunae are present, i.e., in the center region of the cartilage, the matrix is heavily stained.

This figure also shows that the cartilage is surrounded by perichondrium, except where it faces a joint cavity *(JC)*. Here, the bare cartilage forms a surface. Note that the joint cavity is a space between the cartilages whose boundaries are completed by connective tissue *(CT)*. The connective tissue at the surface of the cavity is special. It will constitute the synovial membrane in the adult and contribute to the formation of a lubricating fluid (synovial fluid) that is present in the joint cavity. Therefore, all the surfaces that will enclose the adult joint cavity are derived originally from the mesenchyme. Synovial fluid is a viscous substance containing, among other things, glycosaminoglycans; it can be considered an exudate of interstitial fluid. The synovial fluid could be considered an extension of the extracellular matrix, as the joint cavity is not lined by an epithelium.

Figure 2, fetal finger, human, thionine-picric acid ×30.

This figure shows a developing long bone of the finger and its articulation with the distal and proximal bones. Before the stage shown here, each bone consisted entirely of a hyaline cartilaginous structure similar to the cartilages seen in Figure 1 but shaped like the long bones into which they would develop. Here, only the ends, or epiphyses, of the bone remain as cartilage, the epiphyseal cartilage *(C)*. The shaft, or diaphysis, has become a cylinder of bone tissue *(B)* surrounding the marrow cavity *(MC)*. The dark region at the ends of the marrow cavity is calcified cartilage *(arrowhead)* that is being replaced by bone. The bone at the ends of the marrow cavity constitutes the metaphysis. With this staining method, the calcified cartilage appears dark brown. The newly formed metaphyseal bone, which is admixed with this degenerating calcified cartilage and is difficult to define at this low magnification, has the same yellow-brown color as the diaphyseal bone. By the continued proliferation of cartilage, the bone grows in length. Later, the cartilage becomes calcified; bone is then produced and occupies the site of the resorbed cartilage. With the cessation of cartilage proliferation and its replacement by bone, growth of the bone stops, and only the cartilage at the articular surface remains. The details of this process are explained under endochondral bone formation (Plates 13 and 14).

KEY

B, bone
C, cartilage
CT, connective tissue
JC, joint cavity
L, ligament
MC, marrow cavity
arrowhead, calcified cartilage

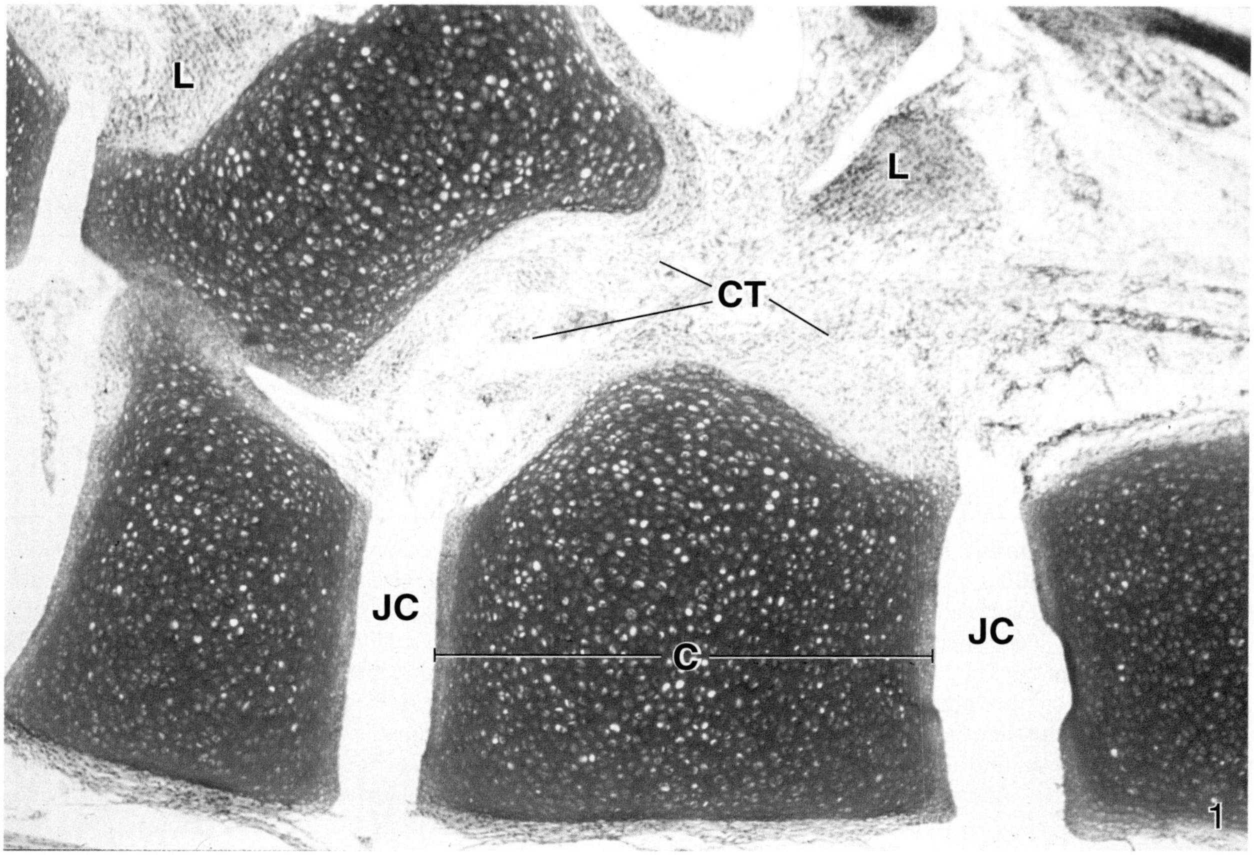
L
L
CT
JC
C
JC
1

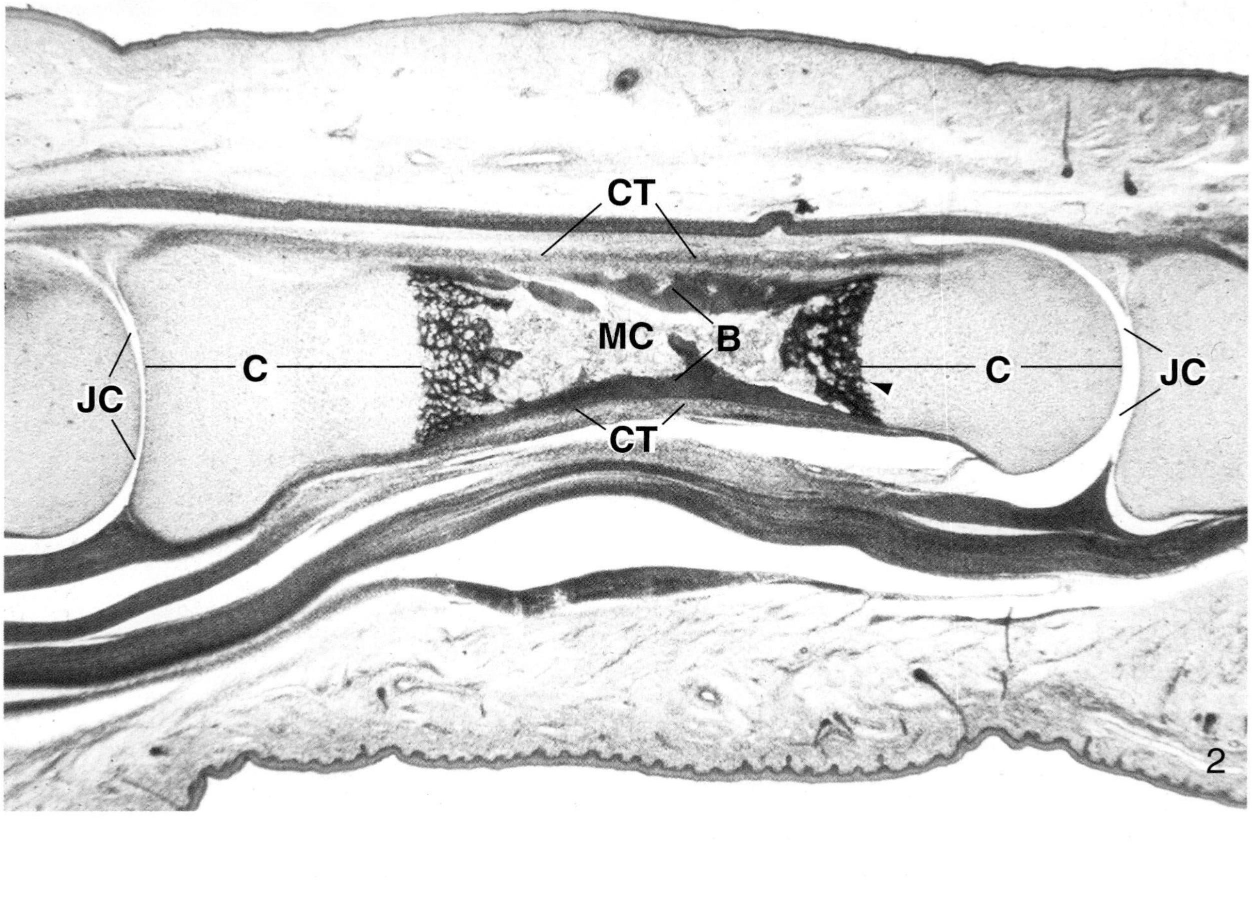
CT
MC
B
JC
C
C
JC
CT
2

PLATE 9. ELASTIC CARTILAGE

Elastic cartilage has a matrix containing elastic fibers and elastic lamellae in addition to type II collagen. It is found in the auricle of the external ear, in the auditory tube, in the epiglottis, and in part of the larynx. The elastic material imparts properties of elasticity, as distinguished from resiliency, which are not shared by hyaline cartilage. Elastic cartilage is surrounded by perichondrium, and it, too, increases in size by both appositional and interstitial growth. Unlike hyaline cartilage, however, elastic cartilage does not normally calcify.

Figure 1, epiglottis, human, H&E and orcein stains ×80.

This section of the epiglottis contains elastic cartilage *(EC)* as the centrally located structure. The essential components of the cartilage, namely, the matrix that stains deep blue and the light, unstained lacunae surrounded by matrix, are evident in this low-magnification micrograph. The perimeter of the cartilage is covered by perichondrium; its fibrous character is just barely visible in this figure. Also note the adipose tissue *(AT)* within the boundaries of the elastic cartilage.

Both above and below the elastic cartilage is connective tissue, and each surface of the epiglottis is formed by stratified squamous epithelium *(SE)*. Mucous glands *(MG)* are in the connective tissue in the bottom of this figure.

Figure 2, epiglottis, human, H&E and orcein stains ×250; inset ×400.

This shows an area of the elastic cartilage at higher magnification. The elastic fibers appear as the blue, elongate profiles within the matrix. They are most evident at the edges of the cartilage, but they are obscured in some deeper parts of the matrix, where they blend with the elastic material that forms a honeycomb about the lacunae. Elastic fibers *(E)* are also in the adipose tissue *(AT)*, between the adipocytes.

Some of the lacunae in the cartilage are arranged in pairs separated by a thin plate of matrix. The plate of matrix appears as a bar between the adjacent lacunae. This is a reflection of interstitial growth by the cartilage, in that the adjacent cartilage cells are derived from the same parent cell. They have moved away from each other and secreted a plate of cartilage matrix between them to form two lacunae. Most chondrocytes shown in this figure occupy only part of the lacuna. This is, in part, due to shrinkage, but it is also due to the fact that older chondrocytes contain lipid in large droplets that is lost during the processing of the tissue. The shrinkage of chondrocytes within the lacunae or their loss due to dropping out of the section during preparation causes the lacunae to stand out as light, unstained areas against the darkly stained matrix.

The *inset* shows the elastic cartilage at still higher magnification. Here, the elastic fibers *(E)* are again evident as elongate profiles, chiefly at the edges of the cartilage. Most chondrocytes in this part of the specimen show little shrinkage. Many of the cells display a typically rounded nucleus, and the cytoplasm is evident. Note, again, that some lacunae contain two chondrocytes, indicating interstitial growth.

KEY

AT, adipose tissue
E, elastic fiber
EC, elastic cartilage
MG, mucous gland
SE, stratified squamous epithelium

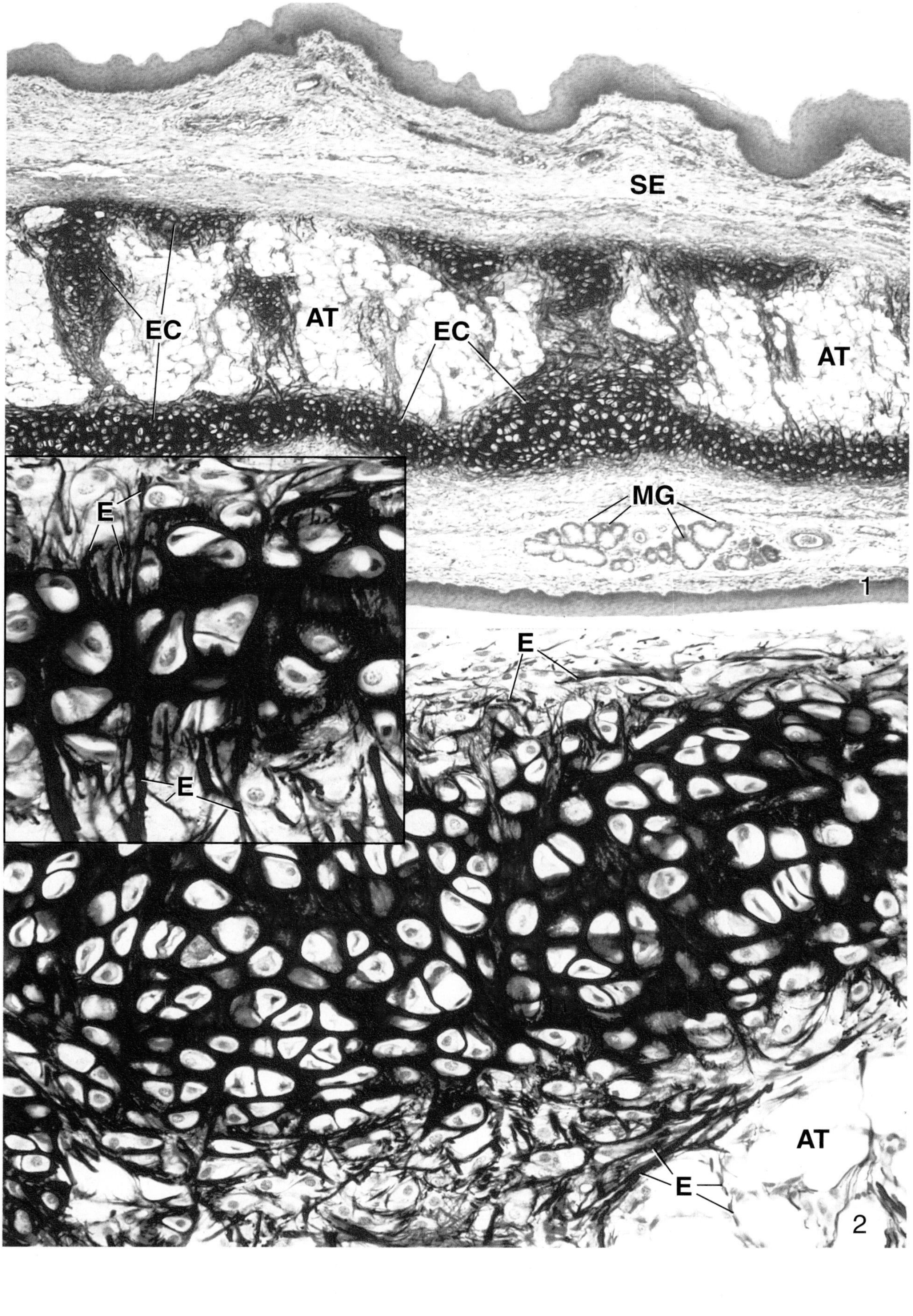
SE
EC
AT
EC
AT
E
MG
1
E
E
E
AT
E
2

PLATE 10. FIBROCARTILAGE

Fibrocartilage is a combination of dense connective tissue and cartilage. It has a matrix with large bundles of type I collagen in addition to type II collagen. The amount of cartilage varies, but in most locations the cartilage cells and their matrix occupy a lesser portion of the tissue mass. Fibrocartilage is found at the intervertebral discs, the symphysis pubis, the knee joint, the mandibular joint, the sternoclavicular joint, and the shoulder joint. It may also be present along the grooves or insertions for tendons and ligaments. Its presence is associated with sites where resilience is required in dense connective tissue to help absorb sudden physical impact, i.e., where resistance to both compressive and shearing forces is required in the tissue. Histologically, fibrocartilage appears as small fields of cartilage blending almost imperceptibly with regions of dense fibrous connective tissue. It is usually identified by the presence of aggregates of rounded cartilage cells (isogenous groups) among bundles of collagen fibers and by the basophilic staining of the capsular matrix material and territorial matrix secreted by these cells. No perichondrium is present.

Figure 1, intervertebral disc, human, Mallory's trichrome ×160.

This is a low-magnification view of fibrocartilage. The Mallory method stains collagen light blue. The tissue has a fibrous appearance, and at this low magnification the nuclei of the fibroblasts *(F)* appear as small, elongate or spindle-shaped bodies. There are relatively few fibroblasts present, as is characteristic of dense connective tissue. The cartilage cells *(C)* are more numerous and exhibit close spatial groupings, i.e., ***isogenous groups***. Some of the cartilage cells appear as elongate clusters of cells, whereas others appear in single-file rows. The matrix material immediately surrounding the cartilage cells has a homogeneous appearance and is, thereby, distinguishable from the fibrous connective tissue.

Figure 2, intervertebral disc, human, Mallory's trichrome ×700.

This figure shows the area circumscribed by the *rectangle* in Figure 1 at higher magnification. The cartilage cells are contained within lacunae *(arrows),* and their cytoplasm stains deeply. The surrounding cartilage matrix material is scant and blends into the dense connective tissue. Cartilage matrix material can be detected best by observing the larger group of cartilage cells at the left of this figure and then observing this same area in Figure 1. Note the light homogeneous area around the cell nest in the lower-power view. This is the region of cartilage matrix. At the greater magnification of Figure 2, it is possible to see that some of the collagen fibers are incorporated in the matrix, where they appear as wispy bundles.

KEY

C, cartilage | **F,** fibroblast | **arrow,** lacuna

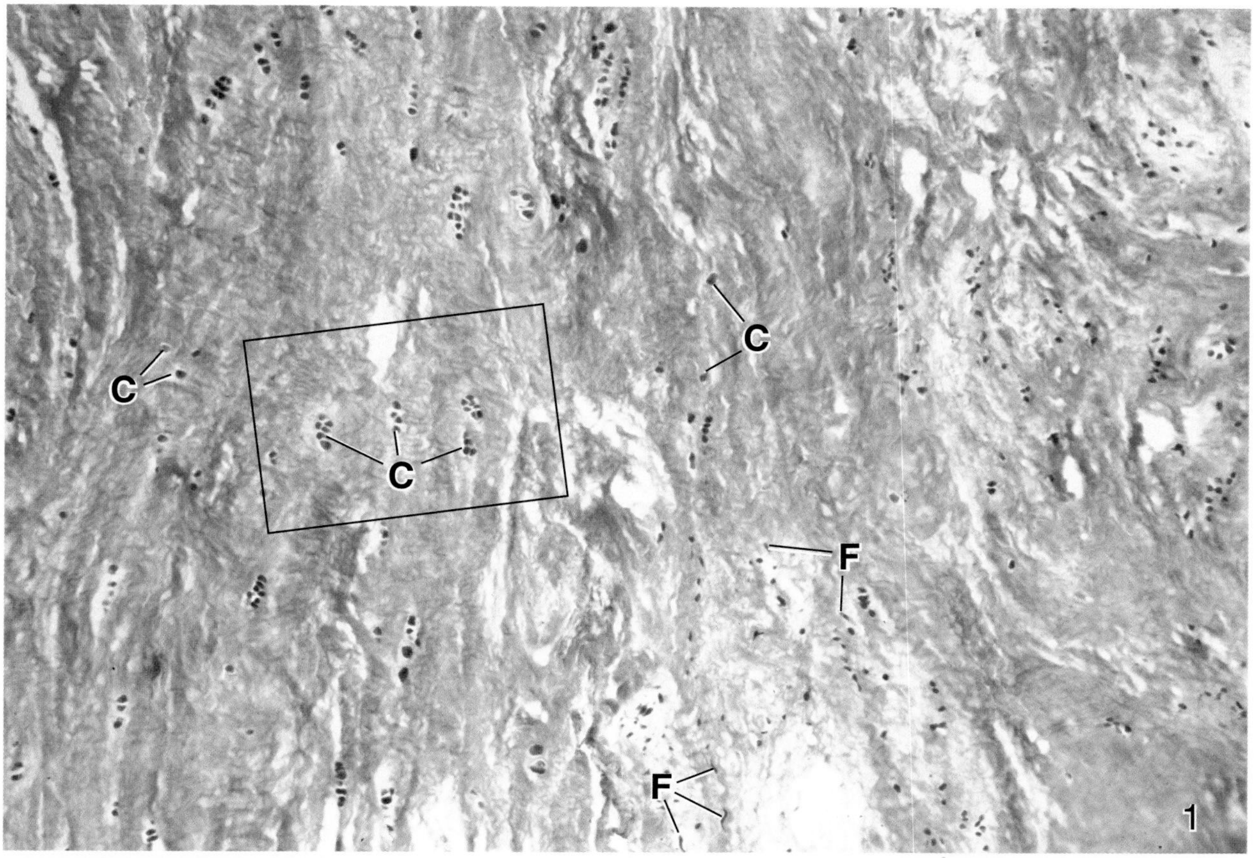
C
C
C
F
F
1

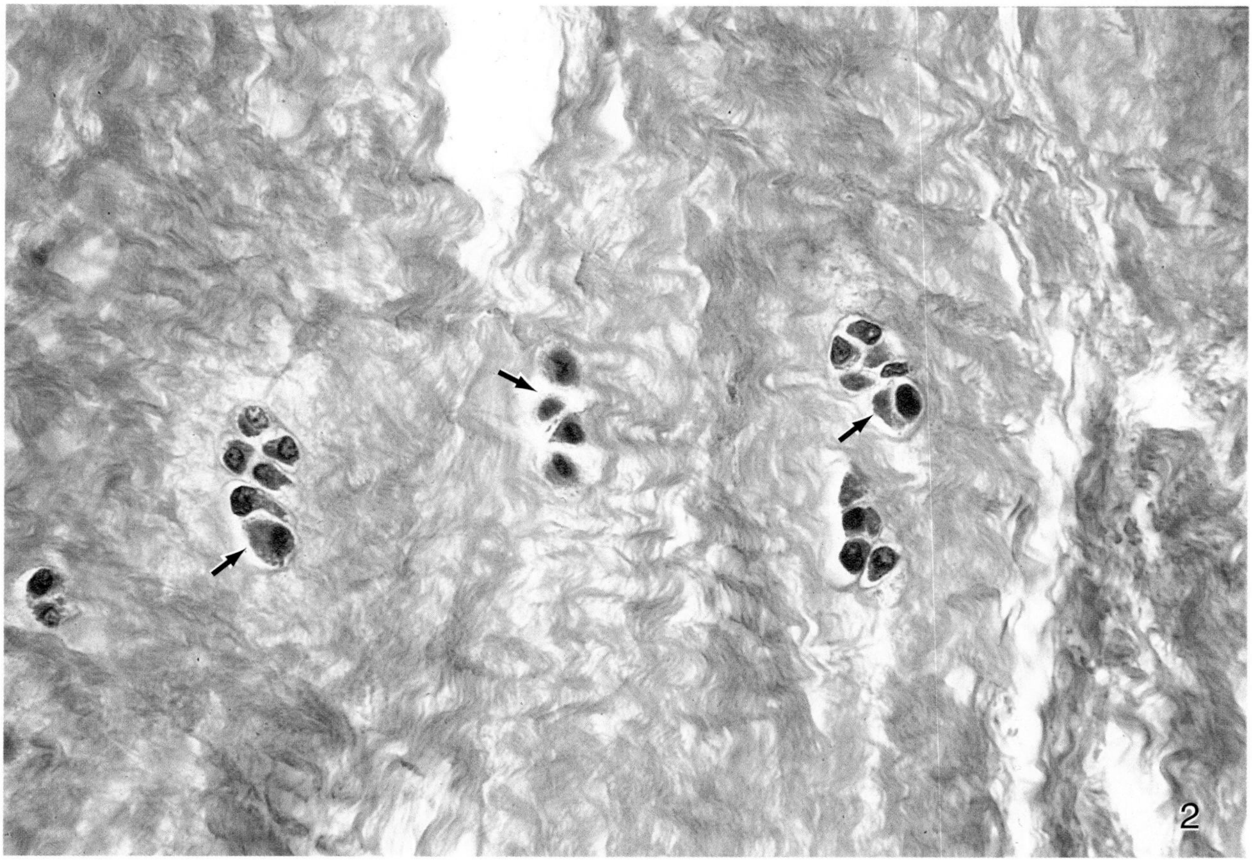
2

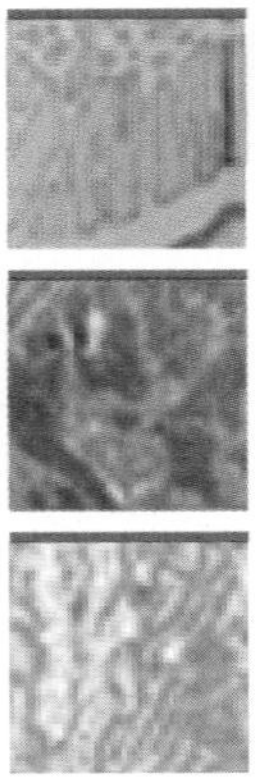

8

Bone

▼ OVERVIEW OF BONE

Bone is a connective tissue characterized by a mineralized extracellular matrix

Bone is a specialized form of connective tissue that, like other connective tissues, consists of cells and extracellular matrix. The feature that distinguishes bone from other connective tissues is the mineralization of its matrix, which produces an extremely hard tissue capable of providing *support* and *protection*. The mineral is calcium phosphate, in the form of ***hydroxyapatite crystals*** [$Ca_{10}(PO_4)_6(OH)_2$].

By virtue of its mineral content, bone also serves as a *storage site* for calcium and phosphate. Both calcium and phosphate can be mobilized from the bone matrix and taken up by the blood as needed to maintain appropriate levels throughout the body. Thus, in addition to support and protection, bone plays an important sec-

ondary role in the homeostatic regulation of blood calcium levels.

Bone matrix contains collagen type I and some collagen type V, along with glycosaminoglycans, glycoproteins, and sialoproteins

The major structural component of bone matrix is type I collagen and, to a lesser extent, type V collagen. These collagens constitute about 90% of the bone matrix. The matrix also contains ground substance in the form of ***glycosaminoglycans*** (hyaluronic acid, chondroitin sulfate, and keratan sulfate); small ***glycoproteins*** such as osteocalcin, osteonectin, and osteopontin; and several ***sialoproteins.*** The glycoproteins and sialoproteins of the ground substance play a role in binding calcium in the mineralization process. Both the collagen and the ground substance components become mineralized to form bone.

Within the bone matrix are spaces called ***lacunae*** (sing., lacuna), each of which contains a bone cell, or ***osteocyte.*** The osteocyte extends numerous processes into small tunnels called ***canaliculi.*** Canaliculi run through the mineralized matrix, connecting adjacent lacunae and allowing contact between the cell processes of neighboring osteocytes. In this manner, a continuous network of canaliculi and lacunae containing cells and their processes is formed throughout the entire mass of mineralized tissue. Electron micrographs show that osteocyte processes communicate by gap junctions. Bone tissue depends on the osteocytes, which are responsible for maintaining its viability.

In addition to the osteocyte, three other cell types are present in bone:

- ***Osteoprogenitor cells*** are cells that give rise to osteoblasts.
- ***Osteoblasts*** are cells that secrete the extracellular matrix of bone; once the cell is surrounded with its secreted matrix, it is referred to as an osteocyte.
- ***Osteoclasts*** are bone-resorbing cells present on bone surfaces where bone is being removed or remodeled (reorganized) or where bone has been damaged.

Osteoprogenitor cells and osteoblasts are developmental precursors of the osteocyte. Osteoclasts are phagocytotic cells derived from bone marrow. Each of these cells is described in more detail below.

▼ BONES AND BONE TISSUE

Bones are the organs of the skeletal system; bone tissue is the structural component of bones

Typically, a bone consists of bone tissue and other connective tissues, including hemopoietic tissue, fat tissue, blood vessels, and nerves. If the bone forms a freely movable (synovial) joint, hyaline cartilage is present. The ability of the bone to perform its skeletal function is due to the bone tissue and, where present, the hyaline or articular cartilage.

Bone tissue is classified as either compact (dense) or spongy (cancellous)

If a bone is cut, two distinct structural arrangements of bone tissue can be recognized (Fig. 8.1). A compact, dense layer forms the outside of the bone; a sponge-like meshwork consisting of ***trabeculae*** (thin, anastomosing spicules of bone tissue) forms the interior of the bone. The spaces within the meshwork are continuous and, in a living bone, are occupied by marrow and blood vessels.

Bones are classified according to shape; the location of spongy and compact bone varies with bone shape

Spongy and compact bone tissues are located in specific parts of bones. It is useful, then, to outline briefly the kinds of bones and survey where the two kinds of bone tissue are located. On the basis of shape, bones can be classified into four groups:

- ***Long bones*** are longer in one dimension than other bones and consist of a shaft and two ends, e.g., the tibia and the metacarpals. A schematic diagram of a long bone sectioned longitudinally through the shaft is shown in Figure 8.2.
- ***Short bones*** are nearly equal in length and diameter, e.g., the carpal bones of the hand.
- ***Flat bones*** are thin and plate-like, e.g., the bones of the calvarium (skull cap) and the sternum. They consist of two layers of relatively thick compact bone with an intervening layer of spongy bone.
- ***Irregular bones*** have a shape that does not fit into any one of the three groups just described; the shape may be complex, e.g., a vertebra, or the bone may contain air spaces or sinuses, e.g., the ethmoid bone.

Long bones have a shaft, called the ***diaphysis,*** and two expanded ends, each called an ***epiphysis*** (see Fig. 8.2). The articular surface of the epiphysis is covered with hyaline cartilage. The flared portion of the bone between the diaphysis and the epiphysis is called the ***metaphysis.*** It extends from the diaphysis to the epiphyseal line. A large cavity filled with bone marrow, called the ***marrow*** or ***medullary cavity,*** forms the inner portion of the bone. In the shaft, almost the entire thickness of the bone tissue is compact; at most, only a small amount of spongy bone faces the marrow cavity. At the ends of the bone, the re-

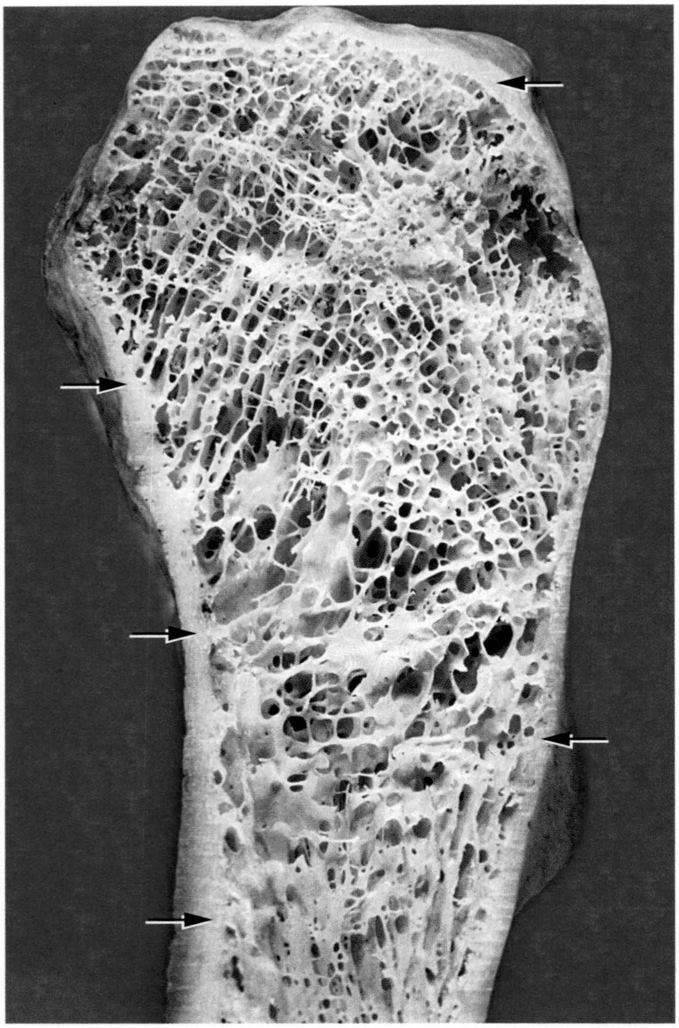

FIGURE 8.1
Epiphysis of an adult long bone. Specimen showing longitudinally sectioned epiphysis of a long bone. The outer portion of the bone has a solid structure *(arrows)* and represents compact (dense) bone. The interior of the bone exhibits a spongy configuration and represents spongy (cancellous) bone. It consists of numerous interconnecting bony trabeculae separated by a labyrinth of interconnecting marrow spaces.

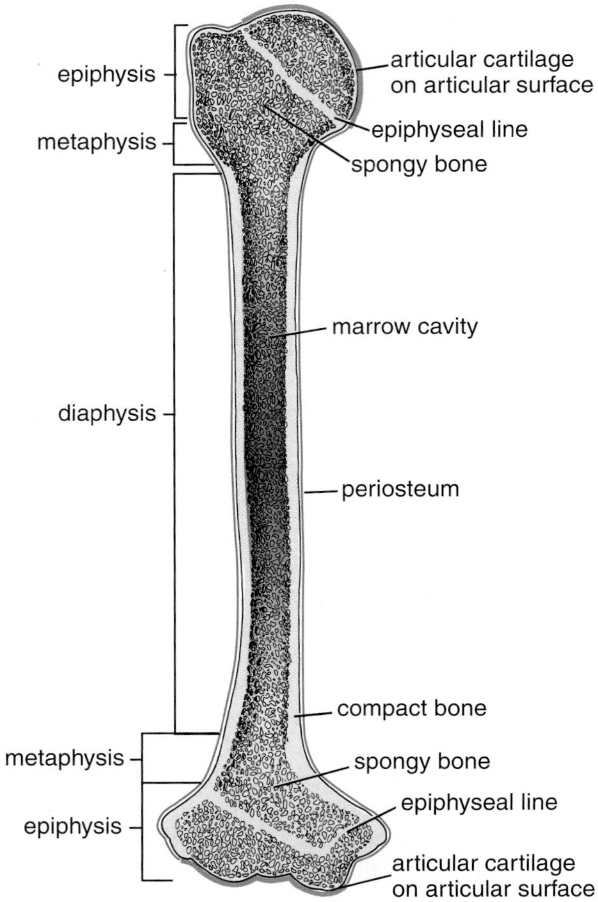

FIGURE 8.2
Structure of a typical long bone. The diaphysis (shaft) of a long bone contains a large marrow cavity surrounded by a thick-walled tube of compact bone. A small amount of spongy bone may line the inner surface of the compact bone. The proximal and distal ends, or epiphyses, of the long bone consist chiefly of spongy bone with a thin outer shell of compact bone. The expanded or flared part of the diaphysis nearest the epiphysis is referred to as the metaphysis. Except for the articular surfaces that are covered by hyaline (articular) cartilage, indicated in *blue,* the outer surface of the bone is covered by a fibrous layer of connective tissue called the periosteum, indicated in *pink.*

verse is true. Here, the spongy bone is extensive, and the compact bone consists of little more than a thin outer shell (see Fig. 8.1).

Short bones possess a shell of compact bone and have spongy bone and a marrow space on the inside. Short bones usually form movable joints with their neighbors; like long bones, their articular surfaces are covered with hyaline cartilage. Elsewhere, ***periosteum,*** a fibrous connective tissue capsule, covers the outer surface of the bone.

▼ GENERAL STRUCTURE OF BONES

Outer Surface of Bones

Bones are covered by periosteum, a sheath of dense fibrous connective tissue containing osteoprogenitor cells

Bones are covered by a periosteum except in areas where they articulate with another bone. In the latter case, the articulating surface is covered by cartilage. The per-

iosteum that covers an actively growing bone consists of an outer fibrous layer that resembles other dense connective tissues and an inner, more cellular layer that contains the osteoprogenitor cells. If active bone formation is not in progress on the bone surface, the fibrous layer is the main component of the periosteum, and the inner layer is not well defined. The relatively few cells that are present, the ***periosteal cells,*** are, however, capable of undergoing division and becoming osteoblasts under appropriate stimulus.

In general, the collagen fibers of the periosteum are arranged parallel to the surface of the bone in the form of a capsule. The character of the periosteum is different where ligaments and tendons attach to the bone. Collagen fibers from these structures extend directly, but at an angle, into the bone tissue, where they are continuous with the collagen fibers of the extracellular matrix of the bone tissue. These fibers are called ***Sharpey's fibers.***

Bones that articulate with neighboring bones possess movable (synovial) joints

Where a bone articulates with a neighboring bone, as in ***synovial joints,*** the contact areas of the two bones are referred to as ***articular surfaces.*** The articular surfaces are covered by hyaline cartilage, also called ***articular cartilage*** because of its location and function; articular cartilage is exposed to the joint cavity. This cartilage is not covered with perichondrium.

Bone Cavities

Bone cavities are lined by endosteum, a layer of connective tissue cells that contains osteoprogenitor cells

The lining tissue of both the compact bone facing the marrow cavity and the trabeculae of spongy bone within the cavity is referred to as ***endosteum.*** The endosteum is often only one cell layer thick and consists of cells that can differentiate into osteoblasts in response to appropriate stimuli. These osteoprogenitor cells, called ***endosteal cells,*** are flattened cells that resemble fibroblasts.

The marrow cavity and the spaces in spongy bone contain bone marrow

Red bone marrow consists of developing blood cells in different stages of development (see page 232) and a network of reticular cells and fibers that serve as a supporting framework for the developing blood cells and vessels. As an individual grows, the amount of red marrow does not increase in proportion to bone growth. In later stages of growth and in the adult, when the rate of blood cell formation has diminished, the tissue in the marrow cavity consists mostly of fat cells; it is then called ***yellow marrow.*** In response to appropriate stimuli, such as extreme blood loss, yellow marrow can revert to red marrow. In the adult, red marrow is normally restricted to the spaces of spongy bone in a few locations such as the sternum and the iliac crest. Diagnostic bone marrow samples and marrow for transplantation are obtained from these sites.

Mature Bone

Mature bone is composed of structural units called osteons (Haversian systems)

Mature bone is largely composed of cylindrical units called ***osteons*** or ***Haversian systems*** (Fig. 8.3). The osteons consist of ***concentric lamellae*** (sing., lamella) of bone matrix, surrounding a central canal, the ***osteonal (Haversian) canal,*** which contains the vascular and nerve supply of the osteon. Canaliculi containing the processes of osteocytes

BOX 8.1

Clinical Correlations: Articular Cartilage and Joint Diseases

Inflammation of the joints ***(arthritis)*** can be caused by many factors and can produce varying degrees of pain and disability, from the pathologic response of articular cartilage to injury.

Simple trauma to a joint by a single incident or by repeated insult can so damage the articular cartilage that it calcifies and begins to be replaced by bone. This process can lead to ***ankylosis,*** i.e., bony fusion in the joint and subsequent loss of motion. The foot and knee joints of runners and football players and hand and finger joints of stringed instrument players are especially vulnerable to this condition.

Immune responses or infectious processes that localize in joints, as in ***rheumatoid arthritis*** or ***tuberculosis,*** can also damage the articular cartilages, producing both severe joint pain and gradual ankylosis. Surgery that replaces the damaged joint with a prosthetic joint can often relieve the pain and restore joint motion in seriously debilitated individuals.

Another common cause of damage to articular cartilages is the deposition of crystals of uric acid in the joints, particularly those of the toes and fingers. This condition is known as ***gouty arthritis*** or, more simply, ***gout.*** Gout has become more common because of the widespread use of thiazide diuretics in the treatment of hypertension. In genetically predisposed individuals, gout is the most common side effect of these drugs. Gout causes severe, unbearable pain because of the sharp crystals in the joint. The irritation also causes the formation of calcareous deposits that deform the joint and limit its motion.

are generally arranged in a radial pattern with respect to the canal. The system of canaliculi that opens to the osteonal canal also serves for the passage of substances between the osteocytes and blood vessels. Between the osteons are remnants of previous concentric lamellae, called ***interstitial lamellae*** (Fig. 8.3). Because of this organization, mature bone is also called ***lamellar bone.***

The long axis of an osteon is usually parallel to the long axis of the bone. The collagen fibers in the concentric lamellae in an osteon are laid down parallel to one another in any given lamella but in different directions in adjacent lamellae. This arrangement gives the cut surface of lamellar bone the appearance of plywood and imparts great strength to the osteon.

Lamellar bone is also found at sites other than the osteon. ***Circumferential lamellae*** follow the entire inner and outer circumferences of the shaft of a long bone, appearing much like the growth rings of a tree (see Fig. 8.3). ***Perforating canals (Volkmann's canals)*** are channels in lamellar bone through which blood vessels and nerves travel from the periosteal and endosteal surfaces to reach the osteonal canal; they also connect osteonal canals to one another. They usually run at approximately right angles to the long axis of the osteons and of the bone (Fig. 8.3). Volkmann's canals are not surrounded by concentric lamellae, a key feature in their histologic identification.

Mature spongy bone is structurally similar to mature compact bone

Mature spongy bone is similar in structure to mature compact bone except that the tissue is arranged as trabeculae or spicules; numerous interconnecting marrow spaces of various size are present between the bone tissue. The matrix of the bone is lamellated. If the trabeculae are sufficiently thick, they will contain osteons.

The blood supply to the shaft of a long bone is chiefly by arteries that enter the marrow cavity through nutrient foramina

Nutrient foramina are openings in the bone through which blood vessels pass to reach the marrow. The greatest numbers of nutrient foramina are found in the diaphysis and epiphysis (Fig. 8.4). Metaphyseal arteries supplement the blood supply to the bone. Drainage of the bone is by veins that leave through the nutrient foramina or through the bone tissue of the shaft and out through the periosteum.

The nutrient arteries that supply the diaphysis and epiphysis arise developmentally as the principal vessel of the periosteal buds. The metaphyseal arteries, in contrast, arise developmentally from periosteal vessels that become incorporated into the metaphysis during the growth process, i.e., through the widening of the bone.

The blood supply to bone tissue is essentially centrifugal

The blood that nourishes bone tissue moves from the marrow cavity into and through the bone tissue and out via periosteal veins; thus its flow is in a centrifugal direction. With respect to nourishment of the bone tissue itself, Volkmann's canals provide the major route of entry for

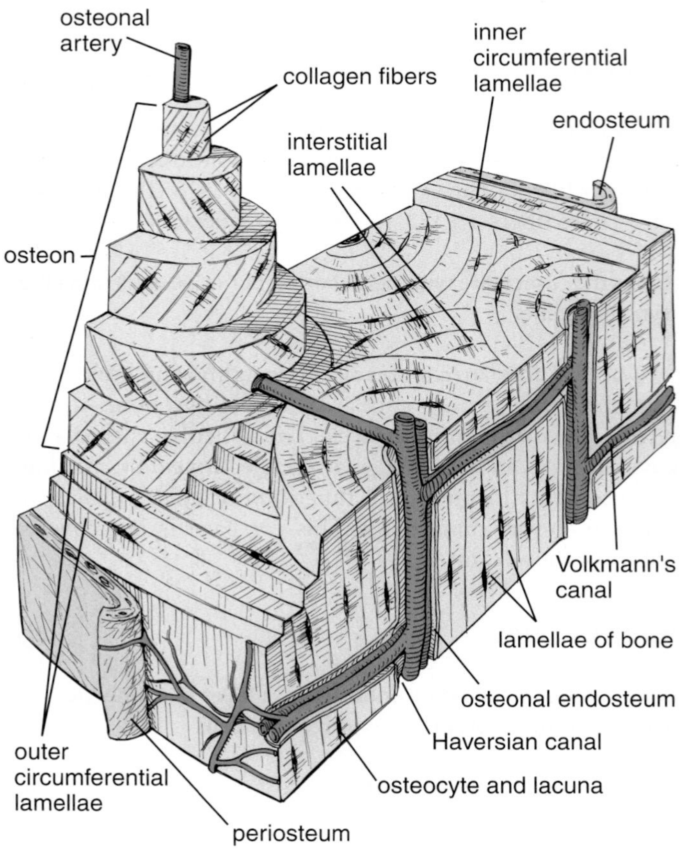

FIGURE 8.3
Diagram of a section of compact bone removed from the shaft of a long bone. The concentric lamellae and the Haversian canal that they surround constitute an osteon (Haversian system). One of the Haversian systems in this diagram is drawn as an elongated cylindrical structure rising above the plane of the bone section. It consists of several concentric lamellae that have been partially removed to show the perpendicular orientation of collagen fibers in adjacent layers. Interstitial lamellae result from bone remodeling and formation of new Haversian systems. The inner and outer surfaces of the compact bone in this diagram show additional lamellae—the outer and inner circumferential lamellae—that are arranged in broad layers. The inner circumferential lamella is covered by a thin layer of endosteum that faces the marrow cavity, similar to the outer surface of the bone, which is covered by periosteum. Branches of nutritional arteries accompanied by small veins are shown within the Haversian and Volkmann's canals. These arteries also supply the periosteum, endosteum, and bone marrow.

vessels to pass through the compact bone. The smaller blood vessels enter the Haversian canals, which contain a single arteriole and a venule or a single capillary. A lesser supply to the bone tissue arises from periosteal vessels, which usually provide for only the outermost portions of the compact bone. Bone tissue lacks lymphatic vessels; only the periosteal tissue is provided with lymphatic drainage.

Immature Bone

Bone tissue initially formed in the skeleton of a developing fetus is called ***immature bone.*** It differs from mature bone in several respects (Fig. 8.5):

- Immature bone does not display an organized lamellated appearance. On the basis of its collagen fiber arrangement, such bone is designated ***nonlamellar.*** Nonlamellar bone is also referred to as ***bundle*** or ***woven bone*** because of the interlacing arrangement of the collagen fibers.
- Immature bone contains relatively more cells per unit area than does mature bone.
- The cells in immature bone tend to be randomly arranged, whereas cells in mature bone tend to be arranged with their long axes in the same direction as the lamellae.

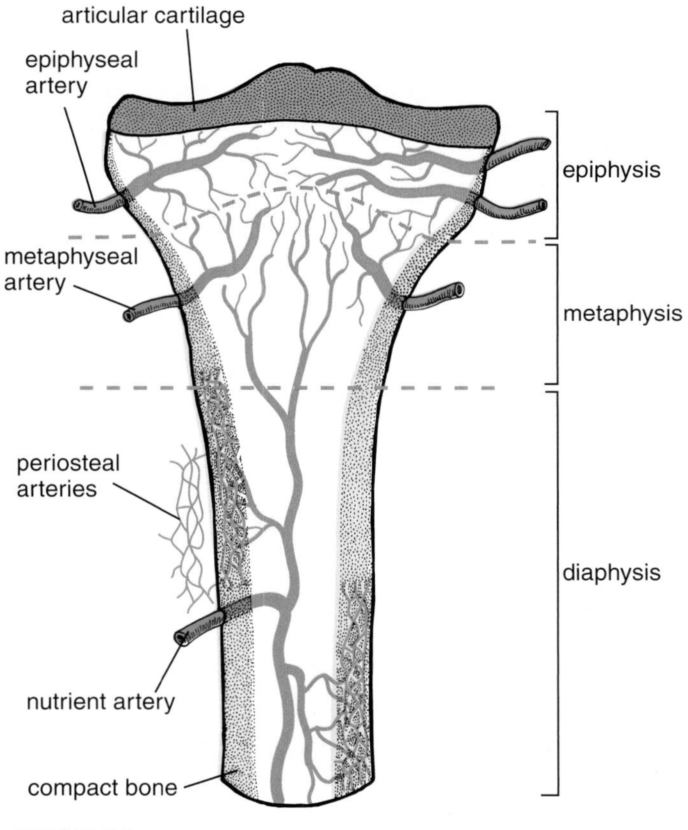

FIGURE 8.4
Diagram showing the blood supply of an adult long bone. The nutrient artery and the epiphyseal arteries enter the bone through nutrient foramina. These openings in the bone arise developmentally as the pathways of the principal vessels of periosteal buds. Metaphyseal arteries arise from periosteal vessels that become incorporated into the metaphysis as the bone grows in diameter.

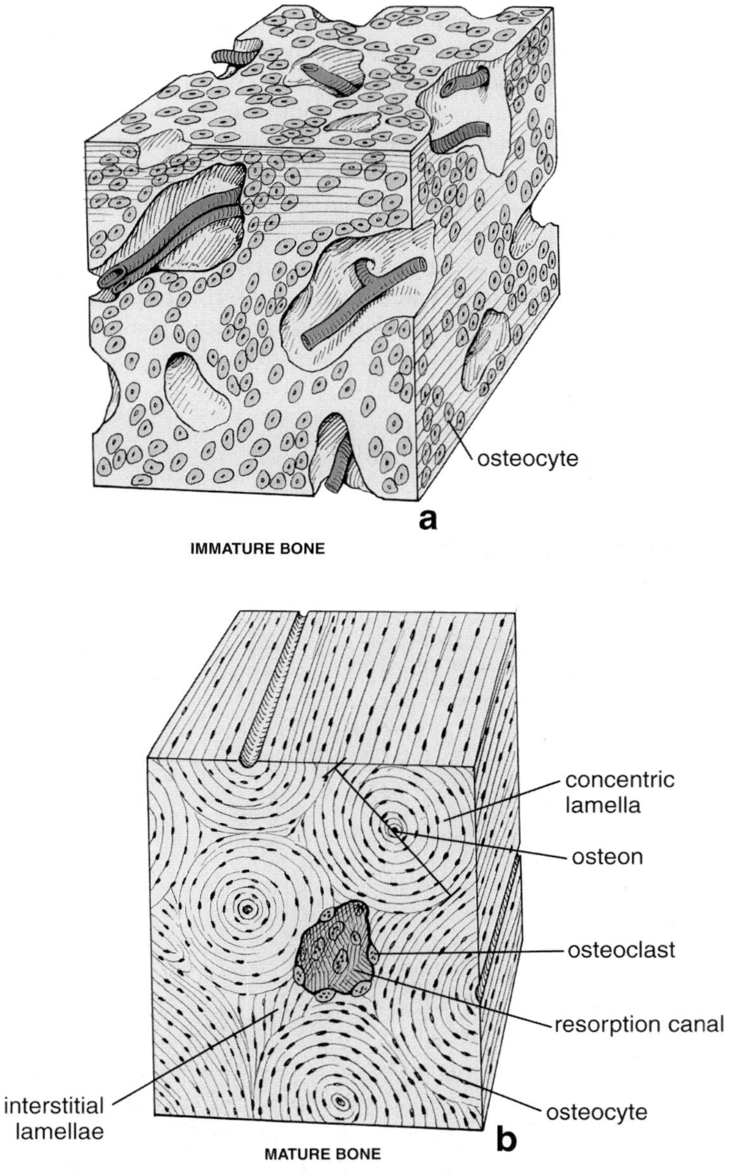

FIGURE 8.5
Diagram of immature and mature bone. Immature bone does not display an organized lamellar appearance because of the interlacing arrangement of the collagen fibers. The cells tend to be randomly arranged, whereas the cells in mature bone are organized in a circular fashion that reflects the lamellar structure of the Haversian system. Resorption canals in mature bone have their long axes in the same direction as the Haversian canals.

- The matrix of immature bone has more ground substance than does the matrix of mature bone. The matrix in immature bone stains more intensely with hematoxylin, whereas the matrix of mature bone stains more intensely with eosin.

Although not evident in typical histologic sections (Fig. 8.6), immature bone is not heavily mineralized when it is initially formed, whereas mature bone undergoes prolonged secondary mineralization. The secondary mineralization of mature bone is evident in microradiographs of ground sections that show younger Haversian systems to be less mineralized than older Haversian systems (see Fig. 8.19).

Immature bone forms more rapidly than mature bone. Although mature bone is clearly the major bone type in the adult, and immature bone is the major bone type in the developing fetus, areas of immature bone are present in adults, especially where bone is being remodeled. Areas of immature bone are also seen regularly in the alveolar sockets of the adult oral cavity and where tendons insert into bones. It is this immature bone in the alveolar sockets that makes it possible to undertake orthodontic corrections even in adults.

▼ CELLS OF BONE TISSUE

As noted above in this chapter, four designated cells are associated with bone tissue: osteoprogenitor cells, osteoblasts, osteocytes, and osteoclasts. With the exception of the osteoclast, each of these cells may be regarded as a differentiated form of the same basic cell type. Each undergoes transformation from a less mature form to a more mature form in relation to functional activity (growth of bone). In contrast, the osteoclast originates from a different cell line and is responsible for bone resorption, an activity associated with bone remodeling.

Osteoprogenitor Cells

The osteoprogenitor cell is a resting cell that can transform into an osteoblast and secrete bone matrix

Osteoprogenitor cells are found on the external and internal surfaces of bones. They comprise the ***periosteal cells*** that form the innermost layer of the periosteum and the ***endosteal cells*** that line the marrow cavities, the osteonal

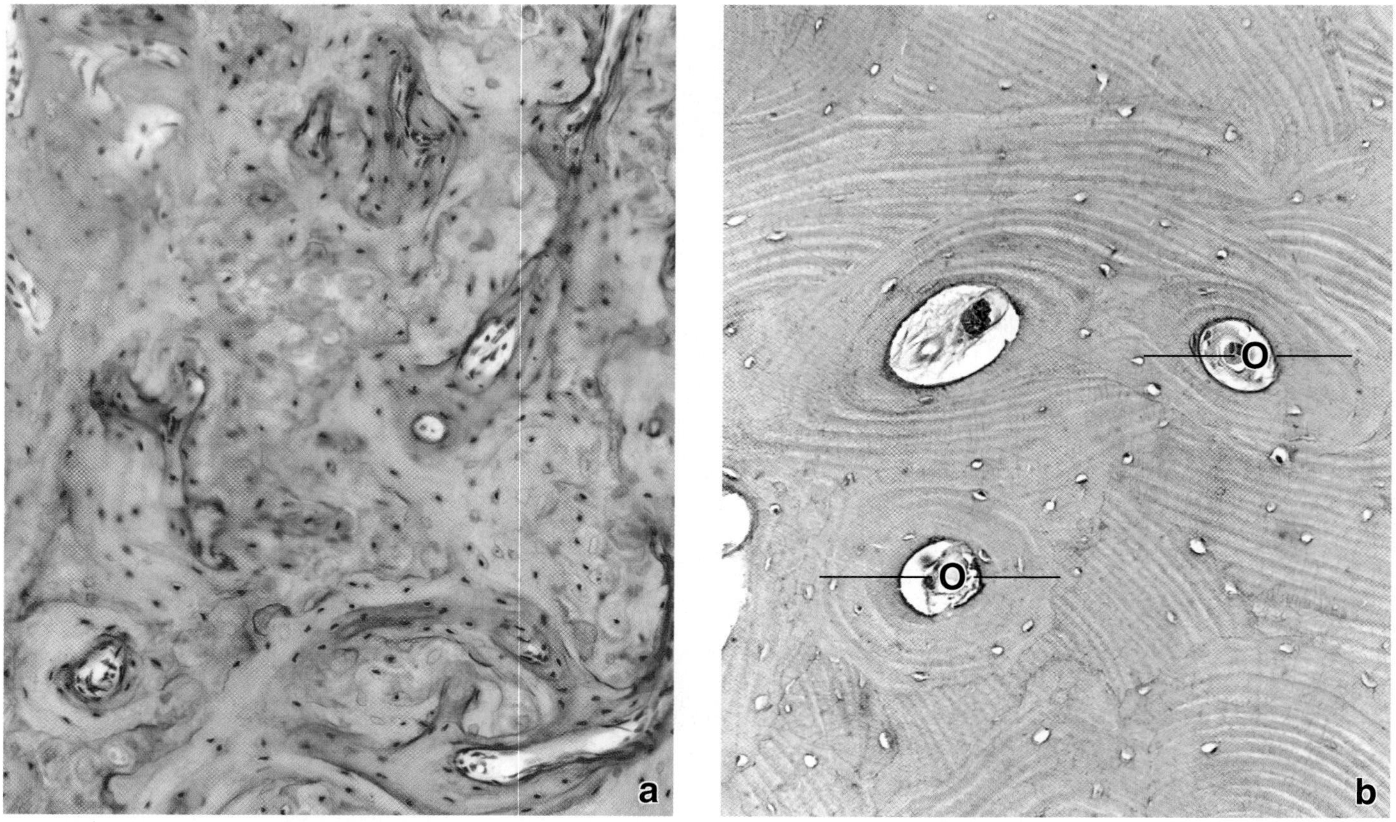

FIGURE 8.6
Photomicrographs of decalcified immature and mature bone. a. Decalcified immature bone, stained with H&E, showing the relationships of cells to the extracellular matrix. The immature bone has more cells, and the matrix is not layered in osteonal arrays. ×130. **b.** This cross section of decalcified mature compact bone stained with H&E shows several osteons *(O)* with concentric lamellae. The Haversian canals contain blood vessels and connective tissue. Osteocytes undergo considerable shrinkage during routine slide preparation, revealing empty lacunae with a small nucleus attached to their walls. Mature bone has fewer osteocytes per unit area than immature bone. Note the presence of interstitial lamellae between neighboring osteons. ×160.

(Haversian) canals, and the perforating (Volkmann's) canals. Osteoprogenitor cells can divide and proliferate, as shown by autoradiographic studies. In growing bones, osteoprogenitor cells appear as flattened cells with lightly staining, elongate or ovoid nuclei and inconspicuous acidophilic or slightly basophilic cytoplasm. Electron micrographs reveal profiles of rough endoplasmic reticulum (rER) and free ribosomes as well as a small Golgi apparatus and other organelles. The morphology of the osteoprogenitor cell is consistent with the finding that its stimulation leads to differentiation into a more active secretory cell, the osteoblast.

Bone-lining cells cover bone that is not remodeling but are analogous to osteoprogenitor cells at sites of bone growth

In sites where remodeling is not occurring in mature bone, the bone surfaces are covered by a layer of flat cells with attenuated cytoplasm and a paucity of organelles beyond the perinuclear region (see Fig. 8.7a). They do not

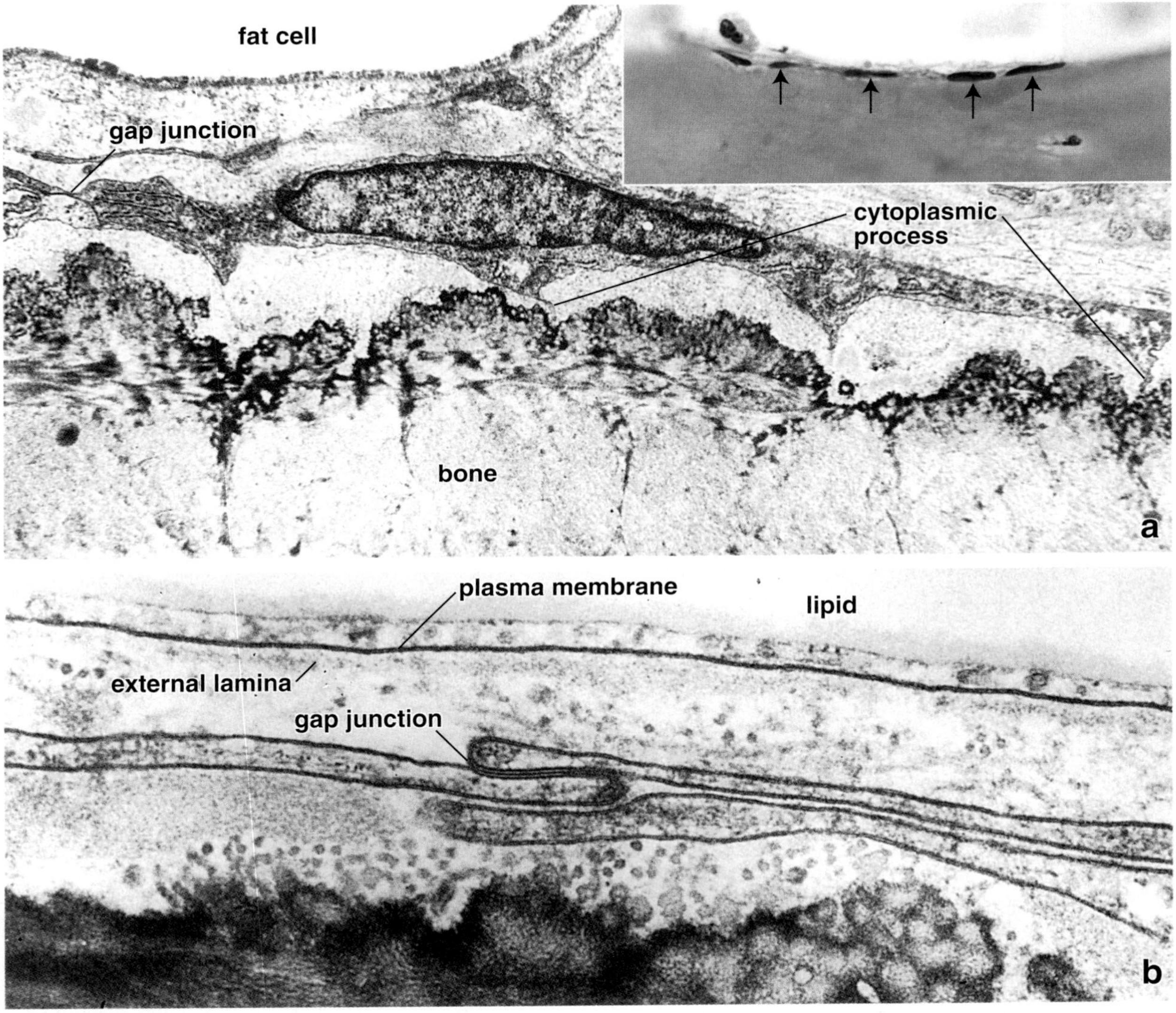

FIGURE 8.7
Electron micrograph of bone-lining cells. a. The cytoplasm of a bone-lining cell located on the surface of a spicule of mature bone is very attenuated and contains small amounts of rER and free ribosomes. A gap junction is seen between the two adjacent bone-lining cells. In addition, cytoplasmic processes are clearly seen where they pass through the matrix of unmineralized bone (osteoid). A fat cell of the marrow is also present. ×8,900. (From Miller SC, et al. *Anat Rec* 1980;198:163–173.) **Inset.** High-magnification photomicrograph of a similar bone spicule stained with H&E, included for orientation purposes. The bone-lining cells on the surface of the spicule are indicated by the *arrows.* ×350. **b.** Electron micrograph of the cytoplasm of two bone-lining cells observed at higher magnification. The gap junction is clearly seen where the two cells are in apposition. The edge of a fat cell is seen at the top of the electron micrograph; its lipid, thin rim of cytoplasm, plasma membrane, and external lamina are also evident. ×27,000.

form a complete cellular lining on the bone surface; gap junctions are present where the lining cell processes contact one another (Fig. 8.7b). These cells, designated simply as ***bone-lining cells,*** are analogous to the osteoprogenitor cells but are probably in a more quiescent state than those located at sites of bone growth. They are also thought to function in the maintenance and nutritional support of the osteocytes embedded in the underlying bone matrix. This suggested role is based on the observation that the cell processes of bone-lining cells extend into the canalicular channels of the adjacent bone (see Fig. 8.7b) and communicate by means of gap junctions with processes of osteocytes.

The degree of differentiation of the osteoprogenitor cell is not entirely clear. Their derivation from mesenchymal cells and their apparent ability to differentiate into three kinds of cells other than osteoblasts (adipose cells, chondroblasts, and fibroblasts) suggest that they, like fibroblasts, can modify their morphologic and functional characteristics in response to specific stimuli. This question is important because the healing of bone fractures involves the formation of new connective tissue and cartilage in the callus that develops around the bone during the repair process (see "Fractures and Bone Repair," page 201). Although the precise origin of the cells in healing bone may still be unclear, some evidence indicates that periosteal cells and endosteal cells participate in all stages of the healing process.

Osteoblasts

The osteoblast is the differentiated bone-forming cell that secretes bone matrix

Like its close relatives, the fibroblast and the chondroblast, the osteoblast is a versatile secretory cell that retains the ability to divide. It secretes both the collagen and the ground substance that constitute the initial unmineralized bone, or ***osteoid.*** The osteoblast is also responsible for the calcification of the matrix. The calcification process appears to be initiated by the osteoblast through the secretion into the matrix of small, 50- to 250-nm, membrane-limited ***matrix vesicles.*** The vesicles are rich in alkaline phosphatase and are actively secreted only during the period in which the cell produces the bone matrix. The role of these vesicles is discussed on page 200 ("Biologic Mineralization and Matrix Vesicles").

Osteoblasts are recognized in the light microscope by their cuboidal or polygonal shape and their aggregation into a single layer of cells lying in apposition to the forming bone (Fig. 8.8). Because the newly deposited matrix is not immediately calcified, it stains lightly or not at all, compared with mature mineralized matrix, which stains heavily with eosin. Because of this staining property of the newly formed matrix, osteoblasts appear to be separated from the bone by a light band. This band represents the osteoid; it is nonmineralized matrix.

The cytoplasm of the osteoblast is markedly basophilic, and the Golgi apparatus, because of its size, is sometimes observed as a clear area adjacent to the nucleus. Small, periodic acid–Schiff (PAS)-positive granules are observed in the cytoplasm, and a strong alkaline phosphatase reaction associated with the cell membrane can be detected by appropriate histochemical staining.

In contrast to the secreting osteoblasts found in active matrix deposition, inactive osteoblasts are flat or attenuated cells that cover the bone surface. These cells resemble osteoprogenitor cells. Osteoblasts respond to mechanical stimuli to mediate the changes in bone growth

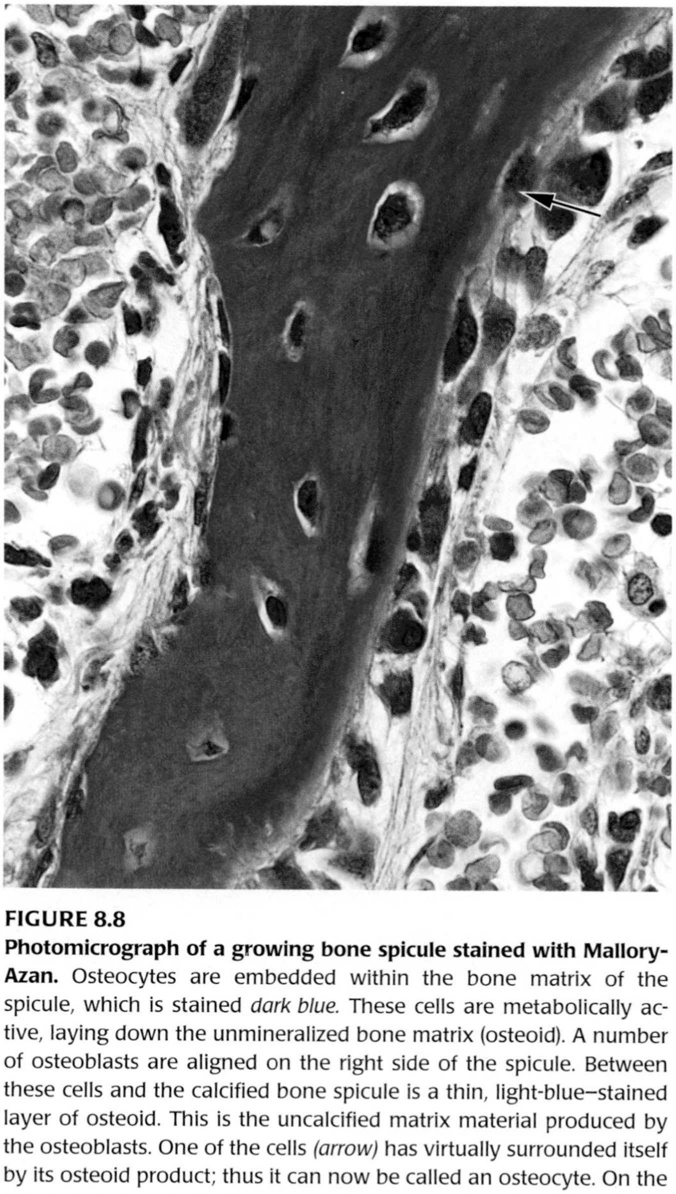

FIGURE 8.8
Photomicrograph of a growing bone spicule stained with Mallory-Azan. Osteocytes are embedded within the bone matrix of the spicule, which is stained *dark blue.* These cells are metabolically active, laying down the unmineralized bone matrix (osteoid). A number of osteoblasts are aligned on the right side of the spicule. Between these cells and the calcified bone spicule is a thin, light-blue–stained layer of osteoid. This is the uncalcified matrix material produced by the osteoblasts. One of the cells *(arrow)* has virtually surrounded itself by its osteoid product; thus it can now be called an osteocyte. On the left side of the spicule, the nongrowing part, are inactive osteoblasts. The cells exhibit flattened nuclei and attenuated cytoplasm. ×550.

and bone remodeling. As osteoid deposition occurs, the osteoblast is eventually surrounded by osteoid matrix and then becomes an osteocyte.

Osteoblast processes communicate with other osteoblasts and with osteocytes by gap junctions

At the electron microscope level, osteoblasts exhibit thin cytoplasmic processes that penetrate the adjacent osteoid produced by the cell and are joined to similar processes of adjacent osteocytes by gap junctions. This early establishment of junctions between an osteoblast and adjacent osteocytes (as well as between adjacent osteoblasts) allows neighboring cells within the bone tissue to communicate.

The osteoblast cytoplasm is characterized by abundant rER and free ribosomes (Fig. 8.9). These features are consistent with its basophilia observed in the light microscope as well as with its role in the production of collagen and proteoglycans for the extracellular matrix. The Golgi apparatus and surrounding regions of the cytoplasm contain numerous vesicles with a flocculent content that is presumed to consist of matrix precursors. These vesicles are the PAS-staining

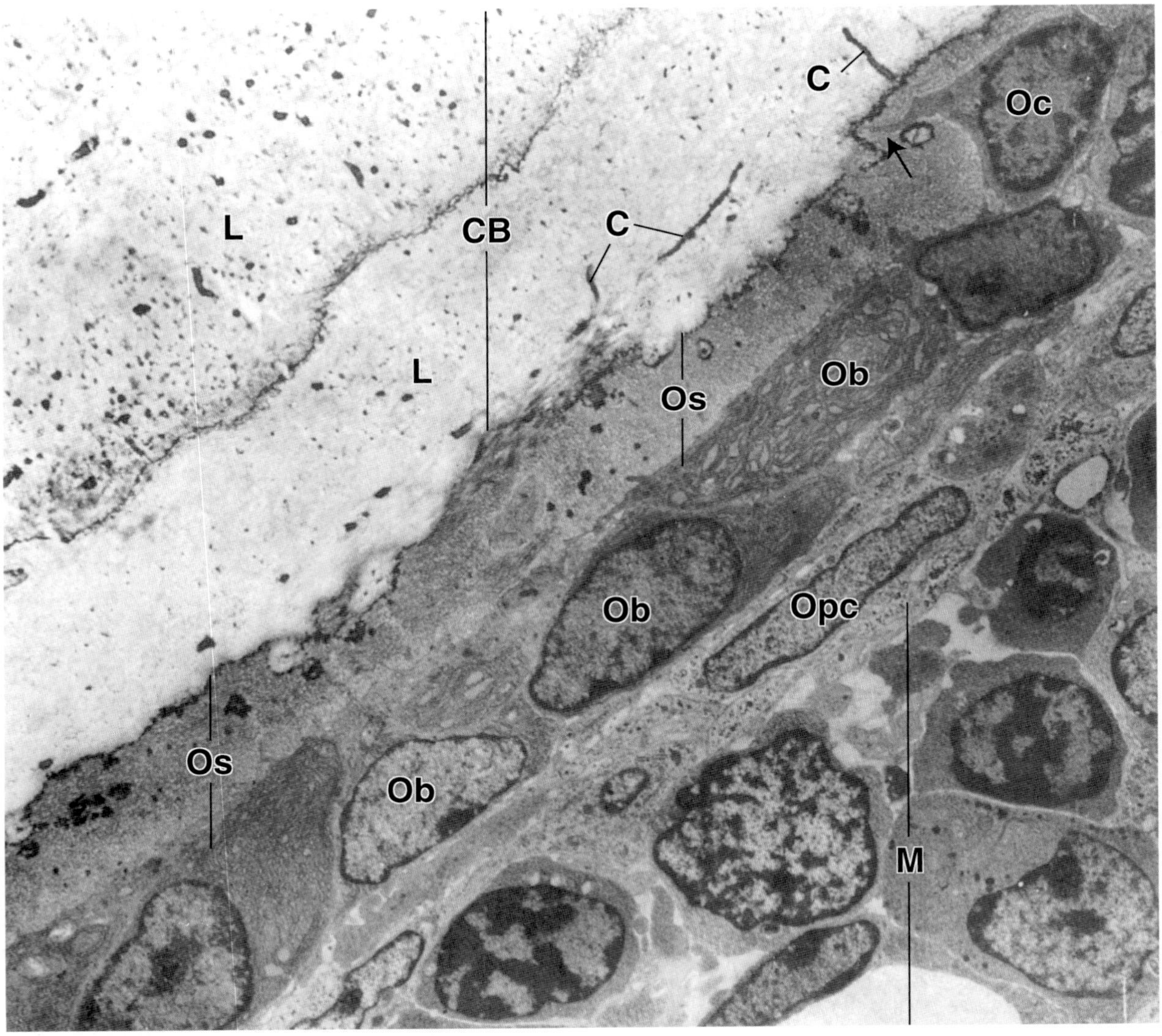

FIGURE 8.9
Electron micrograph showing active bone formation. This electron micrograph is similar to the growing surface of the bone spicule in the preceding light micrograph (Fig. 8.8). The marrow cavity *(M)* with its developing blood cells is seen in the lower right corner. Osteoprogenitor cells *(Opc)* are evident between the marrow and the osteoblasts *(Ob)*. They exhibit elongate or ovoid nuclei. The osteoblasts are aligned along the growing portion of the bone, which is covered by a layer of osteoid *(Os)*. In this same region, one of the cells (upper right corner) embedded within the osteoid exhibits a small process *(arrow)*. This cell, because of its location within the osteoid, can now be called an osteocyte *(Oc)*. The remainder of the micrograph (upper left) is composed of calcified bone matrix *(CB)*. Within the matrix are canaliculi *(C)* containing osteocyte processes. The boundary between two adjacent lamellae *(L)* of previously formed bone is evident as an irregular dark line. ×9,000.

granules seen in light microscopy. The matrix vesicles, also produced by the osteoblast, appear to arise by a different pathway, originating as sphere-like outgrowths that pinch off from the plasma membrane to become free in the matrix. Other cell organelles include numerous rod-shaped mitochondria and occasional dense bodies and lysosomes.

Osteocytes

The osteocyte is the mature bone cell and is enclosed by bone matrix that it previously secreted as an osteoblast

When completely surrounded by osteoid or bone matrix, the osteoblast is referred to as an osteocyte, the cell now responsible for maintaining the bone matrix. Osteocytes can synthesize new matrix, as well as resorb it, at least to a limited extent. Such activities help to maintain the homeostasis of blood calcium. Death of osteocytes, either through trauma, e.g., a fracture, or cell senescence, results in resorption of the bone matrix by *osteoclast* activity, followed by repair or remodeling of the bone tissue by *osteoblast* activity.

Each osteocyte occupies a space, or ***lacuna,*** that conforms to the shape of the cell. Osteocytes extend cytoplasmic processes through the canaliculi in the matrix to contact processes of neighboring cells by means of gap junctions. In hematoxylin and eosin (H&E)–stained sections, the canaliculi and the processes they contain are not discernable. In ground sections, the canaliculi are readily evident (see Fig. 8.11). Osteocytes are typically smaller than their precursors because of their reduced perinuclear cytoplasm. Often, in routinely prepared microscopic specimens, the cell is highly distorted by shrinkage and other artifacts that result from decalcifying the matrix prior to sectioning the bone. In such instances, the nucleus may be the only prominent feature. In well-preserved specimens, osteocytes exhibit less cytoplasmic basophilia than osteoblasts, but little additional cytoplasmic detail can be seen.

Electron microscopy has revealed osteocytes in various functional states. Indeed, there is evidence that the osteocyte can modify the surrounding bone matrix through synthetic and reabsorptive activities. Three functional states, each with a characteristic morphology, have been described:

- ***Quiescent osteocytes*** exhibit a paucity of rER and a markedly diminished Golgi apparatus (Fig. 8.10a). An osmiophilic lamina representing mature calcified matrix is seen in close apposition to the cell membrane.
- ***Formative osteocytes*** show evidence of matrix deposition and exhibit certain characteristics similar to those of osteoblasts. Thus, the rER and Golgi apparatus are more abundant, and there is evidence of osteoid in the pericellular space within the lacuna (Fig. 8.10b).
- ***Resorptive osteocytes,*** like formative osteocytes, contain numerous profiles of endoplasmic reticulum and a well-developed Golgi apparatus. Moreover, secondary lysosomes are conspicuous (Fig. 8.10c).

That the resorptive osteocyte removes matrix is supported by the observation that the pericellular space is devoid of collagen fibrils and may contain a flocculent material suggestive of a breakdown product. The more peripheral, nonresorbed matrix is bounded by an osmiophilic lamina, which presumably represents the boundary of the intact mature calcified matrix. Resorption of bone by this mechanism, called ***osteocytic osteolysis,*** with the concomitant release of calcium ions, allows increases in blood calcium to maintain appropriate levels. The stimulus for the resorption of bone is increased secretion of parathyroid hormone (PTH).

Osteoclasts

The osteoclast is responsible for bone resorption

Osteoclasts are large, multinucleated cells found at sites where bone is being removed. They rest directly on the bone tissue where resorption is taking place (Fig. 8.11). As a result of osteoclast activity, a shallow bay called a ***resorption bay*** **(Howship's lacuna)** can be observed in the bone directly under the osteoclast. The cell is conspicuous not only because of its large size but also because of its marked acidophilia. It also exhibits a strong histochemical reaction for acid phosphatase because of the numerous lysosomes that it contains.

The portion of the cell in direct contact with the bone can be divided into two parts: a central region containing numerous plasma membrane infoldings forming microvillous-type structures, called the ***ruffled border;*** and a ring-like perimeter of cytoplasm, the ***clear zone,*** that demarcates the bone area being resorbed. The clear zone contains abundant microfilaments but essentially lacks other organelles. The ruffled border stains less intensely than the remainder of the cell and often appears as a light band adjacent to the bone at the resorption site (see Fig. 8.11).

At the electron microscopic level, hydroxyapatite crystals from the bone substance are observed between the processes of the ruffled border (Fig. 8.12). Internal to the ruffled border and in close proximity are numerous mitochondria and lysosomes. The nuclei are typically located in the part of the cell more removed from the bone surface. In this same region are profiles of rER, multiple stacks of Golgi saccules, and many vesicles.

Osteoclasts resorb bone by releasing lysosomal hydrolases into the extracellular space

Some, if not most, of the vesicles in the osteoclast are lysosomes that develop from late endosomes. They are

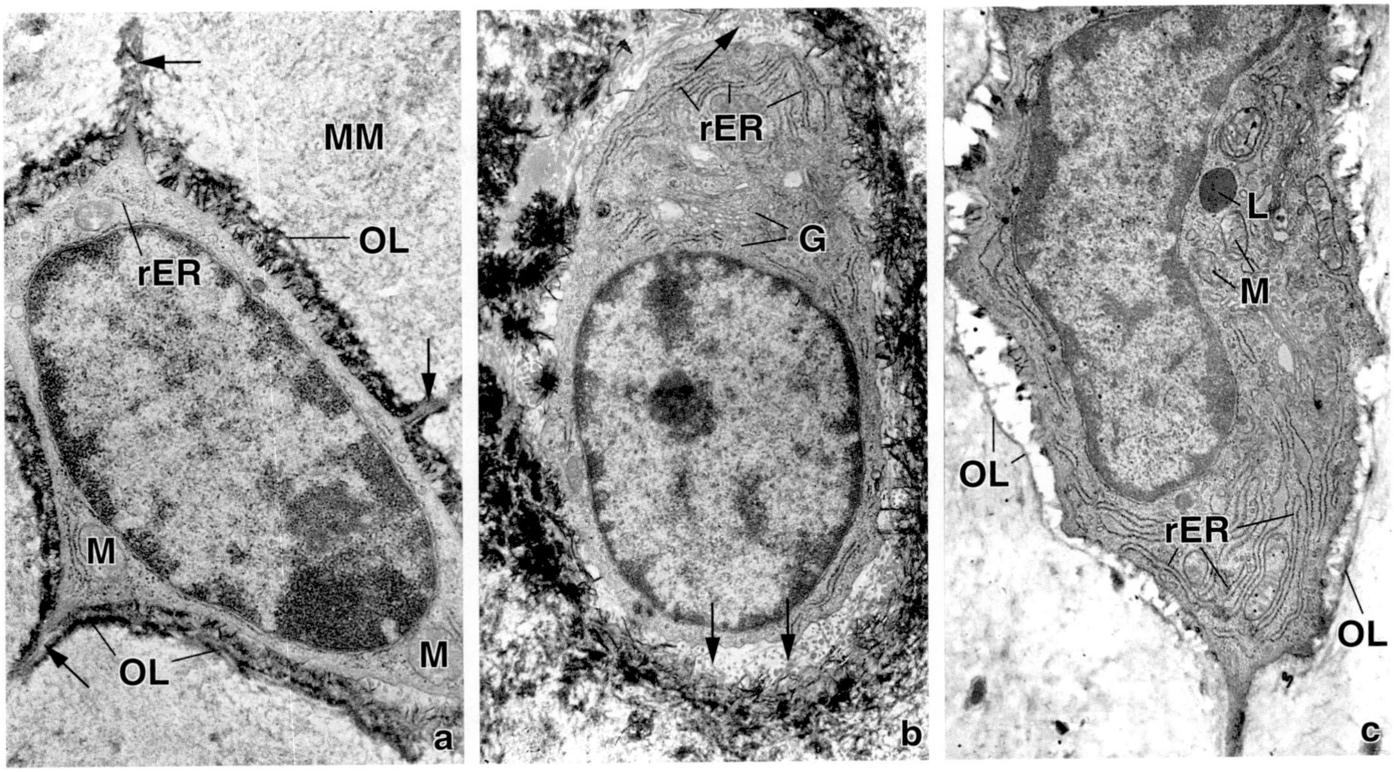

FIGURE 8.10
Electron micrographs of three different functional stages of an osteocyte. a. Relatively quiescent osteocyte that contains only a few profiles of rER and a few mitochondria *(M)*. The cell virtually fills the lacuna that it occupies; the *arrows* indicate where cytoplasmic processes extend into canaliculi. Hydroxyapatite crystals have been lost from the matrix, which is ordinarily mineralized *(MM)*, but some hydroxyapatite crystals fill the pericellular space. The hydroxyapatite crystals obscure the other substances within the pericellular space. The dark band marking the boundary of the lacuna is the osmiophilic lamina *(OL)*. ×25,000. **b.** A formative osteocyte containing larger amounts of rER and a large Golgi apparatus *(G)*. Of equal importance is the presence of a small amount of osteoid in the pericellular space within the lacuna. The osteoid shows profiles of collagen fibrils *(arrows)* not yet mineralized. The lacuna of a formative osteocyte is not bounded by an osmiophilic lamina. ×25,000. **c.** A resorptive osteocyte containing a substantial amount of rER, a large Golgi apparatus, mitochondria *(M)*, and lysosomes *(L)*. The pericellular space is devoid of collagen fibrils and may contain some flocculent material. The lacuna containing a resorptive osteocyte is bounded by a less conspicuous osmiophilic lamina *(OL)*. ×25,000.

released into the extracellular space in the clefts between the cytoplasmic processes of the ruffled border, a clear example of lysosomal hydrolases functioning outside the cell. Once liberated, these hydrolytic enzymes, which include collagenase, digest the organic components of the bone matrix. Before digestion can occur, however, the bone matrix must be decalcified. Current evidence indicates that the dissolution of the calcium salts occurs through secretion of organic acids by the membranes of the ruffled border. Moreover, a low pH favors the action of acid hydrolases. Accordingly, a local acidic environment is created in the extracellular space between the bone and the osteoclast. The clear zone adjacent to the ruffled border seems to form a seal against the bone, thus creating a compartment at the site of the ruffled border where focal decalcification and degradation of the matrix occur. Support for the concept of acid secretion by the osteoclast comes, in part, from the finding that carbonic anhydrase, an enzyme associated with carbonic acid production, is present in the region of the ruffled border.

Osteoclasts are phagocytotic

Numerous coated pits and coated vesicles are also present at the ruffled border, suggesting endocytotic activity. Osteoclasts are observed at sites where bone remodeling is in progress. (The process of remodeling is described in more detail shortly.) Thus, in sites where osteons are being altered or where a bone is undergoing change during the growth process, osteoclasts are relatively numerous. As noted, an increase in PTH level promotes bone resorption and has a demonstrable effect on osteoclast activity, in addition to its ef-

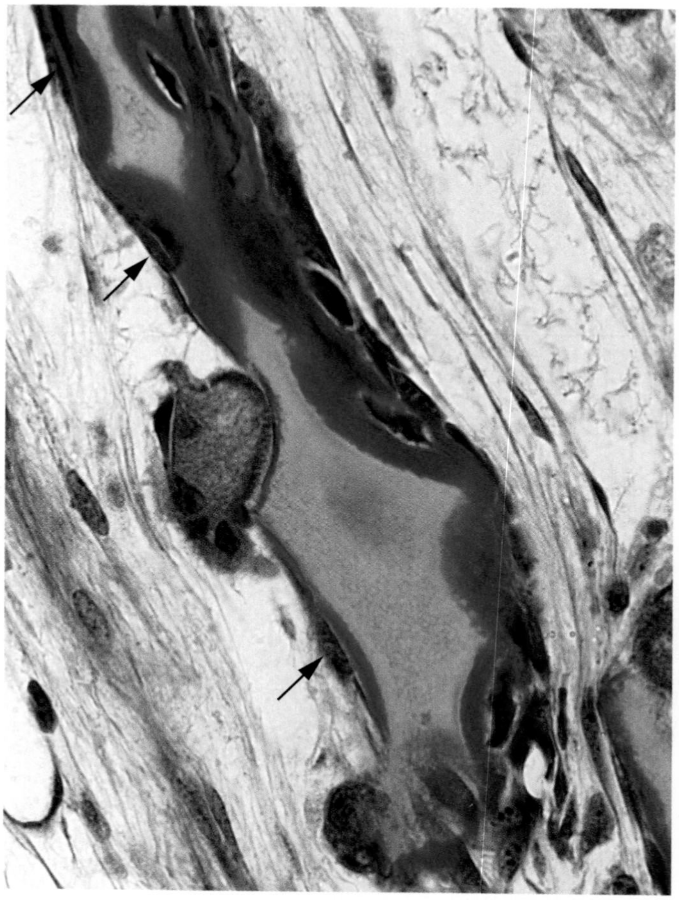

FIGURE 8.11
Photomicrograph of an osteoclast on a bone spicule. This Mallory-stained specimen shows a spicule made of calcified cartilage (stained *light blue*) and a covering of bone tissue (stained *dark blue*). An osteoclast on the left side of the spicule has resorbed bone tissue and lies in a depression (Howship's lacuna) in the spicule. The light band between the osteoclast and the bone spicule corresponds to the ruffled border of the osteoclast. The *arrows* on the nongrowing surface indicate cytoplasm of inactive bone lining cells (osteoprogenitor cells). In contrast, bone is being deposited on the opposite side of the spicule, as evidenced by the presence of osteoblasts on this surface and newly formed osteocytes just below the surface of the spicule. ×550.

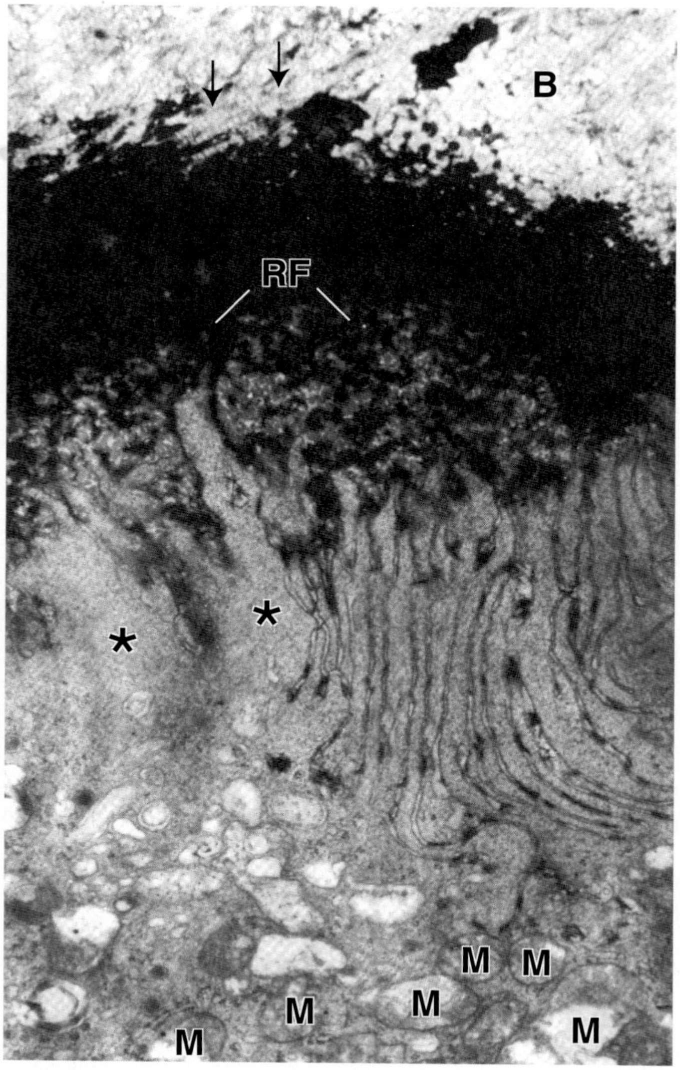

FIGURE 8.12
Electron micrograph of an osteoclast. This micrograph shows a segment of bone surface *(B)* and a portion of an osteoclast that is in apposition to the partially digested bone. The resorption front *(RF)* of the osteoclast possesses numerous infoldings of the plasma membrane. When viewed in the light microscope, these infoldings are evident as the ruffled border. When the plane of section is parallel to the infoldings *(asterisks)*, a broad, nonspecialized expanse of cytoplasm is seen. The cytoplasm of the osteoclast contains numerous mitochondria *(M)*, lysosomes, and Golgi apparatus, all of which are functionally linked with the resorption and degradation of the bone matrix. In the upper part of the figure, some collagen fibrils are evident; the *arrows* indicate where 68-nm cross-banding is visible. ×10,000.

fects on osteocytes, described above. In contrast, calcitonin, secreted by parafollicular cells of the thyroid gland, has a counterbalancing effect, reducing osteoclast activity. Little is known, however, about the role of endocrine activity in normal bone remodeling during growth.

Contrary to what was once thought, osteoclasts are not related to osteoblasts. They are derived from mononuclear hemopoietic progenitor cells, namely, ***CFU-GM,*** a cell that gives rise to the neutrophilic granulocyte and monocyte lineages, and ***CFU-M,*** a cell that gives rise to monocytes. It is thought that osteoclasts arise by fusion of either CFU-GM cells or CFU-M cells. In both origin and function, they are closely related to macrophages. Morphologically, osteoclasts resemble Langhans' giant cells formed by fusion of tissue macrophages (histiocytes).

BONE FORMATION

The development of a bone is traditionally classified as endochondral or intramembranous

The distinction between endochondral and intramembranous formation rests on whether a cartilage model serves as the precursor of the bone (**endochondral ossification**) or the bone is formed by a simpler method, without the intervention of a cartilage precursor (**intramembranous ossification**). The bones of the extremities and those parts of the axial skeleton that bear weight (e.g., vertebrae) develop by endochondral ossification. The flat bones of the skull and face, the mandible, and the clavicle develop by intramembranous ossification.

The existence of two distinct types of ossification does not imply that existing bone is either membrane bone or endochondral bone. These names refer *only* to the mechanism by which a bone is initially formed. Because of the remodeling that occurs later, the initial bone tissue laid down by endochondral formation or by intramembranous formation is soon replaced. The replacement bone is established on the preexisting bone by appositional growth and is identical in both cases. Although the long bones are classified as being formed by endochondral formation, their continued growth involves the histogenesis of both endochondral and intramembranous bone, with the latter occurring through the activity of the periosteal (membrane) tissue.

Intramembranous Ossification

In intramembranous ossification, bone is formed by differentiation of mesenchymal cells into osteoblasts

The first evidence of intramembranous ossification occurs around the eighth week of gestation in humans. Some of the pale-staining, elongate mesenchymal cells within the mesenchyme migrate and aggregate in specific areas, the sites where bone is destined to form. This condensation of cells within the mesenchymal tissue is the membrane referred to in the term *intramembranous ossification* (Fig. 8.13). As the process continues, the newly organized tissue at the presumptive bone site becomes more vascularized, and the aggregated mesenchymal cells become larger and rounded. The cytoplasm of these cells changes from eosinophilic to basophilic, and a clear Golgi area becomes evident. These cytologic changes result in the differentiated osteoblast, which then secretes the collagens and other components of the bone matrix (osteoid). The osteoblasts within the bone matrix become increasingly separated from one another as the matrix is produced, but they remain attached by thin cytoplasmic processes. Because of the abundant collagen content, the bone matrix appears denser than the surrounding mesenchyme, in which the intercellular spaces reveal only delicate connective tissue fibers.

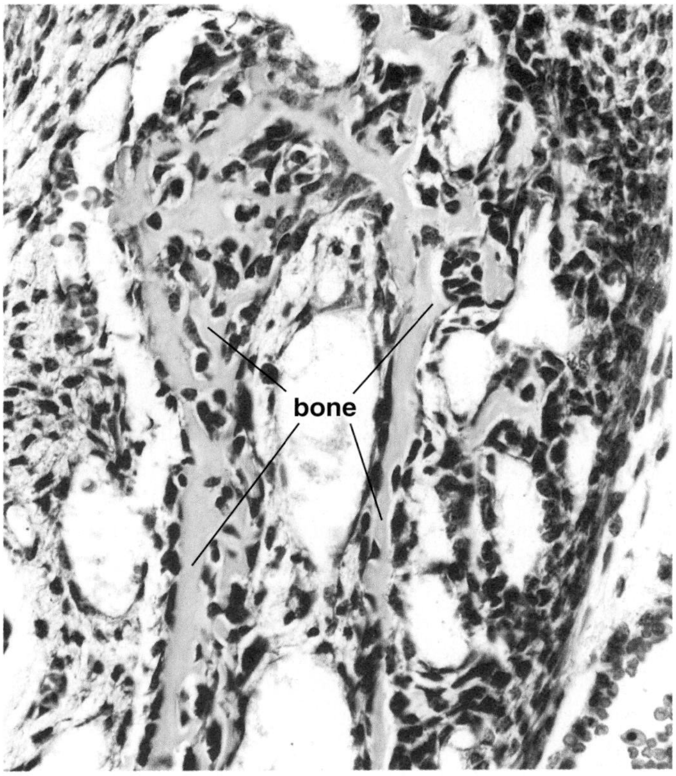

FIGURE 8.13
Section of mandible developing by the process of intramembranous ossification. This photomicrograph shows a section from a developing mandible, stained with H&E. In this relatively early stage of development, the mandible consists of bone spicules of various sizes and shapes. The bone spicules interconnect with each other and form trabeculae, providing the general shape of the developing bone (no cartilage model is present). The numerous osteoblasts responsible for this growing region of spicules are seen at the surface of the newly deposited bone. The older, calcified portion of spicules contains osteocytes surrounded by bone matrix. In the right portion of the figure, adjacent to the bone spicules, the connective tissue is very cellular and is developing into the early periosteum. ×250.

Newly formed bone matrix appears in histologic sections as small, irregularly shaped spicules and trabeculae

With time, the matrix becomes calcified, and the interconnecting cytoplasmic processes of the bone-forming cells, now termed osteocytes, are contained within canaliculi. Concomitantly, more of the surrounding mesenchymal cells in the membrane proliferate, giving rise to a population of osteoprogenitor cells. Some of the osteoprogenitor cells come into apposition with the initially formed spicules, become osteoblasts, and add more matrix. By this process, called ***appositional growth,*** the spicules enlarge and become joined in a trabecular network with the general shape of the developing bone.

Through continued mitotic activity, the osteoprogenitor cells maintain their numbers and thus provide a constant source of osteoblasts for growth of the bone spicules. The new osteoblasts, in turn, lay down bone matrix in successive layers, giving rise to woven bone. This immature bone, discussed on page 185, is characterized internally by interconnecting spaces occupied by connective tissue and blood vessels. Bone tissue formed by the process just described is referred to as ***membrane bone*** or ***intramembranous bone.***

Endochondral Ossification

Endochondral ossification also begins with the proliferation and aggregation of mesenchymal cells at the site of the future bone. However, the mesenchymal cells differentiate into chondroblasts that, in turn, produce cartilage matrix.

Initially, a hyaline cartilage model with the general shape of the bone is formed

Once established, the cartilage model (a miniature version of the future definitive bone) grows by interstitial and appositional growth. The increase in the length of the cartilage model is attributed to interstitial growth. The increase in its width is largely due to the addition of cartilage matrix produced by new chondrocytes that differentiate from the chondrogenic layer of the perichondrium surrounding the cartilage mass. Illustrations *1* and *1a* of Figure 8.14 show an early cartilage model.

The first sign of ossification is the appearance of a cuff of bone around the cartilage model

At this stage, the perichondrial cells in the midregion of the cartilage model no longer give rise to chondrocytes. Instead, bone-forming cells or osteoblasts are produced. Thus, the connective tissue surrounding this portion of the cartilage is *no longer functionally a perichondrium;* rather, because of its altered role, it is *now called periosteum.* Moreover, because the cells within this layer are differentiating into osteoblasts, an osteogenic layer can now be identified within the periosteum. As a result of these changes, a layer of bone is formed around the cartilage model. This bone can be classified as either periosteal bone, because of its location, or intramembranous bone, because of its method of development. In the case of a long bone, a distinctive cuff of periosteal bone, the ***bony collar,*** is established around the cartilage model in the diaphyseal portion of the developing bone. The bony collar is shown in illustrations 2 and *2a* of Figure 8.14.

With the establishment of the periosteal bony collar, the chondrocytes in the midregion of the cartilage model become hypertrophic

As the chondrocytes enlarge, their surrounding cartilage matrix is resorbed, forming thin irregular cartilage plates between the hypertrophic cells. The hypertrophic cells begin to synthesize alkaline phosphatase, and concomitantly, the surrounding cartilage matrix undergoes calcification (see illustrations *3* and *3a* of Fig. 8.14). The calcification of the cartilage matrix should not be confused with calcification that occurs in bone tissue.

The calcified cartilage matrix inhibits diffusion of nutrients, causing death of the chondrocytes in the cartilage model

With the death of the chondrocytes, much of the matrix breaks down, and neighboring lacunae become confluent, producing an increasingly large cavity. While these events are occurring, one or several blood vessels grow through the thin diaphyseal bony collar to vascularize the cavity (see illustrations *4* and *4a* of Fig. 8.14).

Periosteal cells migrate into the cavity along with growing blood vessels

Cells from the periosteum migrate with the penetrating blood vessels and some of the primitive periosteal cells to become osteoprogenitor cells in the cavity. Other primitive cells also gain access to the cavity via the new vasculature, leaving the circulation to give rise to the marrow. As the calcified cartilage breaks down and is partially removed, some remains as irregular spicules. When the osteoprogenitor cells come in apposition to the remaining calcified cartilage spicules, they become osteoblasts and begin to lay down bone (osteoid) on the spicule framework. Thus, the bone formed in this manner may be described as endochondral bone. The combination of bone, which is initially only a thin layer, and the underlying calcified cartilage is described as a ***mixed spicule.***

Histologically, mixed spicules can be recognized by their staining characteristics. Calcified cartilage tends to be basophilic, whereas bone is distinctly eosinophilic. With the Mallory stain, bone stains a deep blue, and calcified cartilage stains light blue (Fig. 8.15). Also, calcified cartilage no longer contains cells, whereas the newly produced bone may reveal osteocytes in the bone matrix. Such spicules persist for a short time before the calcified cartilage component is removed. The remaining bone component of the spicule may continue to grow by appositional growth, thus becoming larger and stronger, or it may undergo resorption as new spicules are formed.

Growth of Endochondral Bone

Endochondral bone growth begins in the second trimester of fetal life and continues into early adulthood

The events described above represent the early stage of endochondral bone formation as seen in the fetus, beginning at about the 12th week of gestation. The continuing growth process, which takes place throughout the growth

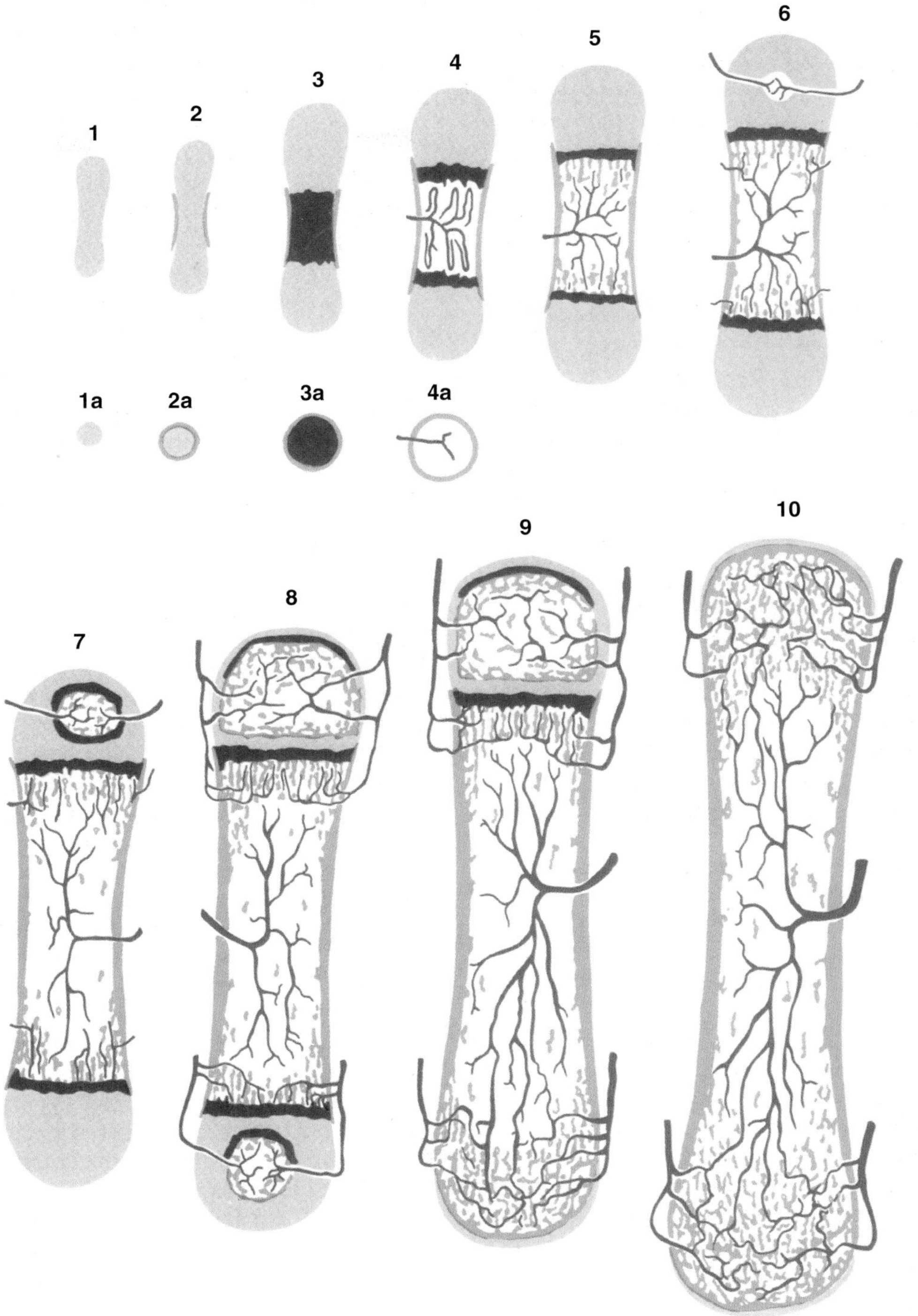

FIGURE 8.14
Schematic diagram of developing long bone. Illustrations **1** to **10** depict longitudinal sections; **1a** to **4a** depict cross sections through the shaft of the long bone. The process begins with the formation of a cartilage model (**1** and **1a**); next, a periosteal (perichondrial) collar of bone forms around the shaft (diaphysis) of the cartilage model (**2** and **2a**); then, the cartilaginous matrix in the shaft begins to calcify (**3** and **3a**). Blood vessels and connective tissue cells then erode and invade the calcified cartilage (**4** and **4a**), creating a primitive marrow cavity in which remnant spicules of calcified cartilage remain at the two ends of the cavity. Endochondral bone forms on these spicules of calcified cartilage. The bone at the ends of the developing marrow cavity constitutes the metaphysis. Periosteal bone continues to form; the periosteal bone is formed as the result of intramembranous ossification. It can be recognized histologically because it is not accompanied by local cartilage erosion, nor is the bone deposited on spicules of calcified cartilage. Blood vessels and perivascular cells invade the proximal epiphyseal cartilage **(6),** and a secondary center of ossification is established in the proximal epiphysis **(7).** A similar epiphyseal (secondary) ossification center forms at the distal end of the bone **(8),** and an epiphyseal cartilage is thus formed between each epiphysis and the diaphysis. With continued growth of the long bone, the distal epiphyseal cartilage disappears **(9),** and finally, with cessation of growth, the proximal epiphyseal cartilage disappears **(10).** The metaphysis then becomes continuous with the epiphysis. Epiphyseal lines remain where the epiphyseal plate last existed. (From Bloom W, Fawcett DW. *A Textbook of Histology.* Philadelphia: WB Saunders, 1975.)

period of the individual into early adulthood, is described below.

Growth of long bones depends on the presence of epiphyseal cartilage throughout the growth period

As the diaphyseal marrow cavity enlarges (see illustration 5 of Fig. 8.14), a distinct zonation can be recognized in the cartilage at both ends of the cavity. This remaining cartilage, referred to as ***epiphyseal cartilage,*** exhibits distinct zones as illustrated in Figure 8.16. The zones in the epiphyseal cartilage, beginning with that most distal to the diaphyseal center of ossification and proceeding toward that center, are

- **Zone of reserve cartilage,** which exhibits no cellular proliferation or active matrix production.

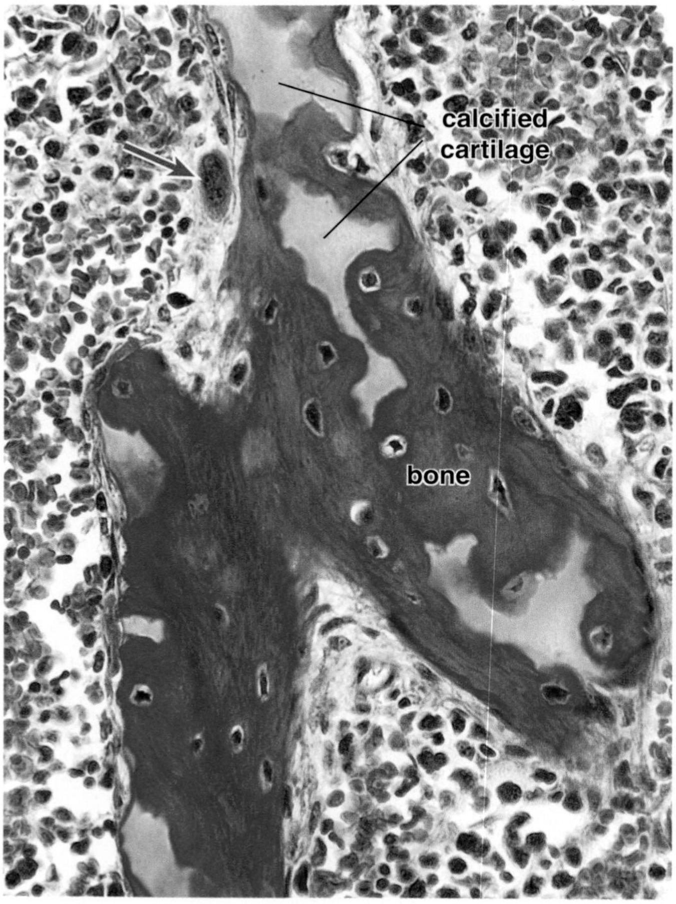

FIGURE 8.15
Photomicrograph of a mixed bone spicule formed during endochondral bone formation. In this Mallory-Azan–stained section, bone has been deposited on calcified cartilage spicules. In the center of the photomicrograph, the spicules have already grown to create an anastomosing trabecula. The initial trabecula still contains remnants of calcified cartilage, as shown by the light-blue staining of the calcified matrix compared with the dark-blue staining of the bone. In the upper part of the spicule, note a lone osteoclast *(arrow)* aligned near the surface of the spicule, where remodeling is about to be initiated. ×275.

- **Zone of proliferation,** which is adjacent to the zone of reserve cartilage in the direction of the diaphysis. In this zone, the cartilage cells undergo division and organize into distinct columns. These cells are larger than those in the reserve zone and actively produce matrix.
- **Zone of hypertrophy,** which contains greatly enlarged cartilage cells. The cytoplasm of these cells is clear, which is a reflection of the glycogen that they normally accumulate (and that is lost during fixation). The matrix is compressed into linear bands between the columns of hypertrophied cartilage cells.
- **Zone of calcified cartilage,** in which the enlarged cells begin to degenerate and the matrix becomes calcified.
- **Zone of resorption,** which is the zone nearest the diaphysis. The calcified cartilage here is in direct contact with the connective tissue of the marrow cavity.

In the zone of resorption, small blood vessels and accompanying connective tissue invade the region occupied by the dying chondrocytes. They form a series of spearheads, leaving the calcified cartilage as longitudinal spicules, at least as seen in longitudinal sections of bone. Actually, in a cross section of the bone, the cartilage appears as a honeycomb because the invading vessels and connective tissue have migrated into the sites previously occupied by the cartilage cells.

Bone deposition occurs on the cartilage spicules in the same manner as described for the formation of the initial ossification center

As bone is laid down on the calcified spicules, the cartilage is resorbed, ultimately leaving a primary spongy bone. This spongy bone undergoes reorganization through osteoclastic activity and addition of new bone tissue, thus accommodating the continued growth and physical stresses placed on the bone.

Shortly after birth, a secondary ossification center develops in the upper epiphysis. The cartilage cells undergo hypertrophy and degenerate. As in the diaphysis, calcification of the matrix occurs, and blood vessels and osteogenic cells from the perichondrium invade the region, creating a new marrow cavity (see illustrations *6* and *7* of Fig. 8.14). Later, a similar epiphyseal ossification center forms at the lower end of the bone (see illustration *8* of Fig. 8.14). This center is also regarded as a secondary ossification center, although it develops later. With the development of the secondary ossification centers, the only cartilage that remains from the original model is the articular cartilage at the ends of the bone and a transverse disc of cartilage, known as the ***epiphyseal plate,*** which separates the epiphyseal and diaphyseal cavities.

Cartilage of the epiphyseal plate is responsible for maintaining the growth process

For a bone to retain proper proportions and its unique shape, both external and internal remodeling must occur as the bone grows in length. The proliferative zone of the epiphyseal plate gives rise to the cartilage on which bone is later laid down.

- The thickness of the epiphyseal plate remains relatively constant during growth.
- The amount of new cartilage produced (zone of proliferation) equals the amount resorbed (zone of resorption).
- The resorbed cartilage is, of course, replaced by spongy bone.

In reviewing the growth process, it is important to realize that

- *Actual lengthening of the bone occurs when new cartilage matrix is produced at the epiphyseal plate.* Production of new cartilage matrix pushes the epiphysis away

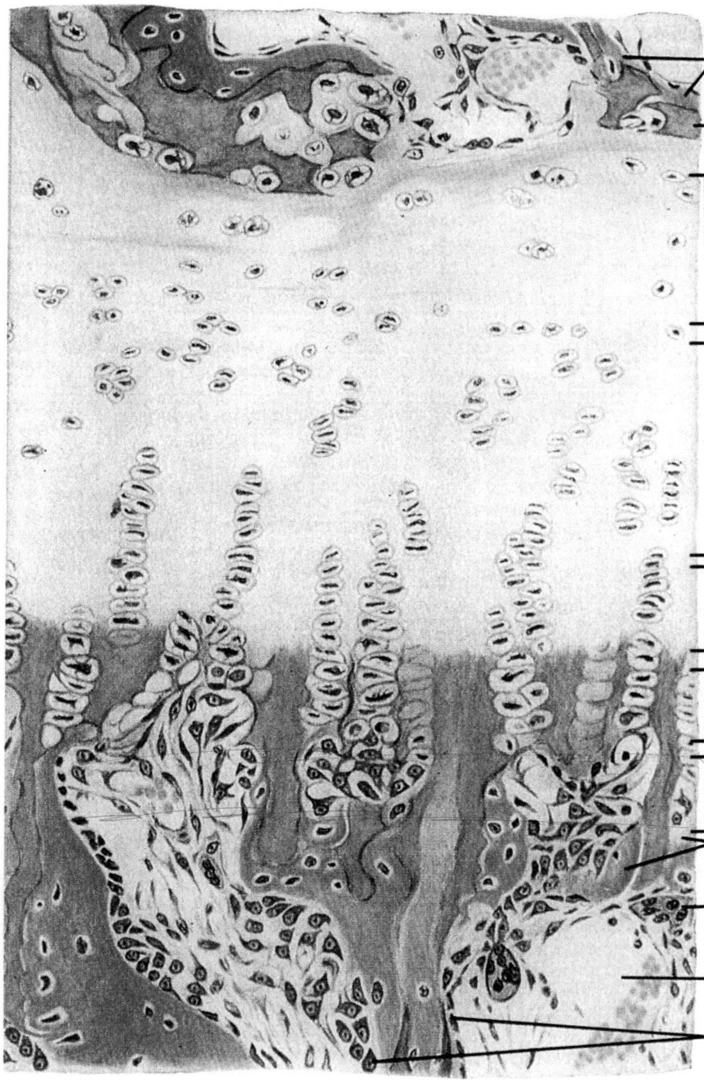

FIGURE 8.16
Longitudinal section through the distal end of a metatarsal bone of a 2-month-old infant. The epiphyseal (secondary) ossification center is well formed. Bone formation is taking place at both the epiphyseal and the diaphyseal surface of the epiphyseal plate. The zonation is apparent on the diaphyseal side because the growth rate there is so much greater than the epiphyseal ossification center. Because both centers are active, the zone of reserve cartilage is relatively narrow. H&E ×280. (From Kelly DE, Wood RL, Enders AC. *Bailey's Textbook of Microscopic Anatomy.* Baltimore: Williams & Wilkins, 1978.)

from the diaphysis, elongating the bone. The events that follow this incremental growth, namely, hypertrophy, calcification, resorption, and ossification, simply involve the mechanism by which the newly formed cartilage is replaced by bone tissue during development.

- *Bone increases in width or diameter when appositional growth of new bone occurs between the cortical lamellae and the periosteum.* The marrow cavity then enlarges by resorption of bone on the endosteal surface of the cortex of the bone.

As bones elongate, remodeling is required

Remodeling consists of preferential resorption of bone in some areas and deposition of bone in other areas, as described above and outlined in Figure 8.17.

When an individual achieves maximal growth, proliferation of new cartilage within the epiphyseal plate terminates

When proliferation of new cartilage ceases, the cartilage that has already been produced in the epiphyseal plate continues to undergo the changes that lead to the deposition of new bone until, finally, there is no remaining cartilage. At this point, the epiphyseal and diaphyseal marrow cavities become confluent. The elimination of the epiphyseal plate is referred to as ***epiphyseal closure.*** In illustration *9* of Figure 8.14, the lower epiphyseal cartilage is no longer present, and in illustration *10,* both epiphyseal cartilages are gone. Growth is now complete, and the only remaining cartilage is found on the articular surfaces of the bone. Vestigial evidence of the site of the epiphyseal plate is reflected by an ***epiphyseal line*** consisting of bone tissue (see Fig. 8.2).

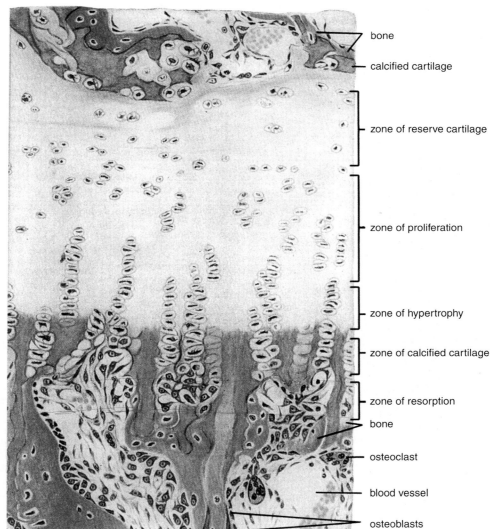

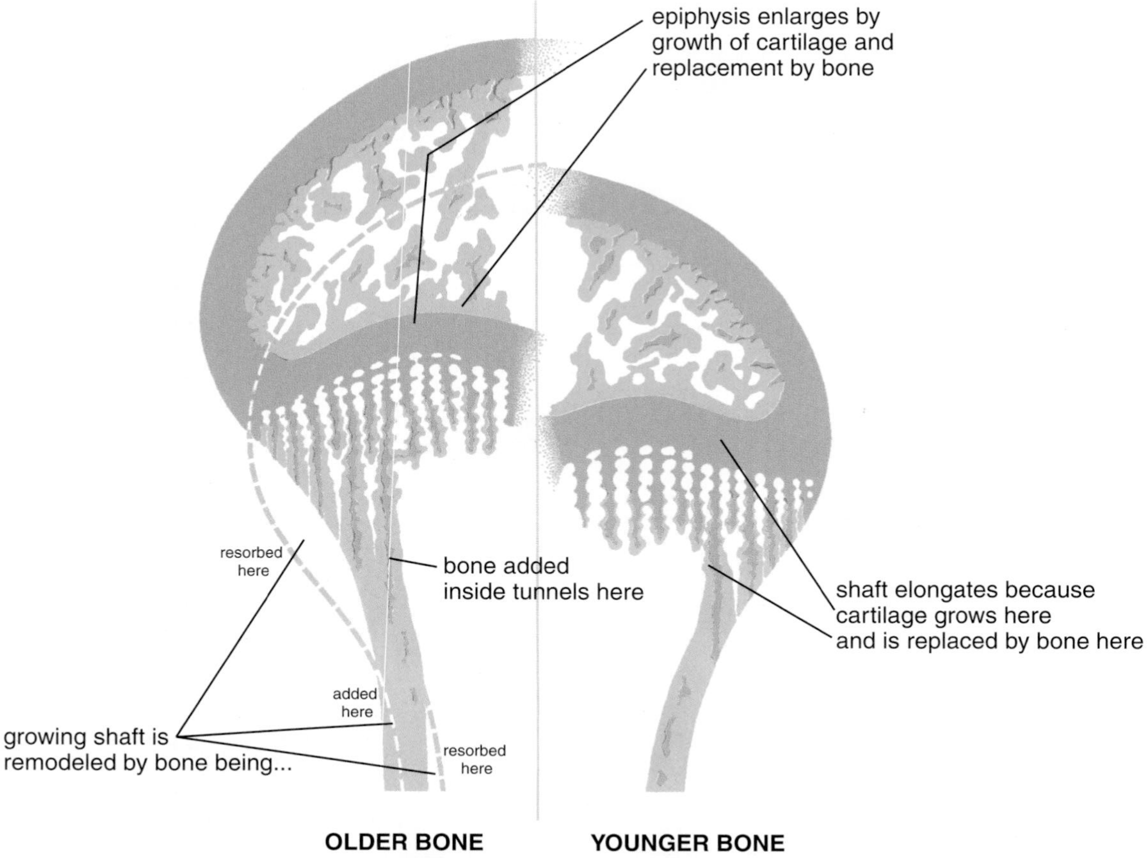

FIGURE 8.17
Diagram of external remodeling of a long bone. This diagram shows two periods during the growth of the bone. The younger bone profile (before remodeling) is shown on the right; the older (after remodeling), on the left. Superimposed on the left side of the figure is the shape of the bone (left half only) as it appeared at an earlier time. The bone is now longer, but it has retained its general shape. To grow in length and retain the general shape of the particular bone, bone resorption occurs on some surfaces, and bone deposition occurs on other surfaces, as indicated in the diagram. (Based on Ham AW. *J Bone Joint Surg Am* 1952;34:701.)

Development of the Osteonal (Haversian) System

Osteons typically develop in preexisting compact bone

Compact bone can take several different forms. Compact bone may be formed from fetal spongy bone by continued deposition of bone on the spongy bone spicules; it may be deposited directly as adult compact bone (e.g., the circumferential lamellae of an adult bone); or it might be older compact bone consisting of osteons and interstitial lamellae. The process in which new osteons are formed is referred to as ***internal remodeling.***

In the development of new osteons, a tunnel is bored through compact bone by osteoclasts

Formation of a new osteon in compact bone involves initially the creation of a tunnel-like space, the resorption cavity, by osteoclast activity. This resorption cavity will have the dimensions of the new osteon. When osteoclasts have produced an appropriately sized cylindrical tunnel by resorption of compact bone, blood vessels and their surrounding connective tissue occupy the tunnel. As the tunnel is occupied, new bone deposition on its wall begins almost immediately. These two aspects of cellular activity, namely, osteoclast resorption and osteoblast synthesis, constitute a ***bone-remodeling*** unit. A bone-remodeling unit consists of two distinct parts: an advancing ***cutting cone*** (also called a ***resorption canal***) and a ***closing cone*** (Fig. 8.18). The cutting cone consists of active osteoclasts followed by an advancing capillary loop and pericytes. It also contains numerous dividing cells that give rise to osteoblasts, additional pericytes, and endothelial cells. (Recall that osteoclasts are derived from blood-borne monocytes.) The osteoclasts cut a canal about 200 μm in diameter. This canal establishes the diameter of the future

BOX 8.2

Clinical Correlations: Nutritional Factors in Bone Formation

Both nutritional and hormonal factors affect the degree of bone mineralization. Calcium deficiency during growth causes ***rickets,*** a condition in which the bone matrix does not calcify normally. Rickets may be due to insufficient amounts of dietary calcium or to insufficient vitamin D (a steroid prohormone), which is needed for absorption of calcium by the intestines. In the adult, the same nutritional or vitamin deficiency leads to ***osteomalacia.***

Although rickets and osteomalacia are no longer major problems where nutrition is adequate, another form of insufficient bone mineralization is regularly seen in the condition known as ***osteoporosis.*** In this condition, bone tissue (both mineral and matrix) is diminished, presumably because resorption by osteoclasts exceeds deposition by osteoblasts. Osteoporosis develops as a consequence of immobilization (as in a bedridden patient) and in postmenopausal women. The factors that cause the imbalance in cellular activity are not known, although some relief appears to result from maintaining hormonal (estrogen) levels and dietary fluoride levels.

In addition to its influence on intestinal absorption of calcium, vitamin D is also needed for normal calcification. Other vitamins known to affect bone are A and C. Vitamin A deficiency suppresses endochondral growth of bone; vitamin A excess leads to fragility and subsequent fractures of long bones. Vitamin C is essential for synthesis of collagen, and its deficiency leads to ***scurvy.*** The matrix produced in scurvy is not calcifiable.

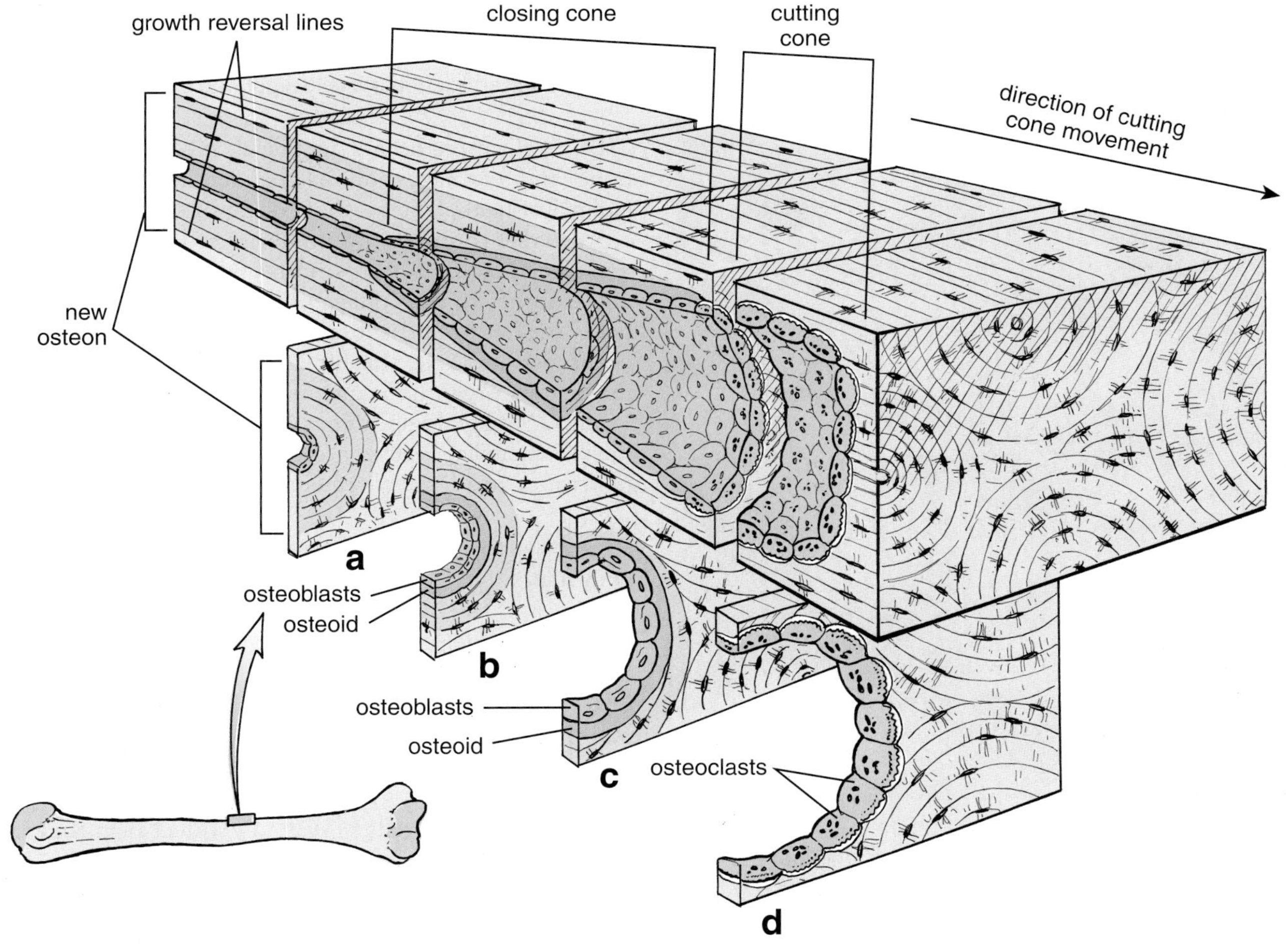

FIGURE 8.18
Diagram of a bone-remodeling unit. A bone-remodeling unit consists of an advancing cutting cone and a closing cone. The cutting cone formed by osteoclasts is responsible for boring the tunnel or resorption cavity through the compact bone. Its action is initiated within the Haversian canal at the left of the diagram (in the area corresponding to section **a**). The cutting cone moves along the Haversian canal, in the direction indicated by the *arrow,* to the area corresponding to section **d**. Section **d** shows the cross section through the cutting cone. The resorption cavity is the site where the future osteon is formed by the action of the closing cone, which consists of osteoblasts. These cells begin to deposit the osteoid on the walls of the canal in successive lamellae. Gradual formation of the new bone fills the resorption cavity. Note the deposition of the osteoid deep to the osteoblasts seen in sections **b** and **c**. As successive lamellae of bone are deposited, the canal ultimately attains the relatively narrow diameter of the mature Haversian canal, like that shown in section **a**. The growth reversal line that appears at the outer limits of a newly formed osteon represents a border between the resorption activity of the cutting cone and the bony matrix not remodeled by this activity.

osteonal (Haversian) system. The cutting cone constitutes only a small fraction of the length of the bone-remodeling unit; thus, it is seen much less frequently than the closing cone.

After the diameter of the future Haversian system is established, osteoblasts begin to deposit the organic matrix (osteoid) of bone on the walls of the canal in successive lamellae. With time, the bone matrix in each of the lamellae becomes mineralized. As the successive lamellae of bone are deposited, *from the periphery inward*, the canal ultimately attains the relatively narrow diameter of the adult osteonal canal.

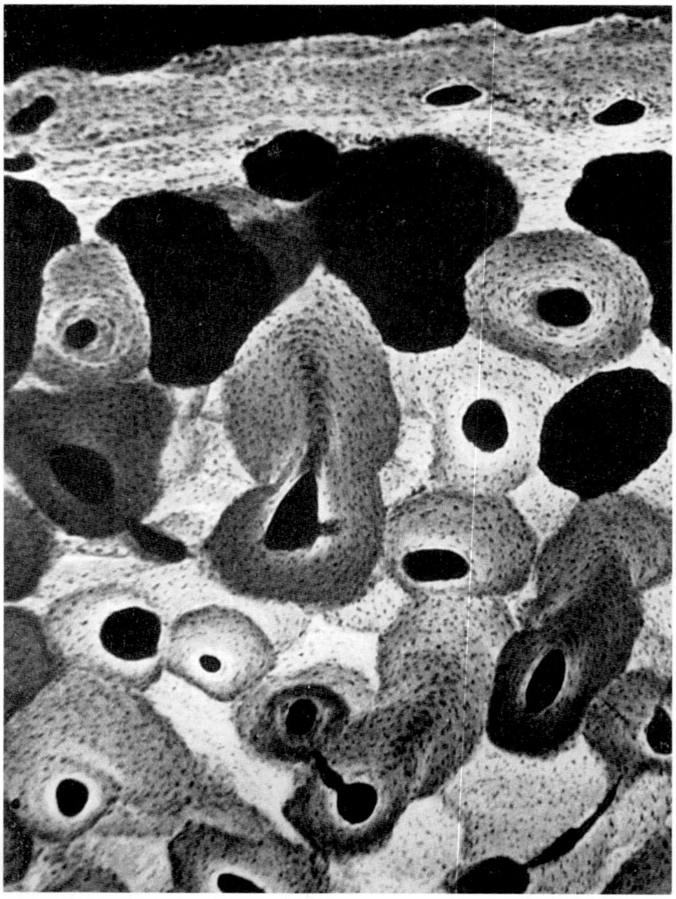

FIGURE 8.19
Microradiograph of the cross section of a bone. This 200-μm-thick cross section of bone from a healthy 19-year-old male shows various degrees of mineralization in different osteons. Mature compact bone is actively replacing immature bone, which is seen on the periosteal (upper) surface. The degree of mineralization is reflected by the shade of light and dark in the microradiograph. Thus, *very light areas* represent the highly mineralized tissue that deflects the x-rays and prevents them from striking the photographic film. Conversely, *dark areas* contain less mineral and, thus, are less effective in deflecting the x-rays. Note that the interstitial lamellae (the older bone) are very light, whereas some of the osteons are very dark (these are the most newly formed). The Haversian canals appear black, as they represent only soft tissue. ×157. (Courtesy of Dr. Jenifer Jowsey.)

Compact adult bone contains Haversian systems of varying age and size

Microradiographic examination of a ground section of bone reveals that younger Haversian systems are less completely mineralized than older systems (Fig. 8.19). They undergo a progressive secondary mineralization that continues (up to a point) even after the osteon has been fully formed. Figure 8.19 also illustrates the dynamic internal remodeling of compact bone. In the adult, deposition balances resorption. In the aged, resorption often exceeds deposition. If this imbalance becomes excessive, osteoporosis develops (see page 199).

BIOLOGIC MINERALIZATION AND MATRIX VESICLES

Biologic mineralization is a cell-regulated extracellular event

Mineralization occurs in the extracellular matrices of bone and cartilage and in the dentin, cementum, and enamel of teeth. The matrices of all of these structures except enamel contain collagen fibrils and ground substance, and mineralization occurs both within the collagen fibrils and external to the collagen fibrils, in relation to components of the ground substance. In enamel, mineralization occurs within the extracellular organic matrix secreted by the enamel organ (see page 441). Despite the extracellular location of biologic mineralization and the fact that physicochemical factors are basic to the process, *biologic mineralization is a cell-regulated event.*

Mineralization involves the secretion of matrix vesicles into the bony matrix

In places where mineralization of bone, cartilage, dentin, and cementum is initiated, the local concentration of Ca^{2+} and PO_4^- ions in the matrix must exceed the normal threshold level. Several events are responsible for this mineralization:

- Binding of extracellular Ca^{2+} by osteocalcin and other sialoproteins creates a high local concentration of this ion.
- The high Ca^{2+} concentration stimulates the osteoblasts to secrete alkaline phosphatase, which increases the local concentration of PO_4^- ions. The high PO_4^- concentration stimulates further increases in Ca^{2+} concentration where mineralization will be initiated.
- At this stage of high extracellular Ca^{2+} and PO_4^- concentration, the osteoblasts release small (50- to 200-nm) matrix vesicles into the bony matrix by exocytosis. The matrix vesicles contain alkaline phosphatase and pyrophosphatase that cleave PO_4^- ions from other molecules of the matrix.

- The matrix vesicles that accumulate Ca^{2+} and cleave PO_4^- ions cause the local isoelectric point to increase, which results in crystallization of $CaPO_4$ in the surrounding matrix vesicles.
- The $CaPO_4$ crystals initiate matrix mineralization by formation and deposition of $[Ca_{10}(PO_4)_6(OH)_2]$ (hydroxyapatite) crystals in the matrix surrounding the osteoblasts.

The osteoblast-derived matrix vesicles are the essential factors in controlling the initial site of mineral deposition in osteoid. Once the initial crystals of hydroxyapatite have precipitated, they grow rapidly by accretion until they join neighboring crystals produced around other matrix vesicles. In this way, a wave of mineralization sweeps through the osteoid. Other cells that produce osteoid are the ameloblasts and odontoblasts of developing teeth.

PHYSIOLOGIC ASPECTS OF BONE

Bone serves as a reservoir for body calcium

The maintenance of normal blood calcium levels is critical to health and life. Calcium may be delivered from the bone matrix to the blood if the circulating blood levels of calcium fall below a critical point (physiologic calcium concentration in the human ranges from 8.9 to 10.1 mg/dL). Conversely, excess blood calcium may be removed from the blood and stored in bone.

These processes are regulated by parathyroid hormone (PTH), secreted by the parathyroid gland (see page 660), and ***calcitonin,*** secreted by the parafollicular cells of the thyroid gland (see page 658).

BOX 8.3

Functional Considerations: Hormonal Regulation of Bone Growth

Hormones other than PTH and calcitonin have major effects on bone growth. One such hormone is ***pituitary growth hormone*** (GH, somatotropin). This hormone stimulates growth in general and, especially, growth of epiphyseal cartilage and bone. Oversecretion in childhood leads to gigantism, an abnormal increase in the length of bones; absence or hyposecretion of somatotropin in childhood leads to failure of growth of the long bones, resulting in pituitary dwarfism. Absence or severe hyposecretion of thyroid hormone during development and infancy leads to failure of bone growth and dwarfism, a condition known as congenital hypothyroidism. Oversecretion of somatotropin in an adult leads to ***acromegaly,*** an abnormal thickening and selective overgrowth of hands, feet, mandible, nose, and intramembranous bones of the skull.

- PTH acts on the bone to *raise low blood calcium levels* to normal.
- ***Calcitonin*** acts to *lower elevated blood calcium levels* to normal.

PTH acts by stimulating both osteocytes and osteoclasts to resorb bone, allowing the release of calcium into the blood. As described above (see page 190), resorption of bone by osteocytes constitutes ***osteocytic osteolysis.*** PTH also reduces excretion of calcium by the kidney and stimulates absorption of calcium by the small intestine. PTH further acts to maintain homeostasis by stimulating the kidney to excrete the excess phosphate produced by bone resorption. Calcitonin inhibits bone resorption, specifically inhibiting the effects of PTH on osteoclasts.

FRACTURES AND BONE REPAIR

The initial response to a fracture is similar to the response to any injury that produces tissue destruction and hemorrhage. Neutrophils are the first cells to arrive on the scene, followed by macrophages that begin to clean up the site of injury. Fibroblasts and capillaries then proliferate and grow into the site of injury. New loose connective tissue, ***granulation tissue,*** is formed, and as this tissue becomes denser, cartilage forms in parts of it. Both fibroblasts and periosteal cells participate in this phase of the healing process. The dense connective tissue and newly formed cartilage grow, covering the bone at the fracture site, producing a ***callus*** (Fig. 8.20). A callus will form whether or not the fractured parts of the bone are in immediate apposition to each other. The callus helps stabilize and bind together the fractured bone.

While the callus is forming, osteoprogenitor cells of the periosteum divide and differentiate into osteoblasts. The newly formed osteoblasts begin to deposit new bone on the outer surface of the bone at some distance from the fracture. This new formation of bone progresses toward the fracture site until new bone forms a bony sheath over the fibrocartilaginous callus. Osteogenic buds from the new bone invade the callus and begin to deposit new bone within the callus, gradually replacing the original fibrous and cartilaginous callus with a ***bony callus.*** The cartilage in the original callus calcifies and is replaced by bone as in endochondral ossification.

Endosteal proliferation and differentiation also occur in the marrow cavity, and medullary bone grows from both ends of the fracture toward the center. When this bone unites, the bony union of the fractured bone produced by the osteoblasts derived from both the periosteum and endosteum consists of spongy bone. As in normal bone formation, the spongy bone is gradually replaced by compact bone. While compact bone is being formed, the bony callus is removed by the action of os-

teoclasts, and gradual remodeling restores the bone to its original shape.

In healthy individuals, this process usually takes from 6 to 12 weeks, depending on the severity of the break and the particular bone that is broken. Setting the bone, i.e., reapproximating the normal structure, and holding the parts in place by internal fixation (by pins, screws, or plates) or by external fixation (by casts or by pins and screws) speeds the healing process and usually results in superior structural and functional restoration.

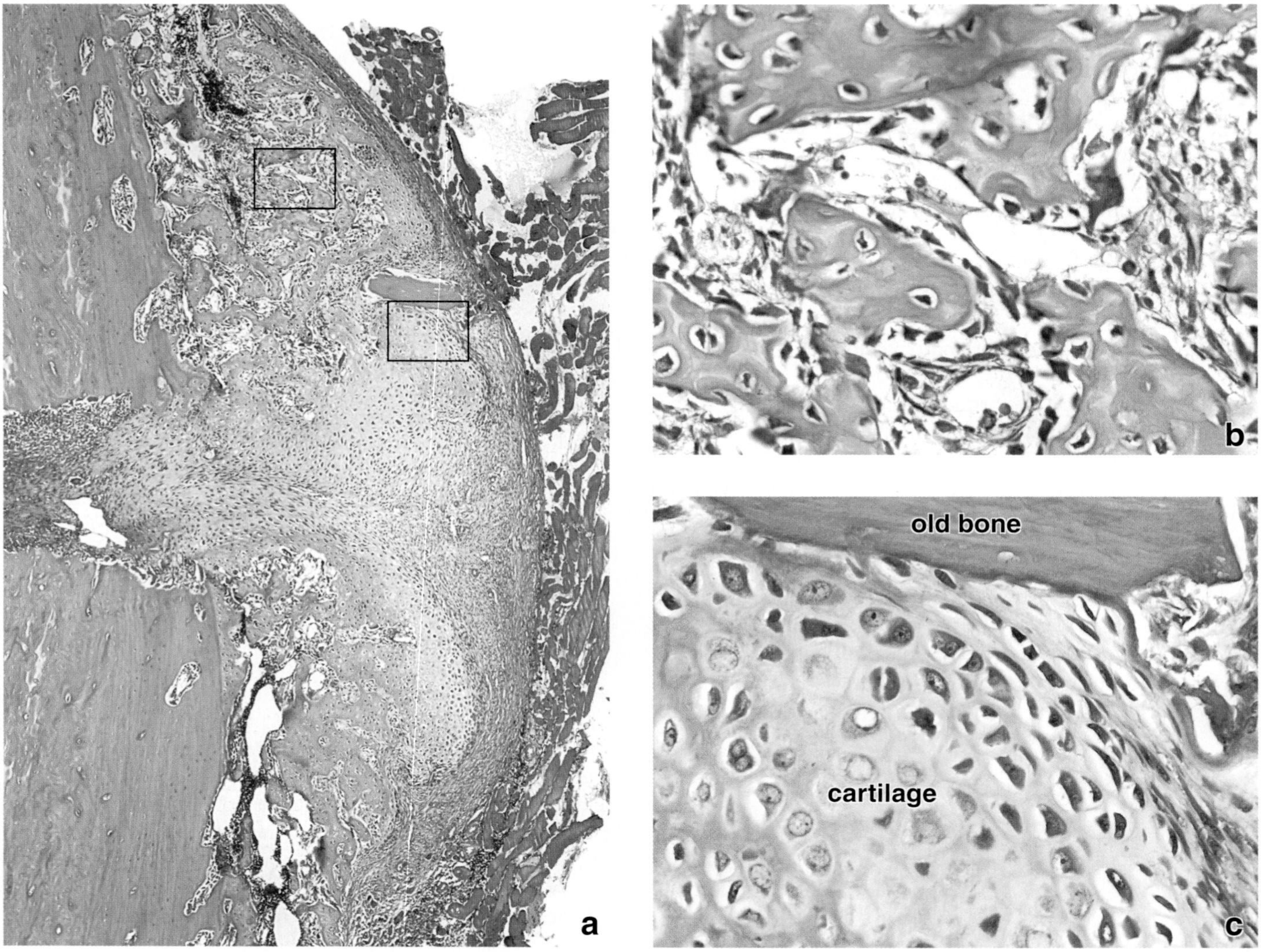

FIGURE 8.20

Photomicrograph of fractured long bone undergoing repair. **a.** This low-magnification photomicrograph of a 3-week-old bone fracture, stained with H&E, shows parts of the bone separated from each other by the fibrocartilaginous callus. At this stage, the cartilage undergoes endochondral ossification. In addition, the osteoblasts of the periosteum are involved in secretion of new bony matrix on the outer surface of the callus. On the right of the microphotograph, the fibrocartilaginous callus is covered by periosteum, which also serves as the attachment site for the skeletal muscle. ×35. **b.** Higher magnification of the callus from the area indicated by the *upper rectangle* in *a* shows osteoblasts lining bone trabeculae. Most of the original fibrous and cartilaginous matrix at this site has been replaced by bone. The early bone is deposited as an immature bone, which is later replaced by mature compact bone. ×300. **c.** Higher magnification of the callus from the area indicated by the *lower rectangle* in *a.* A fragment of old bone pulled away from the fracture site by the periosteum is now adjacent to the cartilage. It will be removed by osteoclast activity. The cartilage will calcify and be replaced by new bone spicules as seen in *b.* ×300.

PLATE 11. BONE, GROUND SECTION

Bone is a specialized connective tissue characterized by a mineralized extracellular matrix. Calcium phosphate, in the form of *hydroxyapatite crystals* ($Ca_{10}(PO_4)_6OH_2$), is deposited along the collagen fibrils and in the proteoglycan ground substance. Bone serves as a storage site for calcium and phosphate, which can be released to the blood to maintain homeostatic levels. *Osteocytes* reside in lacunae in the bone matrix and extend fine cellular processes into canaliculi that connect the lacunae, thus forming a continuous network of cells within the mineralized tissue. Bones are organs of the skeletal system; bone tissue is the structural component of bones.

Ground sections of bone are prepared from bone that has not been fixed but merely allowed to dry. Thin slices of the dried bone are then cut with a saw and further ground to a thinness that allows viewing in a light microscope. Slices may be treated with India ink to fill spaces that were formerly occupied by organic matter, e.g., cells, blood vessels, and unmineralized matrix. A simpler method is to mount the ground specimen on a slide with a viscous medium that traps air in some of the spaces, as in the specimen in this plate. Here, some of the osteonal canals and a perforating canal are filled with the mounting medium, making them translucent instead of black. Specimens prepared in this manner are of value chiefly to display the architecture of the compact bone.

Figure 1, ground bone, human, ×80.

This figure reveals a cross-sectioned area of a long bone at low magnification and includes the outer or peripheral aspect of the bone, identified by the presence of circumferential lamellae *(CL)*. (The exterior or periosteal surface of the bone is not included in the micrograph.) To their right are the osteons *(O)* or Haversian systems that appear as circular profiles. Between the osteons are interstitial lamellae *(IL)*, the remnants of previously existing osteons.

Osteons are essentially cylindrical structures. In the shaft of a long bone, the long axes of the osteons are oriented parallel to the long axis of the bone. Thus, a cross section through the shaft of a long bone would reveal the osteons in cross section, as in this figure. At the center of each osteon is an osteonal (Haversian) canal *(HC)* that contains blood vessels, connective tissue, and cells lining the surface of the bone material. Because the organic material is not retained in ground sections, the Haversian canals and other spaces will appear black, as they do here, if filled with India ink or air. Concentric layers of mineralized substance, the concentric lamellae, surround the Haversian canal and appear much the same as growth rings of a tree. The canal is also surrounded by concentric arrangements of lacunae. These appear as the small, dark, elongate structures.

During the period of bone growth and during adult life, there is constant internal remodeling of bone. This involves the destruction of osteons and formation of new ones. The breakdown of an osteon is usually not complete, however; part of the osteon may remain intact. Moreover, portions of adjacent osteons may also be partially destroyed. The space created by the breakdown process is reoccupied by a new osteon. The remnants of the previously existing osteons become the interstitial lamellae.

Blood vessels reach the Haversian canals from the marrow through other tunnels called perforating (Volkmann's) canals *(VC)*. In some instances, as here, Volkmann's canals travel from one Haversian canal to another. Volkmann's canals can be distinguished from Haversian canals in that they pass through lamellae, whereas Haversian canals are surrounded by concentric rings of lamellae.

Figure 2, ground bone, human, ×300.

This figure shows a higher-magnification micrograph of the labeled osteon from the upper left of Figure 1. It includes some of the circumferential lamellae (here labeled *IL*) that are now seen at the bottom of the micrograph (the micrograph has been reoriented). Note the lacunae *(L)* and the fine thread-like profiles emanating from the lacunae. These thread-like profiles represent the canaliculi, spaces within the bone matrix that contained cytoplasmic processes of the osteocyte. The canaliculi of each lacuna communicate with canaliculi of neighboring lacunae to form a three-dimensional channel system throughout the bone.

Figure 3, ground bone, human, ×400.

In a still higher magnification, the circumferential lamellae are found around the shaft of the long bone at the outer as well as the inner surface of the bone. The osteoblasts that contribute to the formation of circumferential lamellae at these sites come from the periosteum and endosteum, respectively, whereas the osteons are constructed from osteoblasts in the canal of the developing Haversian system. This figure reveals not only the canaliculi but also the lamellae of the bone. The latter are just barely defined by the faint lines *(arrows)* that extend across the micrograph. Collagenous fibers in neighboring lamellae are oriented in different directions. This change in orientation accounts for the faint line or interface between adjacent lamellae.

KEY

CL, circumferential lamellae
HC, Haversian canal
IL, interstitial lamellae
L, lacuna
O, osteon
VC, Volkmann's canal
arrow, lamellar boundary

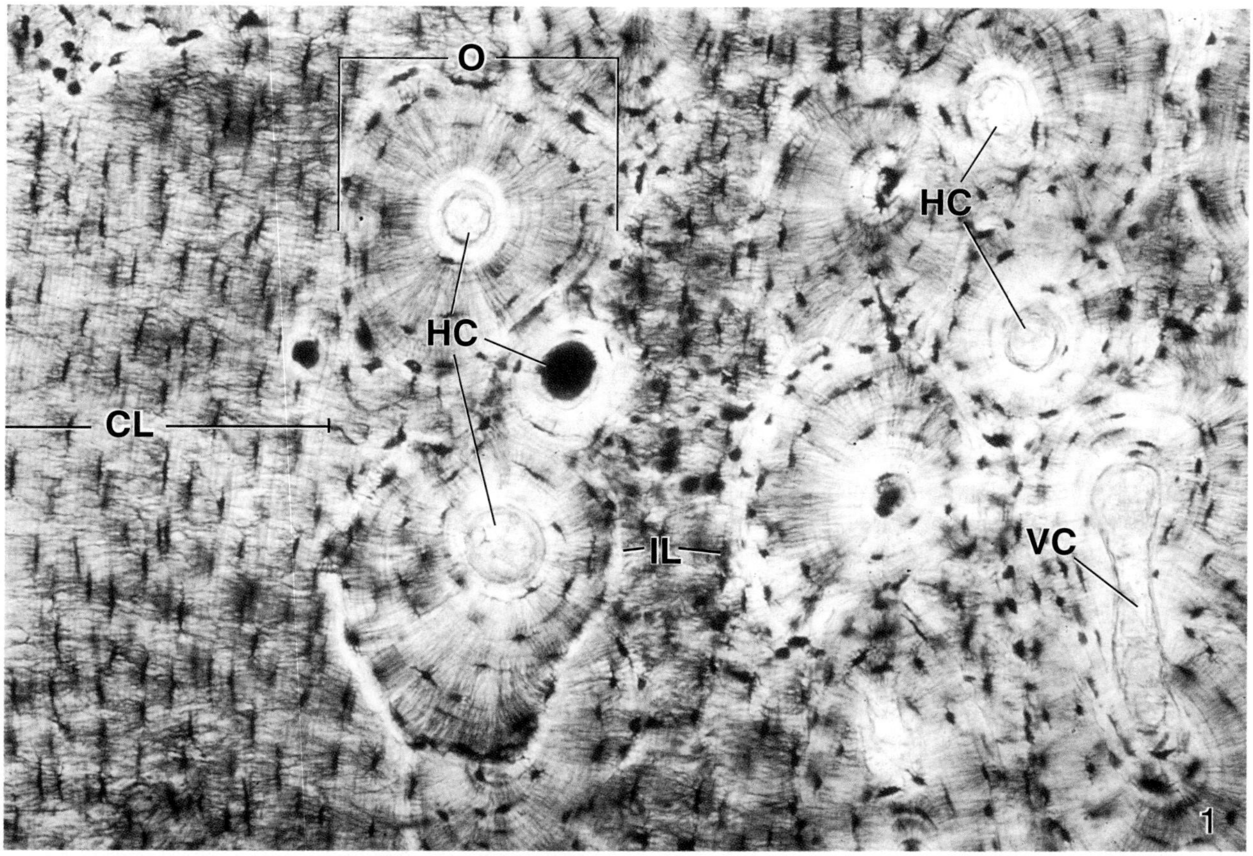
O
HC
HC
HC
CL
IL
VC
1

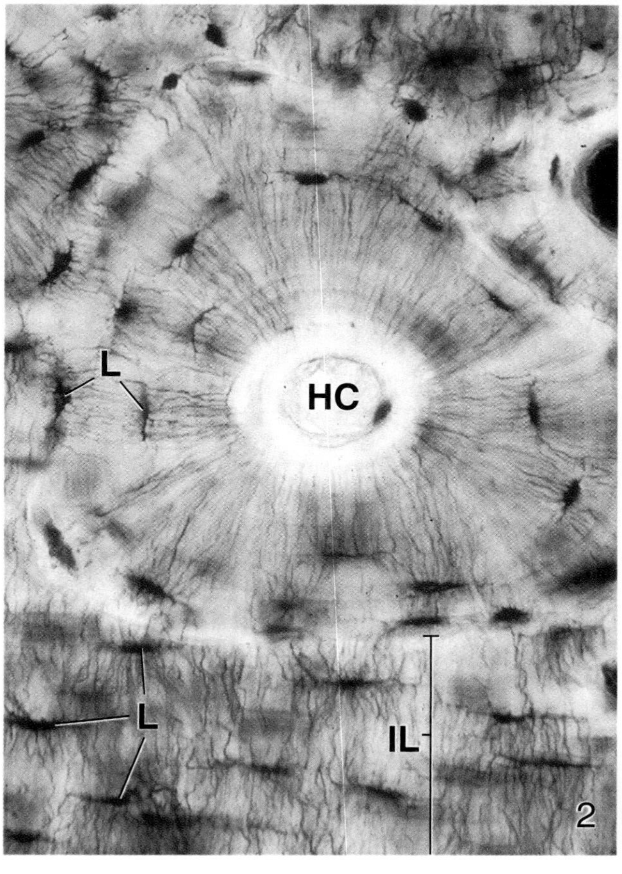
L
HC
L
IL
2

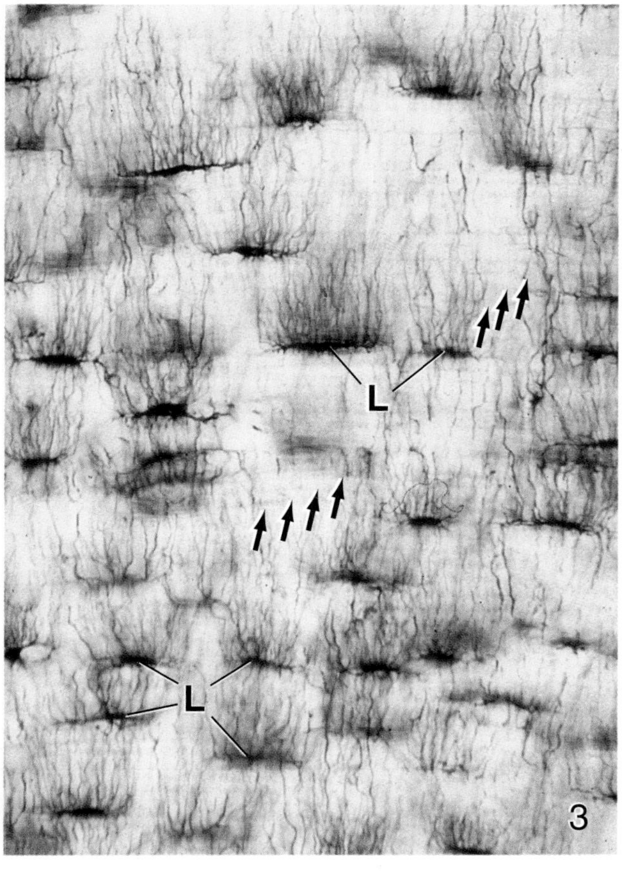
L
L
3

PLATE 12. SPONGY AND COMPACT BONE

Hematoxylin and eosin (H&E)–stained sections of decalcified bone exhibit all of the formed soft tissue components that are seen in other dense connective tissues and allow one to distinguish the several cell types found in developing and mature bone. Such preparations also allow the use of special stains and histochemical methods to study bone development and function in more detail than is possible with H&E sections.

Figure 1, bone, monkey, H&E ×80; upper inset ×175.

This figure shows a decalcified section of two bones framing a joint cavity. Articular cartilage *(AC)* covers the surfaces that contact the neighboring bone. The free surface of each cartilage presents a relatively smooth contour, whereas the junction between the cartilage and the bone *(SB)* is irregular.

The articular cartilage is hyaline **(upper inset).** It shows the characteristic features of hyaline cartilage seen in Plate 7, page 173, namely, chondrocytes in lacunae, a homogeneous avascular matrix (homogeneous in that it presents no formed elements visible in the light microscope), and variable staining of the matrix. At least some of the cartilage cells are in lacunae that are close to each other, suggesting that they are daughter cells of the same parent cell.

The bone under the articular cartilage is spongy bone. It consists of spicules or trabeculae of bone tissue as well as marrow spaces *(M).* In this sample, the marrow consists primarily of adipose tissue. In addition to the marrow spaces, the bone tissue also contains space or tunnels for blood vessels *(BV);* in this respect, bone differs fundamentally from the hyaline cartilage on the articular surface, which is avascular. The essential features of the bone tissue are seen at higher magnification in the **upper inset.** These are osteocytes *(Oc)* in lacunae, an eosinophilic matrix, and blood vessels *(BV).* The spongy bone shown in this figure is nonlamellar; i.e., the matrix is not organized as lamellae, but rather, the collagen fibers are in the form of interwoven bundles. Certain features of woven nonlamellar bone are also displayed in the **upper inset;** namely, the cells are unevenly and randomly dispersed and are not arranged in an oriented pattern around the blood vessels. For comparison, note how the lacunae (and, therefore, also the osteocytes) display an oriented pattern about the Haversian canal in Figure 2 of Plate 11.

Figure 2, bone, monkey, H&E ×80; lower inset ×350.

This figure shows the shaft of a long bone. The center of the bone consists of a large marrow cavity *(M)* filled chiefly with adipose tissue; surrounding the marrow cavity is the bone tissue of the shaft. It is compact bone *(CB).* Although the compact bone tissue contains tunnels for blood vessels *(BV),* it does not contain marrow spaces. On its outer surface, the bone tissue is covered by a periosteum *(Po),* and its inner surface is covered by endosteum (*Eo,* **lower inset**). The endosteum consists of several layers of cells (nuclei of these cells are evident) and collagenous fibers. The endosteal cells have the potential to develop into osteoblasts (as do periosteal cells) if the need should arise, e.g., in fracture repair.

Histologically, the compact bone shown in this figure displays three characteristics: an eosinophilic matrix; lacunae in which osteocytes are located; and vascular tunnels *(BV).* The osteocytes *(Oc)* are identified chiefly by their nuclear staining, which stands out in contrast to the surrounding eosinophilic matrix. The boundaries of the lacunae and the canaliculi radiating from them (see Plate 11) are not evident.

In the adult human, compact bone is organized chiefly as Haversian systems or as other forms of lamellar bone. Although this form of bone tissue is readily seen in well-oriented ground sections, it is not always easy to identify in decalcified sections. It is particularly difficult to make this identification in longitudinal decalcified sections of a long bone as shown in this figure.

KEY

AC, articular cartilage
BV, blood vessel
CB, compact bone
Eo, endosteum
M, marrow spaces
Oc, osteocyte
Po, periosteum
SB, spongy bone

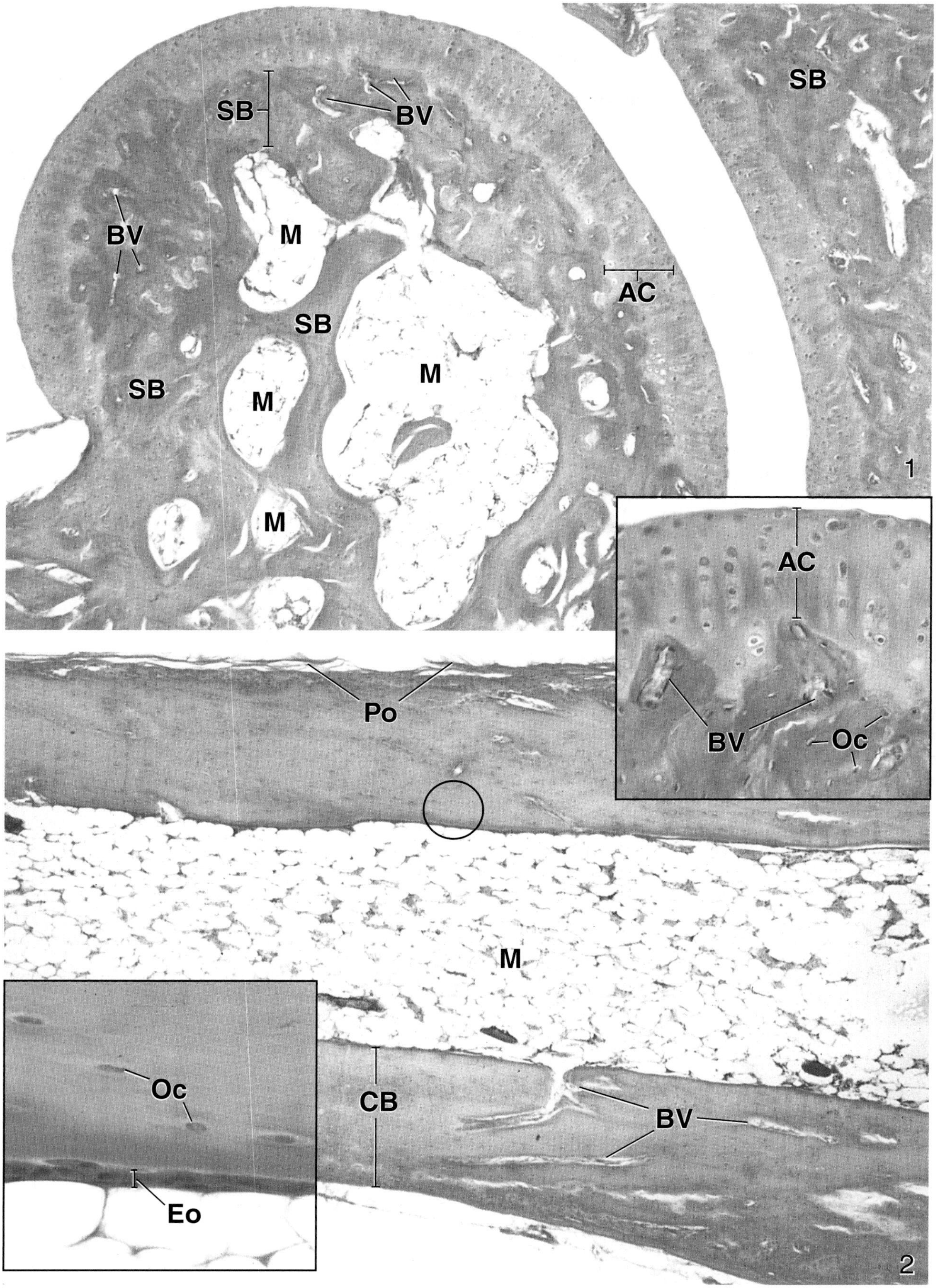
SB
SB
BV
BV
M
AC
SB
M
SB
M
M
1
AC
BV
Oc
Po
M
Oc
CB
BV
Eo
2

PLATE 13. ENDOCHONDRAL BONE FORMATION I

Endochondral bone formation involves the continuing growth of a cartilage precursor, which serves as a fetal skeleton, and the simultaneous removal of the cartilage and its replacement with bone tissue. In addition, as a bone grows, some of the bone tissue is removed while newer bone tissue is being laid down, a process called remodeling. Remodeling that alters the shape of the bone is called *external remodeling;* that which does not alter the shape of the bone, as in the formation of Haversian systems, is called *internal remodeling.*

Two specialized cell types are identified with the process of bone growth and remodeling. The *osteoblast* is engaged in the formation of bone. Although the removal of bone is not as well described as its formation, it has been established that multinucleated cells, called *osteoclasts,* are engaged in the removal of bone. Osteocytes, also, can alter and resorb bone in their immediate vicinity. The process is called *osteocytic osteolysis.* It is important in calcium homeostasis, i.e., the maintenance of normal blood calcium concentrations.

Figure 1, developing bone, monkey, H&E ×240.
The early steps of endochondral bone formation are shown in this figure. The structure seen here is the cartilage model of the bone about to be formed. The steps of bone formation are

1. The cartilage *(C)* cells in the center of the cartilage model become hypertrophic *(HC).*
2. The matrix of the cartilage becomes calcified *(CM).* (The calcified matrix stains intensely with hematoxylin and appears as the darker condensed matrix material between the enlarged cartilage cells.)
3. A collar of bone forms around the circumference of the center of the cartilage model. This bone is called ***periosteal bone*** *(PB)* because the osteoblasts that have produced the bone material develop from the periosteum. (Note that the periosteal bone is, in fact, intramembranous bone [see Plate 15, page 213], because it develops within the connective tissue membrane that immediately surrounds the developing bone and not on a spicule of calcified cartilage.)

Figure 2, developing bone, human, H&E ×60.
The bone in this figure shows later events and a continuation of the earlier ones just described. A vascular bud (not shown) and accompanying perivascular cells from the periosteum have invaded the shaft of the cartilage model, resulting in the formation of a cavity *(Cav).* Examination at higher magnification would reveal that the cavity contains fat cells, hematopoietic tissue (the dark-blue–staining component), and other connective tissue elements. While the new steps of bone formation occur, the earlier steps continue:

1. Cartilage *(C)* cells proliferate at the epiphyses. They are responsible for production of new matrix material. It is this process that creates lengthening of the bone.
2. Periosteal bone *(PB)* continues to form.
3. Cartilage cells facing the cavity become hypertrophic.
4. Cartilage matrix becomes calcified.
5. Erosion of cartilage occurs, creating spicules of cartilage.
6. Bone forms on the spicules of the calcified cartilage at the erosion front; this bone is ***endochondral bone*** *(EB).*

As these processes continue in the shaft of the bone, one end of the cartilage model (the epiphysis) is invaded by blood vessels and connective tissue from the periosteum (periosteal bud), and it undergoes the same changes that occurred earlier in the shaft (except that no periosteal bone forms). This same process then occurs at the other end of the bone. Consequently, at each end of the developing long bone, a cartilaginous plate (epiphyseal plate) is created that lies between two sites of bone formation.

Figure 3, developing bone, human, H&E ×60; inset ×200.
This shows an early stage after the invasion of the epiphysis. A secondary ossification center *(Os)* has formed, and along with this event, the head of the long bone will develop a marrow cavity similar in its content to that of the diaphysis. The cartilage separating the two cavities is the epiphyseal plate *(EP).* At the early stage shown in this figure, the plate is not well defined. Despite the enlargement of the epiphyseal cavity, the remaining cartilage between the two cavities persists as a disc or plate until growth ceases. The **inset** shows some calcified cartilage as well as the deposition of endochondral bone *(EB)* within the secondary ossification center.

KEY

C, cartilage
Cav, marrow cavity
CC, calcified cartilage
CM, calcified matrix
EB, endochondral bone
EP, epiphyseal plate
HC, hypertrophic cartilage cell
JC, joint cavity
Os, secondary ossification center
PB, periosteal bone

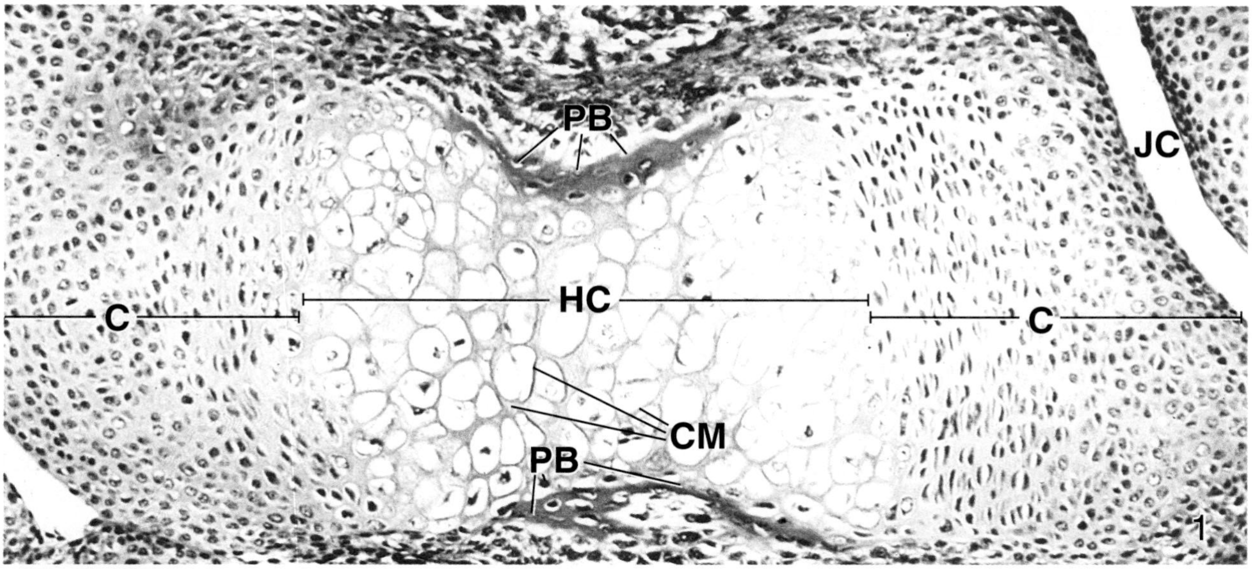
PB
JC
HC
C
C
CM
PB
1

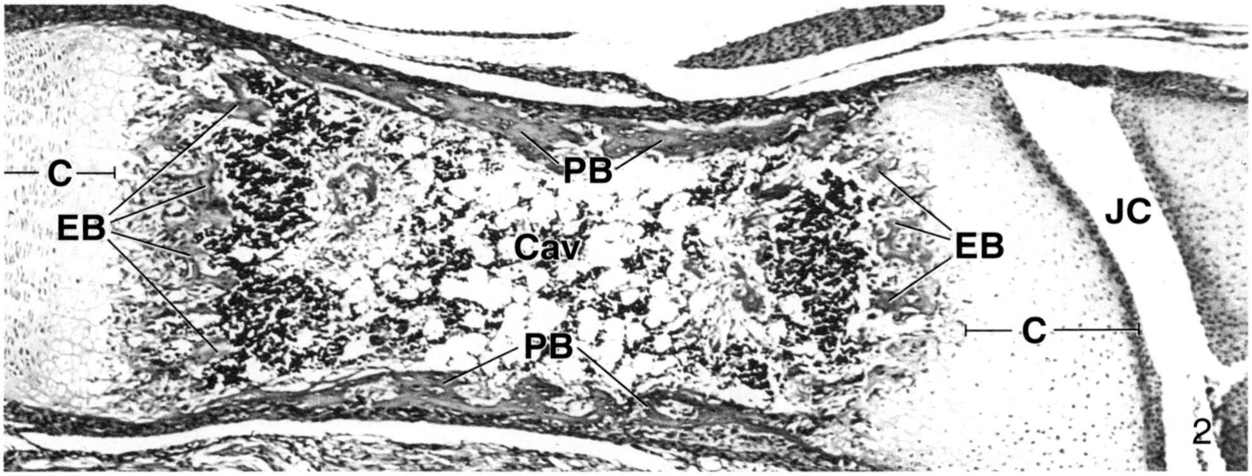
C
EB
PB
Cav
JC
EB
C
PB
2

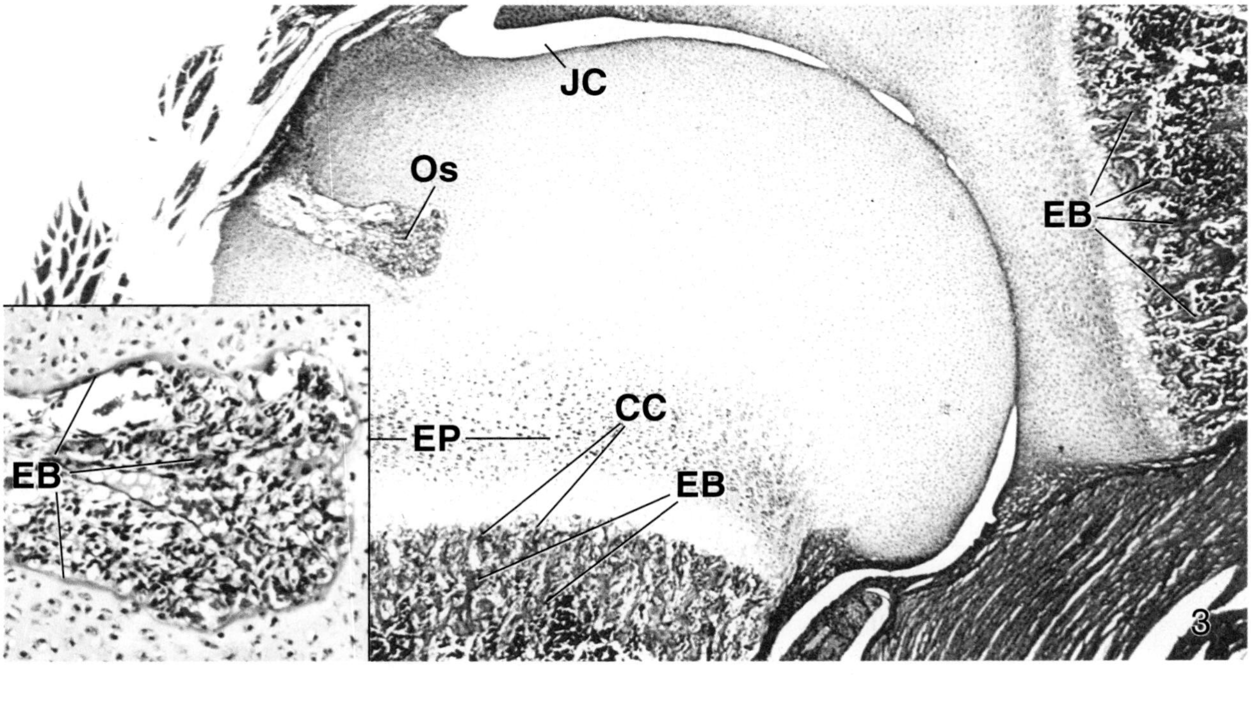
JC
Os
EB
EB
EP
CC
EB
3

PLATE 14. ENDOCHONDRAL BONE FORMATION II

Endochondral bone formation is the principal process by which the long bones, e.g., the bones of the axial skeleton and the appendages and digits, increase in length to achieve their adult dimensions. So long as *epiphyseal cartilage* exists between the diaphyseal and epiphyseal ossification centers, the bone will continue to grow. Cessation of bone growth is the result of the cessation of interstitial growth of the epiphyseal cartilages. X-ray examination of the bones of late adolescents can determine whether there is still an epiphyseal cartilage plate and, therefore, determine the potential for further growth in bone length and body height.

Figure 1, developing bone, human, H&E ×80; inset ×380.

This is a photomicrograph of an epiphysis at higher magnification than that seen in Figure 3 of Plate 13. Different zones of the cartilage of the epiphyseal plate reflect the progressive changes that occur in active growth of endochondral bone. These zones are not sharply delineated, and the boundaries between them are somewhat arbitrary. They lead toward the marrow cavity *(M),* so that the first zone is furthest from the cavity. There are five zones:

- ***Zone of reserve cartilage*** *(RC).* The cartilage cells of this zone have not yet begun to participate in the growth of the bone; thus, they are reserve cells. These cells are small, usually only one to a lacuna, and not grouped. At some time, some of these cells will proliferate and undergo the changes outlined for the next zone.
- ***Zone of proliferating cartilage*** *(PC).* The cells of this zone are increasing in number; they are slightly larger than the reserve cells and close to their neighbors; they begin to form rows.
- ***Zone of hypertrophic cartilage*** *(HC).* The cells of this zone are aligned in rows and are significantly larger than the cells in the preceding zone.
- ***Zone of calcified matrix*** *(C).* In this zone the cartilage matrix is impregnated with calcium salts.
- ***Zone of resorption.*** This zone is represented by eroded cartilage that is in direct contact with the connective tissue of the marrow cavity. Spicules (actually a honeycomb at the level of the advancing blood vessels) of cartilage are formed because the pericapillary cells invade and resorb in spearheads rather than along a straight front. Specifically, the pericapillary cells break into the rows of hypertrophied chondrocytes, temporarily leaving the calcified cartilage between the rows of cells. In this manner, spicules of calcified cartilage are formed. Endochondral bone *(EB)* is then deposited on the surfaces of these calcified cartilage spicules by osteoblasts *(Ob),* thus forming *mixed spicules* as seen in the **inset.**

Figure 2, developing bone, human, H&E ×150; inset ×380.

This is a higher magnification of the lower middle area of Figure 1. It shows calcified cartilage spicules on which bone has been deposited. In the lower portion of the figure, the spicules have already grown to create anastomosing bone trabeculae. These initial trabeculae still contain remnants of calcified cartilage, as shown by the blue color of the cartilage matrix (compared with the red staining of the bone). Osteoblasts *(Ob)* are aligned on the surface of the spicules, where bone formation is active.

The **upper inset** in Figure 1 shows the surface of several spicules from the *left circle* in Figure 2, at higher magnification. Note the osteoblasts *(Ob),* some of which are just beginning to produce bone in apposition to the calcified cartilage *(C).* The lower right of the **inset** shows bone *(EB)* with an osteocyte *(Oc)* already embedded in the bone matrix.

The **lower inset,** an enlargement of the *right circle* in Figure 2, reveals several osteoclasts *(Ocl).* They are in apposition to the spicule, which is mostly cartilage. A small amount of bone is evident, based on the red-staining material in this **inset.** Note the light area *(arrow)* representing the ruffled border of the osteoclast. Examination of Figure 2 reveals a number of other osteoclasts *(Ocl).*

KEY

C, calcified cartilage matrix
EB, endochondral bone
HC, hypertrophic cartilage
M, marrow
Ob, osteoblast
Oc, osteocyte
Ocl, osteoclast
PC, proliferating cartilage
RC, reserve cartilage
arrow, ruffled border of osteoclast

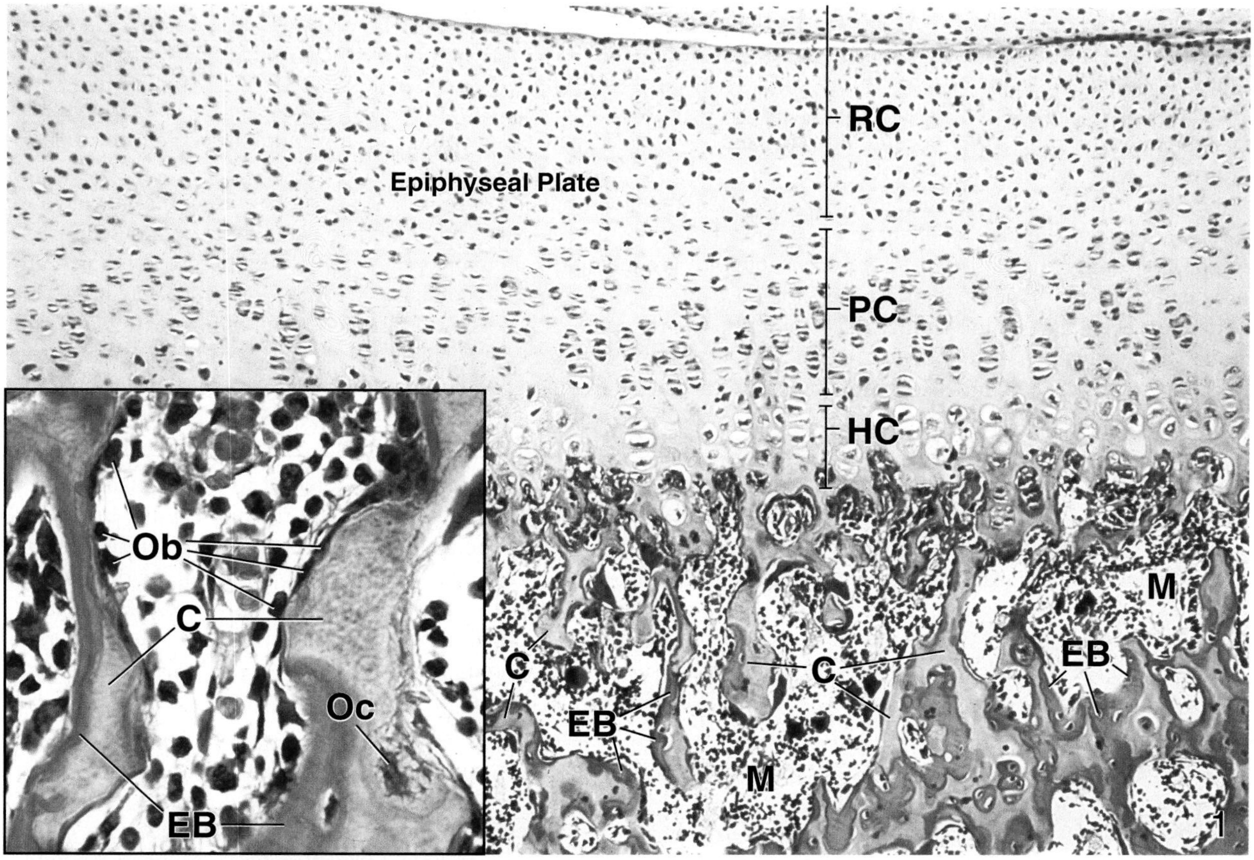
Epiphyseal Plate
RC
PC
HC
Ob
C
Oc
EB
C
EB
C
M
EB
M
1

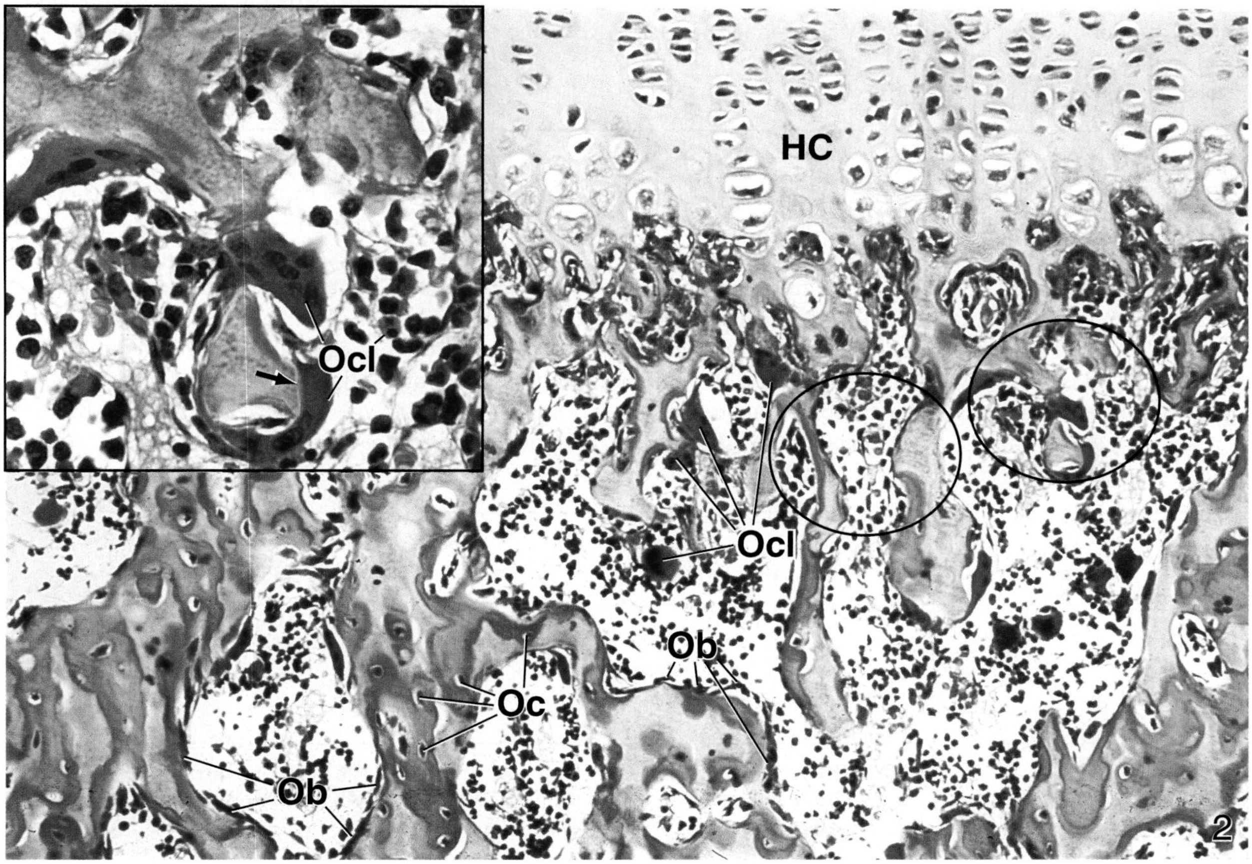
HC
Ocl
Ocl
Ob
Oc
Ob
2

PLATE 15. INTRAMEMBRANOUS BONE FORMATION

Intramembranous bone formation is limited to those bones that are not required to perform an early supporting function, e.g., the flat bones of the skull. This process requires the proliferation and differentiation of cells of the mesenchyme to become *osteoblasts,* the bone-forming cells. They produce ground substance and collagen. This initial matrix, called *osteoid,* calcifies to form bone.

As the osteoblasts continue to secrete their product, some are entrapped within their matrix and are then known as *osteocytes.* They are responsible for maintenance of the newly formed bone tissue. The remaining osteoblasts continue the bone deposition process at the bone surface. They are capable of reproducing to maintain as adequate population for continued growth.

This newly formed bone appears first as *spicules* that enlarge and interconnect as growth proceeds, creating a three-dimensional trabecular structure similar in shape to the future mature bone. The interstices contain blood vessels and connective tissue (mesenchyme). As the bone continues to grow, remodeling occurs. This involves resorption of localized areas of bone tissue by *osteoclasts* in order to maintain appropriate shape in relation to size and to permit vascular nourishment during the growth process.

Figure 1, fetal head, human, Mallory trichrome ×45.

A cross section of the developing lower jaw bone, as seen at this relatively early stage of development, consists of bone spicules *(BS)* of various sizes and shapes. The bone spicules interconnect and, in three dimensions, have the general shape of the mandible. Other structures present that will assist in orientation include developing teeth *(DT),* the tip of Meckel's cartilage *(MC),* also referred to as the mandibular process, seen on the left side, and the oral cavity *(OC).* The bottom surface of the specimen shows the epidermis *(Ep)* of the underside of the chin. A large portion of the developing tongue is seen in the upper half of the figure. The tongue consists largely of developing striated visceral muscle fibers arranged in a three-dimensional orthogonal array that is characteristic of this organ.

Figure 2, fetal head, human, Mallory trichrome ×175.

This higher-magnification view of the *boxed area* in Figure 1 shows the interconnections of the bone spicules *(BS)* of the developing mandible. Within and around the spaces enclosed by the developing spicules is mesenchymal tissue. These mesenchymal cells will give rise to new osteoblasts as well to the cells that will form the vascular components of the bone. The more dense connective tissue *(CT)* will differentiate into the periosteum on one side of the developing mandible. Other structures shown in the field include numerous blood vessels *(BV)* and the enamel organ *(EO)* of a developing tooth.

Figure 3, fetal head, human, Mallory trichrome ×350.

This higher-magnification micrograph of a portion of the field in Figure 2 shows to advantage the distinction between newly deposited osteoid, which stains blue, and mineralized bone, which stains red. Osteoblasts are seen in two different levels of activity. Those that are relatively inactive and are in apposition to well-formed osteoid *(Ob^1)* exhibit elongate nuclear profiles and appear to be flattened on the surface of the osteoid. Those osteoblasts *(Ob^2)* that are actively secreting new osteoid appear as tall, columnar-like cells adjacent to osteoid. One of the spicules shows a cell completely surrounded by bone matrix; this is an osteoblast that has become trapped in its own secretions and is now an osteocyte *(OC).* At this magnification, the very loose connective tissue characteristics of the mesenchyme and the sparseness of the mesenchymal cells *(MC)* are well demonstrated. The highly cellular connective tissue *(CT)* on the right margin of the figure is the developing perichondrium. Some of its cells will also develop into osteoblasts to allow growth of the bone at its surface.

KEY

BS, bone spicules
BV, blood vessels
CT, connective tissue
DT, developing tooth
EO, enamel organ
Ep, epithelium
MC, Meckel's cartilage
Ob^1, inactive osteoblast
Ob^2, active osteoblast
OC, oral cavity (Fig. 1.)
OC, osteocyte (Fig. 3.)

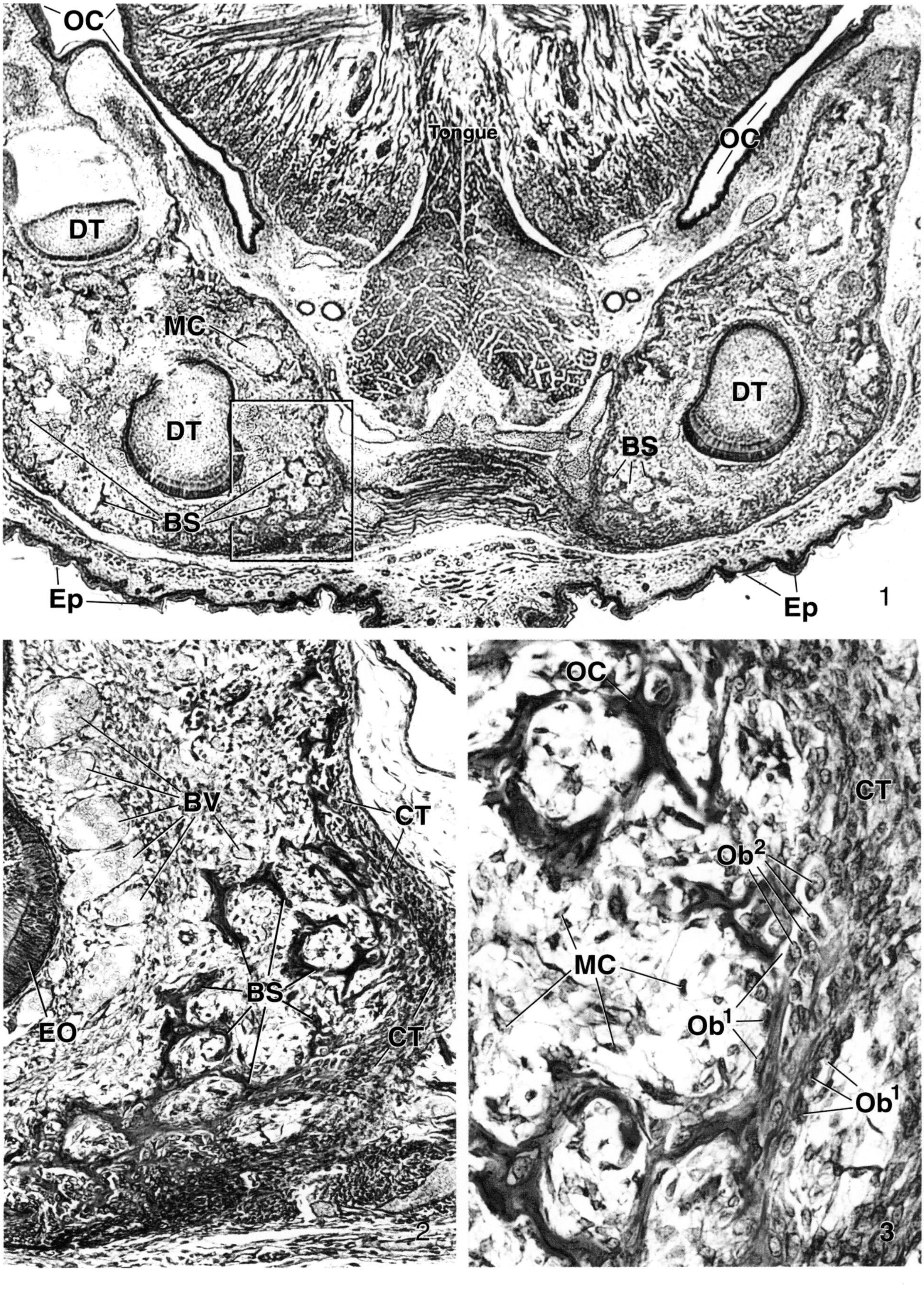
OC
Tongue
OC
DT
MC
DT
DT
BS
BS
Ep
Ep
1
BV
CT
BS
EO
CT
2
OC
CT
Ob²
MC
Ob¹
Ob¹
3

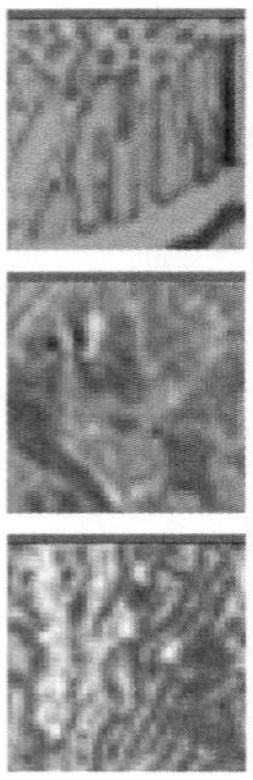

9

Blood

▼ OVERVIEW OF BLOOD

Blood is a fluid connective tissue that circulates through the cardiovascular system

Like the other connective tissues, ***blood*** consists of cells and an extracellular component whose volume exceeds that of the cells. The total volume of blood in the normal adult is about 6 liters, which amounts to 7 to 8% of total body weight. Blood is propelled through the cardiovascular system by the pumping action of the heart to reach the body tissues. Its many functions include

- Transport of nutrients and oxygen directly or indirectly to cells
- Transport of wastes and carbon dioxide away from cells
- Delivery of hormones and other regulatory substances to and from cells and tissues

- Maintenance of homeostasis by acting as a buffer and by participating in coagulation and thermoregulation
- Transport of humoral agents and cells of the immune system that protect the body from pathogenic agents, foreign proteins, and transformed cells, i.e., cancer cells

Blood consists of cells and their derivatives and a protein-rich fluid called plasma

Blood cells and their derivatives include

- ***Erythrocytes,*** also called ***red blood cells (RBCs)***
- ***Leukocytes,*** also called ***white blood cells (WBCs)***
- ***Platelets***

Plasma is the liquid extracellular material that imparts fluid properties to blood. The relative volume of cells and plasma in whole blood is approximately 45 and 55%, respectively. The volume of packed erythrocytes in a sample of blood is called the ***hematocrit.*** It is obtained by centrifuging a blood sample to which anticoagulants have been added. The hematocrit reading is then obtained by measuring the percentage of the centrifuge tube volume occupied by the erythrocytes, compared with the whole blood volume. A normal reading is about 39 to 50 in males and 35 to 45 in females; thus 39 to 50% or 35 to 45% of the blood volume, respectively, consists of erythrocytes.

Leukocytes and platelets constitute only 1% of the blood volume. In a blood sample that has been centrifuged, the cell fraction (the part of the sample that contains the cells) consists mainly of packed erythrocytes (>99%). The leukocytes and platelets are contained in a narrow layer at the upper part of the cell fraction, called the ***buffy coat.*** As Table 9.1 indicates, there are nearly 1000 times more erythrocytes (~5 × 10^{12} cells/L of blood) than leukocytes (~7 × 10^9/L of blood).

▼ PLASMA

Although the blood cells are the major objects of interest in histology, a brief examination of plasma is also useful. The composition of plasma is summarized in Table 9.2. More than 90% of plasma by weight is water, which serves as the solvent for a variety of solutes, including proteins, dissolved gases, electrolytes, nutrients, regulatory substances, and waste materials.

Plasma proteins consist primarily of albumin, globulins, and fibrinogen

Albumin is the main protein constituent of the plasma, accounting for approximately half of the total plasma proteins. It is the smallest plasma protein (about 70 kDa) and is made in the liver. Albumin is responsible for exerting the concentration gradient between blood and extracellular tissue fluid. This major osmotic pressure on the blood vessel wall, called the ***colloid osmotic pressure,*** maintains the correct proportion of blood to tissue fluid volume. If a significant amount of albumin leaks out of the blood vessels into the loose connective tissue or is lost from the blood to the urine in the kidneys, the colloid osmotic pressure of the blood decreases, and fluid accumulates in the tissues. (This increase in tissue fluid is most readily noted by swelling of the ankles at the end of a day.) Albumin also acts as a carrier protein; it binds and transports hormones (thyroxine), metabolites (bilirubin), and drugs (barbiturates).

TABLE 9.1. **Formed Elements of the Blood**

	Cells/L		
Formed Elements	**Male**	**Female**	**%**
Erythrocytes	4.3–5.7 × 10^{12}	3.9–5.0 × 10^{12}	
Leukocytes	3.5–10.5 × 10^9	3.5–10.5 × 10^9	100
Agranulocytes			
Lymphocytes	0.9–2.9 × 10^9	0.9–2.9 × 10^9	25.7–27.6[A]
Monocytes	0.3–0.9 × 10^9	0.3–0.9 × 10^9	8.6[A]
Granulocytes			
Neutrophils	1.7–7.0 × 10^9	1.7–7.0 × 10^9	48.6–66.7[A]
Eosinophils	0.05–0.5 × 10^9	0.05–0.5 × 10^9	1.4–4.8[A]
Basophils	0–0.03 × 10^9	0–0.03 × 10^9	0–0.3[A]
Platelets	150–450 × 10^9	150–450 × 10^9	

[A]Percentage of leukocytes.

TABLE 9.2. **Composition of Blood Plasma**

Component	**%**
Water	91–92
Protein (albumin, globulins, fibrinogen)	7–8
Other solutes:	1–2
Electrolytes (Na^+, K^+, Ca^{2+}, Mg^{2+}, Cl^-, HCO_3^-, PO_4^{3-}, SO_4^{2-})	
• Nonprotein nitrogen substances (urea, uric acid, creatine, creatinine, ammonium salts)	
• Nutrients (glucose, lipids, amino acids)	
• Blood gases (oxygen, carbon dioxide, nitrogen)	
• Regulatory substances (hormones, enzymes)	

Globulins include the ***immunoglobulins (γ-globulins),*** the largest component of the globulin fraction, and ***nonimmune globulins (α- and β-globulins).*** The immunoglobulins are antibodies, a class of functional immune-system molecules secreted by plasma cells. (Antibodies are discussed in Chapter 13.)

Nonimmune globulins are secreted by the liver. They help maintain the osmotic pressure within the vascular system and also serve as carrier proteins for various substances such as copper (by ceruloplasmin), iron (by transferrin), and hemoglobin (by haptoglobin). Nonimmune globulins also include fibronectin, lipoproteins, coagulation factors, and other molecules that may exchange between the blood and the extravascular connective tissue.

Fibrinogen, the largest protein (340 kDa), is made in the liver. In cascade reactions with other coagulation factors, fibrinogen is transformed into fibrin, which forms an insoluble clot that stops blood flow in the event of damage to the blood vessel.

Aside from these large proteins and the regulatory substances, which are small proteins or polypeptides, most of the other plasma constituents are small enough to pass through the blood vessel wall into the extracellular spaces of the adjacent connective tissue.

In general, plasma proteins react with common fixatives; they are often retained within the blood vessels in tissue sections. Plasma proteins do not possess structural form above the molecular level; thus, when they are retained in blood vessels in the tissue block, they appear as a homogeneous substance that stains evenly with eosin in hematoxylin and eosin (H&E)–stained sections.

The interstitial fluid of connective tissues is derived from blood plasma

Interstitial fluid, not surprisingly, has an electrolyte composition that reflects that of blood plasma, from which it is derived. The composition of interstitial fluid in nonconnective tissues, however, is subject to considerable modification by the absorptive and secretory activities of epithelia. Epithelia may create special microenvironments conducive to their function. For example, a blood–brain barrier exists between the blood and nerve tissue. Barriers also exist between the blood and the parenchymal tissue in the testis, thymus gland, eye, and other epithelial compartments. Fluids, barriers, and their functions are discussed in subsequent chapters that describe these particular organs.

Examination of blood cells requires special preparation and staining

The preparation method that best displays the cell types of peripheral blood is the blood smear. This method differs from the usual preparation seen in the histology laboratory in that the specimen is not embedded in paraffin and sectioned. Rather, a drop of blood is placed directly on a slide and spread thinly over the surface of the slide, i.e., "pulled" with the edge of another slide, to produce a monolayer of cells (Fig. 9.1a). The preparation is then air dried and stained. Another difference in the preparation of a blood smear is that instead of H&E, special mixtures of dyes are used to stain the blood cells. The resulting prepa-

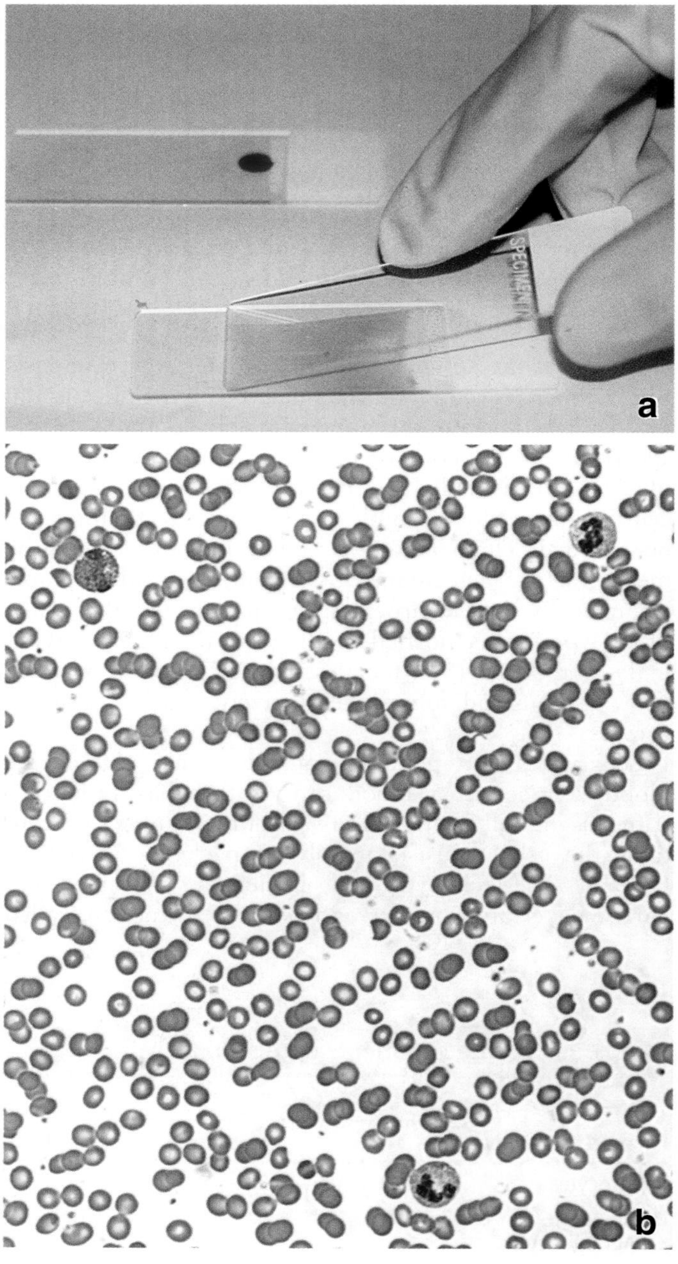

FIGURE 9.1
Blood smear: preparation technique and overview photomicrograph. a. Photograph showing the method of producing a blood smear. A drop of blood is placed directly on a glass slide and spread over its surface with the edge of another slide. **b.** Photomicrograph of smear from peripheral blood, stained with Wright's stain, showing the cells evenly distributed. The cells are mainly erythrocytes. Three leukocytes are present. ×350.

ration may then be examined with a high-power oil-immersion lens, with or without a coverslip (Fig. 9.1b).

The modified Romanovsky-type stain commonly used for blood smears consists of a mixture of methylene blue (a basic dye), related azures (also basic dyes), and eosin (an acidic dye). On the basis of their appearance after staining, leukocytes are traditionally divided into granulocytes and agranulocytes. Although both cell types may contain granules, the granulocytes possess obvious, specifically stained granules in their cytoplasm. In general, the basic dyes stain nuclei, granules of basophils, and the RNA of the cytoplasm, whereas the acidic dye stains the erythrocytes and the granules of eosinophils. It was originally thought that the fine neutrophil granules were stained by a "neutral dye" that formed when methylene blue and its related azures were combined with eosin. However, the mechanism by which the specific neutrophil granules are stained is not clear. Some of the basic dyes (the azures) are metachromatic and may impart a violet to red color to the material they stain.

▼ ERYTHROCYTES

Erythrocytes are anucleate, biconcave disks

Erythrocytes, or ***red blood cells (RBCs),*** are anucleate cells devoid of typical organelles. They function only within the bloodstream to bind oxygen for delivery to the tissues and, in exchange, bind carbon dioxide for removal from the tissues. Their shape is that of a biconcave disk with a diameter of 7.8 μm, an edge thickness of 2.6 μm, and a central thickness of 0.8 μm. This shape maximizes the cell's surface area (~140 μm^2), an important attribute in gas exchange.

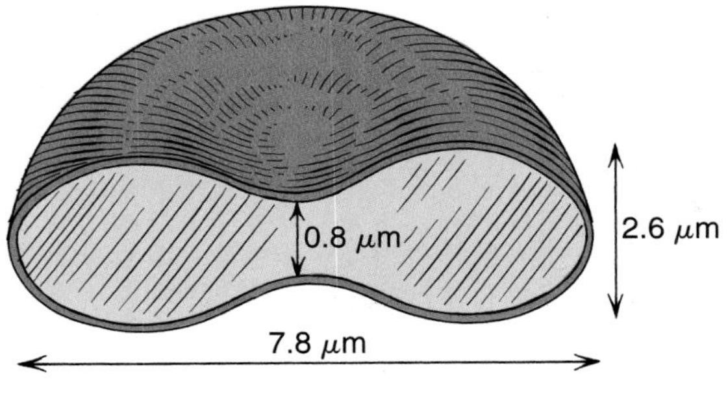

The life span of the erythrocyte is approximately 120 days, after which most (~90%) are phagocytosed by macrophages in the spleen, bone marrow, and liver. The remaining aged erythrocytes (~10%) break down intravascularly, releasing hemoglobin into the blood.

In H&E–stained sections, erythrocytes are usually 7 to 8 μm in diameter. Because their size is relatively consistent in fixed tissue, they can be used to estimate the size of other cells and structures in tissue sections; in this role, erythrocytes are appropriately referred to as the "histologic ruler."

Because both living and preserved erythrocytes usually appear as biconcave disks, they can give the impression that their form is rigid and inelastic (Fig. 9.2). They are, in fact, extremely deformable. They pass easily through the smallest blood vessels by folding upon themselves and can thus pass through even the narrowest capillaries. They stain uniformly with eosin. In thin sections viewed with the transmission electron microscope (TEM), the contents of an erythrocyte appear as a dense, finely granular material (Fig. 9.3).

The shape of the erythrocyte is maintained by membrane proteins

The cell membrane of an erythrocyte is composed of a typical lipid bilayer and contains two functionally significant groups of proteins:

- ***Integral membrane proteins*** represent most of the proteins in the lipid bilayer. They consist of two major families: ***glycophorins*** and ***band 3 protein.*** The extracellular domains of these integral membrane proteins are glycosylated and express specific blood group antigens. ***Glycophorin C,*** a member of the glycophorin family, plays an important role in attaching the underlying cytoskeletal protein network to the cell membrane. ***Band 3 protein*** binds hemoglobin and acts as an additional anchoring site for the cytoskeletal proteins (Fig. 9.4).
- ***Peripheral membrane proteins*** reside on the inner surface of the cell membrane. They are organized into a two-dimensional hexagonal lattice network that laminates the inner layer of the membrane. The lattice itself, which is positioned parallel to the membrane, is composed mainly of ***spectrin*** tetramers, ***actin, band 4.1, adducin, band 4.9,*** and ***tropomyosin*** (see Fig. 9.4). The lattice is anchored to the lipid bilayer by ***ankyrin,*** which interacts with ***band 4.2*** protein as well as with band 3 integral membrane protein.

This unique cytoskeletal arrangement contributes to the shape of the erythrocyte and imparts elastic properties and stability to the membrane. The cytoskeleton is not static; it undergoes continuous rearrangement in response to various physical factors and chemical stimuli as the cell moves through the vascular network. Any defect in the expression of genes that encode these cytoskeleton proteins can result in abnormally shaped and fragile erythrocytes. For instance, ***hereditary spherocytosis*** is caused by a primary defect in spectrin gene expression that results in spherical erythrocytes. ***Hereditary elliptocytosis*** is caused by a deficiency in band 4.1 protein that results in elliptic erythrocytes. In both conditions, erythrocytes are unable to adapt to changes in their environment (e.g., osmotic pressure and mechanical deformations), which results in destruction of the cells, or ***hemolysis.***

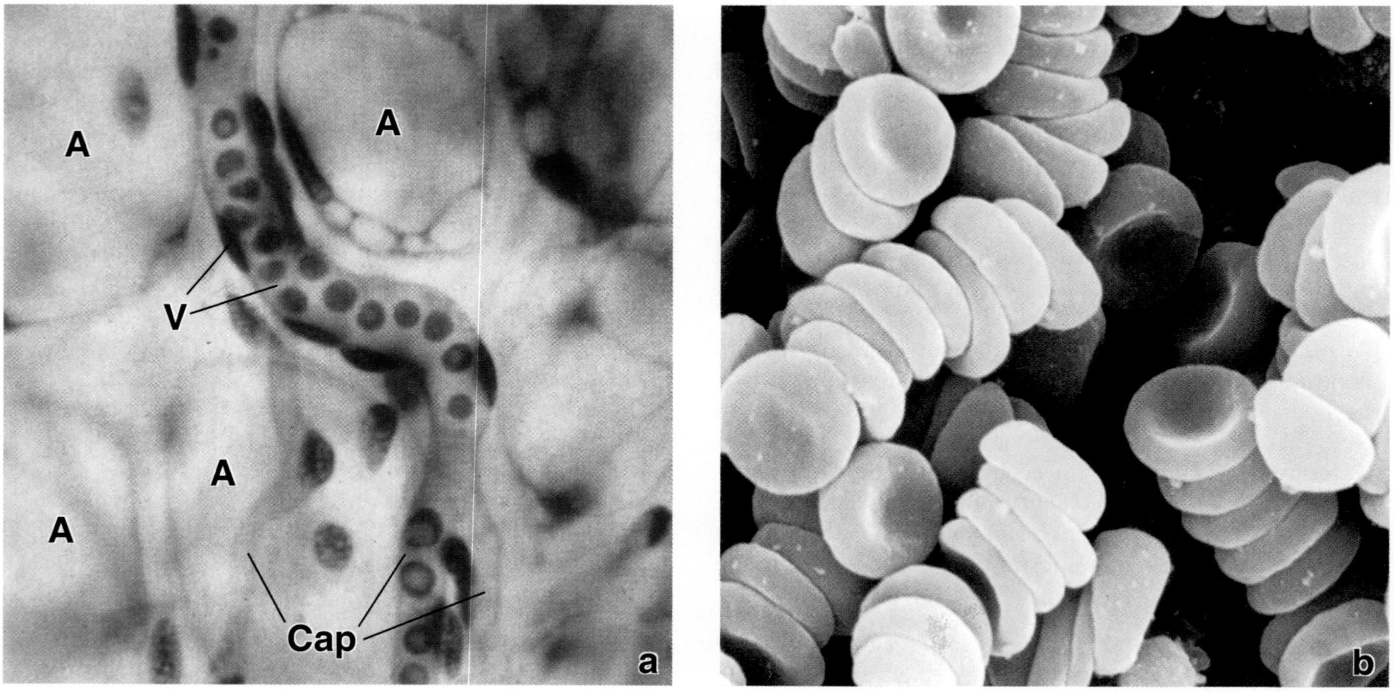

FIGURE 9.2
Erythrocyte morphology. a. Photomicrograph of three capillaries *(Cap)* joining to form a venule *(V)*, as observed in adipose tissue within a full-thickness mesentery spread. The erythrocytes appear in single file in one of the capillaries (the other two are empty). The light center area of some of the erythrocytes is due to their biconcave shape. Erythrocytes are highly plastic and can fold on themselves when passing through very narrow capillaries. The large round structures are adipose cells *(A)*. ×470. **b.** Scanning electron micrograph of erythrocytes collected in a blood tube. Note the concave shape of the cells. The stacks of erythrocytes in these preparations are not unusual and are referred to as rouleau. Such formations in vivo indicate an increased level of plasma immunoglobulin. ×2,800.

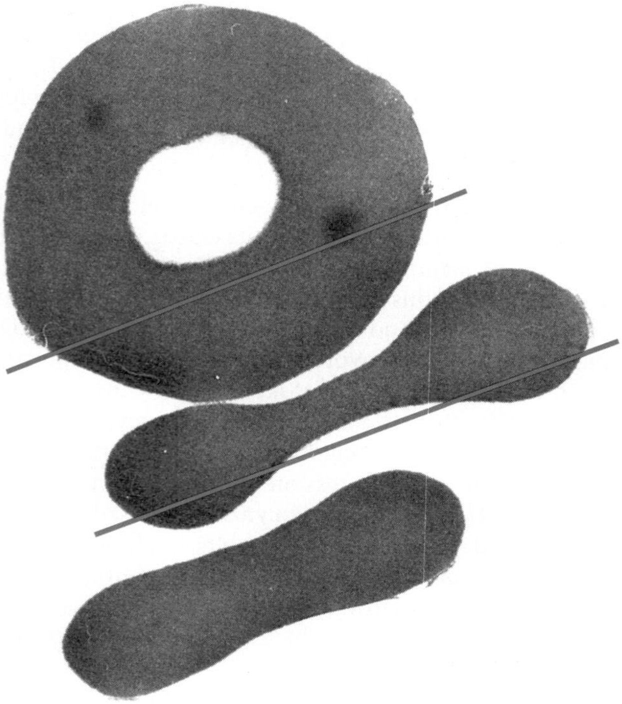

FIGURE 9.3
Electron micrograph of erythrocytes seen in different planes. The donut-shaped erythrocyte represents a section cut in a plane parallel to the diameter of the cell but missing its center. The plane of section is represented by the *blue line* in the adjacent erythrocyte; thus, the "hole in the donut" is the area represented by the segment of the *line* that is outside the cell. The third erythrocyte has a smaller diameter than its neighbor because the section passed in a plane represented by the *line* passing through the donut-shaped erythrocyte. ×8,000.

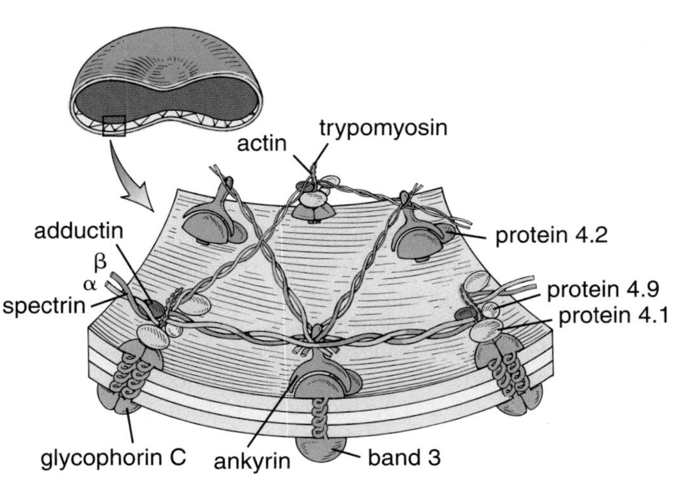

FIGURE 9.4
Erythrocyte membrane organization. The *rectangle* in the sectioned erythrocyte (upper left) represents the area of the membrane in the larger diagram. The large diagram shows the arrangement of the peripheral and integral membrane proteins. The peripheral proteins form a cytoskeletal lattice on the interior surface of the plasma membrane, in which the predominant protein is spectrin. The lattice is anchored to the plasma membrane by a number of protein complexes.

Erythrocytes contain hemoglobin, a protein specialized for the transport of oxygen and carbon dioxide

Erythrocytes transport oxygen and carbon dioxide bound to the protein ***hemoglobin.*** A high concentration of this protein is present within erythrocytes and is responsible for their uniform staining with eosin and the cytoplasmic granularity seen with the TEM. The disk shape of the erythrocyte facilitates gas exchange because more hemoglobin molecules are closer to the plasma membrane than they would be in a spherical cell. Thus, gases have less distance to diffuse within the cell to reach a binding site on the hemoglobin.

Hemoglobin consists of four polypeptide chains, each complexed to an iron-containing heme group (Fig. 9.5). The structure of the polypeptide chains varies. Depending on the particular polypeptides present, hemoglobin is designated as HbA, HbA_2, or HbF. Hemoglobin in the adult is about 96% HbA, 3% HbA_2, and 1% HbF. HbF is the principal form of hemoglobin in the fetus. Although it persists

BOX 9.1

Clinical Correlations: ABO and Rh Blood Group Systems

An important factor in blood transfusion is the ***ABO blood group system,*** which essentially involves two antigens called A antigen and B antigen (Table 9.3). These antigens are present on the surface of the erythrocyte, attached to the extracellular domains of glycophorins, which are integral membrane proteins. Individuals with A antigens possess serum anti-B antibodies that are directed against the B antigen. Individuals with B antigens possess serum anti-A antibodies that are directed against A antigen. The presence of A or B antigens and anti-A or anti-B antibodies determines the four primary ***blood groups: A, B, AB,*** and ***O.*** Individuals with blood group AB do not have antibodies directed against A or B antigens. Thus, they are universal acceptors of any blood type. Group O individuals have both anti-A and anti-B antibodies in their serum and neither A nor B antigens on their erythrocytes. Thus, these individuals are universal blood donors. If an individual is transfused with blood of an incompatible type, the recipient's antibodies will attack the donor erythrocytes, causing a ***hemolytic transfusion reaction,*** or destruction of the transfused erythrocytes.

The other important blood group system, the ***Rh system,*** is based on the ***Rhesus (Rh) antigen.*** In humans, this system is represented by an Rh transmembrane polypeptide that shares antigenic sites with rhesus monkey erythrocytes. Although the Rh polypeptide expresses many antigen sites on its extracellular domain, only three of them—D, C, and E antigens—have clinical significance. An individual who possesses only one of these three antigens is referred to as ***Rh positive (Rh^+).*** All three antigens stimulate production of anti-Rh antibodies in individuals without the same antigens.

Rh incompatibility may induce a hemolytic transfusion reaction and in newborns cause the hemolytic disease ***erythroblastosis fetalis.*** Erythroblastosis fetalis occurs in $Rh(D)^+$ newborns delivered by $Rh(D)^-$ mothers and results from an immune reaction of anti-D immunoglobulins passed across the placenta from the mother. The anti-D antibodies are produced by the mother in response to the D antigen expressed on the fetal erythrocytes that leak into her circulation during pregnancy. Administration of anti-D antibodies (RhoGAM) to the mother during the pregnancy and following parturition destroy any circulating $Rh(D)^+$ fetal erythrocytes that persist in the mother's blood, thus preventing Rh incompatibility reactions in future pregnancies.

TABLE 9.3. **ABO Blood Group System**

Blood Type	Erythrocyte Surface Antigen	Serum Antibody
A	A antigen	Anti-B
B	B antigen	Anti-A
AB	A and B antigens	No antibodies *(universal blood recipient)*
O	No A or B antigens	Anti-A and anti-B *(universal blood donor)*

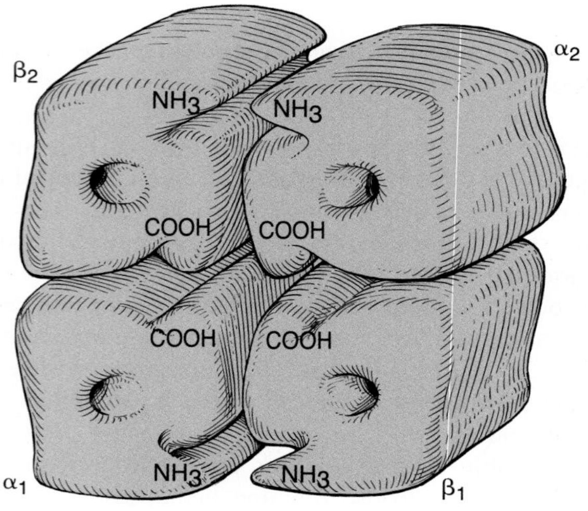

FIGURE 9.5
Structural diagram of the hemoglobin molecule. Each hemoglobin molecule is composed of four subunits. Each subunit contains a heme, the iron-containing portion of hemoglobin, embedded in a hydrophobic cleft of a globin chain. The folding of the globin chain places the heme near the surface of the molecule, where it is readily accessible to oxygen. There are four different types of globin chains: α, β, δ, and γ, which occur in pairs. The types of globin chains present in the molecules determine the type of hemoglobin. The figure illustrates hemoglobin A (HbA), which is composed of two α and two β chains.

BOX 9.2

Clinical Correlations: Hemoglobin Disorders

ANEMIA

Anemia is defined clinically as a decrease in the concentration of hemoglobin in the blood for the age and gender of an individual. While in certain anemias this decreased concentration of hemoglobin is due to a decrease in the amount of hemoglobin in each cell, most anemias are caused by a reduction in the number of erythrocytes. Causes of anemia include loss of blood (hemorrhage), insufficient production of erythrocytes, or accelerated destruction of erythrocytes in the circulation. Insufficient dietary iron or deficiencies of vitamins such as vitamin B_{12} or folic acid can lead to decreased production of erythrocytes. Gastric atrophy, as a result of autoimmune disease, with concomitant destruction of the parietal cells that secrete intrinsic factor, a molecule essential for absorption of vitamin B_{12} by cells in the ileum, is the cause of a form of anemia called ***pernicious anemia.***

SICKLE CELL DISEASE

Sickle cell disease is caused by a single point mutation in the gene that encodes the β-globin chain of hemoglobin A. The result of this mutation is an abnormal β-globin chain in which the amino acid valine is substituted for glutamic acid in position 6. Hemoglobin containing this abnormal β-globin chain is designated sickle hemoglobin (HbS). The substitution of the hydrophobic valine for the hydrophilic glutamic acid causes HbS to aggregate under conditions of reduced oxygen tension. Instead of the normal biconcave disk shape, many of the erythrocytes become sickle-shaped at low oxygen tension, hence the name of this disease (Fig. 9.6). Sickled erythrocytes are more rigid than normal cells and adhere more readily to the endothelial surface. Thus, sickled erythrocytes may pile up in the smallest capillaries, depriving portions of tissues and organs of oxygen and nutrients. Large-vessel obstruction may also occur, which in children frequently leads to stroke. Sickled erythrocytes are also more fragile and break down or are destroyed more quickly than normal erythrocytes.

Sickle cell disease is a homozygous recessive genetic disorder. However, heterozygous individuals may occasionally have clinical consequences at high altitude or under extreme physical stress.

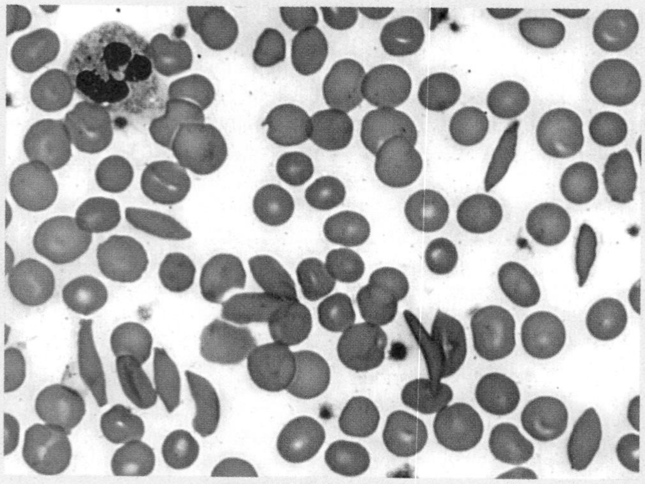

FIGURE 9.6
Photomicrograph of a sickle cell anemia blood smear. Blood smear stained with Wright's stain shows abnormal "boat" and "sickle"-shaped cells from an individual with sickle cell anemia. ×400.

in slightly higher percentages than normal in sickle cell disease and thalassemia, it does not appear to have a pathologic role. A monomer of hemoglobin is similar in composition and structure to myoglobin, the oxygen-binding protein found in striated muscle.

▼ LEUKOCYTES

Leukocytes are subclassified into two general groups. The basis for this division is the presence or absence of prominent ***specific granules*** in the cytoplasm. Cells containing specific granules are classified as ***granulocytes*** (neutrophils, eosinophils, and basophils), and cells that lack specific granules are classified as ***agranulocytes*** (lymphocytes and monocytes). However, both agranulocytes and granulocytes possess small, ***nonspecific azurophilic granules,*** which are lysosomes. The relative number of the various leukocytes is given in Table 9.1.

Neutrophils

Neutrophils are the most numerous WBCs as well as the most common granulocyte

Neutrophils measure 10 to 12 μm in diameter in blood smears and are obviously larger than erythrocytes. Although named for their lack of characteristic cytoplasmic staining, they are also readily identified by their multilobed nucleus; thus, they are also called ***polymorphonuclear neutrophils*** or ***polymorphs.*** Mature neutrophils possess two to four lobes of nuclear material joined by thinner nuclear strands. The arrangement is not static; rather, in living neutrophils the lobes and connecting strands change their shape, position, and even number.

The chromatin of the neutrophil has a characteristic arrangement. Wide regions of heterochromatin are located chiefly at the periphery of the nucleus, in contact with the nuclear envelope. Regions of euchromatin are located chiefly at the center of the nucleus, with relatively smaller regions contacting the nuclear envelope (Fig. 9.7). In females, the ***Barr body*** forms a drumstick-shaped appendage on one of the nuclear lobes.

Neutrophils contain three types of granules

The cytoplasm of a neutrophil contains three kinds of granules. The different types of granules reflect the various phagocytotic functions of the cell:

- ***Specific granules*** (secondary granules) are the smallest granules and are at least twice as numerous as azurophilic granules. They are barely visible in the light microscope; in electron micrographs they are ellipsoidal (see Fig. 9.7). Specific granules contain various enzymes ***(type IV collagenase, phospholipase)*** as well as ***complement activators*** and other bacteriostatic and bactericidal agents ***(lysozyme).***

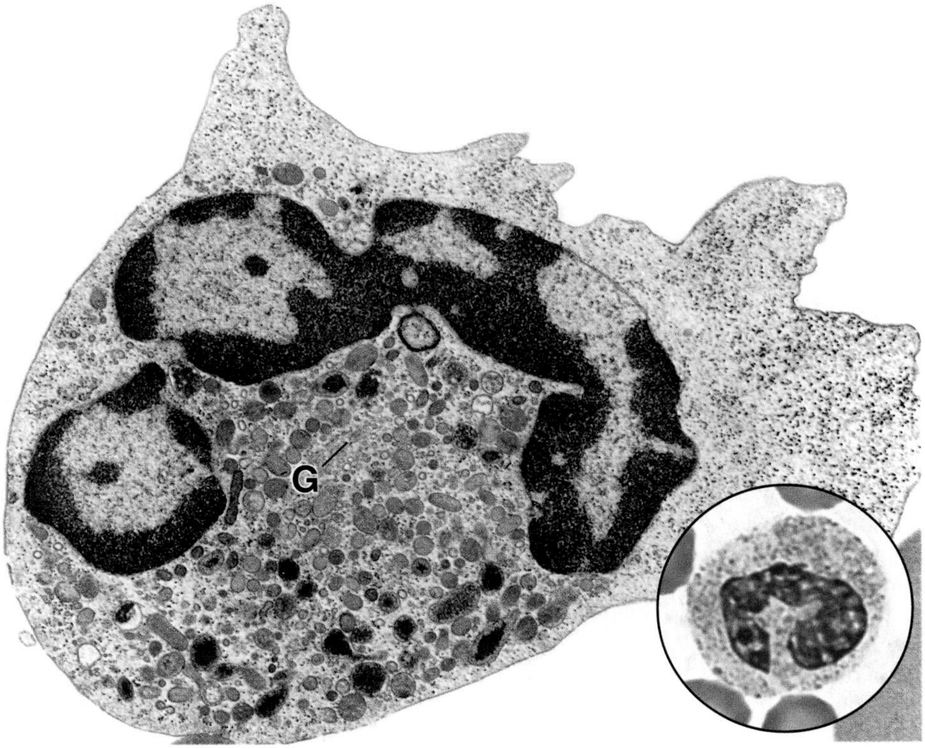

FIGURE 9.7
Electron micrograph of a human mature neutrophil. The nucleus shows the typical multilobed configuration with the heterochromatin at the periphery and the euchromatin more centrally located. A small Golgi apparatus *(G)* is present; other organelles are sparse. The punctate appearance of the cytoplasm adjacent to the convex aspect of the nuclear profile is due to glycogen particles. Adjacent to the concave aspect of the nuclear profile are numerous granules. Specific granules appear less dense and more rounded than azurophilic granules. The latter are fewer in number and are extremely electron dense. ×22,000. (Courtesy of Dr. Dorothea Zucker-Franklin.) For comparison, the **inset** shows a neutrophil from a blood smear observed in the light microscope. ×1,800.

- ***Azurophilic granules*** (primary granules) are larger and less numerous than specific granules. They arise early in granulopoiesis and occur in all granulocytes, as well as in monocytes and lymphocytes. The azurophilic granules are the lysosomes of the neutrophil and contain ***myeloperoxidase,*** which appears as a finely stippled material with the TEM. Myeloperoxidase helps to generate highly reactive bactericidal hypochlorite and chloramines. In addition to a variety of the typical acid hydrolases, azurophilic granules also contain cationic proteins called ***defensins,*** which in function are analogous to antibodies.
- ***Tertiary granules*** in neutrophils are of two types. One type contains ***phosphatases*** and is sometimes called a phosphasome. The other type contains ***metalloproteinases,*** such as gelatinases and collagenases, which are thought to facilitate the migration of the neutrophil through the connective tissue.

Aside from these granules, membrane-bounded organelles are sparse. A small Golgi apparatus is evident in the center of the cell, and mitochondria are relatively few in number (see Fig. 9.7).

Neutrophils are motile cells; they leave the circulation and migrate to their site of action in the connective tissue

An important property of neutrophils and other leukocytes is their motility. Neutrophils are the most numerous of the first wave of cells to enter an area of tissue damage. Their migration is controlled by the expression of adhesion molecules on the neutrophil surface that interact with corresponding ligands on endothelial cells (Fig. 9.8).

The initial phase of neutrophil migration occurs in the postcapillary venules and is regulated by a mechanism involving neutrophil–endothelial cell recognition. ***Selectins*** on the surface of the circulating neutrophil (CD62L) interact with receptors (GlyCAM-1) on the surface of the endothelial cells. The neutrophil becomes partially tethered to the endothelial cell as a result of this interaction, which slows the neutrophil and causes it to roll on the surface of the endothelium. In the second phase, another group of adhesion molecules on the neutrophil surface, called ***integrins*** (VLA 5), are activated by chemokine signals from the endothelial cells. In the third phase, integrins and other adhesion molecules from the ***immunoglobulin superfamily*** (e.g., ICAM, VCAM) expressed on the neutrophil surface engage with their specific receptors on the endothelial cells, attaching the neutrophil to the endothelial cell. The neutrophil then extends a pseudopod to an intercellular junction. Histamine and heparin released at the injury site by perivascular mast cells open the intercellular junction, allowing the neutrophil to migrate into the connective tissue. With the TEM, the cytoplasmic contents of a neutrophil pseudopod appear as an expanse of finely granular cytoplasmic matrix with no membranous organelles (see Fig. 9.7). The finely granular appearance is due to the presence of actin filaments, some microtubules, and glycogen, which are involved in the extension of the cytoplasm to form the pseudopod and the subsequent contraction that pulls the cell forward. Once the neutrophil enters the connective tissue, further migration to the injury site is directed by a process known as ***chemotaxis,*** the binding of chemoattractant molecules and extracellular matrix proteins to specific receptors on the surface of the neutrophil.

Neutrophils are active phagocytes at the site of inflammation

Once at the site of tissue injury, the neutrophil must recognize any foreign substance before phagocytosis can occur. Neutrophils can recognize some bacteria and foreign organisms that have had no modifications made to their surfaces, whereas others must be opsonized (coated with antibodies and/or complement) to make them more attractive to the neutrophil. After recognition and attachment, the antigen is engulfed by extended pseudopods of the neutrophil and internalized to form a phagosome (Fig. 9.9). Specific and azurophilic granules then fuse with the phagosome membrane, and the lysosomal hydrolases of the azurophilic granules digest the foreign material. After digestion, the degraded material is stored in residual bodies or exocytosed. Most neutrophils die in this process; the accumulation of dead bacteria and dead neutrophils constitutes the thick yellowish exudate called ***pus.***

Neutrophils also secrete interleukin-1 (IL-1), a substance known as a ***pyrogen*** (fever-inducing agent). IL-1 induces synthesis of prostaglandins, which in turn act on the thermoregulatory center of the hypothalamus to produce fever. Fever is therefore a consequence of acute inflammation involving a massive neutrophilic response.

Inflammation and wound healing also involve monocytes, lymphocytes, eosinophils, basophils, and fibroblasts

Monocytes also enter the connective tissue as a secondary response to tissue injury. At the site of tissue injury they transform into ***macrophages*** that phagocytose cell and tissue debris, fibrin, remaining bacteria, and dead neutrophils. Normal wound healing depends on the participation of macrophages in the inflammatory response; they become the major cell type in the inflammatory site after the neutrophils are spent. At the same time that the macrophages become active at the site of inflammation, fibroblasts near the site and undifferentiated mesenchymal cells in the adventitia of small vessels at the site begin to divide and differentiate into fibroblasts and myofibroblasts that will secrete the fibers and ground substance of the healing wound. Like neutrophils, monocytes are attracted to the inflammatory site by chemotaxis. Lymphocytes, eosinophils, and basophils also play a role in inflammation, but they are more involved in the immunologic aspects of the process (see Chapter 13).

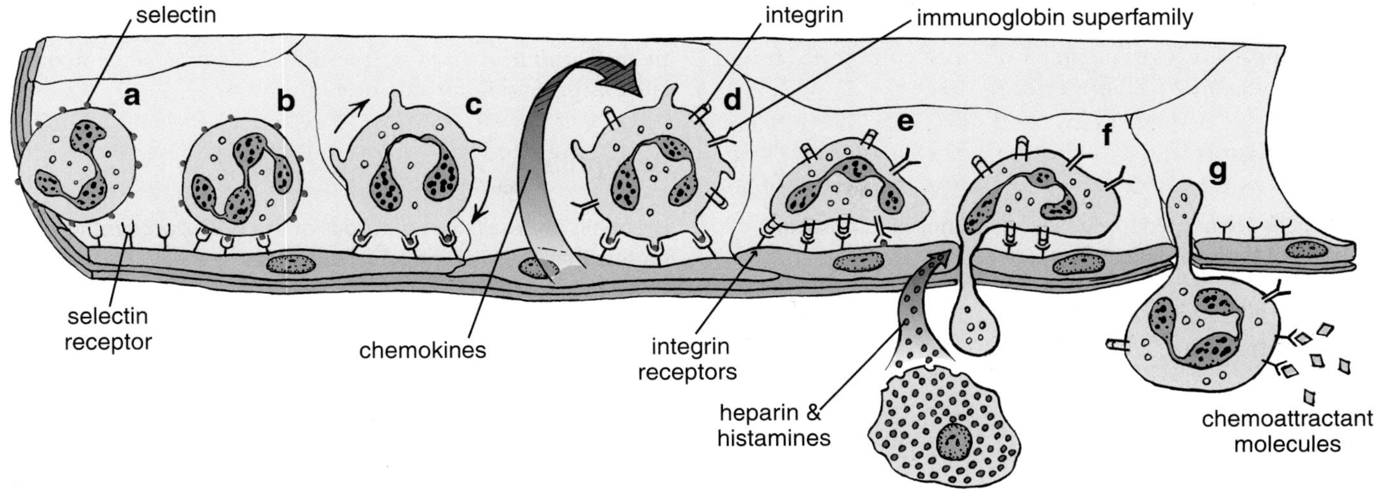

FIGURE 9.8

Diagram of events in the migration of a neutrophil from a postcapillary venule into the connective tissue. a. Circulating neutrophils are slowed down by the interaction of their surface adhesion molecules, selectins (CD62L), with the endothelium of the venule **(b). c.** As the result of this interaction, the cell rolls on the surface of the endothelium. The neutrophil then adheres to the endothelium and responds to chemokines secreted by the endothelial cells. **d.** Their secretion induces the expression of other adhesion molecules on the surface of the neutrophil, such as integrins (VLA-5) and the immunoglobulin superfamily of adhesion molecules (e.g., ICAM, VCAM). **e.** These adhesion molecules allow the neutrophil to bind to adhesion molecule receptors on the endothelial cells. **f.** The neutrophil then extends a pseudopod to an intercellular junction previously opened by histamine and heparin released from the mast cells in the connective tissue, allowing the neutrophil to migrate through the vessel wall **(g).**

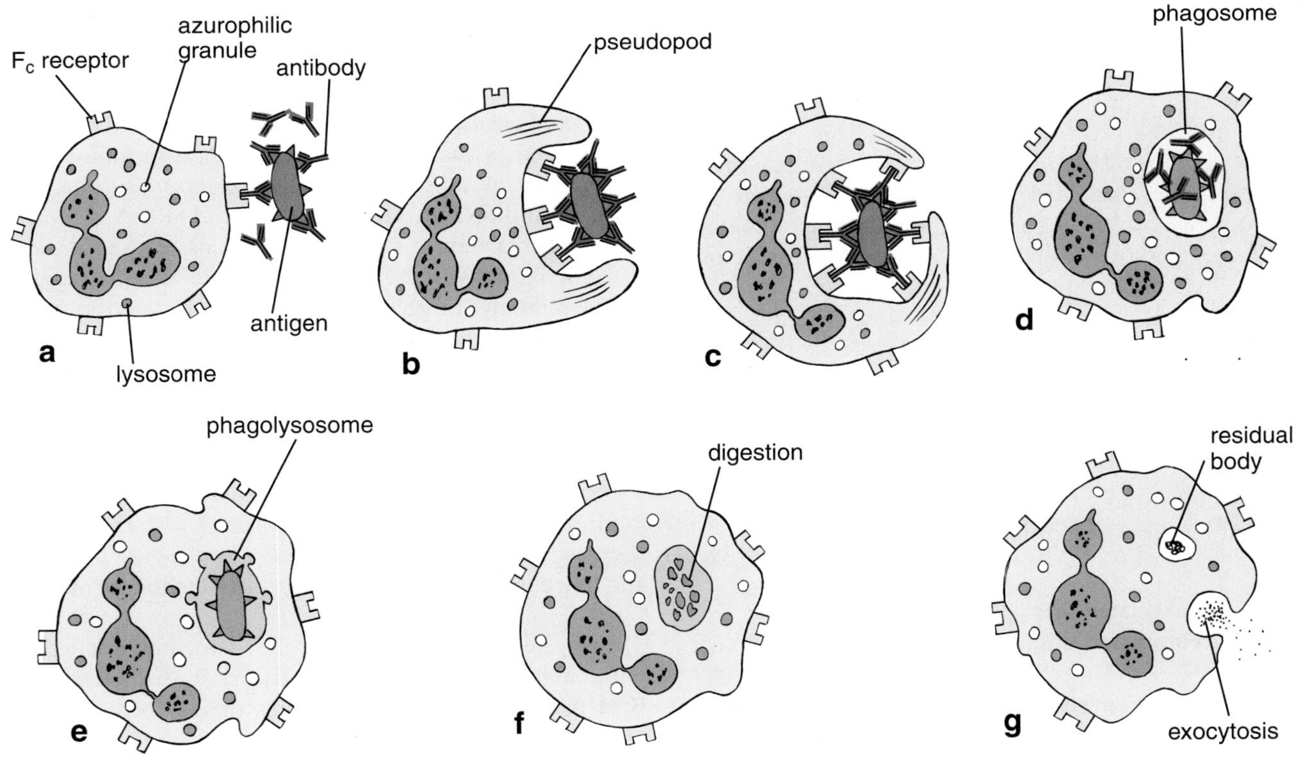

FIGURE 9.9

Neutrophil phagocytosis. a. Phagocytosis begins with recognition and attachment of foreign material (antigen), mainly by F_c receptors that interact with the F_c region of antibodies bound to the antigen. **b.** The antigen is then engulfed by pseudopods of the neutrophil. **c.** As the pseudopods come together and fuse, the antigen is internalized. **d.** Once the phagosome is formed, digestion is initiated by activation of membrane-bounded oxidases of the phagosome. **e.** Next, both specific and azurophilic granules fuse with the phagosome and release their contents, forming a phagolysosome. This fusion and release of granules is called degranulation. **f.** The enzymatic contents of the granules are responsible for killing and digesting the microorganism. The entire digestive process occurs within the phagolysosome, which protects the cell from self-injury. **g.** The digested material is either exocytosed into the extracellular space or stored as residual bodies within the neutrophil.

Eosinophils and lymphocytes are more commonly found at sites of chronic inflammation.

Eosinophils

Eosinophils are named for the large, eosinophilic, refractile granules in their cytoplasm

Eosinophils are about the same size as neutrophils, and their nuclei are typically bilobed (Fig. 9.10). As in neutrophils, the compact heterochromatin of eosinophils is chiefly adjacent to the nuclear envelope, whereas the euchromatin is located in the center of the nucleus. The cytoplasm contains two types of granules: numerous, large, elongated specific granules and azurophilic granules (otherwise, the eosinophil contains only a sparse representation of membranous organelles).

- ***Specific granules*** of eosinophils contain a ***crystalloid body*** that is readily seen with the TEM, surrounded by a less electron-dense matrix. These crystalloid bodies are responsible for the refractivity of the granules in the light microscope. They contain four major proteins: an arginine-rich protein called ***major basic protein (MBP)*** that accounts for the intense acidophilia of the granule, ***eosinophil cationic protein (ECP), eosinophil peroxidase (EPO),*** and ***eosinophil-derived neurotoxin (EDN).*** MBP is localized in the crystalloid body; the other three proteins are found in the granule matrix. Specific granules also contain ***histaminase, arylsulfatase, collagenase,*** and ***cathepsins.*** MBP, ECP, and EPO have a strong cytotoxic effect on protozoans and helminthic parasites; EDN causes nervous system dysfunction in parasitic organisms; histaminase neutralizes the activity of histamine; and arylsulfatase neutralizes slow-reacting substance of anaphylaxis (SRS-A) secreted by basophils (see Chapter 5, page 145).
- ***Azurophilic granules*** are lysosomes. They contain a variety of the usual lysosomal acid hydrolases and other hydrolytic enzymes that function in destruction of parasites and hydrolysis of antigen–antibody complexes internalized by the eosinophil.

Eosinophils are associated with allergic reactions, parasitic infections, and chronic inflammation

The release of arylsulfatase and histaminase by eosinophils at sites of allergic reaction moderates the potentially deleterious effects of inflammatory vasoactive agents. The eosinophil also participates in other immunologic responses, and phagocytoses antigen–antibody complexes. Thus, the count of eosinophils in blood samples of individuals with allergies and parasitic infections is usually high. Eosinophils play a major role is host defense against helminthic parasites. They are also found in large numbers in the lamina propria of the intestinal tract and at other sites of potential chronic inflammation.

Basophils

Basophils are the least numerous of the WBCs, accounting for less than 0.5% of the total leukocytes

Often, several hundred WBCs must be examined in a blood smear before one ***basophil*** is found. Basophils are about the same size as neutrophils and are so named because the numerous large granules in its cytoplasm stain with basic dyes. The lobed basophil nucleus is usually obscured by the granules in stained blood smears, but its characteristics are evident in electron micrographs (Fig. 9.11). Heterochromatin is chiefly in a peripheral location, and euchromatin is chiefly centrally located; typical cytoplasmic organelles are sparse. The basophil plasma membrane possesses numerous F_c receptors for immunoglobulin E (IgE) antibodies. In addition, a specific 39-kDa protein called CD40L is expressed on the basophil's surface. CD40L interacts with a complementary receptor (CD40) on B lymphocytes, which results in increased synthesis of IgE.

The basophil cytoplasm contains two types of granules: specific granules that are larger than the specific granules of the neutrophil and nonspecific azurophilic granules.

- ***Specific granules*** exhibit a grainy texture and myelin figures when viewed with the TEM. These granules contain a variety of substances, namely, ***heparan sulfate, histamine,*** and ***SRS-A.*** Histamine and the SRS-A are vasoactive agents that, among other actions, cause dilation of small blood vessels. Heparan sulfate is a sulfated glycosaminoglycan that is closely related to the heparin found in the granules of tissue mast cells. The amount of sulfate in this molecule accounts for the intense basophilia of the specific granules of the basophil. No role for heparan sulfate in inflammation has yet been elucidated.
- ***Azurophilic granules*** are the lysosomes of basophils and contain a variety of the usual lysosomal acid hydrolases similar to those in other leukocytes.

The function of basophils is closely related to that of mast cells

Basophils are functionally related to, but not identical with, mast cells of the connective tissue (see Table 5.6). Both mast cells and basophils bind an antibody secreted by plasma cells, IgE, through F_c receptors expressed on their cell surface. The subsequent exposure to, and reaction with, the antigen specific for IgE triggers the release of vasoactive agents from the basophil and mast cell granules. These substances are responsible for the severe vascular disturbances associated with hypersensitivity and anaphylaxis. Furthermore, both basophils and mast cells are derived from the same hemopoietic stem cell. Precursors of

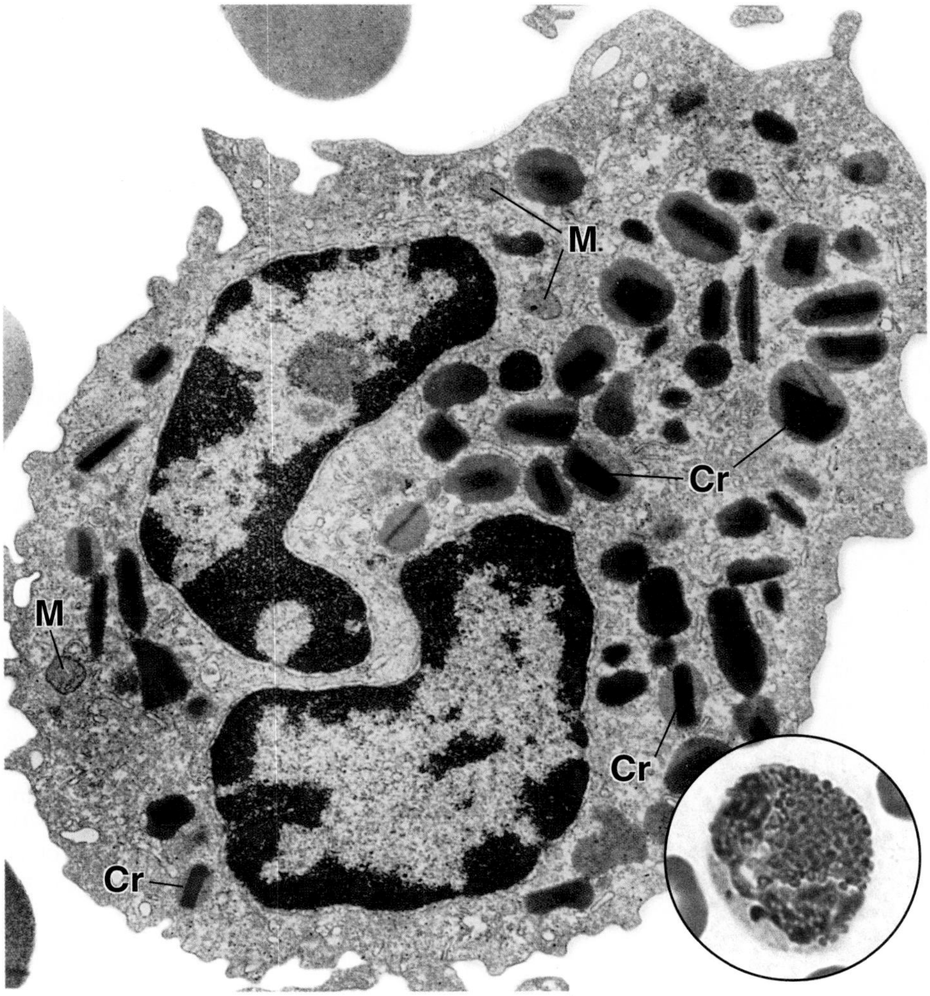

FIGURE 9.10
Electron micrograph of a human eosinophil. The nucleus is bilobed, but the connecting segment is not within the plane of section. The granules are of moderate size, compared with those of the basophil, and show a crystalline body *(Cr)* within the less electron-dense matrix of the granule. *M,* mitochondria. ×26,000. (Courtesy of Dr. Dorothea Zucker-Franklin.) **Inset.** Light microscopic image of an eosinophil from a blood smear. ×1,800.

mast cells are present in blood but do not develop until they leave the circulation and lodge in tissue sites.

Lymphocytes

Lymphocytes are the main functional cells of the lymphatic or immune system

Lymphocytes are the most common agranulocytes and account for about 30% of the total blood leukocytes. In understanding the function of the lymphocytes, one must realize that most lymphocytes found in blood or lymph represent recirculating ***immunocompetent cells,*** i.e., cells that have developed the capacity to recognize and respond to antigens and are in transit from one lymphatic tissue to another. In the tissues associated with the ***immune system*** (Chapter 13), three groups of lymphocytes can be identified according to size: small, medium, and large lymphocytes, ranging in diameter from 6 to 30 μm. The large lymphocytes are either activated lymphocytes, which possess surface receptors that interact with a specific antigen, or natural killer (NK) lymphocytes (see below). In the bloodstream, most lymphocytes are small or medium sized, 6 to 15 μm in diameter. The majority—more than 90%—are small lymphocytes.

In blood smears, the small lymphocyte approximates the size of a erythrocyte

When observed in the light microscope in a blood smear, the small lymphocyte has an intensely staining, slightly indented, spherical nucleus. The cytoplasm appears as a very thin, pale blue rim surrounding the nucleus. In general, there are no recognizable cytoplasmic organelles, other than an occasional fine azurophilic granule. The TEM reveals that the cytoplasm primarily contains free ribosomes and a few mitochondria. Other organelles are so sparse that they are usually not seen in a thin section. Small, dense lysosomes that correspond to the azurophilic granules seen in the light microscope are occasionally observed; a pair of centrioles and a small Golgi apparatus are located in the cell center, the area of the indentation of the nucleus.

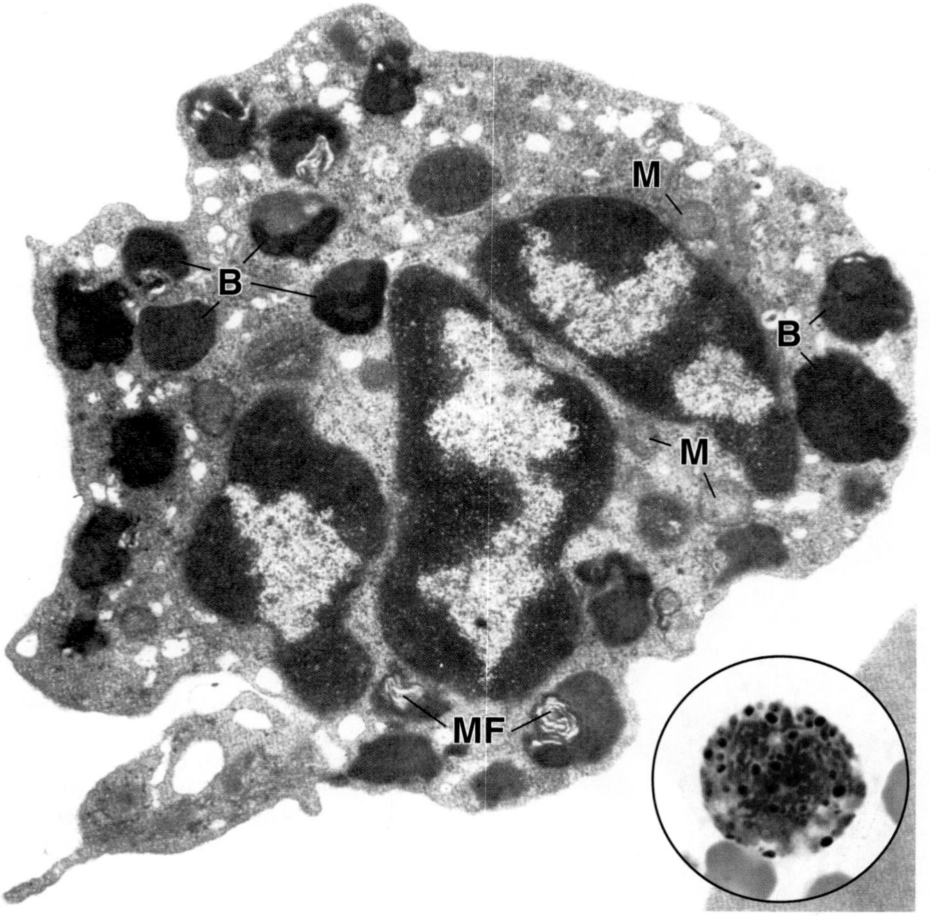

FIGURE 9.11
Electron micrograph of a human basophil. The nucleus appears as three separate bodies; the connecting strands are not in the plane of section. The basophil granules *(B)* are very large and irregularly shaped. Some granules reveal myelin figures *(MF)*. M, mitochondria. ×26,000. (Courtesy of Dr. Dorothea Zucker-Franklin.) **Inset.** Light microscopic appearance of a basophil from a blood smear. ×1,800.

In the medium lymphocyte, the cytoplasm is more abundant, the nucleus is larger and less heterochromatic, and the Golgi apparatus is somewhat more developed (Fig. 9.12). Greater numbers of mitochondria and polysomes and small profiles of rough endoplasmic reticulum are also seen in these medium-sized cells. The ribosomes are the basis for the slight basophilia displayed by lymphocytes in stained blood smears.

Three functionally distinct types of lymphocytes are present in the body: T lymphocytes, B lymphocytes, and NK cells

The characterization of lymphocyte types is based on their function, not on their size or morphology. ***T lymphocytes (T cells)*** are so named because they undergo differentiation in the thymus. ***B lymphocytes (B cells)*** are so named because they were first recognized as a separate population in the bursa of Fabricius in birds or bursa-equivalent organs (e.g., bone marrow) in mammals. ***NK*** cells develop from the same precursor cell as B and T cells and are so named because they are programmed to kill certain types of transformed cells.

- ***T cells*** have a long life span and are involved in cell-mediated immunity. They express CD2, CD3, and CD7 marker proteins on their surface; however, they are subclassified on the basis of the presence or absence of CD4 and CD8 proteins. $CD4^{+}$ T lymphocytes possess the CD4 marker and recognize antigens bound to major histocompatability complex II (MHC II) molecules. $CD8^{+}$ T lymphocytes possess the CD8 marker and recognize antigen bound to MHC I molecules.
- ***B cells*** have variable life spans and are involved in the production of circulating antibodies. Mature B cells in blood express IgM and IgD on their surface as well as MHC II molecules. Their specific markers are CD9, CD19, CD20, and CD24.
- ***NK cells*** are programmed during their development to kill certain virus-infected cells and some types of tumor cells. NK cells are larger than B and T cells (~15 μm in diameter) and have a kidney-shaped nucleus. Because NK cells have several large cytoplasmic granules easily seen by light microscopy, they are also called large granular lymphocytes (LGLs). Their specific markers include CD16, CD56, and CD94.

T and B cells are indistinguishable in blood smears and tissue sections; immunocytochemical staining for different types of markers and receptors on their cell surface must be used to identify them (see below). NK lymphocytes can be identified in the light microscope by size, nuclear shape, and presence of cytoplasmic granules; however, immunocytochemical staining for their specific markers is used to confirm microscopic identification.

T and B lymphocytes express different surface molecules

Although the T and B cells cannot be distinguished on the basis of their morphology, their distinctive surface proteins (CD proteins) can be used to identify the cells with immunolabeling techniques. In addition, immunoglobulin molecules (antibodies) are expressed on the surface of B cells that function as antigen receptors. In contrast, T cells do not have antibodies but express unique cell surface recognition proteins called T cell receptors (TCRs). These recognition proteins appear during discrete stages in the maturation of the cells within the thymus. In general, the surface molecules mediate or augment specific T cell functions and are required for the recognition or binding of T cells to antigens displayed on the surface of target cells.

In human blood, approximately 60 to 80% of the lymphocytes are mature T cells, and 20 to 30% are mature B cells. Approximately 5 to 10% of the cells do not demonstrate the surface markers associated with either T or B cells. These are NK cells and the rare circulating hemopoietic stem cells (see below). The size differences described above may have functional significance; some of the large lymphocytes may be cells that have been stimulated to divide, whereas others may be plasma cell precursors that are undergoing differentiation in response to the presence of antigen.

Three fundamentally different types of T lymphocytes have been identified: cytotoxic, helper, and suppressor

The activities of cytotoxic, helper, and suppressor T lymphocytes are mediated by molecules located on their surface. Immunolabeling techniques have made it possible to identify specific types of T cells and study their function.

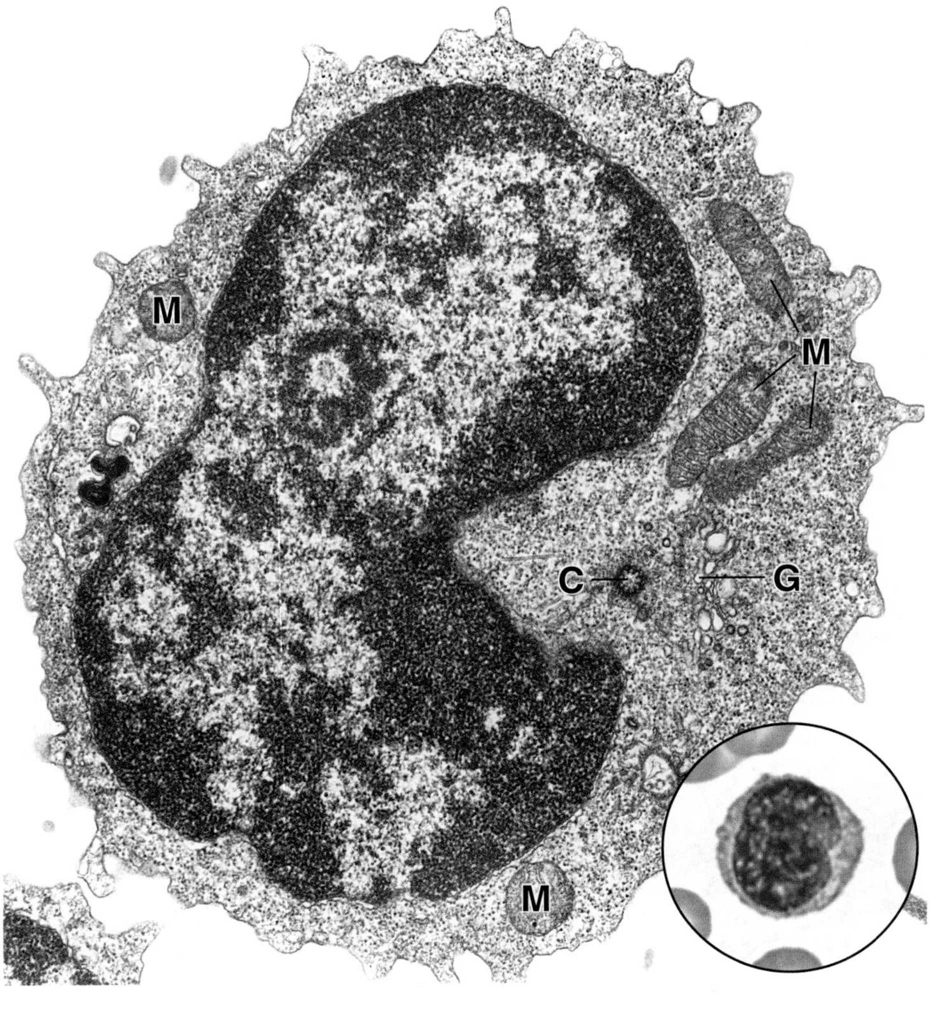

FIGURE 9.12
Electron micrograph of a medium-sized lymphocyte. The punctate appearance of the cytoplasm is due to the presence of numerous free ribosomes. Several mitochondria *(M)* are evident. The cell center or centrosphere region of the cell (the area of the nuclear indentation) also shows a small Golgi apparatus *(G)* and a centriole *(C)*. ×26,000. (Courtesy of Dr. Dorothea Zucker-Franklin.) **Inset.** Light microscopic appearance of a medium-sized lymphocyte from a blood smear. ×1,800.

- ***Cytotoxic CD8⁺ T lymphocytes*** serve as the primary effector cells in cell-mediated immunity. $CD8^+$ cells are specifically sensitized T lymphocytes that recognize antigens through the TCRs on host cells that are infected with viruses or have become neoplastic. Cytotoxic $CD8^+$ T lymphocytes only recognize antigens bound to MHC I molecules. After the TCR binds the antigen–MHC I complex, the cytotoxic $CD8^+$ T lymphocyte secretes lymphokines and perforins that produce ion channels in the membrane of the infected or neoplastic cell, leading to its lysis (see Chapter 13). Cytotoxic $CD8^+$ T lymphocytes play a significant role in rejection of allografts and in tumor immunology.
- ***Helper $CD4^+$ T lymphocytes*** are critical for induction of an immune response to a foreign antigen. Antigen bound to MHC II molecules is presented by antigen-presenting cells such as macrophages to a helper $CD4^+$ T lymphocyte. Binding of the TCR to the antigen–MHC II complex activates the helper $CD4^+$ T lymphocyte. The activated helper $CD4^+$ T lymphocyte then produces interleukins (mainly IL-2), which act in an autocrine mode to simulate the proliferation and differentiation of more helper $CD4^+$ T lymphocytes. Newly differentiated cells synthesize and secrete lymphokines that affect function as well as differentiation of B cells, T cells, and NK cells. B cells differentiate into plasma cells and synthesize antibody.
- ***Suppressor and/or cytotoxic $CD8^+$, $CD45RA^+$, T lymphocytes*** diminish or suppress antibody formation by B cells. They also downregulate the ability of T lymphocytes to initiate a cellular immune response. The suppressor and/or cytotoxic T cells may also function in the regulation of erythroid cell maturation in the bone marrow.

Monocytes

Monocytes are the precursors of the cells of the mononuclear phagocytotic system

Monocytes are the largest of the WBCs in a blood smear (average diameter, 18 µm). They travel from the bone marrow to the body tissues, where they differentiate into the various phagocytes of the mononuclear phagocytotic system, i.e., connective tissue macrophages (histiocytes), osteoclasts, alveolar macrophages, perisinusoidal macrophages in the liver (Kupffer cells), and macrophages of lymph nodes, spleen, and bone marrow, among others (see Chapter 5). Monocytes remain in the blood for only about 3 days.

The nucleus of the monocyte is typically more indented than that of the lymphocyte (Fig. 9.13). The indentation is the site of the cell center where a well-developed Golgi apparatus and centrioles are located. Monocytes also contain smooth endoplasmic reticulum, rough endoplasmic reticulum, and small mitochondria. Although these cells are classified as agranular, they contain small, dense, azurophilic granules. These granules contain typical lysosomal enzymes similar to those found in the azurophilic granules of neutrophils.

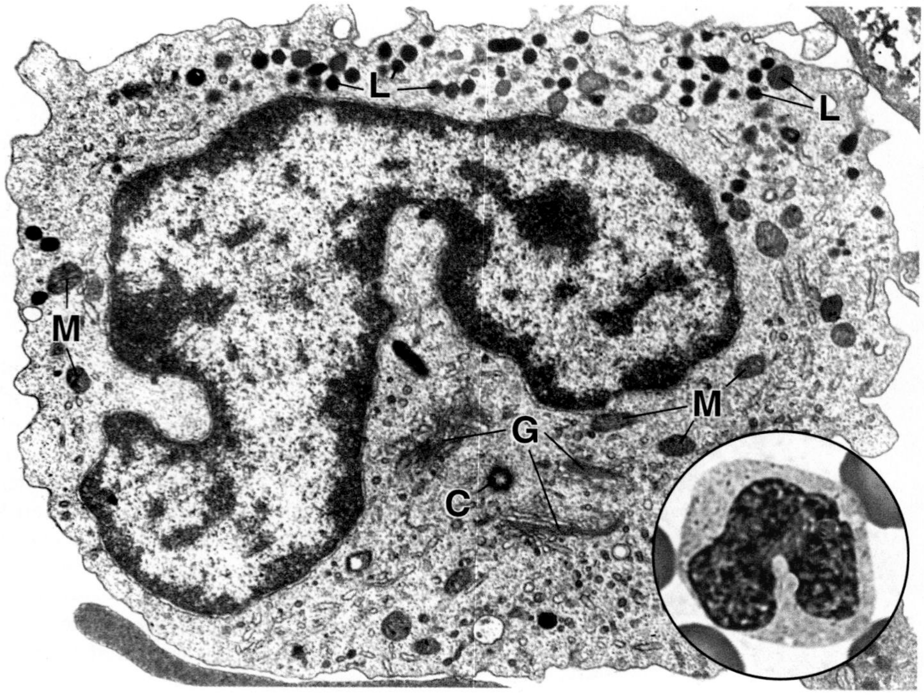

FIGURE 9.13
Electron micrograph of a human mature monocyte. The nucleus is markedly indented, and adjacent to this site, a centriole *(C)* and several Golgi profiles *(G)* are evident. The small dark granules are azurophilic granules, the lysosomes *(L)* of the cell. The slightly larger and less dense profiles are mitochondria *(M)*. ×22,000. (Courtesy of Dr. Dorothea Zucker-Franklin.) **Inset.** Light microscopic appearance of a monocyte from a blood smear. ×1,800.

Monocytes transform into macrophages, which function as antigen-presenting cells in the immune system

During inflammation, as indicated, the monocyte leaves the blood vessel at the site of inflammation, transforms into a tissue macrophage, and phagocytoses bacteria, other cells, and tissue debris. The monocyte-macrophage is an antigen-presenting cell and plays an important role in immune responses by partially degrading antigens and presenting their fragments on the MHC II molecules located on the macrophage surface to helper $CD4^+$ T lymphocytes for recognition.

▼ PLATELETS

Platelets are small, membrane-bounded, anucleate cytoplasmic fragments derived from megakaryocytes

Platelets are derived from large polyploid cells (cells whose nuclei contain multiple sets of chromosomes) in the bone marrow, called ***megakaryocytes*** (Fig. 9.14). In platelet formation, small bits of cytoplasm are separated from the peripheral regions of the megakaryocyte by extensive ***platelet demarcation channels.*** The membrane that

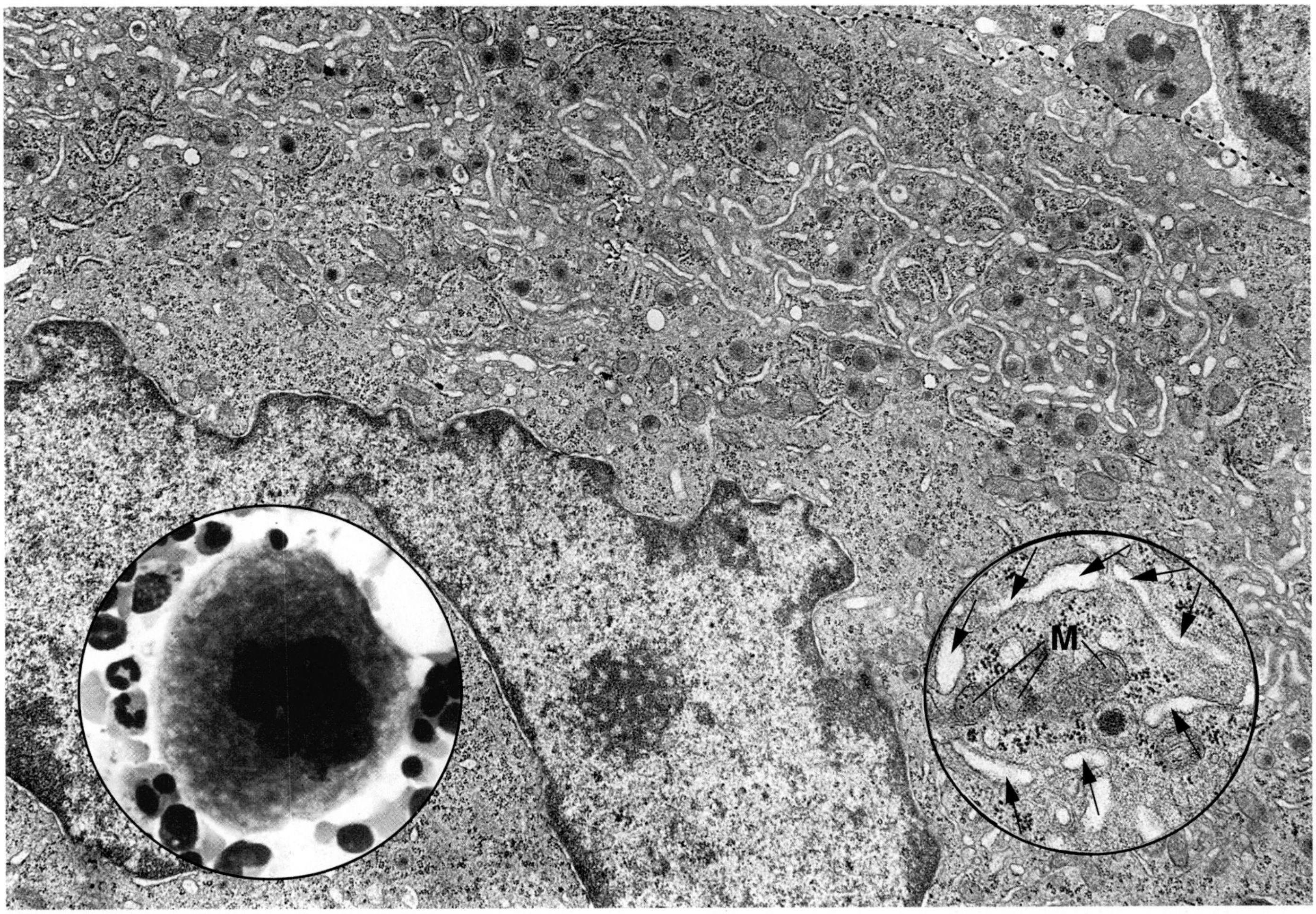

FIGURE 9.14
Electron and light micrographs of a megakaryocyte. This electron micrograph shows a portion of a megakaryocyte from a bone marrow section. Two lobes of the nucleus and the surrounding cytoplasm are visible. The cell border is indicated by the *dotted line* (upper right). The cytoplasm reveals evidence of platelet formation as indicated by the extensive platelet demarcation channels. ×13,000. **Left inset.** Light micrograph showing an entire megakaryocyte from a marrow smear. Its nucleus is multilobed and folded on itself, giving an irregular outline. The "foamy" peripheral cytoplasm of the megakaryocyte represents areas in which segmentation to form platelets is occurring. The smaller surrounding cells are developing blood cells. ×1,000. **Right inset.** Higher-power electron micrograph showing a section of cytoplasm that is almost fully partitioned by platelet demarcation channels *(arrows)*. It also shows mitochondria *(M)*, a very dense δ granule, and glycogen particles. For comparison, Figure 9.15a shows a mature circulating platelet. ×30,000.

lines these channels arises by invagination of the plasma membrane; therefore, the channels are in continuity with the extracellular space. The continued development and fusion of the platelet demarcation membranes result in the complete partitioning of cytoplasmic fragments to form individual platelets. Upon entry into the vascular system from the bone marrow, the platelets circulate as discoid structures about 2 to 3 μm in diameter. Their life span is about 10 days.

Structurally, platelets may be divided into four zones based on organization and function

The TEM reveals a structural organization of the platelet cytoplasm that can be categorized into four zones (Fig. 9.15):

- ***Peripheral zone.*** This zone consists of the cell membrane covered by a thick surface coat of glycocalyx. The glycocalyx consists of glycoproteins, glycosaminoglycans, and several coagulation factors adsorbed from the plasma. The integral membrane glycoproteins function as receptors in platelet function.
- ***Structural zone.*** This zone consists of microtubules, actin filaments, myosin, and actin-binding proteins that form a network supporting the plasma membrane. Approximately 8 to 24 microtubules reside as a bundle immediately below the actin filament network. They are circumferentially arranged and responsible for maintaining the platelet's disk shape.
- ***Organelle zone.*** This zone occupies the center of the platelet. It consists of mitochondria, peroxisomes, glycogen particles, and at least three types of granules dispersed within the cytoplasm. The most numerous granules are ***α granules*** (300 to 500 nm in diameter), which contain mainly fibrinogen, coagulation factors, plasminogen, plasminogen activator inhibitor, and platelet-

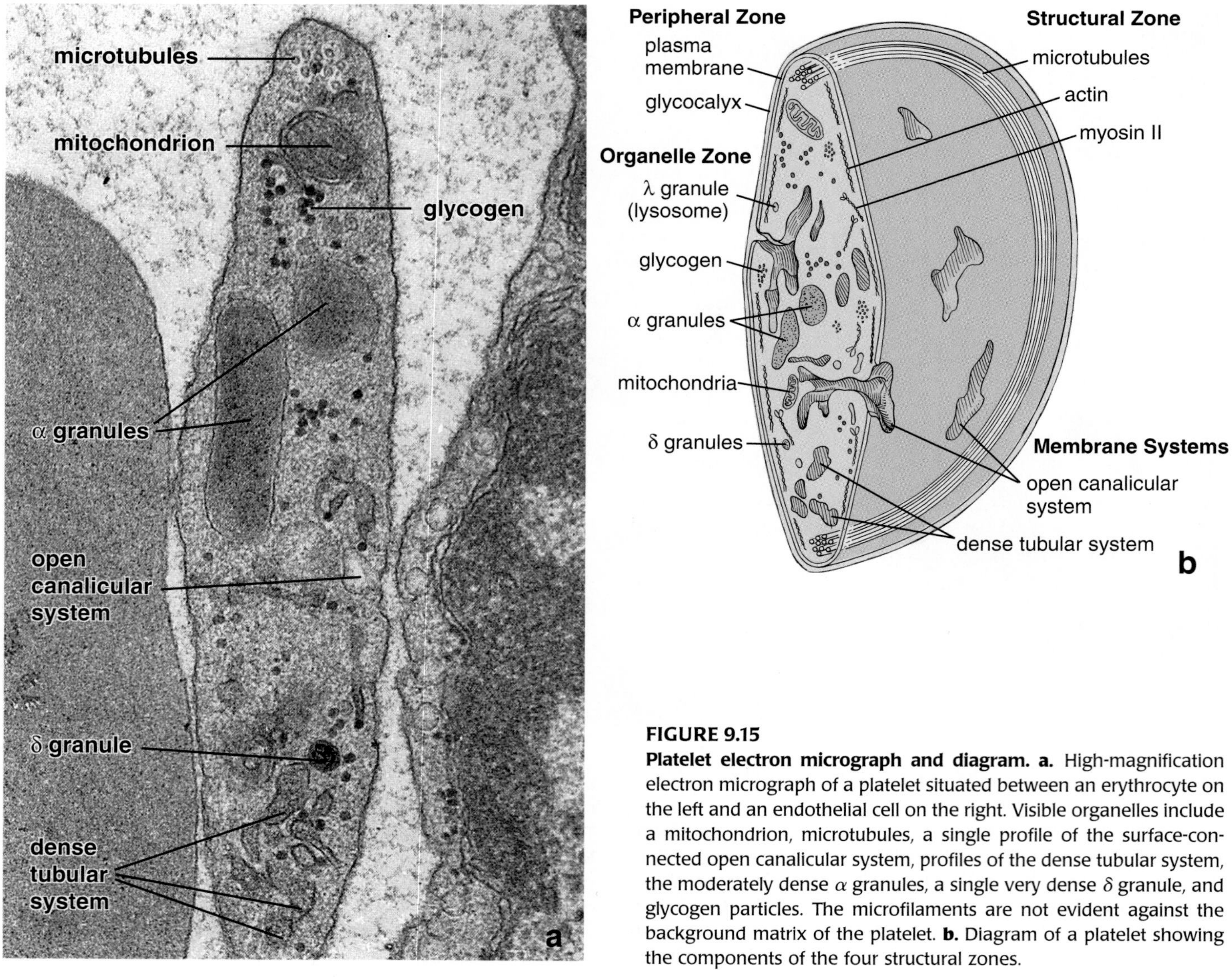

FIGURE 9.15
Platelet electron micrograph and diagram. a. High-magnification electron micrograph of a platelet situated between an erythrocyte on the left and an endothelial cell on the right. Visible organelles include a mitochondrion, microtubules, a single profile of the surface-connected open canalicular system, profiles of the dense tubular system, the moderately dense α granules, a single very dense δ granule, and glycogen particles. The microfilaments are not evident against the background matrix of the platelet. **b.** Diagram of a platelet showing the components of the four structural zones.

derived growth factor. The contents of these granules play an important role in the initial phase of vessel repair, blood coagulation, and platelet aggregation. The smaller, denser, and less numerous ***δ granules*** mainly contain adenosine diphosphate, adenosine triphosphate, serotonin, and histamine, which facilitate platelet adhesion and vasoconstriction in the area of the injured vessel. The ***λ granules*** are similar to lysosomes found in other cells and contain several hydrolytic enzymes. The contents of λ granules function in clot resorption during the later stages of vessel repair.

- *Membrane zone.* This zone consists of two types of membrane channels. The ***open canalicular system (OCS)*** is the first type of membrane channel. The OCS is a developmental remnant of the platelet demarcation channels and is simply membrane that did not participate in subdividing the megakaryocyte cytoplasm. In effect, they are invaginations into the cytoplasm from the plasma membrane. The ***dense tubular system (DTS)*** is the second type of membrane channel. The DTS contains an electron-dense material originating from the rough endoplasmic reticulum of the megakaryocyte, which serves as a storage site for calcium ions. DTS channels do not connect with the surface of the platelet; however, both the OCS and DTS fuse in various areas of the platelet to form membrane complexes that are important in regulation of the intraplatelet calcium concentration.

Platelets function in continuous surveillance of blood vessels, blood clot formation, and repair of injured tissue

Platelets are involved in several aspect of hemostasis. They continuously survey the endothelial lining of blood vessels for gaps and breaks. When a blood vessel wall is injured or broken, platelets adhere to the exposed connective tissue at the damaged site. The adhesion of the platelets triggers a complex process that results in aggregation of platelets into a clot called a ***primary hemostatic platelet plug.*** Extravasation of blood is then stopped by the mass of aggregated platelets. The glycocalyx of the platelets provides a reaction surface for the conversion of soluble fibrinogen into fibrin, which stabilizes the initial plug. At the same time, the activated platelets release their α and δ granules, which contain among other substances coagulation factors and serotonin. Serotonin is a potent vasoconstrictor that causes the vascular smooth muscle cells to contract, thereby reducing local blood flow at the site of injury. In addition, tissue factors secreted by the damaged blood vessel cells aid in the formation of a definitive clot known as a ***secondary hemostatic plug.***

After the definitive clot is formed, platelets cause clot retraction, probably as a function of the actin and myosin found in the structural zone of the platelet. Contraction of the clot permits the return of normal blood flow through the vessel. Finally, after the clot has served its function, it is lysed by plasmin, a fibrinolytic enzyme that circulates in the plasma in an inactive form known as plasminogen. The hydrolytic enzymes released from the λ granules assist in this process. The activator for plasminogen conversion, ***tissue plasminogen activator (TPA),*** is derived principally from endothelial cells. It is currently used as an emergency treatment to minimize the damage caused by strokes due to clots.

An additional role of platelets is to help repair the injured tissues beyond the vessel itself. Platelet-derived growth factor released from the α granules stimulates smooth muscle cells and fibroblasts to divide and allow tissue repair.

▽ FORMATION OF BLOOD CELLS (HEMOPOIESIS)

Hemopoiesis (hematopoiesis) includes both ***erythropoiesis*** and ***leukopoiesis,*** as well as ***thrombopoiesis*** (development of platelets) (Table 9.4). Blood cells have a limited life span; they are continuously produced and destroyed. Both the human erythrocyte (life span of 120 days) and the platelet (life span of 10 days) spend their entire life in the circulating blood. WBCs, however, migrate out of the circulation shortly after entering it from the bone marrow and spend most of their variable life spans (and perform all of their functions) in the tissues.

In the adult, erythrocytes, granulocytes, monocytes, and platelets are formed in the red bone marrow; lymphocytes are also formed in the red bone marrow and in the lymphatic tissues. To study the stages of blood cell formation, a sample of bone marrow is prepared as a stained smear in a manner similar to that described on page 216 for the preparation of a smear of blood.

Hemopoiesis is initiated in early embryonic development

During fetal life, both erythrocytes and leukocytes are formed in several organs before the differentiation of the bone marrow. The first or ***yolk sac phase*** of hemopoiesis begins in the third week of gestation and is characterized by the formation of ***"blood islands"*** in the wall of the yolk sac of the embryo. In the second or ***hepatic phase,*** early in fetal development, hemopoietic centers appear in the liver (Fig. 9.16). Blood cell formation in these sites is largely limited to erythroid cells, although some leukopoiesis occurs in the liver. The liver is the major blood-forming organ in the fetus during the second trimester. The third or ***bone marrow phase*** of fetal hemopoiesis and leukopoiesis involves the bone marrow (and other lymphatic tissues) and begins in the second trimester of pregnancy. After birth, hemopoiesis takes place only in the red bone marrow and lymphatic tissues, as in the adult (Fig. 9.17). The precursors of both the blood cells and germ cells arise in the yolk sac.

TABLE 9.4. **Hemopoiesis**[A]

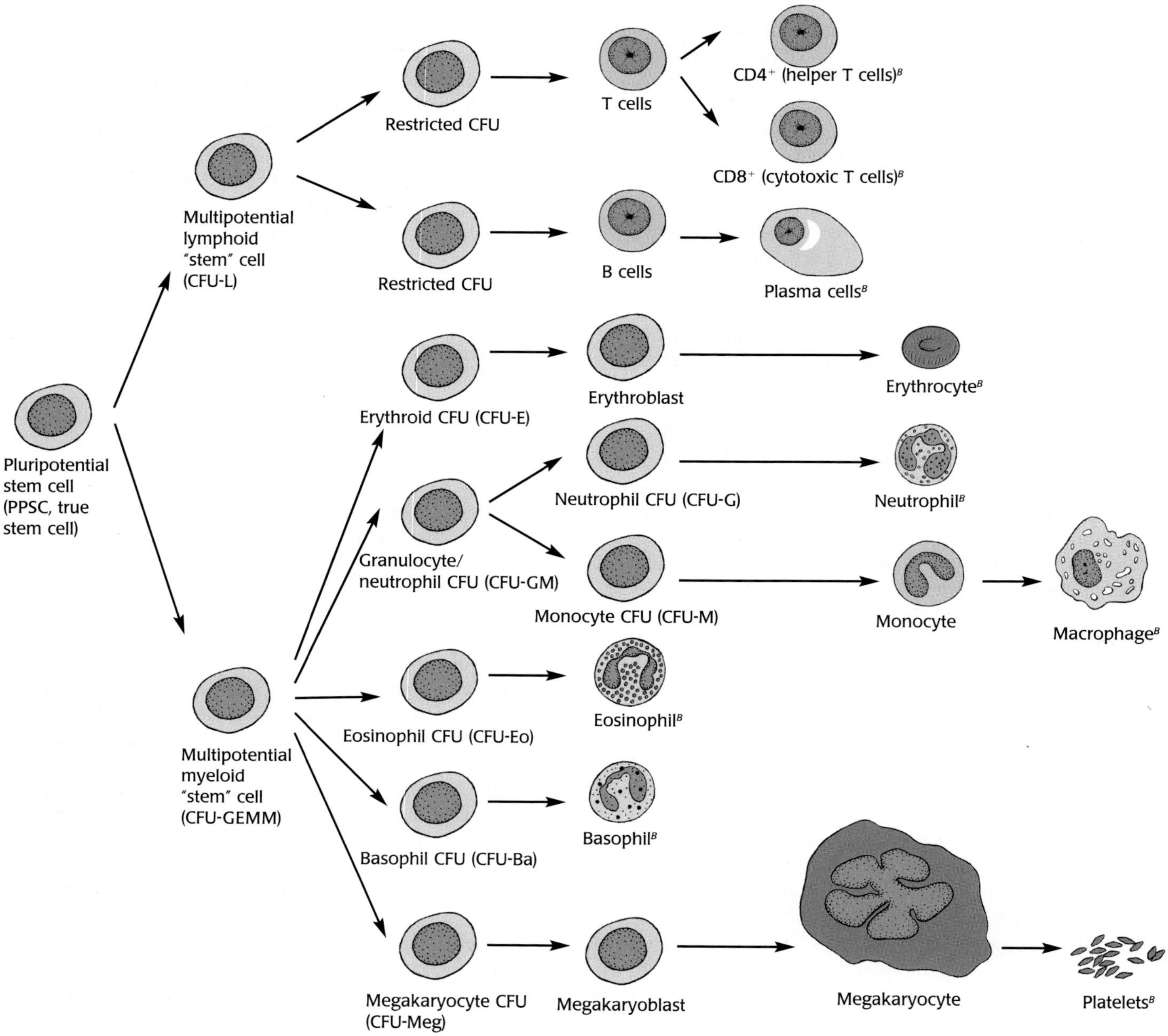

[A]This table includes the most recent concepts of a pluripotential stem cell, multipotential colony-forming units (CFUs), and restricted CFUs. Cytokines (including hemopoietic growth factors) may and do act individually and severally at any point in the process from the first stem cell to the mature blood or connective tissue cell.

[B]Mature functional cells in blood, bone marrow, or connective tissue.

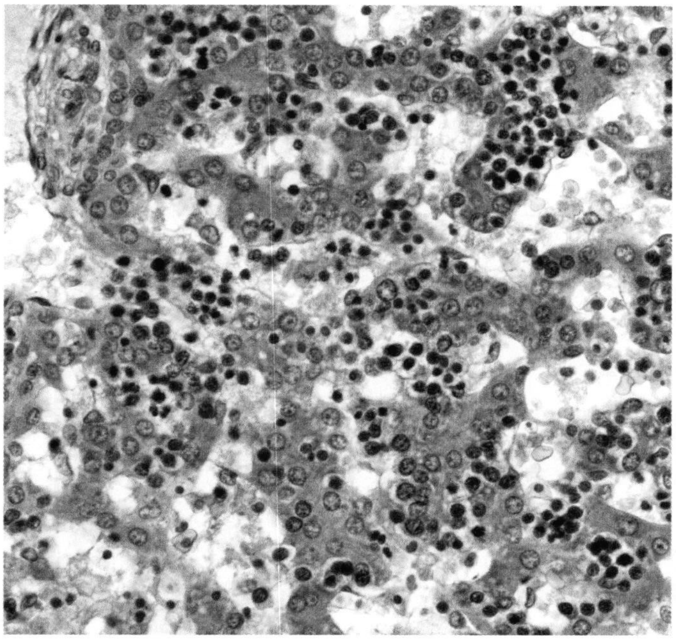

FIGURE 9.16
Hepatic stage of hemopoiesis. Photomicrograph of the fetal liver stained with H&E shows active hemopoiesis. The small round bodies are mostly nuclei of developing erythrocytes. Although it is difficult to discern, these cells are located between developing liver cells and the wall of the vascular sinus. ×350.

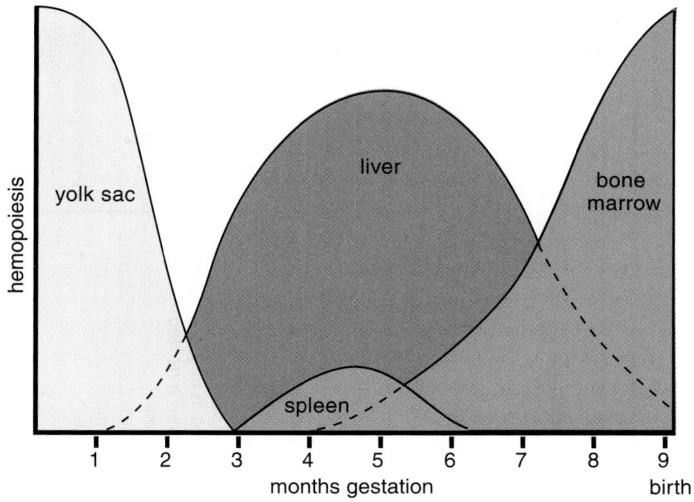

FIGURE 9.17
Dynamics of hemopoiesis in embryonic and fetal life. During embryonic and fetal life, erythrocytes are formed in several organs. Essentially, three major organs involved in hemopoiesis can be sequentially identified: the yolk sac in the early developmental stages of the embryo; the liver during the second trimester of pregnancy; and the bone marrow during the third trimester. The spleen participates to a very limited degree during the second trimester of pregnancy. At birth, most hemopoiesis occurs in the red bone marrow, as in the adult.

Monophyletic Theory of Hemopoiesis

According to the monophyletic theory of hemopoiesis, blood cells are derived from a common stem cell

Considerable circumstantial evidence has for many years supported the ***monophyletic (or unitarian) theory of hemopoiesis,*** in which all blood cells arise from a common stem cell. This theory is in contrast to the polyphyletic theory, in which each blood cell type has its own stem cell. Decisive evidence for the validity of the monophyletic theory has come with the isolation and demonstration of the ***pluripotential stem cell (PPSC),*** a descriptive term used to identify the hemopoietic stem cell that gives rise to all other progenitor stem cells. These progenitor stem cells are defined by the presence of the $CD34^+$ surface marker protein. PPSCs are not identifiable in the microscope.

A PPSC gives rise to multiple colony-forming units (CFUs)

As noted above, PPSC is a term used to designate the basic cell in hemopoiesis. Descendants of this cell differentiate into CFU-GEMM, the multipotential myeloid stem cell, and CFU-L, the multipotential lymphoid stem cell. Ultimately, CFU-GEMM differentiates into specific lineage progenitors: CFU-E, a cell that gives rise to the erythrocyte lineage; CFU-GM, a cell that gives rise to the neutrophilic granulocyte and monocyte lineages; CFU-Eo, a cell that gives rise to eosinophils; CFU-Ba, a cell that gives rise to basophils; and CFU-Meg, a cell that gives rise to megakaryocytes. (Table 9.5). The PPSC is not only capable of differentiating into all the blood cell lineages but it is also capable of self-renewal; i.e., the pool of stem cells is self-sustaining.

Perhaps the easiest way to begin the histologic study of blood cell development is to refer to the illustration in Figure 9.18. This figure shows the stages of blood cell development in which characteristic cell types can be identified in the light microscope in a tissue section or bone marrow smear. Hemopoiesis is initiated in an apparent random manner when individual stem cells begin to differentiate into one of the blood cell lineages. Stem cells have surface receptors for specific cytokines and growth factors that influence and direct their proliferation and maturation into a specific lineage.

Development of Erythrocytes (Erythropoiesis)

Erythrocytes develop from the multipotential myeloid stem cell (CFU-GEMM) under the influence of erythropoietin, GM-CSF, IL-3, and IL-4. The erythropoietin-sensitive erythrocyte progenitor cell CFU-E gives rise to the

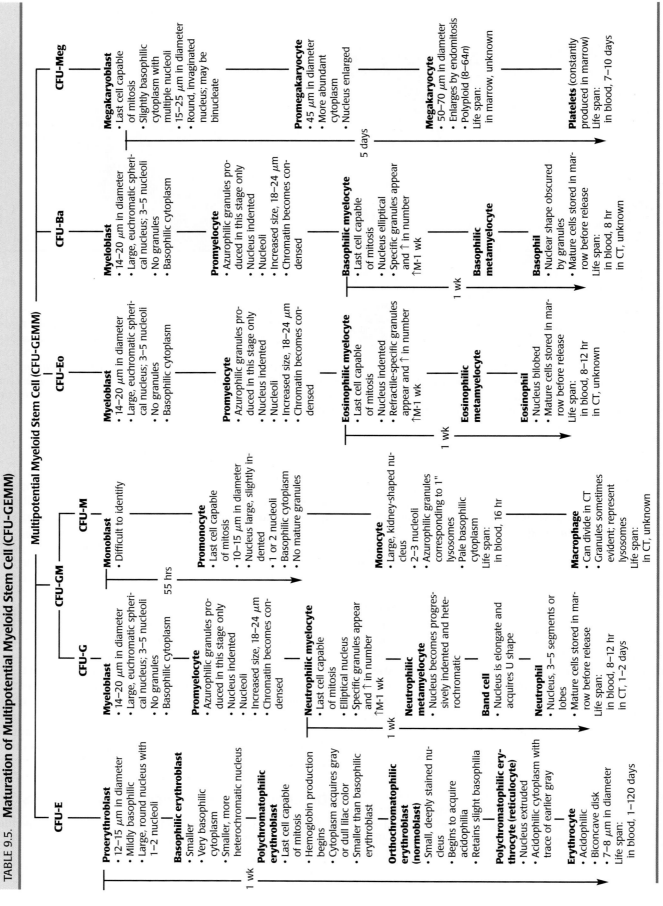

TABLE 9.5. **Maturation of Multipotential Myeloid Stem Cell (CFU-GEMM)**

Multipotential Myeloid Stem Cell (CFU-GEMM)

CFU-E (1 wk)

Proerythroblast
- 12–15 μm in diameter
- Mildly basophilic
- Large, round nucleus with 1–2 nucleoli

Basophilic erythroblast
- Smaller
- Very basophilic cytoplasm
- Smaller, more heterochromatic nucleus

Polychromatophilic erythroblast
- Last cell capable of mitosis
- Hemoglobin production begins
- Cytoplasm acquires gray or dull lilac color
- Smaller than basophilic erythroblast

Orthochromatophilic erythroblast (normoblast)
- Small, deeply stained nucleus
- Begins to acquire acidophilia
- Retains slight basophilia

Polychromatophilic erythrocyte (reticulocyte)
- Nucleus extruded
- Acidophilic cytoplasm with trace of earlier gray

Erythrocyte
- Acidophilic
- Biconcave disk
- 7–8 μm in diameter

Life span:
in blood, 1–120 days

CFU-GM

CFU-G

Myeloblast
- 14–20 μm in diameter
- Large, euchromatic spherical nucleus; 3–5 nucleoli
- No granules
- Basophilic cytoplasm

Promyelocyte
- Azurophilic granules produced in this stage only
- Nucleus indented
- Nucleoli
- Increased size, 18–24 μm
- Chromatin becomes condensed

(1 wk)

Neutrophilic myelocyte
- Last cell capable of mitosis
- Elliptical nucleus
- Specific granules appear and ↑ in number

↑M-1 wk

Neutrophilic metamyelocyte
- Nucleus becomes progressively indented and heterochromatic

Band cell
- Nucleus is elongate and acquires U shape

Neutrophil
- Nucleus, 3–5 segments or lobes
- Mature cells stored in marrow before release

Life span:
in blood, 8–12 hr
in CT, 1–2 days

CFU-M

(55 hrs)

Monoblast
- Difficult to identify

Promonocyte
- Last cell capable of mitosis
- 10–15 μm in diameter
- Nucleus large, slightly indented
- 1 or 2 nucleoli
- Basophilic cytoplasm
- No mature granules

Monocyte
- Large, kidney-shaped nucleus
- 2–3 nucleoli
- Azurophilic granules corresponding to 1" lysosomes
- Pale basophilic cytoplasm

Life span:
in blood, 16 hr

Macrophage
- Can divide in CT
- Granules sometimes evident; represent lysosomes

Life span:
in CT, unknown

CFU-Eo

Myeloblast
- 14–20 μm in diameter
- Large, euchromatic spherical nucleus; 3–5 nucleoli
- No granules
- Basophilic cytoplasm

Promyelocyte
- Azurophilic granules produced in this stage only
- Nucleus indented
- Nucleoli
- Increased size, 18–24 μm
- Chromatin becomes condensed

(1 wk)

Eosinophilic myelocyte
- Last cell capable of mitosis
- Nucleus indented
- Refractile-specific granules appear and ↑ in number

↑M-1 wk

Eosinophilic metamyelocyte

Eosinophil
- Nucleus bilobed
- Mature cells stored in marrow before release

Life span:
in blood, 8–12 hr
in CT, unknown

CFU-Ba

Myeloblast
- 14–20 μm in diameter
- Large, euchromatic spherical nucleus; 3–5 nucleoli
- No granules
- Basophilic cytoplasm

Promyelocyte
- Azurophilic granules produced in this stage only
- Nucleus indented
- Nucleoli
- Increased size, 18–24 μm
- Chromatin becomes condensed

(1 wk)

Basophilic myelocyte
- Last cell capable of mitosis
- Nucleus elliptical
- Specific granules appear and ↑ in number

↑M-1 wk

Basophilic metamyelocyte

Basophil
- Nuclear shape obscured by granules
- Mature cells stored in marrow before release

Life span:
in blood, 8 hr
in CT, unknown

CFU-Meg

(5 days)

Megakaryoblast
- Last cell capable of mitosis
- Slightly basophilic cytoplasm with multiple nucleoli
- 15–25 μm in diameter
- Round, invaginated nucleus; may be binucleate

Promegakaryocyte
- 45 μm in diameter
- More abundant cytoplasm
- Nucleus enlarged

Megakaryocyte
- 50–70 μm in diameter
- Enlarges by endomitosis
- Polyploid (8–64*n*)

Life span:
in marrow, unknown

Platelets (constantly produced in marrow)

Life span:
in blood, 7–10 days

This table summarizes the maturation of blood cells with histologic characteristics at the various stages, maturation time, and life span after leaving the marrow. Times indicated along vertical lines are the approximate time between recognizable stages. ↑M–1 wk indicates increase in number by mitosis for 1 week before differentiation begins. CT means connective tissue.

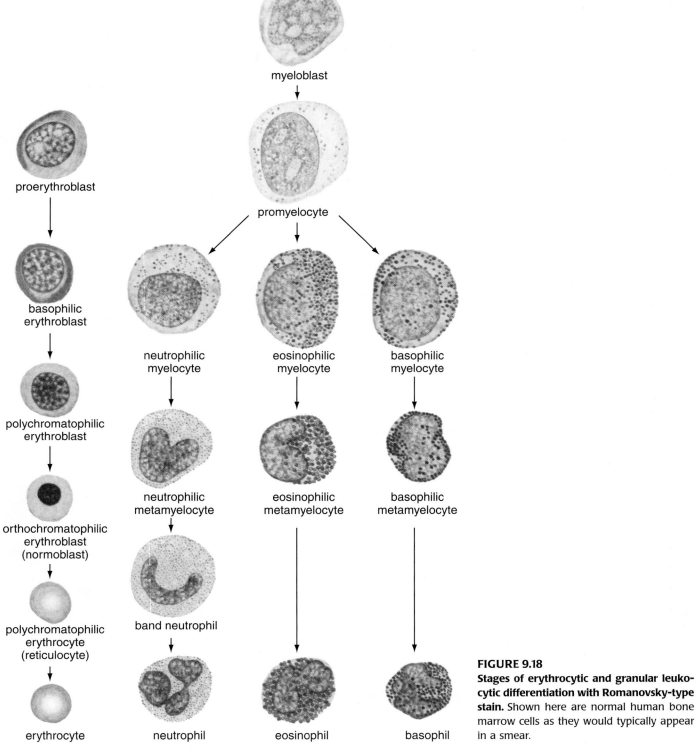

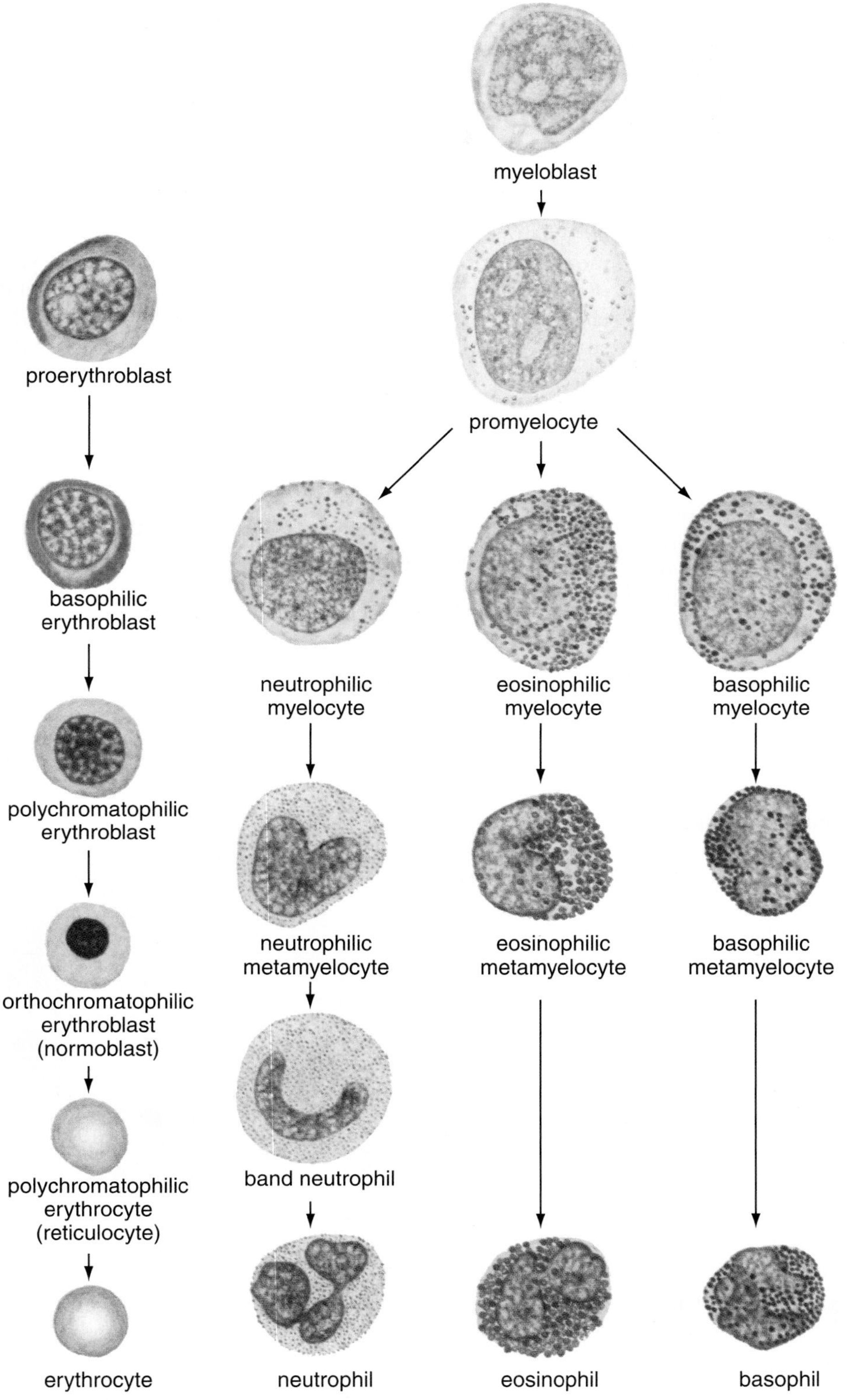

FIGURE 9.18
Stages of erythrocytic and granular leukocytic differentiation with Romanovsky-type stain. Shown here are normal human bone marrow cells as they would typically appear in a smear.

first recognizable erythrocyte precursor, the proerythroblast.

The first recognizable precursor cell in erythropoiesis is called the proerythroblast

The ***proerythroblast*** is a relatively large cell measuring 12 to 20 μm in diameter. It contains a large spherical nucleus with one or two visible nucleoli. The cytoplasm shows mild basophilia because of the presence of free ribosomes. Although recognizable, the proerythroblast is not easily identified in routine bone marrow smears.

The basophilic erythroblast is smaller than the proerythroblast, from which it arises by mitotic division

The nucleus of the ***basophilic erythroblast*** is smaller (10 to 16 µm in diameter) and progressively more heterochromatic with repeated mitoses. The cytoplasm shows strong basophilia because of the large number of free ribosomes (polyribosomes) that synthesize hemoglobin. The accumulation of hemoglobin in the cell gradually changes the staining reaction of the cytoplasm, so that it begins to stain with eosin. At the stage when the cytoplasm displays both acidophilia, because of the staining of hemoglobin, and basophilia, because of the staining of the ribosomes, the cell is called a polychromatophilic erythroblast.

The polychromatophilic erythroblast shows both acidophilic and basophilic staining of cytoplasm

The staining reactions of the ***polychromatophilic erythroblast*** may blend to give an overall gray or lilac color to the cytoplasm, or distinct pink (acidophilic) and purple (basophilic) regions may be resolved in the cytoplasm. The nucleus of the cell is smaller than that of the basophilic erythroblast, and coarse heterochromatin granules form a checkerboard pattern that helps identify this cell type.

The orthochromatophilic erythroblast is recognized by its increased acidophilic cytoplasm and dense nucleus

The next named stage in erythropoiesis is the ***orthochromatophilic erythroblast (normoblast).*** This cell has a small, compact, densely stained nucleus. The cytoplasm is eosinophilic because of the large amount of hemoglobin (Fig. 9.19). It is only slightly larger than a mature erythrocyte. At this stage, the orthochromatophilic erythroblast is no longer capable of division.

The polychromatophilic erythrocyte has extruded its nucleus

The orthochromatic erythroblast loses its nucleus by extruding it from the cell; it is then ready to pass into a blood sinus of the red bone marrow. Some polyribosomes that can still synthesize hemoglobin are retained in the cell. These polyribosomes impart a slight basophilia to the otherwise eosinophilic cells; for this reason, these new cells are called ***polychromatophilic erythrocytes*** (Fig. 9.20). The polyribosomes of the new erythrocytes can also be demonstrated with special stains that cause the polyribosomes to clump and form a reticular network. Consequently, polychromatophilic erythrocytes are also (and more commonly) called ***reticulocytes.*** In normal blood, reticulocytes (new erythrocytes) constitute about 1 to 2% of the total erythrocyte count. However, if increased numbers of erythrocytes enter the bloodstream (as during increased erythropoiesis to compensate for blood loss), the number of reticulocytes increases.

Kinetics of Erythropoiesis

Mitoses occur in proerythroblasts, basophilic erythroblasts, and polychromatophilic erythroblasts

At each of these stages of development, the erythroblast divides several times. It takes about a week for the progeny of a newly formed basophilic erythroblast to reach the cir-

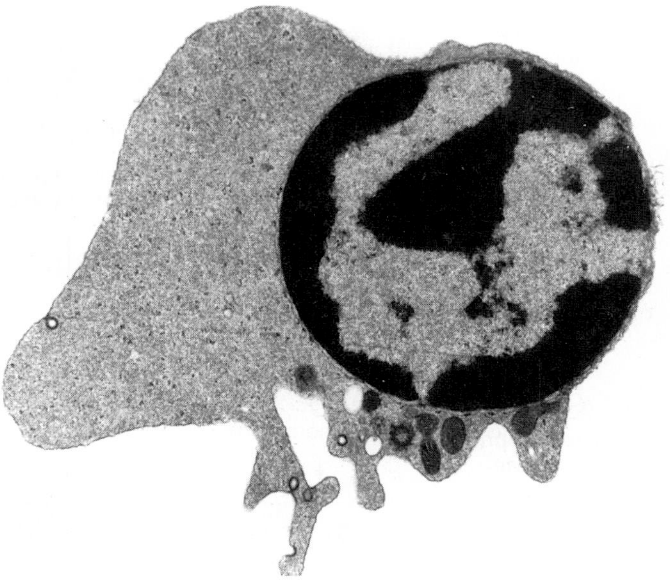

FIGURE 9.19
Electron micrograph of a orthochromatophilic erythroblast (normoblast). The cell is shown just before extrusion of the nucleus. The cytoplasm contains a group of mitochondria located below the nucleus and small cytoplasmic vacuoles. The cytoplasm is relatively dense because of its hemoglobin content. The fine, dense particles scattered in the cytoplasm are ribosomes. ×10,000. (Courtesy of Dr. Dorothea Zucker-Franklin.)

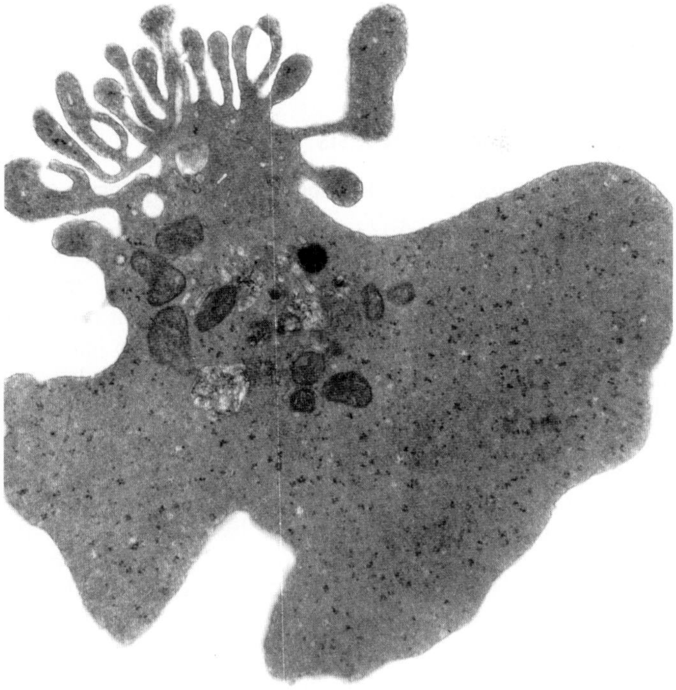

FIGURE 9.20
Electron micrograph of a polychromatophilic erythrocyte (reticulocyte). The nucleus is no longer present, and the cytoplasm shows the characteristic fimbriated processes that occur just after nuclear extrusion. Mitochondria are still present, as are early and late endosomes and ribosomes. ×16,500. (Courtesy of Dr. Dorothea Zucker-Franklin.)

culation. Nearly all erythrocytes are released into the circulation as soon as they are formed; bone marrow is not a storage site for erythrocytes. Erythrocyte formation and release are regulated by ***erythropoietin,*** a 34-kDa glycoprotein hormone synthesized and secreted by the kidney in response to decreased blood oxygen concentration. Erythropoietin acts on the specific receptors expressed on the surface of CFU-E.

Erythrocytes have a life span of about 120 days in humans

When erythrocytes are about 4 months old, they become senescent. The macrophage system of the spleen, bone marrow, and liver phagocytoses and degrades the senescent erythrocytes. The ***heme*** and ***globin*** dissociate, and the globin is hydrolyzed to amino acids, which enter the metabolic pool for reuse. The iron on the heme is released, enters the iron storage pool in the spleen in the form of ***hemosiderin*** or ***ferritin,*** and is stored for reuse in hemoglobin synthesis. The rest of the heme moiety of the hemoglobin molecule is partially degraded to ***bilirubin,*** bound to albumin, released into the bloodstream, and transported to the liver, where it is conjugated and excreted via the gallbladder as the ***bilirubin glucuronide*** of bile.

Development of Granulocytes (Granulopoiesis)

Neutrophils originate from the multipotential CFU-GEMM stem cell, which is induced to differentiate into CFU-GM by cytokines such as GM-CSF, G-CSF, and IL-3. The neutrophil undergoes six morphologically identifiable stages in the process of maturation: myeloblast, promyelocyte, myelocyte, metamyelocyte, band cell, and mature neutrophil. Eosinophils and basophils undergo a morphologic maturation similar to that of neutrophils. All three lineages originate from the multipotential CFU-GEMM cell. This cell is induced by GM-CSF, IL-3, and IL-5 to differentiate into CFU-Eo, which eventually matures into an eosinophil. Lack of IL-5 causes the stem cell to differentiate into CFU-Ba, which matures into a basophil. One cannot differentiate eosinophilic or basophilic precursors from neutrophilic precursors morphologically in the light microscope until the cells reach the myelocyte stage, when the specific granules appear.

Myeloblasts are the first recognizable cells that begin the process of granulopoiesis

The ***myeloblast*** is the earliest recognizable neutrophil precursor cell in the bone marrow. It has a large, euchromatic, spherical nucleus with 3 to 5 nucleoli. It measures 14 to 20 μm in diameter and has a large nuclear-to-cytoplasmic volume. The small amount of agranular cytoplasm stains intensely basophilic. A Golgi area is often seen where the cytoplasm is unstained. The myeloblast matures into a promyelocyte.

BOX 9.3

Clinical Correlations: Hemoglobin Breakdown and Jaundice

If the conjugation of bilirubin or its excretion into bile by the liver cells is inhibited, or if blockage of the bile duct system occurs, bilirubin may reenter the blood, causing a yellow appearance of the sclera of the eye and the skin. This condition is called ***jaundice.*** Jaundice can be caused by an increase in erythrocyte destruction, which is characteristic of ***hemolytic anemia.*** This condition results from either inherited defects in the erythrocyte (e.g., hereditary spherocytosis) or external factors such as pathogenic microorganisms, animal venoms, chemicals, or drugs. Some jaundice is common in newborn infants (physiologic jaundice) because of inefficiency of the bilirubin-conjugating system in the newborn liver.

Promyelocytes are the only cells to produce azurophilic granules

The *promyelocyte* has a large spherical nucleus with azurophilic (primary) granules in the cytoplasm. Azurophilic granules are produced only in promyelocytes; cells in subsequent stages of granulopoiesis do not make azurophilic granules. For this reason, the number of azurophilic granules is reduced with each division of the promyelocyte and its progeny. Promyelocytes do not exhibit subtypes. Recognition of the neutrophil, eosinophil, and basophil lines is possible only in the next stage, the myelocyte, when specific (secondary) and tertiary granules begin to form.

Myelocytes first exhibit specific granules

Myelocytes begin with a more or less spherical nucleus that becomes increasingly heterochromatic and acquires a distinct indentation during subsequent divisions. Specific granules begin to emerge from the convex surface of the Golgi apparatus, whereas azurophilic granules are seen at the concave side. The significance of this separation is unclear. Myelocytes continue to divide and give rise to metamyelocytes.

The metamyelocyte is the stage at which neutrophil, eosinophil, and basophil lines can be clearly identified by the presence of numerous specific granules

A few hundred granules are present in the cytoplasm of each metamyelocyte, and the specific granules of each variety outnumber the azurophilic granules. In the neutrophil, this ratio of specific to azurophilic granules is about 2 to 1. The nucleus becomes more heterochromatic, and the indentation deepens to form a kidney bean–shaped structure. Theoretically, the metamyelocyte stage in granulopoiesis is followed by the band stage and then the segmented stage. Although these stages are obvious in the neutrophil line (see below), they are rarely if ever observed in the eosinophil and basophil lines in which the next easily recognized stages of development are the *mature eosinophil* and *mature basophil,* respectively.

In the neutrophil line, the band (stab) cell precedes development of the first distinct nuclear lobes

The nucleus of the *band (stab) cell* is elongated and of nearly uniform width, giving it a horseshoe-like appearance. Nuclear constrictions then develop in the band neutrophil and become more prominent until two to four nuclear lobes are recognized; the cell is then considered a mature neutrophil, also called a *polymorphonuclear neutrophil (segmented neutrophil).* Although the percentage of band cells in the circulation is almost always low (0 to 3%), it may increase in acute or chronic inflammation and infection.

Kinetics of Granulopoiesis

Cell division in granulopoiesis stops by the late myelocyte stage

The mitotic phase in granulopoiesis lasts about a week. The postmitotic phase—from metamyelocyte to mature granulocyte—also lasts about a week. The time it takes for half of the circulating segmented neutrophils to leave the peripheral blood is about 6 to 8 hours. Neutrophils leave the blood randomly; i.e., a given neutrophil may circulate for only a few minutes or as long as 16 hours before entering the perivascular connective tissue.

Neutrophils live for 1 to 2 days in the connective tissue, after which they are destroyed by apoptosis and are subsequently engulfed by macrophages. Also, large numbers of neutrophils are lost via migration into the lumen of the gastrointestinal tract from which they are discharged with the feces. As a result of the release of neutrophils from the bone marrow, approximately 5 times as many mature and near-mature neutrophils are normally present in the bone marrow as are present in the circulation. This reserve pool constantly releases neutrophils into the circulation and is replenished by maturing cells. The reserve neutrophils can be released abruptly in response to inflammation, infection, or strenuous exercise. The entire hemopoietic process is summarized in Table 9.5.

A reservoir of neutrophils is also present in the vascular compartment. This reserve consists of a freely circulating pool and a marginated pool, with the latter contained in small blood vessels. The neutrophils adhere to the endothelium much as they do prior to leaving the vasculature at sites of injury or infection (see page 222). The normally marginated neutrophils, however, loosely adhere to the endothelium through the action of selectin and can be recruited very quickly. They are in dynamic equilibrium with the circulating pool.

Cytokines are glycoprotein hormones and stimulating factors that regulate all stages of hemopoiesis

In addition to identifying the various types of progenitor and precursor cells, recent studies have identified and begun to characterize numerous glycoproteins that act as both circulating hormones and local mediators to regulate hemopoiesis and the differentiation of specific cell types (Table 9.6). One factor, *erythropoietin,* discussed above, regulates erythrocyte development. Other factors, collectively called *colony-stimulating factors (CSFs),* are subclassified according to the specific cell or groups of cells that they affect. The most completely characterized of the

TABLE 9.6. **Hemopoietic Cytokines, Their Sources, and Target Cells**[A]

Cytokine	Symbol	Source	Target
Granulocyte–macrophage colony-stimulating factor	GM-CSF	T cells, endothelial cells, fibroblasts	CFU-GEMM, CFU-E, CFU-GM, CFU-Eo, CFU-Ba, CFU-Meg, all granulocytes, erythrocytes
Granulocyte colony-stimulating factor	G-CSF	Endothelial cells, monocytes	CFU-E, CFU-GM, CFU-Eo, CFU-Ba, CFU-Meg
Monocyte colony-stimulating factor	M-CSF	Monocytes, macrophages, endothelial cells	CFU-GM, CFU-M, monocytes, macrophages
Erythropoietin	EPO	Kidney, liver	CFU-E, CFU-GEMM
Thrombopoietin	TPO	Bone marrow	CFU-Meg, megakaryocytes
Interferon-γ	IFN-γ	$CD4^+$ T cells, NK cells	B cells, T cells, NK cells, neutrophils, monocytes
Interleukin-1	IL-1	Neutrophils, monocytes, macrophages endothelial cells	$CD4^+$ T cells, B cells
Interleukin-2	IL-2	$CD4^+$ T cells	T cells, B cells, NK cells
Interleukin-3	IL-3	$CD4^+$ T cells	CFU-GEMM, CFU-E, CFU-GM, CFU-Eo, CFU-Ba, CFU-Meg, all granulocytes, erythroid cells
Interleukin-4	IL-4	$CD4^+$ T cells, mast cells	B cells, T cells, mast cells
Interleukin-5	IL-5	$CD4^+$ T cells	CFU-Eo, eosinophils, B cells
Interleukin-6	IL-6	Endothelial cells, neutrophils, macrophages, T cells	CFU-GEMM, CFU-E, CFU-GM, B cells, T cells, macrophages, hepatocytes
Interleukin-7	IL-7	Adventitial cells of bone marrow	Early pre-B, pre-T cells
Interleukin-8	IL-8	Macrophages, endothelial cells	T cells, neutrophils
Interleukin-9	IL-9	$CD4^+$ T cells	$CD4^+$ T cells, CFU-GEMM, CFU-E
Interleukin-10	IL-10	Macrophages, T cells	T cells, B cells, NK cells
Interleukin-11	IL-11	Macrophages	CFU-GEMM, CFU-E, CFU-GM, T cells, B cells, macrophages, megakaryocytes

[A]Hemopoietic cytokines include colony-stimulating factors (CSFs), interleukins, and inhibitory factors. They are almost all glycoproteins with a basic polypeptide chain of about 20 kDa. Nearly all of them act on stem cells, colony-forming units (CFUs), colony-forming cells (CFCs), committed cells, maturing cells, and mature cells. Therefore, the targets listed above are target lines rather than individual target cells.

recently isolated factors are several that stimulate granulocyte and macrophage formation, *GM-CSF, G-CSF,* and *M-CSF.* ***Interleukins,*** produced by lymphocytes, act on other leukocytes and their progenitors. *IL-3* is a cytokine that appears to affect most CFUs and even terminally differentiated cells. Any particular cytokine may act at one or more stages in hemopoiesis, affecting cell division, differentiation, or cell function. These factors are synthesized by many different cell types, including kidney cells (erythropoietin), T lymphocytes (IL-3), endothelial cells (IL-6), adventitial cells in the bone marrow (IL-7), and macrophages (the CSFs that affect granulocyte and macrophage development).

The isolation, characterization, manufacture, and clinical testing of cytokines in the treatment of human disease is a major activity of the burgeoning biotechnology industry. Several hemopoietic and lymphopoietic cytokines have been manufactured by recombinant DNA technology and are already used in clinical settings. These include recombinant erythropoietin, G-CSF, GM-CSF, and IL-3; others are under active development.

Monocyte Development

The multipotential myeloid stem cell (CFU-GEMM) also gives rise to the cells that develop along the monocyte-macrophage pathway

Monocytes are produced in the bone marrow from a bipotential stem cell (CFU-GM) that can mature into either monocytes or neutrophils. The differentiation and growth of CFU-GM into monocytes is stimulated by GM-CSF, IL-3, and M-CSF. The monocyte precursors in bone marrow are ***monoblasts*** and ***promonocytes.*** Rapidly dividing promonocytes constitute about half of the progenitor cells of this line in the bone marrow. The other half appear to be promonocytes that divide slowly and serve as a reserve population of progenitor cells. The transformation of CFU-M to monocyte takes about 55 hours, and the monocytes remain in the circulation for only about 16 hours before emigrating to the tissues, where they differentiate into macrophages. The subsequent life span is not yet fully elucidated.

Megakaryocyte Development

Platelets also develop from the multipotential myeloid stem cell (CFU-GEMM), which differentiates into the CFU-Meg cell committed to developing into a megakaryocyte

Platelets are produced in the bone marrow from the same multipotential stem cells (CFU-GEMM) as the erythroid and myeloid series. Under the influence of GM-CSF and IL-3, this stem cell differentiates into CFU-Meg, which is committed to further development into the ***megakaryoblast (megakaryocytoblast)***. The megakaryoblast that develops from this CFU-Meg is a large cell (about 30 µm in diameter) with a nonlobed nucleus. No evidence of platelet formation is seen at this stage. Successive ***endomitoses*** occur in the megakaryoblast; i.e., chromosomes replicate, but neither karyokinesis nor cytokinesis occurs. Under hormonal stimulation by ***thrombopoietin,*** ploidy increases from $8n$ to $64n$ before chromosomal replication ceases. The cell then becomes a platelet-producing megakaryocyte, a cell measuring 50 to 70 µm in diameter with a complex multilobed nucleus and scattered azurophilic granules. Both the nucleus and the cell increase in size in proportion to the ploidy of the cell. With the TEM, multiple centrioles and multiple Golgi apparatus are also seen in these cells.

When bone marrow is examined in a smear, platelet fields are seen to fill much of the peripheral cytoplasm of the megakaryocyte. When examined with the TEM, the peripheral cytoplasm of the megakaryocyte appears to be divided into small compartments by invagination of the plasma membrane. As described above, these invaginations are the platelet demarcation channels (see Fig. 9.14).

Lymphopoiesis

Multipotential lymphoid stem cells (CFU-L) also originate in the bone marrow

Although lymphocytes continuously proliferate in the peripheral lymphatic organs, the bone marrow remains a source of lymphocytes. Progeny of the ***multipotential lymphoid stem cells*** (CFU-L) that are destined to become T cells leave the bone marrow and travel to the thymus, where they complete their differentiation and thymic cell education (see Chapter 13). They then enter the circulation as long-lived, small T lymphocytes. In mammals, cells destined to become B cells originate in bursa-equivalent organs such as the bone marrow, gut-associated lymphatic tissue (GALT), and spleen. Bone marrow, however, remains the primary site of lymphopoiesis in mammals. Lymphocytes constitute as much as 30% of all nucleated cells in the bone marrow.

The precursors of the small lymphocytes in bone marrow are called ***transitional cells.*** Slightly larger than small lymphocytes, they also have a thin rim of cytoplasm and few organelles. The nucleus has a fine, lightly staining chromatin network. Although figures are unavailable for humans, it is calculated that as many as 10^8 small lymphocytes are produced daily in the mouse bone marrow. The production and differentiation of lymphocytes are discussed in more detail in Chapter 13.

▼ BONE MARROW

Red bone marrow lies entirely within the spaces of bone, in the medullary cavity of young long bones and the spaces of spongy bone

Bone marrow consists of blood vessels, specialized units of blood vessels called ***sinusoids,*** and a sponge-like network of hemopoietic cells. In sections, the hemopoietic cells appear to lie in "cords" between sinusoids or between sinusoids and bone.

The sinusoid of red bone marrow is a unique vascular unit. It occupies the position normally occupied by a capillary; i.e., it is interposed between arteries and veins. It is believed to be derived from vessels that have just nourished the cortical bone tissue. The sinusoids arise from these vessels at the corticomedullary junction. The sinusoid wall consists of an endothelial lining, a basal lamina, and an outer adventitial cell layer (Fig. 9.21). The endothelium is a simple squamous epithelium.

The ***adventitial cell,*** also called a ***reticular cell,*** sends sheet-like extensions into the substance of the hemopoietic cords, which provide some support for the developing blood cells. In addition, adventitial cells produce reticular fibers. They also play a role in stimulating the differentiation of developing progenitor cells into blood cells by secreting several CSFs (e.g., IL-7). When blood cell formation and the passage of mature blood cells into the sinusoids are active, adventitial cells and the basal lamina become displaced by mature blood cells as they approach the endothelium to enter the sinusoid from the bone marrow cavity.

The bone marrow sinusoidal system is a closed circulation; newly formed blood cells must penetrate the endothelium to enter the circulation

As a maturing blood cell or a megakaryocyte process pushes against an endothelial cell, the abluminal plasma membrane is pressed against the luminal plasma membrane until they fuse, thus forming a transitory opening, or ***aperture.*** The migrating cell or the megakaryocyte process literally pierces the endothelial cell. Each blood cell must squeeze through such an aperture to enter the lumen of a sinusoid. Similarly, a megakaryocyte process must protrude through an aperture so that the platelets can be released directly into the sinusoid lumen. The aperture is lined by the fused plasma membrane, thus maintaining the

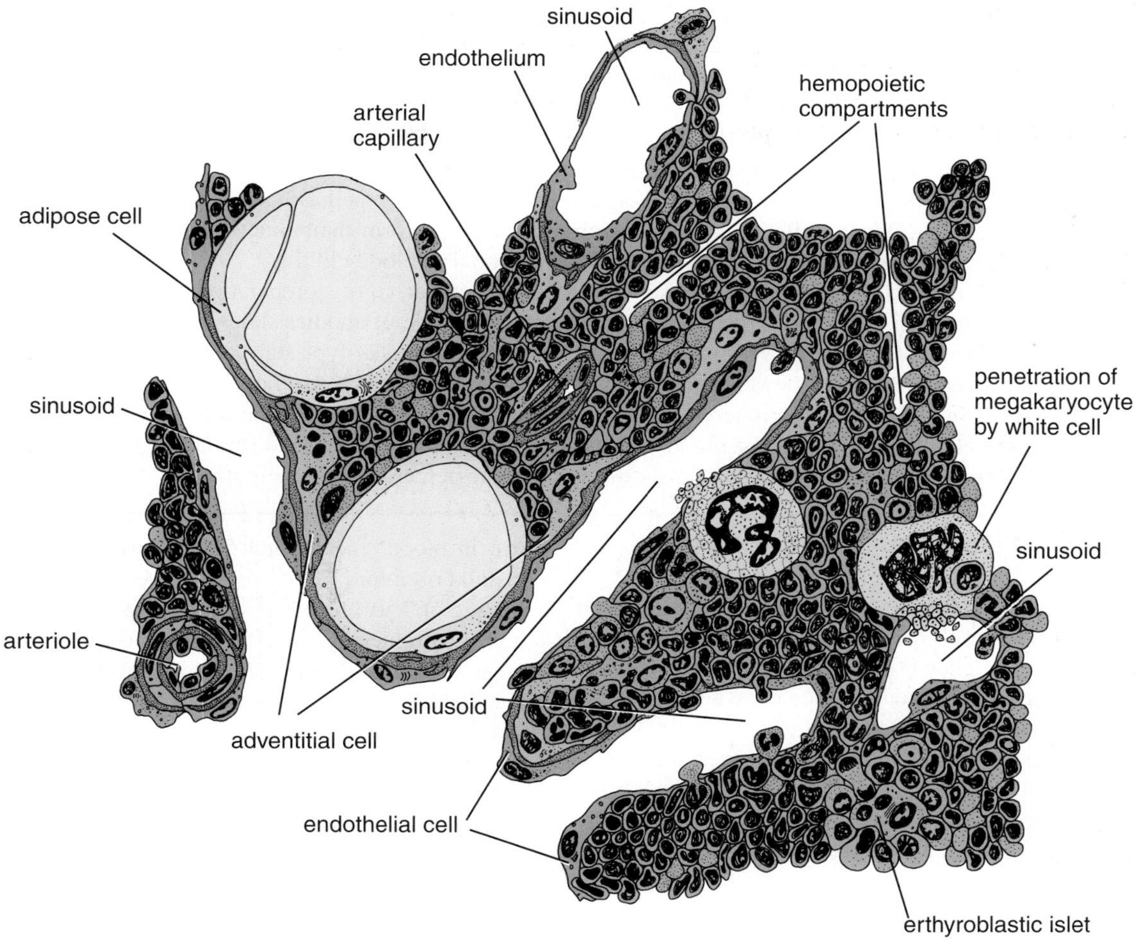

FIGURE 9.21
Diagram of the marrow with active hemopoiesis. Note the erythroblastic islets engaged in the formation of erythrocytes, megakaryocytes discharging platelets into the sinusoids, endothelial cells adjacent to a basal lamina that is sparse in places and absent where blood cells are entering the sinusoids, and adventitial or reticular cells extending from the basal lamina into the hemopoietic compartment. (Modified from Weiss L, ed. *Cell and Tissue Biology: A Textbook of Histology.* 6th ed. Baltimore: Urban & Schwarzenberg, 1988.)

integrity of the endothelial cell during the transcellular passage. As the blood cell completes its passage through the aperture or the megakaryocyte that has extruded its platelets withdraws its process, the endothelial cell "repairs itself," and the aperture disappears.

In active ***red bone marrow,*** the cords of hemopoietic cells contain predominately developing blood cells and megakaryocytes. The cords also contain macrophages, mast cells, and some adipose cells. Although the cords of hemopoietic tissue appear to be unorganized, specific types of blood cells develop in nests or clusters. Each nest in which erythrocytes develop contains a macrophage. These nests are located near the sinusoid wall. Megakaryocytes are also located adjacent to the sinusoid wall, and they discharge their platelets directly into the sinusoid through apertures in the endothelium. Granulocytes develop in cell nests farther from the sinusoid wall. When mature, the granulocyte migrates to the sinusoid and enters the bloodstream.

Bone marrow not active in blood cell formation contains predominately adipose cells, giving it the appearance of adipose tissue

Inactive bone marrow is called yellow bone marrow. It is the chief form of bone marrow in the medullary cavity of bones in the adult that are no longer hemopoietically active, such as the long bones of the arms, legs, fingers, and toes. In these bones, the red bone marrow has been replaced completely by fat. Even in hemopoietically active bone marrow in adult humans, such as that in the ribs, vertebrae, pelvis, and shoulder girdle, about half of the bone marrow space is occupied by adipose tissue and half by hemopoietic tissue. The yellow bone marrow retains its hemopoietic potential, however, and when necessary, as after severe loss of blood, it can revert to red bone marrow, both by extension of the hemopoietic tissue into the yellow bone marrow and by repopulation of the yellow bone marrow by circulating stem cells.

PLATE 16. ERYTHROCYTES AND AGRANULOCYTES

Blood is a fluid connective tissue that circulates through the cardiovascular system. It consists of formed elements, cells and their derivatives, and a protein-rich fluid matrix called *plasma.* The formed elements include *red cells (erythrocytes), white cells (leukocytes),* and *platelets.* Cells constitute approximately 45% of the blood volume, and red blood cells constitute about 99% of the cells. Red blood cells function in the transport and exchange of oxygen and carbon dioxide in the other tissues of the body. White cells consist of *agranulocytes* and *granulocytes,* and each white cell type has a specific function in immune and protective responses in the body. Most white cells leave the circulation to perform their functions in the connective tissue, whereas red cells function within the vascular system. Platelets are essential in blood clotting.

The relative distribution of cells in blood is usually studied in a blood smear. In this preparation, a small drop of blood is placed on a microscope slide and is smeared across the slide with the short edge of another slide. The preparation is then air-dried and stained with a mixture of dyes (e.g., Wright's stain, a modified Romanovsky-type stain). In examining a blood smear, it is useful to survey the smear with a low-power objective in order to ascertain which parts of the preparation show an even distribution of blood cells. In general, the periphery of the smear should be avoided, since the cells are either distorted, too close to each other (at the end where the drop of blood was placed), or too widely dispersed (at the opposite end, where the smear ended). Furthermore, the edges of a blood smear do not show a true percent distribution of white cells.

Figure 1, blood smear, human, Wright's stain ×400.

This is a low-magnification photomicrograph of a smear with the blood cells well distributed. Most of the cells are erythrocytes (RBC). They are readily identified because of their number and lack of a nucleus. Scattered among the red cells are three white blood cells that can be distinguished from the erythrocytes without difficulty by their larger size and their staining characteristics. Interspersed among the cells are numerous small speck-like objects. These are blood platelets that have aggregated into small groups and, thus, can be readily observed even at this low magnification. They can be visualized better at higher magnification in Figures 2 to 4 *(arrows).*

Erythrocytes have a biconcave shape. They measure about 8.0 μm in diameter in the circulating blood, about 7.5 μm in blood smears, and 6 to 10 μm, depending on the method used for preserving the tissue, in sectioned material. (A size of 7 μm for the erythrocyte in sectioned material is useful to remember. It enables one to estimate the size of other structures in a histologic section by comparison with the RBC without resorting to a micrometer.) Erythrocytes stain uniformly with eosin, a component of the usual dye mixture (e.g., Wright's) used to stain blood smears. Because of the biconcave form of the erythrocyte, however, its center is thinner and appears lighter than the periphery.

To distinguish the different kinds of leukocytes in a blood smear, it is advantageous to use the highest available magnification, usually an oil-immersion lens. This enables one to use the morphologic features of the cytoplasm in addition to nuclear morphology and cytoplasmic staining in identifying the cell type.

Figures 2–7, blood smear, white blood cells, human, Wright's stain ×1800.

Figures 2 to 4 illustrate characteristic features of lymphocytes. The nucleus stains intensely, generally has a rounded shape, and, as illustrated in Figure 2, may possess a slight indentation. These cells measure about 8, 10, and 12 μm in diameter, respectively (circulating lymphocytes range from 6 to 12 μm). In a small lymphocyte (Fig. 2), only a small amount of cytoplasm is evident, and the nucleus seems to constitute most of the cellular volume. In large lymphocytes of circulating blood (Figs. 3 and 4), there is a larger amount of cytoplasm. (Large lymphocytes of circulating blood are equivalent to the medium-sized lymphocytes of lymphatic tissue. The large lymphocytes of lymphatic tissue are not a characteristic feature of circulating blood except in certain abnormal conditions.) The cytoplasm of lymphocytes may stain a pale blue; sometimes, a distinct, lightly stained Golgi area is evident. In addition, lymphocyte cytoplasm may contain azurophilic granules, as shown in Figures 3 and 4.

Figures 5 to 7 show characteristic features of monocytes. These cells measure approximately 12 and 15 μm in diameter, respectively (monocytes range from 9 to 18 μm). The nucleus is somewhat less "compact" than the nucleus of lymphocytes. The cytoplasm, like that of lymphocytes, stains lightly but tends to have a grayer or duller blue tint. Azurophilic granules are also present in the cytoplasm. Lymphocytes and monocytes are classified as agranulocytes; i.e., they are usually free of specific cytoplasmic granules. Moreover, their nuclei are nonlobed, although monocyte nuclei may occasionally show a deep indentation (Fig. 6). Thus, they are distinguished from granulocytes, which possess specific cytoplasmic granules as well as a lobed or segmented nucleus.

KEY

arrows, blood platelets

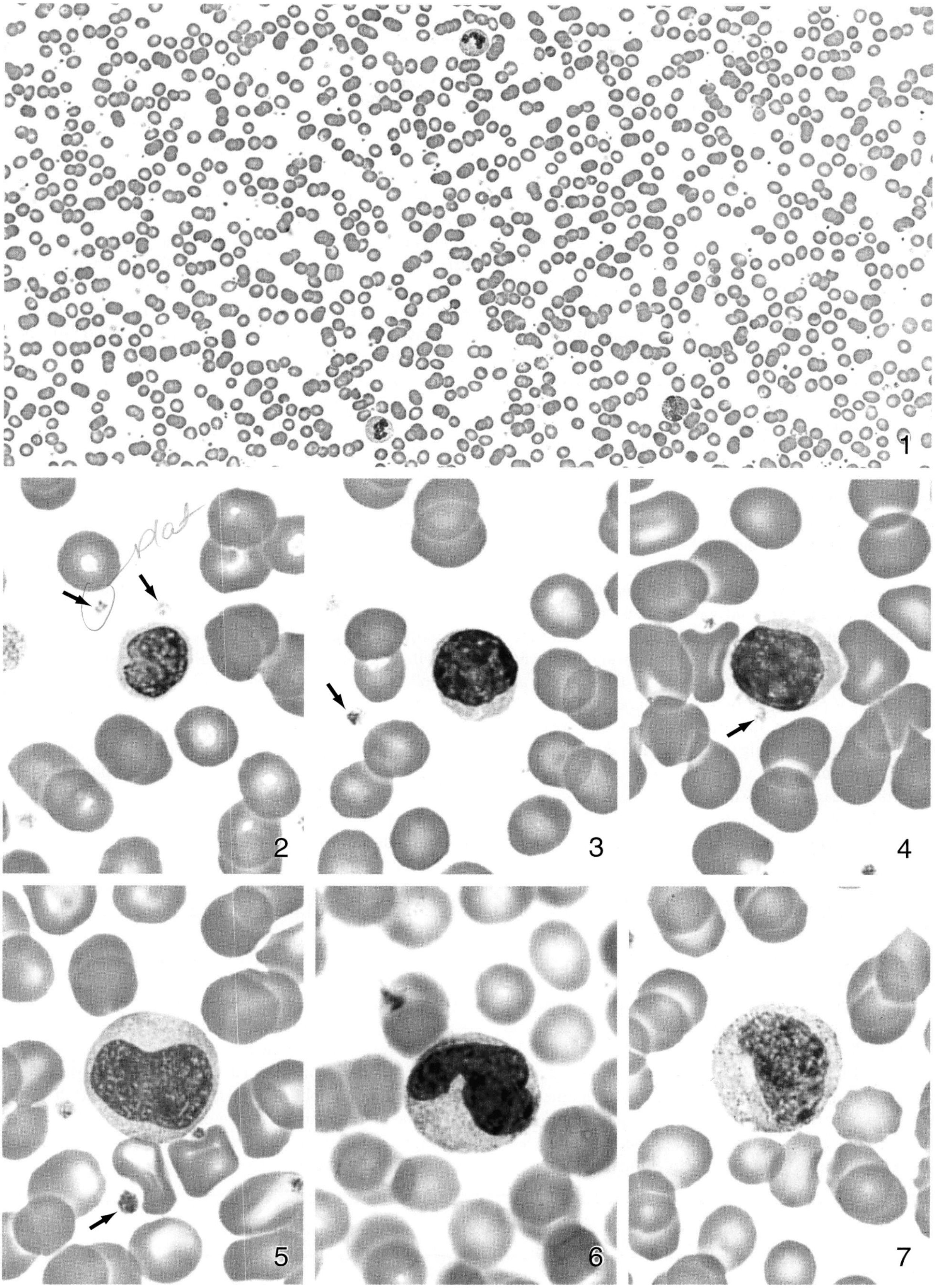
1
2
3
4
5
6
7

PLATE 17. GRANULOCYTES

Granulocytes are characterized by a lobed nucleus and by the specific staining characteristics of granules in the cytoplasm. Three kinds of granulocytes are present in a peripheral blood smear: *neutrophils (polymorphonuclear leukocytes),* 55 to 60%; *eosinophils,* ~2 to 5%; and *basophils,* 1% or less. All of the granulocytes leave the bloodstream and enter the connective tissue to perform their specific functions.

Neutrophils are actively phagocytic cells that have both *specific granules* and *azurophilic granules*. The azurophilic granules are the lysosomes of the neutrophil; the specific granules contain bacteriostatic and bactericidal agents, such as *lysozyme.* At sites of injury or infection, neutrophils engage in active phagocytosis of bacteria and other foreign organisms and passive phagocytosis of damaged connective tissue cells, red blood cells, and fibrin. Many neutrophils die in this process. The accumulation of dead neutrophils and dead bacteria constitutes *pus.* Eosinophils contain numerous large specific granules characterized by the presence of a *crystalloid inclusion* containing *major basic protein,* the material responsible for the intense acidophilia. The granules also contain *histaminase* and *arylsulfatase,* the actions of which serve to moderate the potentially deleterious effects of the inflammatory vasoactive agents *histamine* and *slow-reacting substance (SRS) of anaphylaxis.* Eosinophils are commonly found at sites of chronic infection and inflammation, and their number is elevated in individuals with allergies and parasitic infections. They phagocytize antigen–antibody complexes.

Basophils have specific granules that contain hydrolytic enzymes, *heparan sulfate,* histamine, and SRS. The intense basophilia is due to the anionic nature of the heparan sulfate. Basophils bind immunoglobulin E (secreted by plasma cells) on their surface; when subsequently exposed to the specific antigen that stimulated synthesis of that antibody, the basophils release their vasoactive agents, causing the severe vascular disturbances associated with hypersensitivity reactions and anaphylaxis.

Figures 1–6, blood smears, human, Wright's stain ×1800.

Neutrophils develop in the red bone marrow from cells that have a rounded nucleus. During their maturation, the nucleus changes from a rounded to a segmented or lobed form. A fully developed neutrophil nucleus may have as many as five lobes. The configuration and number of lobes vary from one cell to another (Figs. 1 and 2), and on the basis of the variable nuclear morphology, these cells are sometimes called polymorphonuclear leukocytes. It should be understood, however, that each cell has only one nucleus, with each lobe being joined to its neighbor by a strand of nuclear material.

Neutrophils usually measure 9 to 14 μm in diameter. The cytoplasm of these cells contains granules that range from 0.1 to 0.4 μm in diameter and stain variably, either azure, light blue, or violet. Although neutrophils contain specific granules, the identification of these cells can usually be accomplished on the basis of the distinctive lobulation of the nucleus. Moreover, because these cells are the most numerous of the leukocytes in a smear of normal blood, their number is an aid in their identification.

The neutrophil in Figure 2 shows a small projection from one of the nuclear lobes *(arrow).* This is referred to as a drumstick. It is the inactive female X chromosome. Its presence is sufficient to identify the blood as having come from a female, assuming that the normal complement of chromosomes is present. Because the visualization of the drumstick requires a fortuitous orientation of the nuclear lobes, many cells usually need to be examined before a recognizable drumstick profile is found.

Eosinophils are shown in Figures 3 and 4. These cells measure about 13 μm in diameter (eosinophils range from 10 to 14 μm). The most conspicuous feature of eosinophils is the presence of numerous cytoplasmic granules that stain with eosin. The granules virtually fill the cytoplasm. The eosinophilic granules have specific morphologic characteristics that can be used in the identification of the cells. They are relatively uniform in size within a particular cell, are about 0.6 μm in diameter, significantly larger than granules of neutrophils, and are typically closely packed. In going "through focus," eosinophilic granules often display a marked refractility. The nucleus of the eosinophil is usually bilobed, as seen in Figures 2 and 3.

Basophils are shown in Figures 5 and 6. They measure about 8 and 12 μm in diameter, respectively (range of basophil size is 8 to 14 μm). These cells contain cytoplasmic granules of variable size that stain intensely with the methylene blue of the blood stain. The granules are randomly distributed throughout the cell, usually superimposed over the nucleus and obscuring it to such a degree that its boundaries barely can be distinguished. In Figure 6, some of the granules are larger than the eosinophilic granules, others are smaller than the eosinophilic granules, and some are as small as those found in the neutrophils. The range in size of basophil granules (in contrast to the more uniform size of granules in eosinophils) is another characteristic that may aid in the identification of these cells. Because the basophil is so rare, it may be necessary to examine a large area of a blood smear before one can be found.

KEY

arrow, drumstick (inactive X chromosome)

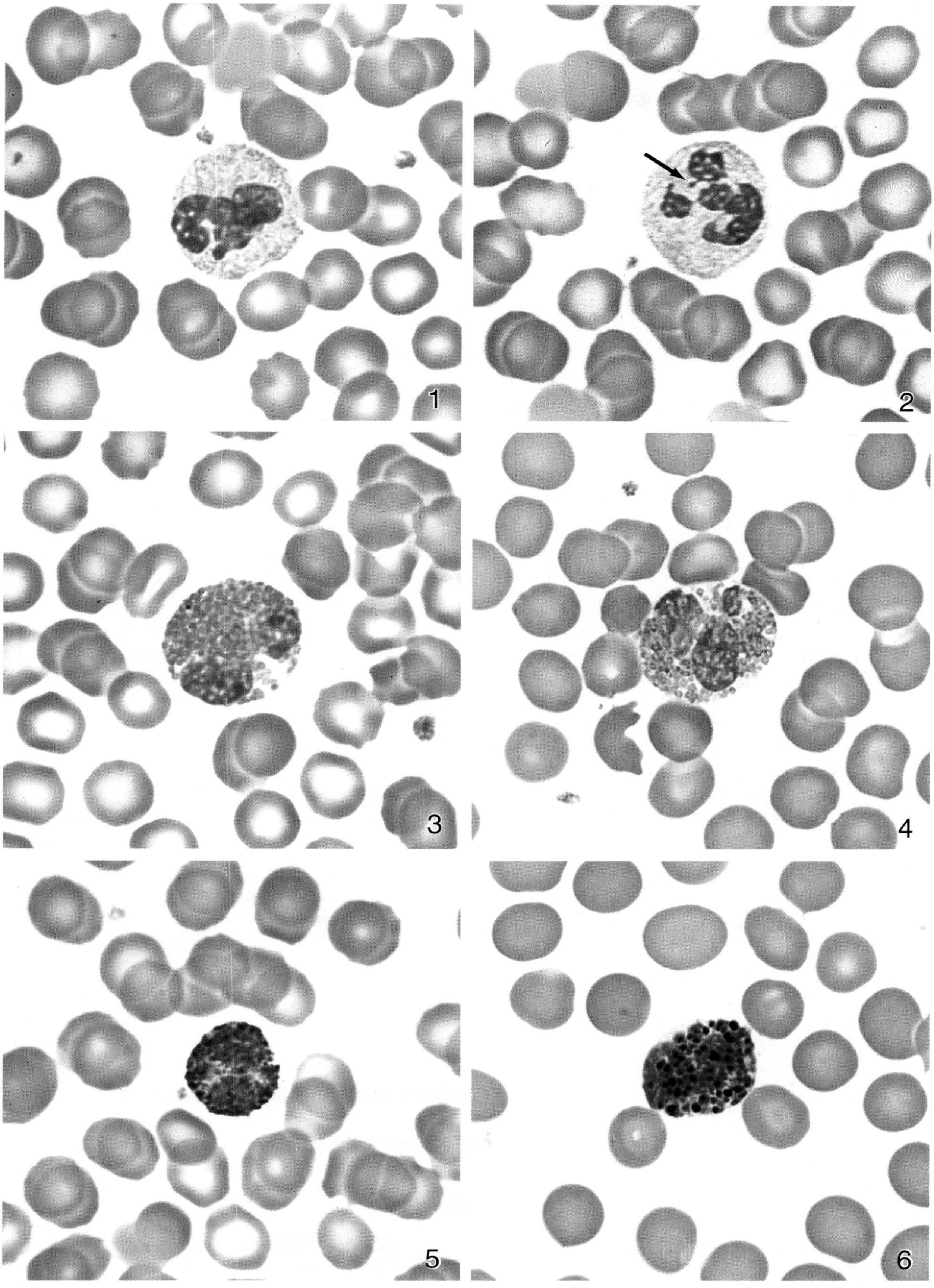
1
2
3
4
5
6

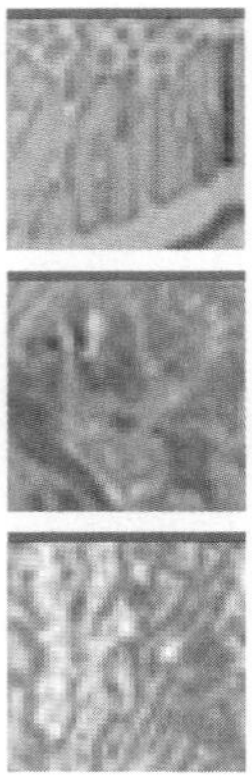

10

Muscle Tissue

▽ OVERVIEW AND CLASSIFICATION OF MUSCLE

Muscle tissue is responsible for movement of the body and its parts and for changes in the size and shape of internal organs. This tissue is characterized by aggregates of specialized, elongated cells arranged in parallel array, whose primary role is contraction (Fig. 10.1).

Myofilament interaction is responsible for muscle cell contraction

Two types of myofilaments are associated with cell contraction:

- ***Thin filaments*** (6 to 8 nm in diameter, 1.0 μm long), composed primarily of the protein **actin.** Each thin filament of fibrous actin ***(F-actin)*** is a polymer formed from globular actin molecules ***(G-actin)***.

- ***Thick filaments*** (~15 nm in diameter, 1.5 μm long), composed of the protein ***myosin II.*** Each thick filament consists of 200 to 300 myosin II molecules. The long, rod-shaped tail portion of each molecule aggregates in a regular parallel but staggered array, while the head portions project out in a regular helical pattern.

The two types of myofilaments occupy the bulk of the cytoplasm, which in muscle cells is also called ***sarcoplasm*** *[Gr. sarcos, flesh; plasma, thing].* Actin and myosin are also present in most other cell types (although in considerably smaller amounts), where they play a role in cellular activities such as cytokinesis, exocytosis, and cell migration. In contrast, muscle cells contain a large number of aligned contractile filaments that the cells use for the single purpose of producing mechanical work.

Muscle is classified on the basis of the appearance of the contractile cells

Two principal types of muscle are recognized:

- ***Striated muscle,*** in which the cells exhibit cross-striations at the light microscope level
- ***Smooth muscle,*** in which the cells do not exhibit cross-striations

Striated muscle tissue is further subclassified on the basis of its location:

- ***Skeletal muscle*** is attached to bone and is responsible for movement of the axial and appendicular skeleton and for maintenance of body position and posture. In addition, skeletal muscles of the eye (extraocular muscles) provide precise eye movement.

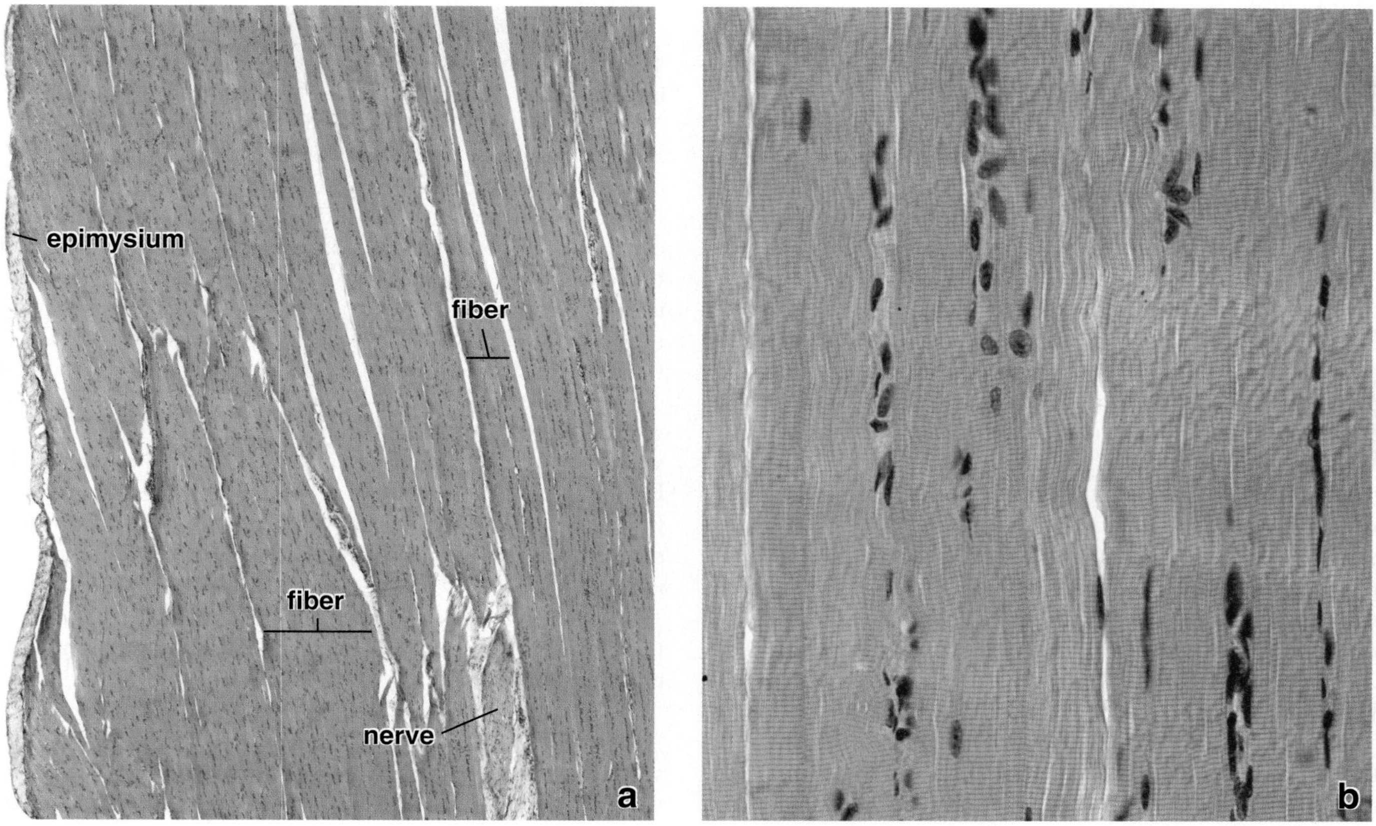

FIGURE 10.1
Photomicrograph of a skeletal muscle. a. This low-magnification photomicrograph shows skeletal muscle in longitudinal section. Muscle fibers (cells) are arranged in parallel; they are vertically oriented, and the length of each fiber extends beyond the upper and lower edge of the micrograph. The fibers appear to be of different thicknesses. This is largely a reflection of the plane of section through the muscle fibers. Note on the left the epimysium, the sheath of dense connective tissue surrounding the muscle. ×160. **b.** At higher magnification, cross-striations of the muscle fibers are readily seen. The nuclei of skeletal muscle fibers are located in the cytoplasm immediately beneath the plasma membrane. ×360.

- ***Visceral striated muscle*** is morphologically identical with skeletal muscle but is restricted to the soft tissues, namely, the tongue, pharynx, lumbar part of the diaphragm, and upper part of the esophagus. These muscles play essential roles in speech, breathing, and swallowing.
- ***Cardiac muscle*** is a type of striated muscle found in the wall of the heart and in the base of the large veins that empty into the heart.

The cross-striations in striated muscle are produced largely by the specific cytoarchitectural arrangement of both thin and thick myofilaments. This arrangement is the same in all types of striated muscle cells. The main differences between skeletal muscle cells and cardiac muscle cells are in their size, shape, and organization relative to one another.

Smooth muscle cells do not exhibit cross-striations because the myofilaments do not achieve the same degree of order in their arrangement. In addition, the myosin-containing myofilaments in smooth muscle are highly labile. Smooth muscle is restricted to the viscera and vascular system, the arrector pili muscles of the skin, and the intrinsic muscles of the eye.

SKELETAL MUSCLE

A skeletal muscle cell is a multinucleated syncytium

In skeletal muscle, each muscle cell, more commonly called a ***muscle fiber,*** is actually a multinucleated ***syncytium.*** A muscle fiber is formed during development by the fusion of small, individual muscle cells called ***myoblasts.*** When viewed in cross section, the mature multinucleated muscle fiber reveals a polygonal shape with a diameter of 10 to 100 μm. Their length varies from almost a meter, as in the sartorius muscle of the lower limb, to as little as a few millimeters, as in the stapedius muscle of the middle ear. (*Note:* A muscle fiber should not be confused with a connective tissue fiber; muscle fibers are cellular elements, whereas connective tissue fibers are extracellular products of connective tissue cells.)

The nuclei of a skeletal muscle fiber are located in the cytoplasm immediately beneath the plasma membrane, also called the ***sarcolemma.*** In the past, the term *sarcolemma* was used to describe a thick "membrane" that was thought to be the cytoplasmic boundary of the muscle cell. It is now known that the thick sarcolemma actually represents the plasma membrane of the cell, its external lamina, and the surrounding reticular lamina.

A skeletal muscle consists of striated muscle fibers held together by connective tissue

The connective tissue that surrounds both individual muscle fibers and bundles of muscle fibers is essential for force transduction. At the end of the muscle, the connective tissue continues as a tendon or some other arrangement of collagen fibers that attaches the muscle, usually, to bone. A rich supply of blood vessels and nerves travels in the connective tissue.

The connective tissue associated with muscle is named according to its relationship with the muscle fibers:

- ***Endomysium*** is the delicate layer of reticular fibers that immediately surrounds individual muscle fibers. Only small-diameter capillaries and the finest neuronal branches are present within the endomysium, running parallel to the muscle fibers.
- ***Perimysium*** is a thicker connective tissue layer that surrounds a group of fibers to form a ***bundle*** or ***fascicle.*** Fascicles are functional units of muscle fibers that tend to work together to perform a specific function. Larger blood vessels and nerves travel in the perimysium.
- ***Epimysium*** is the sheath of dense connective tissue that surrounds a collection of fascicles that constitutes the muscle (see Fig. 10.1a). The major vascular and nerve supply of the muscle penetrates the epimysium.

There are three types of skeletal muscle fibers: red, white, and intermediate

Skeletal muscle fibers differ in diameter and in their natural color in vivo. The color differences are not apparent in hematoxylin and eosin (H&E)–stained sections. However, special cytologic and histochemical reactions based on oxidative enzyme activity, specifically the succinic dehydrogenase and nicotinamide adenine dinucleotide–tetrazolium (NADH–TR) reactions, confirm the observations of fresh tissue and reveal several types of skeletal muscle fibers (Fig. 10.2). The most obvious are red fibers, white fibers, and intermediate fibers. The histochemical staining and enzyme activity of these three types of muscle fibers reflect their functional differences. Typically, all three fiber types are present in any given muscle. The proportion of each type varies according to the functional role of the muscle.

Fiber type is mainly attributable to myoglobin content and mitochondrial number

Myoglobin is an oxygen-binding protein that closely resembles hemoglobin found in erythrocytes and occurs in varying amounts in muscle fibers. It provides a ready source of oxygen for muscle metabolic reactions. Classification of skeletal muscle fibers into red, white, and intermediate fibers reflects the myoglobin content and the number of mitochondria with their constituent cytochrome electron transport complexes. These complexes are essential for oxidative phosphorylation to produce adenosine triphosphate (ATP), the energy source for muscle.

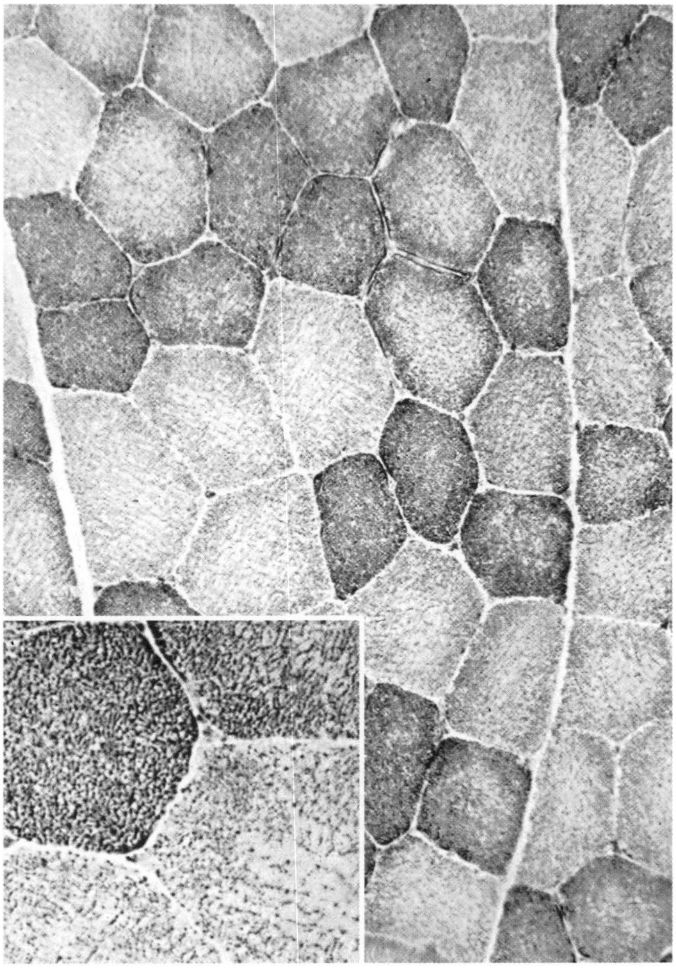

FIGURE 10.2
Cross section of white and red skeletal muscle fibers. This cross section of muscle fibers stained with the NADH–TR reaction demonstrates two fiber types. The deeply stained, smaller muscle fibers exhibit strong oxidative enzyme activity and correspond to the red muscle fibers. The lighter-staining, larger fibers correspond to the white fibers. ×280. **Inset.** Portions of the two fiber types at higher magnification. The reaction also reveals the mitochondria that contain the oxidative enzymes. The contractile components, the myofibrils, are unstained. ×550. (Original slide specimen courtesy of Dr. Scott W. Ballinger.)

- ***Red fibers*** are small fibers with large amounts of myoglobin and cytochrome complexes and many mitochondria. They make up ***slow-twitch motor units*** (a *twitch* is a single, brief contraction of the muscle). Red fibers have great resistance to fatigue but generate relatively less muscle tension than white fibers. Myosin adenosine triphosphatase (ATPase) activity, essential for contraction, is greatest in red muscle fibers. The large numbers of mitochondria in red fibers are characterized by high levels of oxidative enzymes, as demonstrated by strong succinic dehydrogenase and NADH–TR histochemical staining reactions (see Fig. 10.2). Red fibers are typically found in the limb muscles of mammals and in the breast muscle of migrating birds. More importantly, they are the principal fibers of the long muscles of the back in humans, where they are particularly adapted to the long, slow contractions needed to maintain erect posture.
- ***White fibers*** are large fibers with less myoglobin and fewer cytochromes and mitochondria. They make up ***fast-twitch motor units,*** fatigue rapidly, and generate a large peak muscle tension. Thus, white fibers are adapted for rapid contraction and precise, fine movements. They constitute most fibers of the extraocular muscles and the muscles that control the movements of the digits. White fibers have a greater number of neuromuscular junctions than do red fibers, thus allowing more precise neuronal control of movements in these muscles.
- ***Intermediate fibers*** are of intermediate size. The amount of myoglobin and the number of mitochondria they contain are also intermediate between those of red and white fibers.

Myofibrils and Myofilaments

The structural and functional subunit of the muscle fiber is the myofibril

Skeletal muscles are composed of ***fascicles,*** which in turn are composed of individual muscle fibers. The muscle fiber is filled with longitudinally arrayed subunits called ***myofibrils*** (Fig. 10.3). Myofibrils are visible in favorable histologic preparations and are best seen in cross sections of muscle fibers. In these sections they give the fiber a stippled appearance. Myofibrils extend the entire length of the muscle cell.

Myofibrils are composed of bundles of myofilaments

Myofilaments are the individual filamentous polymers of myosin II (thick filaments) and actin and its associated proteins (thin filaments). Myofilaments are the actual contractile elements of striated muscle. The bundles of myofilaments that make up the myofibril are surrounded by a well-developed smooth endoplasmic reticulum (sER), also called the ***sarcoplasmic reticulum.*** This reticulum forms a highly organized tubular network around the contractile elements in all striated muscle cells. Mitochondria and glycogen deposits are located between the myofibrils in association with the sER.

Cross-striations are the principal histologic feature of striated muscle

Cross-striations are evident in H&E–stained preparations of longitudinal sections of muscle fibers. They may also be

BOX 10.1

Functional Considerations: Muscle Metabolism and Ischemia

Like all cells, muscle cells depend on the energy source contained in the high-energy phosphate bonds of ATP and phosphocreatine. The energy stored in these high-energy phosphate bonds comes from the metabolism of ***fatty acids*** and ***glucose.*** Glucose is the primary metabolic substrate in actively contracting muscle. It is derived from the general circulation as well as from the breakdown of glycogen, which is normally stored in the muscle fiber cytoplasm. As much as 1% of the dry weight of skeletal and cardiac muscle may be glycogen.

In rapidly contracting muscles, such as the leg muscles in running or the extraocular muscles, most of the energy for contraction is supplied by anaerobic glycolysis of stored glycogen. The buildup of intermediary metabolites from this pathway, particularly lactic acid, can produce an oxygen deficit that causes ischemic pain (cramp) in cases of extreme muscular exertion.

Most of the energy used by muscle recovering from contraction or by resting muscle is derived from oxidative phosphorylation. This process closely follows the β-oxidation of fatty acids in mitochondria that liberates two carbon fragments. The oxygen needed for oxidative phosphorylation and other terminal metabolic reactions is derived from hemoglobin in circulating erythrocytes and from oxygen bound to myoglobin stored in the muscle cells.

seen in unstained preparations of living muscle fibers examined with a phase contrast or polarizing microscope, in which they appear as alternating light and dark bands. These bands are termed the ***A band*** and the ***I band*** (Fig. 10.3).

In polarizing microscopy, the dark bands are ***birefringent;*** i.e., they alter the polarized light in two planes. Therefore, the dark bands, being doubly refractive, are ***anisotropic*** and are given the name ***A band.*** The light bands are ***monorefringent;*** i.e., they do not alter the plane of polarized light. Therefore, they are ***isotropic*** and are given the name ***I band.***

Both the A and I bands are bisected by narrow regions of contrasting density (see Fig. 10.3). The light I band is bisected by a dense line, the ***Z line,*** also called the ***Z disk*** *[Ger. **Z**wischenscheibe, between disks]*. The dark A band is bisected by a less dense, or light, region called the ***H band*** *[Ger. **H**ell, light]*. Furthermore, bisecting the light H band is a narrow dense line called the ***M line*** *[Ger. **M**itte, middle]*. The M line is best demonstrated in electron micrographs (Fig 10.4), although in ideal H&E preparations it can be detected in the light microscope.

As noted above, the cross-banding pattern of striated muscle is due to the arrangement of the two kinds of myofilaments. To understand the mechanism of contraction, this banding pattern must be considered in functional terms.

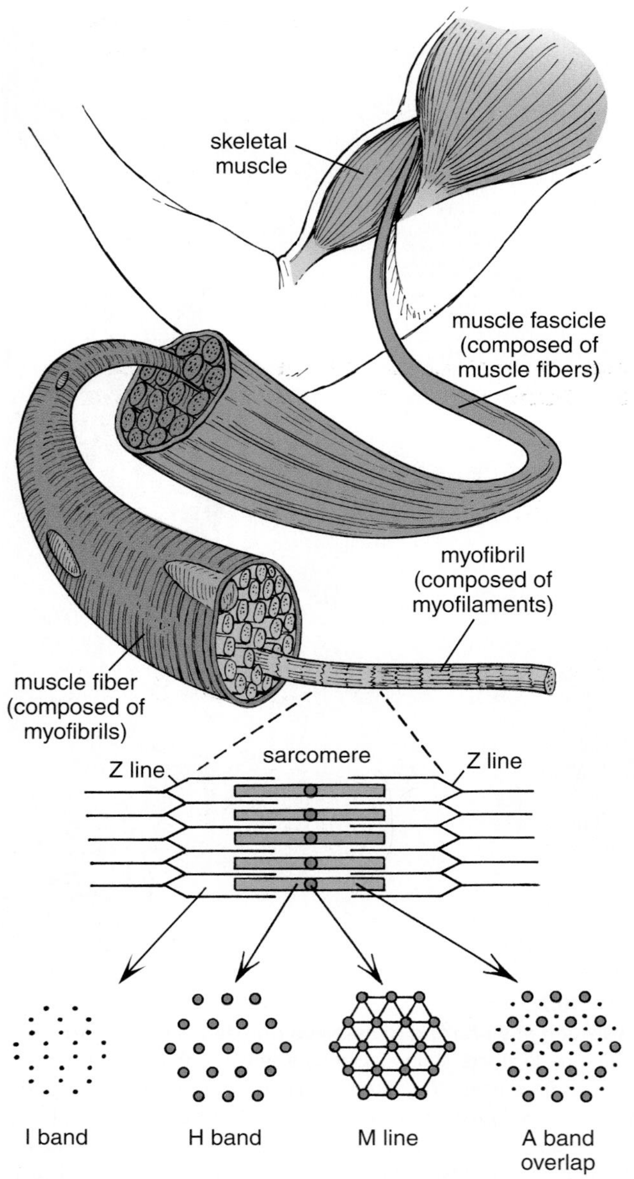

FIGURE 10.3
Organization of a skeletal muscle. A skeletal muscle consists of bundles of muscle fibers called fascicles. In turn, each fascicle consists of a bundle of elongate muscle fibers (cells). The muscle fiber represents a collection of longitudinal units, the myofibrils, which in turn are composed of myofilaments of two types: thick (myosin) filaments and thin (actin) filaments. The myofilaments are organized in a specific manner that imparts a cross-striated appearance to the myofibril and to the fiber. The functional unit of the myofibril is the sarcomere; it extends in both directions from one Z line to the next Z line. The A band marks the extent of the myosin filaments. Actin filaments extend from the Z line into the region of the A band, where they interdigitate with the myosin filaments as shown. The cross sections through different regions of the sarcomere are also shown *(from left to right):* through thin filaments of the I band; through thick filaments of the H band; through the center of the A band, where adjacent thick filaments are linked to form the M line; and through the A band, where thin and thick filaments overlap. Note that each thick filament is within the center of a hexagonal array of thin filaments.

The functional unit of the myofibril is the sarcomere, the segment of the myofibril between two adjacent Z lines

The *sarcomere* is the basic contractile unit of striated muscle. It is the portion of a myofibril between two adjacent Z lines. A sarcomere measures 2 to 3 μm in relaxed mammalian muscle. It may be stretched to more than 4 μm and, during extreme contraction, may be reduced to as little as 1 μm (Fig. 10.5). The entire muscle cell exhibits cross-striations because sarcomeres in adjacent myofibrils are in register.

The arrangement of thick and thin filaments gives rise to the density differences that produce the cross-striations of the myofibril

The myosin-containing thick filaments are about 1.5 μm long and are restricted to the central portion of the sarcomere, i.e., the A band. The thin filaments attach to the Z line and extend into the A band to the edge of the H band. Portions of two sarcomeres, on either side of a Z line, constitute the I band and contain only thin filaments. In a longitudinal section of a sarcomer[illegible] ine appears as a zigzag structure, with matrix m[illegible] *matrix,* bisecting the zigzag. The Z line a[illegible] material anchor the thin filaments from adja[illegible]es to the angles of the zigzag by the actin-b[illegible] *α-actinin.* These features are illustrated in [illegible]

F-actin, troponin, and tropomyosin in thin filaments and myosin II in thick filaments are the primary proteins in the contractile apparatus

Thin filaments contain F-actin, tropomyosin, and troponin. Thick filaments contain only myosin II.

G-actin is a small, 42-kDa molecule that polymerizes to form a double-stranded helix, the ***F-actin*** filament. These

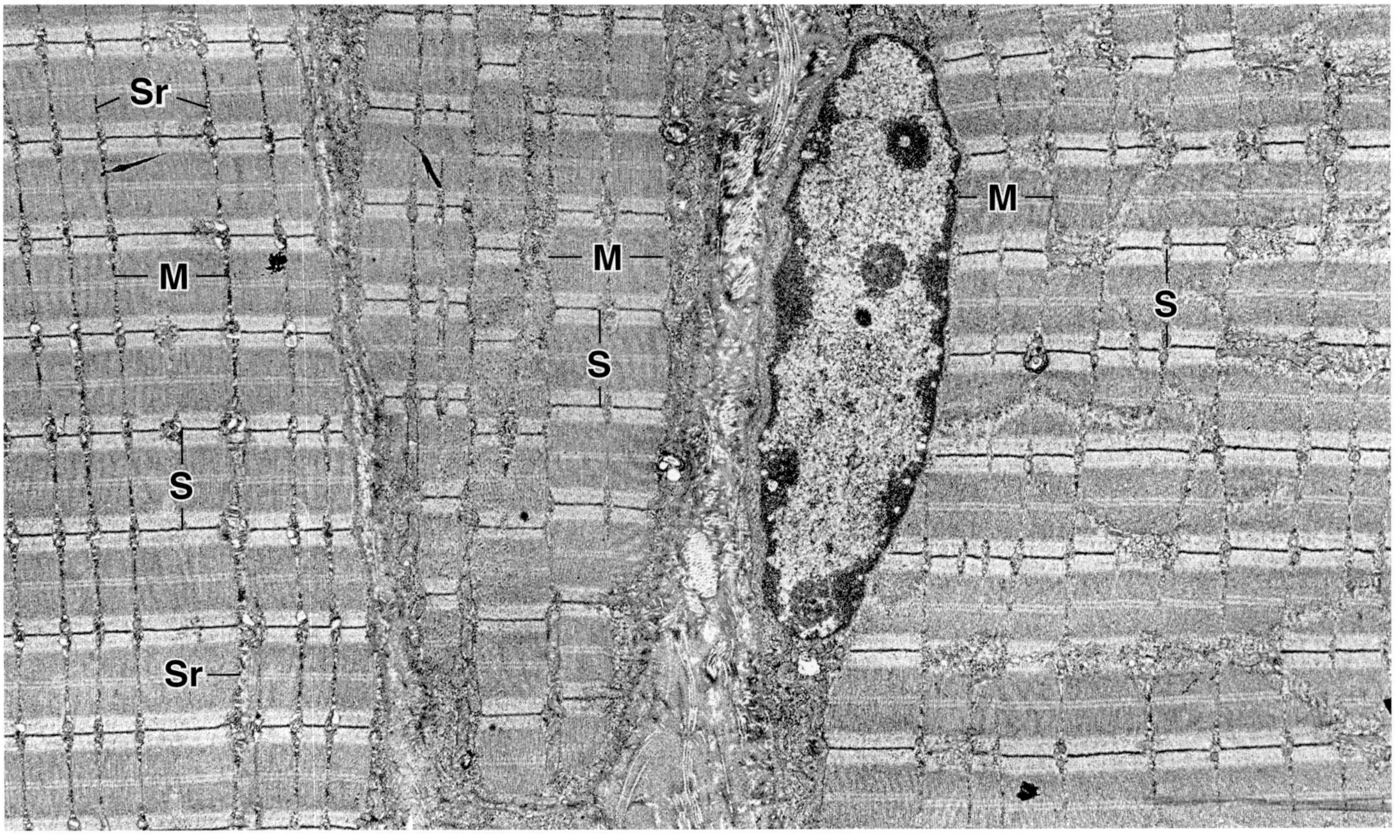

FIGURE 10.4
Electron micrograph of skeletal muscle fiber. This low-magnification electron micrograph shows the general organization of skeletal muscle fibers. Small portions of three muscle fibers in longitudinal profile are included in this micrograph. The muscle fiber on the right reveals a nucleus at its periphery. Two fibers—one in the middle and another on the left—exhibit regular profiles of myofibrils separated by a thin layer of surrounding sarcoplasm *(Sr)*. Each repeating part of the myofibril between adjacent Z lines is a sarcomere *(S)*. The cross-banded pattern visible on this micrograph reflects the arrangement, in register, of the individual myofibrils *(M)*; a similar pattern found in the myofibril reflects the arrangement of myofilaments. The detailed features of a sarcomere are shown at higher magnification in Figure 10.6a. The presence of the connective tissue in the extracellular space between the fibers constitutes the endomysium of the muscle. ×6,500.

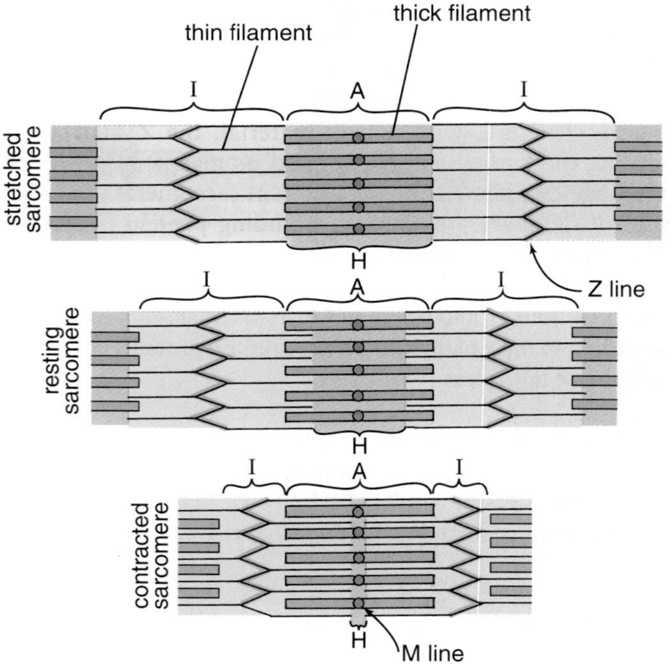

FIGURE 10.5
Sarcomeres in different functional stages. In the resting state *(middle)*, interdigitation of thin (actin) and thick (myosin) filaments is not complete; the H and I bands are relatively wide. In the contracted state *(bottom)*, the interdigitation of the thin and thick filaments is increased according to the degree of contraction. In the stretched state *(top)*, the thin and thick filaments do not interact; the H and I bands are very wide. The length of the A band always remains the same and corresponds to the length of the thick filaments; the lengths of the H and I bands change, again in proportion to the degree of sarcomere relaxation or contraction.

actin filaments are polar; all G-actin molecules are oriented in the same direction. The plus end of each filament is bound to the Z line by α-actinin; the minus end extends toward the M line. Each G-actin molecule of the thin filament has a binding site for myosin.

Tropomyosin is a 64-kDa protein that also consists of a double helix of two polypeptides. It forms filaments that run in the groove between the F-actin molecules in the thin filament. In resting muscle, tropomyosin and the troponins mask the myosin-binding site on the actin molecule.

Troponin actually consists of a complex of three globular subunits. Each tropomyosin molecule contains one troponin complex. ***Troponin-C (TnC)*** is the smallest subunit of the troponin complex (18 kDa). It binds Ca^{2+}, the essential step in the initiation of contraction (see below). ***Troponin-T (TnT),*** a 30-kDa subunit, binds to tropomyosin, anchoring the troponin complex. ***Troponin-I (TnI),*** also a 30-kDa subunit, binds to actin, thus inhibiting actin–myosin interaction.

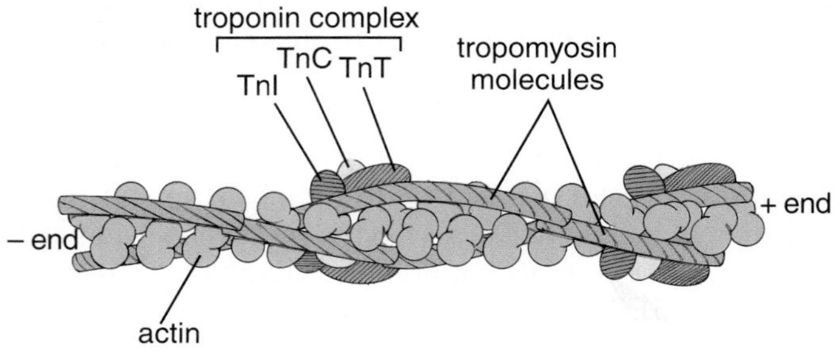

Myosin II, a 510-kDa protein, is composed of ***two polypeptide heavy chains*** (222 kDa each) and ***four light chains.*** Light chains are of two types (18 kDa and 22 kDa), and one molecule of each type is present in association with each myosin head. The phosphorylation by myosin light chain kinase of one of the two types of myosin light chains initiates contraction in smooth muscles (see page 267). Each heavy chain has a small globular head that projects at an approximately right angle at one end of the long rod-shaped molecule. This globular head has two specific binding sites, one for ATP and one for actin. It also demonstrates ATPase and motor activity. The myosin molecules aggregate tail to tail to form the thick filaments; the rod-shaped segments overlap, so that the globular heads project from the thick filament. The "bare" zone in the middle of the filament, i.e., the portion of the filament that does not have globular projections, is the H band. The projecting globular heads of the myosin molecules form cross-bridges between the thick and thin filaments on either side of the H band (see Fig. 10.5).

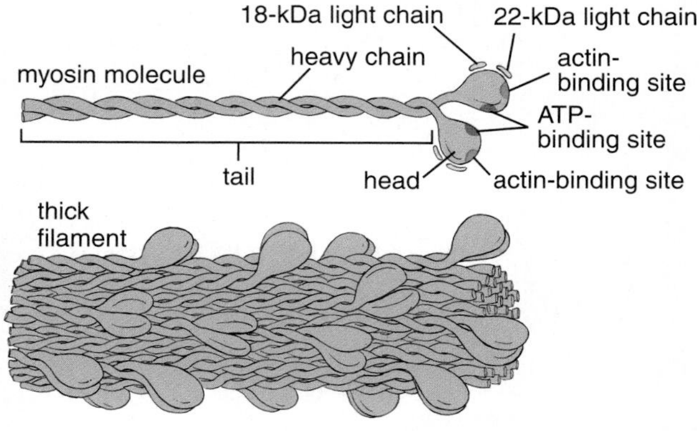

Accessory proteins maintain precise alignment of thin and thick filaments

To maintain efficiency and speed of muscle contraction, both thin and thick filaments in each myofibril must be aligned precisely and kept at an optimal distance from one another. Proteins known as ***accessory proteins*** are essential in regulating the spacing, attachment, and alignment of the myofilaments. These structural protein components of skeletal muscle fibrils constitute less than 25% of the total protein of the muscle fiber. They include (Fig. 10.6)

- ***Titin,*** a large (2500-kDa) protein, forms an elastic lattice that anchors thick filaments in the Z lines. Two spring-

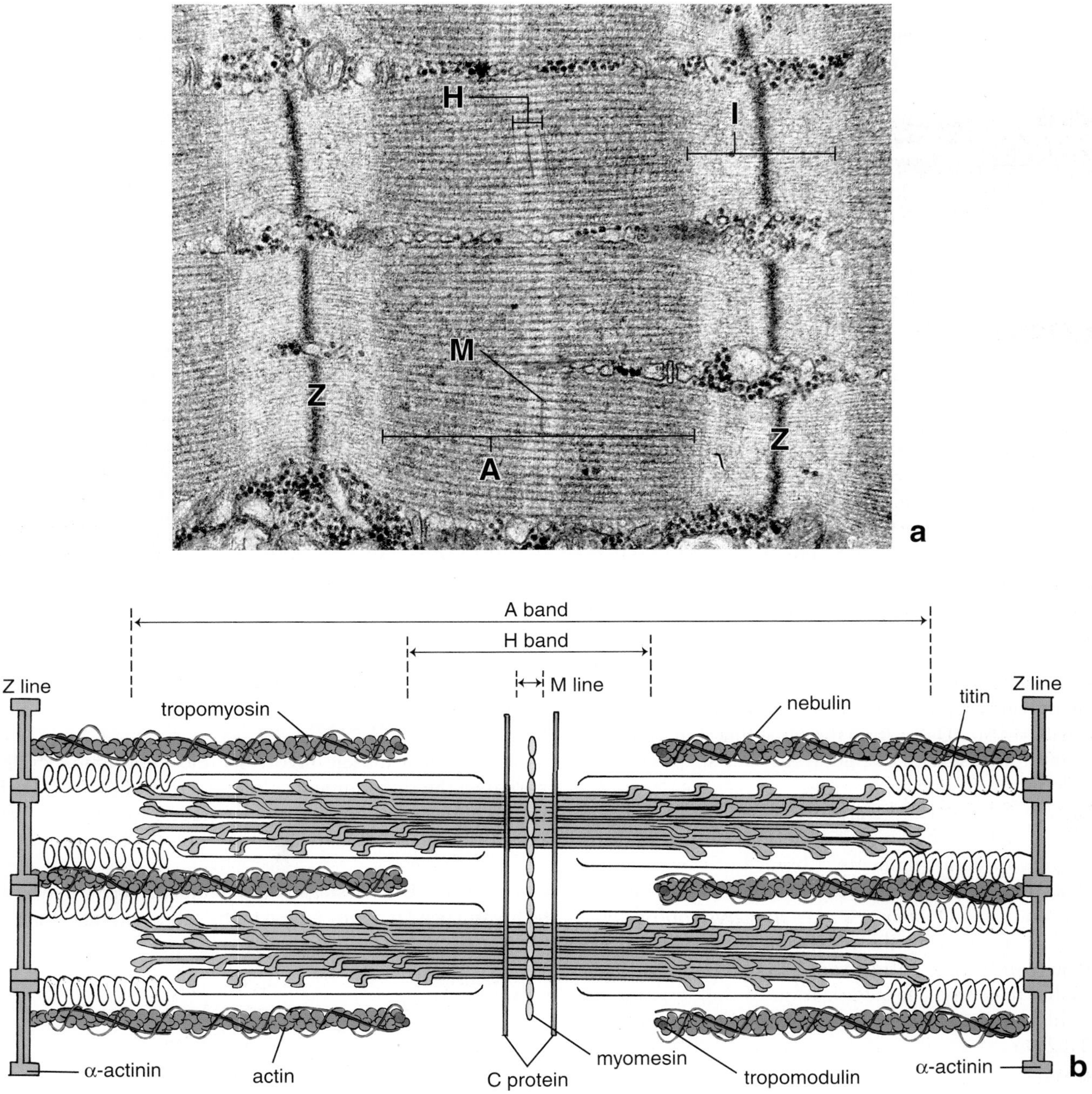

FIGURE 10.6

Electron micrograph of skeletal muscle and corresponding molecular structure of a sarcomere. a. This high-magnification electron micrograph shows a longitudinal section of the myofibrils. The I band, which is bisected by the Z line, is composed of barely visible, thin (actin) filaments. They are attached to the Z line and extend across the I band into the A band. The thick filaments, composed of myosin, account for the full width of the A band. Note that in the A band there are additional bands and lines. One of these, the M line, is seen at the middle of the A band; another, the less electron dense H band, consists only of thick filaments. The lateral parts of the A band are more electron dense and represent areas where the thin filaments interdigitate with the thick filaments. ×35,000. **b.** Diagram illustrating the distribution of myofilaments and accessory proteins within a sarcomere. The accessory proteins are titin, a large elastic molecule that anchors the thick (myosin) filaments to the Z line; α-actinin, which bundles thin (actin) filaments into parallel arrays and anchors them at the Z line; nebulin, an elongated inelastic protein attached to the Z lines that wraps around the thin filaments and assists α-actinin in anchoring the thin filament to Z lines; tropomodulin, an actin-capping protein that maintains and regulates the length of the thin filaments; tropomyosin, which stabilizes thin filaments and, in association with troponin, regulates binding of calcium ions; and myomesin and C proteins, myosin-binding proteins that hold thick filaments in register at the M line. The interactions of these various proteins maintain the precise alignment of the thin and thick filaments in the sarcomere.

like portions of the protein adjacent to the thin filaments help stabilize the centering of the myosin-containing thick filament, preventing excessive stretching of the sarcomere.

- ***α-Actinin,*** a short, bipolar, rod-shaped, 190-kDa actin-binding protein, bundles thin filaments into parallel arrays and anchors them at the Z line.
- ***Nebulin,*** an elongated, inelastic, 600-kDa protein, is attached to the Z lines and runs parallel to the thin filaments. It helps α-actinin anchor thin filaments to Z lines and is thought to regulate the length of thin filaments during muscle development.
- ***Tropomodulin,*** a small, ~40-kDa actin-binding protein, is attached to the free portion of the thin filament. This actin-capping protein maintains and regulates the length of the sarcomeric actin filament. Variations in thin filament length (such as those in white and red muscle fibers) affect the length–tension relationship during muscle contraction and therefore influence the physiologic properties of the muscle.
- ***Desmin,*** a type of 53-kDa intermediate filament, forms a lattice that surrounds the sarcomere at the level of the Z lines, attaching them to one another and to the plasma membrane, thus forming stabilizing cross-links between neighboring myofibrils.
- ***Myomesin,*** a 185-kDa myosin-binding protein, holds thick filaments in register at the M line.
- ***C protein,*** one of possibly several myosin-binding proteins (140 to 150 kDa), serves the same function as myomesin and forms several distinct transverse stripes on either side of the M line.
- ***Dystrophin,*** a large 427-kDa protein, is thought to link laminin, which resides in the external lamina of the muscle cell, to actin filaments. Absence of this protein is associated with progressive muscular weakness, a condition called ***Duchenne's muscular dystrophy.*** Dystrophin is encoded on the X chromosome, which explains why only boys suffer from Duchenne's muscular dystrophy. Recently, characterization of the dystrophin gene and its product has been clinically important (see Box 10.2)

When a muscle contracts, each sarcomere shortens and becomes thicker, but the myofilaments remain the same length

The light microscope reveals that during contraction the sarcomere and I band shorten, while the A band remains the same length. To maintain the myofilaments at a constant length, the shortening of the sarcomere must be due to an increase in the overlap of the thick and thin filaments. This overlap can readily be seen by comparing electron micrographs of resting and contracted muscle. The H band narrows, and the thin filaments penetrate the H band during contraction. These observations indicate that the thin filaments slide past the thick filaments during contraction.

BOX 10.2

Clinical Correlations: Muscular Dystrophy—Dystrophin and Dystrophin-Associated Proteins

Dystrophin is a rod-shaped cytoskeletal protein with a short head and a long tail that is located just beneath the skeletal muscle cell membrane. F-actin is bound at the end portion of the tail. Two groups of transmembrane proteins—α- and β-***dystroglycans*** and α-, β-, γ-, and δ-***sarcoglycans***—participate in a ***dystrophin–glycoprotein complex*** that links dystrophin to the extracellular matrix proteins laminin and agrin. Dystroglycans form the actual link between dystrophin and laminin; sarcoglycans are merely associated with the dystroglycans in the membrane.

Recent research has successfully characterized the dystrophin gene and its products. Several forms of muscular dystrophy are attributed to mutations of single genes encoding several proteins of the dystrophin–glycoprotein complex. Duchenne's and Becker-type muscular dystrophy are associated with mutations that affect dystrophin expression; different forms of limb girdle muscular dystrophy are caused by mutations in the genes encoding the four different sarcoglycans; and another form of congenital muscular dystrophy is caused by a mutation in the gene encoding the α_2 chain of muscle laminin.

The Contraction Cycle

Shortening of a muscle involves rapid contraction cycles that move the thin filaments along the thick filament. Each contraction cycle consists of five stages: attachment, release, bending, force generation, and reattachment.

***Attachment* is the initial stage of the contraction cycle, in which the myosin head is tightly bound to the actin molecule of the thin filament**

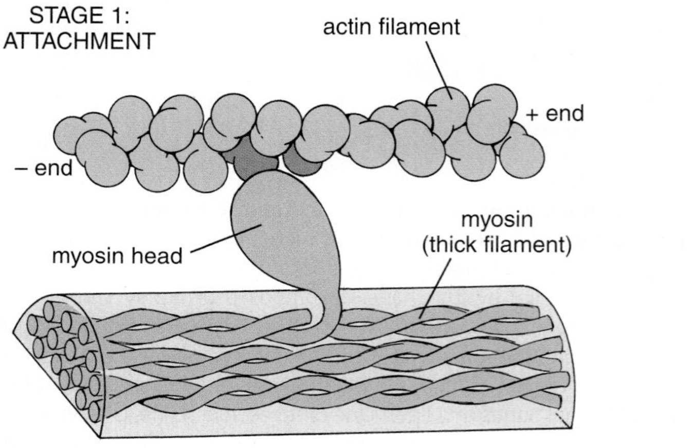

At the beginning of the contraction cycle, the myosin head is tightly bound to the actin molecule of the thin filament, and ATP is absent. This arrangement is known as the ***rigor configuration.*** The muscular stiffening and rigid-

ity that begins at the moment of death is due to lack of ATP and is known as ***rigor mortis.*** In an actively contracting muscle, this step ends with the binding of ATP to the myosin head.

Release is the second stage of the cycle, in which the myosin head is uncoupled from the thin filament

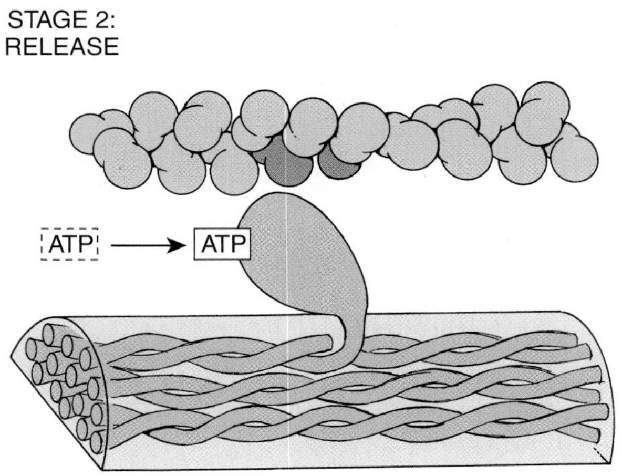

In this stage of the contraction cycle, ATP binds to the myosin head and induces conformational changes of the actin-binding site. This change reduces the affinity of the myosin head for the actin molecule of the thin filament, causing the myosin head to uncouple from the thin filament.

Bending is the third stage of the cycle, in which the myosin head, as a result of hydrolysis of ATP, advances a short distance in relation to the thin filament

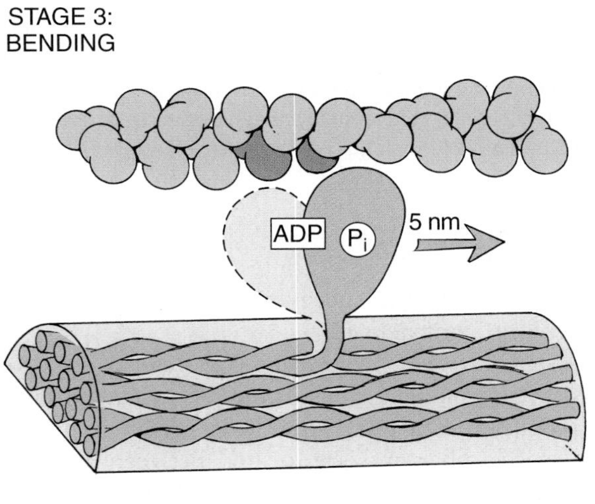

The ATP-binding site on the myosin head undergoes further conformational changes, causing the myosin head to bend. This movement is initiated by the breakdown of ATP into adenosine diphosphate (ADP) and inorganic phosphate; both products, however, remain bound to the myosin head. In this stage of the cycle, the linear displacement of the myosin head relative to the thin filament is approximately 5 nm.

Force generation is the fourth stage of the cycle, in which the myosin head releases inorganic phosphate and the power stroke occurs

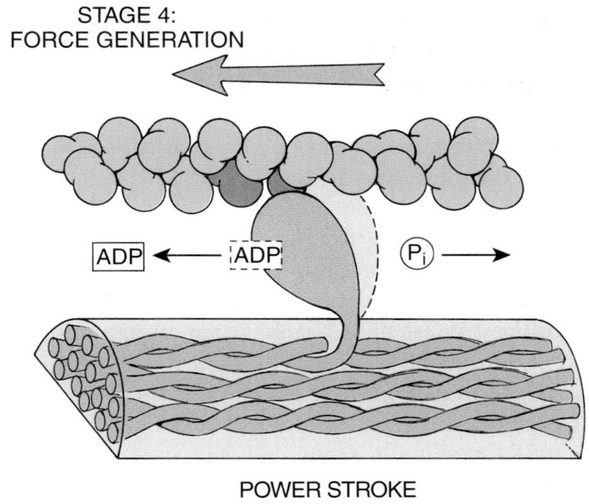

The myosin head binds weakly to its new binding site on the neighboring actin molecule of the thin filament, causing release of the inorganic phosphate. This release has two effects. First, the binding affinity between the myosin head and its new attachment site increases. Second, a force is generated by the myosin head as it returns to its original unbent position. Thus, as the myosin head straightens, it forces movement of the thin filament along the thick filament. This is the ***"power stroke"*** of the cycle. During this stage, ADP is lost from the myosin head.

Reattachment is the fifth and last stage of the cycle, in which the myosin head binds tightly to a new actin molecule

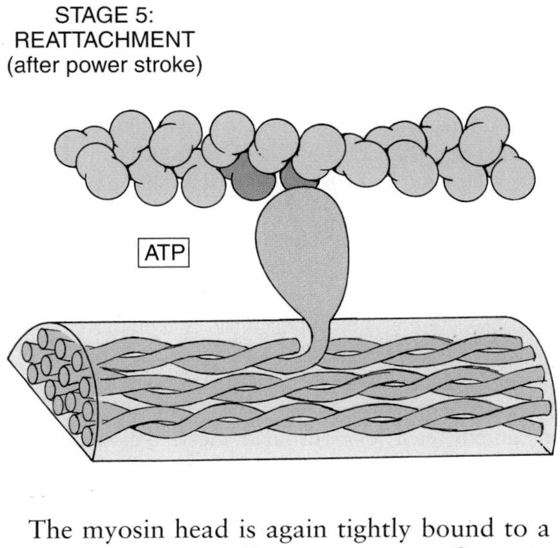

The myosin head is again tightly bound to a new actin molecule of the thin filament (rigor configuration), and the cycle can repeat.

Although an individual myosin head may detach from the thin filament during the cycle, other myosin heads in the same thick filament will attach to actin molecules, thereby resulting in movement. Because the myosin heads are arranged as mirror images on either side of the H band, this action pulls the thin filaments into the A band, thus shortening the sarcomere.

Regulation of contraction involves Ca^{2+}, sarcoplasmic reticulum, and the transverse tubular system

Ca^{2+} must be available for the reaction between actin and myosin. After contraction, Ca^{2+} must be removed. This rapid delivery and removal of Ca^{2+} is accomplished by the combined work of the sarcoplasmic reticulum and the transverse tubular system.

The ***sarcoplasmic reticulum*** is arranged as a repeating series of networks around the myofibrils. Each network of the reticulum extends from one A–I junction to the next A–I junction within a sarcomere. The adjacent network of sarcoplasmic reticulum continues from the A–I junction to the next A–I junction of the neighboring sarcomere. Therefore, one network of sarcoplasmic reticulum surrounds the A band, and the adjacent network surrounds the I band (Fig. 10.7). Where the two networks meet, at the junction between A and I bands, the sarcoplasmic reticulum forms a slightly more regular ring-like channel called the ***terminal cisterna.*** The terminal cisternae serve as reservoirs for Ca^{2+}. To release Ca^{2+} into the sarcoplasm, the plasma membrane of the terminal cisternae contains an abundance of ***gated Ca^{2+}-release channels.*** Also located around the myofibrils in association with the sarcoplasmic reticulum are large numbers of mitochondria and glycogen granules, both of which are involved in providing the energy necessary for the reactions involved in contraction.

The ***transverse tubular system,*** or ***T system,*** consists of numerous tubular invaginations of the plasma membrane; each one is called a ***T tubule.*** T tubules penetrate to all levels of the muscle fiber and are located between adjacent terminal cisternae at the A–I junctions (see Fig. 10.7). They contain ***voltage sensor proteins,*** depolarization-sensitive transmembrane channels that are activated when the plasma membrane depolarizes. Conformational changes of these proteins affect gated Ca^{2+}-release channels located in the adjacent plasma membrane of the terminal cisternae. The complex of T tubule and the two adjacent terminal cisternae is called a ***triad.***

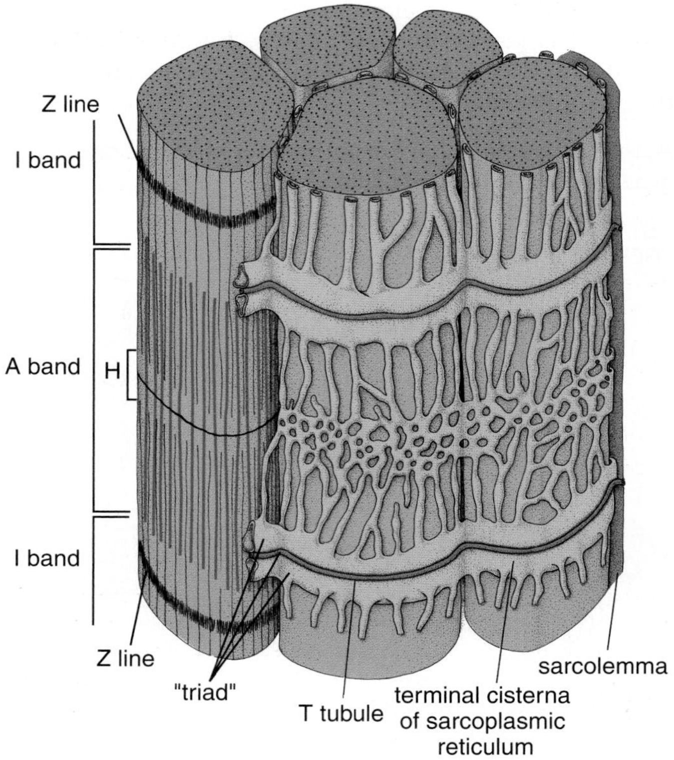

FIGURE 10.7
Diagram of the organization of striated muscle fiber. This diagram illustrates the organization of the sarcoplasmic reticulum and its relationship to the myofibrils. Note that in striated muscle fibers, two transverse (T) tubules supply a sarcomere. Each T tubule is located at an A–I band junction and is formed as an invagination of the sarcolemma of striated muscle. It is associated with two terminal cisternae of the sarcoplasmic reticulum that surrounds each myofibril, one cisterna on either side of the T tubule. The triple structure as seen in cross section, where the two terminal cisternae flank a transverse tubule at the A–I band junction, is called a "triad." Depolarization of the T tubule membrane initiates the release of calcium ions from the sarcoplasmic reticulum and eventually triggers muscle contraction. (Courtesy of Dr. Charles P. Leblond.)

BOX 10.3

Functional Considerations: The Sliding Filament Model

The sliding filament model postulates that the ratchet-like movements of the myosin heads bound to actin produce the movement of the thin filaments relative to the thick filaments, which in turn causes the sarcomere to shorten. Although the sliding filament model can explain contraction in a single sarcomere, it cannot adequately explain the shortening of a myofibril of a muscle fiber. Obviously, if the activity just described were to occur simultaneously in adjacent sarcomeres, no contraction could occur. Equal and opposite forces would be exerted on either side of the Z line, and the contraction of any given sarcomere would be prevented by the contraction of its two immediate serial neighbors. Recent studies with ultrahigh-speed photography have demonstrated that an extremely small temporal delay occurs between the contraction of adjacent sarcomeres, so that a wave-like contraction actually occurs in each muscle fibril and, consequently, in each muscle fiber.

The depolarization of the T-tubule membrane triggers the release of Ca^{2+} from the terminal cisternae to initiate muscle contraction

When a nerve impulse arrives at the neuromuscular junction, the release of neurotransmitter (acetylcholine) from the nerve ending triggers a localized plasma membrane depolarization of the muscle cell. The depolarization, in turn, causes ***voltage-gated Na^+ channels*** in the plasma membrane to open, allowing an influx of Na^+ from the extracellular space into the muscle cell. The influx of Na^+ results in general depolarization, which spreads rapidly over the entire plasma membrane of the muscle fiber. When the depolarization encounters the opening of the T tubule, it is transmitted along the membranes of the T system into the depths of the cell. Electrical charges activate ***voltage sensor proteins*** located in the membrane of the T tubule. The activation of these sensors, in turn, opens ***gated Ca^{2+}-release channels*** in adjacent terminal sacs of the sarcoplasmic reticulum, causing the massive, rapid release of Ca^{2+} into the sarcoplasm. The increased concentration of Ca^{2+} in the sarcoplasm initiates contraction of the myofibril by binding to the TnC portion of the troponin complex on the thin filaments (see page 252). The change in molecular conformation of TnC causes the TnI to dissociate from the actin molecules, allowing the troponin complex to uncover myosin-binding sites on the actin molecules. The myosin heads are now free to interact with actin molecules to initiate the muscle contraction cycle.

Simultaneously, a Ca^{2+}-activated ATPase pump in the membrane of the sarcoplasmic reticulum transports Ca^{2+} back into the terminal cisternae. The resting concentration of Ca^{2+} is restored in the cytosol in less than 30 msec. This restoration of resting Ca^{2+} concentration near the myofilaments normally causes contraction to stop. Contraction will continue, however, as long as nerve impulses continue to depolarize the plasma membrane of the T tubules.

Motor Innervation

Skeletal muscle fibers are richly innervated by motor neurons that originate in the spinal cord or brain stem. The axons of the neurons branch as they near the muscle, giving rise to twigs or terminal branches that end on individual muscle fibers (Fig. 10.8).

The neuromuscular junction is the contact made by the terminal branches of the axon with the muscle

At the ***neuromuscular junction (motor end plate),*** the myelin covering ***(myelin sheath)*** of the axon ends, and the terminal portion of the axon is covered by only a thin portion of the ***neurilemmal (Schwann) cell*** and its external lamina. The end of the axon ramifies into a number

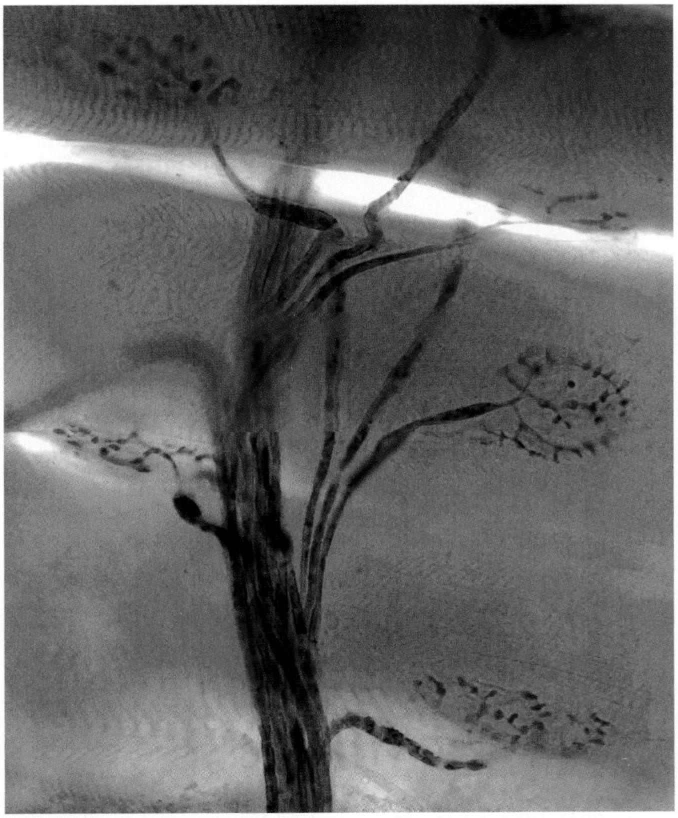

FIGURE 10.8
Photomicrograph of neuromuscular junction. This silver preparation shows a motor nerve and its final branches that lead to the neuromuscular junctions (motor end plates). The skeletal muscle fibers are oriented horizontally in the field and are crossed perpendicularly by the motor nerve fibers. Note that these fibers distally lose their myelin sheath and divide extensively into small swellings forming a cluster of neuromuscular junctions. ×620.

of end branches, each of which lies in a shallow depression on the surface of the muscle fiber, the receptor region (Fig. 10.9). The axon ending is a typical presynaptic structure and contains numerous mitochondria and synaptic vesicles that contain the neurotransmitter ***acetylcholine.***

Release of acetylcholine into the synaptic cleft initiates depolarization of the plasma membrane, which leads to muscle cell contraction

The muscle fiber plasma membrane that underlies the synaptic cleft has many deep ***junctional folds*** (subneural folds). Specific ***acetylcholine receptors*** are limited to the plasma membrane immediately bordering the cleft and at the top of the folds. The external lamina extends into the subneural folds (see Fig. 10.9). The synaptic vesicles of the axon terminal release acetylcholine into the cleft, which

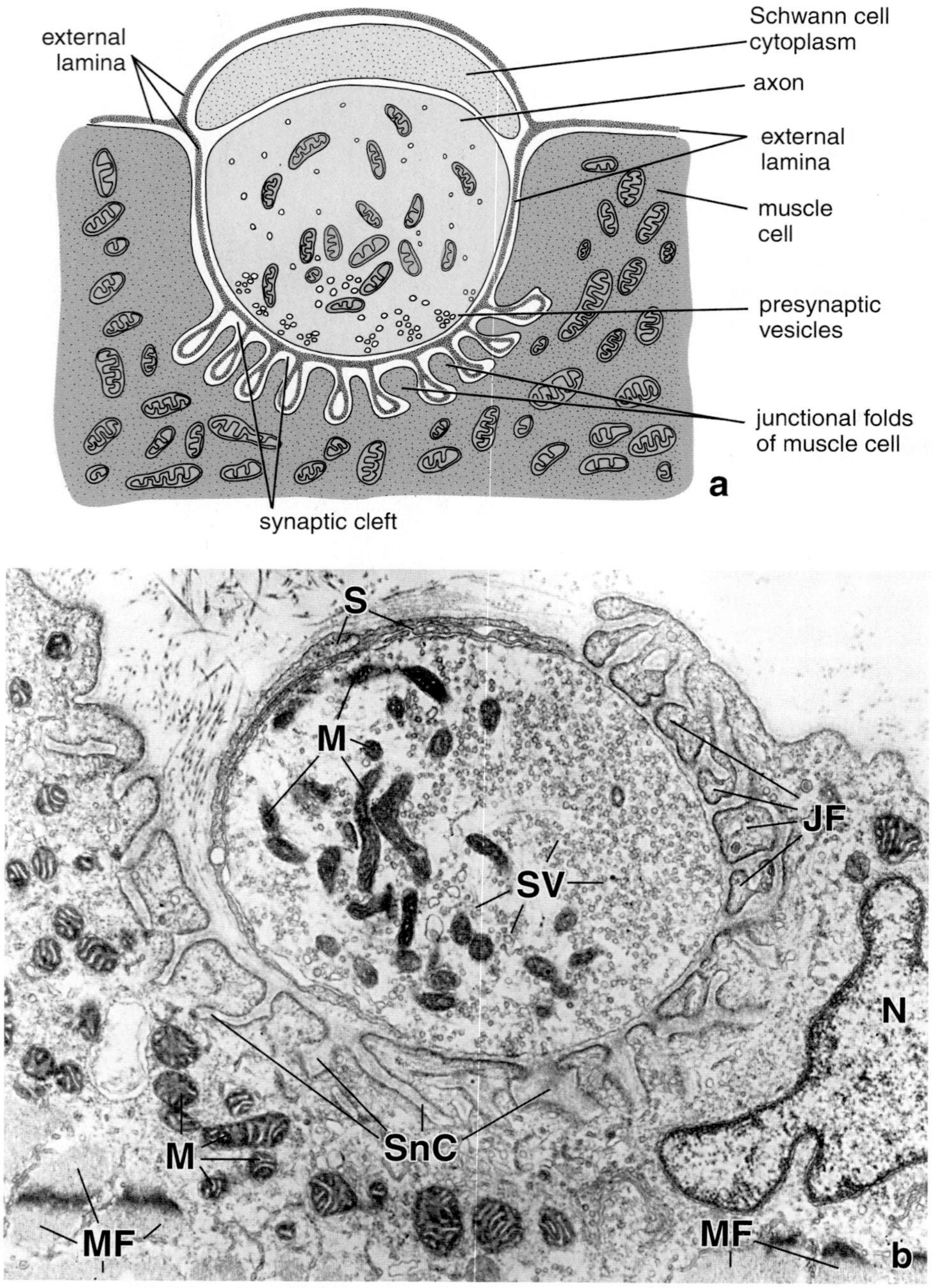

FIGURE 10.9
Neuromuscular junction. a. Diagram of a neuromuscular junction. An axon is shown making contact with a muscle cell. Note how the junctional folds of the muscle cell augment the surface area within the synaptic cleft. The external lamina extends throughout the cleft area. The cytoplasm of the Schwann cell is shown covering the axon terminal. (Modified from Kelly DE, Wood RL, Enders AC, eds. *Bailey's Textbook of Microscopic Anatomy.* Baltimore: Williams & Wilkins, 1984.) **b.** Electron micrograph of a neuromuscular junction shows the axon ending within the synaptic cleft of a skeletal muscle fiber. An aggregation of mitochondria *(M)* and numerous synaptic vesicles *(SV)* is visible. The portion of the motor axon ending that is not in apposition to the muscle fiber is covered by Schwann cell cytoplasm *(S)*, but no myelin is present. The muscle fiber shows the junctional folds *(JF)* and the subneural clefts *(SnC)* between them. The external lamina of the muscle fiber is barely evident within the subneural clefts. Other structures present are the aggregated mitochondria of the muscle fiber *(M)* in the region of the neuromuscular junction, the nucleus *(N)* of the muscle fiber, and some myofibrils *(MF)*. ×32,000. (Courtesy of Dr. George D. Pappas.)

then binds to acetylcholine receptors on the sarcolemma. This binding opens cation channels associated with the acetylcholine receptors, causing an influx of Na^+. The influx of Na^+ results in a localized membrane depolarization, which in turn leads to the events described above. An enzyme called ***acetylcholinesterase*** quickly breaks down the acetylcholine to prevent continued stimulation.

The muscle fiber cytoplasm that underlies the junctional folds contains nuclei, many mitochondria, rough endoplasmic reticulum (rER), free ribosomes, and glycogen. These cytoplasmic organelles are believed to be involved in the synthesis of specific acetylcholine receptors in the membrane of the cleft, as well as acetylcholinesterase.

A neuron along with the specific muscle fibers that it innervates is called a motor unit

A single neuron may innervate several to a hundred or more muscle fibers. Muscles capable of the most delicate movements have the fewest muscle fibers per motor neuron in their motor units. For example, in eye muscles, the innervation ratio is about one neuron to three muscle

fibers; in the postural muscles of the back, a single neuron may innervate hundreds of muscle fibers.

The nature of muscle contraction is determined by the number of motor neuron endings as well as by the number of specific type of muscle fibers that are depolarized. Although depolarization of a muscle fiber at a single neuromuscular junction is characterized as an "all-or-none" phenomenon, not all nerve terminals discharge at once, which allows a graded response to the contractile stimulus. Loss of innervation produces muscle fiber (and muscle) ***atrophy*** as well as total loss of function in the denervated muscle.

Innervation is necessary for muscle cells to maintain their structural integrity

The motor nerve cell not only instructs the muscle cells to contract but also exerts a trophic influence on the muscle cells. If the nerve supply to a muscle is disrupted, the muscle cell undergoes regressive changes known as tissue atrophy. The most conspicuous indication of this atrophy is thinning of the muscle and its cells. If innervation is reestablished surgically or by the slower process of natural regeneration of the nerve, the muscle can regain normal shape and strength.

The events leading to contraction of skeletal muscle can be summarized as a series of steps

The events involved in contraction can be summarized as follows (the numbers refer to the numbers in Fig. 10.10):

1. The contraction of a skeletal muscle fiber is initiated when a nerve impulse traveling along the axon of a motor neuron arrives at the neuromuscular junction.
2. The nerve impulse prompts the release of acetylcholine into the synaptic cleft, which causes local depolarization of sarcolemma.

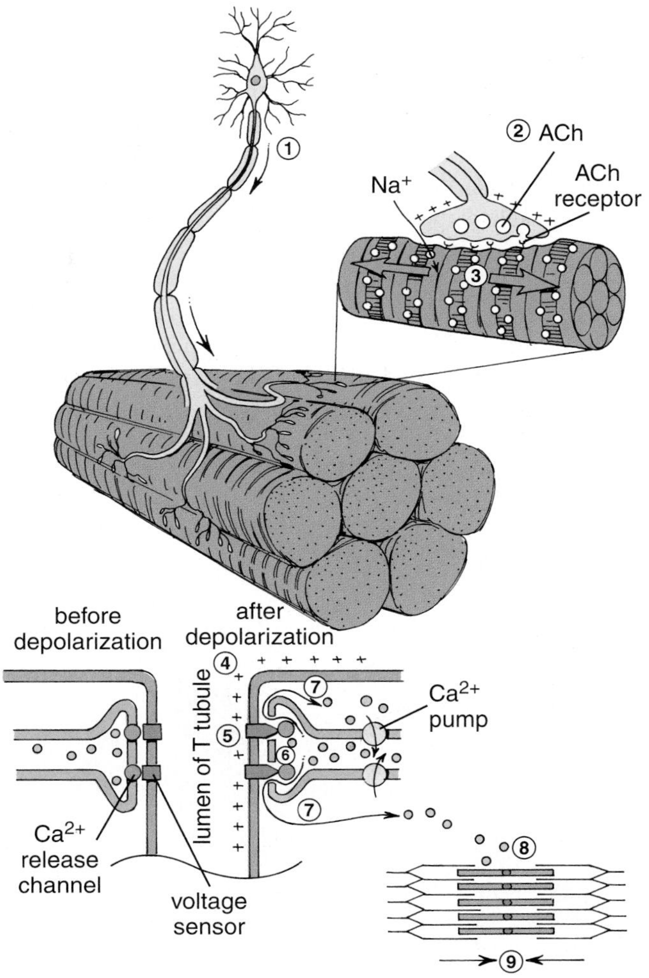

FIGURE 10.10
Summary of events leading to contraction of skeletal muscle. See the text for a description of the events indicated by the *numerals*.

3. Voltage-gated Na^+ channels open, and Na^+ enters the cell.
4. General depolarization spreads over the plasma membrane of the muscle cell and continues via membranes of the T tubules.
5. Voltage sensor proteins in the plasma membrane of T tubules change their conformation.
6. At the muscle cell triads, the T tubules are in close contact with the lateral enlargements of the sarcoplasmic reticulum, where gated Ca^{2+}-release channels are activated by conformational changes of voltage sensor proteins.
7. Ca^{2+} is rapidly released from the sarcoplasmic reticulum into the sarcoplasm.
8. Ca^{2+} binds to the TnC portion of the troponin complex.
9. The contraction cycle is initiated, and Ca^{2+} is returned to the terminal cisternae of the sarcoplasmic reticulum.

BOX 10.4

Clinical Correlations: Myasthenia Gravis

Myasthenia gravis is an autoimmune disease characterized by extreme muscle weakness. In this disease, the acetylcholine receptors on the sarcolemma are blocked by antibodies to the receptor protein. Thus, the number of functional receptor sites is reduced, weakening the muscle fiber response to the nerve stimulus. As the disease progresses, the number of neuromuscular junctions is reduced. Abnormalities within the synaptic cleft (e.g., widening of the synaptic cleft, disappearance of junctional folds) also occur, further reducing the effectiveness of the muscle fibers.

Sensory Innervation

Encapsulated sensory receptors in muscles and tendons provide information about the degree of tension in a muscle and its position.

The muscle spindle is the specialized stretch receptor located within the skeletal muscle

The ***muscle spindle*** is a specialized receptor unit in muscle; it consists of two types of modified muscle fibers called ***spindle cells*** and neuron terminals (Fig. 10.11). Both types of modified muscle fibers are surrounded by an ***internal capsule.*** A fluid-filled space separates the internal capsule from an outer ***external capsule.*** One type of spindle cell, the ***nuclear bag fiber,*** contains an aggregation of nuclei in an expanded midregion; the other type, called a ***nuclear chain fiber,*** has many nuclei arranged in a chain. The muscle spindle transmits information about the degree of stretching in a muscle. The sensory (afferent) nerve fibers carrying information from the muscle spindle have endings that are spirally arranged around the midregion of both types of spindle cells. In addition, spindle cells receive motor (efferent) innervation from the spinal cord and brain by γ efferent nerve fibers, which are thought to regulate the sensitivity of the

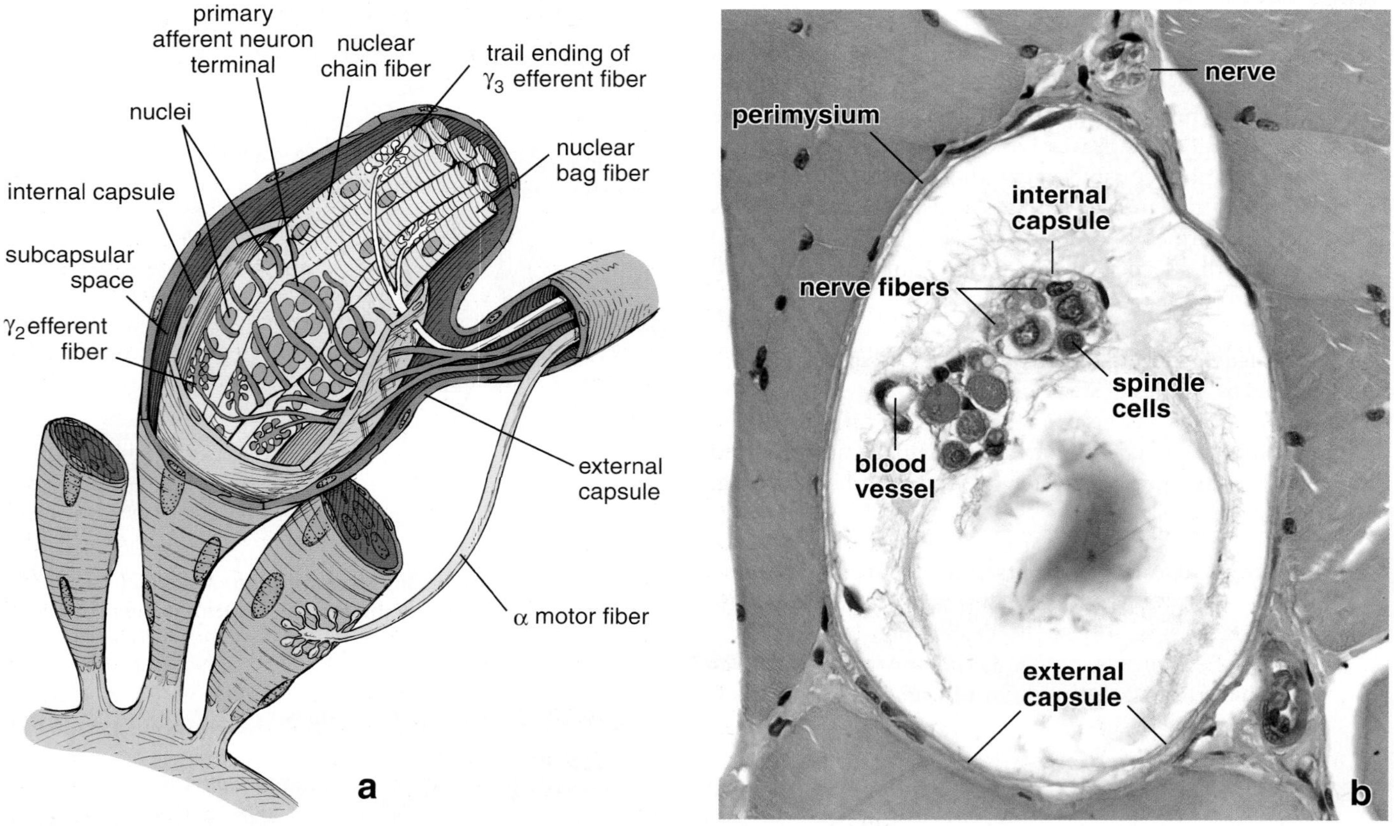

FIGURE 10.11

Muscle spindle. a. Schematic diagram of a muscle spindle. The diameter of the spindle is expanded to illustrate structural details. Each spindle contains approximately two to four nuclear bag fibers and six to eight nuclear chain fibers. In the nuclear bag fibers, the muscle fiber nuclei are clumped in the expanded central portion of the fiber, hence the name *bag.* In contrast, the nuclei concentrated in the central portion of the nuclear chain fibers are arranged in a chain. Both afferent (sensory) and efferent (motor) nerve fibers supply muscle spindle cells. The afferent nerve fibers respond to excessive stretching of the muscle, which in turn inhibits the somatic motor stimulation of the muscle. The efferent nerve fibers regulate the sensitivity of the afferent endings in the muscle spindle. **b.** Photomicrograph of a cross section of a muscle spindle, showing two bundles of spindle cells in the encapsulated, fluid-filled receptor. In one bundle, several of the spindle cells are cut at the level that reveals their nuclei. An internal capsule surrounds the spindle cells. The external capsule of the muscle spindle and the adjacent perimysium can be seen as a faint double-layer boundary of the receptor. Immediately above and outside of the muscle spindle is a nerve that may be supplying the spindle. The several types of nerves associated with the spindle cells as well as the type of spindle cells cannot be distinguished in this H&E–stained section. Near one of the bundles of spindle cells is a small blood vessel. The flocculent material within the capsule consists of precipitated proteoglycans and glycoproteins from the fluid that filled the spindle before fixation. ×550.

stretch receptor. When skeletal muscle is stretched, nerve endings of sensory nerves become activated. They convey their impulses to the central nervous system, which in turn modulates the activity of motor neurons innervating that particular muscle.

Recent real-time studies with computed tomography (CT) scans of living muscle in different states of contraction suggest that muscle spindles may also represent the axes of functional units within large skeletal muscles. Such functional units precisely regulate contractions of portions of the muscle by creating "fixation points" within the muscle substance.

Similar encapsulated receptors, ***tendon organs,*** are found in the tendons of muscle and also respond to stretch. These receptors contain only afferent fibers.

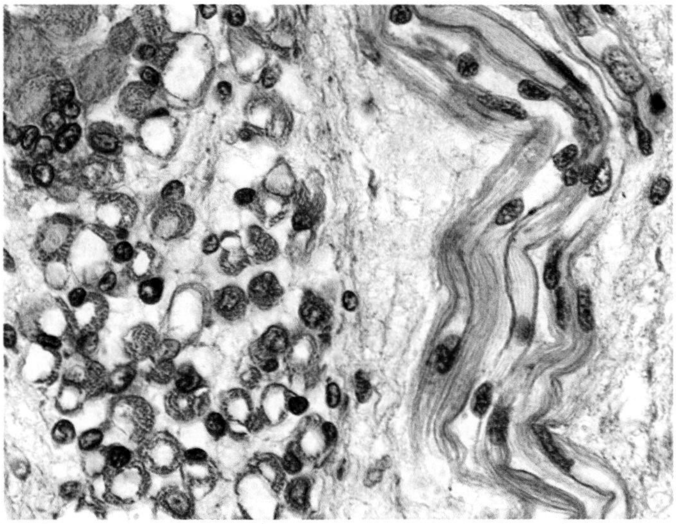

FIGURE 10.12
Photomicrograph of developing skeletal muscle myotubes. This photomicrograph shows a cross section (on the left) and a longitudinal section (on the right) of developing skeletal muscle fibers in the stage of secondary myotubes. These myotubes are formed by sequential fusion of myoblasts forming elongated tubular structures. Note that the myotubes have a small diameter and widely spaced, centrally positioned nuclei that gradually become displaced into the cell periphery by the increased number of newly synthesized myofilaments. In the mature multinucleated muscle fiber (upper left), all nuclei are positioned in the peripheral sarcoplasm, just inside the plasma cell membrane. ×220.

Development, Repair, Healing, and Renewal

In skeletal muscle development, myoblasts fuse to form multinucleated myofibers

Myoblasts are derived from a self-renewing population of multipotential myogenic stem cells that originate in the embryo from unsegmented paraxial mesoderm (cranial muscle progenitors) or segmented mesoderm of somites (epaxial and hypaxial muscle progenitors). Developing muscle contains two types of myoblasts:

- ***Early myoblasts*** are responsible for the formation of ***primary myotubes,*** chain-like structures that extend between tendons of the developing muscle. Primary myotubes are formed by nearly synchronous fusion of early myoblasts. Myotubes undergo further differentiation into mature skeletal muscle fibers. Primary myotubes observed in the light microscope exhibit a chain of multiple central nuclei containing myofilaments.
- ***Late myoblasts*** give rise to ***secondary myotubes,*** which are formed in the innervated zone of developing muscle where the myotubes have direct contact with nerve terminals. Secondary myotubes continue to be formed by sequential fusion of myoblasts into the already-formed secondary myotubes at random positions along their length. Secondary myotubes are characterized by a smaller diameter, more widely spaced nuclei, and an increased number of myofilaments (Fig. 10.12). In the mature multinucleated muscle fiber, the nuclei are all in the peripheral sarcoplasm, just inside the plasma membrane.

Some nuclei that appear to belong to the skeletal muscle fiber are nuclei of satellite cells

Satellite cells are interposed between the plasma membrane of the muscle fiber and its external lamina. They are small cells with scant cytoplasm. The cytoplasm typically blends in with the muscle cell sarcoplasm when viewed in the light microscope, thus making them difficult to identify. Each satellite cell has a single nucleus with a chromatin network denser and coarser than that of muscle cell nuclei. The regenerative capacity of skeletal muscle is limited. Satellite cells function as stem cells that, after injury, proliferate to give rise to new myoblasts. As long as the external lamina remains intact, the myoblasts fuse within the external lamina to form myotubes, which then mature into a new fiber. In contrast, if the external lamina is disrupted, fibroblasts repair the injured site, with subsequent scar tissue formation.

Muscular dystrophies are characterized by progressive degeneration of skeletal muscle fibers, which places a constant demand on the satellite cells to replace the degenerated fibers. Ultimately, the satellite cell pool is exhausted. New experimental data indicate that during this process, additional myogenic cells are recruited from the bone marrow and supplement the available satellite cells. The rate of degeneration exceeds the rate of regeneration, however, resulting in loss of muscle function. A future treatment strategy for muscular dystrophies may include the transplantation of satellite cells or their myogenic bone marrow counterparts into damaged muscle.

CARDIAC MUSCLE

Cardiac muscle has the same types and arrangement of contractile filaments as skeletal muscle. Therefore, cardiac muscle cells and the fibers they form exhibit cross-striations evident in routine histologic sections. In addition, cardiac muscle fibers exhibit densely staining cross-bands, called ***intercalated disks,*** that cross the fibers in a linear fashion or frequently in a way that resembles the risers of a stairway (Fig. 10.13). The intercalated disks represent highly specialized attachment sites between adjacent cells. This linear cell-to-cell attachment of the cardiac muscle cells results in "fibers" of variable length. Thus, unlike skeletal and visceral striated muscle fibers that represent multinucleated single cells, cardiac muscle fibers consist of numerous cylindrical cells arranged end to end. Furthermore, some cardiac muscle cells in a fiber may join with two or more cells through intercalated disks, thus creating a branched fiber.

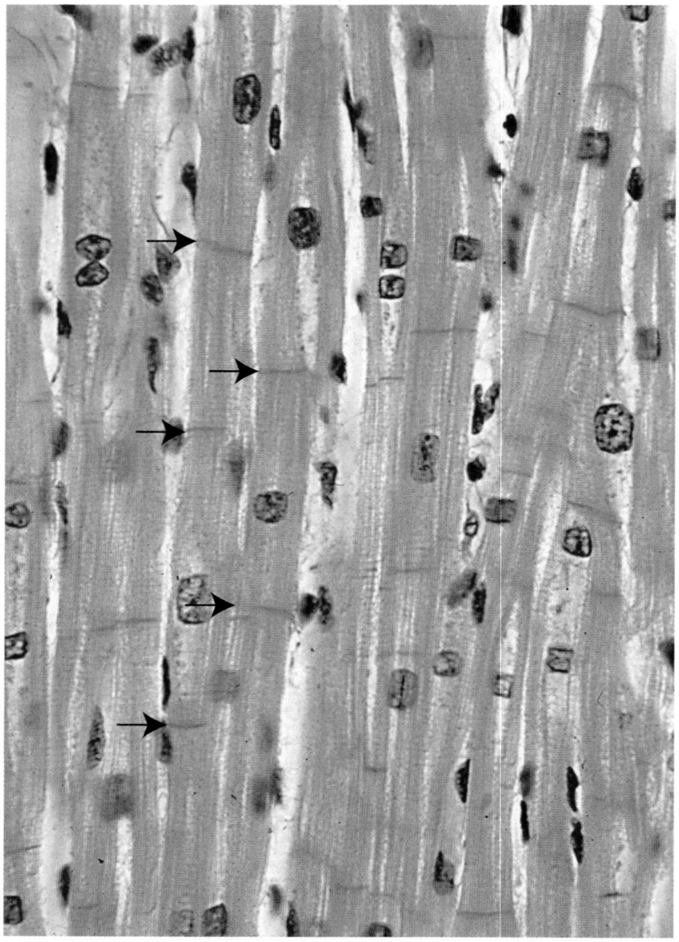

FIGURE 10.13
Photomicrograph of longitudinally sectioned cardiac muscle. The *arrows* point to the intercalated disks. The disks represent specialized cell-to-cell attachments of the cardiac muscle cells. Also note the apparent branching of the muscle fibers. ×360.

Structure of Cardiac Muscle

The cardiac muscle nucleus lies in the center of the cell

The central location of the nucleus in cardiac muscle cells is one feature that helps distinguish them from multinucleated skeletal muscle fibers, whose nuclei lie immediately under the plasma membrane. The transmission electron microscope (TEM) reveals that the myofibrils of cardiac muscle separate to pass around the nucleus, thus outlining a biconical juxtanuclear region in which the cell organelles are concentrated. This region is rich in mitochondria and contains the Golgi apparatus, lipofuscin pigment granules, and glycogen. In the atria of the heart, ***atrial granules*** measuring 0.3 to 0.4 μm in diameter are also concentrated in the juxtanuclear cytoplasm. These granules contain two polypeptide hormones: ***atrial natriuretic factor (ANF)*** [L. natrium, sodium] and ***brain natriuretic factor (BNF).*** Both hormones are diuretics, affecting urinary excretion of sodium. They inhibit renin secretion by the kidney and aldosterone secretion by the adrenal gland (see pages 622 and 671). They also inhibit contractions of vascular smooth muscle. In congestive heart failure, levels of circulating BNF increase.

Numerous large mitochondria and glycogen stores are adjacent to each myofibril

In addition to the juxtanuclear mitochondria, cardiac muscle cells are characterized by large mitochondria that are densely packed between the myofibrils. These large mitochondria often extend the full length of a sarcomere and contain numerous, closely packed cristae (Fig. 10.14). Concentrations of glycogen granules are also located between the myofibrils. Thus, the structures that store energy (glycogen granules) and the structures that release and recapture energy (mitochondria) are located adjacent to the structures (myofibrils) that use the energy to drive contraction.

The intercalated disks represent junctions between cardiac muscle cells

As previously noted, the ***intercalated disk*** represents the attachment site between cardiac muscle cells. In the light microscope, the disk appears as a densely staining linear structure that is oriented transversely to the muscle fiber. Often it consists of short segments arranged in a step-like fashion (Fig. 10.15). When the site of the intercalated disk is examined with the TEM, the densely staining structure seen in the light microscope can be attributed to the presence of a ***transverse component*** that

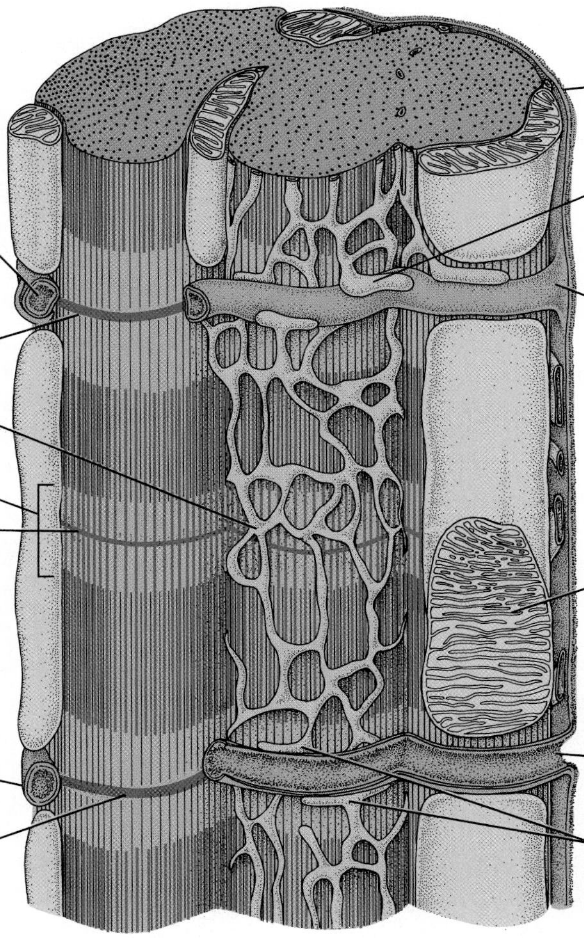

FIGURE 10.14
Diagram of the organization of cardiac muscle fiber. The T tubules of cardiac muscle are much larger than the T tubules of skeletal muscle and carry an investment of external lamina material into the cell. They also differ in that they are located at the level of the Z disk. The portion of the sarcoplasmic reticulum adjacent to the T tubule is not in the form of an expanded cisterna but rather is organized as an anastomosing network. (Redrawn from Fawcett DW, McNutt NS. *J Cell Biol* 1969;42:1–45.)

crosses the fibers at a right angle to the myofibrils. The transverse component is analogous to the risers of the stairway. A ***lateral component*** (not visible in the light microscope) occupies a series of surfaces perpendicular to the transverse component and lies parallel to the myofibrils. The lateral component is analogous to the steps of the stairway. Both components of the intercalated disk contain specialized cell-to-cell junctions between adjoining cardiac muscle cells:

- ***Fascia adherens (adhering junction)*** is the major constituent of the transverse component of the intercalated disk and is responsible for its staining in routine H&E preparations. It holds the cardiac muscle cells at their ends to form the functional cardiac muscle fiber (see Fig. 4.12, page 101). It always appears as a transverse boundary between the cardiac muscle cells. The TEM reveals an intercellular space between the adjacent cells that is filled with electron-dense material that resembles the material found in the zonula adherens of epithelia. The fascia adherens serves as the site at which the thin filaments in the terminal sarcomere anchor onto the plasma membrane. In this way, the fascia adherens is functionally similar to the epithelial zonula adherens, where actin filaments of the terminal web are also anchored.
- ***Maculae adherentes (desmosomes)*** bind the individual muscle cells to one another. Maculae adherentes help prevent the cells from pulling apart under the strain of regular repetitive contractions. They reinforce the fascia adherens and are found in both the transverse and lateral components of the intercalated disks.
- ***Gap junctions (communicating junctions)*** constitute the major structural element of the lateral component of the intercalated disk. Gap junctions provide ionic continuity between adjacent cardiac muscle cells, thus allowing informational macromolecules to pass from cell to cell. This exchange permits cardiac muscle fibers to behave as a syncytium while retaining cellular integrity and individuality. The position of the gap junctions on the lateral surfaces of the intercalated disk protects them from the forces generated during contraction.

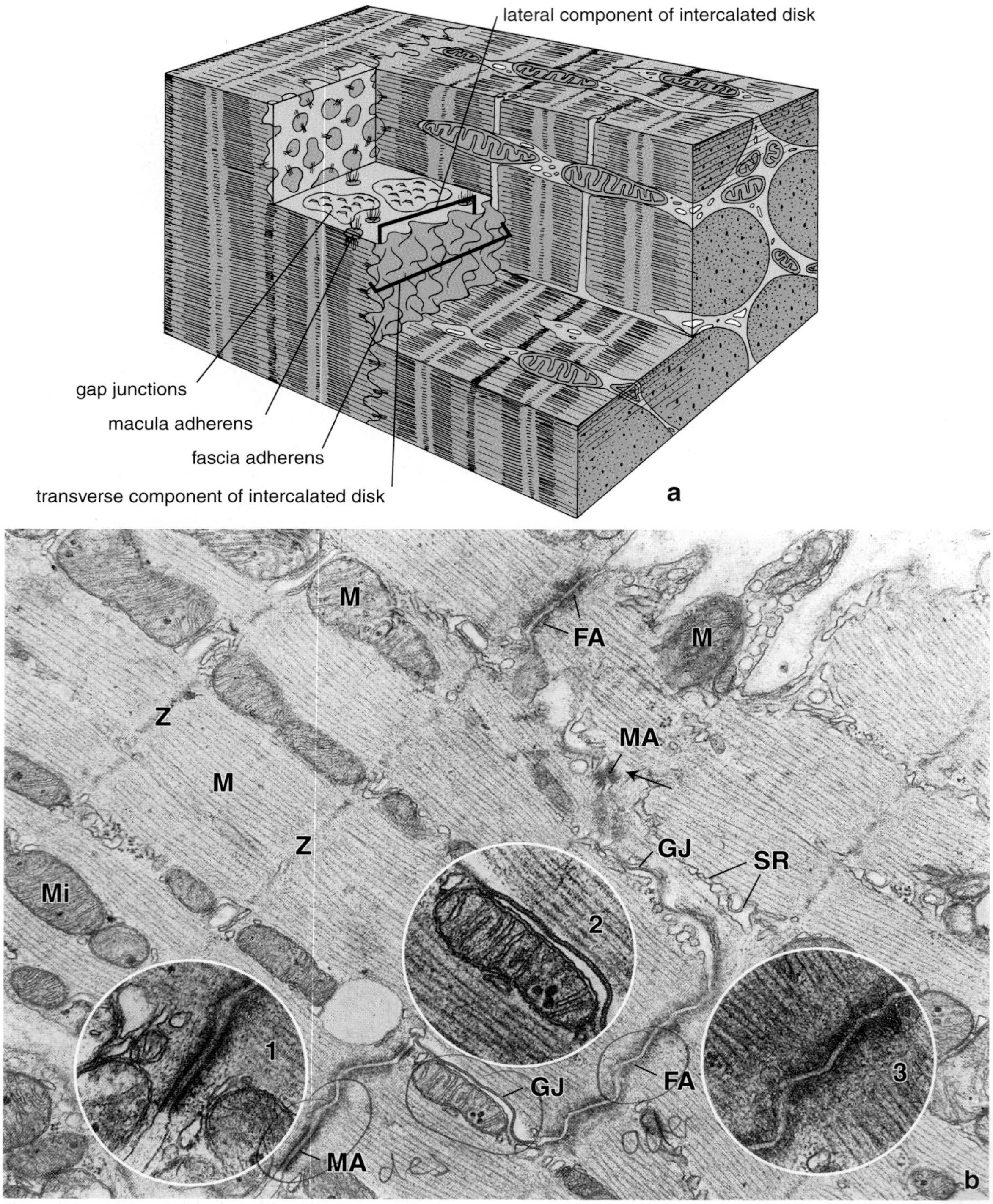

FIGURE 10.15

Structure of cardiac muscle fiber. a. Three-dimensional view of an intercalated disk, which represents a highly specialized attachment site between adjacent cardiac muscle cells. The intercalated disk is composed of the transverse component *(blue area)* that crosses the fibers at a right angle to the myofibrils (analogous to the risers of a stairway) and a lateral component *(pink area)* that occupies a series of surfaces perpendicular to the transverse component and parallel to the myofibrils (analogous to the steps of a stairway). The fascia adherens is the major constituent of the transverse component. It holds the cardiac muscle cells at their ends and serves as the attachment site for thin filaments. The maculae adherentes reinforce the fascia adherens and are also found in the lateral components. The gap junctions are found only in the lateral component of the intercalated disk. **b.** This electron micrograph reveals portions of two cardiac muscle cells joined by an intercalated disk. The line of junction between the two cells takes an irregular, step-like course, making a number of nearly right-angle turns. In its course, different parts of the intercalated disk are evident. These include the transverse components (fascia adherens and maculae adherentes) and lateral components (gap junctions and maculae adherentes). The macula adherens *(MA)* is enlarged in **inset 1** (×62,000). The fascia adherens *(FA)* is more extensive than the macula adherens, being disposed in a larger area of irregular outline. The fascia adherens is enlarged in **inset 3** (×62,000). The fascia adherens of the intercalated disk corresponds to the zonula adherens of other tissues. The gap junction *(GJ)* is enlarged in **inset 2** (×62,000). Other features typical of cardiac muscle are also present: mitochondria *(Mi),* sarcoplasmic reticulum *(SR),* and components of the sarcomere, including Z lines *(Z),* M line *(M),* and myofilaments. This particular specimen is in a highly contracted state, and consequently, the I band is practically obscured. ×30,000.

The sER in cardiac muscle cells is organized into a single network along the sarcomere, extending from Z line to Z line

The sER of cardiac muscle is not as well organized as that of skeletal muscle. It does not separate bundles of myofilaments into discrete myofibrils. The T tubules in cardiac muscle penetrate into the myofilament bundles at the level of the Z line, between the ends of the sER network. Thus, there is only one T tubule per sarcomere in cardiac muscle. Small terminal cisternae of the sER interact with the T tubules to form a *diad* at the level of the Z line (see Fig. 10.14). The external lamina adheres to the invaginated plasma membrane of the T tubule as it penetrates into the cytoplasm of the muscle cell. The T tubules are larger and more numerous in cardiac ventricular muscle than in skeletal muscle. They are less numerous, however, in cardiac atrial muscle.

Cardiac muscle cells exhibit a spontaneous rhythmic contraction

The intrinsic spontaneous contraction or beat of cardiac muscle is evident in embryonic cardiac muscle cells as well as in cardiac muscle cells in tissue culture. The heartbeat is initiated, locally regulated, and coordinated by specialized, modified cardiac muscle cells called ***cardiac conducting cells.*** These cells are organized into nodes and highly specialized conducting fibers ***(Purkinje fibers)*** that generate and rapidly transmit the contractile impulse to various parts of the myocardium in a precise sequence. Both parasympathetic and sympathetic nerve fibers terminate in the nodes. Sympathetic stimulation accelerates the heartbeat by increasing the frequency of impulses to the cardiac conducting cells. Parasympathetic stimulation slows down the heartbeat by decreasing the frequency of the impulses. The impulses carried by these nerves do not initiate contraction but only modify the rate of intrinsic cardiac muscle contraction by their effect at the nodes. The structure and functions of the conducting system of the heart are described in Chapter 12.

Injury and Repair

Mature cardiac muscle cells do not divide under normal conditions

In the past, it was thought that destroyed cardiac muscle cells could not be replaced by new muscle cells. A localized injury to cardiac muscle tissue that results in the death of cells is repaired by the formation of fibrous connective tissue. Consequently, cardiac function is lost at the site of injury. This pattern of injury and repair is seen in nonfatal ***myocardial infarction*** (heart attack). However, recent studies of hearts removed from individuals who had received transplants reveal nuclei undergoing mitosis. While the number of dividing nuclei in these hearts is low (0.1%), it suggests that damaged cells can potentially be replaced. This finding suggests that in the future, a method might be developed that could induce human cardiac muscle to regenerate into healthy tissue.

▼ SMOOTH MUSCLE

Smooth muscle generally occurs as bundles or sheets of elongate fusiform cells with finely tapered ends (Fig. 10.16). The cells, also called fibers, range in length from 20 μm in the walls of small blood vessels to about 200 μm in the wall of the intestine; they may be as large as 500 μm in the wall of the uterus during pregnancy. Smooth muscle cytoplasm stains rather evenly with eosin in routine H&E preparations because of the concentrations of actin and myosin that these cells contain. The nuclei of smooth muscle cells are located in the center of the cell and often have a corkscrew appearance in longitudinal section. This characteristic is due to contraction of the cell during fixation and is often useful in distinguishing smooth

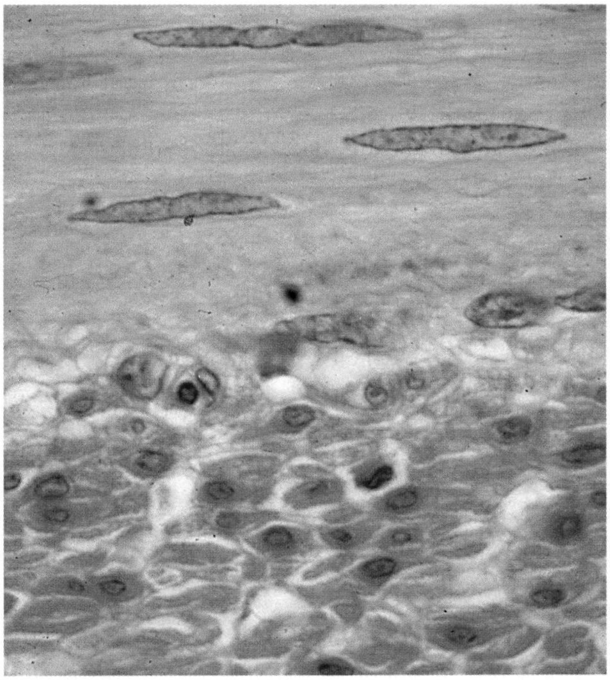

FIGURE 10.16
Photomicrograph of smooth muscle from the small intestine. The muscle is arranged in two layers. The upper portion of the micrograph shows the muscle cells cut in longitudinal section. Note that at the point of cross section, some cells have the nucleus included in the plane of section, whereas others do not. This observation reflects the much greater length than width of the cell. Note that it is usually the smaller cross-sectional profiles that lack the nucleus; they represent the tapering ends of the muscle cells. Also note that the longitudinal smooth muscle cells are not easily delineated from one another, which is due to the way they lie over one another within the thickness of the section. ×600.

muscle cells from fibroblasts in routine histologic sections. In the noncontracted cell, the nucleus appears as an elongated structure with tapering ends, lying in the center axis of the cell. When the nucleus is included in a cross section of a smooth muscle fiber, it appears as a round or circular profile whether the cell is contracted or relaxed. The TEM shows that most of the cytoplasmic organelles are concentrated at each end of the nucleus. These include numerous mitochondria, some cisternae of the rER, free ribosomes, glycogen granules, and a small Golgi apparatus.

Structure of Smooth Muscle

Smooth muscle cells possess a contractile apparatus of thin and thick filaments and a cytoskeleton of actin and desmin intermediate filaments

The remaining sarcoplasm is filled with thin filaments that form a part of the contractile apparatus. The myosin component of the smooth muscle cell is extremely labile and tends to be lost during tissue preparation. Special techniques can be used, however, to retain the structural integrity of the thick myosin filaments and thus demonstrate them with the TEM. Interspersed with the thin filaments are intermediate filaments containing the protein ***desmin*** (vascular smooth muscle contains ***vimentin*** filaments in addition to desmin filaments) and actin filaments, which are part of the cytoskeleton of the cell (Fig. 10.17). In addition, the cytoskeleton contains ***cytoplasmic densities*** or ***dense bodies*** that are visible among the filaments. The thin filaments of the contractile apparatus along with the actin and desmin filaments attach to the dense bodies, which in turn anchor to the sarcolemma.

The components of the contractile apparatus in smooth muscle cells are

- ***Thin filaments*** containing ***actin, tropomyosin,*** and ***caldesmon.*** Actin and tropomyosin are involved in the force-generating interaction with myosin II molecules. Caldesmon is a 120- to 150-kDa protein that binds to F-actin, blocking the myosin-binding site. The action of tropomyosin and caldesmon is controlled by the Ca^{2+}-dependent action of regulatory molecules.
- ***Thick filaments*** containing ***myosin II,*** which is similar to myosin II found in skeletal muscle. It, too, is composed of two polypeptide heavy chains and four light chains. Phosphorylation by myosin light chain kinase of one of the two types of myosin light chains initiates the contraction of smooth muscle.

Myosin light chain kinase, a-actinin, and ***calmodulin*** are other smooth muscle proteins also associated with the contractile apparatus. Calmodulin, a 17-kDa, Ca^{2+}-binding protein, is related to the TnC found in skeletal muscle, which regulates the intracellular concentration of Ca^{2+}. A ***Ca^{2+}–calmodulin complex*** binds to the caldesmon, causing its phosphorylation and release from F-actin.

Dense bodies provide an attachment site for thin filaments and intermediate filaments

Dense bodies contain a variety of attachment plaque proteins, including α-actinin, that anchor both thin filaments and intermediate filaments either directly or indirectly to the sarcolemma. Dense bodies are intracellular analogs of the striated muscle Z lines. In support of this concept is the finding that dense bodies, although frequently appearing as small, isolated, irregular, electron-

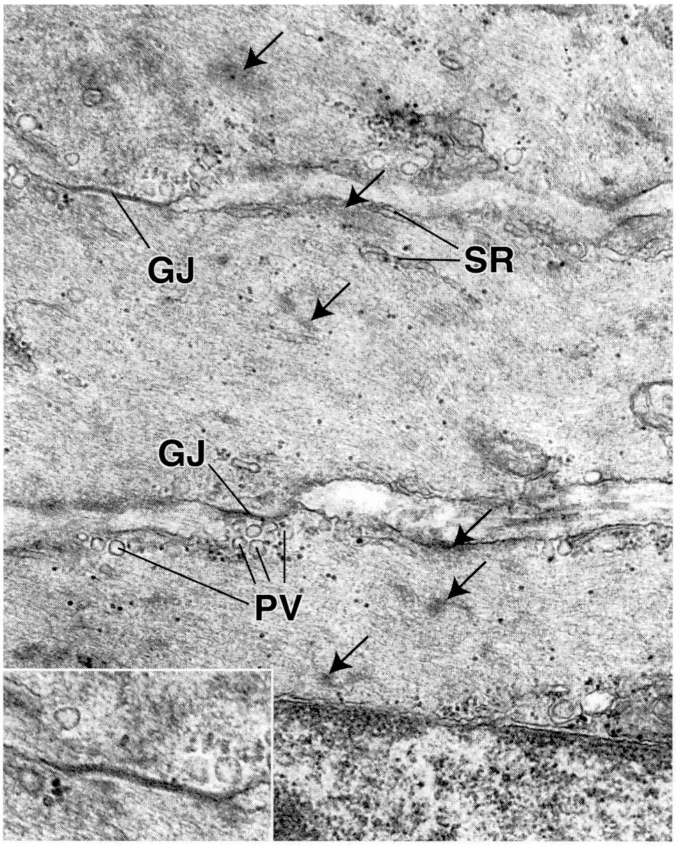

FIGURE 10.17
Electron micrograph of smooth muscle cells. This electron micrograph shows parts of three smooth muscle cells. The nucleus of one cell is in the lower part of the micrograph. The bulk of the cytoplasm is occupied by thin (actin) filaments, which are just recognizable at this magnification. The α-actinin–containing cytoplasmic densities, or dense bodies, are visible among the myofilaments *(arrows)*. Elements of the sarcoplasmic reticulum *(SR)* and the pinocytotic vesicles *(PV)* are also indicated. The other two cells in the middle and upper part of the micrograph possess visible gap junctions *(GJ)* that allow communication between adjacent cells. The small dark particles are glycogen. ×25,000. **Inset.** Enlargement of the gap junction. Note the presence of pinocytotic vesicles. ×35,000.

dense bodies, may also appear as irregular linear structures. In fortuitous sections, they exhibit a branching configuration consistent with a three-dimensional anastomosing network that extends from the sarcolemma into the interior of the cell (Fig. 10.18).

Contraction of smooth muscle is regulated by the Ca^{2+}–calmodulin/myosin light chain kinase system

A modified version of the sliding filament model described on page 256 can explain contraction in both striated and smooth muscle (Fig. 10.19). As in striated muscle, contraction is initiated by an increase in the Ca^{2+} concentration in the cytosol, but the contraction does not act through a troponin–tropomyosin complex on the thin filament. Rather, in smooth muscle, an increase in Ca^{2+} concentration stimulates a myosin light chain kinase to phosphorylate one of the two light chains of myosin. The phosphorylation reaction is regulated by a ***Ca^{2+}–calmodulin complex.*** When the light chain of myosin is phosphorylated, the myosin head attaches to actin and produces contraction. When it is dephosphorylated, the

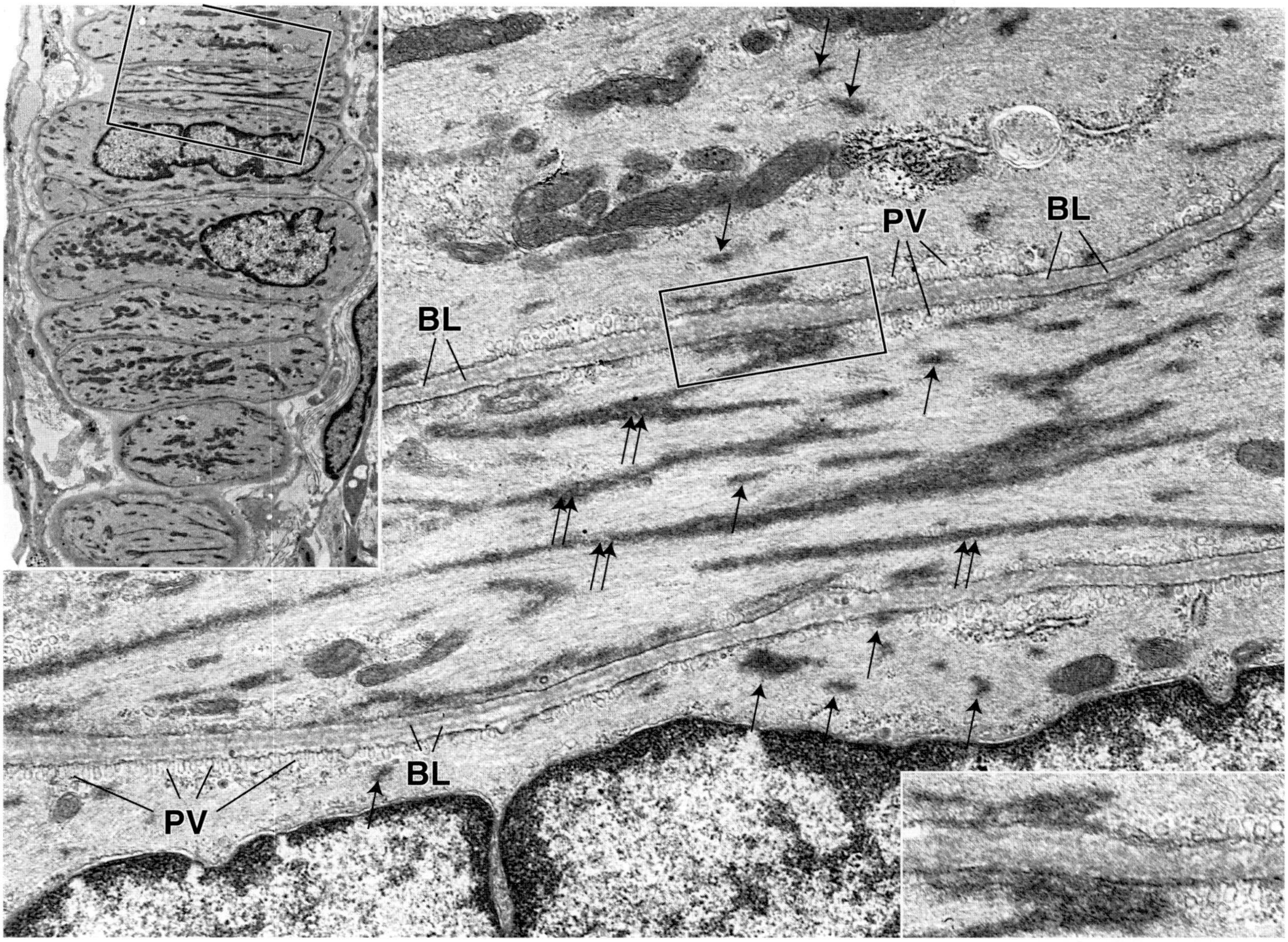

FIGURE 10.18
Electron micrographs showing the cytoplasmic densities in vascular smooth muscle cells. Upper inset. The plane of section includes only the smooth muscle cells in the vascular wall. The *rectangle in the inset* shows portions of three smooth muscle cells that appear at higher magnification in the large electron micrograph. The α-actinin–containing cytoplasmic densities *(single arrows)* usually appear as irregular masses, some of which are in contact with, and attached to, the plasma membrane. The cell in the center of the micrograph has been cut in a plane closer to the cell surface and reveals these same densities as a branching structure *(double arrows).* A three-dimensional model of the cytoplasmic densities would reveal an anastomosing network. *BL,* basal (external) lamina; *PV,* pinocytotic vesicles. ×27,000. **Lower inset.** Higher magnification of cytoplasmic densities attached to the plasma membrane from the area indicated by the *rectangle.* Note that each cell possesses a basal (external) lamina. In addition, the pinocytotic vesicles can be observed in different stages of their formation. ×49,500.

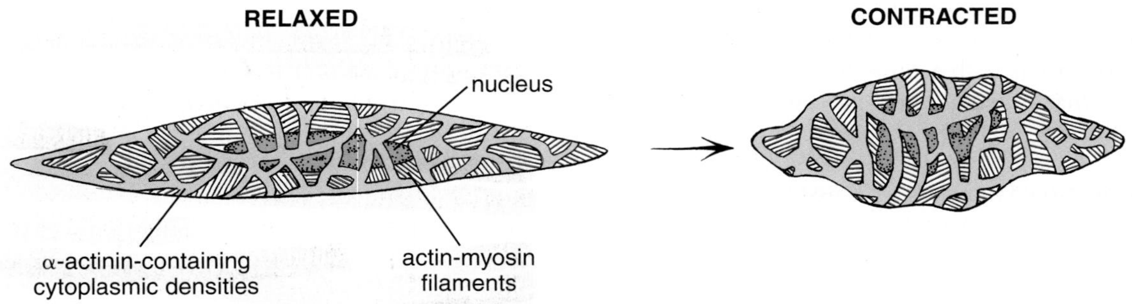

FIGURE 10.19
A suggested model for smooth muscle cell contraction. Bundles of myofilaments containing thin and thick filaments, shown in *dark brown,* anchor on cytoplasmic densities, shown in *beige.* These densities, in turn, anchor to the sarcolemma. Cytoplasmic densities are intracellular analogs of striated muscle Z lines. They contain the actin-binding protein α-actinin. Because the contractile filament bundles are oriented obliquely to the long axis of the cell, their contraction shortens the cell and produces the "corkscrew" shape of the nucleus.

myosin head dissociates from actin. This phosphorylation occurs slowly, with maximum contraction often taking up to a second to achieve.

Smooth muscle cell myosin hydrolyzes ATP at about 10% of the rate of skeletal muscle, producing a slow cross-bridging cycle that results in slow contraction of these cells. Thus, smooth muscle cells, and nonmuscle cells that contract by this same mechanism, are capable of sustained contractions over long periods of time while using only 10% of the ATP that would be used by a striated muscle cell performing the same work.

Smooth muscle cells have a membrane system of sarcolemmal invaginations, vesicles, and sER but lack a T system

A characteristic feature of smooth muscle cells is the presence of large numbers of invaginations of the cell membrane that resemble caveolae (see page 266). Beneath the plasma membrane and often in proximity to the sparse profiles of the sER are cytoplasmic vesicles. It is thought that the invaginations of the cell membrane and the underlying vesicles along with the sER function in a manner analogous to the T system of striated muscle to deliver Ca^{2+} to the cytoplasm. The vesicles and the sER sequester Ca^{2+} from the extracellular matrix and release it during cell depolarization. The Ca^{2+} binds to calmodulin, which activates phosphorylation of the myosin light chain kinase to initiate contraction.

Functional Aspects of Smooth Muscle

Smooth muscle is specialized for slow, prolonged contraction

As noted above, smooth muscle cells may remain contracted for long periods of time without fatiguing. They may contract in a wave-like manner, producing peristaltic movements such as those in the gastrointestinal tract and the male genital tract, or contraction may occur along the entire muscle, producing extrusive movements, e.g., those in the urinary bladder, gallbladder, and uterus. Smooth muscle exhibits a ***spontaneous contractile activity*** in the absence of nerve stimuli.

Contraction of smooth muscle is usually regulated by postganglionic neurons of the ***autonomic nervous system*** *(ANS);* most smooth muscle is directly innervated by both sympathetic and parasympathetic nerves. In the gastrointestinal tract, the third component of the ANS, the ***enteric division,*** is the primary source of nerves to the muscular layers.

Although most Ca^{2+} enters the cytoplasm during depolarization by voltage-gated Ca^{2+} channels, some Ca^{2+} channels, called ***ligand-gated Ca^{2+} channels,*** are activated by hormones. Thus, smooth muscle contraction may also be initiated by certain hormones secreted from the posterior pituitary gland (e.g., oxytocin and, to a lesser extent, antidiuretic hormone, ADH [see page 657]). In addition, smooth muscle cells may be stimulated or inhibited by hormones secreted by the adrenal medulla (e.g., epinephrine and norepinephrine). Oxytocin is a potent stimulator of smooth muscle contraction, and its release by the posterior pituitary plays an essential role in uterine contraction during parturition. It is often used to induce or enhance labor. Many peptide secretions of enteroendocrine cells also stimulate or inhibit smooth muscle contraction, particularly in the alimentary canal and its associated organs.

Nerve terminals in smooth muscle are observed only in the connective tissue adjacent to the muscle cells

Nerve fibers pass through the connective tissue within the bundles of smooth muscle cells; enlargements in the

passing nerve fiber, or ***bouton en passant*** (see page 289), occur adjacent to the muscle cells to be innervated. The enlargements contain synaptic vesicles with neuromuscular transmitters. However, the neuromuscular site is not comparable to the neuromuscular junction of striated muscle. Rather, a considerable distance, usually 10 to 20 μm (in some locations, up to 200 μm), may separate the nerve terminal and the smooth muscle. The neurotransmitter released by the nerve terminal must diffuse across this distance to reach the muscle.

Not all smooth muscle cells are exposed directly to the neurotransmitter, however. As discussed above, smooth muscle cells make contact with neighboring cells by ***gap junctions.*** As in cardiac muscle, contraction is propagated from cell to cell via gap junctions, thus producing coordinated activity within a smooth muscle bundle or layer. The gap junction between two smooth muscle cells was originally designated a ***nexus,*** a term still in use.

Smooth muscle cells also secrete connective tissue matrix

Smooth muscle cells have organelles typical of secretory cells. A well-developed rER and Golgi apparatus are found in the perinuclear zone. Smooth muscle cells synthesize both type IV (basal lamina) collagen and type III (reticular) collagen as well as laminin, elastin, and proteoglycans. Except at the gap junctions, smooth muscle cells are surrounded by an external lamina. In some locations, such as the walls of blood vessels and the uterus, smooth muscle cells secrete large amounts of both type I collagen and elastin.

Renewal, Repair, and Differentiation

Smooth muscle cells are capable of dividing to maintain or increase their number

Smooth muscle cells may respond to injury by undergoing mitosis. In addition, smooth muscle contains regularly replicating populations of cells. Smooth muscle in the uterus proliferates during the normal menstrual cycle and during pregnancy; both activities are under hormonal control. The smooth muscle cells of blood vessels also divide regularly in the adult, presumably to replace damaged or senile cells; the smooth muscle of the muscularis externa of the stomach and colon regularly replicates and may even slowly thicken during life (Fig. 10.20).

New smooth muscle cells have been shown to develop from undifferentiated mesenchymal cells in the adventitia of blood vessels. Smooth muscle cells have also been shown to develop from the division and differentiation of endothelial cells and pericytes in developing vessels. Pericytes are stellate cells located within the basal lamina of capillaries and postcapillary venules. In capillaries, their cytoplasmic morphology is difficult to distinguish from that of the endothelial cell. In postcapillary venules and pericytic venules, they may form a nearly complete investment of the vessel with cells that resemble smooth muscle cells (see Chapter 12).

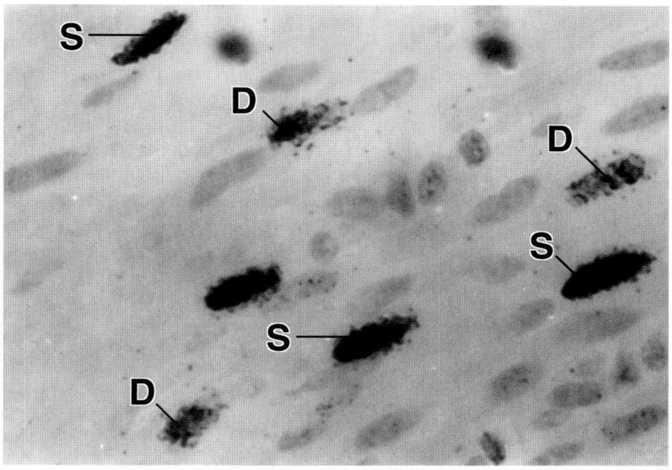

FIGURE 10.20
Autoradiograph of rabbit smooth muscle from the wall of the colon. The animal was injected with tritiated thymidine 21 days before the tissue was sampled. In this nest of labeled cells, both heavily labeled stem cells *(S)* and lightly labeled daughter cells *(D)* are visible. These are frequently adjacent to each other. ×700.

BOX 10.5

Functional Considerations: Complexity of Smooth Muscle Innervation

The description of autonomic innervation of smooth muscle according to the sympathetic and parasympathetic classification and their respective adrenergic and cholinergic transmitters may be more complex than traditionally thought. Viewed with the TEM, nerve terminals with synaptic vesicles that appear to be empty are considered ***cholinergic*** (i.e., secreting the neurotransmitter ***acetylcholine);*** nerve terminals with synaptic vesicles filled with dense granular material are considered ***adrenergic*** (i.e., secreting the neurotransmitter ***norepinephrine).*** Other neurotransmitters have been identified and are collectively called ***purinergic.*** They are likely to be contained in large vesicles with an opaque content.

Nerve endings in smooth muscle tissue that contain primarily mitochondria and no vesicles are considered sensory. Both sympathetic and parasympathetic fibers innervate smooth muscle, and it is difficult to distinguish between the fibers. In some smooth muscle, the adrenergic neurotransmitters stimulate and the cholinergic transmitters inhibit contraction; in other smooth muscle, the reverse is true.

BOX 10.6

Functional Considerations: Comparison of the Three Muscle Types

Cardiac muscle shares structural and functional characteristics with skeletal muscle and smooth muscle. In both cardiac and skeletal muscle, the contractile elements—thick and thin filaments—are organized into sarcomeres surrounded by sER and mitochondria. Both cardiac and smooth muscle cells retain their individuality, although both are in functional communication with their neighbors through gap junctions. In addition, cardiac and smooth muscle cells have a spontaneous beat that is regulated but not initiated by autonomic or hormonal stimuli. Both have centrally located nuclei and perinuclear organelles. These common characteristics suggest that cardiac muscle may have evolved in the direction of skeletal muscle from the smooth muscle of primitive circulatory systems. A summary of major characteristics of all three muscle types is provided in Table 10.1.

TABLE 10.1. **Comparison of the Three Muscle Types**

	Skeletal	**Cardiac**	**Smooth**
	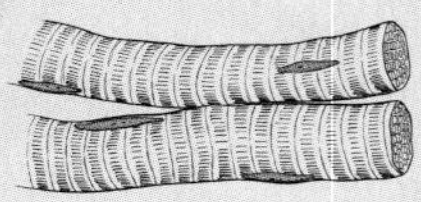	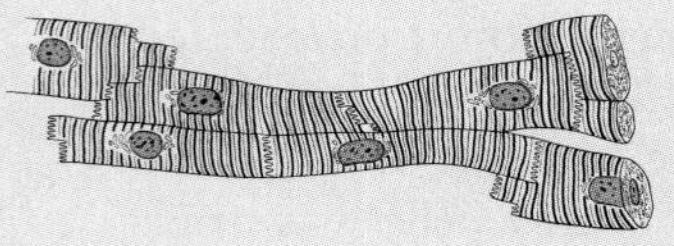	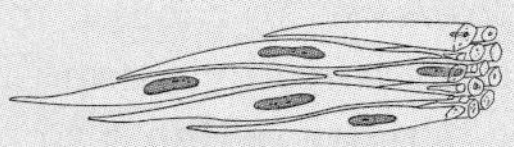
Structural features			
Muscle cell	Large, elongate cell, 10–100 μm in diameter, up to 100 cm in length (sartorius m.)	Short, narrow cell, 10–15 μm in diameter, 80–100 μm in length	Short, elongate, fusiform cell, 0.2–2 μm in diameter, 20–200 μm in length
Location	Muscles of skeleton visceral striated (e.g., tongue, esophagus, diaphragm)	Heart, superior and inferior vena cava, pulmonary veins	Vessels, organs, and viscera
Connective tissue components	Epimysium, perimysium, endomysium	Endomysium (subendocardial and subpericardial connective tissue)	Endomysium, sheaths and bundles
Fiber	Single skeletal muscle cell	Linear, branched arrangement of several cardiac muscle cells	Single smooth muscle cell
Striation	Present	Present	None
Nucleus	Many peripheral	Single central, surrounded by juxtanuclear region	Single central
T tubules	Present at A–I junction (triad: with two terminal cisternae), two T tubules/sarcomere	Z lines (diad: with small terminal cisternae), one T tubule/sarcomere	Replaced by invagination and vesicle similar to caveolae
Cell-to-cell junctions	None	Intercalated disks containing 1. Fasciae adherentes 2. Macula adherens (desmosome) 3. Gap junctions	Gap junction (nexus)
Special features	Well-developed sER and T tubules	Intercalated disks	Dense bodies, caveolae, and cytoplasmic vesicles
Functions			
Type of innervation	Voluntary	Involuntary	Involuntary
Efferent innervation	Somatic	Autonomic	Autonomic
Type of contraction	"All or none" (red and white fibers)	"All or none" rhythmic (pacemakers, conductive system of the heart)	Slow, partial, rhythmic, spontaneous contractions (pacemakers of stomach)
Regulation of contraction	By binding of Ca^{2+} to TnC, causes tropomyosin movement and exposes myosin-binding sites on actin filaments	By binding of Ca^{2+} to TnC, causes tropomyosin movement and exposes myosin-binding sites on actin filaments	By phosphorylation of myosin light chain by myosin light chain kinase in the presence of Ca^{2+}–calmodulin complex
Growth and regeneration			
Mitosis	None	None (in normal condition)	Present
Response to demand	Hypertrophy	Hypertrophy	Hypertrophy and hyperplasia
Regeneration	Limited (satellite cells and myogenic cells from bone marrow)	None (in normal condition)	Present

Fibroblasts in healing wounds may develop morphologic and functional characteristics of smooth muscle cells (***myofibroblasts;*** see page 141). Epithelial cells in numerous locations, particularly sweat glands, mammary glands, salivary glands, and the iris of the eye, may acquire the characteristics of smooth muscle cells ***(myoepithelial cells)***. ***Myoid cells*** of the testis have a contractile function in the seminiferous tubules, and cells of the ***perineurium,*** a concentric layer of connective tissue that surrounds groups of nerve fibers and partitions peripheral nerves into distinct fascicles, function as contractile cells as well as transport barrier cells.

PLATE 18. SKELETAL MUSCLE

Muscle tissue is composed of cells that contain large amounts of the contractile proteins *actin* and *myosin* in particular arrangements that facilitate contraction of the cells and the tissue. Muscle is classified on the basis of the appearance of the contractile cells; two principal types are recognized: striated muscle and smooth muscle. Striated muscle is further subclassified as skeletal muscle, visceral striated muscle, and cardiac muscle. Skeletal and visceral striated muscle cells, also called *fibers,* are long multinucleated protoplasmic units arranged in parallel with their neighbors. The multiple nuclei are at the periphery of the cell, just under the plasma membrane; contractile elements fill the rest of the cell. The highly ordered arrangement of the contractile filaments of actin and myosin accounts for the *cross-striations* characteristic of a longitudinal section of skeletal muscle fibers. The same arrangement is seen in cardiac muscle cells, and thus, both are called striated muscle. Skeletal muscle has a rich blood supply, and each fiber is usually close to several capillaries.

Figure 1, skeletal muscle, H&E ×400.
A section of skeletal muscle fibers in longitudinal profile is shown in this figure. Note the parallel alignment of the fibers *(M);* they are vertically oriented in the illustration. The fibers appear to be of different thickness. This is largely a reflection of the plane of section through the muscle fibers. For example, note the polygonal shape of the fibers when cross-sectioned, as in Figures 2 and 3. A random imaginary line drawn across either micrograph, as if the line were the plane of a longitudinal section, would result in considerable variation in the width of each fiber included in the section. Some fibers might be sectioned along their broadest dimension; some, at their narrowest dimension; and others, at some intermediate dimension.

The cross-striations are the bands that appear at right angles to the long axis of the fibers. They are seen at higher magnification in the **inset.** Two major bands, the darker or more heavily stained *A* band and the lighter *I* band, have been labeled. In addition, the **inset** shows a thin line that bisects the I band; this is the *Z* line. The distance between adjacent Z lines constitutes the *sarcomere.* The other bands, i.e., the M and H bands, are not evident despite the relaxed state of the muscle fibers. The relatively wide I band indicates the relaxed state of the muscle.

Examination of the cytoplasm about the nucleus in the **inset** reveals that the cross-striations do not extend into the areas adjacent to the nuclear poles. This cytoplasm stains lightly *(asterisks)* and contains a concentration of organelles not directly involved in the contractile process.

Between the muscle fibers is a small amount of delicate connective tissue, the ***endomysium.*** There are also two capillaries *(C)* within the endomysium. Although they do not display the structural features of the vessel walls, they can be identified by virtue of the red blood cells in the lumen. The nuclei directly associated with the capillary belong to endothelial cells. Note how they appear to bulge into the lumen **(inset).**

Figure 2, skeletal muscle, H&E ×260.
A cross section of striated muscle cells is shown here. As noted, the muscle fibers *(M)* appear as polygonal profiles. They are partially outlined by numerous nuclei; at the relatively low magnification shown in this figure, however, it is not easy to ascertain if these nuclei belong to the muscle cells, to the capillary endothelial cells, to satellite cells, or to fibroblasts in the endomysium that surrounds the individual muscle cells. A larger amount of connective tissue *(CT)* separates bundles of muscle fibers; this connective tissue is called ***perimysium;*** it contains small arteries and veins *(BV).*

Figure 3, skeletal muscle, H&E ×640.
Several cross-sectioned muscle cells are shown at higher magnification in this figure. The nuclei *(N)* that bulge into the cytoplasm belong to the muscle cell. (However, some nuclei in this position may belong to satellite cells; undifferentiated cells on the muscle side of the basal lamina cannot be identified definitely in H&E sections.) The striated muscle cells contain longitudinal units called myofibrils. The cut ends of the myofibrils account for the stippled appearance often seen in cross-sectioned muscle cells, as in this figure. Numerous ring-like structures *(asterisks)* are seen in the endomysium; these are "empty" capillaries. Other capillaries, cut obliquely or longitudinally, contain red blood cells *(arrows).* During maximal muscular activity, the capillaries are all patent; at lower activity levels, only some of the capillaries are patent.

KEY

A, A band
BV, blood vessels (small artery and vein)
C, capillary
CT, connective tissue (perimysium surrounding muscle fascicles)
I, I band
M, muscle fiber
N, nuclei of muscle cells
Z, Z line
arrows, red blood cells in capillaries
asterisks: Fig. 1, myofibril-free region of cytoplasm; Fig. 3, empty capillaries

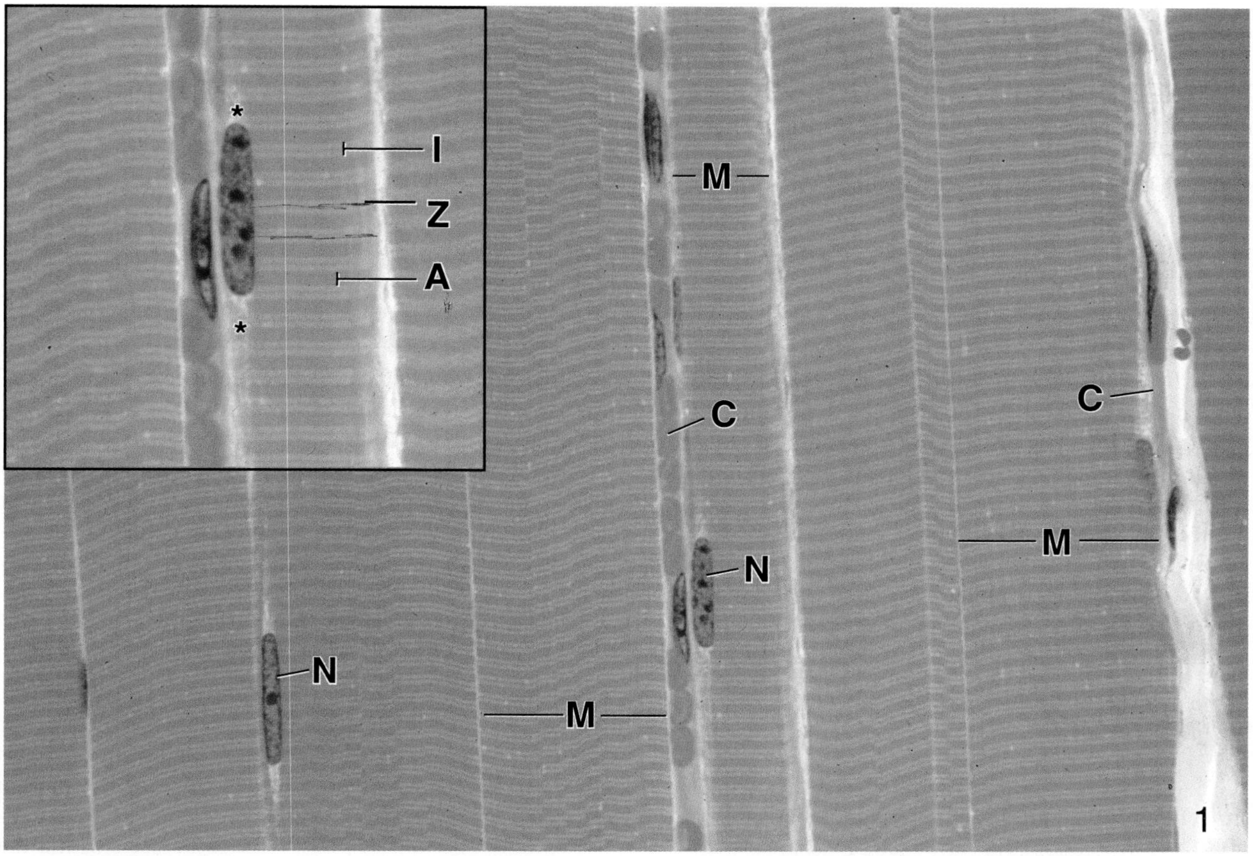
*
I
Z
A
*
M
C
C
M
N
N
M
1

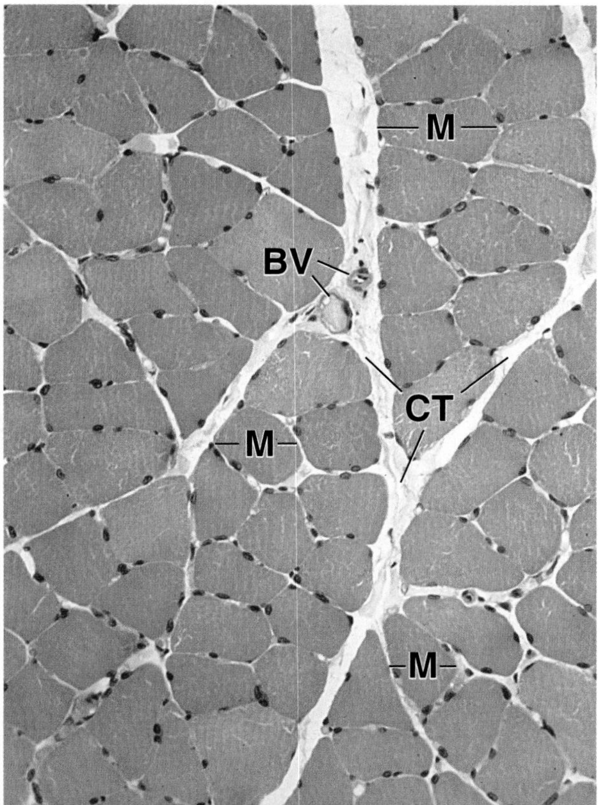
M
BV
CT
M
M
2

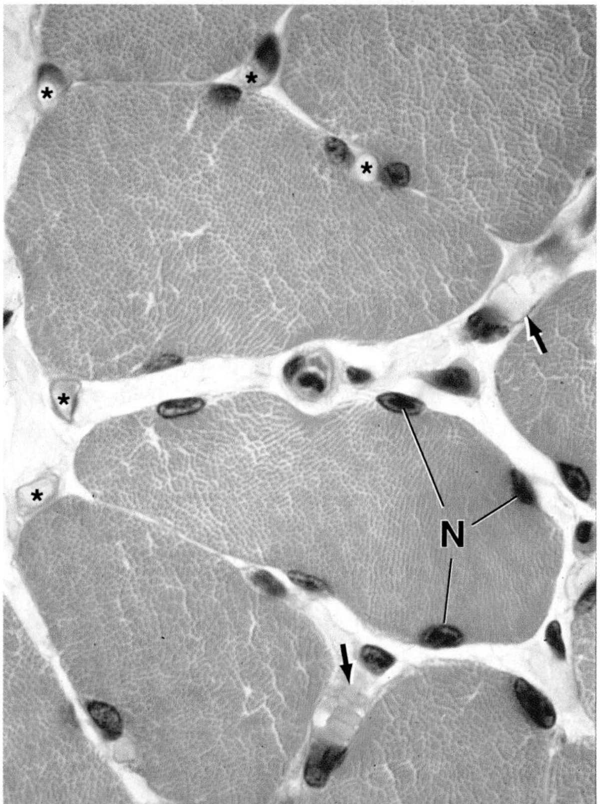
*
*
*
*
*
N
3

PLATE 19. MUSCLULOTENDINOUS JUNCTION AND NEUROMUSCULAR JUNCTION

Skeletal muscle fibers attach at their ends to collagen fibers. The latter may be part of a tendon, a fibrous sheet (aponeurosis), the periosteum, or a raphe. It is by these attachments that the contractile activity of the muscle fibers is translated into useful work in moving or stabilizing parts of the body.

Skeletal muscle fibers are richly innervated by motor neurons that originate in the spinal cord or brain stem. The axons of the neuron branch as they near the muscle, giving rise to twigs that end on individual muscle fibers. The *motor unit* or *neuromotor unit* is the name given to a neuron and the specific muscle cells it innervates; a single neuron may innervate from several to a hundred or more muscle fibers.

Figure 1, musculotendinous junction, H&E ×350.

In this figure, the muscle fibers appear to terminate directly on the tendon. The muscle fibers *(M)* are in the left half of the figure. They stain redder than the tendon *(T),* which typically stains pale pink with eosin. The skeletal muscle fibers have been cut obliquely, and the boundaries between individual muscle cells are not distinct. In many places, however, there is a slight separation of the muscle fibers, and along with the orientation of the muscle cell nuclei, this separation tends to show their general direction. Cross-striations can be identified at right angles to the direction of the fibers. In contrast, the tendon gives no obvious indication of how the collagen fibers are arranged. This needs to be surmised from the orientation of the fibroblast nuclei, which usually have their long axes parallel to the direction of the fibers. Although the nuclei of the fibroblasts are readily identified, the cytoplasm of these cells is not distinguishable from the collagen of the tendon.

Figure 2, musculotendinous junction, electron micrograph ×24,600.

At the actual junction between the muscle cell and tendon, the end of the cell becomes serrated, and the cytoplasmic projections of the muscle cell interdigitate with the collagen fibrils of the tendon. This arrangement is, at best, only suggested in Figure 1, but it is evident in an electron micrograph of the junction, such as that shown here.

This figure shows four finger-like projections of the muscle cell. The external lamina *(BL)* is directly adjacent to the plasma membrane *(PM)* of the muscle cell and follows the finger-like projections. Actin filaments *(arrows)* of the terminal sarcomeres extend into the finger-like projections and insert into densities on the inner face of the plasma membrane *(arrowheads).* Note that the terminal sarcomeres possess only one Z disk *(ZD).* Also to be seen within the muscle cell cytoplasm are triads *(Tr),* glycogen granules *(G),* and mitochondria *(Mi).* External to the cell are fibrils of the tendon *(T).*

Figure 3, neuromuscular junction, Golgi stain ×280.

In the neuromuscular junction shown here, a special stain has been used to visualize the neural elements. This staining procedure does not reveal the skeletal muscle cells to best advantage. They are horizontally disposed in the illustration; cross-striations *(arrows)* are visible in some muscle fibers. The nerve *(N)* enters the field from the left, initially dips downward, then turns in an upward direction. As it does, it can be seen to divide into smaller branches, and finally, as it nears the muscle cells, the nerve fiber branches to make contact with several muscle cells. At the terminal between nerve fiber and each muscle cell, the nerve fiber arborizes to form a disk-like structure, the motor end plate *(MEP),* on the surface of the muscle cells. The motor end plate is the physiologic contact between nerve and muscle; it is, in fact, a neuromuscular synapse at which the neurotransmitter acetylcholine is liberated. This transmitter initiates the sequence of muscle membrane events that leads to contraction of the muscle.

KEY

BL, basal lamina
G, glycogen
M, striated muscle
MEP, motor end plate
Mi, mitochondria
N, nerve
PM, plasma membrane (sarcolemma)
T, tendon
Tr, triad
ZD, Z disk
arrowheads, attachment of actin filaments into plasma membrane
arrows, actin filaments (Fig. 2.)
arrows, cross-striations (Fig. 3.)

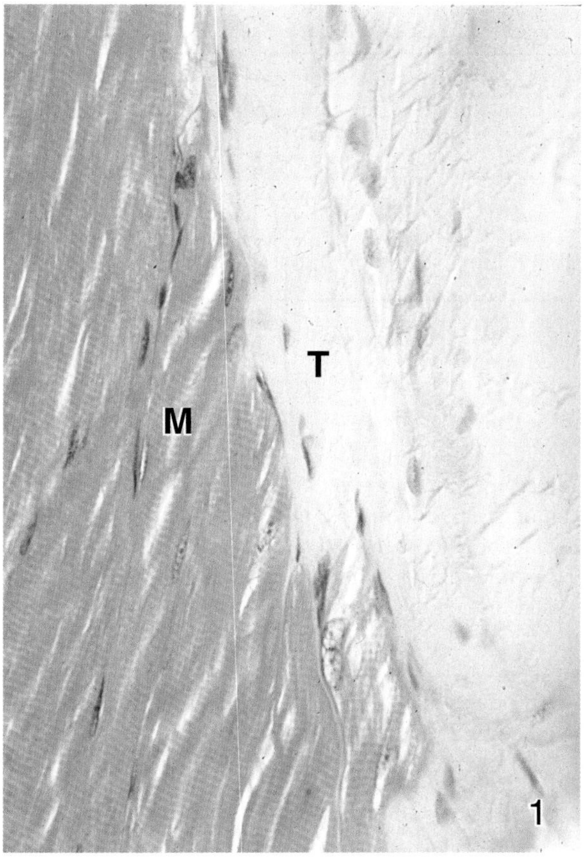
M
T
1

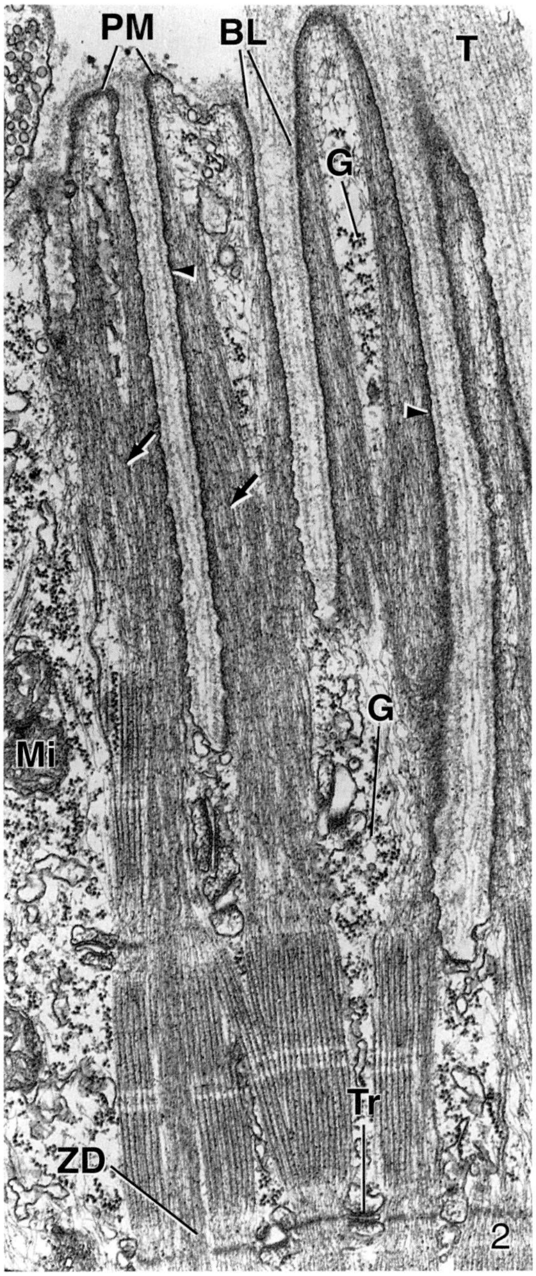
PM
BL
T
G
Mi
G
Tr
ZD
2

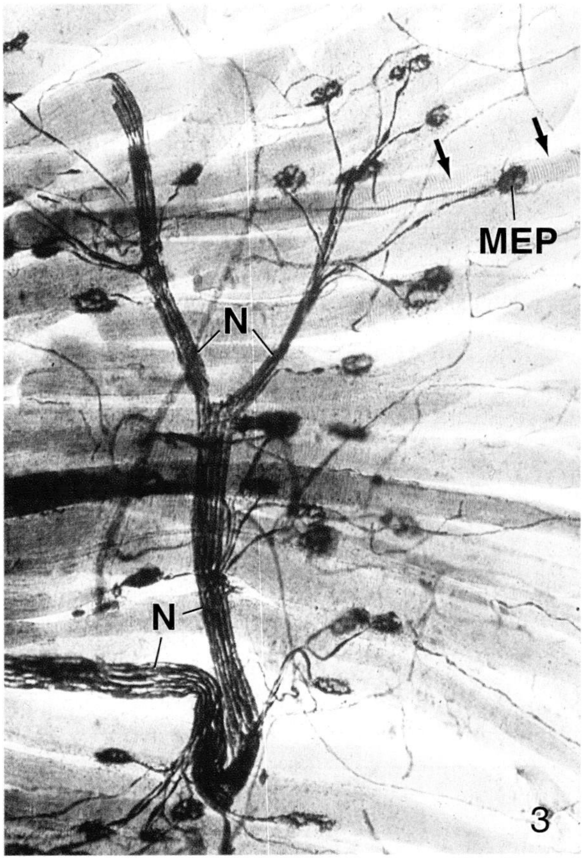
MEP
N
N
3

PLATE 20. CARDIAC MUSCLE

Cardiac muscle consists of fibers that possess the same arrangement of contractile filaments and thus the same cross-banding patterns that are present in striated skeletal and visceral muscle. Although cardiac muscle is, therefore, also striated, it differs in many significant respects from skeletal and striated visceral muscle. Cardiac muscle consists of individual cells that are joined by complex junctions to form a functional unit (fiber). The histologically obvious differences between cardiac and the other striated muscle fibers are the presence in cardiac muscle of *intercalated disks* (the light microscopic representation of the complex junctions), the location of cardiac muscle cell nuclei in the center of the fiber, and the branching of the cardiac muscle fibers. All of these characteristics are evident in a well-prepared longitudinal section of the muscle.

Figure 1, heart, H&E ×160.

This figure shows a longitudinal section of cardiac muscle. The muscle fibers are disposed horizontally in the illustration and show cross-striations. In addition to the regular cross-striations (those of greater frequency), however, there is another group of very pronounced cross-bands, namely, the intercalated disks *(ID)*. Intercalated disks most often appear as a straight band, but sometimes they are arranged in a stepwise manner (see also Fig. 2). These disks are not always displayed in routine H&E sections; therefore, one may not be able to depend on these structures for identifying cardiac muscle. Intercalated disks are opposing cell-to-cell contacts. Thus, cardiac muscle fibers differ in a very fundamental respect from fibers of skeletal muscle. The cardiac muscle fiber consists of an end-to-end alignment of individual cells; in contrast, the skeletal muscle fiber is a single multinucleated protoplasmic unit. In examining a longitudinal section of cardiac muscle, it is useful to scan specific fibers along their long axes. By doing so, one can find places where the fibers obviously branch. Two such branchings are indicated by the *arrows* in this figure.

Figure 2, heart, H&E ×400.

Like skeletal muscle, the cardiac muscle is composed of linear contractile units, the ***myofibrils***. These are evident in this figure as the longitudinally disposed linear structures that extend through the length of the cell. The myofibrils separate to bypass the nuclei, and in doing so, they delineate a perinuclear region of cytoplasm that is free of myofibrils and their cross-striations. These perinuclear cytoplasmic areas *(asterisks)* contain the cytoplasmic organelles that are not directly involved in the contractile process. Many cardiac muscle cells are binucleate; both nuclei typically occupy the myofibril-free region of cytoplasm, as shown in the cell marked by the *asterisks*. The third nucleus in this region appears to belong to the connective tissue either above or below the "in-focus" plane of section. Often, the staining of muscle cell nuclei in a specific specimen is very characteristic, especially when seen in face view as here. Notice, in the nucleus between the *asterisks*, the well-stained nucleolus and the delicate pattern of the remainder of the nucleus. Once such features have been characterized for a particular specimen, it becomes easy to identify nuclei with similar staining characteristics throughout the specimen. For example, survey the field in Figure 1 for nuclei with similar features. Having done this, it is substantially easier to identify nuclei of connective tissue cells *(CT)*, which display different staining properties and are not positioned in the same relationship to the muscle cells.

Figure 3, heart, H&E ×160.

This figure shows cross-sectioned cardiac muscle fibers. Many have rounded or smooth-contoured polygonal profiles. Some fibers, however, are generally more irregular and elongate in profile. These probably reflect a profile of both a fiber and a branch of the fiber. The more lightly stained region in the center of many fibers represents the myofibril-free region of the cell already referred to above and indicated by the *asterisks* in Figure 2. Delicate connective tissue surrounds the individual muscle fibers. This contains capillaries and sometimes larger vessels, such as the venule *(V)* in the center of the bundle of muscle fibers. Larger amounts of connective tissue *(CT)* surround bundles of fibers, and this tissue contains larger blood vessels, such as the arteriole *(A)* marked in the figure.

Figure 4, heart, H&E ×400.

At higher magnification, it is possible to see the cut ends of the myofibrils. These appear as the numerous red areas that give the cut face of the muscle cell a stippled appearance. The nuclei *(N)* occupy a central position surrounded by myofibrils. Remember, in contrast, that nuclei of skeletal muscle fibers are located at the periphery of the cell. Note, also, that as mentioned, the nucleus-free central area of the cell, devoid of myofibrils, shows areas of perinuclear cytoplasm similar to that marked with *asterisks* in Figure 2.

KEY

A, arteriole
C, capillaries
CT, connective tissue
ID, intercalated disks
N, nuclei of cardiac muscle cells
V, venule
arrows, sites where fibers branch
asterisks, perinuclear cytoplasmic areas

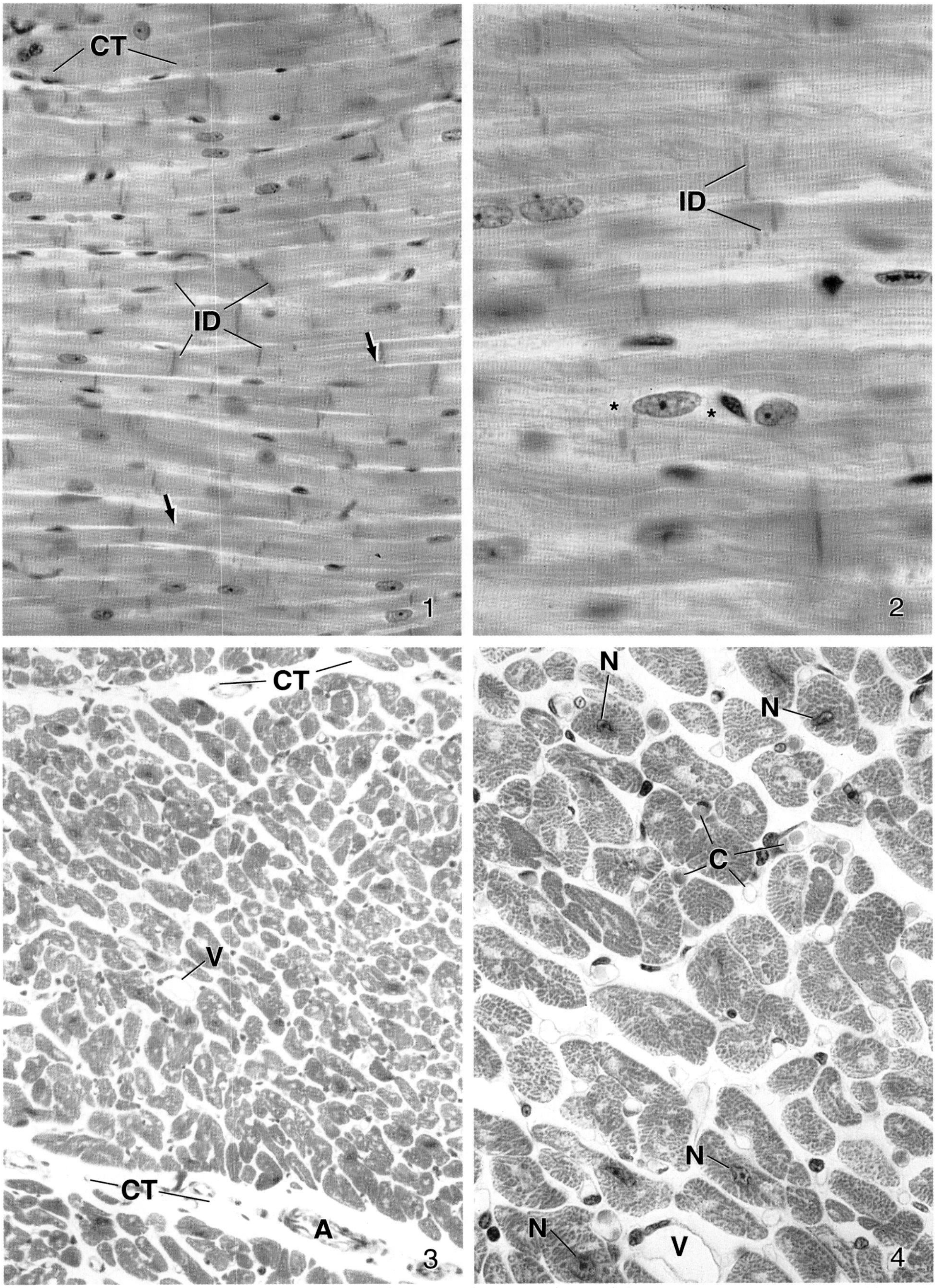
CT
ID
1
ID
*
*
2
CT
V
CT
A
3
N
N
C
N
N
V
4

PLATE 21. CARDIAC MUSCLE, PURKINJE FIBERS

All cardiac muscle cells exhibit a spontaneous rhythmic contraction or beat. This beat is evident in embryonic cardiac muscle cells as well as in isolated cardiac muscle cells in tissue culture. In the heart, this beat is initiated, locally regulated, and coordinated by specialized, modified cardiac muscle cells that are organized into nodes and bundles to transmit the contractile impulse to various parts of the myocardium in a precise sequence. The beat of the heart is initiated at the *sinuatrial (SA) node,* a group of specialized cardiac muscle cells located near the junction of the superior vena cava and the right atrium. The impulse then spreads along the cardiac muscle fibers of the atria and through internodal tracts composed of modified cardiac muscle cells. The impulse is then picked up at the *atrioventricular (AV) node.* Again, some of the cardiac muscle cells are specialized to conduct impulses from the AV node through the ventricular septum into the ventricular walls. Within the ventricular septum, the cells are grouped into a bundle, the *AV bundle (of His*). The bundle divides into two main branches, the left and right bundle branches, going to the left and right ventricles, respectively. These specialized conducting fibers, which carry the impulse at a rate approximately 4 times faster than the cardiac muscle fibers, are responsible for the final distribution of the electrical stimulus to the myocardium. As the bundles ramify in the ventricles, the specialized conducting cells are given the name *Purkinje fibers.*

Figure 1, heart, sheep, H&E ×160.

A section of cardiac muscle and Purkinje fibers is shown in a relatively low-magnification view in this figure. The cardiac muscle fibers *(CM)* appear in the left of the figure; the Purkinje fibers *(PF)* occupy much of the remainder of the field. Connective tissue separates groups of Purkinje fibers from each other and from the cardiac muscle. Small blood vessels *(BV)* and nerves *(NF)* are also present within the connective tissue.

Figure 2, heart, sheep, H&E ×350.

The nature of the Purkinje fibers and their architecture are seen more advantageously here at higher magnification. The fibers are made up of individual cells of irregular shape that maintain extensive contact with one another. Intercalated disks are not observed, but maculae adherentes are present, joining adjacent cells of the fiber.

The cytoplasm of a Purkinje cell contains a large amount of glycogen that is usually extracted during fixation and dehydration of the tissue. Thus, the glycogen-rich areas *(G)* appear as homogeneous, pale-staining regions that usually occupy the center portion of the cell. The periphery of the cell contains the myofibrils *(Mf).* The nucleus *(N)* is round and much larger than the nucleus of the cardiac muscle cell. Because of the considerable size of the Purkinje cells, the nuclei are often not included in the section, and one may get a misleading impression of the disposition and number of cells that make up a fiber. On the other hand, because the myofibrils tend to be located at the periphery of the cell, they can be used to locate the cell boundaries and, thus, help delineate the individual cells of the bundle. The Purkinje fibers ultimately terminate by joining cardiac muscle fibers, thereby permitting direct passage of the impulse to the cardiac muscle fiber.

The connective tissue *(CT)* through which the Purkinje fibers course may also contain nerves *(NF)* and ganglion cells *(GC).* These neural elements belong to the autonomic nervous system, which regulates the activity of the Purkinje fibers and heart muscle.

KEY

BV, blood vessel
CM, cardiac muscle fibers
CT, connective tissue
G, glycogen-rich area
GC, ganglion cell
Mf, myofibrils
N, nucleus of Purkinje cell
NF, nerve fibers
PF, Purkinje fibers

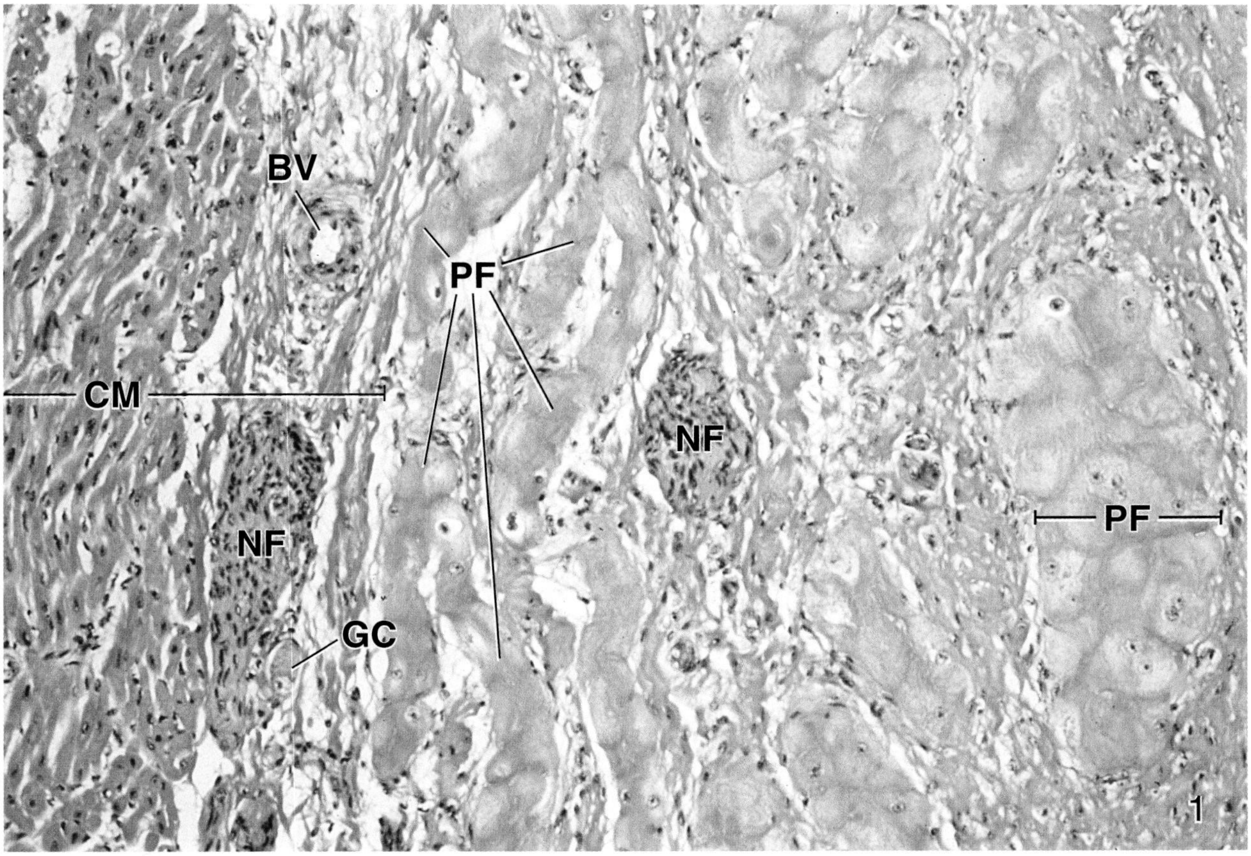
BV
PF
CM
NF
NF
PF
GC
1

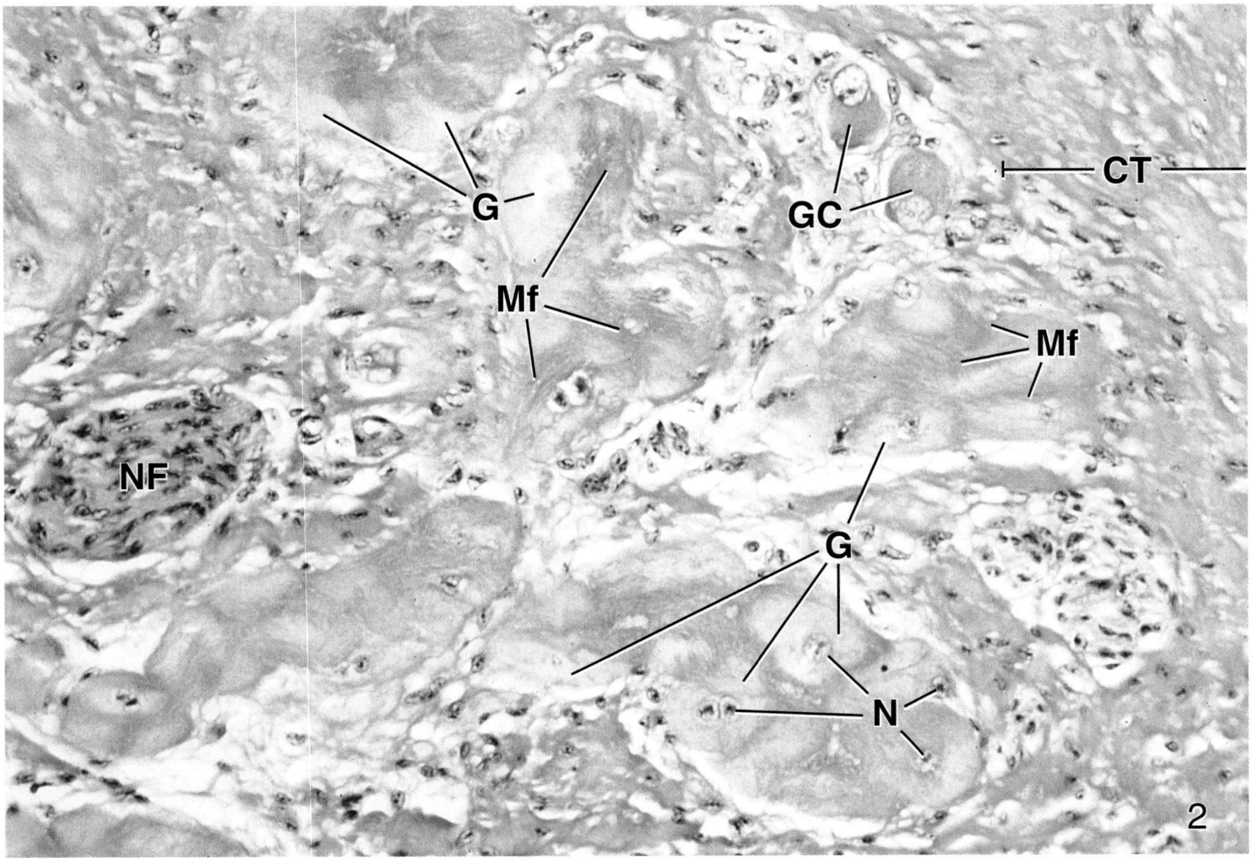
G
GC
CT
Mf
Mf
NF
G
N
2

PLATE 22. SMOOTH MUSCLE

Smooth muscle is the simplest appearing muscle tissue and is the intrinsic muscle of the alimentary canal, blood vessels, genitourinary tract, respiratory tract, and other hollow and tubular organs. Smooth muscle generally occurs as bundles or sheets of elongated fusiform cells, also called fibers. Smooth muscle is specialized for slow, prolonged contraction. There are no direct neural endings on smooth muscle cells; nerve terminals in smooth muscle are in the immediately adjacent connective tissue, and the neurotransmitter diffuses to the muscle cells. Gap junctions between smooth muscle cells allow propagation of the contraction within the muscle.

Figure 1, intestine, monkey, H&E ×900.
Smooth muscle tissue is composed of cells that are typically fusiform or spindle-shaped and organized in parallel arrangements. In this longitudinal section, smooth muscle cells appear elongate. Their nuclei *(N)* are also elongated and conform to the general shape of the cell. In this preparation, the nuclei appear slightly twisted, like a corkscrew; this is characteristic of contracted cells. In this specimen, the cells are sufficiently separated from one another to allow one to delineate the cell boundaries. However, the boundaries cannot always be seen in H&E sections (see Fig. 4).

Figure 2, intestine, monkey, H&E ×900.
This is a cross section through smooth muscle cells from the same specimen shown in Figure 1. The cells now appear as circular or polygonal profiles with variations in size. The nuclei *(N)* also appear as circular profiles and are included in some cells. In most of the cells, however, the nuclei have not been included in the section, and only the eosinophilic cytoplasm appears. Because the cells are staggered, some are cut through the thick central portion, in which case the nucleus is included, whereas others are cut through the tapering ends, in which case only the cytoplasm is seen *(asterisks)*. The differences in diameter between neighboring cells and the variable nuclear profiles are characteristic features of cross-sectioned smooth muscle. Typically, smooth muscle cells are grouped in ill-defined bundles. Note the connective tissue *(CT)* surrounding part of the bundle. Small amounts of extracellular connective tissue fibers and, occasionally, a fibroblast *(F)* are seen between the individual muscle cells within a bundle.

Figure 3, artery, human, H&E ×425.
The smooth muscle cells *(SM)* of a blood vessel (arterial) wall are shown here. These cells are arranged in a circular pattern, forming part of the vessel wall. When the blood vessel is bisected longitudinally, as it is in the upper part of the figure, the smooth muscle cells are cut in cross section, and the nuclei appear rounded *(arrows)*, as they are in Figure 2. In addition, most of the cells display cross-sectioned profiles of only cytoplasm, for the reasons given above. In the bottom of the figure, the blood vessel presents a different profile. It has turned and is leaving the plane of section. Here, the blood vessel is cut essentially in a cross section. The smooth muscle cells are now seen as longitudinal curved profiles, as evidenced by the elongate profiles of the nuclei *(arrowheads)*. The vertically disposed nuclei between the two luminal profiles *(L)* are nuclei of endothelial cells. Connective tissue *(CT)* is external to the smooth muscle cells.

Figure 4, uterus, human, H&E ×160.
Interlacing bundles of smooth muscle cells from the uterus are shown here. These bundles are separated from each other by connective tissue. However, it is not always easy to distinguish between connective tissue and the smooth muscle. Three bundles of smooth muscle cells have been delineated by the *interrupted lines*. In each, there are smooth muscle cells that are arranged in predominately one direction: longitudinal, oblique, and cross section. Careful examination of these areas will reveal nuclei whose profile can be used to determine the orientation of the cells. After noting the orientation of the cells and the nuclei, now note their number per given area of tissue. Comparing the smooth muscle with the connective tissue *(CT)*, note that the connective tissue shows far fewer nuclear profiles per given area of tissue. The lumen in the upper part of the figure belongs to a blood vessel *(BV)* whose mural components blend imperceptibly with the surrounding connective tissue.

KEY

BV, blood vessel
CT, connective tissue
F, nucleus of fibroblast
L, lumen of arteriole
N, nuclei of smooth muscle cells
SM, smooth muscle cell
arrows, nuclei of cross-sectioned smooth muscle cells
arrowheads, nuclei of longitudinally sectioned smooth muscle cells
asterisks, cytoplasm of smooth muscle cell
interrupted lines, boundaries of bundles of smooth muscle cells

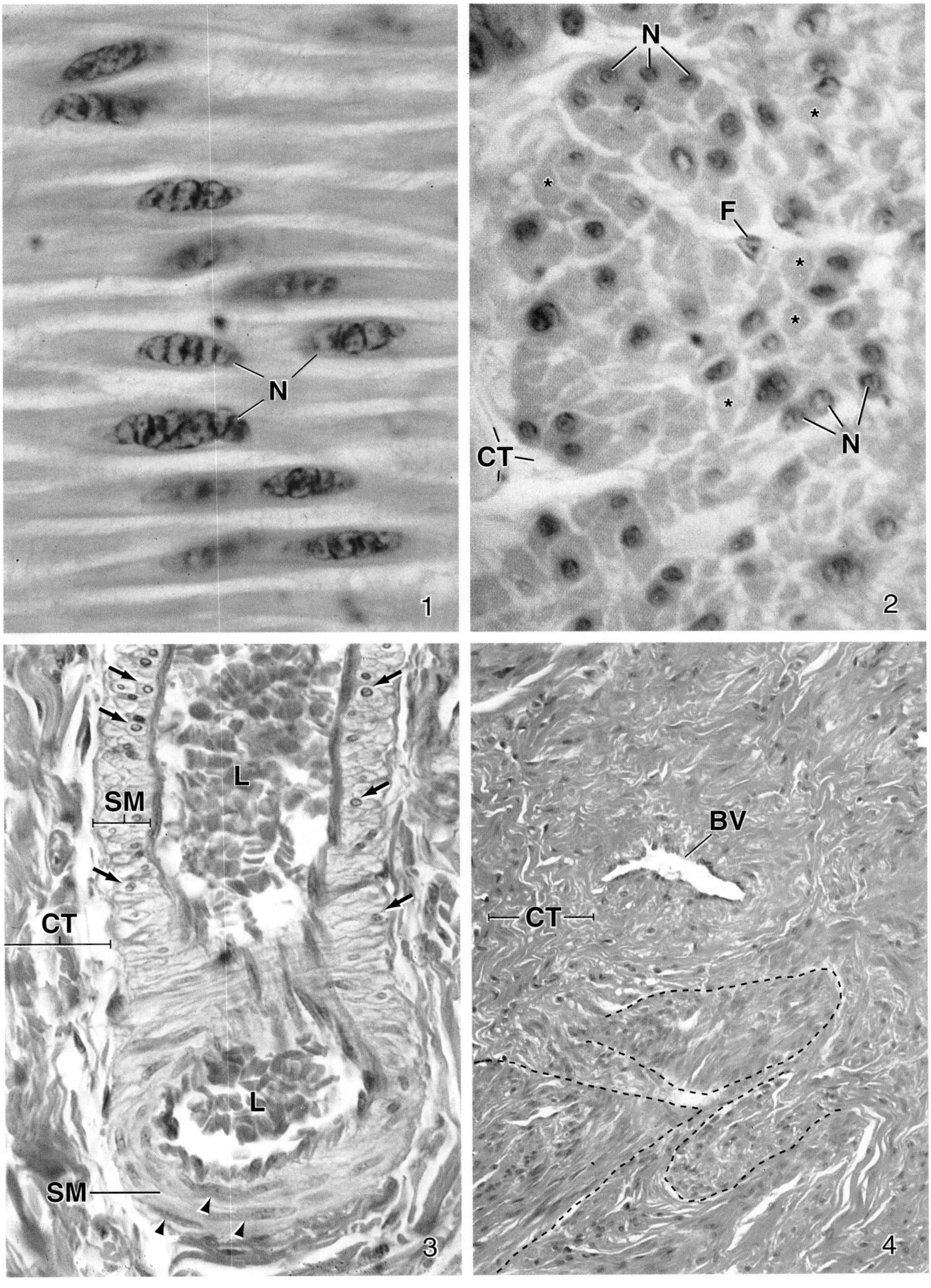
N
1
N
*
F
CT
N
2
SM
L
CT
L
SM
3
BV
CT
4

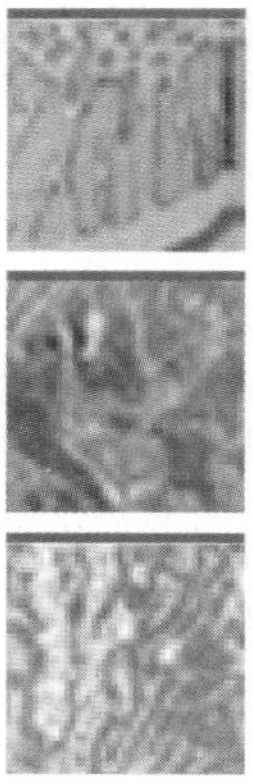

11

Nerve Tissue

BOXES

OVERVIEW OF THE NERVOUS SYSTEM

The nervous system enables the body to respond to continuous changes in its external and internal environment. It controls and integrates the functional activities of the organs and organ systems. Anatomically, the nervous system is divided into the

- *Central nervous system (CNS),* consisting of the brain and the spinal cord, located in the cranial cavity and spinal canal, respectively.
- *Peripheral nervous system (PNS),* consisting of cranial, spinal, and peripheral nerves that conduct impulses from (efferent or motor nerves) and to (afferent or sensory nerves) the CNS, collections of nerve cell bodies outside the CNS called ***ganglia,*** and specialized nerve endings (both motor and sensory).

Functionally, the nervous system is divided into the

- *Somatic nervous system (SNS),* consisting of somatic *[Gr. soma, body]* parts of the CNS and PNS. It provides sensory and motor innervation to all parts of the body except viscera, smooth muscle, and glands.
- *Autonomic nervous system (ANS),* consisting of autonomic parts of the CNS and PNS. It provides efferent involuntary motor innervation to smooth muscle, the conducting system of the heart, and glands. It also provides afferent sensory innervation from the viscera (pain and autonomic reflexes). The ANS is further subdivided into a *sympathetic division* and a *parasympathetic division.* A third element, the *enteric division,* is sometimes incorporated into the ANS subdivision (see page 310).

COMPOSITION OF NERVE TISSUE

Nerve tissue consists of two principal types of cells, neurons and supporting cells

The ***neuron,*** or ***nerve cell,*** is the functional unit of the nervous system; it consists of a cell body, containing the nucleus, and several processes of varying length. Nerve cells are specialized to receive stimuli from other cells and to conduct electrical impulses to other parts of the system via their processes. They are arranged as an integrated communications network, with several neurons in a chain-like fashion typically involved in sending impulses from one part of the system to another. Specialized contacts between neurons that provide for transmission of information from one neuron to the next are called *synapses.*

Supporting cells are nonconducting cells that are in intimate apposition to the neurons. In the CNS they are called ***neuroglia*** or, simply, ***glia.*** In the PNS they are called ***Schwann cells*** and ***satellite cells.*** Schwann cells surround the processes of nerve cells and isolate them from adjacent cells and extracellular matrix. Within ganglia the supporting cells are called ***satellite cells.*** They surround the nerve cell bodies, the part of the cell that contains the nucleus, and are analogous to the Schwann cells.

Supporting cells provide

- Physical support (protection) for delicate neuronal processes
- Electrical insulation for nerve cell bodies and processes
- Metabolic exchange pathways between the vascular system and the neurons of the nervous system

In addition to neurons and supporting cells, an extensive vasculature is present in both the CNS and the PNS. The blood vessels are separated from the nerve tissue by the basal laminae and variable amounts of connective tissue, depending on vessel size. The boundary between blood vessels and nerve tissue in the CNS excludes many substances that normally leave blood vessels to enter other tissues. This selective restriction of blood-borne substances in the CNS is called the ***blood–brain barrier,*** which is discussed on page 313.

The nervous system allows rapid response to external stimuli

The nervous system evolved from the simple neuroeffector system of invertebrate animals. In primitive nervous systems, only simple receptor–effector reflex loops exist to respond to external stimuli. In higher animals and humans, the SNS retains the ability to respond to stimuli from the external environment through the action of effector cells (such as skeletal muscle), but the neuronal responses are infinitely more varied. They range from simple reflexes that require only the spinal cord to complex operations of the brain, including memory and learning.

The autonomic part of the nervous system regulates the function of internal organs

The specific effectors in the internal organs that respond to the information carried by autonomic neurons include

- *Smooth muscle,* whose contraction modifies the diameter or shape of tubular or hollow viscera such as the blood vessels, gut, gallbladder, and urinary bladder.
- *Cardiac conducting cells (Purkinje fibers)* located within the conductive system of the heart. The inherent frequency of Purkinje fiber depolarization regulates the rate of cardiac muscle contraction and can be modified.

- ***Glandular epithelium,*** in which the synthesis, composition, and release of secretions can be modified.

The regulation of the function of internal organs involves close cooperation between the nervous system and the endocrine system. Neurons in several parts of the brain and other sites behave as secretory cells and are referred to as ***neuroendocrine tissue.*** The varied roles of neurosecretions in regulating the functions of the endocrine, digestive, respiratory, urinary, and reproductive systems are described in subsequent chapters.

▼ THE NEURON

The neuron is the structural and functional unit of the nervous system

The human nervous system contains over 10 billion neurons. Although neurons show the greatest variation in size and shape of any group of cells in the body, they fall into three general categories:

- ***Sensory neurons*** convey impulses from receptors to the CNS. Processes of these neurons are included in ***somatic afferent*** and ***visceral afferent*** nerve fibers. ***Somatic afferent fibers*** convey sensations of pain, temperature, touch, and pressure from the body surface. In addition, these fibers convey pain and proprioception (nonconscious sensation) from organs within the body (e.g., muscles, tendons, and joints) to provide the brain with information related to the orientation of the body and limbs. ***Visceral afferent fibers*** transmit impulses of pain and other sensations from mucous membranes, glands, and blood vessels.
- ***Motor neurons*** convey impulses from the CNS or ganglia to effector cells. Processes of these neurons are included in ***somatic efferent*** and ***visceral efferent*** nerve fibers. Somatic efferent neurons send voluntary impulses to skeletal muscles. Visceral efferent neurons transmit involuntary impulses to smooth muscle, cardiac conducting cells (Purkinje fibers), and glands (Fig. 11.1).
- ***Interneurons,*** also called ***intercalated neurons,*** form a communicating and integrating network between the sensory and motor neurons. It is estimated that more than 99.9% of all neurons belong to this integrating network.

The functional components of a neuron include the cell body, axon, dendrites, and synaptic junctions

The ***cell body*** of a neuron contains the nucleus and those organelles that maintain the cell. The processes extending from the cell body constitute the single common structural characteristic of all neurons. Most neurons have only one ***axon,*** usually the longest process extending from the cell, which transmits impulses away from the cell body to a specialized terminal ***(synapse),*** that makes contact with another neuron or an effector cell (e.g., a muscle cell or glandular epithelial cell). A neuron usually has many ***dendrites,*** shorter processes that transmit impulses from the periphery (i.e., other neurons) toward the cell body.

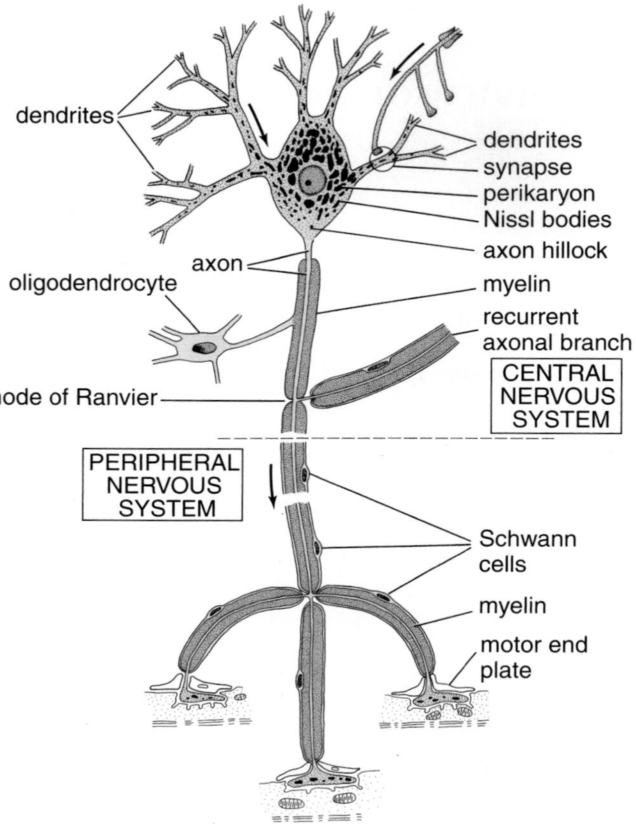

FIGURE 11.1
Diagram of a motor neuron. The perikaryon, dendrites, and initial part of the axon are within the CNS. The axon leaves the CNS and, while in the PNS, is part of a nerve (not shown) as it courses to its effectors (striated muscle). In the CNS, the myelin for the axon is produced by, and is part of, an oligodendrocyte; in the PNS, the myelin is produced by, and is part of, a Schwann cell. (Adapted from Junqueira LC, Carneiro J, Kelley RO. *Basic Histology.* 9th ed. Norwalk, CT: Appleton & Lange, 1998.)

Neurons are classified on the basis of the number of processes extending from the cell body (Fig. 11.2):

- ***Multipolar*** neurons have one axon and two or more dendrites.
- ***Bipolar*** neurons have one axon and one dendrite.
- ***Unipolar*** (actually ***pseudounipolar***) neurons have one process, the axon, which divides close to the cell body into two long processes. The vast majority of unipolar neurons are located in the dorsal root ganglia and cranial nerve ganglia.

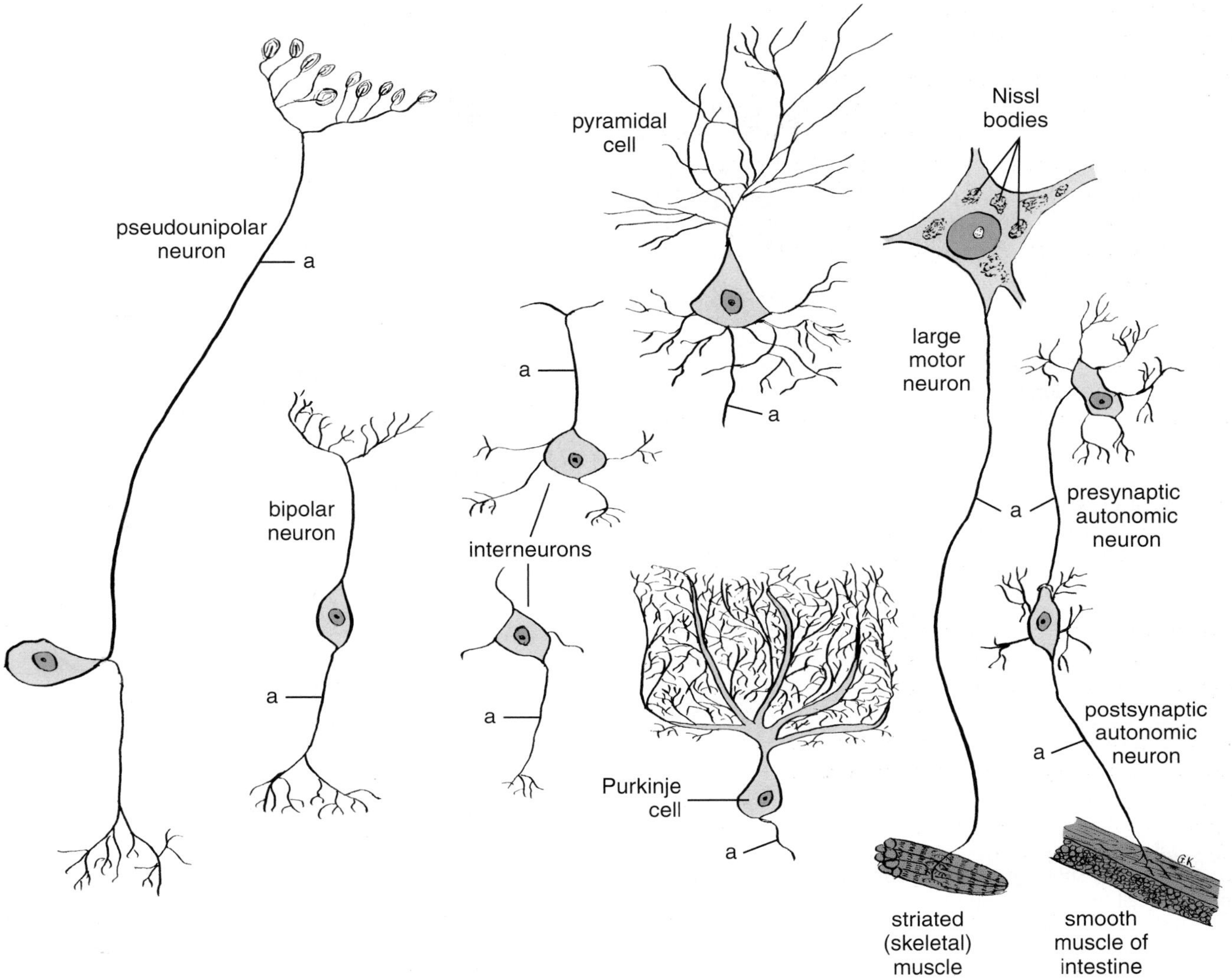

FIGURE 11.2
Diagram illustrating different types of neurons. The cell bodies of pseudounipolar (unipolar), bipolar, and postsynaptic autonomic neurons are located outside the CNS. Integrative neurons are restricted to the CNS; many of them have elaborate dendritic arborizations that facilitate their identification. *a,* axon.

Motor neurons and interneurons are multipolar

Interneurons constitute most of the neurons in the nervous system. The direction of impulses is from dendrite to cell body to axon or from cell body to axon. Thus, functionally, the dendrites and cell body of multipolar neurons are the receptor portions of the cell, and their plasma membrane is specially adapted for impulse generation. The axon is the conducting portion of the cell, and its plasma membrane is specialized for impulse conduction. The terminal portion of the axon, the synaptic ending, contains various neurotransmitters, i.e., small molecules whose release at the synapse affects other neurons as well as muscle cells and glandular epithelium.

Sensory neurons are unipolar

The cell body of a sensory neuron is situated in a dorsal root ganglion close to the CNS (Fig. 11.3); one axonal branch extends to the periphery, and one extends to the CNS. The two axonal branches are the conducting units. Functionally, impulses are generated in the peripheral arborizations (branches) of the neuron; these arborizations are the receptor portion of the cell. Unipolar neurons are also sometimes called pseudounipolar because during development they exist as bipolar neurons. They become unipolar as their processes migrate around the cell body and fuse into a single process as the cell matures.

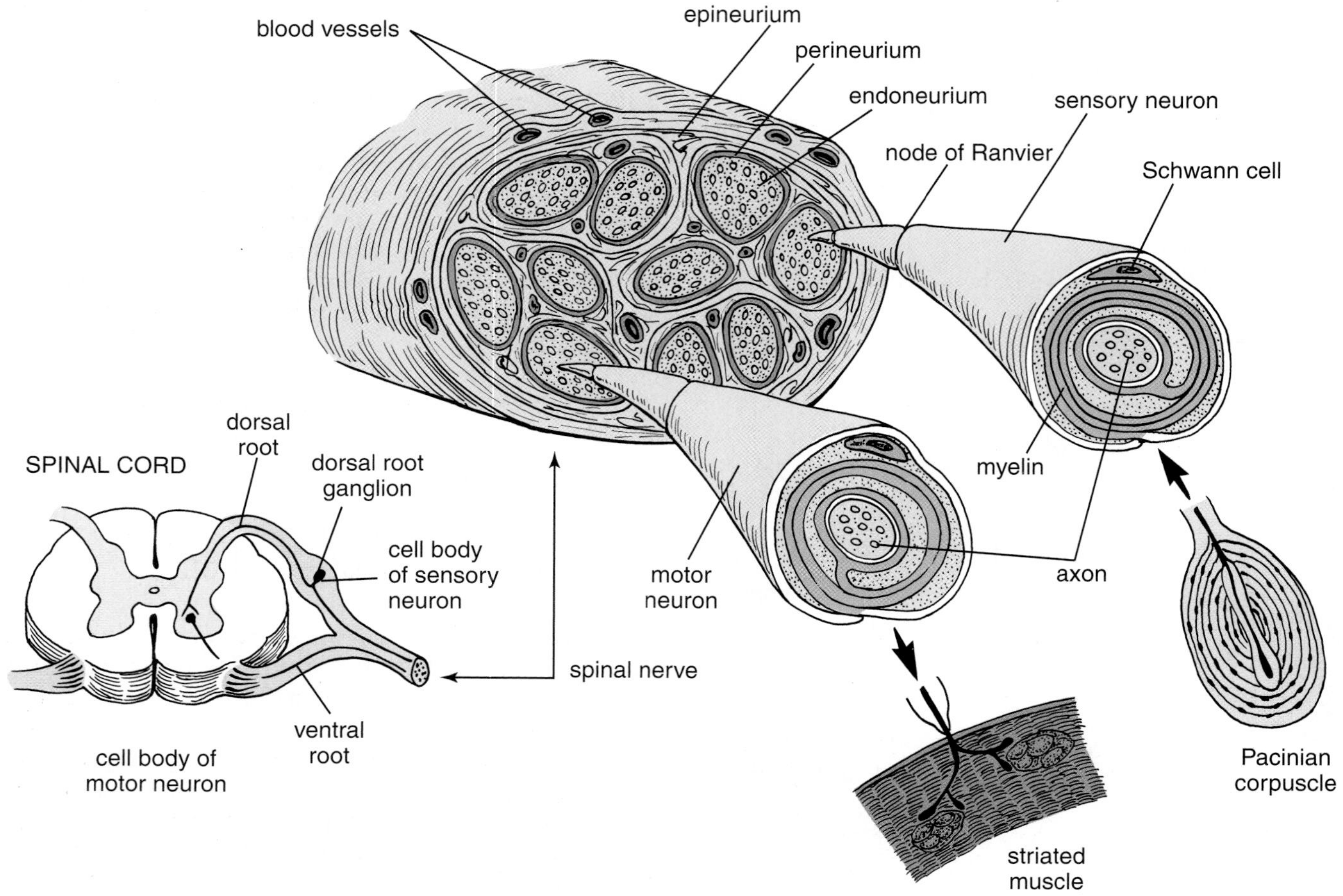

FIGURE 11.3
Schematic diagram showing arrangement of motor and sensory neurons. The cell body of a motor neuron is located in the ventral (anterior) horn of the gray matter of the spinal cord. Its axon, surrounded by myelin, leaves the spinal cord via a ventral (anterior) root and becomes part of a spinal nerve that carries it to its destination on striated (skeletal) muscle fibers. The sensory neuron originates in the skin within a receptor (here, a Pacinian corpuscle) and continues as a component of a spinal nerve, entering the spinal cord via the dorsal (posterior) root. Note the location of its cell body in the dorsal root ganglion (sensory ganglion). A segment of the spinal nerve is enlarged to show the relationship of the nerve fibers to the surrounding connective tissue (endoneurium, perineurium, and epineurium). In addition, segments of the sensory and motor neurons have been enlarged to show the relationship of the axons to the Schwann cells and myelin. (Autonomic nerve fibers are not shown in the diagram.)

True bipolar neurons are limited to the retina of the eye and the ganglia of the vestibulocochlear nerve (cranial nerve VIII) of the ear

Neurons associated with the receptors for the special senses (taste, smell, hearing, sight, and equilibrium) often do not fit the above generalizations. For example, the amacrine cells of the retina have no axons, and the olfactory receptors resemble neurons of primitive neural systems, in that they retain a surface location and remain a slowly renewing cell population.

Cell Body

The cell body of a neuron has characteristics of a protein-producing cell

The cell body, or ***perikaryon,*** is the dilated region of the neuron that contains a large, euchromatic nucleus with a prominent nucleolus and surrounding ***perinuclear cytoplasm.*** The perinuclear cytoplasm reveals abundant rough endoplasmic reticulum (rER) and free ribosomes when observed with the transmission electron microscope (TEM), a

feature consistent with its protein synthetic activity. In the light microscope the ribosomal content appears as small bodies, called ***Nissl bodies,*** that stain intensely with basic dyes and metachromatically with thionine dyes (Fig. 11.4). Each Nissl body corresponds to a stack of rER. The perinuclear cytoplasm also contains numerous mitochondria, a large perinuclear Golgi apparatus, lysosomes, microtubules, neurofilaments (intermediate filaments), transport vesicles, and inclusions (Fig. 11.5). Nissl bodies, free ribosomes, and, occasionally, the Golgi apparatus extend into the dendrites but not into the axon. This area of the cell body, called the ***axon hillock,*** is free of large cytoplasmic organelles and serves as a landmark to distinguish between axons and dendrites in both light microscope and TEM preparations.

The euchromatic nucleus, large nucleolus, prominent Golgi apparatus, and Nissl substance indicate the high level of anabolic activity needed to maintain these large cells.

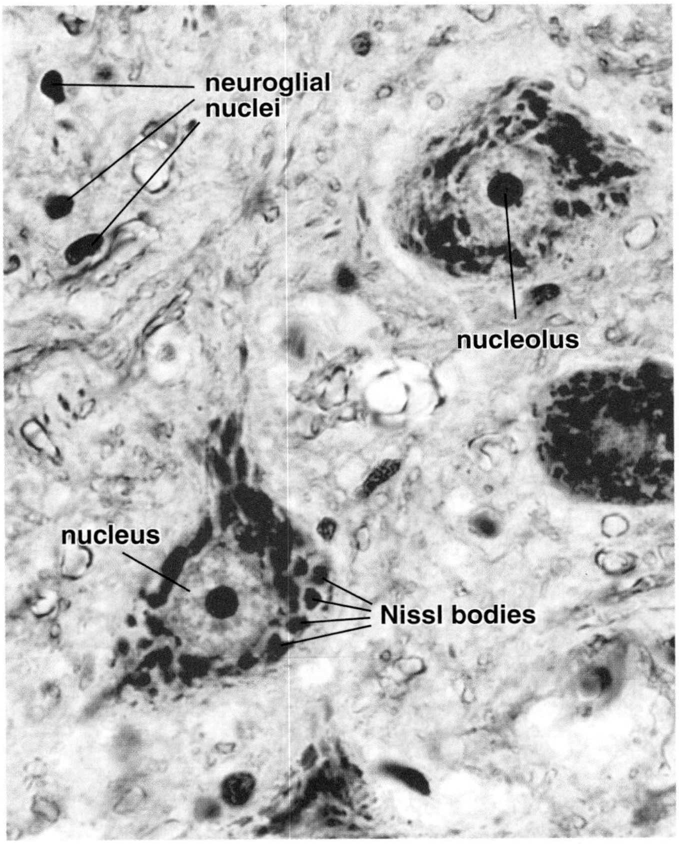

FIGURE 11.4
Photomicrograph of nerve cell bodies. This photomicrograph shows a region of the ventral (anterior) horn of a human spinal cord stained with toluidine blue. Typical features of the nerve cell bodies visible in this photomicrograph include large, spherical, pale-stained nuclei with a single prominent nucleolus and abundant Nissl bodies within the cytoplasm of the perikaryon. Most of the small nuclei belong to neuroglial cells. The remainder of the field consists of nerve fibers and cytoplasm of neuroglial cells. ×640.

Neurons do not divide; they must last for a lifetime

Although neurons do not replicate, the subcellular components of the neurons turn over regularly and have molecular lifespans measured in hours, days, and weeks. The constant need to replace enzymes, transmitter substances, membrane components, and other complex molecules explains the morphologic features characteristic of a high level of synthetic activity. Newly synthesized protein molecules are transported to distant locations within a neuron in a process referred to as ***axonal transport*** (page 293).

Dendrites and Axons

Dendrites are receptor processes that receive stimuli from other neurons or from the external environment

The main function of dendrites is to receive information from other neurons or from the external environment and carry that information to the cell body. Generally, dendrites are located in the vicinity of the cell body. They have a greater diameter than axons, are unmyelinated, are usually tapered, and form extensive arborizations called ***dendritic trees.*** Dendritic trees significantly increase the receptor surface area of a neuron. Many neuron types are characterized by the extent and shape of their dendritic trees (see Fig. 11.2). In general, the contents of the cell body and dendrites are similar, with the exception of the Golgi apparatus. Whereas the Golgi network remains close to the nucleus, other organelles characteristic of the cell body proper, including ribosomes and rER, are found in the dendrites, especially in the base of the dendrites.

Axons are effector processes that transmit stimuli to other neurons or effector cells

The main function of the axon is to convey information away from the cell body to another neuron or to an effector cell, such as a muscle cell. *Each neuron has only one axon,* and it may be extremely long. Axons that originate from neurons in the motor nuclei of the CNS (***Golgi type I neurons***) may travel more than a meter to reach their effector targets, skeletal muscle. In contrast, interneurons of the CNS (***Golgi type II neurons***) have a very short axon. Although an axon may give rise to a ***recurrent branch*** near the cell body (i.e., one that turns back toward the cell body; see Fig. 11.1) and to other collateral branches, the branching of the axon is most extensive in the vicinity of its targets.

The axon originates from the axon hillock. As mentioned, it usually lacks large cytoplasmic organelles such as Nissl bodies and Golgi cisternae. Microtubules, neurofila-

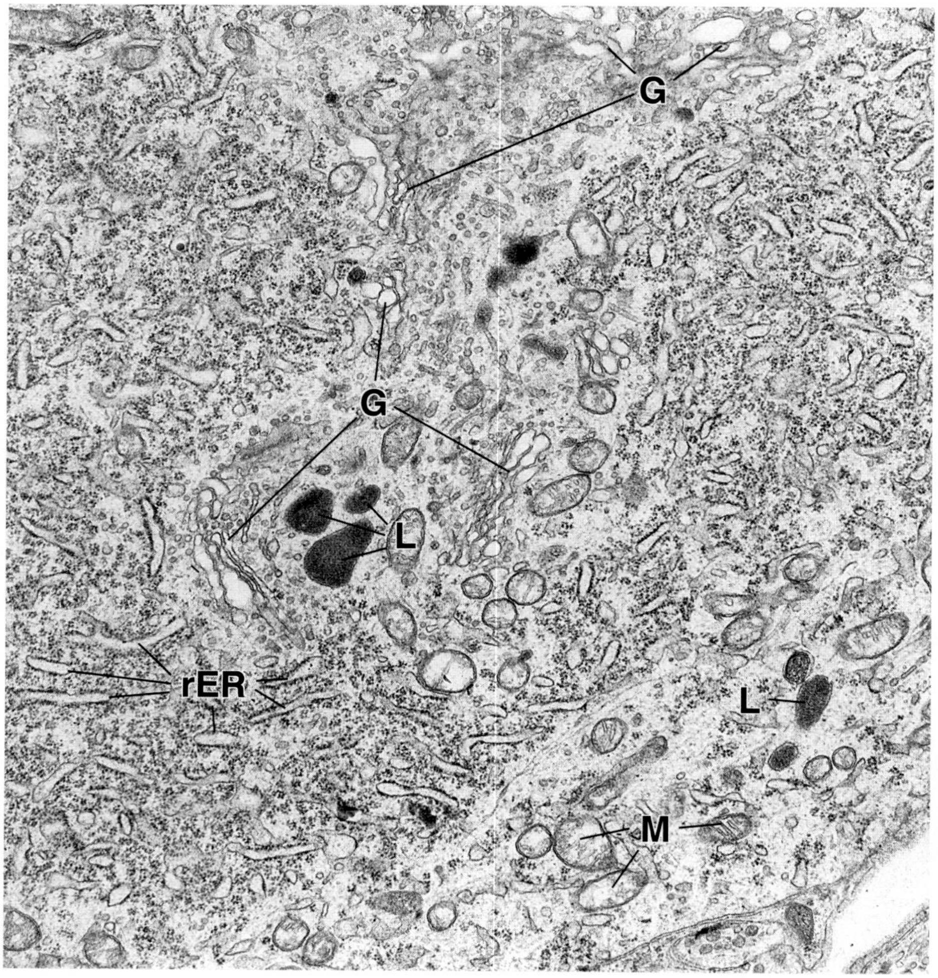

FIGURE 11.5
Electron micrograph of a nerve cell body. The cytoplasm is occupied by aggregates of free ribosomes and profiles of rough endoplasmic reticulum *(rER)* that constitute the Nissl bodies of light microscopy. The Golgi apparatus *(G)* appears as isolated areas containing profiles of flattened sacs and vesicles. Other characteristic organelles include mitochondria *(M)* and lysosomes *(L)*. The neurofilaments and microtubules are difficult to discern at this relatively low magnification. ×15,000.

ments, mitochondria, and vesicles, however, pass through the axon hillock into the axon. The region of the axon between the apex of the axon hillock and the beginning of the myelin sheath (see below) is called the ***initial segment.*** The initial segment is the site at which an ***action potential*** is generated in the axon. The action potential (described in more detail below) is stimulated by impulses carried to the axon hillock on the membrane of the cell body after other impulses are received on the dendrites or the cell body itself.

Some large axon terminals are capable of local protein synthesis, which may be involved in memory processes

Almost all of the structural and functional protein molecules are synthesized in the perikaryon. These molecules are distributed to the axons and dendrites via ***axonal transport systems*** (described on page 293). However, contrary to the common view that the perikaryon is the only site of protein synthesis, recent studies provide evidence of local synthesis of axonal proteins in some large nerve terminals. Some vertebral axon terminals (i.e., from the retina) contain polyribosomes with complete translational machinery for protein synthesis. These discrete areas within the axon terminals, called ***periaxoplasmic plaques,*** possess biochemical and molecular characteristics of active protein synthesis. Protein synthesis within the periaxoplasmic plaques is modulated by neuronal activity. These proteins may be involved in the processes of neuronal cell memory.

Synapses

Neurons communicate with other neurons and with effector cells by synapses

Synapses are specialized junctions between neurons that facilitate transmission of impulses from one (presynaptic) neuron to another (postsynaptic) neuron. Synapses also occur between axons and effector (target) cells, such as muscle and gland cells. Synapses between neurons may be classified morphologically as

- ***Axodendritic,*** occurring between axons and dendrites
- ***Axosomatic,*** occurring between axons and the cell body
- ***Axoaxonic,*** occurring between axons and axons
- ***Dendrodendritic,*** occurring between dendrites and dendrites (Fig. 11.6)

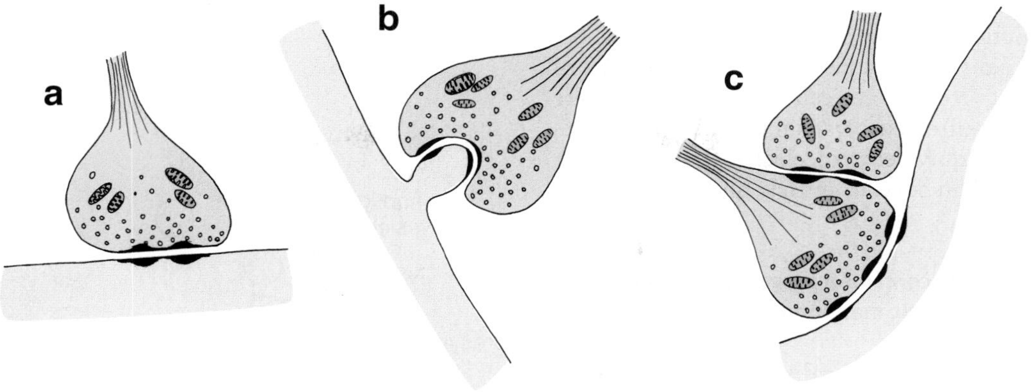

FIGURE 11.6
Schematic diagram of different types of synapses. a. Axodendritic or axosomatic. **b.** Axodendritic, in which an axon terminal synapses with a dendritic spine. **c.** Axoaxonic. The axoaxonic synapse may enhance or inhibit the axodendritic (or axosomatic) synapse. (Modified from Barr ML. *The Human Nervous System.* New York: Harper & Row, 1979.)

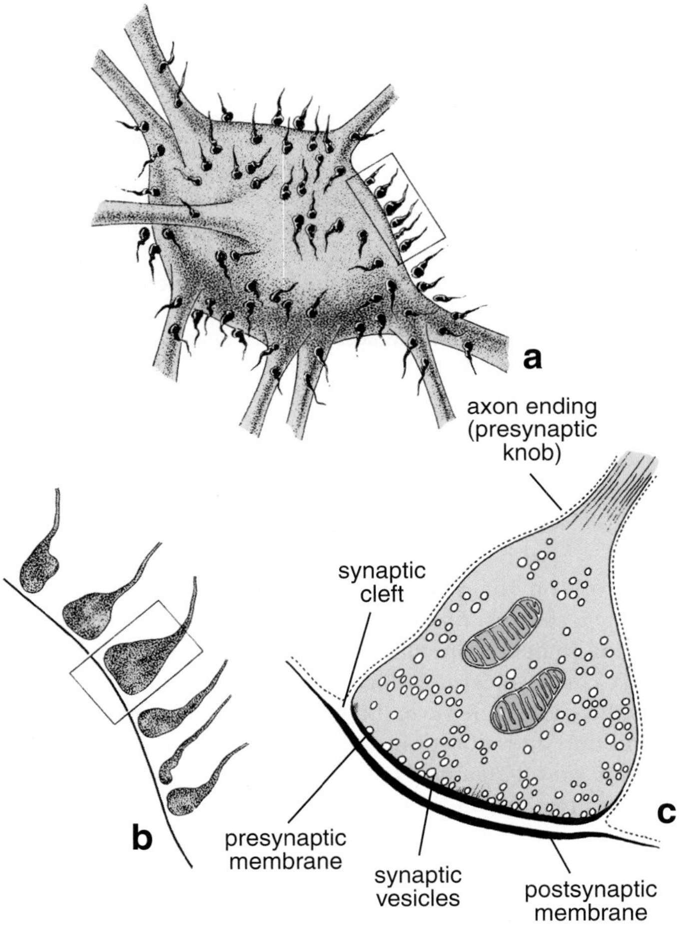

FIGURE 11.7
Representation of a neuron cell body in the CNS. a. This drawing illustrates the cell body of a neuron. Axon endings forming synapses are shown as the numerous ovoid bodies with tail-like appendages. Each represents an axon terminal from a different neuron making contact with the cell body or its dendrites. **b.** A drawing of the area within the *rectangle* in *a.* The drawing shows the axon endings and their synapses with the neuron cell body. **c.** Enlargement of the axon ending within the *rectangle* in *b,* illustrating its appearance with the transmission electron microscope, which reveals its significant structural features. (From DeRobertis EDP, Nowinsky WW, Saez FA. *Biologia Celular.* Buenos Aires: El Ateneo, 1970.)

Synapses are not resolvable in routine hematoxylin and eosin (H&E) preparations. However, silver precipitation staining methods (e.g., Golgi method) not only demonstrate the overall shape of some neurons but also show synapses as oval bodies on the surface of the receptor neuron (Fig. 11.7). Typically, an axon makes several of these button-like contacts with the receptor portion of the neuron. Often, the incoming neuron travels along the surface of the neuron, making several synaptic contacts called ***boutons en passant*** *(Fr., buttons in passing)*. The axon then continues, to end finally as a terminal twig with an enlarged tip, a ***bouton terminal*** *(Fr., terminal button)*,or ***end bulb.*** The number of synapses on a neuron or its processes, which may vary from a few to *tens of thousands* per neuron, appears to be directly related to the number of impulses that a neuron is receiving and processing.

Synapses are classified as chemical or electrical

Classification depends on the mechanism of conduction of the nerve impulses and the way the action potential is generated in the target cells. Synapses may also be classified as

- *Chemical synapses,* in which conduction of impulses is achieved by the release of chemical substances (neurotransmitters) from the presynaptic neuron. Neurotransmitters then diffuse across the narrow intercellular space that separates a presynaptic neuron from a postsynaptic neuron or target cell.

- ***Electrical synapses,*** which are common in invertebrates, contain gap junctions that permit movement of ions between cells and consequently permit the direct spread of electrical current from one cell to another. These synapses do not require neurotransmitters for their function. Mammalian equivalents of electrical synapses include ***gap junctions*** in smooth muscle and cardiac muscle cells.

A typical chemical synapse contains a presynaptic knob, synaptic cleft, and postsynaptic membrane

Components of a typical chemical synapse include

- ***Presynaptic knob (presynaptic component),*** the end of the neuron process from which neurotransmitters are released. The presynaptic component, i.e., the bouton terminal, is characterized by the presence of ***synaptic vesicles,*** membrane-limited structures that range from 30 to 100 nm in diameter and contain neurotransmitters (Fig. 11.8). A specific ATP-binding protein called **N-*ethylmaleimide–sensitive factor (NSF)*** found on the membrane of synaptic vesicles is required for formation, targeting, and fusion of these vesicles with the presynaptic membrane. Numerous small mitochondria and a layer of dense material, the ***presynaptic density,*** are present on the cytoplasmic side of the plasma membrane.
- ***Synaptic cleft,*** the 20- to 30-nm space that separates the presynaptic neuron from the postsynaptic neuron or target cell, which the neurotransmitter must cross.
- ***Postsynaptic membrane (postsynaptic component),*** which contains receptor sites with which the neurotransmitter interacts. This component is formed from a portion of the plasma membrane of the postsynaptic neuron (Fig. 11.9) and is characterized by a layer of dense material, the ***postsynaptic density,*** on the cytoplasmic side of the membrane.

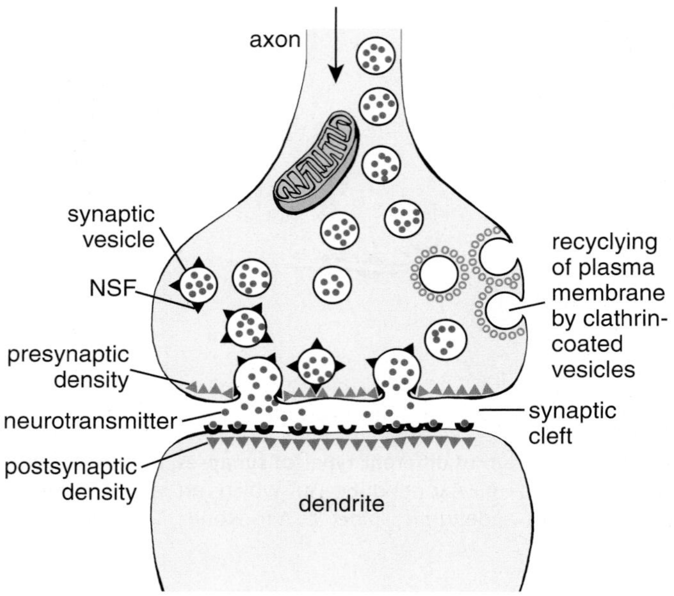

FIGURE 11.8
Diagram of a chemical axodendritic synapse. This diagram illustrates three components of a typical synapse. (1) The presynaptic knob is located at the distal end of the axon from which neurotransmitters are released. The presynaptic knob is characterized by the presence of numerous neurotransmitter-containing synaptic vesicles. Synaptic vesicles contain *N*-ethylmaleimide–sensitive factor *(NSF)* on their membrane; NSF is required for vesicle formation, targeting, and fusion with the presynaptic membrane. The plasma membrane of the presynaptic knob is recycled by the formation of clathrin-coated endocytotic vesicles. (2) The synaptic cleft separates the presynaptic knob of the axon from the postsynaptic membrane of the dendrite. (3) The postsynaptic membrane of the dendrite is frequently characterized by a postsynaptic density and contains receptors with an affinity for the neurotransmitters.

SYNAPTIC TRANSMISSION

Voltage-gated Ca^{2+} channels in the membrane of the bouton regulate transmitter release

When a nerve impulse reaches the bouton, the voltage reversal across the membrane produced by the impulse (called ***depolarization***) causes ***voltage-gated Ca^{2+} channels*** to open in the plasma membrane of the bouton. The influx of Ca^{2+} from the extracellular space causes the synaptic vesicles to migrate to, and fuse with, the presynaptic membrane, thereby releasing the neurotransmitter into the synaptic cleft by exocytosis. The neurotransmitter then diffuses across the synaptic cleft. At the same time, the presynaptic membrane of the bouton that released the neurotransmitter quickly forms endocytotic vesicles that return to the endosomal compartment of the bouton for reloading with neurotransmitter. Meanwhile, specific receptors on the postsynaptic membrane bind neurotransmitter, causing ***ligand-gated Na^+ channels*** in that membrane to open, allowing Na^+ to enter the neuron. This ion flux causes local depolarization in the postsynaptic membrane, which in turn, in favorable conditions (sufficient amount and duration of neurotransmitter release), can cause ***voltage-gated Na^+ channels*** that are present in the same area to open, thereby generating a nerve impulse. The firing of impulses in the postsynaptic neuron is due to the summative action of hundreds of synapses.

The chemical nature of the neurotransmitter determines the type of response at that synapse in the generation of neuronal impulses

The release of neurotransmitter by the presynaptic component can cause either ***excitation*** or ***inhibition*** at the postsynaptic membrane.

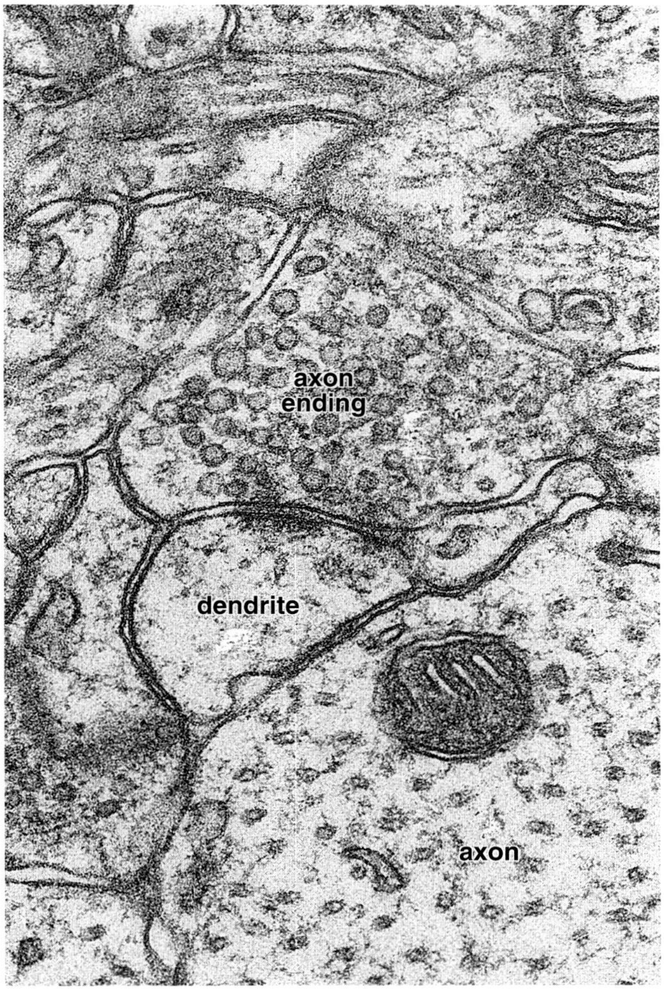

FIGURE 11.9
Electron micrograph of nerve processes in the cerebral cortex. A synapse can be seen in the center of the micrograph, where an axon ending is apposed to a dendrite. The ending of the axon exhibits numerous neurotransmitter-containing synaptic vesicles that appear as circular profiles. The postsynaptic membrane of the dendrite shows a postsynaptic density. A substance of similar density is also present in the synaptic cleft (intercellular space) at the synapse. ×76,000. (Courtesy of Drs. George D. Pappas and Virginia Kriho.)

- In ***excitatory synapses,*** release of neurotransmitters such as ***acetylcholine, glutamine,*** or ***serotonin*** opens cation channels, prompting an influx of Na^+ that causes local reversal of voltage of the postsynaptic membrane to a threshold level (depolarization). This leads to initiation of an action potential and generation of a nerve impulse.
- In ***inhibitory synapses,*** release of neurotransmitters such as ***γ-aminobutyric acid*** (GABA) or ***glycine,*** opens anion channels, causing Cl^- to enter the cell and hyperpolarize the postsynaptic membrane, making it even more negative. In these synapses, the generation of an action potential then becomes more difficult.

The ultimate generation of a nerve impulse in a postsynaptic neuron (firing) depends on the summation of excitatory and inhibitory impulses reaching that neuron. This allows precise regulation of the reaction of a postsynaptic neuron (or muscle or gland cell). The function of synapses is not simply to transmit impulses in an unchanged manner from one neuron to another. Rather, synapses allow for the processing of neuronal input. Typically, the impulse passing from the presynaptic to the postsynaptic neuron is modified at the synapse by other neurons that, although not in the direct pathway, nevertheless have access to the synapse (see Fig. 11.6). These other neurons may influence the membrane of the presynaptic neuron or the postsynaptic neuron and facilitate or inhibit the transmission of impulses.

NEUROTRANSMITTERS

A number of molecules that serve as neurotransmitters have been identified in various parts of the nervous system. The most common neurotransmitters are

- ***Acetylcholine (ACh).*** ACh is the neurotransmitter between axons and striated muscle at the neuromuscular junction (see page 257). ACh also serves as a neurotransmitter between axons and effectors in the ANS. Neurons that use ACh as their neurotransmitter are called ***cholinergic neurons.*** The receptors for ACh in the postsynaptic membrane are known as ***cholinergic receptors*** and are divided into two classes on the basis of their interactions with muscarine, isolated from poisonous mushrooms ***(muscarinic ACh receptor),*** and nicotine, isolated from tobacco plants ***(nicotinic ACh receptor).*** Various drugs affect release of ACh into the synaptic cleft as well as affect its binding to its receptors. For instance, in ***botulism,*** the botulinum toxin produced by the bacteria that grow in improperly canned meat and vegetable products inhibits ACh release. Inhibition of ACh release leads to decreasing receptor stimulation, causing respiratory distress and other skeletal muscle paralysis.
- ***Catecholamines*** such as ***norepinephrine (NE), epinephrine (EPI),*** and ***dopamine (DA).*** These neurotransmitters are synthesized in a series of enzymatic reactions from the amino acid tyrosine. NE serves as a transmitter between axons and effectors in the ANS. Neurons that use NE as their neurotransmitter are called ***adrenergic neurons.*** EPI is secreted by some cells in the CNS as well as the endocrine cells (chromaffin cells) of the adrenal medulla during the fight-or-flight response (page 665).
- ***Serotonin*** or ***5-hydroxytryptamine (5-HT), GABA, glutamate (GLU), aspartate (ASP),*** and ***glycine (GLY)*** are other common neurotransmitters.

Several small peptides also have been shown to act as synaptic transmitters. Among these are ***substance P*** (so named because it was originally found in a *p*owder of ace-

tone extracts of brain and intestine), ***hypothalamic releasing hormones, enkephalins, vasoactive intestinal peptide (VIP), cholecystokinin (CCK),*** and ***neurotensin.*** Many of these same substances are synthesized and released by enteroendocrine cells of the intestinal tract. They may act immediately on neighboring cells *(paracrine secretion)* or be carried in the bloodstream as ***hormones*** to act on distant target cells (**endocrine secretion**). They are also synthesized and released by endocrine organs and by the ***neurosecretory neurons*** of the ***hypothalamus***.

In the past decade, ***nitric oxide (NO),*** a simple gas with free radical properties, also has been identified as a neurotransmitter. At low concentrations, NO carries nerve impulses from one neuron to another. Unlike other neurotransmitters, which are synthesized in the nerve cell body and stored in synaptic vesicles, NO is synthesized within the synapse and used immediately. It is postulated that excitatory neurotransmitter GLU induces a chain reaction in which ***NO synthase*** is activated to produce NO, which in turn diffuses from the presynaptic knob via the synaptic cleft and postsynaptic membrane to the adjacent cell, resulting ultimately in generation of an action potential.

Neurotransmitters released into the synaptic cleft may be degraded or recaptured

The most common process of removal of the neurotransmitter following its release into the synaptic cleft is called ***high-affinity reuptake.*** About 80% of released neurotransmitters are removed by this mechanism. These and other transmitters are reincorporated into vesicles in the presynaptic component by endocytosis and are available for recycling. Enzymes associated with the postsynaptic membrane degrade the remaining 20% of neurotransmitters. For example, ***acetylcholinesterase (AChE)*** degrades ACh; ***catechol-o-methyltransferase*** (**COMT**) as well as ***monoamine oxidase (MAO)*** rapidly degrade NE. The degradation or recapture of neurotransmitters is necessary to limit the duration of stimulation or inhibition of the postsynaptic membrane.

Normally, membrane added to the plasma membrane of the nerve ending by exocytosis when synaptic vesicles fuse with it is retrieved by endocytosis and is reprocessed into synaptic vesicles by the smooth endoplasmic reticulum (sER) located in the nerve ending.

BOX 11.1

Clinical Correlations: Parkinson's Disease

Parkinson's disease is a slowly progressive neurologic disorder caused by the loss of dopamine (DA)-secreting cells in the substantia nigra and basal ganglia of the brain. DA is a neurotransmitter responsible for synaptic transmission in the nerve pathways coordinating smooth and focused activity of skeletal muscles. Loss of DA-secreting cells is associated with a classic pattern of symptoms, including

- Resting tremor in the limb, especially of the hand when in a relaxed position; tremor usually increases during stress and is often more severe on one side of the body
- Rigidity or increased tone (stiffness) in all muscles
- Slowness of movement (bradykinesia) and inability to initiate movement (akinesia)
- Lack of spontaneous movements
- Loss of postural reflexes, which leads to poor balance and abnormal walking (festinating gait)
- Slurred speech; slowness of thought; and small, cramped handwriting

The etiology of ***idiopathic Parkinson's disease,*** in which DA-secreting neurons in the substantia nigra are damaged and lost by degeneration or apoptosis is not known. However, some evidence suggests a hereditary predisposition; about 20% of Parkinson's patients have a family member with similar symptoms.

Symptoms that resemble idiopathic Parkinson's disease may also result from infections (e.g., encephalitis), toxins (e.g., MPTP), drugs used in the treatment of neurologic disorders (e.g., neuroleptics used to treat schizophrenia); and repetitive trauma. Symptoms with these causes are called ***secondary parkinsonism.***

On the microscopic level, degeneration of neurons in the substantia nigra is very evident. This region loses its typical pigmentation, and an increase in the number of glial cells is noticeable ***(gliosis).*** In addition, nerve cells in this region display characteristic intracellular inclusions called ***Lewy bodies,*** which represent accumulation of intermediate neurofilaments in association with proteins α-synuclein and ubiquitin.

Treatment of Parkinson's disease is primarily symptomatic and must strike a balance between relieving symptoms and minimizing psychotic side effects. L-Dopa is a precursor of DA that can cross the blood–brain barrier and is then converted to DA. It is often the primary agent used to treat Parkinson's disease. Other drugs that are used include a group of cholinergic receptor blockers and amantadine, a drug that stimulates release of DA from neurons.

If drug therapies are not effective, several surgical options can be considered. Stereotactic surgery, in which nuclei in selective areas of the brain (globus pallidus, thalamus) are destroyed by a thermocoagulative probe inserted into the brain, can be effective in some cases. Several new surgical procedures are being developed and are still in experimental stages. These include transplantation of DA-secreting neurons into the substantia nigra to replace lost neurons.

Axonal Transport Systems

Substances needed in the axon and dendrites are synthesized in the cell body and require transport to those sites

Most neurons in the body possess elaborate axonal and dendritic processes. Because the synthetic activity of the neuron is concentrated in the perikaryon, ***axonal transport*** is required to convey newly synthesized material to the processes. Axonal transport is a bidirectional mechanism. It serves as a mode of intercellular communication, carrying molecules and information along the microtubules and intermediate filaments from the axon terminal to the perikaryon and from the perikaryon to the axon terminal. Axonal transport is described as

- ***Anterograde transport*** carries material from the perikaryon to the periphery. ***Kinesin,*** a microtubule-associated motor protein that uses ATP, is involved in anterograde transport.
- ***Retrograde transport*** carries material from the axon terminal and the dendrites to the perikaryon. This transport is mediated by another microtubule-associated motor protein, ***dynein.***

The transport systems may also be distinguished by the rate at which substances are transported:

- A ***slow transport system*** conveys substances from the cell body to the terminal bouton at the speed of 0.2 to 4 mm/day. It is only an anterograde transport system. Structural elements such as tubulin molecules (microtubule precursors), actin molecules, and the proteins that form neurofilaments are carried from the perikaryon by the slow transport system. So, too, are cytoplasmic matrix proteins, such as actin, calmodulin, and various metabolic enzymes.
- A ***fast transport system*** conveys substances in both directions at a rate of 20 to 400 mm/day. Thus, it is both an anterograde and a retrograde system. The ***fast anterograde transport system*** carries to the axon terminal different membrane-limited organelles, such as sER components, synaptic vesicles, mitochondria; and low-molecular-weight materials such as sugars, amino acids, nucleotides, some neurotransmitters, and calcium. The ***fast retrograde transport system*** carries to the perikaryon many of the same materials as well as proteins and other molecules endocytosed at the axon terminal. Fast transport in either direction requires ATP, which is used by microtubule-associated motor proteins, and depends on the microtubule arrangement that extends from the perikaryon to the termination of the axon. Retrograde transport is the pathway followed by toxins and viruses that enter the CNS at nerve endings. Retrograde transport of exogenous enzymes, such as horseradish peroxidase, and of radiolabeled or immunolabeled tracer materials is now used to trace neuronal pathways and to identify the perikarya related to specific nerve endings.

Dendritic transport appears to have the same characteristics and to serve the same functions for the dendrite as axonal transport does for the axon.

▼ SUPPORTING CELLS OF THE NERVOUS SYSTEM

Schwann Cells and the Myelin Sheath

Axons in the peripheral nervous system are described as myelinated or unmyelinated

Myelinated axons are surrounded by a lipid-rich layer called the ***myelin sheath.***

External to, and contiguous with, the myelin sheath is a thin layer of Schwann cell cytoplasm called the ***sheath of Schwann,*** or the ***neurilemma*** (Fig. 11.10). This layer contains the nucleus and most of the organelles of the ***Schwann cell.*** Surrounding the Schwann cell is a basal or external lamina.

Functionally, the myelin sheath with its external lamina and the neurilemma *isolates* the axon from the surrounding extracellular compartment. The axon hillock and the terminal arborizations where the axon synapses with its target cells do not have a myelin sheath.

The myelin sheath is composed of multiple layers of Schwann cell membrane wrapped concentrically around the axon

To produce the myelin sheath, each Schwann cell wraps in a spiral around a short (0.08 to 0.1 mm) segment of the axon. During the wrapping of the axon, cytoplasm is squeezed out from between the membrane of the concentric layers of the Schwann cell. The inner leaflets of the plasma membrane then fuse. With the TEM, these fused inner leaflets are electron opaque, appearing as the ***major dense lines*** in the TEM image of the myelin. These concentric dense lamellae alternate with the slightly less dense ***intraperiod lines*** that are formed by fusion of the outer membrane leaflets (Fig. 11.11).

The myelin sheath is segmented because it is formed by numerous Schwann cells arrayed sequentially along the axon. The junction where two adjacent Schwann cells meet is devoid of myelin. This site is called the ***node of Ranvier.*** Therefore, the myelin between two sequential nodes of Ranvier is called an ***internodal segment.***

During formation of the myelin sheath, the axon initially lies in a groove on the surface of the Schwann cell (Fig. 11.11a). Fusion of the edges of the groove to enclose the axon produces the ***inner mesaxon,*** the narrow intercellular space of the innermost rings. The first few lamellae are not compactly arranged; i.e., some cyto-

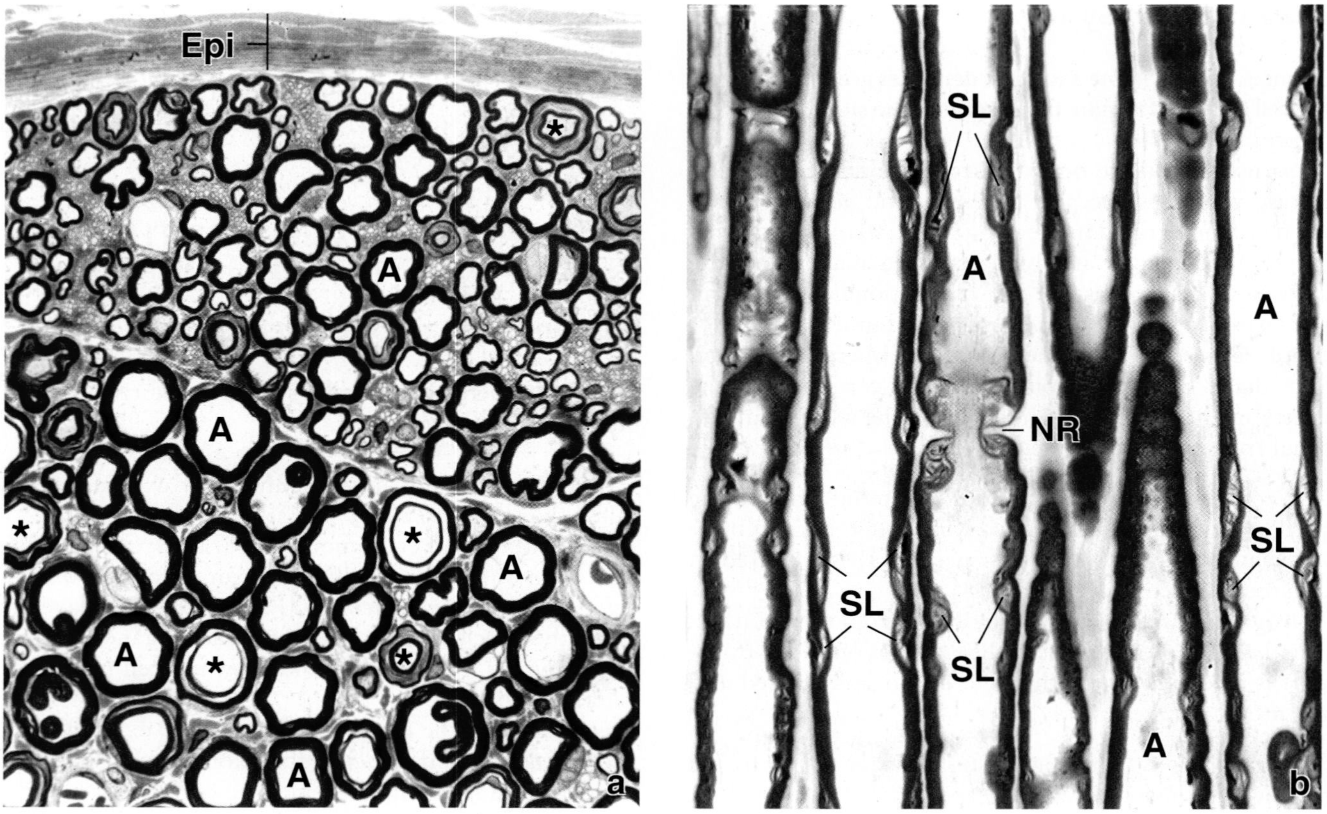

FIGURE 11.10

Photomicrographs of a peripheral nerve in cross and longitudinal sections. a. Photomicrograph of an osmium-fixed, toluidine blue–stained peripheral nerve cut in cross section. The axons *(A)* appear clear. The myelin is represented by the *dark ring* surrounding the axons. Note the variation in diameter of the individual axons. In some of the nerves the myelin appears to consist of two separate rings *(asterisks)*. This is due to the section passing through a Schmidt-Lanterman cleft. *Epi*, epineurium. ×640. **b.** Photomicrograph showing longitudinally sectioned myelinated nerve axons *(A)* in the same preparation as above. A node of Ranvier *(NR)* is seen near the center of the micrograph. In the same axon, a Schmidt-Lanterman cleft *(SL)* is seen on each side of the node. In addition, a number of Schmidt-Lanterman clefts can be seen in the adjacent axons. The perinodal cytoplasm of the Schwann cell at the node of Ranvier and the Schwann cell cytoplasm at the Schmidt-Lanterman cleft appear virtually unstained. ×640.

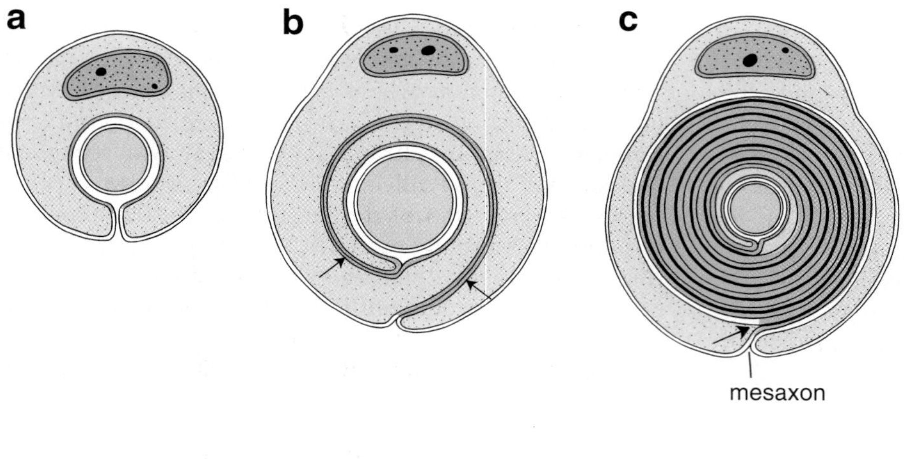

FIGURE 11.11

Diagram showing successive stages in the formation of myelin by a Schwann cell. a. The axon is initially surrounded by a Schwann cell. **b.** The Schwann cell then wraps around the axon, forming multiple Schwann cell layers. **c.** During the wrapping process the cytoplasm is extruded from between the two apposing plasma membranes of the Schwann cell, which then fuse, inner leaflet to inner leaflet, to form the major dense line in the myelin *(arrows)*. The outer opposing leaflets also fuse to form the less conspicuous intraperiod line. The outer mesaxon represents invaginated plasma membrane extending from the outer surface of the Schwann cell to the myelin. The inner mesaxon extends from the inner surface of the Schwann cell (the part facing the axon) to the myelin. (From Barr ML, Kiernan JA. *The Human Nervous System.* New York: Harper & Row, 1983.)

plasm is left in the first few concentric layers (Fig. 11.11b). Similarly, the outermost layer contains some cytoplasm as well as the Schwann cell nucleus (Fig. 11.11c). The apposition of the plasma membrane of the last layer to itself as it closes the ring produces the ***outer mesaxon,*** the narrow intercellular space adjacent to the external lamina.

Myelin is rich in lipid because as the Schwann cell winds around the axon, its cytoplasm, as noted, is extruded from between the opposing layers of the plasma

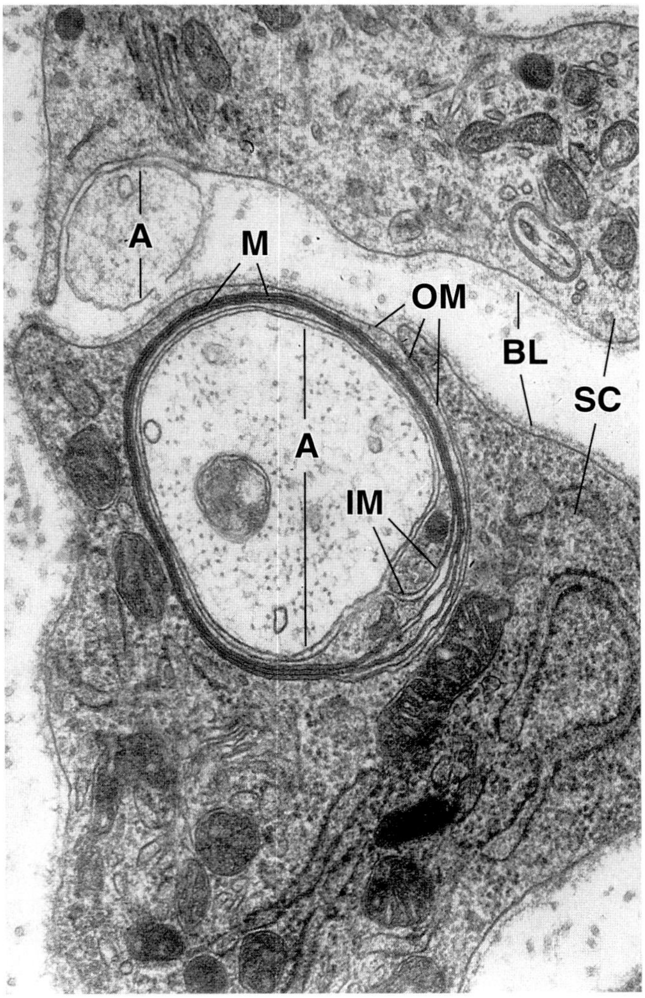

FIGURE 11.12
Electron micrograph of an axon in the process of myelination. At this stage of development, the myelin *(M)* consists of about six membrane layers. The inner mesaxon *(IM)* is represented by the apposition of the internal opposing processes of the Schwann cell *(SC)*. Similarly, the outer mesaxon *(OM)* is represented by the outer fold or lip of the Schwann cell where it meets itself. Another axon (see *upper left A*) is present that has not yet been enwrapped by a Schwann cell. Other notable features include the Schwann cell basal (external) lamina *(BL)* and the considerable amount of Schwann cell cytoplasm associated with the myelination process. ×50,000. (Courtesy of Dr. Stephen G. Waxman.)

membranes. Electron micrographs, however, typically show small amounts of cytoplasm in several locations (Figs. 11.12 and 11.13): the ***inner collar of Schwann cell cytoplasm,*** between the axon and the myelin; the ***Schmidt-Lanterman clefts,*** small islands within successive lamellae of the myelin; ***perinodal cytoplasm,*** at the node of Ranvier; and the ***outer collar of perinuclear cytoplasm,*** around the myelin (Fig. 11.14). These areas of cytoplasm are what light microscopists identified as the Schwann sheath. If one conceptually unrolls the Schwann cell, as shown in Figure 11.15, its full extent can be appreciated, and the inner collar of Schwann cell cytoplasm can be seen to be continuous with the body of the Schwann cell through the Schmidt-Lanterman clefts and through the perinodal cytoplasm. Cytoplasm of the clefts contains lysosomes, occasional mitochondria and microtubules, as well as cytoplasmic inclusions, or dense bodies. The number of Schmidt-Lanterman clefts correlates with the diameter of the axon; larger axons have more clefts.

Unmyelinated axons in the peripheral nervous system are enveloped by Schwann cells and their external lamina

The nerves in the PNS that are described as ***unmyelinated*** are nevertheless enveloped by Schwann cell cytoplasm as shown in Figure 11.16. The Schwann cells are elongated in parallel to the long axis of the axons, and the axons fit into grooves in the surface of the cell. The lips of the groove may be open, exposing a portion of the axolemma (axon plasma membrane), the cell membrane of the axon, to the adjacent external lamina of the Schwann cell, or the lips may be closed, forming a mesaxon.

A single axon or a group of axons may be enclosed in a single invagination of the Schwann cell surface. Large Schwann cells in the PNS may have 20 or more grooves, each containing one or more axons. In the ANS, it is common for bundles of unmyelinated axons to occupy a single groove.

Satellite Cells

The neuronal cell bodies of ganglia are surrounded by a layer of small cuboidal cells called ***satellite cells.*** Although they form a complete layer around the cell body, only their nuclei are typically visible in routine H&E preparations (Fig. 11.17, a and b). In paravertebral and peripheral ganglia, neural cell processes must penetrate between the satellite cells to establish a synapse (there are no synapses in sensory ganglia). They help to establish and maintain a controlled microenvironment around the neuronal body in the ganglion, providing electrical insulation as well as a pathway for metabolic exchanges. Thus, in its functional role the satellite cell is analogous to the Schwann cell except that it does not make myelin.

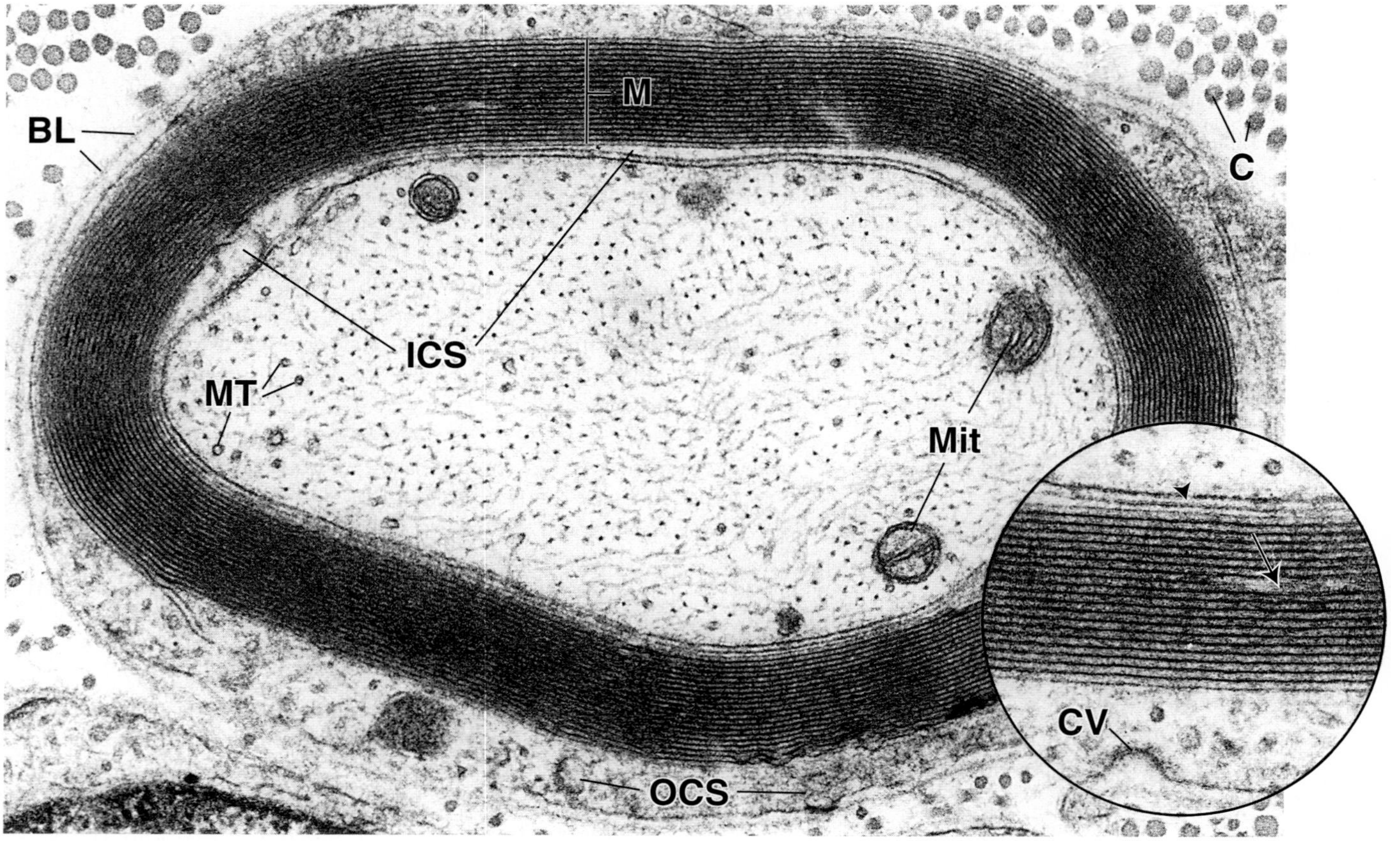

FIGURE 11.13

Electron micrograph of a mature myelinated axon. The myelin sheath *(M)* shown here consists of 19 paired layers of Schwann cell membrane. The pairing of membranes in each layer is due to the extrusion of the Schwann cell cytoplasm. The axon displays an abundance of neurofilaments, most of which have been cross-sectioned, giving the axon a stippled appearance. Also evident in the axon are microtubules *(MT)* and several mitochondria *(Mit).* The outer collar of Schwann cell cytoplasm *(OCS)* is relatively abundant, compared with the inner collar of Schwann cell cytoplasm *(ICS).* The collagen fibrils *(C)* constitute the fibrillar component of the endoneurium. *BL,* basal (external) lamina. ×70,000. **Inset.** Higher magnification of the myelin. The *arrow* points to cytoplasm within the myelin that would contribute to the appearance of the Schmidt-Lanterman cleft as seen in the light microscrope. It appears as an isolated region here because of the thinness of the section. The intercellular space between axon and Schwann cell is indicated by the *arrowhead.* A coated vesicle *(CV)* in an early stage of formation appears in the outer collar of the Schwann cell cytoplasm. ×130,000. (Courtesy of Dr. George D. Pappas.)

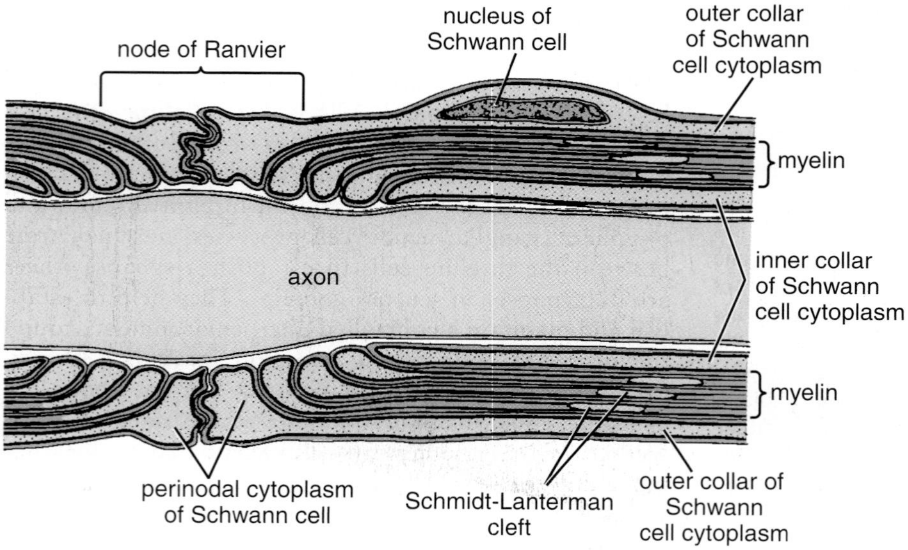

FIGURE 11.14

Diagram of an axon and its covering sheaths. This diagram shows a longitudinal section of the axon and its relationships to the myelin, cytoplasm of the Schwann cell, and node of Ranvier. Schwann cell cytoplasm is present at four locations. These are (1) the inner and (2) the outer cytoplasmic collar of the Schwann cell, (3) the nodes, and (4) the Schmidt-Lanterman clefts. Note that the cytoplasm throughout the Schwann cell is continuous; it is not a series of cytoplasmic islands as it appears in the diagram (see Fig. 11.15). The node of Ranvier is the site at which successive Schwann cells meet. The adjacent plasma membranes of the Schwann cells are not tightly apposed at the node, and extracellular fluid has free access to the neuronal plasma membrane. Also, the node is the site of depolarization of the neuronal plasma membrane during nerve impulse transmission. (Courtesy of Dr. Charles P. Leblond.)

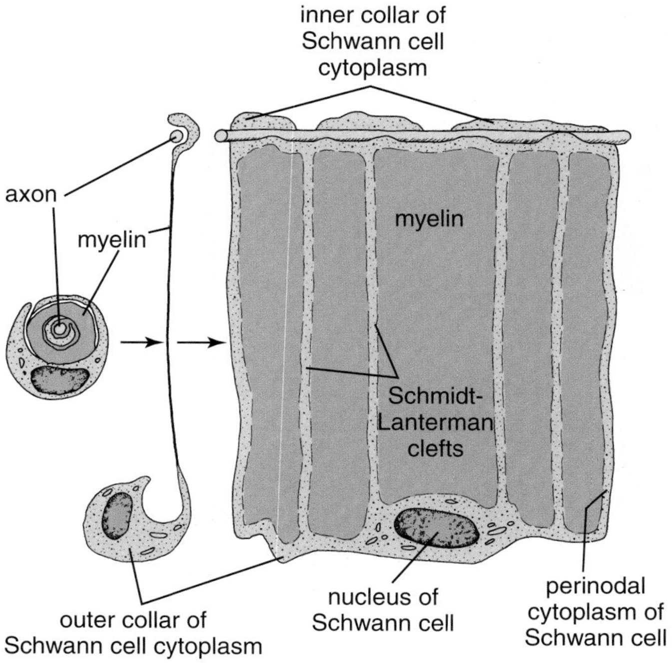

FIGURE 11.15
Diagrams conceptualizing the relationship of myelin and cytoplasm of a Schwann cell. A cross section of a myelinated axon is shown on the left next to a hypothetically uncoiled Schwann cell viewed on edge. The same uncoiled Schwann cell viewed en face is shown on the right. Note how the cytoplasm of the Schwann cell is continuous. (Modified from Webster HD. *J Cell Biol* 1971;48:348–367.)

Neuroglia

Within the CNS, supporting cells are designated ***neuroglia,*** or ***glial cells.*** The four types of glial cells are

- ***Oligodendrocytes,*** small cells that are active in the formation and maintenance of myelin in the CNS
- ***Astrocytes,*** morphologically heterogeneous cells that provide physical and metabolic support for the neurons of the CNS
- ***Microglia,*** inconspicuous cells with small, dark, elongated nuclei that possess phagocytotic properties
- ***Ependymal cells,*** column-shaped cells that line the ventricles of the brain and the central canal of the spinal cord

Only the nuclei of glial cells are seen in routine histologic preparations of the CNS. Heavy-metal staining or immunocytochemical methods are necessary to demonstrate the shape of the entire glial cell.

Although glial cells have long been described as supporting cells of nerve tissue in the purely physical sense, current concepts emphasize the functional interdependence of neuroglial cells and neurons. The most obvious example of physical support occurs during development. The brain and spinal cord develop from the embryonic neural tube. In the head region, the neural tube undergoes remarkable thickening and folding, leading ultimately to the final structure, the brain. During the early stages of the process, embryonic glial cells extend through the entire thickness of the neural tube in a radial manner. These radial glial cells serve as the physical scaffolding that directs the migration of neurons to their appropriate position in the brain.

BOX 11.2

Clinical Correlations: Demyelinating Diseases

In general, ***demyelinating diseases*** are characterized by preferential damage to the myelin sheath. Clinical symptoms of these diseases are related to decreased or lost ability to transmit electrical impulses along nerve fibers. Several immune-mediated diseases affect the myelin sheath.

Guillain-Barré syndrome, known also as ***acute inflammatory demyelinating polyradiculoneuropathy,*** is one of the most common life-threatening diseases of the PNS. Microscopic examination of nerve fibers obtained from patients affected by this disease shows a large accumulation of lymphocytes, macrophages, and plasma cells around nerve fibers within nerve fascicles. Large segments of the myelin sheath are damaged, leaving the axons exposed to the extracellular matrix. These findings are consistent with a T cell–mediated immune response directed against myelin, which causes its destruction and slows or blocks nerve conduction. Patients exhibit symptoms of ascending muscle paralysis, loss of muscle coordination, and loss of cutaneous sensation.

Multiple sclerosis (MS) is a disease that attacks myelin in the CNS. MS is also characterized by preferential damage to myelin, which becomes detached from the axon and is eventually destroyed. In addition, destruction of oligodendroglia, which are responsible for the synthesis and maintenance of myelin, is also evident. Chemical changes in the lipid and protein constituents of myelin produce irregular, multiple ***plaques*** throughout the white matter of the brain. Symptoms of MS depend on the area in the CNS where myelin is damaged. MS is usually characterized by distinct episodes of neurologic deficits such as unilateral vision impairment, loss of cutaneous sensation, lack of muscle coordination and movement, and loss of bladder and bowel control.

Treatment of both diseases is related to diminishing the causative immune response by immunomodulatory therapy with interferon as well as administrating adrenal steroids. For more severe, progressive forms, immunosuppressive drugs may be used.

Microglia possess phagocytotic properties

Microglia are phagocytotic cells. They are normally present only in small numbers in the adult CNS but proliferate and become actively phagocytotic in regions of injury and disease. They are considered part of the mononuclear phagocytotic system (see page 144) and are believed to originate in the bone marrow. Microglia cells enter the CNS parenchyma from the vascular system. Evidence also sug-

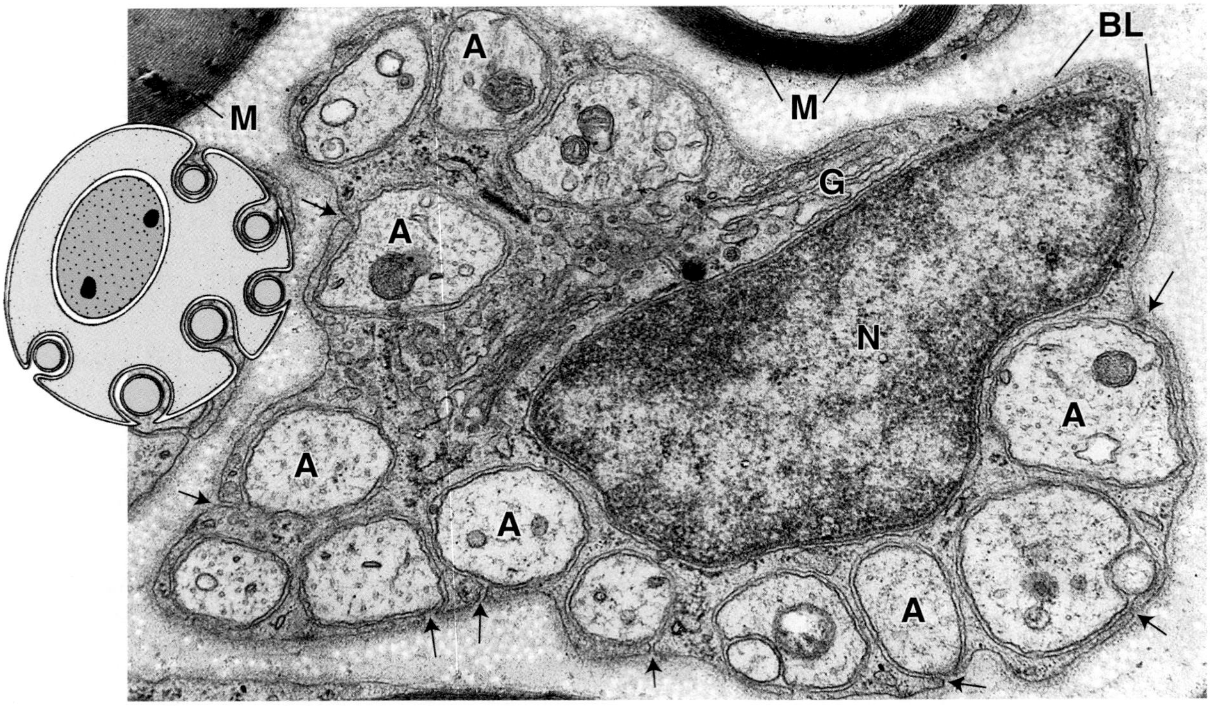

FIGURE 11.16

Electron micrograph of unmyelinated nerve fibers. The individual fibers or axons *(A)* are engulfed by the cytoplasm of a Schwann cell. The *arrows* indicate the site of mesaxons. In effect, each axon is enclosed by the Schwann cell cytoplasm, except for the intercellular space of the mesaxon. Other features evident in the Schwann cell are its nucleus *(N),* the Golgi apparatus *(G),* and the surrounding basal (external) lamina *(BL).* In the upper part of the micrograph, myelin *(M)* of two myelinated nerves is also evident. ×27,000. **Inset.** Schematic diagram showing the relationship of axons engulfed by the Schwann cell. (Barr ML, Kiernan JA. *The Human Nervous System.* New York: Harper & Row, 1983.)

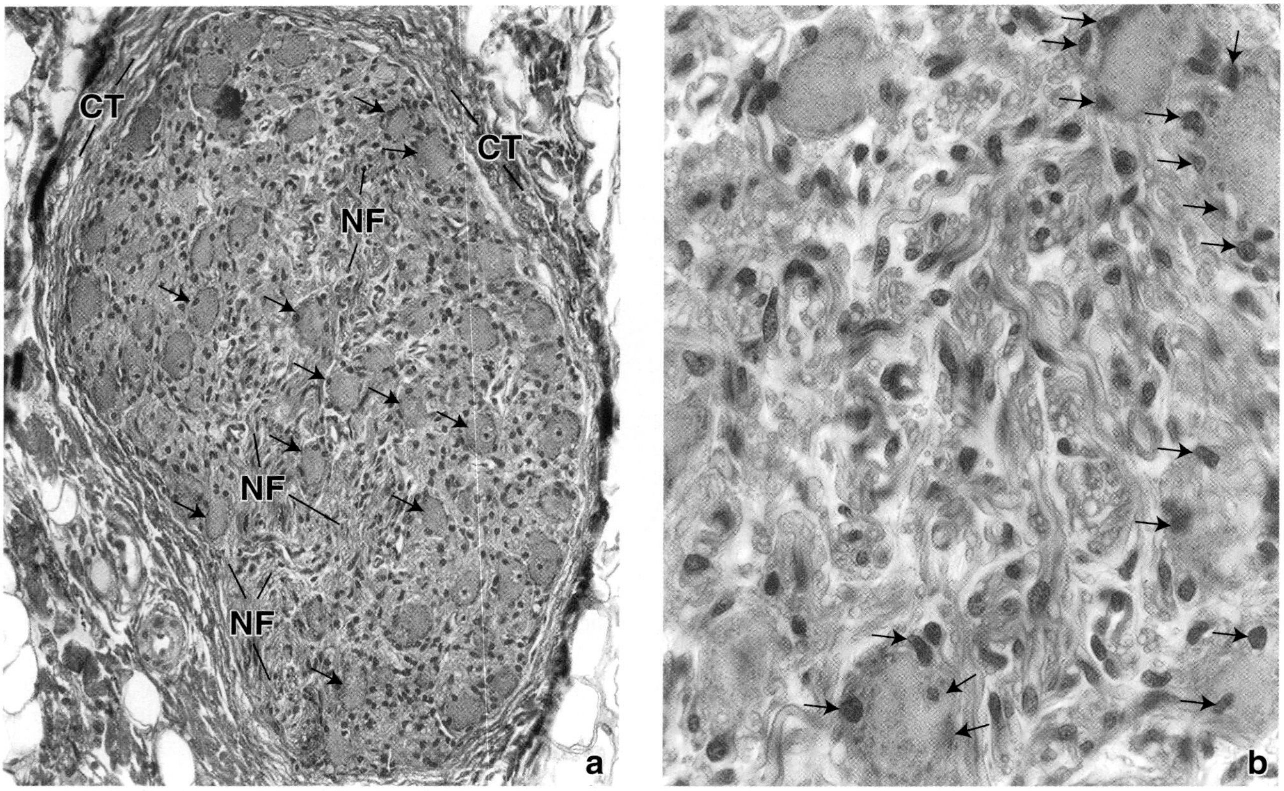

FIGURE 11.17

Photomicrograph of a nerve ganglion. a. Photomicrograph showing a ganglion stained by the Mallory-Azan method. Note the large nerve cell bodies *(arrows)* and nerve fibers *(NF)* in the ganglion. Satellite cells are represented by the very small nuclei at the periphery of the neuronal cell bodies. The ganglion is surrounded by a dense irregular connective tissue capsule *(CT)* that is comparable to, and continuous with, the epineurium of the nerve. ×200. **b.** Higher magnification of the ganglion, showing individual axons and a few neuronal cell bodies with their satellite cells *(arrows).* The nuclei in the region of the axons are mostly Schwann cell nuclei. ×640.

gests that they remove debris of cells that die during development of the nervous system.

Microglia are the smallest of the neuroglial cells and have relatively small, elongated nuclei (Fig. 11.18.) When stained with heavy metals, microglia exhibit short, twisted processes. Both the processes and the cell body are covered with numerous spikes. The spikes may be the equivalent of the ruffled border seen on other phagocytotic cells. The TEM reveals numerous lysosomes, inclusions, and vesicles. However, microglia contain little rER and few microtubules or actin filaments.

Astrocytes are of two types, protoplasmic and fibrous

Astrocytes are the largest of the neuroglial cells. Two kinds of astrocytes are identified:

- ***Protoplasmic astrocytes,*** which are more prevalent in gray matter. These astrocytes have numerous, short, branching cytoplasmic processes (Fig. 11.19).
- ***Fibrous astrocytes,*** which are more common in white matter. These astrocytes have fewer processes, and they are relatively straight (Fig. 11.20).

Both types of astrocytes contain prominent bundles of intermediate filaments composed of ***glial fibrillary acidic protein (GFAP).*** The filaments are much more numerous in the fibrous astrocytes, however, hence the name. Antibodies to GFAP are used as specific stains to identify astrocytes in sections and tissue cultures (see Fig. 11.20b). Tumors arising from fibrous astrocytes, ***fibrous astrocytomas,*** account for about 80% of adult primary brain tumors. They are also characterized by microscopic examination and GFAP specificity.

Astrocyte processes extend between the blood vessels and neurons. The ends of the processes expand, forming *end feet* that cover large areas of the outer surface of the vessel or of the axolemma. It is now thought that astrocytes play a role in the movement of metabolites and wastes to and from neurons and regulate ionic concentrations in the intercellular compartment, thus maintaining the microenvironment of the neurons. They also have a role in maintaining tight junctions of the capillaries that form the blood–brain barrier (page 313).

In addition, astrocytes provide a covering for the "bare areas" of myelinated axons, e.g., at the nodes of Ranvier and at synapses. They may confine neurotransmitters to the synaptic cleft and may remove excess neurotransmitters by pinocytosis. Protoplasmic astrocytes at the brain and spinal cord surfaces extend their processes (subpial feet) to the basal lamina of the pia mater to form the ***glia***

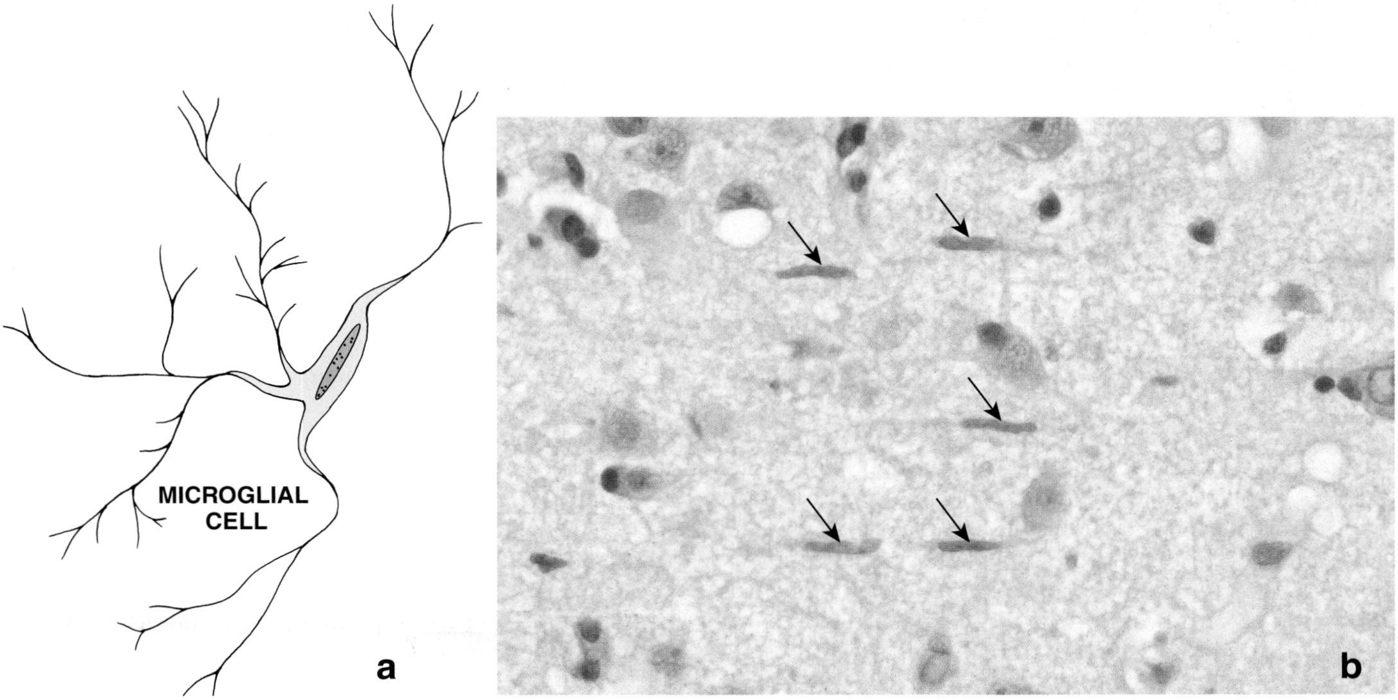

FIGURE 11.18
Microglial cell in the gray matter of the brain. a. This diagram shows the shape and characteristics of a microglial cell. Note the elongated nucleus and relatively few processes emanating from the body. **b.** Photomicrograph of microglial cells *(arrows)* showing their characteristic elongated nuclei. The specimen was obtained from an individual with diffuse microgliosis. In this condition, the microglial cells are present in large numbers and are readily visible in a routine H&E preparation. ×420. (From Fuller GN, Burger PC. Central nervous system. In: Sternberg SS, ed. *Histology for Pathologists.* Philadelphia: Lippincott-Raven, 1997.)

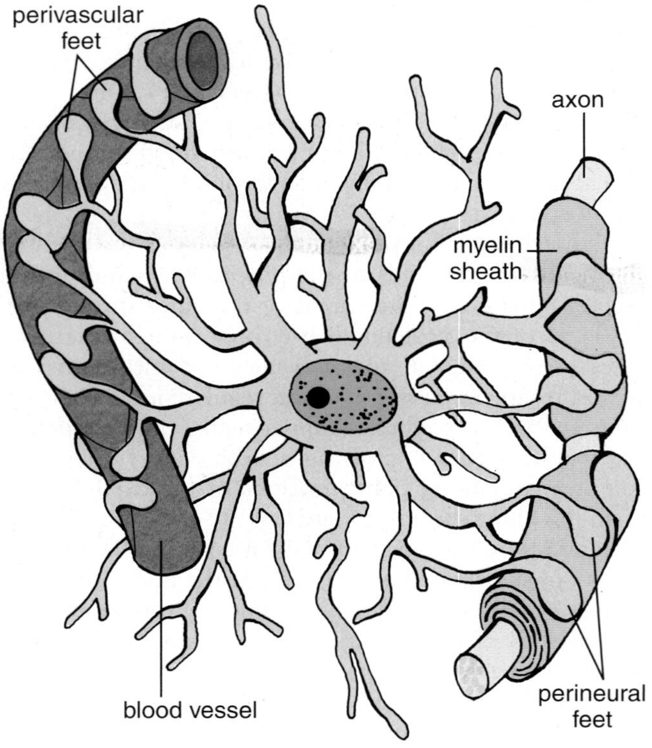

FIGURE 11.19
Protoplasmic astrocyte in the gray matter of the brain. This schematic drawing shows the foot processes of the protoplasmic astrocyte terminating on a blood vessel and the axonal process of a nerve cell. The foot processes terminating on the blood vessel contribute to the blood–brain barrier. The bare regions of the vessel as shown in the drawing would be covered by processes of neighboring astrocytes, thus forming the overall barrier.

limitans, a relatively impermeable barrier surrounding the CNS (Fig. 11.21).

Oligodendrocytes produce and maintain the myelin sheath in the CNS

The oligodendrocyte is the cell responsible for producing CNS myelin. The myelin sheath in the CNS is formed by concentric layers of oligodendrocyte plasma membrane. The formation of the sheath in the CNS is more complex, however, than the simple wrapping that occurs in the PNS.

Oligodendrocytes appear in specially stained preparations in the light microscope as small cells with relatively few processes compared with astrocytes. They are often aligned in rows between axons. Each oligodendrocyte gives off several tongue-like processes that find their way to the axons, where each process wraps itself around a portion of an axon, forming an internodal segment of myelin. The multiple processes of a single oligodendrocyte may myelinate one axon or several nearby axons (Fig. 11.22). The nucleus-containing region of the oligodendrocyte may be at some distance from the axons it myelinates.

The precise manner by which oligodendrocyte plasma membrane becomes concentrically wrapped around a portion of a CNS neuron is not as clearly understood as the parallel process in the PNS. Because a single oligodendrocyte may myelinate several nearby axons simultaneously, the cell cannot spiral around each axon in an independent manner, as the Schwann cell does in the PNS. Instead, each tongue-like process appears to spiral around the axon, always staying in proximity to it, until the myelin sheath is formed. Thus, PNS myelin can be described as forming centrifugally by the movement of the Schwann cell around the outer surface of the newly formed myelin. CNS myelin, on the other hand, can be described as forming centripetally by the continued insinuation of the leading edge of the growing process between the inner surface of the newly formed myelin and the axon.

The myelin sheath in the CNS differs from that in the PNS

There are several other important differences between the myelin sheaths in the CNS and those in the PNS. Myelin in the CNS exhibits fewer Schmidt-Lanterman clefts because the astrocytes provide metabolic support for CNS neurons. Unlike Schwann cells of the PNS, oligodendrocytes do not have an external lamina. Furthermore, because of the manner in which oligodendrocytes form CNS myelin, little or no cytoplasm may be present in the outermost layer of the myelin sheath, and with the absence of external lamina, the myelin of adjacent axons may come into contact. Thus, where myelin sheaths of adjacent axons touch, they may share an intraperiod line. Finally, the nodes of Ranvier in the CNS are larger than those in the PNS. The larger areas of exposed axolemma thus make ***saltatory conduction*** (see below) even more efficient in the CNS.

Another difference between the CNS and the PNS in regard to the relationships between supporting cells and neurons is that unmyelinated neurons in the CNS are often found to be bare; i.e., they are not embedded in glial cell processes. The lack of supporting cells around unmyelinated axons as well as the absence of basal lamina material and connective tissue within the substance of the CNS help to distinguish the CNS from the PNS in histologic sections and in TEM specimens.

Ependymal cells form the epithelial lining of the ventricles of the brain and spinal canal

Ependymal cells form the simple epithelial lining of the fluid-filled cavities of the CNS. They are cuboidal-to-columnar cells that have the morphologic and physiologic characteristics of fluid-transporting cells (Fig. 11.23). They are tightly bound by junctional complexes located at the apical surfaces. Unlike a typical epithelium, ependymal

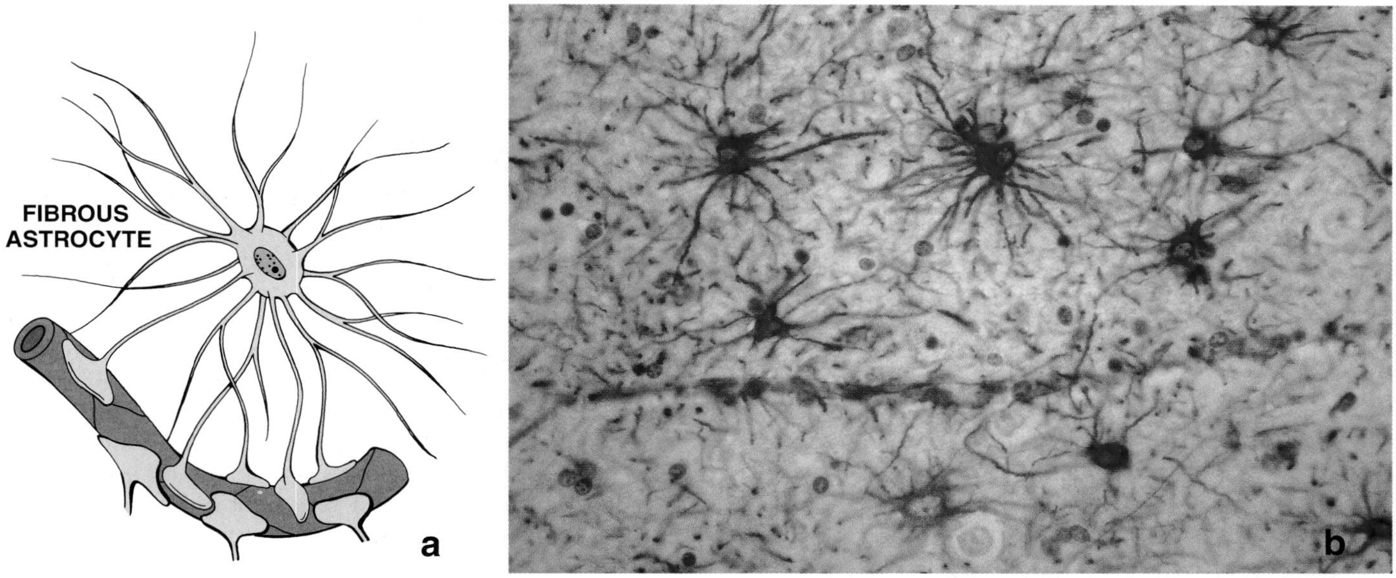

FIGURE 11.20
Fibrous astrocytes in the white matter of the brain. a. Schematic drawing of a fibrous astrocyte in the white mater of the brain. **b.** Photomicrograph of the white matter of the brain, showing the extensive radiating cytoplasmic processes for which astrocytes are named. They are best visualized, as shown here, with immunostaining methods that use antibodies against GFAP. ×220. (From Fuller GN, Burger PC. Central nervous system. In: Sternberg SS, ed. *Histology for Pathologists*. Philadelphia: Lippincott-Raven, 1997.)

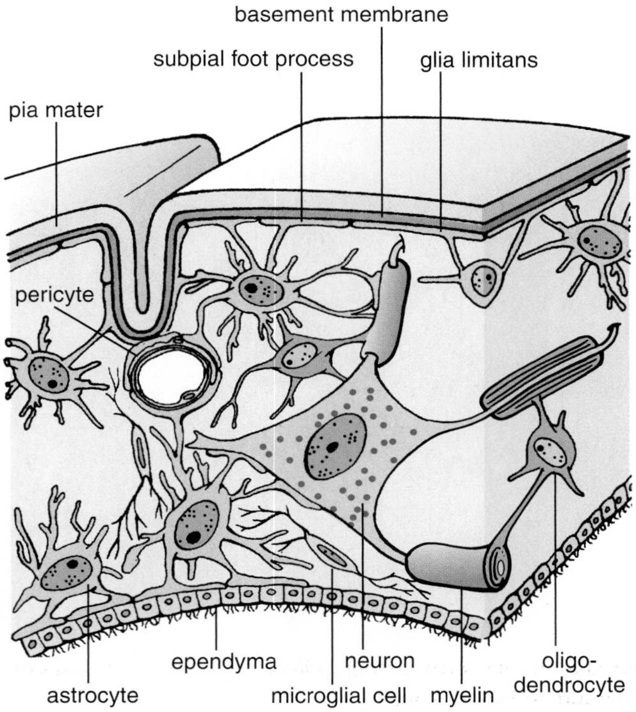

FIGURE 11.21
Distribution of glial cells in the brain. This diagram shows the three types of glial cells—astrocytes, oligodendrocytes, and microglial cells—interacting with several structures and cells found in the brain tissue. Note that the astrocytes and their processes interact with the blood vessels as well as with axons and dendrites. Note that astrocytes also send their processes toward the brain surface, where they contact the basement membrane of the pia mater, forming the glia limitans. In addition, processes of astrocytes extend toward the fluid-filled spaces in the CNS, where they contact the ependymal lining cells. Oligodendrocytes are involved in myelination of the nerve fibers in the CNS. Microglia exhibit phagocytotic functions.

cells lack an external lamina. At the TEM level, the basal cell surface exhibits numerous infoldings that interdigitate with adjacent astrocyte processes. The apical surface of the cell possesses cilia and microvilli. The latter are involved in absorbing cerebrospinal fluid.

Within the system of the brain ventricles, this lining epithelium is further modified to produce the cerebrospinal fluid by transport and secretion of materials derived from adjacent capillary loops. The modified ependymal cells and associated capillaries are called the ***choroid plexus.***

Impulse Conduction

An action potential is an electrochemical process triggered by impulses carried to the axon hillock after other impulses are received on the dendrites or the cell body itself

A nerve impulse is conducted along an axon much as a flame travels along the fuse of a firecracker. This electrochemical process involves the generation of an **action potential,** a wave of membrane depolarization that is initi-

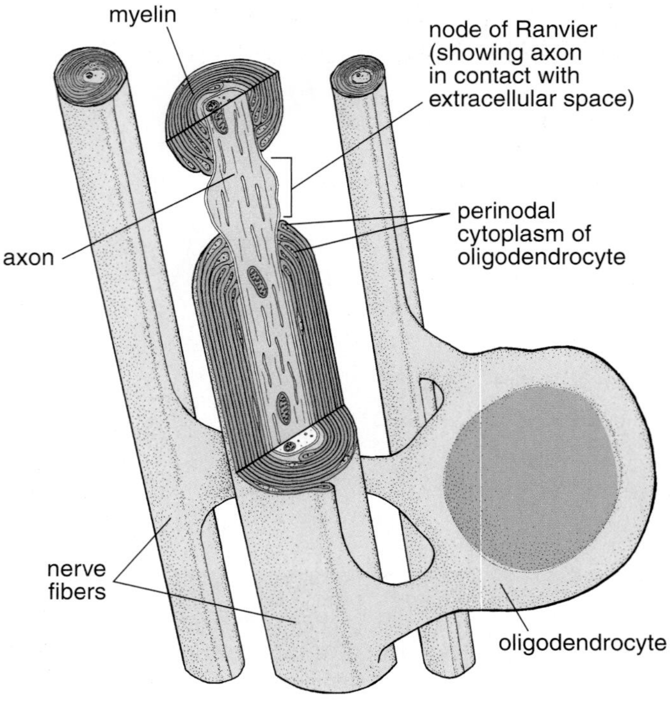

FIGURE 11.22
Three-dimensional view of an oligodendrocyte as it relates to three axons. Cytoplasmic processes from the oligodendrocyte cell body form flattened cytoplasmic sheaths that wrap around each of the axons. The relationship of cytoplasm and myelin is essentially the same as that of Schwann cells. (Modified from Bunge MR, Bunge RP, Ris H. *J Biophys Biochem Cytol* 1961;10:67–94.)

ated at the initial segment of the axon hillock. Its membrane contains a large number of voltage-gated Na^+ and K^+ channels. In response to a stimulus, voltage-gated Na^+ channels in the initial segment of the axon membrane open, causing an influx of Na^+ into the axoplasm. This influx of Na^+ briefly reverses ("depolarizes") the negative membrane potential of the resting membrane (–70 mV) to positive (+30 mV). Following depolarization, the voltage-gated Na^+ channels close and voltage-gated K^+ channels open. K^+ rapidly exits the axon, returning the membrane to its resting potential. Depolarization of one part of the membrane sends electrical current to neighboring portions of unstimulated membrane, which is still positively charged. This local current stimulates adjacent portions of the axon's membrane and repeats depolarization along the membrane. The entire process takes less than one thousandth of a second. After a very brief (refractory) period, the neuron can repeat the process of generating an action potential once again.

Rapid conduction of the action potential is due to the nodes of Ranvier

Myelinated axons conduct impulses more rapidly than unmyelinated axons. Physiologists describe the nerve impulse as "jumping" from node to node along the myelinated axon. This process is called ***saltatory*** *(L. saltus, to jump)*, or ***discontinuous conduction.*** In myelinated nerves, the myelin sheath around the nerve does not conduct an elec-

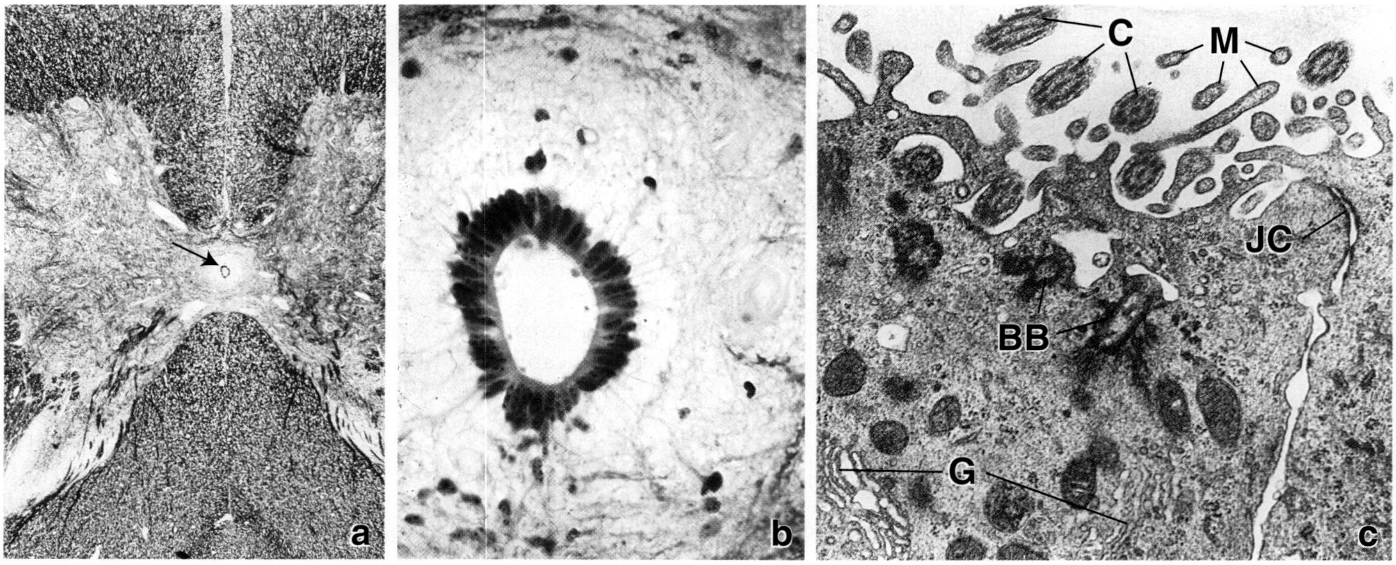

FIGURE 11.23
Ependymal lining of the spinal canal. a. Photomicrograph of the center region of the spinal cord stained with toluidine blue. The *arrow* points to the central canal. ×20. **b.** At higher magnification, ependymal cells, which line the central canal, can be seen to consist of a single layer of columnar cells. ×340. (Courtesy of Dr. George D. Pappas.) **c.** Transmission electron micrograph showing a portion of the apical region of two columnar ependymal cells. They are joined by a junctional complex *(JC)* that separates the lumen of the canal from the lateral intercellular space. The apical surface of the ependymal cells has both cilia *(C)* and microvilli *(M)*. Basal bodies *(BB)* and a Golgi apparatus *(G)* within the apical cytoplasm are also visible. ×20,000. (Courtesy of Dr. Paul Reier.)

tric current and forms an insulating layer around the axon. However, the voltage reversal can ***only*** occur at the nodes of Ranvier, where the axolemma is lacking a myelin sheath. Here, the axolemma is exposed to extracellular fluids and possesses a high concentration of voltage-gated Na^+ and K^+ channels (see Figs. 11.14 and 11.22). Because of this, the voltage reversal (and, thus, the impulse) jumps as "current flow" from one node of Ranvier to the next. The speed of saltatory conduction is related not only to the thickness of the myelin but also to the diameter of the axon. Conduction is more rapid along axons of greater diameter.

In unmyelinated axons, Na^+ and K^+ channels are distributed uniformly along the length of the fiber. The nerve impulse is conducted more slowly and moves as a continuous wave of voltage reversal along the axon.

▼ ORIGIN OF NERVE TISSUE CELLS

CNS neurons are derived from neuroectodermal cells of the neural tube

After developing neurons have migrated to their predestined locations in the neural tube and have differentiated into mature neurons, they no longer divide. Astrocytes and oligodendrocytes are also derived from cells of the neural tube, but studies with tritiated thymidine indicate that these neuroglial cells undergo a slow turnover.

As noted above, microglia are derived from mononuclear phagocytotic cells of blood (mononuclear phagocytotic system [MPS]) along with other macrophages of the body. It is still not known whether they are able to divide after they have reached the CNS. As the only glial cells of mesenchymal origin, microglia possess the vimentin class of intermediate filaments, which can be useful in identifying these cells by using immunocytochemical methods.

The ependymal cells are derived from the proliferation of neuroepithelial cells that immediately surround the canal of the developing neural tube.

PNS ganglion cells are derived from the neural crest

The development of the ganglion cells of the PNS involves the proliferation and migration of ganglion precursor cells from the neural crest to their future ganglionic sites, where they undergo further proliferation. There, the cells develop processes that reach the cells' target tissues (e.g., glandular tissue or smooth muscle cells) and sensory territories. Initially, more cells are produced than are needed. Those that do not make functional contact with a target tissue undergo apoptosis.

Schwann cells also arise originally from the neural crest but undergo mitosis along the growing nerve. Most Schwann cells are formed by mitosis of parent Schwann cells in the peripheral nerves rather than by the migration of cells from the neural crest.

▼ ORGANIZATION OF THE PERIPHERAL NERVOUS SYSTEM

Peripheral Nerves

A peripheral nerve is a bundle of nerve fibers held together by connective tissue

The nerves of the PNS are made up of many nerve fibers that carry sensory and motor (effector) information between the organs and tissues of the body and the brain and spinal cord. Unfortunately, the term ***nerve fiber*** is used in different ways that can be confusing. It can connote the axon with all of its covers (myelin and Schwann cell), as used above, or it can connote the axon alone. It is also used to refer to any process of a nerve cell, either dendrite or axon, especially if insufficient information is available to identify the process as either an axon or a dendrite.

The cell bodies of peripheral nerves may be located within the CNS or outside the CNS in ***peripheral ganglia.*** Ganglia contain clusters of neuronal cell bodies and the nerve fibers leading to and from them (see Fig. 11.17). The cell bodies in dorsal root ganglia as well as ganglia of cranial nerves belong to sensory neurons (*somatic* and *visceral afferents*), whose distribution is restricted to specific locations (Table 11.1 and Fig. 11.3). The cell bodies in the paravertebral, prevertebral, and terminal ganglia belong to postsynaptic "motor" neurons *(visceral efferents)* of the ANS (see Table 11.1 and Fig. 11.17).

To understand the PNS, it is also necessary to describe some parts of the CNS.

Motor neuron cell bodies of the PNS lie in the CNS

The cell bodies of motor neurons that innervate skeletal muscle *(somatic efferents)* are located in the brain, brain stem, and spinal cord. The axons leave the CNS and travel in peripheral nerves to the skeletal muscles that they innervate. A *single neuron* conveys impulses from the CNS to the effector organ.

In the ANS, a chain of *two neurons* connects the CNS to smooth muscle, cardiac muscle, and glands *(visceral efferents).* The cell bodies of ***presynaptic,*** or ***preganglionic, neurons*** of the ANS are located in specific parts of the CNS. Their axons leave the CNS and travel in peripheral nerves to synapse with the ***postsynaptic,*** or ***postganglionic, neurons*** in peripheral ganglia (see Table 11.1).

Sensory neuron cell bodies are located in ganglia outside of, but close to, the CNS

In the sensory system, both the *somatic* and the *visceral afferent* components, a single neuron connects the receptor, through a sensory ganglion, to the spinal cord or brain

TABLE 11.1. Peripheral Ganglia[A]

Ganglia that contain cell bodies of sensory neurons; these are not synaptic stations

- Dorsal root ganglia of all spinal nerves
- Sensory ganglia of all cranial nerves
  - Trigeminal (semilunar, Gasserian) ganglion of the cochlear division of the trigeminal (V) nerve
  - Geniculate ganglion of the facial (VII) nerve
  - Spiral ganglion (contains bipolar neurons) of the cochlear division of the vestibulocochlear (VIII) nerve
  - Vestibular ganglion (contains bipolar neurons) of the vestibular division of the vestibulocochlear (VIII) nerve
  - Superior and inferior ganglia of the glossopharyngeal (IX) nerve
  - Superior and inferior ganglia of the vagus (X) nerve

Ganglia that contain cell bodies of autonomic (postsynaptic) neurons; these are synaptic stations

- Sympathetic ganglia
  - Sympathetic trunk (paravertebral) ganglia (the highest of these is the superior cervical ganglion)
  - Prevertebral ganglia (adjacent to origins of large branches of abdominal aorta), including celiac, superior mesenteric, inferior mesenteric, and aorticorenal ganglia
  - Adrenal medulla, which may be considered a modified sympathetic ganglion (each of the secretory cells of the medulla, as well as the recognizable ganglion cells, is innervated by cholinergic presynaptic sympathetic nerves fibers)
- Parasympathetic ganglia
  - Head ganglia
    - Ciliary ganglion associated with the oculomotor (III) nerve
    - Submandibular ganglion associated with the facial (VII) nerve
    - Pterygopalatine (sphenopalatine) ganglion of the facial (VII) nerve
    - Otic ganglion associated with the glossopharyngeal (IX) nerve
  - Terminal ganglia (near or in wall of organs), including ganglia of the submucosal (Meissner's) and myenteric (Auerbach's) plexuses of the gastrointestinal tract (these are also ganglia of the enteric division of the ANS) and isolated ganglion cells in a variety of organs

[A]*Practical note:* Neuron cell bodies seen in tissue sections such as tongue, pancreas, urinary bladder, and heart are invariably terminal ganglia or "ganglion cells" of the parsympathetic nervous system.

stem. Sensory ganglia are located along the dorsal roots of the spinal nerves and in association with cranial nerves V, VII, VIII, IX, and X (see Table 11.1).

Connective Tissue Components of a Peripheral Nerve

The bulk of a peripheral nerve consists of nerve fibers and their supporting Schwann cells. The individual nerve fibers and their associated Schwann cells are held together by connective tissue organized into three distinctive components, each with specific morphologic and functional characteristics (Fig. 11.24; also, see Fig. 11.3). These components are

- ***Endoneurium,*** which includes loose connective tissue surrounding each individual nerve fiber
- ***Perineurium,*** which includes specialized connective tissue surrounding each nerve fascicle
- ***Epineurium,*** which includes dense irregular connective tissue that surrounds a peripheral nerve and fills the spaces between nerve fascicles

Endoneurium constitutes the loose connective tissue associated with individual nerve fibers

The endoneurium is not conspicuous in routine light microscope preparations, but special connective tissue stains permit its demonstration. At the electron microscope level, collagen fibrils that constitute the endoneurium are readily apparent (see Figs. 11.12 and 11.13). The fibrils run both parallel to, and around, the nerve fibers, functionally binding them together into a fascicle, or bundle. Because fibroblasts are relatively sparse in the interstices of the nerve fibers, it is likely that most of the collagen fibrils are secreted by the Schwann cells. This conclusion is supported by tissue culture studies in which collagen fibrils are formed in pure cultures of Schwann cells and dorsal root neurons. Other than occasional fibroblasts, the only other connective tissue cell normally found within the endoneurium is the mast cell. In general, most of the nuclei (90%) found in cross sections of peripheral nerves belong to Schwann cells; the remaining 10% is equally distributed between the occasional fibroblasts and other cells such as endothelial cells of capillaries and mast cells.

Perineurium is the specialized connective tissue surrounding a nerve fascicle

Surrounding the nerve bundle is a sheath of unique connective tissue cells that constitute the ***perineurium.*** The perineurium serves as a metabolically active diffusion barrier that contributes to the formation of a ***blood–nerve barrier.*** This barrier maintains the ionic milieu of the ensheathed nerve fibers. In a manner similar to the properties exhibited by the endothelial cells of brain capillaries form-

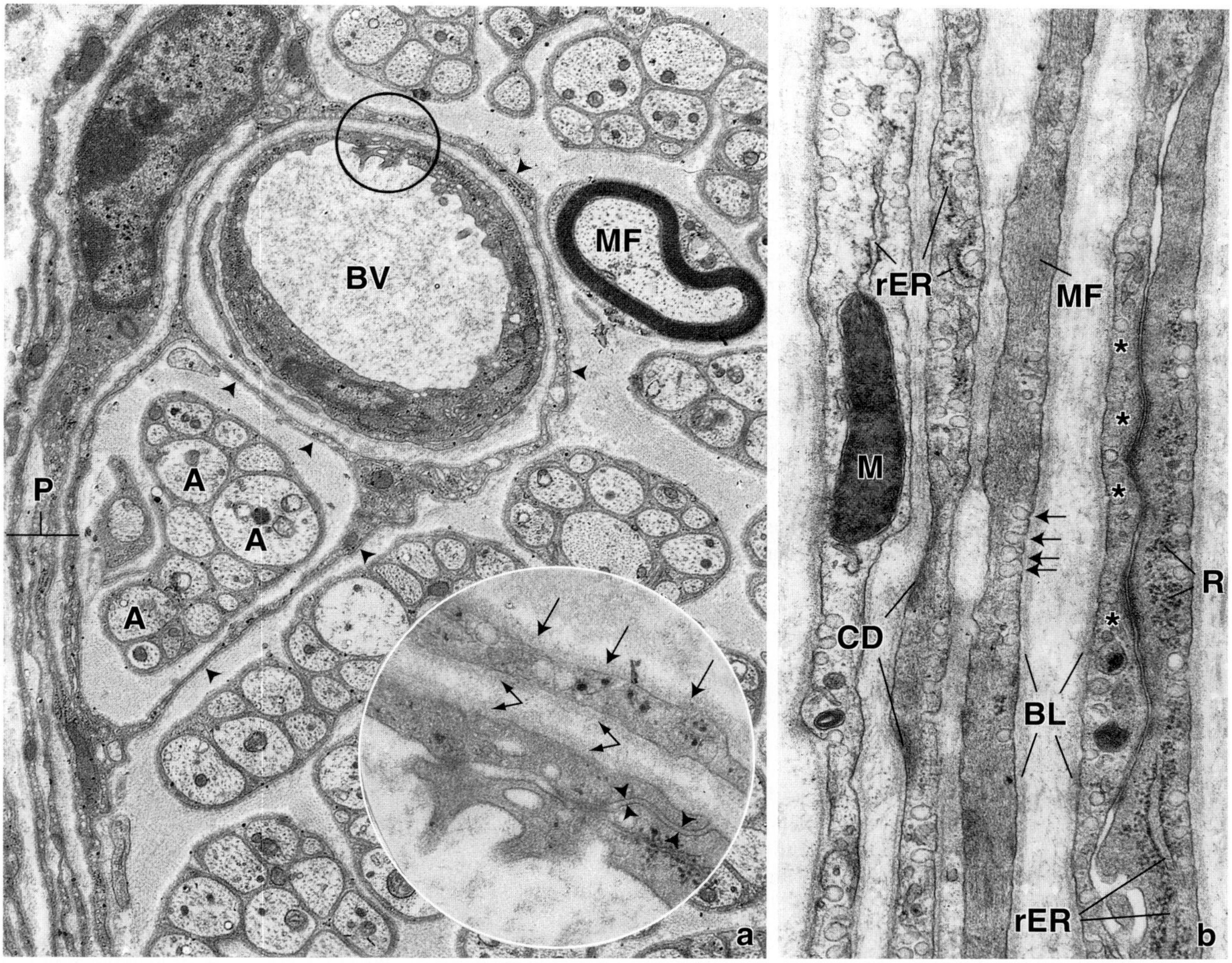

FIGURE 11.24

Electron micrograph of a peripheral nerve and its surrounding perineurium. a. Electron micrograph of unmyelinated nerve fibers and a single myelinated fiber (MF). The perineurium *(P)*, consisting of several cell layers, is seen at the left of the micrograph. Perineurial cell processes *(arrowheads)* have also extended into the nerve to surround a group of axons *(A)* and their Schwann cell as well as a small blood vessel *(BV)*. The enclosure of this group of axons represents the root of a small nerve branch that is joining or leaving the larger fascicle. ×10,000. The area within the *circle* encompassing the endothelium of the vessel and the adjacent perineurial cytoplasm is shown in the **inset** at higher magnification. Note the basal (external) laminae of the vessel and the perineurial cell *(arrows)*. The junction between endothelial cells of the blood vessel is also apparent *(arrowheads)*. ×46,000. **b.** Electron micrograph showing the perineurium of a nerve. Four cellular layers of the perineurium are present. Each layer has a basal (external) lamina *(BL)* associated with it on both surfaces. Other features of the perineurial cell include an extensive population of actin microfilaments *(MF)*, pinocytotic vesicles *(arrows)*, and cytoplasmic densities *(CD)*. These features are characteristic of smooth muscle cells. The innermost perineurial cell layer *(right)* exhibits tight junctions *(asterisks)* where one cell is overlapping a second cell in forming the sheath. Other features seen in the cytoplasm are mitochondria *(M)*, rough endoplasmic reticulum *(rER)*, and free ribosomes *(R)*. ×27,000.

ing the brain–blood barrier (see page 313), perineurial cells possess receptors, transporters, and enzymes that provide for the active transport of substances across the perineurial cells. The perineurium may be one or more cell layers thick, depending on the nerve diameter. The cells that compose this layer are squamous; each layer exhibits an external (basal) lamina on both surfaces (Fig. 11.24b). The cells are contractile and contain an appreciable number of actin filaments, a characteristic of smooth muscle cells and other contractile cells. Moreover, when there are two or more perineurial cell layers (as many as five of six layers may be present in larger nerves), collagen fibrils are present be-

tween the perineurial cell layers, but fibroblasts are absent. Tight junctions, providing the basis for the blood–nerve barrier, are present between the cells located within the same layer of the perineurium. In effect, the arrangement of these cells as a barrier—the presence of tight junctions and basal (external) lamina material—liken them to an epithelioid tissue. On the other hand, their contractile nature and their apparent ability to produce collagen fibrils also liken them to smooth muscle cells and fibroblasts. The limited number of connective tissue cell types within the endoneurium undoubtedly reflects the protective role that the perineurium plays. Typical immune system cells (i.e., lymphocytes, plasma cells) are not found within the endoneurial and perineurial compartments. This absence of immune cells (other than the mast cell) is accounted for by the protective barrier created by the perineurial cells. Typically only fibroblasts and occasional mast cells are present within the nerve compartment.

Epineurium consists of dense irregular connective tissue that surrounds and binds nerve fascicles into a common bundle

The epineurium forms the outermost tissue of the peripheral nerve. It is a typical dense connective tissue that surrounds the fascicles formed by the perineurium. Adipose tissue is often associated with the epineurium in larger nerves.

The blood vessels that supply the nerves travel in the epineurium, and their branches penetrate into the nerve and travel within the perineurium. Tissue at the level of the endoneurium is poorly vascularized; metabolic exchange of substrates and wastes in this tissue depends on diffusion from and to the blood vessels through the perineurial sheath (see Fig. 11.24).

Organization of the Spinal Cord

The spinal cord is a flattened cylindrical structure that is directly continuous with the brain. It is divided into 31 segments (8 cervical, 12 thoracic, 5 lumbar, 5 sacral, and 1 coccygeal), and each segment is connected to a pair of spinal nerves. Each spinal nerve is joined to its segment of the cord by a number of roots or rootlets grouped as dorsal (posterior) or ventral (anterior) roots (Fig. 11.25; see also Fig. 11.3).

In cross section, the spinal cord exhibits a butterfly-shaped grayish tan inner substance, the ***gray matter*** surrounding the central canal, and a whitish peripheral substance, the ***white matter.*** The white matter (see Fig. 11.3) contains only myelinated and unmyelinated axons traveling to and from other parts of the spinal cord and to and from the brain. Functionally related bundles of axons in the white matter are called ***tracts.***

The ***gray matter*** contains neuronal cell bodies and their dendrites, along with axons and neuroglia. Functionally related groups of nerve cell bodies in the gray matter are

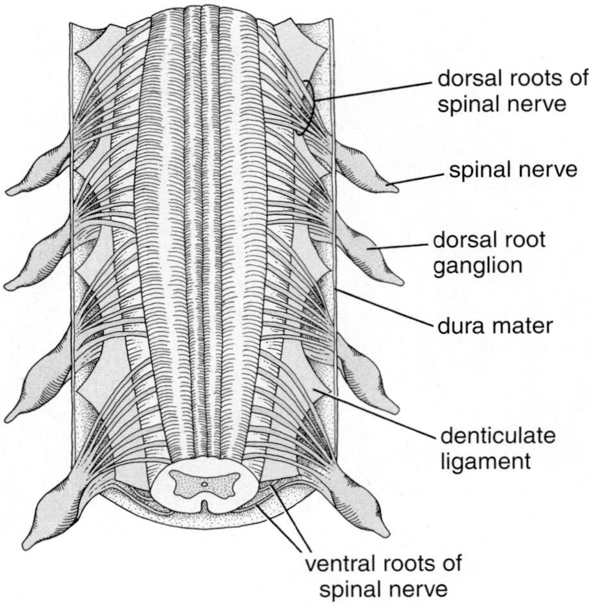

FIGURE 11.25
Posterior view of exposed spinal cord. Note that each spinal nerve emerges from the cord by a number of dorsal (posterior) and ventral (anterior) roots. Note the dura mater (the outer layer of the meninges) and the denticulate ligaments of the pia mater, which anchor the spinal cord to the wall of the spinal canal. (From Barr ML, Kiernan JA. *The Human Nervous System.* New York: Harper & Row, 1983.)

called ***nuclei.*** In this context, the term *nucleus* means a cluster or group of neuronal cell bodies plus fibers and neuroglia. Nuclei of the CNS are the morphologic and functional equivalents of the ganglia of the PNS. Synapses occur only in the gray matter.

The cell bodies of motor neurons that innervate striated muscle are located in the ventral (anterior) horn of the gray matter

Ventral motor neurons, also called ***anterior horn cells,*** are large basophilic cells and are easily recognized in routine histologic preparations (Fig. 11.26). Because the motor neuron conducts impulses away from the CNS, it is called an ***efferent neuron.***

The axon of a motor neuron leaves the spinal cord, passes through the ventral (anterior) root, becomes a component of the spinal nerve of that segment, and, as such, is conveyed to the muscle. The axon is myelinated except at its origin and termination. Near the muscle cell, the axon divides into numerous terminal branches that form neuromuscular synapses with the muscle cell (see page 257).

The cell bodies of sensory neurons are located in ganglia that lie on the dorsal root of the spinal nerve

Sensory neurons in the dorsal root ganglia are pseudounipolar. They have a single process that divides into a pe-

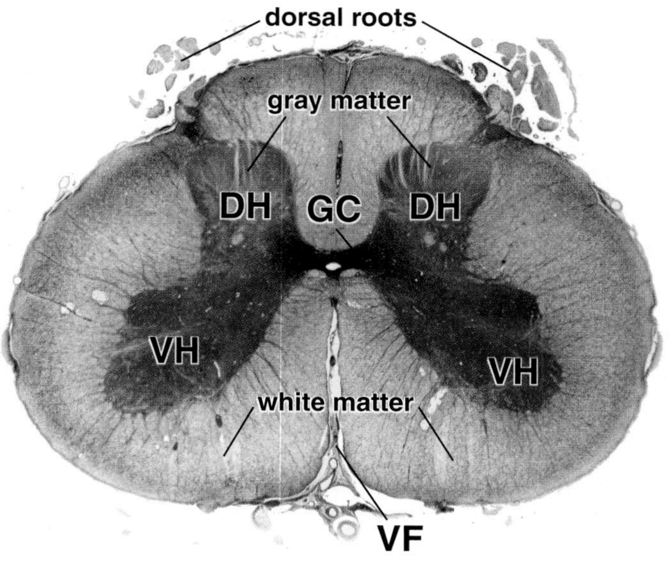

FIGURE 11.26
Cross section of the human spinal cord. The photomicrograph shows a cross section through the lower lumbar (most likely L4-L5) level of the spinal cord stained by the Bielschowsky silver method. The spinal cord is organized into an outer part, the white matter, and an inner part, the gray matter that contains nerve cell bodies and associated nerve fibers. The gray matter of the spinal cord appears roughly in the form of a butterfly. The anterior and posterior prongs are referred to as ventral horns *(VH)* and dorsal horns *(DH)*, respectively. They are connected by the gray commissure *(GC)*. The white matter contains nerve fibers that form ascending and descending tracts. The outer surface of the spinal cord is surrounded by the pia mater. Blood vessels of the pia mater, ventral fissure *(VF)*, and some dorsal roots of the spinal nerves are visible in the section. ×5.

ripheral segment that brings information from the periphery to the cell body and a central segment that carries information from the cell body into the gray matter of the spinal cord. Because the sensory neuron conducts impulses to the CNS, it is called an ***afferent neuron.*** Impulses are generated in the terminal receptor arborization of the peripheral segment.

Afferent (Sensory) Receptors

Afferent receptors are specialized structures located at the distal tips of the peripheral processes of sensory neurons

Although ***receptors*** may have many different structures, they have one basic characteristic in common: They can initiate a nerve impulse in response to a stimulus. Receptors may be classified as

- *Exteroceptors,* which react to stimuli from the external environment, e.g., temperature, touch, smell, sound, or vision
- *Enteroceptors,* which react to stimuli from within the body, e.g., the degree of filling or stretch of the alimentary canal, bladder, and blood vessels
- *Proprioceptors,* which also react to stimuli from within the body, providing sensation of body position and muscle tone and movement

The simplest receptor is a bare axon, called a ***nonencapsulated (free) ending.*** This ending is found in epithelia, in connective tissue, and in close association with hair follicles.

Most sensory nerve endings acquire connective tissue capsules or sheaths of varying complexity

Sensory nerve endings with connective tissue sheaths are called ***encapsulated endings.*** Many encapsulated endings are mechanoreceptors located in the skin and joint capsules (Krause's end bulb, Ruffini's corpuscles, Meissner's corpuscles, and Pacinian corpuscles) and are described in Chapter 14, "Integumentary System" (page 400).

Muscle spindles are encapsulated sensory endings located in skeletal muscle; they are described in Chapter 10, "Muscle Tissue" (page 260). Functionally related Golgi tendon organs are encapsulated tension receptors found at musculotendinous junctions.

Autonomic Nervous System

Although the ANS was introduced early in this chapter, it is useful here to describe some of the salient features of its organization and distribution. The ANS is classified into three divisions:

- *Sympathetic division*
- *Parasympathetic division*
- *Enteric division*

The ANS is that portion of the PNS that conducts impulses to smooth muscle, cardiac muscle, and glandular epithelium. These effectors are the functional units in the organs that respond to regulation by nerve tissue. The term *visceral* is sometimes used to refer to the ANS or its neurons, which are, therefore, called ***visceral efferent neurons.***

Sensory neurons also leave the organs to convey impulses to the CNS. These ***visceral afferent neurons*** have the same arrangement as other sensory neurons; i.e., their cell bodies are located in sensory ganglia, and they possess long peripheral and central axons, as described above.

The main organizational difference between the efferent flow of impulses to skeletal muscle (somatic effectors) and the efferent flow to smooth muscle, cardiac muscle, and glandular epithelium (visceral effectors) is that one neuron conveys the impulses from the CNS to the somatic effector (Fig. 11.27a), whereas a chain of two neurons conveys the impulses from the CNS to the visceral effectors

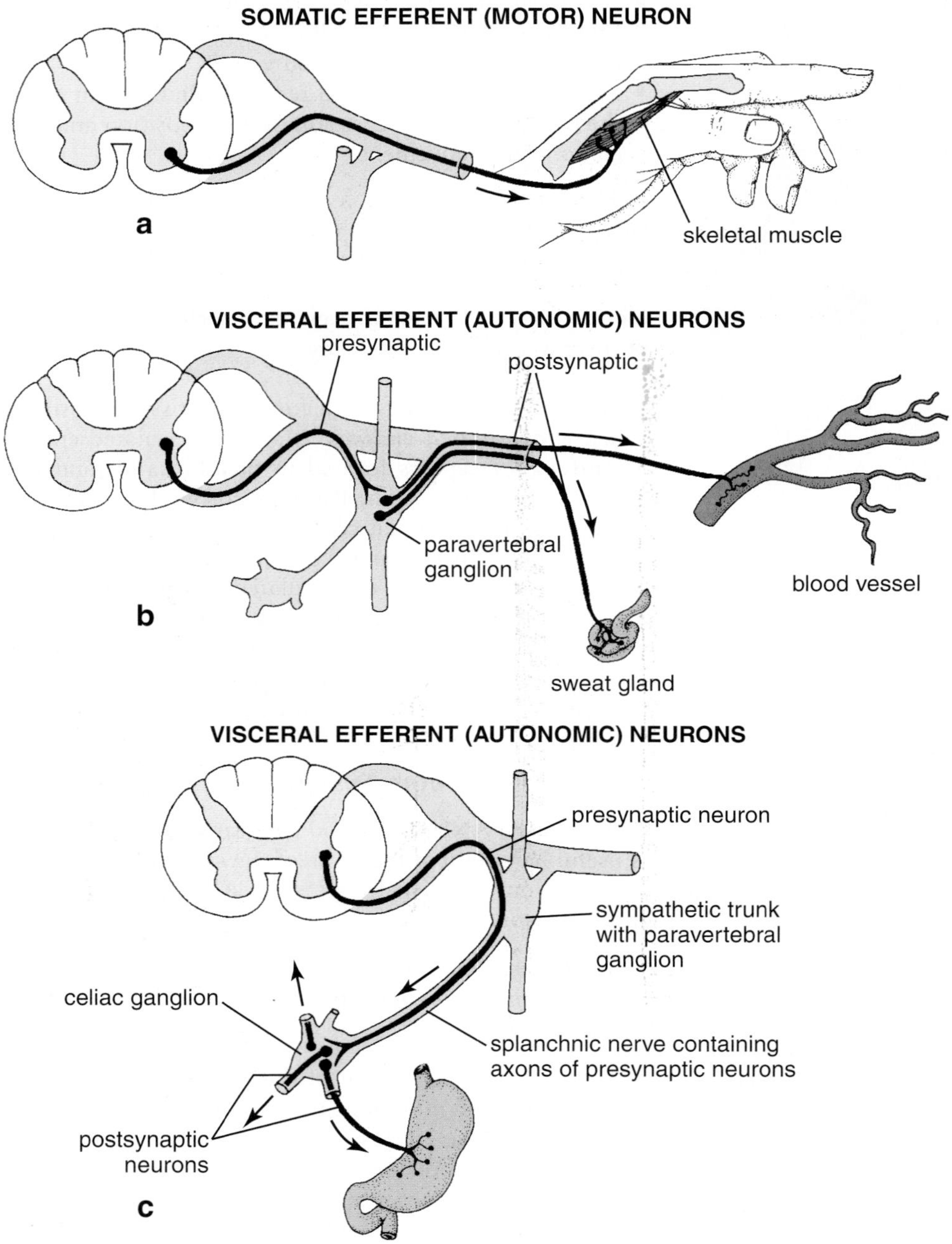

FIGURE 11.27
Schematic diagram comparing somatic efferent and visceral efferent neurons. a. In the somatic efferent (motor) system, one neuron conducts the impulses from the CNS to the effector (skeletal muscle). **b.** In the visceral efferent system (represented in this diagram by the sympathetic division of the ANS), a chain of two neurons conducts the impulses: a presynaptic neuron located within the CNS and a postsynaptic neuron located in the paravertebral or prevertebral ganglia. Moreover, each presynaptic neuron makes synaptic contact with more than one postsynaptic neuron. Postsynaptic sympathetic fibers supply smooth muscles (as in blood vessels) or glandular epithelium (as in sweat glands). **c.** Neurons of the ANS that supply organs of the abdomen reach these organs by way of the splanchnic nerves. In this example, the splanchnic nerve joins with the celiac ganglion, where most of the synapses of the two-neuron chain occur. Note that one presynaptic neuron makes contact with several postsynaptic neurons. (From Reith EJ, Breidenbach B, Lorenc M. *Textbook of Anatomy and Physiology.* St. Louis: CV Mosby, 1978.)

(Fig. 11.27b). Thus, there is a synaptic station in a ganglion outside the CNS, where a ***presynaptic*** neuron makes contact with ***postsynaptic*** neurons. Each presynaptic neuron synapses with several postsynaptic neurons.

The presynaptic neurons of the sympathetic division are located in the thoracic and upper lumbar portions of the spinal cord

The presynaptic neurons send axons from the thoracic and upper lumbar spinal cord to the vertebral and paravertebral ganglia. The ganglia in the paravertebral and vertebral *sympathetic trunk* contain the cell bodies of the postsynaptic effector neurons of the ***sympathetic division*** (Figs. 11.27b and 11.28).

The presynaptic neurons of the parasympathetic division are located in the brain stem and sacral spinal cord

The presynaptic parasympathetic neurons send axons from the brain stem, i.e., the midbrain, pons, and medulla,

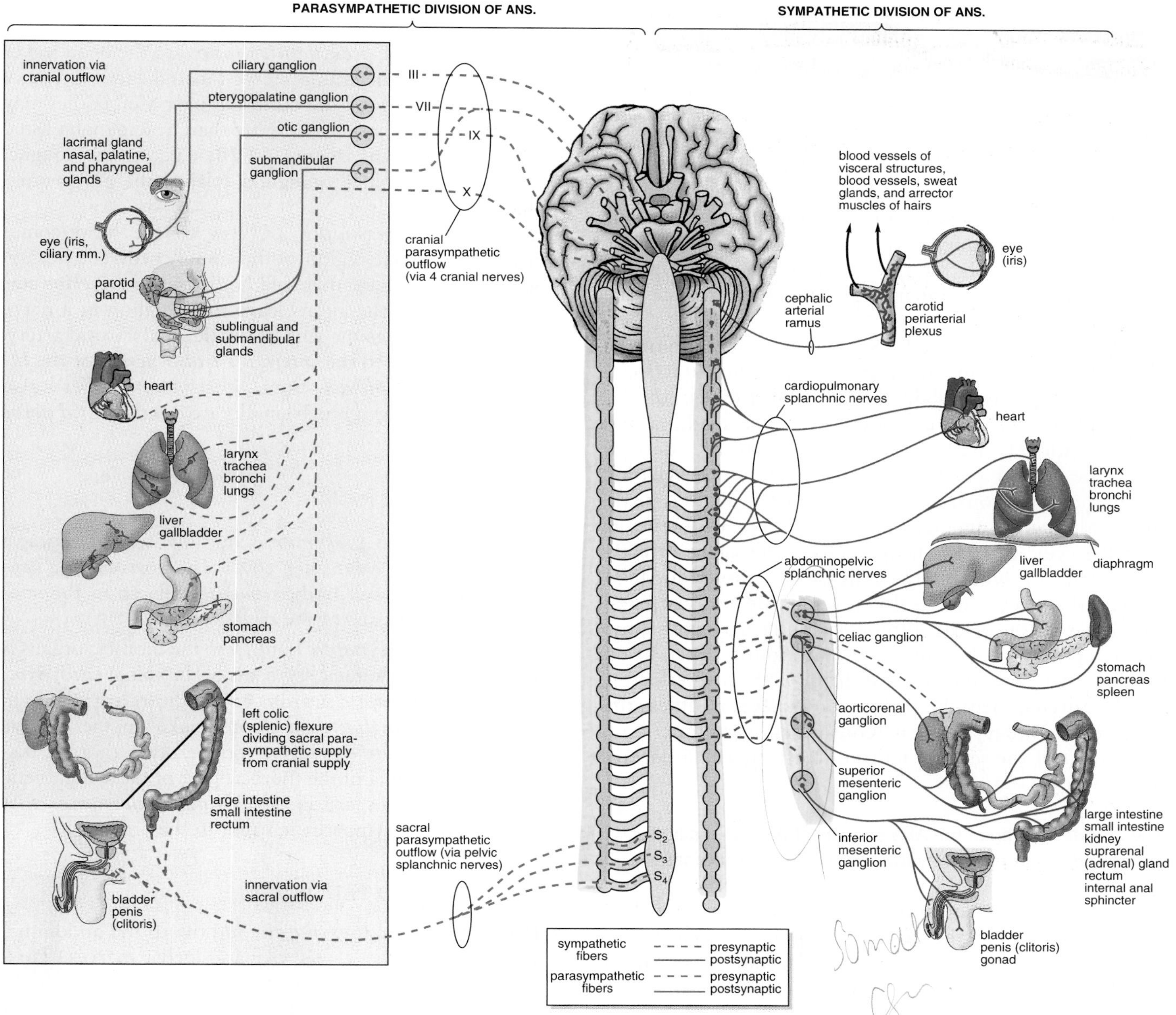

FIGURE 11.28

Schematic diagram showing the general arrangement of sympathetic and parasympathetic neurons of the ANS. The sympathetic outflow is shown on the right; the parasympathetic, on the left. The sympathetic (thoracolumbar) outflow leaves the CNS from the thoracic and upper lumbar segments (T1-L2 or L3) of the spinal cord. These presynaptic fibers communicate with postsynaptic neurons in two locations, the paravertebral and prevertebral ganglia. Paravertebral ganglia are linked together and form two sympathetic trunks *(yellow columns on each side of the spinal cord).* Prevertebral ganglia are associated with the main branches of the abdominal aorta *(yellow circles).* Note the distribution of postsynaptic sympathetic nerve fibers to the viscera. The parasympathetic (craniosacral) outflow leaves the CNS from the gray matter of the brainstem within cranial nerves III, VII, IX, and X and the gray matter of sacral segments (S2-S4) of the spinal cord and is distributed to the viscera. The presynaptic fibers traveling with cranial nerves III, VII, and IX communicate with postsynaptic neurons in various ganglia located in the head and neck region *(yellow circles).* The presynaptic fibers traveling with cranial nerve X and with pelvic splanchnic nerves have their synapses with postsynaptic neurons in the wall of visceral organs (terminal ganglia). The viscera, thus, contain both sympathetic and parasympathetic innervation. Note that a two-neuron chain carries impulses to all viscera except the adrenal medulla. (Modified from Moore KL, Dalley AF. *Clinically Oriented Anatomy.* Baltimore: Lippincott Williams & Wilkins, 1999:48–50.)

and the sacral segments of the spinal cord (S2 through S4) to visceral ganglia. The ganglia in or near the wall of abdominal and pelvic organs and the visceral motor ganglia of cranial nerves III, VII, IX, and X contain cell bodies of the postsynaptic effector neurons of the ***parasympathetic division*** (Figs. 11.27c and 11.28).

The sympathetic and parasympathetic divisions of the ANS often supply the same organs. In these cases, the actions of the two are usually antagonistic. An obvious example of this antagonistic action is that sympathetic stimulation increases the rate of cardiac muscle contractions, whereas parasympathetic stimulation reduces the rate.

Many functions of the SNS are similar to those of the adrenal medulla, an endocrine gland. This functional similarity is partly explained by the developmental relationships between the cells of the adrenal medulla and postsynaptic sympathetic neurons. Both are derived from the neural crest, are innervated by presynaptic sympathetic neurons, and produce closely related physiologically active agents, EPI and NE. The difference is that the sympathetic neurons deliver the agent directly to the effector, whereas the cells of the adrenal medulla deliver the agent indirectly through the bloodstream. The innervation of the adrenal medulla may constitute an exception to the rule that autonomic innervation consists of a two-neuron chain from CNS to an effector; for the adrenal medulla, it is only one neuron, unless the adrenal medullary cell is considered the functional equivalent of the second neuron, in effect, a neurosecretory neuron.

The enteric division of the ANS consists of the ganglia and postsynaptic neuronal networks of the alimentary canal

Ganglia and postsynaptic neurons of the enteric division are located in the lamina propria, muscularis mucosae, submucosa, muscularis externa, and subserosa of the alimentary canal from the esophagus to the anus (see page 476). The enteric division can function independently of presynaptic input from the vagus nerve and sacral outflow; e.g., the intestine will continue peristaltic movements even after the vagus nerve is cut. There are many millions more ganglion cells in the enteric division than could be supplied by the presynaptic neurons of the vagal and sacral outflows.

A Summarized View of Autonomic Distribution

Figures 11.27 and 11.28 summarize diagrammatically the origins and distribution of the ANS. Refer to these figures as you read the descriptive sections. Note that the diagrams indicate both the paired innervation (parasympathetic and sympathetic) common to the ANS as well as the important exceptions to this general characteristic.

HEAD

- ***Parasympathetic presynaptic*** outflow to the head leaves the brain with the cranial nerves, as indicated in Figure 11.28, but the routes are quite complex. Cell bodies may also be found in structures other than head ganglia listed in Table 11.1 and Figure 11.28, e.g., in the tongue. These are "terminal" ganglion cells of the parasympathetic system.
- ***Sympathetic presynaptic*** outflow to the head comes from the thoracic region of the spinal cord. The *postsynaptic neurons* have their cell bodies in the ***superior cervical ganglion;*** the axons leave the ganglion in a nerve network that hugs the wall of the internal carotid artery. The nerve is called the ***internal carotid nerve,*** or the ***internal carotid plexus.*** Some postsynaptic fibers also reach the head by a much smaller ***external carotid nerve*** and ***plexus.***

THORAX

- ***Parasympathetic presynaptic*** outflow to the thoracic viscera is via the vagus nerve (X). The *postsynaptic neurons* have their cell bodies in the walls or in the substance of the organs of the thorax.
- ***Sympathetic presynaptic*** outflow to the thoracic organs is from the upper thoracic segments of the spinal cord. *Sympathetic postsynaptic neurons* for the heart are mostly in the ***cervical ganglia;*** their axons make up the ***cardiac nerves.*** *Postsynaptic neurons* for the other thoracic viscera are in ganglia of the thoracic part of the sympathetic trunk. The axons are in small ***splanchnic nerves*** that travel from the sympathetic trunk to the organs.

ABDOMEN AND PELVIS

- ***Parasympathetic presynaptic*** outflow to the abdominal viscera is via the vagus (X) and pelvic nerves. *Postsynaptic neurons* of the parasympathetic system to abdominopelvic organs are in terminal ganglia that generally are in the walls of the organs, such as the ganglia of the submucosal (Meissner's) plexus and the myenteric (Auerbach's) plexus in the alimentary canal.
- ***Sympathetic presynaptic*** outflow to the abdominopelvic organs is from the thoracic and upper lumbar segments of the spinal cord. *Postsynaptic neurons* have their cell bodies mostly in the prevertebral ganglia (see Fig. 11.27c), although some are in paravertebral ganglia of the sympathetic trunk, and their neurons enter the splanchnic nerves.

EXTREMITIES AND BODY WALL

There is no parasympathetic outflow to the body wall and extremities. Anatomically, the autonomic innervation in

the body wall is only sympathetic (see Fig. 11.27b). Each spinal nerve contains postsynaptic sympathetic fibers, i.e., unmyelinated visceral efferents, of neurons whose cell bodies are in paravertebral ganglia of the sympathetic trunk. For sweat glands, the neurotransmitter released by the "sympathetic" neurons is ACh instead of the usual NE.

ORGANIZATION OF THE CENTRAL NERVOUS SYSTEM

In the brain, the gray matter forms an outer covering or cortex; the white matter forms an inner core or medulla

The *cortex* of gray matter in the brain contains nerve cell bodies, axons, dendrites, and glial cells and is the site of synapses. In addition to the gray matter of the cortex, islands of gray matter, called *nuclei* (see page 306), are found in the deep portions of the cerebrum and cerebellum.

The white matter contains only axons of nerve cells plus the associated glial cells and blood vessels. These axons travel from one part of the nervous system to another. Whereas many of the axons going to, or coming from, a specific location are grouped into bundles called ***tracts,*** the tracts themselves do not stand out as delineated bundles. The demonstration of a tract in white matter of the CNS requires a special procedure, such as the destruction of cell bodies that contribute fibers to the tract. The damaged fibers can be displayed by the use of appropriate staining or labeling methods and then traced. Even in the spinal cord, where the grouping of tracts is most pronounced, there are no sharp boundaries between adjacent tracts.

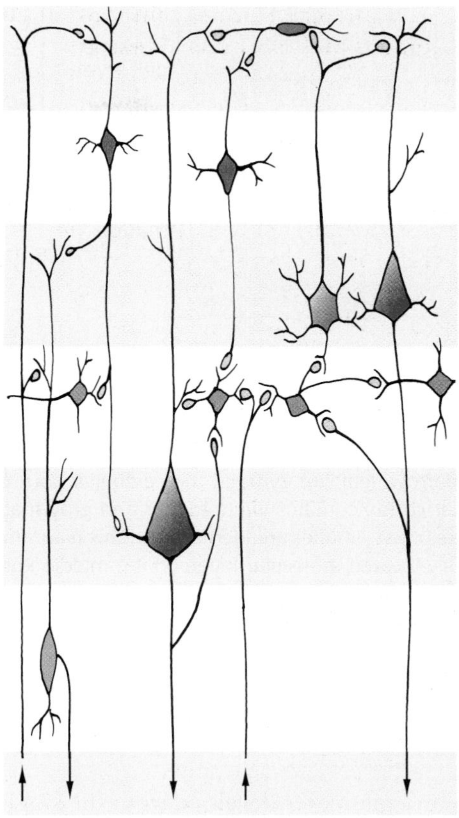

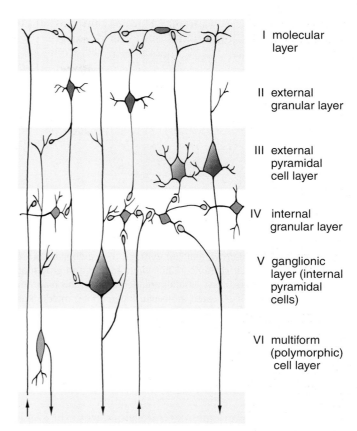

FIGURE 11.29
Nerve cells in intracortical circuits. This simple diagram shows the organization and connections between cells in different layers of the cortex contributing to cortical afferent fibers *(arrows pointing up)* and cortical efferent fibers *(arrows pointing down).* The small interneurons are indicated in *yellow.*

Cells of the Gray Matter

The types of cell bodies found in the gray matter vary according to which part of the brain or spinal cord is being examined.

Each functional region of the gray matter has a characteristic variety of cell bodies associated with a meshwork of axonal, dendritic, and glial processes

The meshwork of axonal, dendritic, and glial processes associated with the gray matter is called the ***neuropil.*** The organization of the neuropil is not demonstrable in H&E–stained sections. It is necessary to use methods other than H&E histology to decipher the cytoarchitecture of the gray matter.

Although general histology programs usually do not deal with the actual arrangements of the neurons in the CNS, the presentation of two examples will add to the appreciation of H&E sections that students usually examine. These examples present a region of the cerebral cortex (Fig. 11.29) and the cerebellar cortex (Fig. 11.30), respectively.

The ***brain stem*** is not clearly separated into regions of gray matter and white matter. The nuclei of the cranial nerves located in the brain stem, however, appear as islands surrounded by more or less distinct tracts of white matter. The nuclei contain the cell bodies of the motor neurons of the cranial nerves and are both the morphologic and functional counterparts of the anterior horns of the spinal cord. In other sites in the brain stem, as in the ***reticular formation,*** the distinction between white matter and gray matter is even less evident.

Connective Tissue of the Central Nervous System

Three sequential connective tissue membranes, the ***meninges,*** cover the brain and spinal cord:

- The ***dura mater*** is the outermost layer.
- The ***arachnoid*** layer lies beneath the dura.
- The ***pia mater*** is a delicate layer resting directly on the surface of the brain and spinal cord.

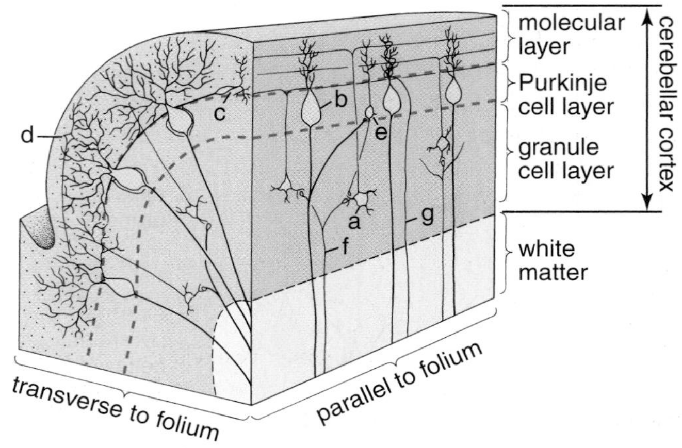

FIGURE 11.30
Cytoarchitecture of the cerebellar cortex. This diagram shows a section of the folium, a narrow, leaf-like gyrus of the cerebellar cortex. Note that the cerebellar cortex contains white matter and gray matter. Three distinct layers of gray matter are identified on this diagram. They are (1) superficially located molecular layer, (2) the middle Purkinje cell layer, and (3) the granule cell layer adjacent to the white matter. *a,* granule cell; *b,* Purkinje cell; *c,* basket cell; *d,* stellate cell; *e,* Golgi cell; *f,* mossy fiber; and *g,* climbing fiber. (Based on Barr ML, Kiernan JA. *The Human Nervous System.* New York: Harper & Row, 1983.)

Because arachnoid and pia mater develope from the single layer of mesenchyme surrounding the developing brain, they are commonly referred as the ***pia-arachnoid.*** In adults, pia mater represents the visceral portion and arachnoid represents the parietal portion of the same layer. This common origin of pia-arachnoid is evident in gross dissection of adult meninges in which numerous strands of connective tissue (arachnoid trabeculae) pass between pia mater and arachnoid.

The dura mater is a relatively thick sheet of dense connective tissue

In the cranial cavity, the thick layer of connective tissue that forms the dura mater *(L., tough mother)* is continuous at its outer surface with the periosteum of the skull. Within the dura mater are spaces lined by endothelium (and backed by periosteum and dura mater, respectively) that serve as the principal channels for blood returning from the brain. These ***venous sinuses*** receive blood from the principal cerebral veins and carry it to the internal jugular veins.

Sheet-like extensions of the inner surface of the dura mater form partitions between parts of the brain, supporting those parts within the cranial cavity and carrying the arachnoid to some of the deeper parts of the brain. In the spinal canal, the vertebrae have their own periosteum, and the dura mater forms a separate tube surrounding the spinal cord (see Fig. 11.25).

The arachnoid is a delicate sheet of connective tissue adjacent to the inner surface of the dura

The arachnoid abuts on the inner surface of the dura and extends delicate ***arachnoid trabeculae*** to the pia mater on the surface of the brain and spinal cord. The web-like trabeculae of the arachnoid give this tissue its name *(Gr., resembling a spider's web)*. Trabeculae are composed of loose connective tissue fibers containing elongated fibroblasts. The space bridged by these trabeculae is the ***subarachnoid space;*** it contains ***cerebrospinal fluid*** (Fig. 11.31).

The ***pia mater*** *(L., tender mother)* is also a delicate connective tissue layer. It lies directly on the surface of the brain and spinal cord and is continuous with the perivascular connective tissue sheath of the blood vessels of the brain and spinal cord. Both surfaces of the arachnoid, the inner surface of the pia mater, and the trabeculae are covered with a thin squamous epithelial layer. Both the arachnoid and pia mater fuse around the opening for the cranial and spinal nerves as they exit the dura mater.

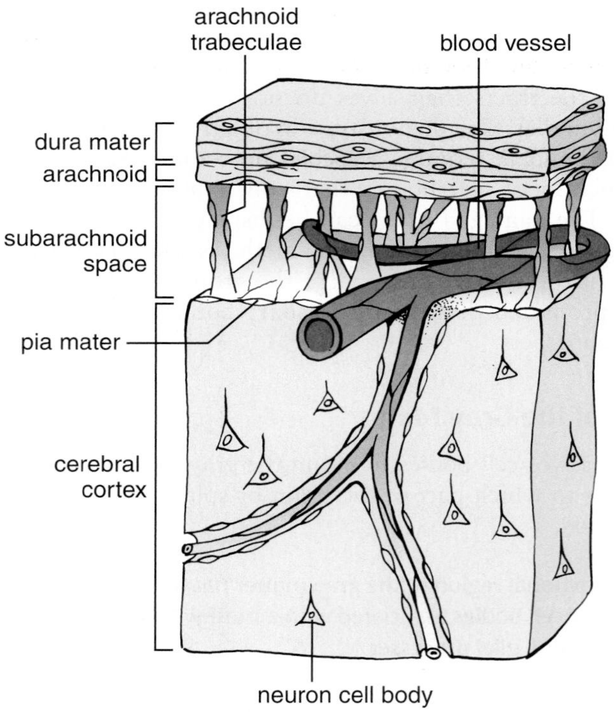

FIGURE 11.31
Schematic diagram of the cerebral meninges. The outer layer, the dura mater, is joined to adjacent bone of the cranial cavity (not shown). The inner layer, the pia mater, adheres to the brain surface and follows all its contours. Note that the pia mater follows the branches of the cerebral arteries as they enter cerebral cortex. The intervening layer, the arachnoid, is adjacent but not attached to the dura mater. The arachnoid sends numerous, web-like arachnoid trabeculae to the pia mater. Located between the arachnoid and the pia mater is the subarachnoid space; it contains cerebrospinal fluid. The space also contains the larger blood vessels (cerebral arteries) that send branches into the substance of the brain.

Blood–Brain Barrier

The blood–brain barrier restricts passage of certain substances from the bloodstream to tissues of the CNS

The observation over 100 years ago that vital dyes injected into the bloodstream can penetrate and stain nearly all organs except the brain provided the first description of the blood–brain barrier. More recently, advances in microscopy and molecular biology techniques have revealed the precise location of this unique barrier and the role of endothelial cells in transporting essential substances to the brain tissue.

The blood–brain barrier develops early in the embryo through an interaction between glial astrocytes and capillary endothelial cells. The barrier is created largely by the elaborate tight junctions between the endothelial cells, which form continuous-type capillaries. Studies with the TEM, using electron-opaque tracers, show complex tight junctions between the endothelial cells. Morphologically, these junctions are more similar to epithelial tight junctions than to those found in other endothelial cells. In addition, TEM studies reveal a close association of astrocytes and their end foot processes with the endothelial basal lamina (Fig. 11.32). The tight junctions eliminate gaps between endothelial cells and prevent simple diffusion of solutes and fluid into the neural tissue.

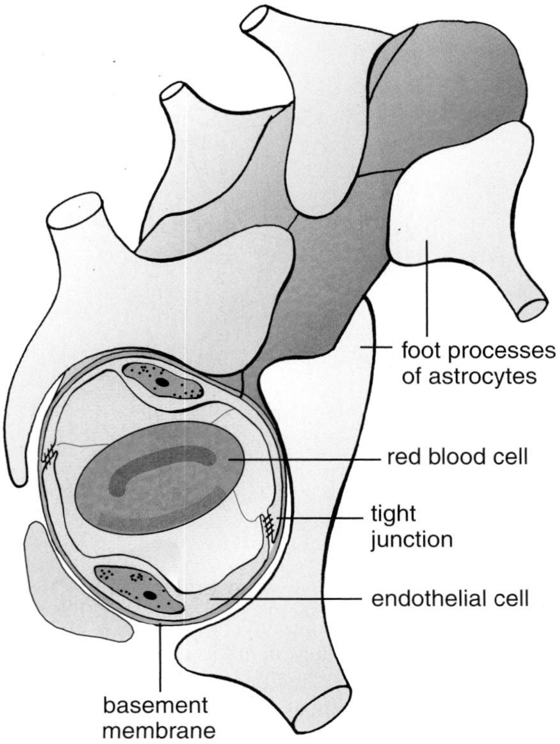

FIGURE 11.32
Schematic drawing of blood–brain barrier. This drawing shows the blood–brain barrier, which consists of endothelial cells joined together by elaborate, complex tight junctions, endothelial basement membrane, and the end foot processes of astrocytes.

Evidence suggests that the tight junction depends on the normal functioning of the astrocyte. In several brain diseases, the blood–brain barrier loses effectiveness. Examination of brain tissue in these conditions by TEM reveals loss of the tight junctions as well as alterations in the morphology of the astrocytes. Other experimental evidence has revealed that astrocytes release soluble factors that increase barrier properties and tight junction protein content.

The presence of only a few small vesicles indicates that pinocytosis across the brain endothelial cells is severely restricted. The substances that do cross the capillary wall are actively transported by specific receptor-mediated endocytosis. Thus, the low permeability of the blood–brain barrier to macromolecules is due to a low level of expression of specific receptors on the endothelial cell surface.

Substances that are required for neuronal integrity must leave and enter the blood capillaries through the endothelial cells. Thus, certain lipid-soluble molecules as well as O_2 and CO_2 easily penetrate the endothelial cell. Other substances such as glucose (which the neuron depends on almost exclusively for energy), amino acids, nucleosides, and vitamins are actively transported by specific transmembrane carrier proteins. In addition, several other proteins that reside within the plasma membrane of the endothelial cells protect the brain by rejecting drugs, foreign proteins, and other disruptive molecules from crossing the barrier.

Recent studies indicate that the end feet of astrocytes also play an important role in maintaining water homeostasis in brain tissue. Water channels (aquaporin AQP4) are found in end feet processes where water crosses the blood–brain barrier. In pathologic conditions such as brain edema, these channels play a key role in reestablishing osmotic equilibrium in the brain.

Some parts of the CNS, however, are not isolated from substances carried in the bloodstream. The barrier is ineffective or absent in the neurohypophysis (posterior pituitary), substantia nigra, and locus ceruleus. In these areas of the brain, sampling of materials circulating in the blood may be necessary to regulate neurosecretory control of parts of the nervous system and of the endocrine system.

RESPONSE OF NEURONS TO INJURY

Degeneration

The portion of a nerve fiber distal to a site of injury degenerates because of interrupted axonal transport

Degeneration of an axon distal to a site of injury is called ***anterograde (Wallerian) degeneration.*** In the PNS, the axon distal to the injury becomes beaded and frag-

ments into discontinuous segments within a few days (Fig. 11.33, a and b). In the CNS, breakdown of the isolated axon segments takes several weeks.

The myelin sheath also fragments, and the myelin fragments enclose the axon fragments. Phagocytotic cells, derived from the Schwann cells in the PNS, microglia in the CNS, and blood monocytes that migrate to the site of injury, remove the myelin and axon fragments. Some retrograde degeneration also occurs but extends for only a few internodal segments. In the PNS, the Schwann cells and their external laminae remain as tubular structures distal to the injury (Fig. 11.33c).

The cell body of an injured nerve swells, its nucleus moves peripherally, and there is loss of Nissl substance

Nerve injury leads to a loss of Nissl substance from the cell body, called ***chromatolysis.*** Chromatolysis is first observed within 1 to 2 days after injury and reaches a peak at about 2 weeks (Fig. 11.33b). The changes in the cell body are proportional to the amount of axoplasm lost by the injury; extensive loss of axoplasm can lead to death of the cell. When a motor fiber is cut, the muscle innervated by that fiber undergoes atrophy (Fig. 11.33c).

Before the development of modern dye and radioisotope tracer techniques, Wallerian degeneration and chromatolysis were used as research tools. These tools allowed researchers to trace the pathways and destination of axons and the localization of the cell bodies of experimentally injured nerves.

Scar Formation

In the PNS, connective tissue and Schwann cells form scar tissue in the gap between the ends of a severed or crushed nerve. If the amount of scar tissue is not too great or if sur-

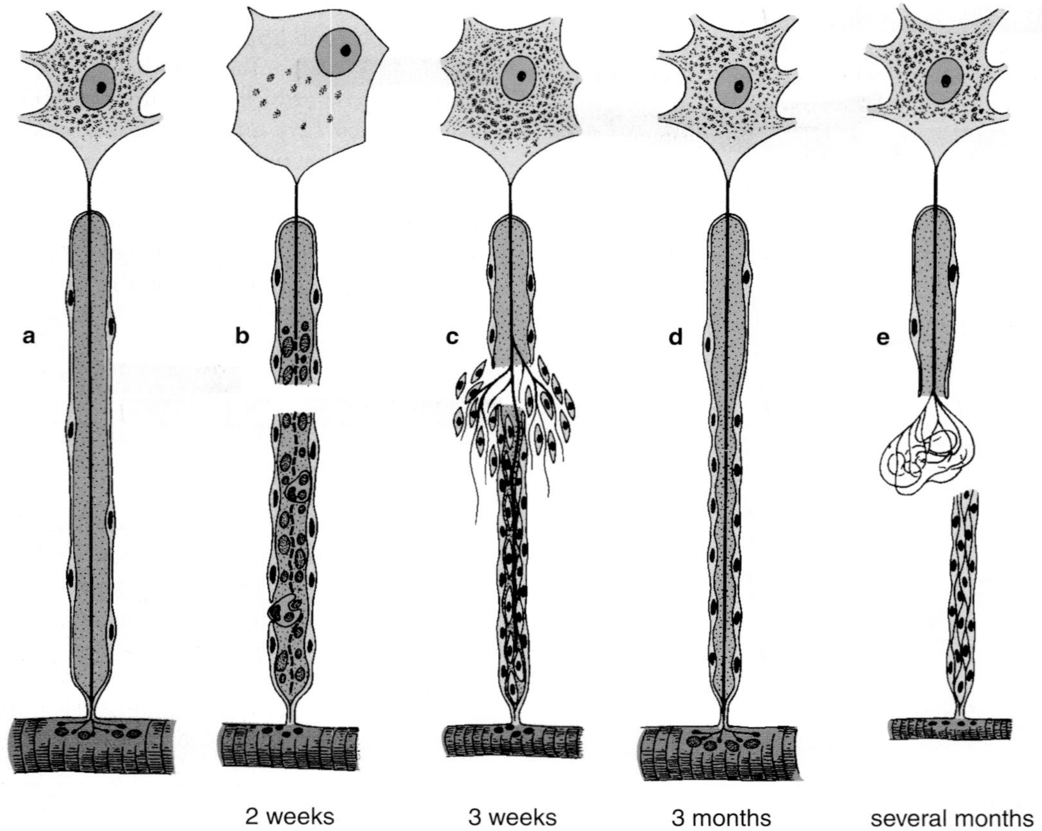

FIGURE 11.33
Response of a nerve fiber to injury. a. A normal nerve fiber, with its perikaryon and the effector cell (striated skeletal muscle). Note the position of the neuron nucleus and the number and distribution of Nissl bodies. **b.** When the fiber is injured, the neuronal nucleus moves to the cell periphery, and the number of Nissl bodies is greatly reduced. The nerve fiber distal to the injury degenerates along with its myelin sheath. Debris is phagocytosed by macrophages. **c.** The muscle fiber shows a pronounced disuse atrophy. Schwann cells proliferate, forming a compact cord penetrated by the growing axon. The axon grows at a rate of 0.5 to 3 mm/day. **d.** In this example, nerve fiber regeneration was successful. Note that the muscle fiber was also regenerated after receiving nerve stimuli. **e.** Regeneration of the nerve may be complicated by misalignment of individual portions of the nerve fibers proximal and distal to the injury. When the axon does not penetrate the cord of Schwann cells, its growth is not organized, resulting in a mass of tangled axonal processes known as traumatic neuroma. (Based on Willis RA, Willis AT. *The Principles of Pathology and Bacteriology.* Woburn, MA: Butterworth, 1972.)

gical apposition of the cut ends of the nerve is possible, the severed nerve will probably regenerate.

In the CNS, scar tissue derived from proliferating glial cells appears to prevent regeneration. Current research on CNS regeneration is, therefore, focused on preventing or inhibiting glial scar formation.

Regeneration

In the PNS, Schwann cells divide and develop cellular bands that bridge a newly formed scar

Division of Schwann cells is the first step in the regeneration of a severed or crushed peripheral nerve. The Schwann cells then bridge the scar. In the second step in regeneration, large numbers of new nerve processes ***(neurites)*** sprout from the proximal stump (Fig. 11.33c). The Schwann cell bridges then serve as guides for the regenerating axons to grow across the scar, thus maintaining the normal pathways of the growing axons.

Although many of the new nerve processes degenerate, their large number increases the probability of reestablishing sensory and motor connections. Successful sprouts grow at about 3 mm/day. After crossing the scar, neurites enter the surviving Schwann tubes in the distal stump. These tubes will then guide the neurites to their destination as well as provide the microenvironment for continued growth (Fig. 11.33d).

If physical contact is reestablished between a motor neuron and its muscle, function is usually reestablished

Microsurgical techniques that rapidly reestablish intimate apposition of severed nerve and vessel ends have made reattachment of severed limbs and digits, with subsequent reestablishment of function, a relatively common procedure.

If the axonal sprouts do not reestablish contact with the bridge of Schwann cells, the sprouts grow in a disorganized manner, and the muscle remains atrophic (Fig. 11.33e).

PLATE 23. SYMPATHETIC AND DORSAL ROOT GANGLIA

Ganglia are clusters of neuronal cell bodies located outside the central nervous system (CNS); nerve fibers lead to and from them. Sensory ganglia lie just outside the CNS and contain the cell bodies of sensory nerves that carry impulses into the CNS. Autonomic ganglia are peripheral motor ganglia of the *autonomic nervous system* (ANS) and contain the cell bodies of postsynaptic neurons that conduct nerve impulses to smooth muscle, cardiac muscle, and glands. Synapses between presynaptic neurons (all of which have their cell bodies in the CNS) and postsynaptic neurons occur in autonomic ganglia. *Sympathetic ganglia* constitute a major subclass of autonomic ganglia; *parasympathetic ganglia* and *enteric ganglia* constitute the other subclasses.

Sympathetic ganglia are located in the paravertebral and vertebral sympathetic chain and send long postsynaptic axons to the viscera. Parasympathetic ganglia are located in, or close to, the organs innervated by their postsynaptic neurons. The enteric ganglia are located in the *submucosal plexus* and the *myenteric plexus* of the alimentary canal. They receive parasympathetic presynaptic input as well as intrinsic input from other enteric ganglia and innervate smooth muscle of the gut wall.

Figure 1, ganglion, human, silver and H&E stains ×160.

A sympathetic ganglion stained with silver and counterstained with H&E is illustrated here. Shown to advantage are several discrete bundles of nerve fibers *(NF)* and numerous large circular structures, namely, the cell bodies *(CB)* of the postsynaptic neurons. Random patterns of nerve fibers are also seen. Moreover, careful examination of the cell bodies shows that some display several processes joined to them. Thus, these are multipolar neurons (one contained within the *rectangle* is shown at higher magnification in Figure 2). Generally, the connective tissue is not conspicuous in a silver preparation, although it can be identified by virtue of its location about the larger blood vessels *(BV),* particularly in the upper part of this figure.

Figure 2, ganglion, human, silver and H&E stains ×500.

The cell bodies of the sympathetic ganglion are typically large, and the one labeled here shows several processes *(P).* In addition, the cell body contains a large, pale-staining spherical nucleus *(N);* this, in turn, contains a spherical, intensely staining nucleolus *(Nl).* These features, namely, a large pale-staining nucleus (indicating much-extended chromatin) and a large nucleolus, reflect a cell active in protein synthesis. Also shown in the cell body are accumulations of lipofuscin *(L),* a yellow pigment that is darkened by the silver. Because of the large size of the cell body, the nucleus is not always included in the section; in that case, the cell body appears as a rounded cytoplasmic mass.

Figure 3, ganglion, cat, H&E ×160.

Dorsal root ganglia differ from autonomic ganglia in a number of ways. Whereas the latter contain multipolar neurons and have synaptic connections, dorsal root ganglia contain pseudounipolar sensory neurons and have no synaptic connections in the ganglion.

Part of a dorsal root ganglion stained with H&E is shown in this figure. The specimen includes the edge of the ganglion, where it is covered with connective tissue *(CT).* The dorsal root ganglion contains large cell bodies *(CB)* that are typically arranged as closely packed clusters. Also, between and around the cell clusters, there are bundles of nerve fibers *(NF).* Most of the fiber bundles indicated by the label have been sectioned longitudinally.

Figure 4, ganglion, cat, H&E ×350.

At higher magnification of the same ganglion, the constituents of the nerve fiber show their characteristic structure, namely, a centrally located axon *(A)* surrounded by a myelin space (not labeled), which, in turn, is bounded on its outer border by the thin cytoplasmic strand of the neurilemma *(arrowheads).*

The cell bodies of the sensory neurons display large, pale-staining spherical nuclei *(N)* and intensely staining nucleoli *(Nl).* Also seen in this H&E preparation are the nuclei of satellite cells *(Sat C)* that completely surround the cell body and are continuous with the Schwann cells that invest the axon. Note how much smaller these cells are than the neurons. Clusters of cells *(asterisks)* within the ganglion that have an epithelioid appearance are en face views of satellite cells where the section tangentially includes the satellite cells but barely grazes the adjacent cell body.

KEY

A, axon
BV, blood vessels
CB, cell body of neuron
CT, connective tissue
L, lipofuscin
N, nucleus of nerve cell
NF, nerve fibers
Nl, nucleolus
P, processes of nerve cell body
Sat C, satellite cells
arrowheads, neurilemma
asterisks, clusters of satellite cells

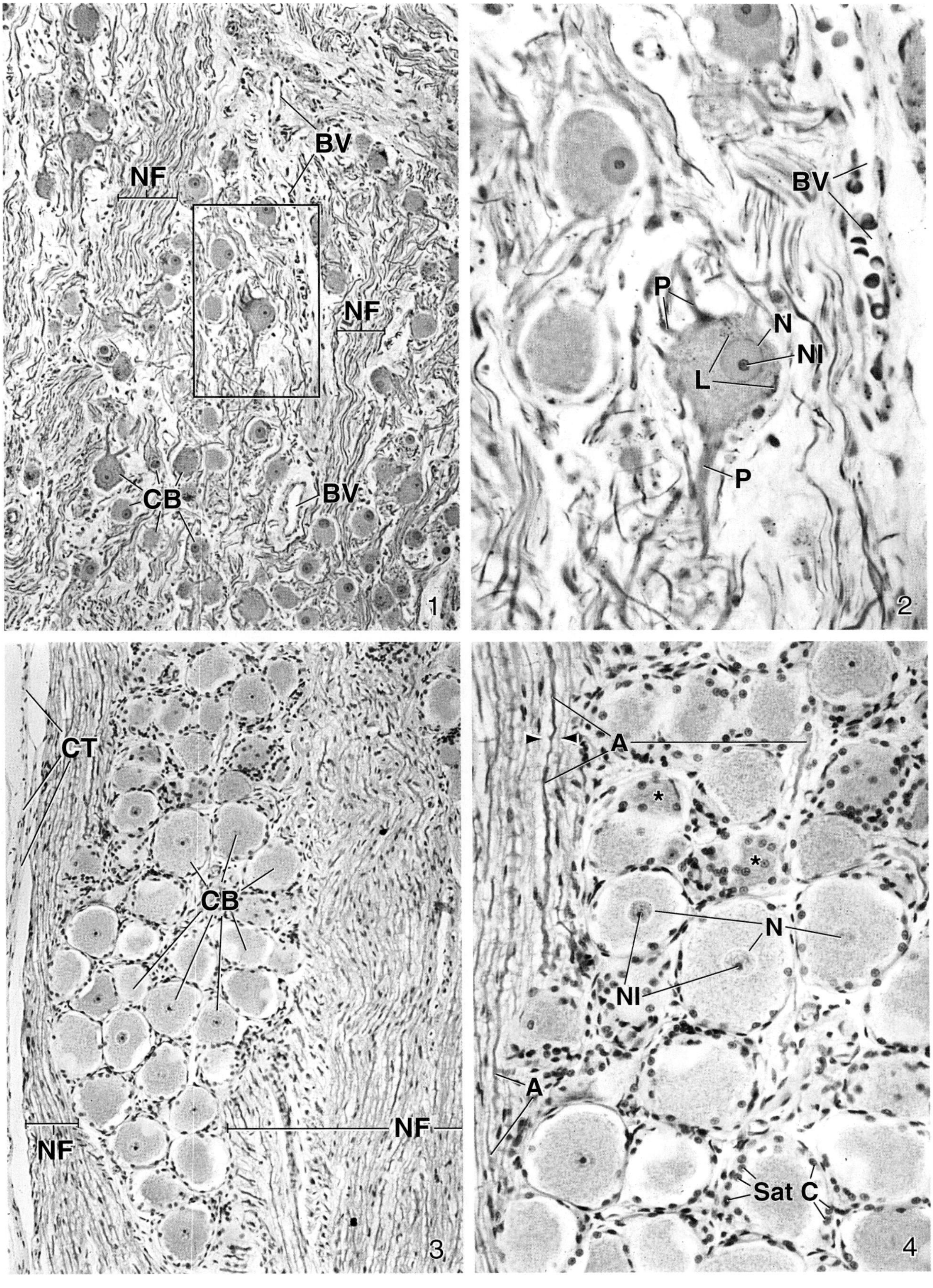
BV
NF
NF
CB
BV
1
BV
P
N
NI
L
P
2
CT
CB
NF
NF
3
A
*
*
N
NI
A
Sat C
4

PLATE 24. PERIPHERAL NERVE

Peripheral nerves are composed of bundles of nerve fibers held together by connective tissue and a specialized layer (or layers) of cells, the *perineurium.* The connective tissue consists of an outer layer, the *epineurium,* surrounding the whole nerve; the perineurium, surrounding bundles of nerve fibers; and the *endoneurium,* associated with individual neurons. Each nerve fiber consists of an axon that is surrounded by a cellular investment called the *neurilemma,* or the *sheath of Schwann.* The fiber may be myelinated or *unmyelinated.* The myelin, if present, is immediately around the axon and is formed by the concentric wrapping of the Schwann cell around the axon. This, in turn, is surrounded by the major portion of the cytoplasm of the Schwann cell, forming the neurilemma. Unmyelinated axons rest in grooves in the Schwann cell.

Figures 1 and 2, femoral nerve, H&E.

This cross section (Fig. 1) shows several bundles of nerve fibers *(BNF).* The external cover for the entire nerve is the epineurium *(Epn),* the layer of dense connective tissue that one touches when a nerve has been exposed during a dissection. The epineurium may also serve as part of the outermost cover of individual bundles. It contains blood vessels *(BV)* and may contain some fat cells. Typically, adipose tissue *(AT)* is found about the nerve.

Figure 2 shows, at higher magnification, an area from the upper left of Figure 1. The illustration has been rotated, and the septum (marked with *arrows* in Fig. 1) is now vertically disposed *(arrows).*

The layer under the epineurium that directly surrounds the bundle of nerve fibers is the perineurium *(Pn).* As seen in the cross section through the nerve, the nuclei of the perineurial cells appear flat and elongate; they are actually being viewed on edge and belong to flat cells that are also being viewed on edge. Again, as noted by the distribution of nuclei, it can be ascertained that the perineurium is only a few cells thick. The perineurium is a specialized layer of cells and extracellular material whose arrangement is not evident in H&E sections. The perineurium *(Pn)* and epineurium *(Epn)* are readily distinguished in the triangular area formed by the diverging perineurium of the two adjacent nerve bundles.

The nerve fibers included in Figure 2 are mostly myelinated, and because the nerve is cross-sectioned, the nerve fibers are also seen in this plane. They have a characteristic cross-sectional profile. Each nerve fiber shows a centrally placed axon *(A);* this is surrounded by a myelin space *(M)* in which some radially disposed precipitate may be retained, as in this specimen. External to the myelin space is a thin cytoplasmic rim representing the neurilemma. On occasion, a Schwann cell nucleus *(SS)* appears to be perched on the neurilemma. As shown in the illustration, the upper edge of the nuclear crescent appears to occupy the same plane as that occupied by the neurilemma *(N).* These features enable one to identify the nucleus as belonging to a Schwann (neurilemma) cell. Other nuclei are not related to the neurilemma but, rather, appear to be between the nerve fibers. Such nuclei belong to the rare fibroblasts *(F)* of the endoneurium. The latter is the delicate connective tissue between the individual nerve fibers; it is extremely sparse and contains the capillaries *(C)* of the nerve bundle.

Figures 3 and 4, femoral nerve, H&E.

The edge of a longitudinally sectioned nerve bundle is shown here; a portion of the same nerve bundle is shown at higher magnification in Figure 4. The boundary between the epineurium *(Epn)* and perineurium is ill-defined. Within the nerve bundle, the nerve fibers show a characteristic wavy pattern. Included among the wavy nerve fibers are nuclei belonging to Schwann cells and to cells within the endoneurium. Higher magnification allows one to identify certain specific components of the nerve. Note that the nerve fibers *(NF)* are now shown in longitudinal profile. Moreover, each myelinated nerve fiber shows a centrally positioned axon *(A)* surrounded by a myelin space *(M),* which, in turn, is bordered on its outer edge by the thin cytoplasmic band of the neurilemma cell *(Nl).* Another diagnostic feature of myelinated nerve fibers is also seen in longitudinal section, namely, the node of Ranvier *(NR).* This is where the ends of the two Schwann cells meet. Histologically, the node appears as a constriction of the neurilemma, and sometimes, the constriction is marked by a cross-band, as in Figure 4. It is difficult to determine whether the nuclei *(N)* shown in Figure 4 belong to Schwann cells or to endoneurial fibroblasts.

KEY

A, axon
AT, adipose tissue
BNF, bundle of nerve fibers
BV, blood vessels
C, capillary
Epn, epineurium
F, fibroblast
M, myelin
N: Fig. 2, neurilemma; Fig. 4, nucleus of Schwann cell
NF, nerve fiber
Nl, neurilemma
NR, node of Ranvier
Pn, perineurium
SS, Schwann cell nucleus
arrows (Figs. 1 and 2), septum formed by perineurium

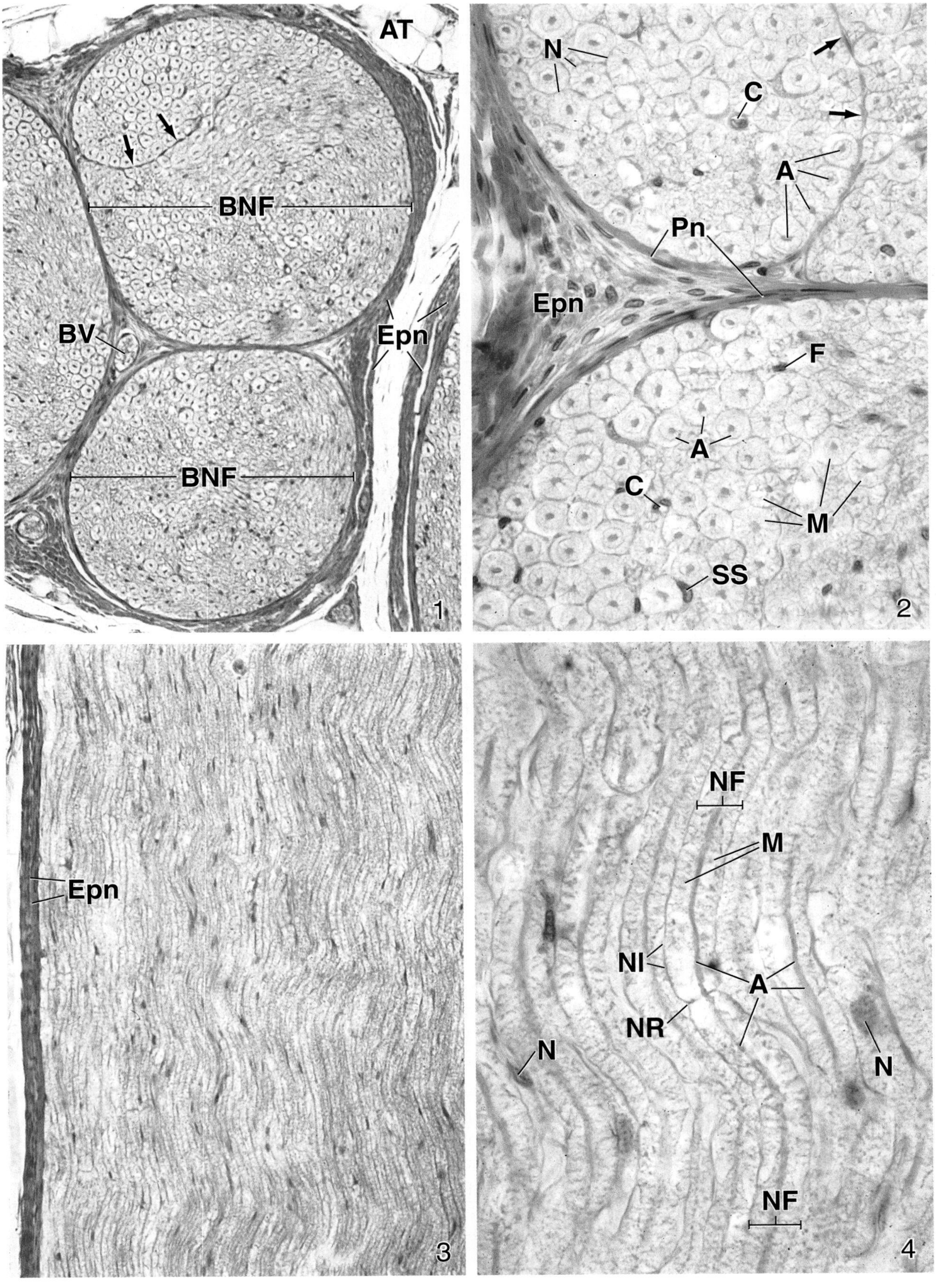
AT
BNF
BV
Epn
BNF
1
N
C
A
Pn
Epn
F
A
C
M
SS
2
Epn
3
NF
M
NI
A
NR
N
N
NF
4

PLATE 25. CEREBRUM

The cerebrum is the principal portion of the brain and contains the cell bodies of nerves that receive and store sensory information, nerves that control voluntary motor activity, and nerves that integrate and coordinate the activity of other nerves, as well as the nerves and neural pathways that constitute memory.

Figure 1, brain, human, Luxol fast blue–PAS ×65. This micrograph shows a low-magnification view of the cerebral cortex (*CC*). It includes the full thickness of the gray matter and a small amount of white matter at the bottom of the micrograph (*WM*). The white matter contains considerably fewer cells per unit area; these are neuroglial cells rather than nerve cell bodies that are present in the cortex. Covering the cortex is the pia mater (*PM*). A vein (*V*) can be seen enclosed by the pia mater. Also, a smaller blood vessel (*BV*) can be seen entering the substance of the cortex. The six layers of the cortex are marked by *dashed lines,* which represent only an approximation of the boundaries. Each layer is distinguished on the basis of predominant cell types and fiber (axon and dendrite) arrangement. Unless the fibers are specifically stained, they cannot be utilized to further aid in identification of the layers. Rather, the delineation of the layers, as they are identified here, is based on cell types, and more specifically, the shape and appearance of the cells.

The six layers of the cortex are named and described as follows:

I: The plexiform layer (or molecular layer) consists largely of fibers, most of which travel parallel to the surface, and relatively few cells, mostly neuroglial cells and occasional horizontal cells of Cajal.

II: The small pyramidal cell layer (or outer granular layer) consists mainly of small pyramidal cells, and granule cells, also called stellate cells.

III: The layer of medium pyramidal cells (or layer of outer pyramidal cells) is not sharply demarcated from layer II. However, the pyramidal cells are somewhat larger and possess a typical pyramidal shape.

IV: The granular layer (or inner granular layer) is characterized by the presence of many small granule cells (stellate cells).

V: The layer of large pyramidal cells (or inner layer of pyramidal cells) contains pyramidal cells that, in many parts of the cerebrum, are smaller than the pyramidal cells of layer III but in the motor area are extremely large and are called Betz cells.

VI: The layer of polymorphic cells contains cells with diverse shapes, many of which have a spindle of fusiform shape. These cells are called fusiform cells.

In addition to pyramidal cells, granule cells, and fusiform cells, two other cell types are also present in the cerebral cortex but are not recognizable in this preparation: the horizontal cells of Cajal, which are present only in layer I and send their processes laterally, and the cells of Martinotti, which send their axons toward the surface (opposite to that of pyramidal cells).

Figure 2, brain, human, Luxol fast blue–PAS ×350. This micrograph is a higher power of layer I, the plexiform layer. It consists of nerve fibers, numerous neuroglial cells (*NN*) and occasional horizontal cells of Cajal. The neuroglial cells appear as naked nuclei, with the cytoplasm being indistinguishable from the nerve fibers that make up the bulk of this layer. Also present is a small capillary (*Cap*). The pink outline of the vessel is due to the PAS staining reaction of its basement membrane.

Figure 3, brain, human, Luxol fast blue–PAS ×350. This micrograph shows layer II, the small pyramidal cell layer. Many small pyramidal cells (*PC*) are present. Granule cells (*GC*) are also numerous, though difficult to identify here.

Figure 4, brain, human, Luxol fast blue–PAS ×350. This micrograph shows layer IV, the granular layer. Many of the cells here are granule cells, but neuroglial cells are also prominent. The micrograph also reveals a number of capillaries. Note how they travel in various directions.

Figure 5, brain, human, Luxol fast blue–PAS ×350. This micrograph shows layer VI, the layer of polymorphic cells, so named because of the diverse shape of the cells in this region. Pyramidal cells (*PC*) are readily recognized. Other cell types present include fusiform cells (*FC*), granule cells and Martinotti cells.

Figure 6, brain, human, Luxol fast blue–PAS ×350. This micrograph shows the outer portion of the white matter. The small round nuclei (*NN*) belong to neuroglial cells. As in the cortex, the cytoplasm of the cell is not distinguishable. Thus, they appear as naked nuclei in the bed of nerve processes. The neuropil is essentially a densely packed aggregation of nerve fibers and neuroglial cells.

KEY

BV, blood vessel
Cap, capillary
CC, cerebral cortex
FC, fusiform cells
GC, granule cells
NN, neuroglial nuclei
PC, pyramidal cells
PM, pia mater
V, vein
WM, white matter

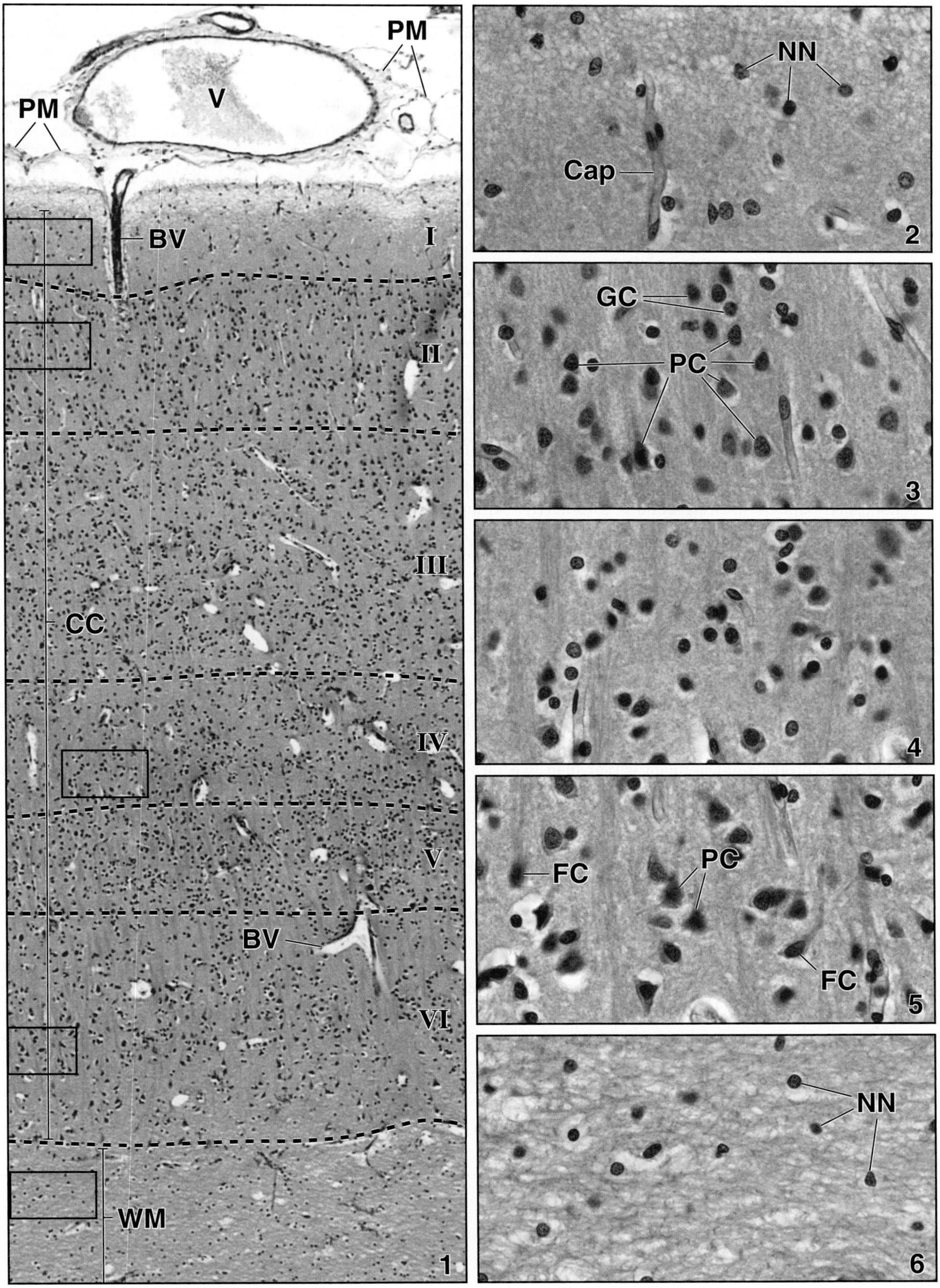
PM
PM
V
BV
I
II
III
CC
IV
V
BV
VI
WM
1
NN
Cap
2
GC
PC
3
4
FC
PC
FC
5
NN
6

PLATE 26. CEREBELLUM

The cerebellum is a portion of the brain lying behind and below the cerebrum; it serves to coordinate both voluntary movements and muscle function in the maintenance of normal posture.

Figure 1, cerebellum, human, H&E ×40.

The cerebellar cortex has the same appearance regardless of which region is examined. In this low-magnification view of the cerebellum, the outermost layer, the molecular layer *(Mol),* is lightly stained with eosin. Under this is the granular layer *(Gr),* which stains intensely with hematoxylin. Together, these two layers constitute the cortex of the cerebellum. Deep in the granular layer is another region that stains lightly with H&E and, except for location, shows no distinctive histologic features. This is the white matter *(WM).* As in the cerebrum, it contains nerve fibers, supporting neuroglial cells, and small blood vessels, but no neuronal cell bodies. The fibrous cover on the cerebellar surface is the pia mater *(Pia).* Cerebellar blood vessels *(BV)* travel in this layer. (Shrinkage artifact has separated the pia mater from the cerebellar surface.) The *rectangular area* is shown at higher magnification in Figure 2.

Figure 2, cerebellum, human, H&E ×400.

At the junction between the molecular and granular layers are the extremely large flask-shaped cell bodies of the Purkinje cells *(Pkj).* These cells are characteristic of the cerebellum. Each possesses numerous dendrites *(D)* that arborize in the molecular layer. The Purkinje cell has a single axon that is not usually evident in H&E sections. This nerve fiber represents the beginning of the outflow from the cerebellum.

The figure shows relatively few neuron cell bodies, those of the basket cells *(BC),* in the molecular layer; they are widely removed from each other and, at best, show only a small amount of cytoplasm surrounding the nucleus. In contrast, the granular layer presents an overall spotted-blue appearance due to the staining of numerous small nuclei with hematoxylin. These small neurons, called granule cells, receive incoming impulses from other parts of the CNS and send axons into the molecular layer, where they branch in the form of a T, so that the axons contact the dendrites of several Purkinje cells and basket cells. Incoming (mossy) fibers contact granule cells in the lightly stained areas called glomeruli *(arrows).* Careful examination of the granular layer where it meets the molecular layer will reveal a group of nuclei *(G)* that are larger than the nuclei of granule cells. These belong to Golgi type II cells.

Figure 3, cerebellum, human, silver stain ×40.

The specimen in this figure has been stained with a silver procedure. Such procedures do not always color the specimen evenly, as do H&E. Note that the part of the molecular layer on the right is much darker than that on the left. A *rectangular area* on the left has been selected for examination at higher magnification in Figure 4. Even at the relatively low magnification shown here, however, the Purkinje cells can be recognized in the silver preparation because of their large size, characteristic shape, and location between an outer molecular layer *(Mol)* and an inner granular layer *(Gr).* The main advantage of this silver preparation is that the white matter *(WM)* can be recognized as being composed of fibers; they have been blackened by the silver-staining procedure. The pia mater *(Pia)* and cerebellar blood vessels are also evident in the preparation.

Figure 4, cerebellum, human, silver stain ×400.

At higher magnification, the Purkinje cell bodies *(Pkj)* stand out as the most distinctive and conspicuous neuronal cell type of the cerebellum, and numerous dendritic branches *(D)* can be seen. Note, also, the blackened fibers within the granular layer *(Gr),* about the Purkinje cell bodies, and in the molecular layer *(Mol)* disposed in a horizontal direction (relative to the cerebellar surface). The *arrow* indicates a T turn characteristic of the turn made by axons of granule cells. As these axonal branches travel horizontally, they make synaptic contact with numerous Purkinje cells.

KEY

BC, basket cells
BV, blood vessels
D, dendrites
F, fibers
G, Golgi type II cells
Gr, granular layer
Mol, molecular layer
Pia, pia mater
Pkj, Purkinje cells
WM, white matter
arrows: Fig. 2, glomeruli; Fig. 4, T branching of axon in molecular layer
rectangular area (Figs. 1 and 3), areas shown at higher magnification in Figures 2 and 4, respectively

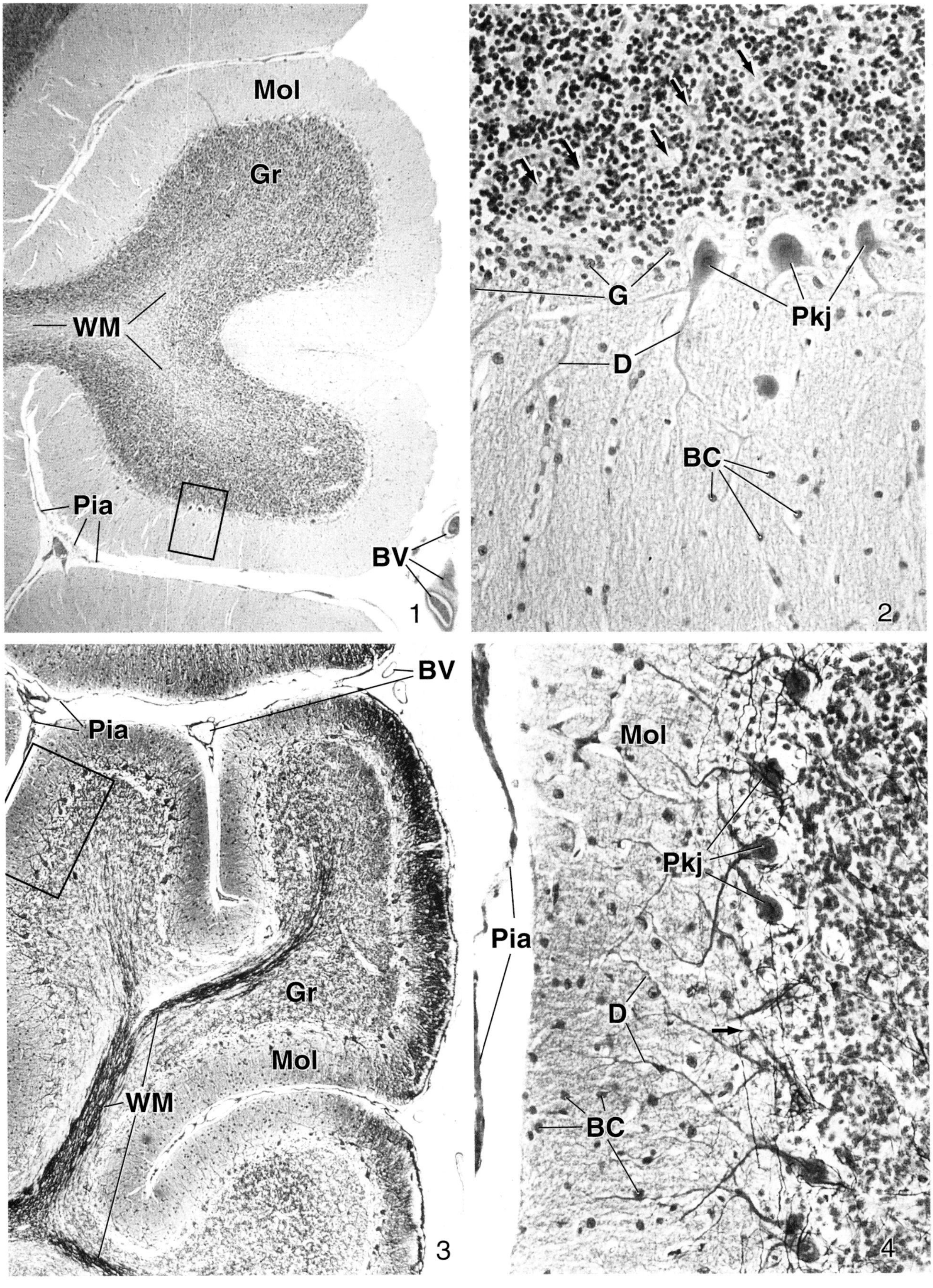
Mol
Gr
WM
Pia
BV
1
G
Pkj
D
BC
2
BV
Pia
Gr
Mol
WM
3
Mol
Pkj
Pia
D
BC
4

PLATE 27. SPINAL CORD

The spinal cord is organized into two discrete parts. The outer part, called the *white matter* of the cord because of its appearance in unfixed specimens, contains ascending and descending nerve fibers. Some of the fibers go to and from the brain, whereas others connect different levels of the spinal cord. The inner part of the spinal cord, called the *gray matter* because of its appearance in unfixed specimens, contains the cell bodies of neurons as well as nerve fibers. The gray matter forms an H- or butterfly-shaped pattern surrounding the central canal. The gray matter is described as having dorsal (posterior) horns and ventral (anterior) horns. The ventral horns contain the large cell bodies of motor neurons, whereas the dorsal horns contain neurons that receive, process, and retransmit information from the sensory neurons whose cell bodies are located in the dorsal root ganglia. The size of the gray matter (and, therefore, the size of the spinal cord) is different at different levels. Where the gray matter contains many large motor nerve cells that control the movement of the appendages, the arms and legs, the gray matter and the spinal cord are considerably larger than where the gray matter contains only the motor neurons for the muscle of the torso.

Figure 1, spinal cord, human, silver stain ×16.
A cross section through the lumbar region of the spinal cord is shown here. The preparation is designed to stain the gray matter that is surrounded by the ascending and descending nerve fibers. Although the fibers that have common origins and destinations in the physiologic sense are arranged in tracts, these tracts cannot be distinguished unless they have been marked by special techniques, such as causing injury to the cell bodies from which they arise or by using special dyes or radioisotopes to label the axons.

The gray matter of the spinal cord appears roughly in the form of a butterfly. The anterior and posterior prongs are referred to as ventral horns *(VH)* and dorsal horns *(DH)*, respectively. The connecting bar is called the gray commissure *(GC)*. The neuron cell bodies that are within the anterior horns (anterior horn cells) are so large that they can be seen even at this extremely low magnification *(arrows)*. The pale-staining fibrous material that surrounds the spinal cord is the pia mater *(Pia)*. It follows the surface of the spinal cord intimately and dips into the large ventral fissure *(VF)* and into the shallower sulci. Blood vessels *(BV)* are present in the pia mater. Some dorsal roots *(DR)* of the spinal nerves are included in the section.

Figure 2, spinal cord, human, silver stain ×640.
This preparation shows a region of a ventral horn. The nucleus *(N)* of the ventral horn cell is the large, spherical, pale-staining structure within the cell body. It contains a spherical, intensely staining nucleolus. The ventral horn cell has many processes, two of which are obvious. A number of other nuclei *(NN)* belong to neuroglial cells. The cytoplasm of these cells is not evident. The remainder of the field consists of nerve fibers and neuroglial cells whose organization is hard to interpret. This is called the neuropil *(Np)*. A capillary crosses through the field below the cell body.

Figure 3, spinal cord, human, toluidine blue ×640.
This preparation of the spinal cord is from an area comparable to that of Figure 2. The toluidine blue reveals the Nissl bodies *(NB)* that appear as the large, dark-staining bodies in the cytoplasm. Nissl bodies do not extend into the axon hillock. The axon leaves the cell body at the axon hillock. The nuclei of neuroglial cells *(NN)* are also evident here, but their cytoplasm is not. The neuropil stains very faintly.

KEY

BV, blood vessels
DH, dorsal (posterior) horn
DR, dorsal root
GC, gray commissure
N, nucleus of ventral horn cell
NB, Nissl bodies
NN, nucleus of neuroglial cell
Np, neuropil
Pia, pia mater
VF, ventral fissure
VH, ventral (anterior) horn
arrows (Fig. 1), cell body of anterior (ventral) horn cell

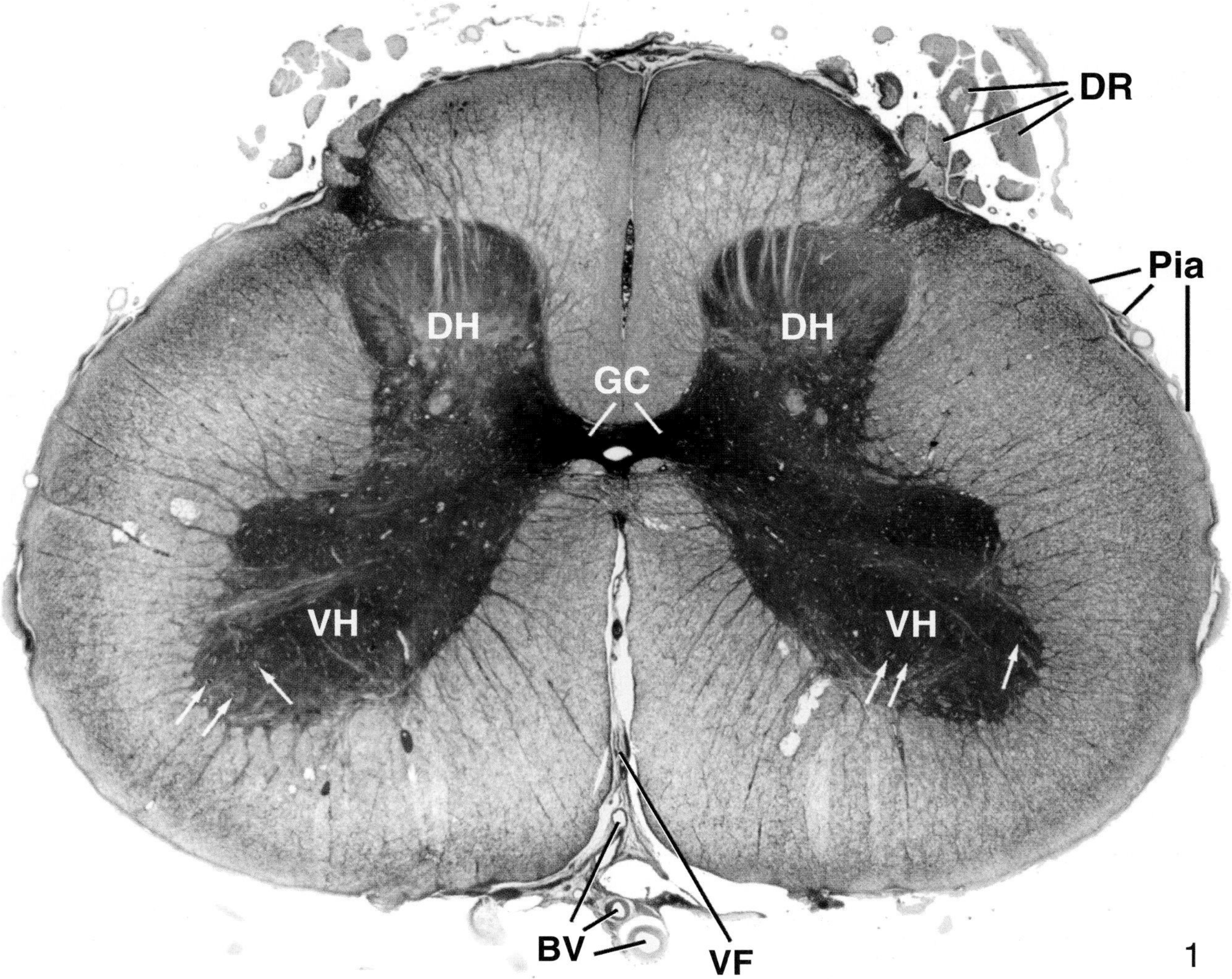

1

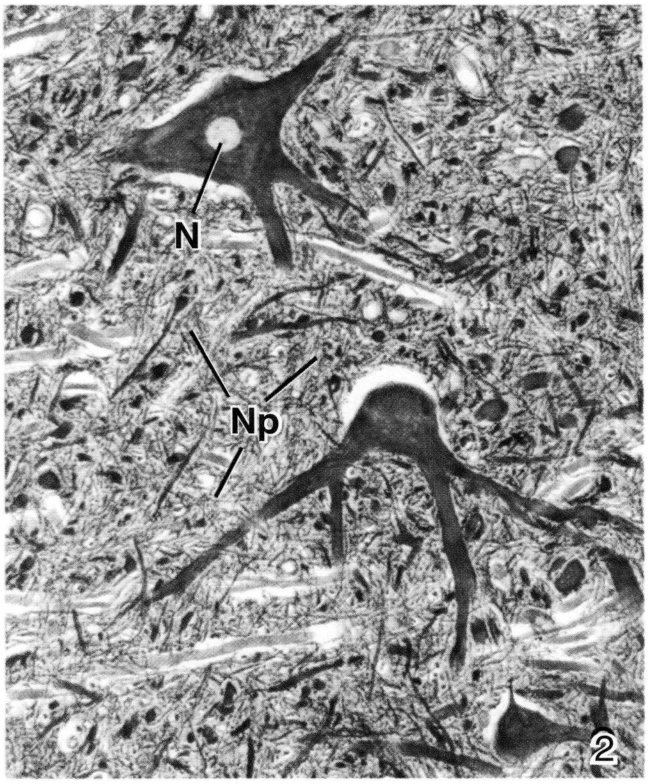

2

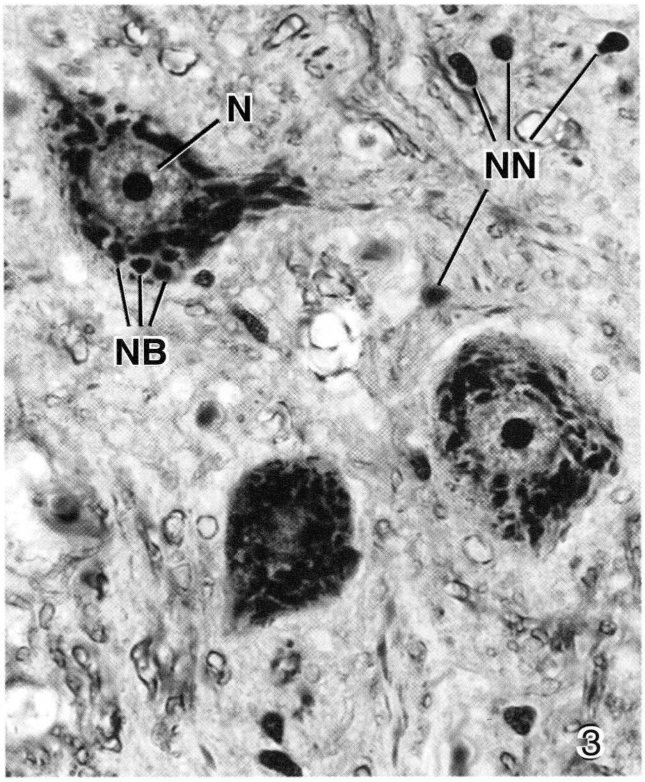

3

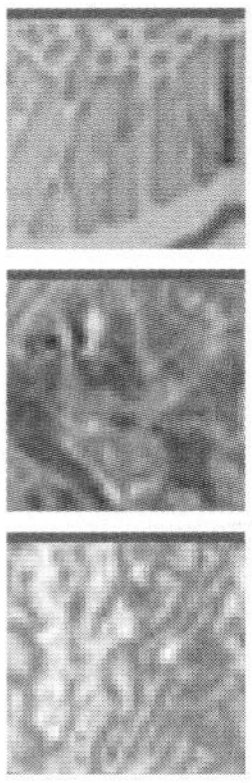

12

Cardiovascular System

▼ OVERVIEW OF THE CARDIOVASCULAR SYSTEM

The cardiovascular system is a transport system that carries blood and lymph to and from the tissues of the body. The constitutive elements of these fluids include cells, nutrients, waste products, hormones, and antibodies.

The cardiovascular system includes the heart, blood vessels, and lymphatic vessels

Blood vessels provide the route by which blood circulates to and from all parts of the body. The heart pumps the blood through the arterial system under significant pressure; blood is returned to the heart under low pressure

with the assistance of negative pressure in the thoracic cavity during inspiration and compression of the veins by skeletal muscle. The blood vessels are arranged so that blood delivered from the heart quickly reaches a network of narrow, thin-walled vessels, the blood **capillaries,** within or in proximity to the tissues in every part of the body.

In the capillaries, a two-directional exchange of fluid occurs between the blood and tissues. The fluid, called **blood filtrate,** carrying oxygen and metabolites, passes through the capillary wall. In the tissues, these molecules are exchanged for carbon dioxide and waste products. Most of the fluid reenters the distal or venous end of the blood capillaries. The remaining fluid enters lymphatic capillaries as lymph and is ultimately returned to the bloodstream through a system of lymphatic vessels that join the blood system at the junction of the internal jugular veins with the subclavian veins. Normally, many of the white blood cells conveyed in the blood leave the blood vessels to enter the tissues. This occurs at the level of the **postcapillary venules.** When pathologic changes occur in the body, as in the inflammatory reaction, large numbers of white blood cells emigrate from these venules.

Arteries are the vessels that deliver blood to the capillaries. The smallest arteries, called ***arterioles,*** are functionally associated with networks of capillaries into which they deliver blood. The arterioles regulate the amount of blood that enters these capillary networks. Together, the arterioles, associated capillary network, and postcapillary venules form a functional unit called the ***microcirculatory*** or ***microvascular bed*** of that tissue (Fig. 12.1). ***Veins,*** beginning with the postcapillary venule, collect blood from the microvascular bed and carry it away.

Two circuits distribute blood in the body: the systemic and the pulmonary circulation

Two pathways of circulation are formed by the blood vessels and the heart:

- ***Pulmonary circulation*** conveys blood from the heart to the lungs and from the lungs to the heart (Fig. 12.2).
- ***Systemic circulation*** conveys blood from the heart to other tissues of the body and from other tissues of the body to the heart.

Although the general arrangement of blood vessels in both circulations is from arteries to capillaries to veins, in some parts of the systemic circulation it is modified so that a vein or an arteriole is interposed between two capillary networks; these vessels constitute ***portal systems.*** Venous portal systems occur in vessels carrying blood to the liver, namely, the ***hepatic portal system (portal vein)*** and, in vessels leading to the pituitary, the ***hypothalamic-hypophyseal portal system.***

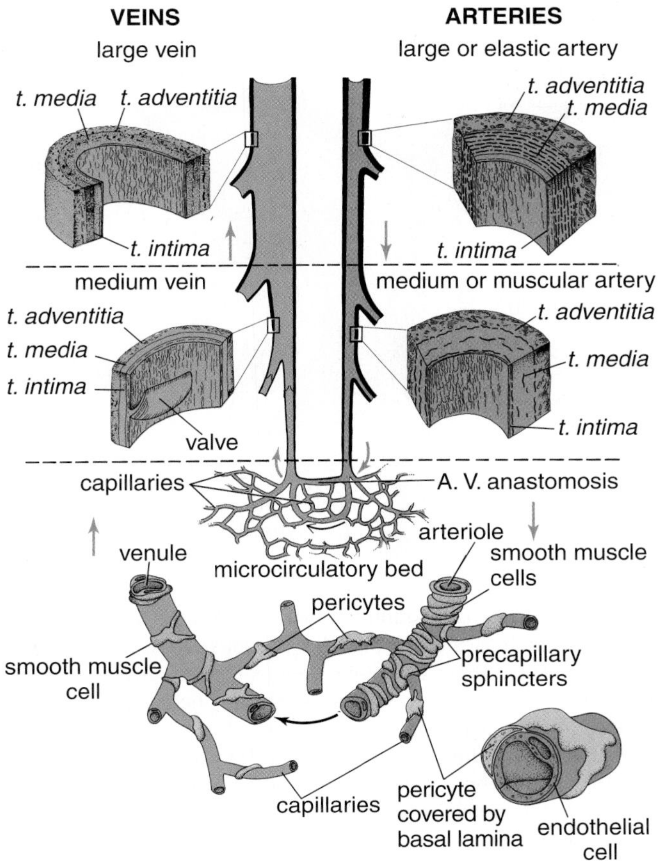

FIGURE 12.1
Schematic diagram of the major structural features of blood vessels. The layers or tunics of the blood vessel walls are labeled in the *upper two panels.* The arrangement of the microcirculatory bed in certain parts of the body is shown in the *lowest panel.* Note the location of pericytes and their relationship to the basal lamina. Also, an arteriovenous *(A.V.)* anastomosis is shown within the microcirculatory bed. *t.,* tunica. (Based on Rhodin JAG. *Handbook of Physiology.* New York: Oxford University Press, 1980.)

GENERAL FEATURES OF ARTERIES AND VEINS

The walls of arteries and veins are composed of three layers called tunics

The three layers of the vascular wall, from the lumen outward (see Fig. 12.1), are

- ***Tunica intima,*** the innermost layer of the vessel. It consists of three components: *(a)* a single layer of squamous epithelial cells, the ***endothelium;*** *(b)* the ***basal lamina*** of the endothelial cells; and *(c)* the ***subendothelial layer,*** consisting of loose connective tissue. Occasional smooth muscle cells are found in the loose connective tissue. The

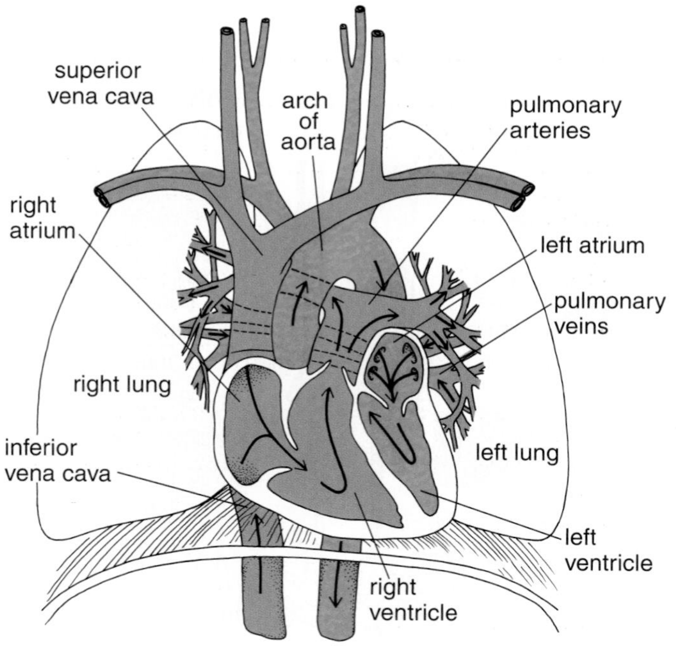

FIGURE 12.2
Diagram depicting circulation of blood through the heart. Blood returns from the tissues of the body via the superior vena cava and inferior vena cava. These two major venous vessels carry the blood to the right atrium. Blood then passes into the right ventricle and is pumped into the pulmonary trunk and next flows into pulmonary arteries that convey the blood to the lungs. The blood is oxygenated in the lungs and is then returned to the left atrium via the pulmonary veins. Blood then passes to the left ventricle and is pumped into the aorta, which conveys the blood to the tissues of the body. From the heart to the lungs and from the lungs to the heart constitutes the pulmonary circulation from the heart to the tissues and from the tissues to the heart constitutes the systemic circulation.

subendothelial layer of the intima in arteries and arterioles contains a sheet-like layer or lamella of fenestrated elastic material called the ***internal elastic membrane.*** Fenestrations enable substances to diffuse readily through the layer and reach cells deep within the wall of the vessel.

- ***Tunica media,*** the middle layer. This layer consists primarily of circumferentially arranged layers of smooth muscle cells. In arteries, it is relatively thick and extends from the ***internal elastic membrane*** to the ***external elastic membrane.*** The external elastic membrane is a layer of elastin that separates the tunica media from the tunica adventitia. Variable amounts of elastin, reticular fibers, and proteoglycans are interposed between the smooth muscle cells of the tunica media. The sheets or lamellae of elastin are fenestrated and are arranged in circular concentric layers. All of the extracellular components of the tunica media are produced by the smooth muscle cells.
- ***Tunica adventitia,*** the outermost connective tissue layer. It is composed primarily of longitudinally arranged collagenous tissue and a few elastic fibers. These connective tissue elements gradually merge with the loose connective tissue surrounding the vessels. The tunica adventitia ranges from relatively thin in most of the arterial system to quite thick in the venules and veins, where it is the major component of the vessel wall. In addition, the tunica adventitia of large arteries and veins contains a system of vessels, called ***vasa vasorum,*** that supply blood to the vascular walls themselves, as well as a network of autonomic nerves, called ***nervi vascularis,*** that control contraction of the smooth muscle in the vessel walls.

Histologically, the various types of arteries and veins are distinguished from each other on the basis of the thickness of the vascular wall and differences in the composition of the layers. Table 12.1 summarizes the features of the various types of blood vessels.

Contraction and relaxation of smooth muscle cells in the tunica media influence blood flow and pressure

Contraction of smooth muscle in the tunica media of small arteries and arterioles reduces the luminal diameter of these vessels ***(vasoconstriction),*** increasing the ***vascular resistance.*** Vasoconstriction leads to an increase in the systemic blood pressure. Generally, vasoconstriction is induced by nerve impulses or circulating hormones. The relaxation of smooth muscle cells increases the luminal diameter of the vessels ***(vasodilation),*** decreasing vascular resistance and systemic blood pressure. Vasodilation occurs in response to substances produced by the endothelial cells, called ***endothelial-derived relaxing factors (EDRFs).*** The most important EDRFs are ***nitric oxide (NO)*** and its related compounds, which are released by epithelial cells in arteries, blood capillaries, and even lymphatic capillaries.

ARTERIES

Traditionally, arteries are classified into three types on the basis of size and the characteristics of the tunica media:

- ***Large*** or ***elastic arteries***
- ***Medium*** or ***muscular arteries*** (most of the "named" arteries of the body)
- ***Small arteries*** and ***arterioles***

Elastic Arteries

Elastic arteries have multiple sheets of elastic lamellae in their walls

The largest elastic arteries, the aorta and pulmonary arteries, convey blood from the heart to the systemic and pulmonary circulations, respectively (see Fig. 12.2). These arteries, as well as their main branches, the brachiocephalic, common carotid, subclavian, and common iliac arteries, are classified as elastic arteries.

From a functional standpoint, elastic arteries serve primarily as conduction tubes; however, they also facilitate

TABLE 12.1. **Characteristics of Blood Vessels**

Arteries

Vessel	*Diameter*	*Inner Layer (Tunica Intima)*	*Middle Layer (Tunica Media)*	*Outer Layer (Tunica Adventitia)*
Elastic artery	>1 cm	Endothelium Connective tissue Smooth muscle	Smooth muscle Elastic lamellae	Connective tissue Elastic fibers Thinner than tunica media
Muscular artery –Large	2–10 mm	Endothelium Connective tissue Smooth muscle Prominent internal elastic membrane	Smooth muscle Collagen fibers Relatively little elastic tissue	Connective tissue Some elastic fibers Thinner than tunica media
–Small	0.1–2 mm	Endothelium Connective tissue Smooth muscle Internal elastic membrane	Smooth muscle (8–10 cell layers) Collagen fibers	Connective tissue Some elastic fibers Thinner than tunica media
Arteriole	10–100 μm	Endothelium Connective tissue Smooth muscle	Smooth muscle (1–2 cell layers)	Thin, ill-defined sheath of connective tissue
Capillary	4–10 μm	Endothelium	None	None

Veins

Vessel	*Diameter*	*Inner Layer (Tunica Intima)*	*Middle Layer (Tunica Media)*	*Outer Layer (Tunica Adventitia)*
Postcapillary venule	10–50 μm	Endothelium Pericytes	None	None
Muscular venule	50–100 μm	Endothelium Pericytes	Smooth muscle (1–2 cell layers)	Connective tissue Some elastic fibers Thicker than tunica media
Small vein	0.1–1 mm	Endothelium Connective issue Smooth muscle (2–3 layers)	Smooth muscle (2–3 layers continuous with tunica intima)	Connective tissue Some elastic fibers Thicker than tunica media
Medium vein	1–10 mm	Endothelium Connective tissue Smooth muscle Internal elastic membrane in some cases	Smooth muscle Collagen fibers	Connective tissue Some elastic fibers Thicker than tunica media
Large vein	>1 mm	Endothelium Connective tissue Smooth muscle	Smooth muscle (2–15 layers) Cardiac muscle near heart Collagen fibers	Connective tissue Some elastic fibers Much thicker than tunica media

the continuous and uniform movement of blood along the tube. Blood flow occurs as follows: The ventricles of the heart pump blood into the elastic arteries during the contraction phase *(systole)* of the cardiac cycle. The pressure generated by contraction of the ventricles moves the blood through the elastic arteries and along the arterial tree. Simultaneously, it also causes the wall of the large elastic arteries to distend. The distension is limited by the network of collagenous fibers in the tunica media and tunica adventitia (Fig. 12.3). During the relaxation phase *(diastole)* of the cardiac cycle, when no pressure is generated by the heart, the recoil of the distended elastic arteries serves to maintain arterial blood pressure and the flow of blood within the vessels. Initial elastic recoil forces blood both away from, and back toward, the heart. The flow of blood toward the heart causes the aortic and pulmonary valves to close. Continued elastic recoil then maintains continuous flow of blood away from the heart.

The tunica intima of the elastic artery consists of endothelium, subendothelial connective tissue, and an inconspicuous internal elastic membrane

The tunica intima of elastic arteries is relatively thick and consists of

- ***Endothelial lining*** with its ***basal lamina.*** The cells are typically flat and elongate, with their long axes ori-

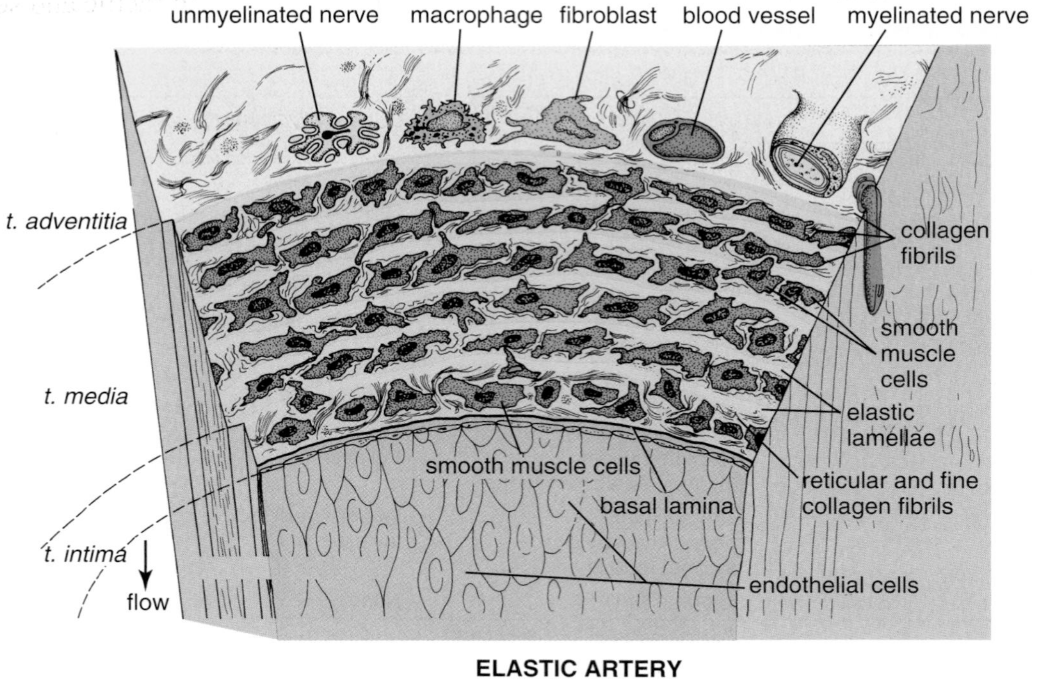

FIGURE 12.3

Schematic diagram of an elastic artery showing its cellular and extracellular components. This diagram shows a section of the wall of a typical elastic artery. Note the organization of smooth muscle cells and the distribution of elastic lamellae. *t.,* tunica. (Based on Rhodin JAG. *Handbook of Physiology.* New York: Oxford University Press, 1980.)

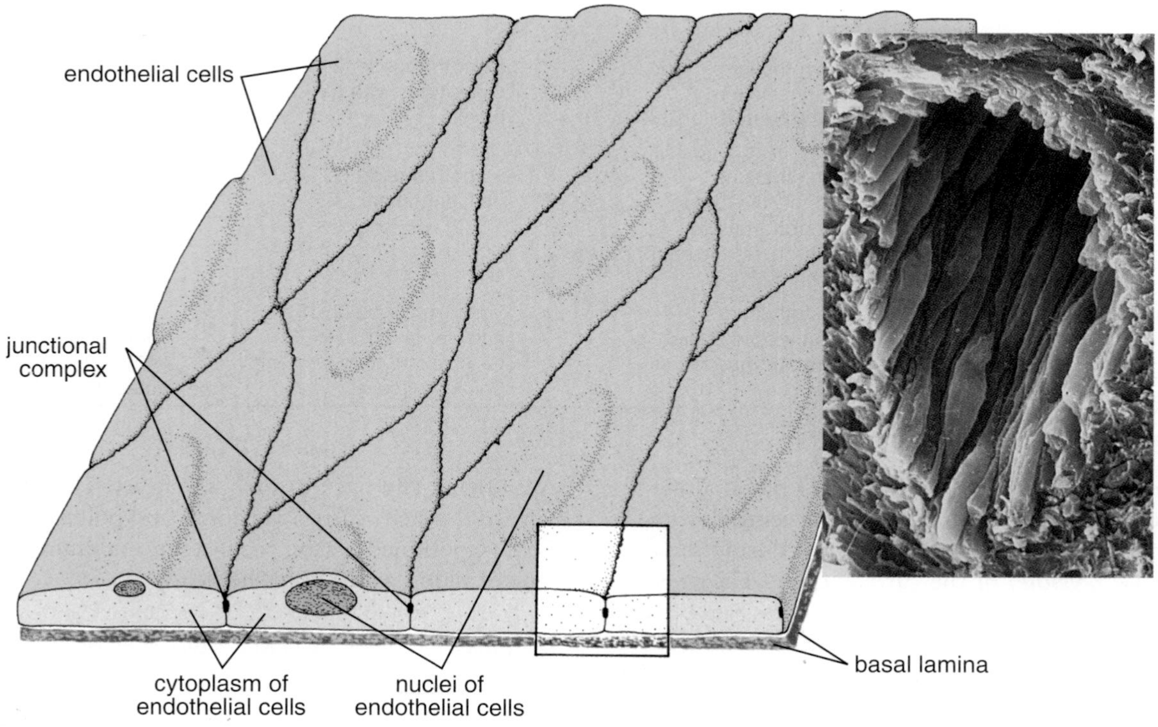

FIGURE 12.4

Diagram and scanning electron micrograph of the endothelium. This schematic drawing shows the luminal surface and cut edge of the endothelium. The cells are elongated with their long axis parallel to the direction of blood flow. Nuclei of endothelial cells are also elongated in the direction of blood flow. The *rectangular area* is shown in Figure 12.5. (Based on Rhodin JAG. *Handbook of Physiology.* New York: Oxford University Press, 1980.) **Inset.** Scanning electron micrograph of a small vein, showing the cells of the endothelial lining. Note the spindle shape with the long axis of the cells running parallel to the vessel. ×1,100.

ented parallel to the direction of blood flow in the artery (Fig. 12.4). In forming the epithelial sheet, the cells are joined by tight junctions (zonulae occludentes) and gap junctions (Fig. 12.5). Endothelial cells possess rod-like inclusions, called ***Weibel-Palade bodies,*** which are present in the cytoplasm. These specific endothelial organelles are electron-dense structures and contain ***von Willebrand factor*** (also called ***coagulating factor VIII***). Studies indicate that most von Willebrand factor is synthesized by arterial endothelial cells and secreted into the blood. The antibody to von Willebrand factor is commonly used as an immunohistochemical marker for identification of endothelium-derived tumors.

- ***Subendothelial layer*** of connective tissue, which in larger elastic arteries consists of connective tissue with both collagen and elastic fibers. The main cell type in this layer is the smooth muscle cell. It is contractile and secretes extracellular ground substance as well as collagen and elastic fibers. Occasional macrophages may also be present.
- The ***internal elastic membrane (lamina),*** which in elastic arteries is not conspicuous because it is one of many elastic layers in the wall of the vessel. It is usually identified only because it is the innermost elastic layer of the arterial wall.

Endothelial cells participate in the structural and functional integrity of the vascular wall

Endothelial cells play an important role in blood homeostasis. The functional properties of these cells change in response to various stimuli. This process, known as an ***endothelial activation,*** is also responsible for the pathogenesis of many vascular diseases (e.g., atherosclerosis). Inducers of endothelial activation include bacterial and viral antigens, cytotoxins, complement products, lipid products, and hypoxia. Activated endothelial cells exhibit new surface adhesion molecules and produce different classes of cytokines, lymphokines, growth factors, vasoconstrictor and vasodilator molecules as well molecules controlling blood coagulation. Therefore, endothelial cells are active participants in a variety of interactions between the blood and underlying connective tissue and are responsible for many properties of the vessels (Table 12.2). These properties include

- ***Maintenance of a selective permeability barrier,*** which allows selective movement of small and large molecules from the blood to the tissues and from the tissues to the blood. This movement is related to the size and charge of the molecules. Small hydrophilic and hydrophobic molecules (e.g., oxygen, carbon dioxide, glucose, amino

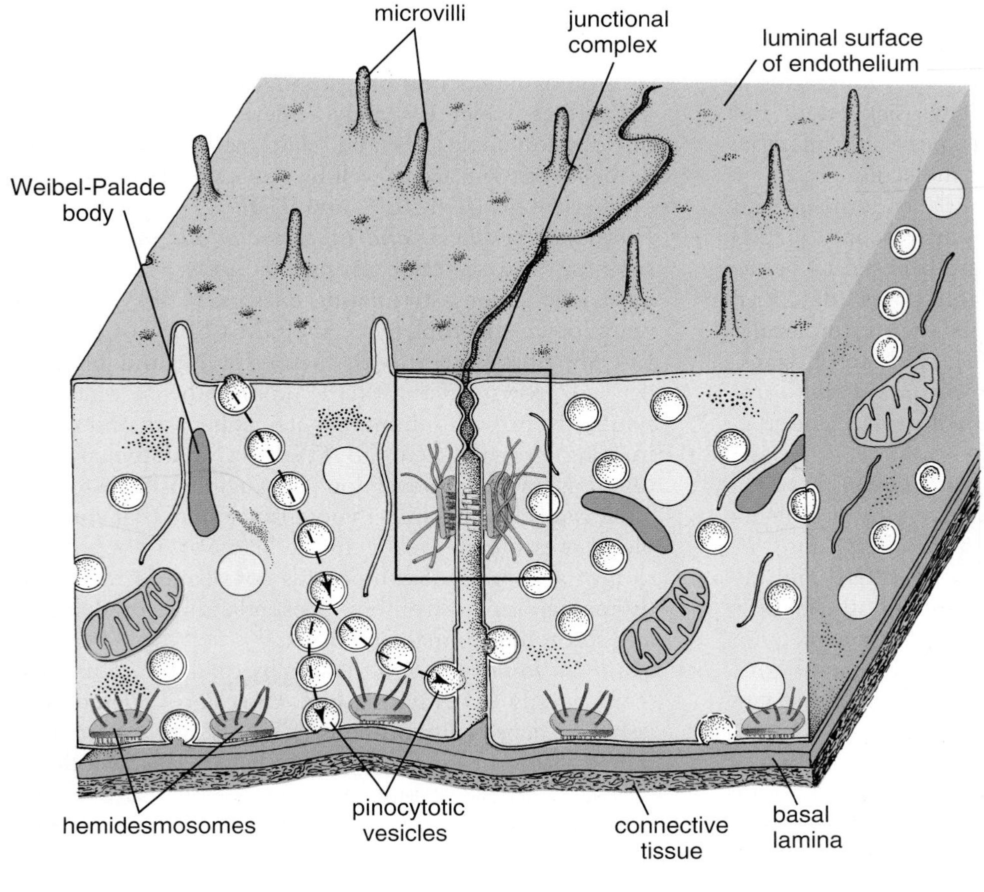

FIGURE 12.5
Diagram depicting segments of two adjacent endothelial cells. This diagram shows cell-to-cell and cell-to-extracellular matrix junctions represented here by the junctional complex and hemidesmosomes, respectively. Observe the organization of the cytoplasm and cytoplasmic inclusion, the Weibel-Palade bodies that are characteristic of endothelial cells. Pinocytotic vesicles in the cell on the left have been positioned to suggest the pathway of vesicles from the lumen of the blood vessel to the basal cell membrane or to the lateral cell membrane as indicated by the *dashed arrows.* Various markers have been traced through pinocytotic pathways across the endothelial cell. (Modified from Rhodin JAG. *Handbook of Physiology.* New York: Oxford University Press, 1980.)

TABLE 12.2. **Summary of Endothelial Cell Properties and Functions**

Major Properties	Associated Functions	Active Molecules Involved
Maintenance of selective permeability barrier	Simple diffusion	Oxygen, carbon dioxide
	Active transport	Glucose, amino acids, electrolytes
	Pinocytosis	Water, small molecules, soluble proteins
	Receptor-mediated endocytosis	LDL, cholesterol, transferrin, growth factors, antibodies, MHC complexes
Maintenance of nonthrombogenic barrier	Secretion of anticoagulants	Thrombomodulin,
	Secretion of antithrombogenic agents	Prostacyclin (PGI_2), tissue plasminogen activator (TPA), antithrombin III, heparin
	Secretion of prothrombogenic agents	Tissue thromboplastin, von Willebrand factor, plasminogen activator inhibitor
Modulation of blood flow and vascular resistance	Secretion of vasoconstrictors	Endothelin, angiotensin-converting enzyme (ACE)
	Secretion of vasodilators	Endothelial derived relaxation factor (EDRF)/nitric oxide (NO), prostacyclin
Regulation of cell growth	Secretion of growth-stimulating factors	Platelet-derived growth factor (PDGF), hemopoietic colony stimulating factors (GM-CSF, G-CSF, M-CSF)
	Secretion of growth-inhibiting factors	Heparin, transforming growth factor β (TGFβ)
Regulation of immune responses	Regulation of leukocyte migration by expression of adhesion molecules	Selectins, integrins, CD marker molecules
	Regulation of immune functions	Interleukin molecules (IL-1, IL-6, IL-8), MHC molecules
Maintenance of extracellular matrix	Synthesis of basal lamina	Type IV collagen, laminin
	Synthesis of glycocalyx	Proteoglycans
Involvement in lipoprotein metabolism	Production of free radicals	LDL, cholesterol, VLDL

Modified from Cotran S, Kumar V, Collins T, Robbins SL, eds. *Robbins Pathologic Basis of Disease.* Philadelphia: WB Saunders, 1999.

acids, and electrolytes) can diffuse or are actively transported across the plasma membrane and released into the extracellular space. Small molecules, water, and soluble proteins are transported by ***pinocytotic vesicles*** (a clathrin-independent form of endocytosis). Small but numerous, pinocytotic vesicles transport bulk material from the blood into the cell. Larger molecules are transported through ***fenestrations*** within the endothelial cells visible in transmission electron microscope (TEM) preparations. These fenestrations are believed to be the morphologic equivalents of the "large pores" described by physiologists. In addition, some specific molecules (e.g., low-density lipoprotein (LDL), cholesterol, transferrin) are transported via ***receptor-mediated endocytosis*** (a clathrin-dependent process), which uses endothelial specific surface receptors.

- ***Maintenance of a nonthrombogenic barrier*** between blood platelets and subendothelial tissue by producing ***anticoagulants*** (thrombomodulin and others) and ***antithrombogenic*** substances (prostacyclin [PGI_2] and tissue plasminogen activator). Damage to endothelial cells causes them to release prothrombogenic agents (von Willebrand factor, plasminogen activator inhibitor). These agents cause platelets to aggregate and release factors that result in the formation of clots or masses, called ***thrombi,*** that potentially prevent blood loss.
- ***Modulation of blood flow and vascular resistance*** by secretion of vasoconstrictors (endothelin, angiotensin-converting enzyme) and vasodilators (EDRF/NO, prostacyclin).
- ***Regulation and modulation of immune responses*** by controlling interaction of lymphocytes with the endothelial surface, which is mainly achieved by the expression of adhesion molecules and their receptors on the endothelial free surface as well by secretion of three classes of interleukins (IL-1, IL-6, and IL-8).
- ***Hormonal synthesis and other metabolic activities*** by synthesis and secretion of various growth factors (hemopoietic colony-stimulating factors [CSFs], such as granulocyte–macrophage CSF [GM-CSF], G-CSF, and M-CSF; fibroblast growth factor (FGF); and platelet-derived growth factor (PDGF)]. Endothelial cells also synthesize growth inhibitors such as heparin and transforming growth factor β (TGF-β). Endothelial cells function in the conversion of angiotensin I to angiotensin II in the renin–angiotensin system that controls blood pressure, as well as in the inactivation or conversion of a number of compounds conveyed in the blood (norepinephrine, thrombin, prostaglandins, bradykinin, and serotonin) to inactive forms.
- ***Modification of the lipoproteins*** by oxidation. Lipoproteins, mainly LDLs with a high cholesterol content and very low density lipoproteins (VLDLs), are oxidized by free radicals produced by endothelial cells. Modified LDLs, in turn, are rapidly endocytosed by macrophages, forming ***foam cells*** (Fig. 12.6). Foam cells are a charac-

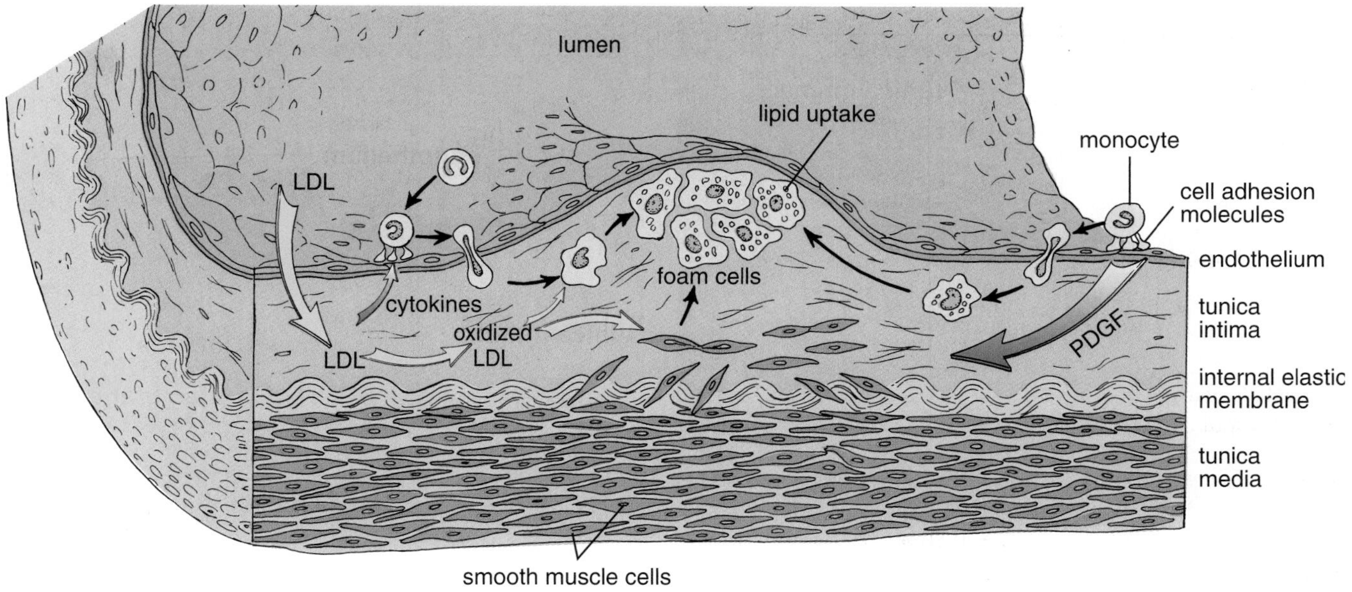

FIGURE 12.6

Schematic diagram of cellular interactions in the formation of an atherosclerotic plaque. Endothelial cells express cell adhesion molecules that initiate monocyte migration through the endothelium. Platelet-derived growth factor *(PDGF)* and other growth factors *(blue arrow)* released from endothelial cells stimulate migration of the smooth muscle cells from the tunica media to the tunica intima. In the tunica intima, smooth muscle cells produce large amounts of extracellular matrix (proteoglycans, collagen) that increase the thickness of the tunica intima. Foam cells derived from both macrophages and smooth muscle cells accumulate LDLs, which cross the endothelial barrier *(yellow arrows)*, and are oxidized by free radicals produced by the endothelial cells.

teristic feature in the formation of atherosclerotic plaques.

The tunica media of elastic arteries consists of multiple layers of smooth muscle cells separated by elastic lamellae

The tunica media is the thickest of the three layers of elastic arteries and consists of

- *Elastin* in the form of fenestrated sheets or lamellae between the muscle cell layers. These lamellae are arranged in concentric layers (Fig. 12.7a). As noted, fenestrations in the lamellae facilitate the diffusion of substances within the arterial wall. The number and thickness of these lamellae are related to blood pressure and age. At birth, the aorta is almost devoid of lamellae; in the adult, the aorta has 40 to 70 lamellae. In individuals with hypertension, both the number and the thickness of the lamellae are increased.
- *Smooth muscle cells* arranged in layers. The smooth muscle cells are arranged in a low-pitch spiral relative to the long axis of the vessel; thus, in cross sections of the artery they appear in a circular array. The smooth muscle cells are spindle shaped with an elongated nucleus. They are invested with an external (basal) lamina except where they are joined by gap junctions. Fibroblasts are not present in the tunica media. Smooth muscle cells synthesize the collagen, elastin, and other molecules of the extracellular matrix. In addition, in response to growth factors (i.e., PDGF, FGF) produced by endothelial cells they may proliferate and migrate to the adjacent intima. This characteristic is important in normal repair of the vascular wall as well in pathologic processes similar to those occurring in atherosclerosis.
- *Collagen fibers* and *ground substance* (proteoglycans), which are synthesized and secreted by the smooth muscle cells.

The tunica adventitia in the elastic artery is a relatively thin connective tissue layer

In elastic arteries, the tunica adventitia is usually less than half the thickness of the tunica media. It consists of

- *Collagen* and *elastic fibers* in the form of a loose network of elastic fibers (not lamellae) that are less organized than those in the tunica media. The collagen fibers help prevent the expansion of the arterial wall beyond physiologic limits during systole of the cardiac cycle.
- *Fibroblasts* and *macrophages,* the principal cells of the tunica adventitia.
- *Blood vessels (vasa vasorum)* and *nerves (nervi vascularis).* Branches of the vasa vasorum partially enter the tunica media and provide nutrients to the outer portion of the arterial wall. The inner part of the wall is supplied by nutrients from the lumen of the vessel.

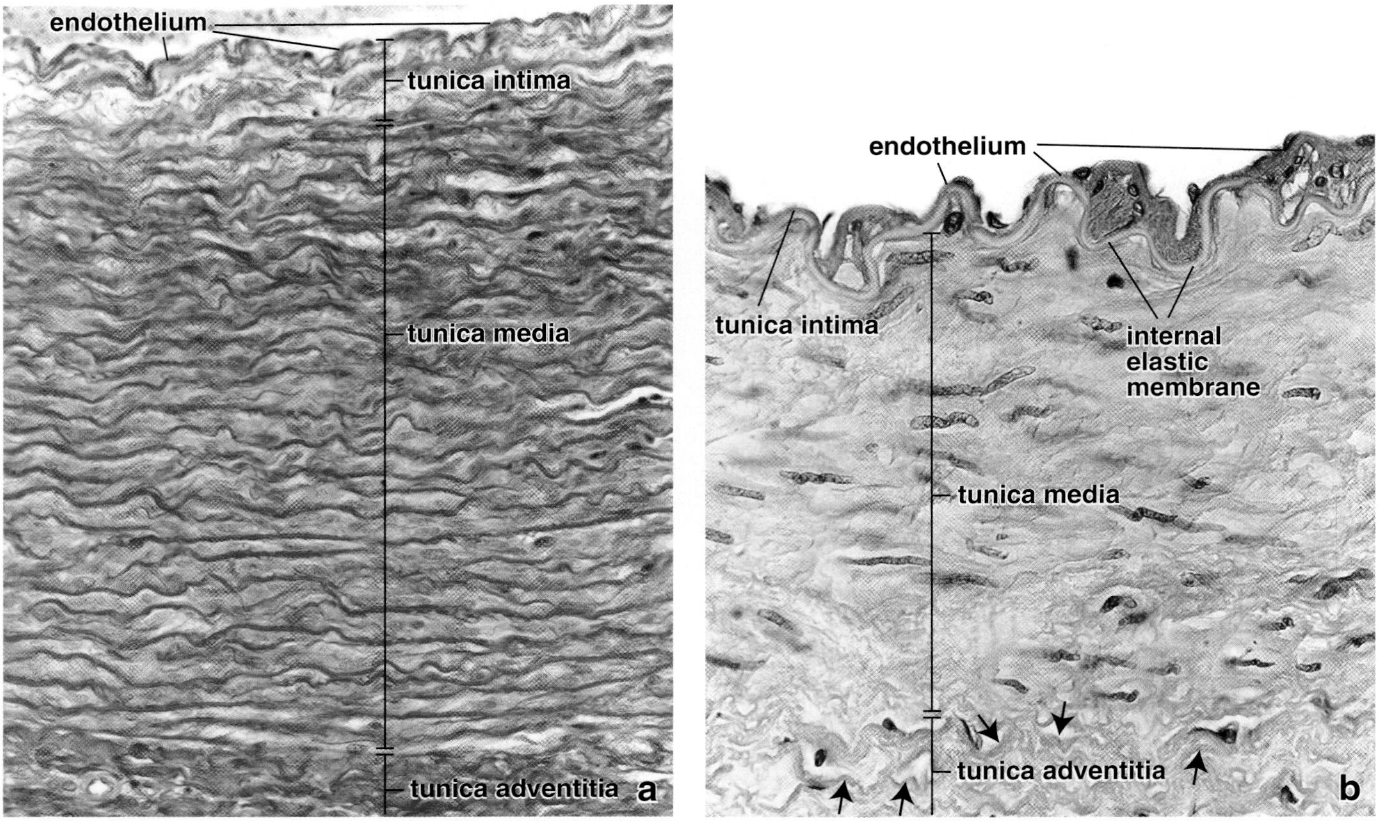

FIGURE 12.7
Photomicrographs of the wall of elastic and muscular types of arteries. a. This photomicrograph shows a cross section of the human aorta stained with resorcin-fuchsin to demonstrate elastic material. Three layers can be recognized: the tunica intima, tunica media, and tunica adventitia. The tunica intima consists of a lining of endothelial cells that rest on a thin layer of connective tissue containing smooth muscle cells, occasional macrophages, and collagen and elastic fibers. The boundary between it and the tissue below, the tunica media, is not sharply defined. The tunica media contains an abundance of smooth muscle cells (note the blue staining nuclei) and numerous elastic fenestrated membranes (the red, wavy lamellae). The tunica adventitia, the outermost part, lacks elastic laminae, consists mainly of connective tissue, and contains the blood vessels and nerves that supply the aortic wall. ×300. **b.** Photomicrograph of a cross section through a muscular artery in a routine H&E preparation shows that the wall of the muscular artery is also divided into the same three layers as in the elastic artery. The tunica intima consists of an endothelial lining, a small amount of connective tissue, and the internal elastic membrane. This structure has a scalloped appearance when the vessel is constricted and is highly refractile. Constriction also causes the endothelial cell nuclei to appear rounded. The tunica media consists mainly of circularly arranged smooth muscle cells and collagen and elastic fibers. The nuclei of the smooth muscle cells, when contracted, have a corkscrew appearance. The tunica adventitia consists mostly of connective tissue. A well-defined external elastic membrane is not apparent in this vessel, but profiles of elastic material *(arrows)* are present. ×360.

Muscular Arteries

Muscular arteries have more smooth muscle and less elastin in the tunica media than do elastic arteries

There is no sharp dividing line between elastic arteries and large muscular arteries (Fig. 12.8). Some of these arteries are difficult to classify because they have features that are intermediate between the two types. Generally, in the region of transition, the amount of elastic material decreases, and smooth muscle cells become the predominant constituent of the tunica media. Also, a prominent ***internal elastic membrane*** becomes apparent, helping to distinguish muscular arteries from elastic arteries. In many instances, a recognizable ***external elastic membrane*** is also evident.

The tunica intima is thinner in muscular arteries and contains a prominent internal elastic membrane

The tunica intima is relatively thinner in muscular arteries than in elastic arteries and consists of an endothelial lining with its basal lamina, a sparse subendothelial layer of connective tissue, and a prominent ***internal elastic membrane.*** In some muscular arteries, the subendothelial layer is so scanty that the basal lamina of the endothelium appears to make contact with the internal elastic membrane.

In histologic sections, the internal elastic membrane usually appears as a well-defined, undulating or wavy structure because of contraction of the smooth muscle (Fig. 12.7b).

The thickness of the tunica intima varies with age and other factors. In young children, it is very thin. In muscular arteries of young adults, the tunica intima accounts for about one sixth of the total wall thickness. In older adults, the tunica intima may be expanded by lipid deposits, often in the form of irregular "fatty streaks."

The tunica media of muscular arteries is composed almost entirely of smooth muscle, with little elastic material

The tunica media of muscular arteries consists of smooth muscle cells amid collagen fibers and relatively little elastic material. The smooth muscle cells are arranged in a spiral fashion in the arterial wall. Their contraction helps maintain blood pressure. As in elastic arteries, there are no fibroblasts in this layer. The smooth muscle cells possess an external (basal) lamina except at the sites of gap junctions and produce extracellular collagen, elastin, and ground substance.

The tunica adventitia of muscular arteries is relatively thick and is often separated from the tunica media by a recognizable external elastic membrane

The tunica adventitia of muscular arteries consists of fibroblasts, collagen fibers, elastic fibers, and in some vessels scattered adipose cells. Compared with elastic arteries, the tunica adventitia of muscular arteries is relatively thick, about the same thickness as the tunica media. Collagen fibers are the principal extracellular component. However, a concentration of elastic material immediately adjacent to the tunica media is often present and as such constitutes the ***external elastic membrane.*** Nerves and small vessels travel in the adventitia and give off branches that penetrate into the tunica media in the large muscular arteries as the vasa vasorum.

Small Arteries and Arterioles

Small arteries and arterioles are distinguished from one another by the number of smooth muscle cell layers in the tunica media

By definition, arterioles have only one or two layers of smooth muscle in their tunica media (Fig. 12.9); a small artery may have up to about eight layers. Typically, the tunica intima of a small artery has an internal elastic membrane, whereas this layer may or may not be present in the arteriole. The endothelium in both is essentially similar to endothelium in other arteries, except that at the EM level, gap junctions may be found between endothelial cells and the smooth muscle cells of the tunica media. Lastly, the tunica adventitia is a thin, ill-defined sheath of connective tissue that blends with the connective tissue in which these vessels travel.

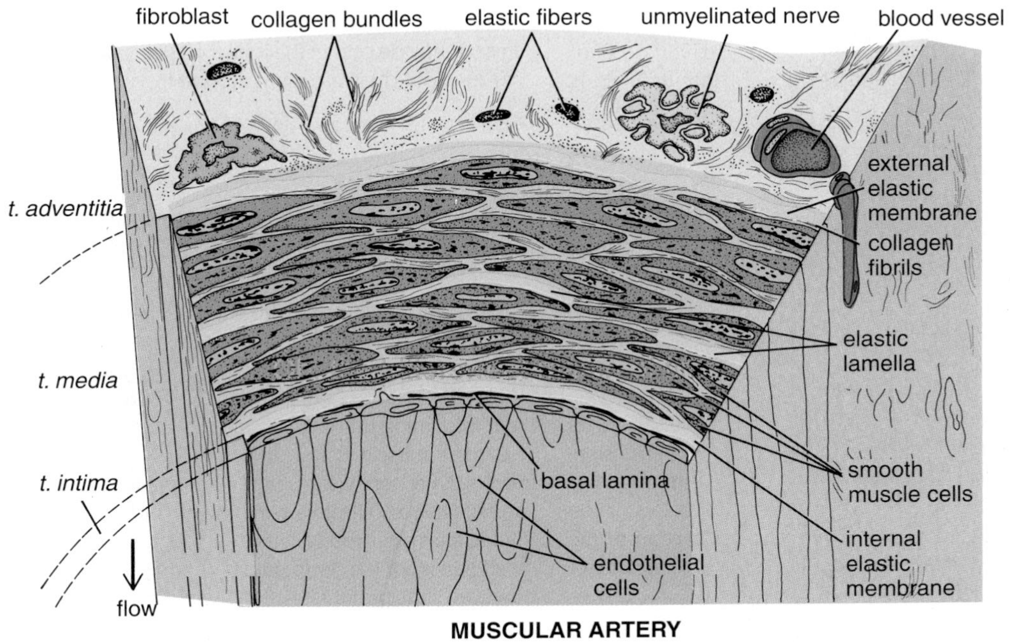

FIGURE 12.8
Schematic diagram of a muscular artery. The cellular and extracellular components are labeled. Note the locations of external and internal elastic membranes. In certain locations, the muscle cells in the tunica media are shown in contact to represent the presence of gap junctions between cells. *t.*, tunica. (Based on Rhodin JAG. *Handbook of Physiology.* New York: Oxford University Press, 1980.)

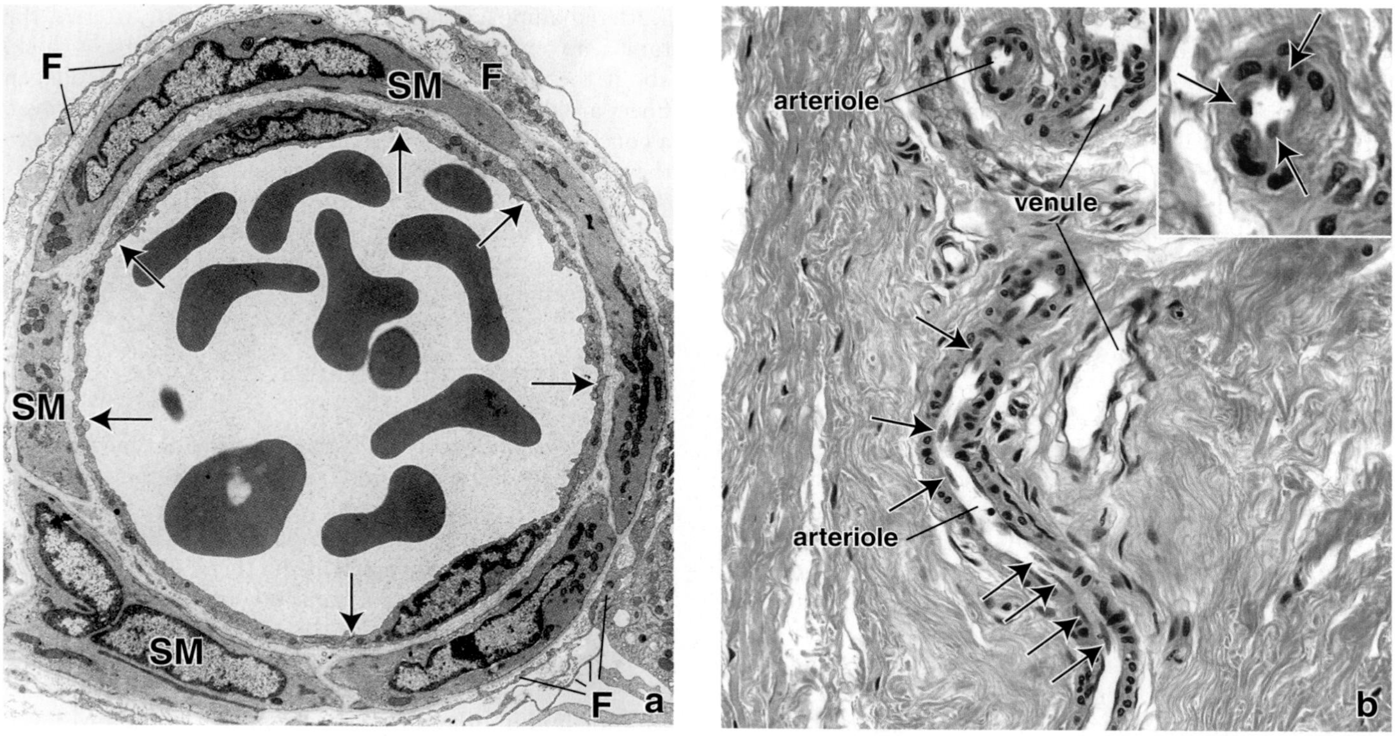

FIGURE 12.9

Electron micrograph and photomicrograph of arterioles. a. This electron micrograph shows a cross section of an arteriole. The tunica intima of the vessel is composed of an endothelium and a very thin layer of subendothelial connective tissue (collagen fibrils and ground substance). The *arrows* indicate the site of junction between adjoining endothelial cells. The tunica media consists of a single layer of smooth muscle cells *(SM)*. The tunica adventitia is composed of collagen fibrils and several layers of fibroblasts *(F)* with extremely attenuated processes. Red blood cells are visible in the lumen. ×6,000. **b.** Photomicrograph of arteriole and venule in the dermis. One arteriole is seen in longitudinal section, while another is seen in cross section. The round and ovoid nuclei in the wall of the longitudinally sectioned arteriole belong to the smooth muscle cells of the tunica media. Their round to ovoid shape indicates that these cells have been cut in cross section. The elongated nuclei *(arrows)* belong to endothelial cells. ×320. **Inset.** The cross-sectioned arteriole is shown here at higher magnification and reveals the endothelial cell nuclei bulging into the lumen *(arrows)*. They reflect a cross-sectional cut. The nuclei of the smooth muscle cells in the tunica media appear as elongate profiles reflecting their circular pattern around the vessel. ×600.

BOX 12.1

Clinical Correlations: Hypertension

Hypertension, or high blood pressure, occurs in about 25% of the population and is defined by a sustained diastolic pressure greater than 90 mm Hg or a sustained systolic pressure in excess of 140 mm Hg. Hypertension is often associated with atherosclerotic vascular disease and with an increased risk of cardiovascular disorders such as stroke and angina pectoris. In most cases of hypertension, the size of the lumen of the small muscular arteries and arterioles is reduced, which leads to increased vascular resistance. Restriction in the luminal size may also result from active contraction of the smooth muscle in the vessel wall, an increase in the amount of smooth muscle in the wall, or both.

In individuals with hypertension, multiplication of smooth muscle cells occurs. The additional smooth muscle then adds to the thickness of the tunica media. Concomitantly, some of the smooth muscle cells accumulate lipid. This is one reason why hypertension is a major risk factor for atherosclerosis. In fat-fed animals, hypertension accelerates the rate of lipid accumulation in the vessel wall. In the absence of a fatty diet, hypertension increases the rate of intimal thickening that occurs naturally with age.

Cardiac muscle is also affected by chronic hypertension. Ventricular hypertrophy, caused by an increase in number and size of cardiac muscle cells, is a common manifestation of hypertension. Ventricular hypertrophy makes the wall less elastic and the heart must then work harder to pump blood. Recent studies have shown, however, that prolonged reduction of blood pressure in patients with ventricular hypertrophy due to chronic hypertension can actually reduce the degree of hypertrophy.

Arterioles control blood flow to capillary networks by contraction of the smooth muscle cells

Arterioles serve as flow regulators for the capillary beds. In the normal relationship between an arteriole and a capillary network, contraction of the smooth muscle in the wall of an arteriole increases the vascular resistance and reduces or shuts off the blood going to the capillaries. The slight thickening of the smooth muscle at the origin of a capillary bed from an arteriole is called the ***precapillary sphincter.*** Most arterioles can dilate 60 to 100% from their resting diameter, and they can maintain up to 40% constriction for a long time. Therefore, a large decrease or increase in vascular resistance has a direct effect on blood flow and systemic arterial pressure. This regulation directs blood to where it may be most needed. For instance, during strenuous physical exertion, such as running, blood flow to skeletal muscle is increased by dilation of arterioles, and blood flow to the intestine is reduced by arteriole constriction. After ingestion of a large meal, however, the reverse is true.

BOX 12.2

Clinical Correlations: Atherosclerosis

Atherosclerotic lesions are the most common acquired abnormality of blood vessels. More than half of the annual deaths in the United States are related to complications of atherosclerotic disease, which includes ischemic heart disease, myocardial infarction, stroke, and gangrene of the limbs. The lesions develop in the intima and consist of a thick layer of fibrous connective tissue containing scattered smooth muscle cells, macrophages, foam cells, lymphocytes, cholesterol crystals, and cell debris. It is believed that both macrophages and smooth muscle cells accumulate lipid, particularly LDL (Fig. 12.10). Progression of the lesion is marked by accumulation of lipid and loss of integrity of the endothelium. In advanced lesions, blood stasis and clotting (thrombosis) may lead to occlusion of the vessel. Other changes seen in advanced lesions include thinning of the tunica media, calcifications, and a necrotic mass within the lesion. Progression from simple to complicated lesions can be found in some people in their 20s and in most individuals by age 50 or 60 years.

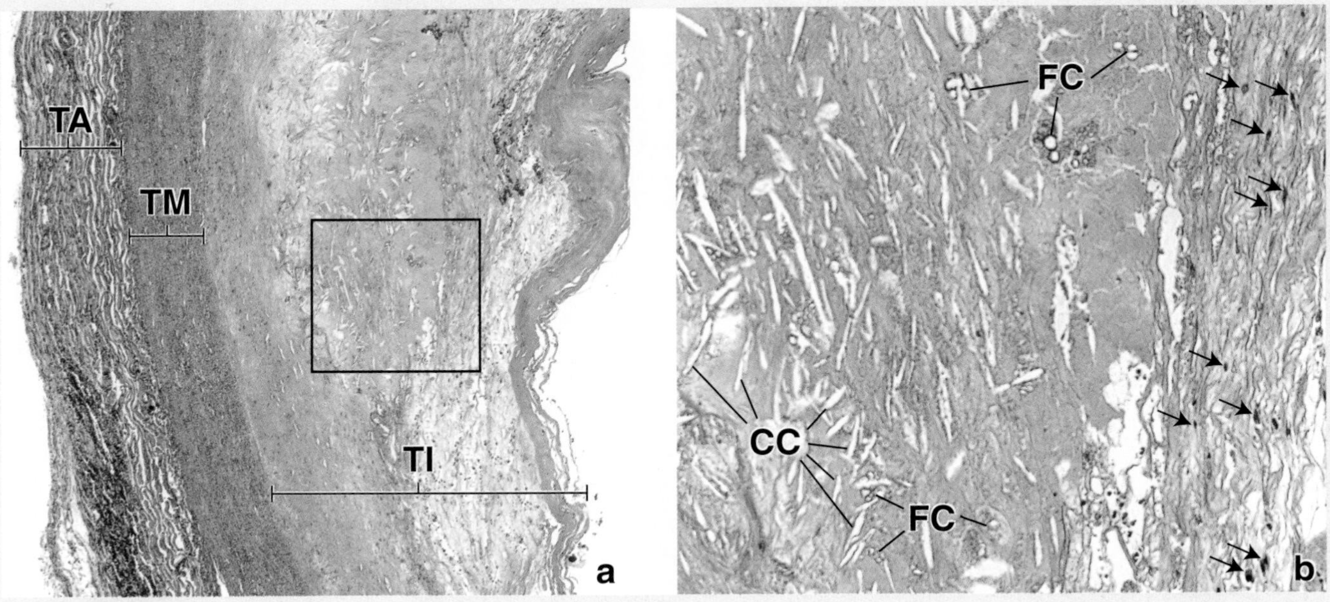

FIGURE 12.10
Photomicrographs of an atherosclerotic lesion. a. This specimen is from a human aorta stained by the Masson trichrome method. The lesion, referred to as a fibrous plaque, consists of connective tissue fibers, smooth muscle cells, fat-containing macrophages (foam cells), and a necrotic material. It occupies the site of the tunica intima *(TI)*, which is greatly expanded in thickness. *TM*, tunica media; *TA*, tunica adventitia. ×40. **b.** A higher power of the area in the *rectangle* in *a*. On the right, some of the fibrous connective tissue of the plaque is evident. The *arrows* point to smooth muscle cell nuclei that have produced the collagen fibers of the fibrous plaque. Also evident are the foam cells *(FC)* and the characteristic cholesterol clefts *(CC)*. The latter are spaces occupied previously by cholesterol crystals that have been dissolved during specimen preparation. The remainder of the plaque consists of necrotic material and lipid. ×240.

CAPILLARIES

Capillaries are the smallest diameter blood vessels, often smaller than the diameter of an erythrocyte

Capillaries form blood vascular networks that allow fluids containing gases, metabolites, and waste products to move through their thin walls. The human body contains approximately 50,000 miles of capillaries. Each consists of a single layer of endothelial cells and their basal lamina. The endothelial cells form a tube just large enough to allow the passage of red blood cells one at a time. In many capillaries the lumen is so narrow that the red cells literally fold upon themselves to pass through the vessel. The passing red blood cells fill virtually the entire capillary lumen, minimizing the diffusion path for gases and nutrients between the capillary and the extravascular tissue. In cross sections and with the TEM, the tube appears to be formed by only one cell or portions of several cells. Because of their thin walls and close physical association with metabolically active cells and tissues, capillaries are particularly well suited for the exchange of gases and metabolites between cells and the bloodstream. The ratios of capillary volume to endothelial surface area and thickness also favor movement of substances across the vessel wall.

Classification of Capillaries

Capillary structure varies in different tissues and organs. Based on their morphology, three types of capillaries are

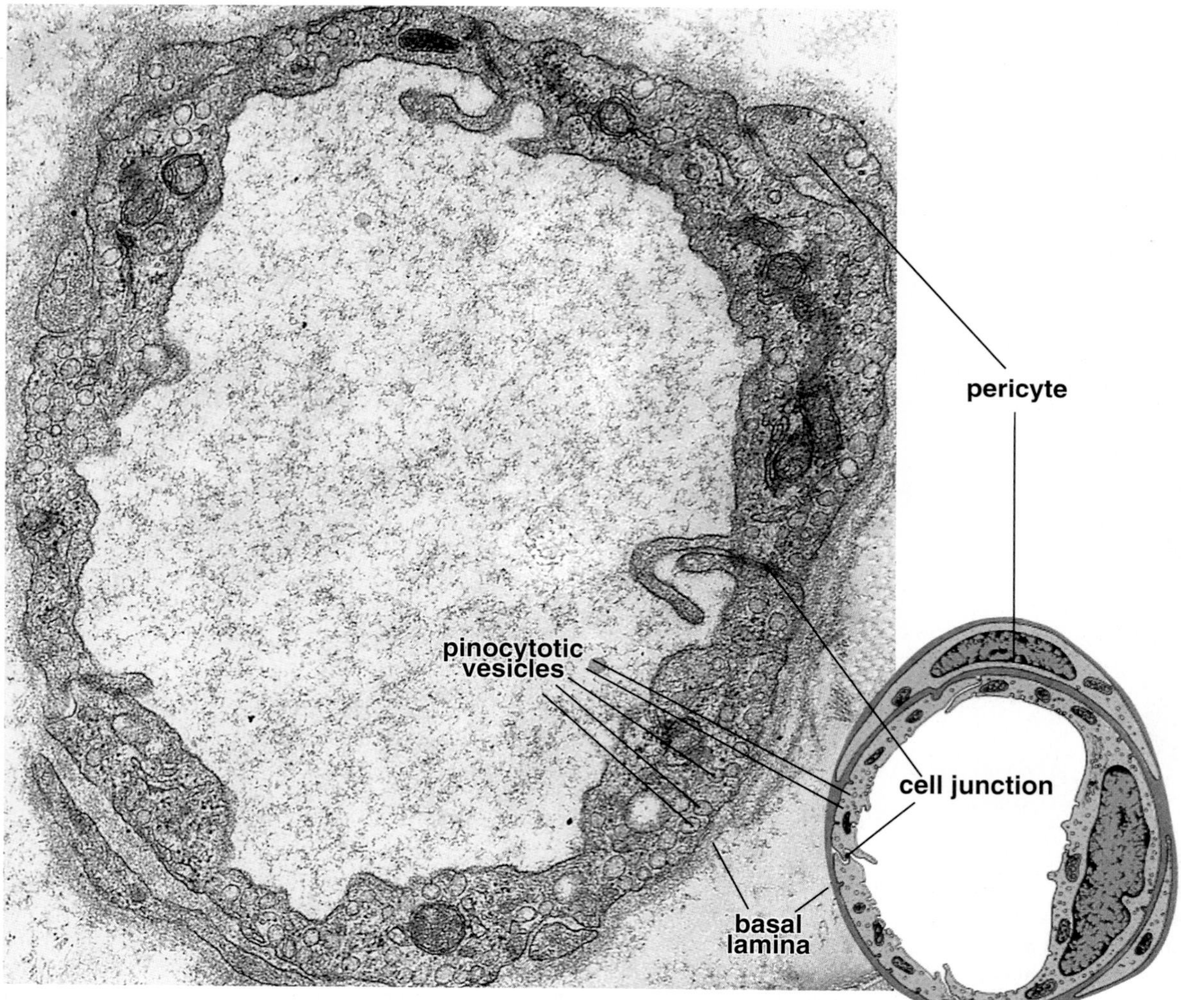

FIGURE 12.11

Electron micrograph and diagram of a continuous capillary. The endothelial cells that make up the wall of a continuous capillary contain numerous pinocytotic vesicles. The cell junctions are frequently marked by cytoplasmic (marginal) folds that protrude into the lumen. The endothelial cell nuclei are not included within the plane of section in the micrograph, but an endothelial cell with its nucleus is shown in the diagram. Similarly, the electron micrograph shows only a small amount of pericyte cytoplasm; a nucleus is not seen but is shown in the diagram (see the upper right and lower left of the micrograph). Note that the pericyte cytoplasm is enclosed by basal lamina. ×30,000.

described: continuous capillaries, fenestrated capillaries, and discontinuous capillaries.

Continuous capillaries are typically found in muscle, lung, and the central nervous system (CNS). With the TEM, they appear in cross sections as two plasma membranes enclosing a ribbon of cytoplasm that may include the nucleus (Fig. 12.11). Occluding junctions can be seen in a typical cross section of a continuous capillary. Numerous pinocytotic vesicles underlie both the luminal and basal plasma membrane surfaces. The vesicles are approximately 70 nm in diameter and function in transport of materials between the lumen and the connective tissue and vice versa.

In some continuous capillaries and postcapillary venules, ***pericytes (Rouget cells)*** may be associated with the endothelium (Fig. 12.11). The pericyte, when present, intimately surrounds the capillary, with branching cytoplasmic processes, and is enclosed by a basal lamina that is continuous with that of the endothelium. The pericyte displays features of a relatively unspecialized cell with a large nucleus rich in heterochromatin. It is derived from the same precursor cell that forms endothelial cells in new vessels. It can also give rise to smooth muscle cells during vessel growth (as in development and wound healing).

Fenestrated capillaries are typically found in endocrine glands and sites of fluid and metabolite absorption, such as the gallbladder and intestinal tract. They are characterized by fenestrations, 80 to 100 nm in diameter, which provide channels across the capillary wall (Fig. 12.12). Fenestrated capillaries also have pinocytotic vesicles. Some research suggests that fenestrations are formed when a forming pinocytotic vesicle spans the narrow cytoplasmic layer and simultaneously opens on the opposite surface. A fenestration may have a thin, nonmembranous diaphragm across its opening. This diaphragm has a central thickening and may be the remnant of the glycocalyx formerly enclosed in the pinocytotic vesicle from which the fenestration may have formed.

Fenestrated capillaries in the gastrointestinal tract and gallbladder have fewer fenestrations and a thicker wall

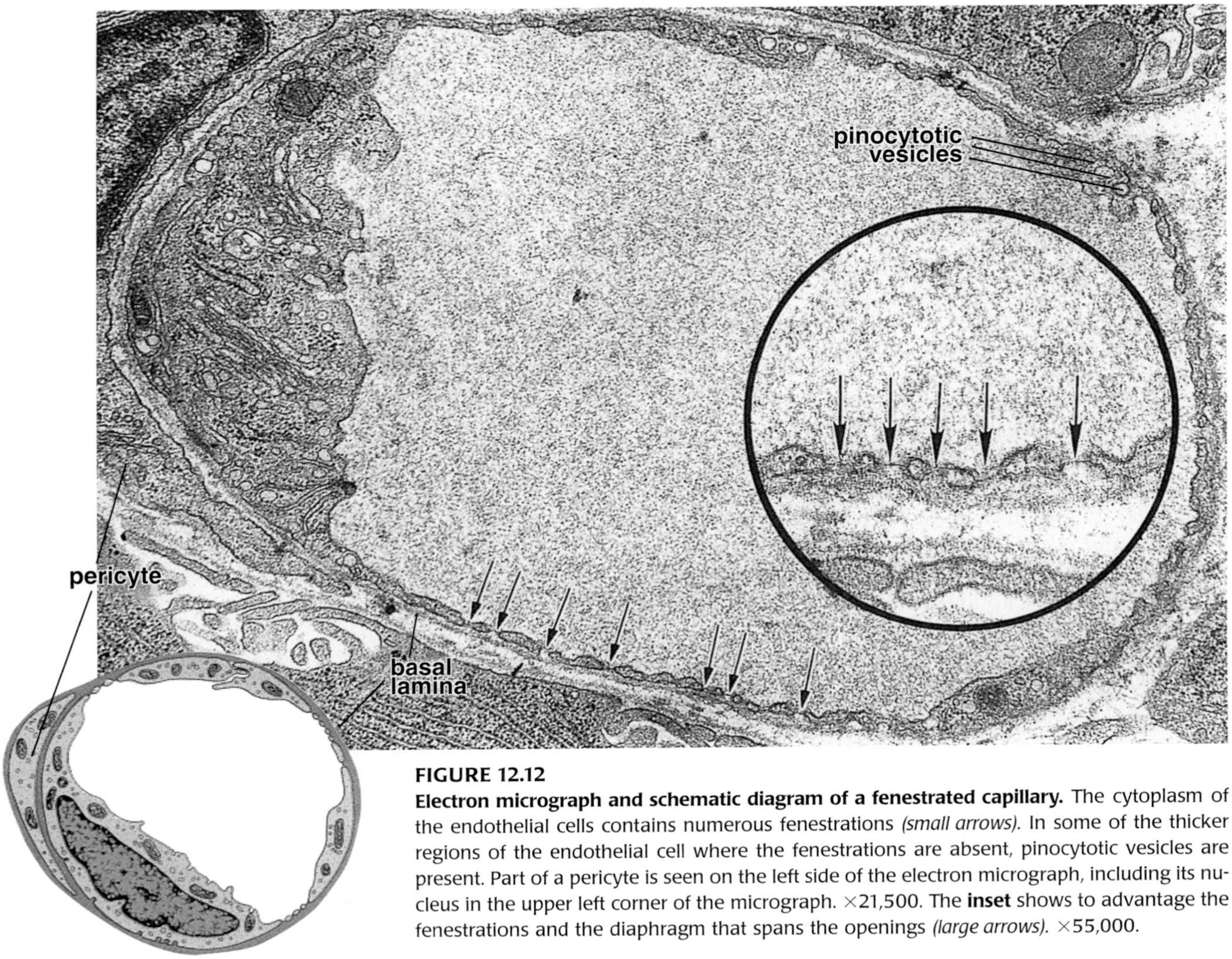

FIGURE 12.12
Electron micrograph and schematic diagram of a fenestrated capillary. The cytoplasm of the endothelial cells contains numerous fenestrations *(small arrows)*. In some of the thicker regions of the endothelial cell where the fenestrations are absent, pinocytotic vesicles are present. Part of a pericyte is seen on the left side of the electron micrograph, including its nucleus in the upper left corner of the micrograph. ×21,500. The **inset** shows to advantage the fenestrations and the diaphragm that spans the openings *(large arrows)*. ×55,000.

when no absorption is occurring. When absorption takes place, the walls thin, and the number of pinocytotic vesicles and fenestrations increases rapidly. The ionic changes in the perivascular connective tissue, caused by the absorbed solutes, stimulate pinocytosis. These observations support the suggested mode of formation of the fenestrations described above.

Discontinuous capillaries (***sinusoidal capillaries,*** or ***sinusoids***) are typically found in the liver, spleen, and bone marrow. They are larger in diameter and more irregularly shaped than other capillaries. Structural features of these capillaries vary from organ to organ and include specialized cells. ***Stellate sinusoidal macrophages (Kupffer cells)*** and vitamin A–storing ***hepatic stellate cells (Ito cells)*** in the liver occur in association with the endothelial cells. In the spleen, endothelial cells exhibit a unique spindle shape with gaps between the neighboring cells; the basal lamina underlying the endothelium may be partially or even completely absent.

Functional Aspects of Capillaries

To understand capillary function, two important points, blood flow and extent or richness of the capillary network, should be considered. Blood flow is controlled through local and systemic signals. In response to vasodilating agents (e.g., EDRFs, NO, low O_2 tension), the smooth muscle in the walls of the arterioles relaxes, resulting in vasodilation and increased blood flow through the capillary system. Pressure within the capillaries increases, and much of the plasma fluid is driven into the tissue. This process occurs in ***peripheral edema.*** Systemic signals carried by the autonomic nervous system and release of norepinephrine by the adrenal gland cause the smooth muscle of the arterioles to contract (vasoconstriction), resulting in decreased blood flow through the capillary bed. In this condition, capillary pressure can decrease and greatly increase absorption of tissue fluid. This situation occurs during loss of blood volume and can add approximately 1 L of fluid into the blood, preventing hypovolemic shock.

The richness of the capillary network is related to the metabolic activity of the tissue. The liver, kidney, cardiac muscle, and skeletal muscle have rich capillary networks. Dense connective tissue is less metabolically active and has less extensive capillary networks.

▼ ARTERIOVENOUS SHUNTS

Arteriovenous shunts allow blood to bypass capillaries by providing direct routes between arteries and veins

Generally, in a microvascular bed, arteries convey blood to the capillaries, and veins convey blood away from the capillaries. However, all the blood does not necessarily pass from arteries to capillaries and thence to veins. In many tissues, there are direct routes between the arteries and veins that divert blood from the capillaries. These routes are called ***arteriovenous (AV) anastomoses,*** or ***shunts*** (see Fig. 12.1). AV shunts are commonly found in the skin of the fingertips, nose, and lips and in the erectile tissue of the penis and clitoris. The arteriole of AV shunts is often coiled, has a relatively thick smooth muscle layer, is enclosed in a connective tissue capsule, and is richly innervated. Contrary to the ordinary precapillary sphincter, contraction of the arteriole smooth muscle of the AV shunt sends blood to a capillary bed; relaxation of the smooth muscle sends blood to a venule, bypassing the capillary bed. AV shunts serve in thermoregulation at the body surface. Closing an AV shunt in the skin causes blood to flow through the capillary bed, enhancing heat loss. Opening an AV shunt in the skin reduces the blood flow to the skin capillaries, conserving body heat. In erectile tissue, such as the penis, closing the AV shunt directs blood flow into the corpora cavernosa, initiating the erectile response (see page 711).

In addition, preferential thoroughfares, whose proximal segment is called a ***metarteriole*** (Fig. 12.13), also allow some blood to pass more directly from artery to vein. Capillaries arise from both arterioles and metarterioles. Although capillaries themselves have no smooth muscle in their walls, a sphincter of smooth muscle, called the ***precapillary sphincter,*** is located at their origin from either an arteriole or a metarteriole. These sphincters control the amount of blood passing through the capillary bed.

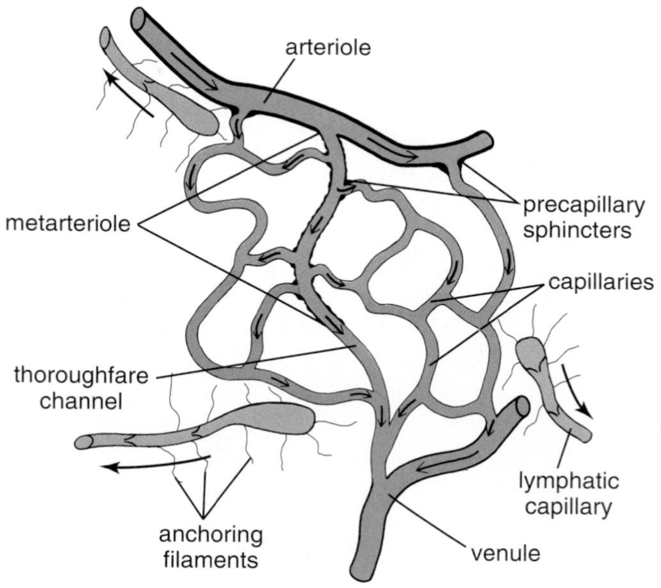

FIGURE 12.13
Diagram of microcirculation. This schematic diagram shows a metarteriole (initial segment of a thoroughfare channel) giving rise to capillaries. The precapillary sphincters of the arteriole and metarteriole control the entry of blood into the capillaries. The distal segment of the thoroughfare channel receives capillaries from the microcirculatory bed, but no sphincters are present where the afferent capillaries enter the thoroughfare channels. Blind-ending lymphatic vessels are shown in association with the capillary bed. Note the presence of anchoring filaments and the valve system within the lymphatic capillaries.

VEINS

The tunics of veins are not as distinct or well defined as the tunics of arteries. Traditionally, veins are divided into three types on the basis of size:

- ***Small veins*** or ***venules***, further subclassified as ***postcapillary*** and ***muscular venules***
- ***Medium veins***
- ***Large veins***

Although large and medium veins have three layers, also designated tunica intima, tunica media, and tunica adventitia, these layers are not as distinct as they are in arteries. Large- and medium-sized veins usually travel with large- and medium-sized arteries; arterioles and muscular venules also sometimes travel together, thus allowing comparison in histologic sections. Typically, veins have thinner walls than their accompanying arteries, and the lumen of the vein is larger than that of the artery. The arteriole lumen is usually patent; that of the vein is often collapsed. Many veins, especially those that convey blood against gravity, such as those of the limbs, contain valves that allow blood to flow in only one direction, back toward the heart. The valves are semilunar flaps consisting of a thin connective tissue core covered by endothelial cells.

Venules

Muscular venules are distinguished from postcapillary venules by the presence of a tunica media

Postcapillary venules receive blood from capillaries and have a diameter as small as 0.2 mm or slightly larger. They possess an endothelial lining with its basal lamina and pericytes. The endothelium of postcapillary venules is the principal site of action of vasoactive agents such as histamine and serotonin. Response to these agents results in extravasation of fluid and emigration of white blood cells from the vessel during inflammation and allergic reactions. Postcapillary venules of lymph nodes also participate in the transmural migration of lymphocytes from the vascular lumen into the lymphatic tissue. The postcapillary venules in the lymph nodes are also called ***high endothelial venules*** *(HEVs)* because of the prominent cuboidal appearance of their endothelial cells and their ovoid nuclei.

Muscular venules are located distal to the postcapillary venules in the returning venous network and have a diameter up to 1 mm. Whereas postcapillary venules have no true tunica media, the muscular venules have one or two layers of smooth muscle that constitute a tunica media. These vessels also have a thin tunica adventitia.

Medium Veins

Medium veins have a diameter of up to 10 mm. Most named veins are in this category. Valves are a characteristic feature of these vessels and are most numerous in the inferior portion of the body, particularly the legs, to prevent retrograde movement of blood because of gravity. The three tunics of the venous wall are most evident in medium-sized veins (Fig. 12.14):

- The ***tunica intima*** consists of an endothelium with its basal lamina, a thin subendothelial layer with occasional smooth muscle cells scattered in the connective tissue elements, and, in some cases, a thin internal elastic membrane.

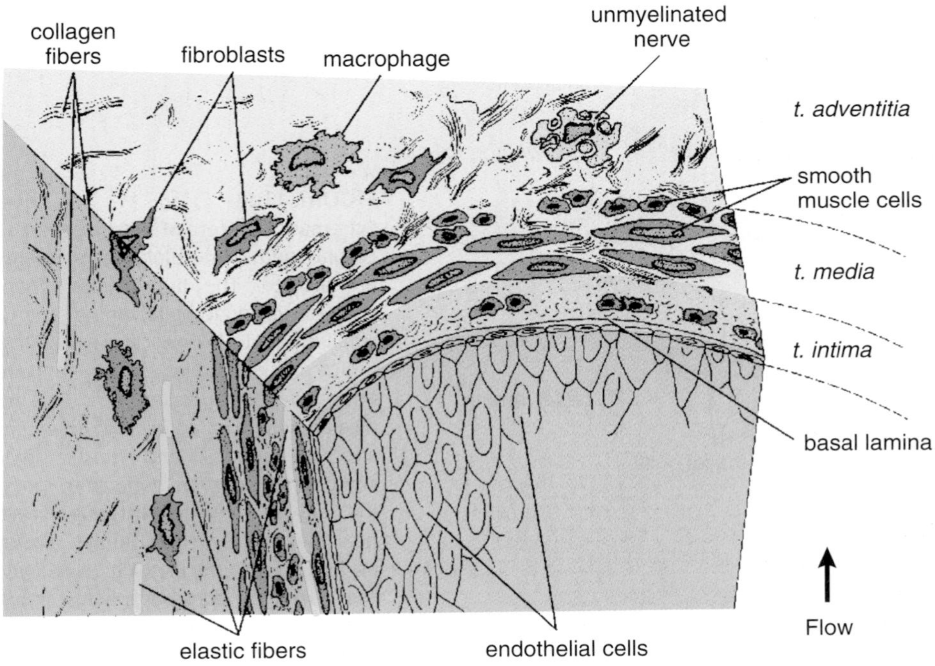

FIGURE 12.14
Schematic diagram of a medium-sized vein. The cellular and extracellular components are labeled. Note that the tunica media contains several layers of circularly arranged smooth muscle cells with interspersed collagen and elastic fibers. Also, a longitudinally arranged smooth muscle layer is present at the junction with the tunica adventitia. *t.*, tunica. (Based on Rhodin JAG. *Handbook of Physiology.* New York: Oxford University Press, 1980.)

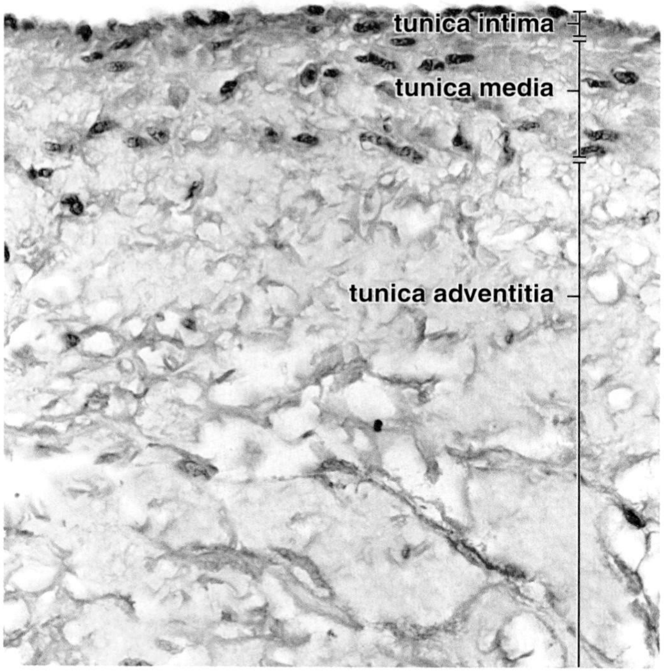

FIGURE 12.15
Photomicrograph of the wall of a medium-sized vein. This photomicrograph shows the three tunics in a section through the wall of a medium-sized vein. The tunica intima consists of endothelium and a very thin subendothelial layer of connective tissue containing some smooth muscle cells. The tunica media contains circularly and spirally arranged smooth muscle cells with collagen and elastic fibers. Note the tunica adventitia, which contains an abundance of collagen and some elastic fibers. The few nuclei seen in this layer belong to fibroblasts. ×360.

- The ***tunica media*** of medium-sized veins is much thinner than the same layer in medium-sized arteries. It contains several layers of circularly arranged smooth muscle cells with interspersed collagen and elastic fibers. In addition, longitudinally arranged smooth muscle cells may be present just beneath the tunica adventitia
- The ***tunica adventitia*** is typically thicker than the tunica media and consists of collagen fibers and networks of elastic fibers (Fig. 12.15).

Large Veins

In large veins, the tunica media is relatively thin, and the tunica adventitia relatively thick

Veins with a diameter greater than 10 mm are classified as large veins. The tunica intima of these veins (Fig. 12.16) consists of an endothelial lining with its basal lamina, a small amount of subendothelial connective tissue, and some smooth muscle cells. Often, the boundary between the tunica intima and tunica media is not clear, and it is not always easy to decide if the smooth muscle cells close to the intimal endothelium belong to the tunica intima or to the tunica media.

The tunica media is relatively thin and contains circumferentially arranged smooth muscle cells, collagen fibers, and some fibroblasts. In some animals, but not in humans, cardiac muscle cells extend into the tunica media of the venae cavae and the pulmonary veins, near their junction with the heart.

The tunica adventitia of large veins (e.g., the subclavian veins and the venae cavae) is the thickest layer of the ves-

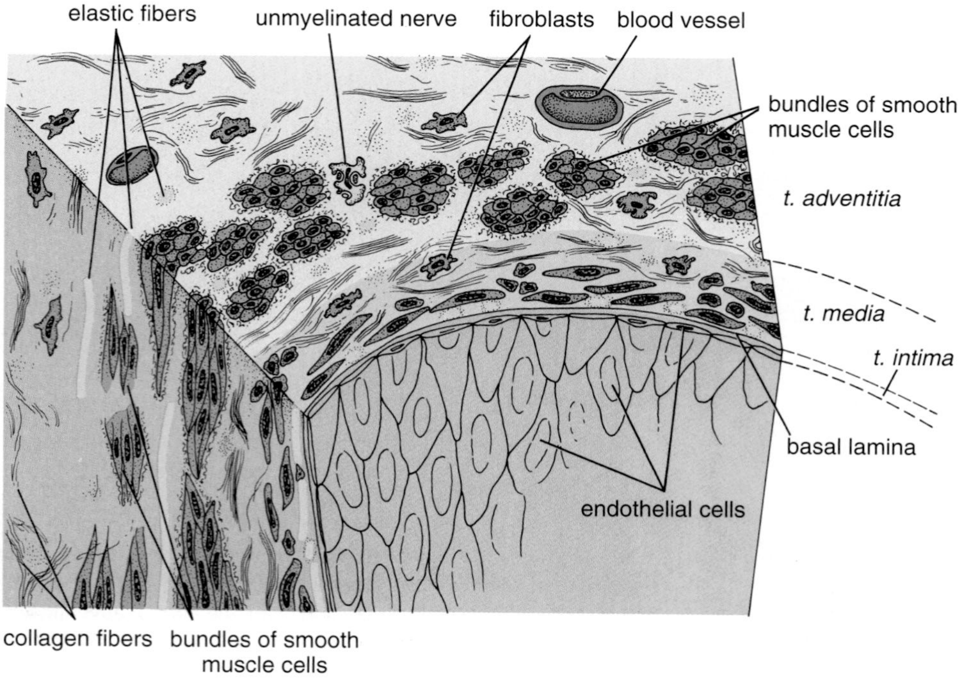

FIGURE 12.16
Schematic diagram of a large vein. The cellular and extracellular components are labeled. The tunica intima consists of an endothelial lining and a small amount of connective tissue. The tunica media contains circumferentially arranged smooth muscle cells. The tunica adventitia, in addition to an extensive collagenous and elastic fiber component, contains bundles of longitudinally arranged smooth muscle cells near the tunica media. *t.*, tunica. (Based on Rhodin JAG. *Handbook of Physiology*. New York: Oxford University Press, 1980.)

sel wall. Along with the usual collagen and elastic fibers and fibroblasts, the tunica adventitia also contains longitudinally disposed smooth muscle cells.

Atypical Veins

In several locations, veins with a highly atypical structure are present. For example, venous channels in the cranial cavity, called ***venous*** or ***dural sinuses,*** are essentially broad spaces in the dura mater that are lined with endothelial cells. Veins in certain other locations (e.g., retina, placenta, trabeculae of the spleen) also have atypical walls and are discussed in the chapters that describe these organs.

▽ HEART

The heart is a muscular pump that maintains unidirectional flow of blood

The heart contains four chambers, the right and left atria and right and left ventricles, through which blood is pumped (see Figs. 12.2 and 12.17). Valves guard the exits of the chambers, preventing backflow of blood. An ***interatrial septum*** and an ***interventricular septum*** separate the right and left sides of the heart. The ***right atrium*** receives blood returning from the body via the inferior and superior venae cavae, the two largest veins of the body. The ***right ventricle*** receives blood from the right atrium and pumps it to the lungs for oxygenation via the pulmonary arteries. The ***left atrium*** receives the oxygenated blood returning from the lungs via the four pulmonary veins. The ***left ventricle*** receives blood from the left atrium and pumps it into the aorta for distribution into the systemic circulation.

The walls of the heart contain

- A musculature of ***cardiac muscle*** for contraction to propel the blood.
- A ***fibrous skeleton,*** which consists of four fibrous rings surrounding the valve orifices, two fibrous trigones connecting the rings, and the membranous part of the interventricular and interatrial septa. The fibrous rings are composed of dense irregular connective tissue. They encircle the base of the two arteries leaving the heart (aorta and pulmonary trunk) and the openings between the atria and the ventricles (right and left A-V orifices) (Fig. 12.18). These rings provide the attachment site for the leaflets of all four valves of the heart that allow blood flow in only one direction through the openings. The membranous part of the interventricular septum is devoid of cardiac muscle; it consists of dense connective tissue that contains a short length of the un-

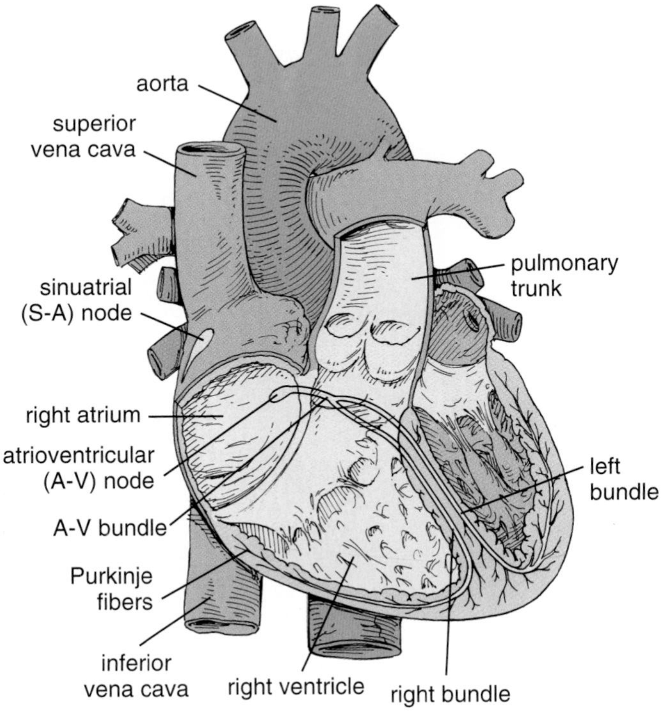

FIGURE 12.17
Chambers of the heart and the impulse-conducting system. The heart has been cut open in the coronal plane to expose its interior and the main parts of its impulse-conducting system *(indicated in yellow).* Impulses are generated in the sinuatrial (S-A) node; they are transmitted through the atrial wall to the atrioventricular (A-V) node and then along the A-V bundle to the Purkinje fibers.

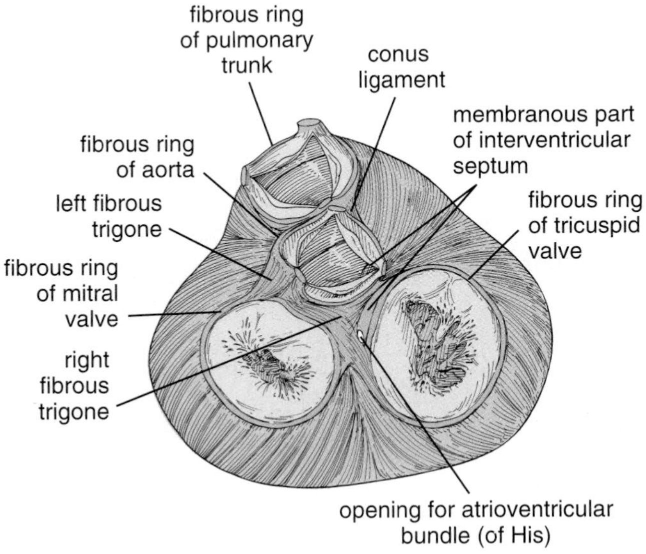

FIGURE 12.18
Fibrous skeleton of the heart as seen with the two atria removed. This fibrous network *(indicated in blue)* serves for the attachment of cardiac muscle; it also serves for the attachment of the cuspid valves between the atria and ventricles and for the semilunar valves of the aorta and the pulmonary artery. The atrioventricular bundle passes from the right atrium to the ventricular septum via the membranous septum of the fibrous skeleton.

branched atrioventricular (A-V) bundle of the cardiac conduction system. The fibrous skeleton provides independent attachments for the atrial and ventricular myocardium. It also acts as an electrical insulator by preventing the free flow of electrical impulses between atria and ventricles.

- An ***impulse-conducting system*** for initiation and propagation of electrical impulses for cardiac muscle contraction. It is formed by highly specialized cardiac muscle cells, which generate and conduct electrical impulses rapidly through the heart.

The wall of the heart is composed of three layers: epicardium, myocardium, and endocardium

The structural organization of the wall of the heart is continuous within the atria and ventricles (see Fig. 12.19). The wall of the heart is composed of three layers. From the outside to the inside they are

- ***Epicardium,*** consisting of a layer of mesothelial cells on the outer surface of the heart and its underlying connective tissue. The blood vessels and nerves that supply the heart lie in the epicardium and are surrounded by adipose tissue that cushions the heart in the pericardial cavity.
- ***Myocardium,*** consisting of cardiac muscle, the principal component of the heart. The myocardium of the ventricles is substantially thicker than that of the atria because of the large amount of cardiac muscle in the walls of the two pumping chambers.
- ***Endocardium,*** consisting of an inner layer of endothelium and subendothelial connective tissue, a middle layer of connective tissue and smooth muscle cells, and a deeper layer of connective tissue, also called the ***subendocardial layer,*** which is continuous with the connective tissue of the myocardium. The impulse-conducting system of the heart (see below) is located in the subendocardial layer of the endocardium.

The ***interventricular septum*** is the wall between the right and left ventricles. It contains cardiac muscle except in the membranous portion. Endocardium lines each surface of the interventricular septum. The ***interatrial septum***

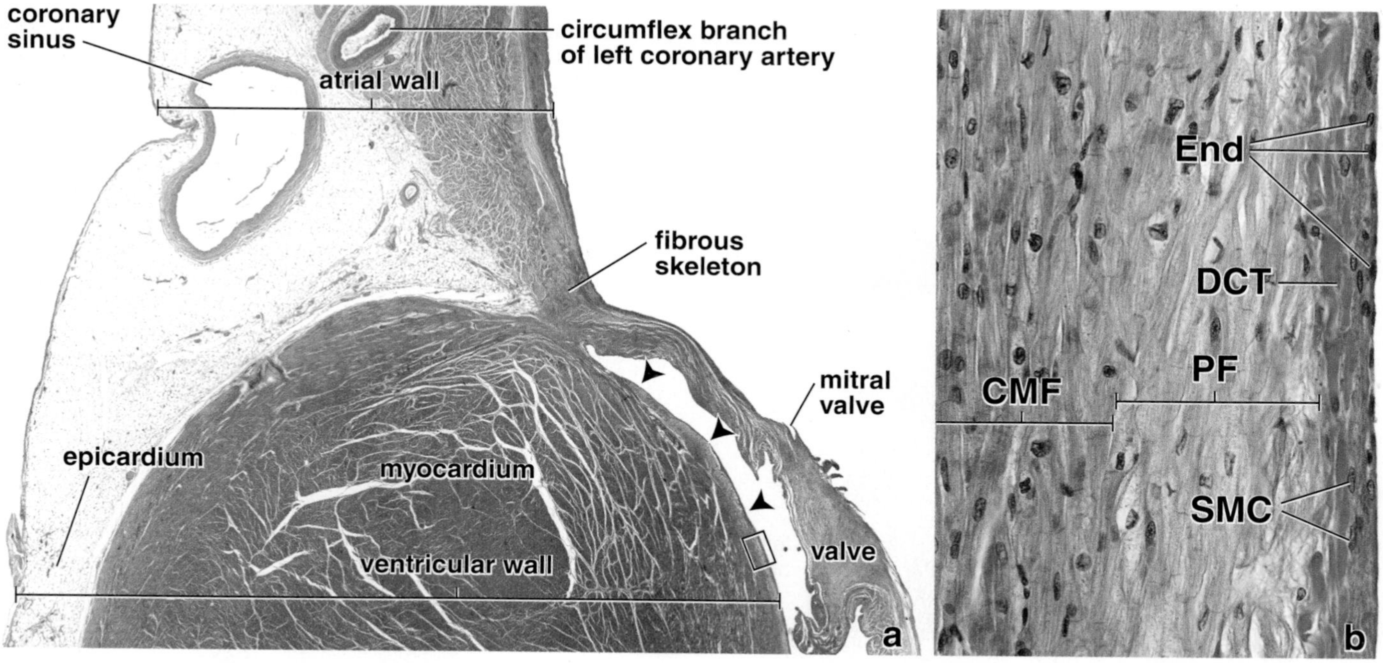

FIGURE 12.19
Photomicrograph of the left atrial and left ventricular wall. a. This photomicrograph shows a sagittal section of the posterior wall of the left atrium and left ventricle. The line of section crosses the coronary (A-V) groove containing the coronary sinus and circumflex branch of the left coronary artery. Note that the section has cut through the fibrous A-V ring of the mitral valve, which provides the attachment site for the muscle of the left atrium and the left ventricle and the cusp of the mitral valve. The ventricular wall consists of three layers: (1) endocardium *(arrowheads);* (2) myocardium; and (3) epicardium. The visible blood vessels lie in the epicardium and are surrounded by adipose tissue. The layers of the mitral valve are shown at higher magnification in Figure 12.20. ×35. **b.** This high magnification of the area indicated by the *rectangle* in *a* shows the characteristic features of the inner surface of the heart. Note that the endocardium consists of a squamous inner layer of endothelium *(End),* a middle layer of subendothelial dense connective tissue *(DCT)* containing smooth muscle cells *(SMC),* and a deeper subendocardial layer containing Purkinje fibers *(PF).* The myocardium contains cardiac muscle fibers *(CMF)* and is seen on the left. ×120.

is much thinner than the interventricular septum. Except in certain localized areas that contain fibrous tissue, it has a center layer of cardiac muscle and a lining of endocardium facing each chamber.

Heart valves are vascular structures composed of connective tissue with overlying endocardium

The heart valves attach to the complex framework of dense irregular connective tissue that forms the fibrous rings and surrounds the orifices containing the valves. Each valve is composed of three layers (Fig. 12.20):

- ***Fibrosa*** forms the core of the valve and contains fibrous extensions from the dense irregular connective tissue of the skeletal rings of the heart.
- ***Spongiosa*** represents loose connective tissue located on the atrial and/or blood vessel side of each valve. It is composed of loosely arranged collagen and elastic fibers infiltrated with a large amount of proteoglycans. The spongiosa acts as a shock absorber as it dampens vibrations associated with the closing of the valve. It also confers flexibility and plasticity to the valve cusps. In the aortic and pulmonary valves, spongiosa located on the blood vessel side is called ***arterialis.*** It corresponds to the loose connective tissue located on the atrial side of the A-V (tricuspid and mitral) valves, called the ***auricularis.***
- ***Ventricularis*** is immediately adjacent to the ventricular and/or atrial surface of each valve and is covered with endothelium. It contains dense connective tissue with many layers of elastic fibers. In the A-V valves, the ventricularis continues into the ***chordae tendineae,*** which are fibrous, thread-like cords also covered with endothelium. They extend from the free edge of the A-V valves to muscular projections from the wall of the ventricles, called ***papillary muscles.***

Valve cusps are normally avascular. Small blood vessels and smooth muscle can be found only in the base of the cusp. The surfaces of the valve are exposed to blood, and the cusps are thin enough to allow nutrients and oxygen to diffuse from the blood.

Several diseases affect the valves of the heart, causing their degeneration (e.g., calcification, fibrosis) and resulting in heart malfunction due to insufficiency or stenosis of valvular orifices. These conditions, known collectively as valvular heart disease, include rheumatic heart disease, vegetative endocarditis, degenerative calcific aortic valve stenosis, and mitral annular calcification. Rheumatic fever, e.g., causes inflammation of the heart valves (valvulitis). Inflammation induces angiogenesis in the valve and vascularization in the normally avascular layers of the valve. These changes most commonly affect the mitral valve (65 to 70%) and aortic valve (20 to 25%). This inflammation can lead to progressive replacement of elastic tissue by irregular masses of collagen fibers, causing the valve to thicken. The valves become rigid and inflexible, which affects their ability to open and close.

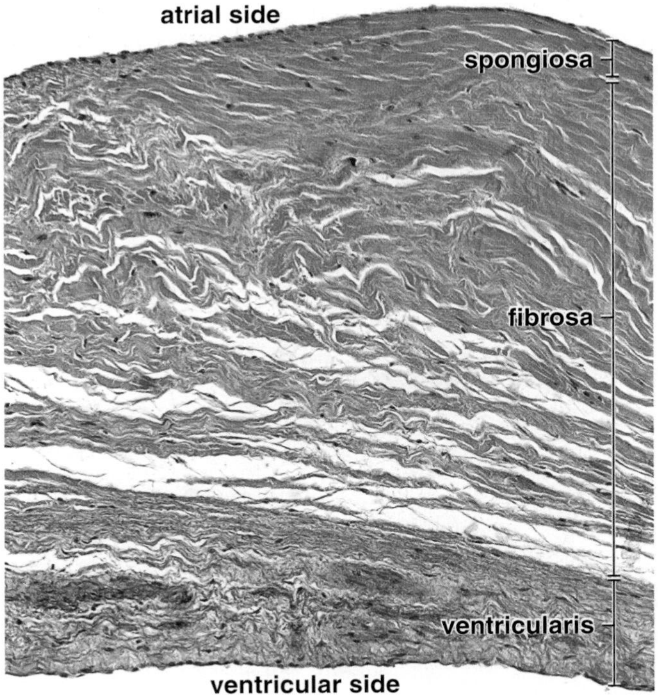

FIGURE 12.20
Photomicrograph of a mitral valve. This photomicrograph shows a section through one of the two cusps of the mitral valve near its attachment to the fibrous ring. Both sides of the cusp are covered by the endothelium. Note that the valve exhibits a layered architecture. Beginning at the atrial side *(top of the image),* the first layer underlying the endothelium is the spongiosa—not well developed in this part of the cusp. The second layer is the fibrosa, which forms the majority of the dense connective tissue in the core of the valve. The third layer, the ventricularis, is formed by dense connective tissue containing layers of elastic and collagen fibers. ×125.

Intrinsic Regulation of Heart Rate

Contraction of the heart is synchronized by specialized cardiac muscle fibers

Cardiac muscle can contract in a rhythmic manner without any direct stimulus from the nervous system. The pace of the beating action in the heart is initiated at the ***sinuatrial (S-A) node,*** a group of specialized cardiac muscle cells located near the junction of the superior vena cava and the right atrium (see Fig. 12.17). The S-A node is also referred to as the ***pacemaker.*** The pacemaker rate of the S-A node is about 60 to 100/min. The S-A node initiates an impulse that spreads along the cardiac muscle fibers of the atria and along internodal tracts composed of modified cardiac muscle fibers. The impulse is then picked up at the ***atrioventricular (A-V) node*** and conducted across the fi-

brous skeleton to the ventricles by the ***atrioventricular (A-V) bundle (of His)***. The bundle divides into smaller ***right*** and ***left bundle branches*** and then into ***subendothelial branches*** commonly called ***Purkinje fibers***.

The A-V bundle, the bundle branches, and the Purkinje fibers are modified cardiac muscle cells that are specialized to conduct impulses (Fig. 12.21). The nodes and A-V bundle and its branches are modified cardiac muscle fibers that are smaller than normal. The Purkinje fibers are modified cardiac muscle fibers that are larger than normal. The components of the conducting system convey the impulse at a rate approximately 4 times faster than the cardiac muscle fibers and are the only elements that can convey impulses across the fibrous skeleton. The conducting system also coordinates the contractions of the atria and ventricles. The contraction is initiated in the atria, forcing blood into the ventricles. A wave of contraction in the ventricles then begins at the apex of the heart, forcing blood from the heart through the aorta and pulmonary trunk.

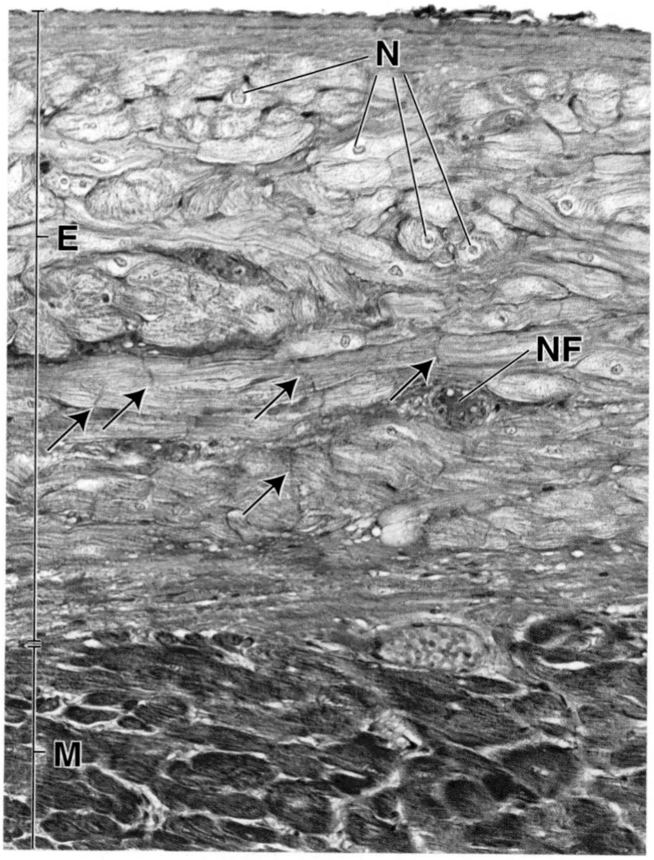

FIGURE 12.21
Photomicrograph of the ventricular wall containing the conducting system. This photomicrograph shows a Mallory-Azan–stained section of the ventricular wall of a human heart. The upper two thirds of the micrograph is occupied by the endocardium *(E)* containing a thick layer of Purkinje fibers. The free luminal surface of the ventricle *(top)* is covered by endothelium and an underlying layer of subendothelial connective tissue *(stained blue)*. The deep layer of endocardium contains the Purkinje fibers. Note the intercalated disks in the fibers *(arrows)*. The Purkinje fibers contain large amounts of glycogen, which appear as homogeneous, pale-staining regions that occupy the center portion of the cell surrounded by the myofibrils. The nuclei *(N)* are round and are larger than the nuclei of the cardiac muscle cells in the myocardium *(M)*. They are frequently surrounded by the lighter-stained cytoplasm that represents the juxtanuclear region of the cell. Because of the considerable size of the Purkinje cells, the nuclei are often not included in the section. Among the Purkinje fibers course nerves *(NF)* that belong to the autonomic nervous system. ×320.

Systemic Regulation of Heart Function

The heart is innervated by both divisions of the autonomic nervous system. The autonomic nerves do not initiate contraction of the cardiac muscle but rather regulate the heart rate according to the body's immediate needs. Parasympathetic fibers terminate chiefly at the S-A and A-V nodes but also extend into the myocardium. Sympathetic fibers supply the S-A and A-V nodes, extend into the myocardium, and also pass through the epicardium to reach the coronary arteries that supply the heart. The autonomic fibers regulate only the rate of impulses emanating from the S-A node. The sympathetic component causes the rate of contraction to increase; the parasympathetic component causes the rate of contraction to decrease.

BOX 12.3

Clinical Correlations: Ischemic Heart Disease

Ischemic heart disease is defined as the imbalance between the supply and demand of the heart for oxygenated blood. The most common cause of ischemic heart disease is ***atherosclerosis.*** In atherosclerosis, the lumina of the coronary arteries progressively narrow because of accumulation of ***fibrofatty intimal plaques*** (see Fig. 12.10). Plaques are formed by lipid deposition, smooth muscle proliferation, and increased synthesis of proteoglycans and collagen within the intima. Blood flow becomes critical when it is reduced by 90%. A sudden occlusion of the narrowed lumen by a thrombus, or clot, released from the surface of an atheromatous plaque precipitates an acute ischemic event. Ischemic events are characterized by ***anginal pain*** associated with the loss of oxygenated blood to the region of the heart supplied by the affected coronary vessel. Coronary artery thrombosis usually precedes and precipitates a myocardial infarct, i.e., a sudden insufficiency of blood supply that results in an area of muscle cell death. With time, a scar forms and replaces the damaged tissue, but the area of infarction loses contractile function. Multiple infarctions over time can produce sufficient loss of cardiac function to cause death. Infarction also commonly occurs in the brain, spleen, kidney, lung, intestine, testes, and tumors (especially of the ovaries and uterus). The risk of developing atherosclerosis increases with age, family history, hypertension, cigarette smoking, hypercholesterolemia, and diabetes.

Specialized receptors monitor heart function

Specialized sensory nerve receptors for physiologic reflexes are located in the walls of large blood vessels near the heart. They function as

- ***Baroreceptors,*** which sense general blood pressure. These receptors are located in the carotid sinus and aortic arch.
- ***Chemoreceptors,*** which detect alterations in oxygen and carbon dioxide tension and in pH. These receptors are the ***carotid*** and ***aortic bodies*** located at the bifurcation of the carotid arteries and in the aortic arch, respectively.

The carotid body consists of cords and irregular groups of epithelioid cells. A rich supply of nerve fibers is associated with these cells. The neural elements are both afferent and efferent. The structure of the aortic bodies is essentially similar to that of the carotid bodies. Both receptors function in neural reflexes that adjust cardiac output and respiratory rate.

▽ LYMPHATIC VESSELS

Lymphatic vessels convey fluids from the tissues to the bloodstream

In addition to blood vessels, another set of vessels circulates fluid, called ***lymph,*** through most parts of the body. These ***lymphatic vessels*** serve as adjuncts to the blood vessels. Unlike the blood vessels, which convey blood to and from tissues, the lymphatic vessels are unidirectional, conveying fluid only from tissues. The smallest lymphatic vessels are called ***lymphatic capillaries.*** They are especially numerous in the loose connective tissues under the epithelium of the skin and mucous membranes. The lymphatic capillaries begin as "blind-ending" tubes in the microcapillary beds (see Fig. 12.13). Lymphatic capillaries converge into increasingly larger vessels, called ***lymphatic vessels,*** which ultimately unite to form two main channels that empty into the blood vascular system by draining into the large veins in the base of the neck. They enter the vascular system at the junctions of the internal jugular and subclavian veins. The largest lymphatic vessel, draining most of the body and emptying into the veins on the left side, is the ***thoracic duct.*** The other main channel is the ***right lymphatic trunk.***

Lymphatic capillaries are more permeable than blood capillaries and collect excess protein-rich tissue fluid

Lymphatic capillaries are a unique part of the circulatory system that form a network of small vessels within the tissues. Because of their greater permeability, lymphatic capillaries are more effective than blood capillaries in removing protein-rich fluid from the intercellular spaces. Once the collected fluid enters the lymphatic vessel it is called lymph. Lymphatic vessels also serve to convey proteins and lipids that are too large to cross the fenestrations of the absorptive capillaries in the small intestine.

Before lymph is returned to the blood, it passes through ***lymph nodes,*** where it is exposed to the cells of the immune system. Thus, the lymphatic vessels serve not only as an adjunct to the blood vascular system but also as an integral component of the immune system.

Lymphatic capillaries are essentially tubes of endothelium that, unlike the typical blood capillary, lack a continuous basal lamina. This incomplete basal lamina can be correlated with their high permeability. ***Anchoring filaments*** extend between the incomplete basal lamina and the perivascular collagen. These filaments may help maintain the patency of the vessels during times of increased tissue pressure, as in inflammation.

As lymphatic vessels become larger, the wall becomes thicker. The increasing thickness is due to connective tissue and bundles of smooth muscle. Lymphatic vessels possess valves that prevent backflow of the lymph, thus aiding unidirectional flow. There is no central pump in the lymphatic system. Lymph moves sluggishly, driven primarily by compression of the lymphatic vessels by adjacent skeletal muscles.

PLATE 28. HEART

The cardiovascular system is a transport system that carries blood and lymph to and from the tissues of the body. The cardiovascular system includes the heart, blood vessels, and lymphatic vessels. Blood vessels provide the route by which blood circulates to and from all parts of the body. The heart pumps the blood. Lymphatic vessels carry tissue-derived fluid, called lymph, back to the blood vascular system.

The heart is a four-chambered organ consisting of a right and left atrium and a right and left ventricle. Blood from the body is returned to the right atrium from which it is delivered to the right ventricle. Blood is pumped from the right ventricle to the lungs for oxygenation and returns to the left atrium. Blood from the left atrium is delivered to the left ventricle from which it is pumped to the rest of the body, i.e., the systemic circulation.

The heart, which differentiates from a straight vascular tube in the embryo, has the same basic three-layered structure in its wall as do the blood vessels above the level of capillaries and postcapillary venules. In the blood vessels, the three layers are called the *tunica intima,* including the vascular endothelium and its underlying connective tissue; the *tunica media,* a muscular layer that varies in thickness in arteries and veins; and the *tunica adventitia,* the outermost layer of relatively dense connective tissue. In the heart, these layers are called the *endocardium,* the *myocardium,* and the *epicardium,* respectively.

Figure 1, heart, atrioventricular septum, human, H&E ×45; inset ×125.

This micrograph of the field shows portions of the atrial *(A)* and ventricular *(V)* walls at the level of the atrioventricular septum and the root of the mitral valve *(MV).* Both chambers and the valve are lined with the squamous endothelium of the endocardium *(En).* Purkinje fibers *(PF)* of the cardiac conduction system are seen in the atrial wall between the relatively thin subendocardial connective tissue *(CT)* and the underlying modified cardiac muscle cells *(CM)* of the atrioventricular node *(AVN).* Some of the adipose tissue *(AT)* that forms a major component of the septum and serves to cushion the heart is seen near the lower left corner of the *image.* Dense fibrous connective tissue *(DCT)* that is continuous with that of the septum and the subendocardial layers of the atrium and ventricle extends from the root of the valve into the leaflet. Thin cardiac muscle fibers can also be seen extending from the wall of the atrium into the upper portion of the valve. **Inset.** This higher-magnification view of the field outlined by the *rectangle* (turned ~90°) shows more clearly the endothelial layer of the endocardium *(En)* and the dense fibrous connective tissue of the endocardium *(DCT)* and subendocardial layer. A thin layer of smooth muscle *(SM)* appears between the more densely packed fibrous tissue immediately subjacent to the endothelium and the more loosely packed dense fibrous tissue of the subendocardium. Particularly evident are the longitudinally sectioned Purkinje fibers *(PF)* of the cardiac conduction system. These modified cardiac muscle cells contain the same fibrillar contractile system as their smaller counterparts in the myocardium, but the fibrils are fewer, are more loosely packed, and often surround what appear to be vacuolated areas. Intercalated disks *(ID),* typical of cardiac muscle cell organization, are evident in some areas.

Figure 2, Heart, atrioventricular septum, coronary artery and cardiac vein, human, H&E ×30.

This micrograph shows cross sections of a coronary artery and cardiac vein in the atrioventricular septum. The coronary artery *(CA)* in the lower left of this micrograph is surrounded by small bundles of small cardiac muscle cells *(CM)* that are part of the atrioventricular node *(AVN).* A loop of the conduction bundle *(CB)* containing Purkinje fibers is evident to the right of the artery. The darkly stained tunica intima *(TI)* is delimited by an internal elastic membrane *(IEM)* that is easily distinguished even at this relatively low magnification. The thick muscular tunica media *(TM)* is also easily distinguished from the thinner, fibrous tunica adventitia *(TA).* A smaller arterial vessel *(A′)* is seen in the adipose tissue near the upper left edge of the figure. The cardiac vein *(CV)* is much larger than the corresponding artery and occupies most of the field. In this vessel, the tunica intima *(TI)* appears denser than either of the other two layers, which are, themselves, impossible to distinguish at this magnification. The fibrous nature of the media and adventitia of the vein is evident, however. In this particular preparation, remnants of fixed blood *(B)* are evident in all three vessels. A small lymph node *(LN)* is seen adjacent to the coronary artery.

KEY

A, atrium
A′, artery
AT, adipose tissue
AVN, atrioventricular node
B, blood
CA, coronary artery
CB, conduction bundle
CM, cardiac muscle
CT, connective tissue
CV, cardiac vein
DCT, dense connective tissue
En, endothelium
ID, intercalated disk
IEM, internal elastic membrane
LN, lymph node
MF, muscle fibers
MV, mitral valve
PF, Purkinje fibers
SM, smooth muscle
TA, tunica adventitia
TM, tunica media
TI, tunica intima
V, ventricle

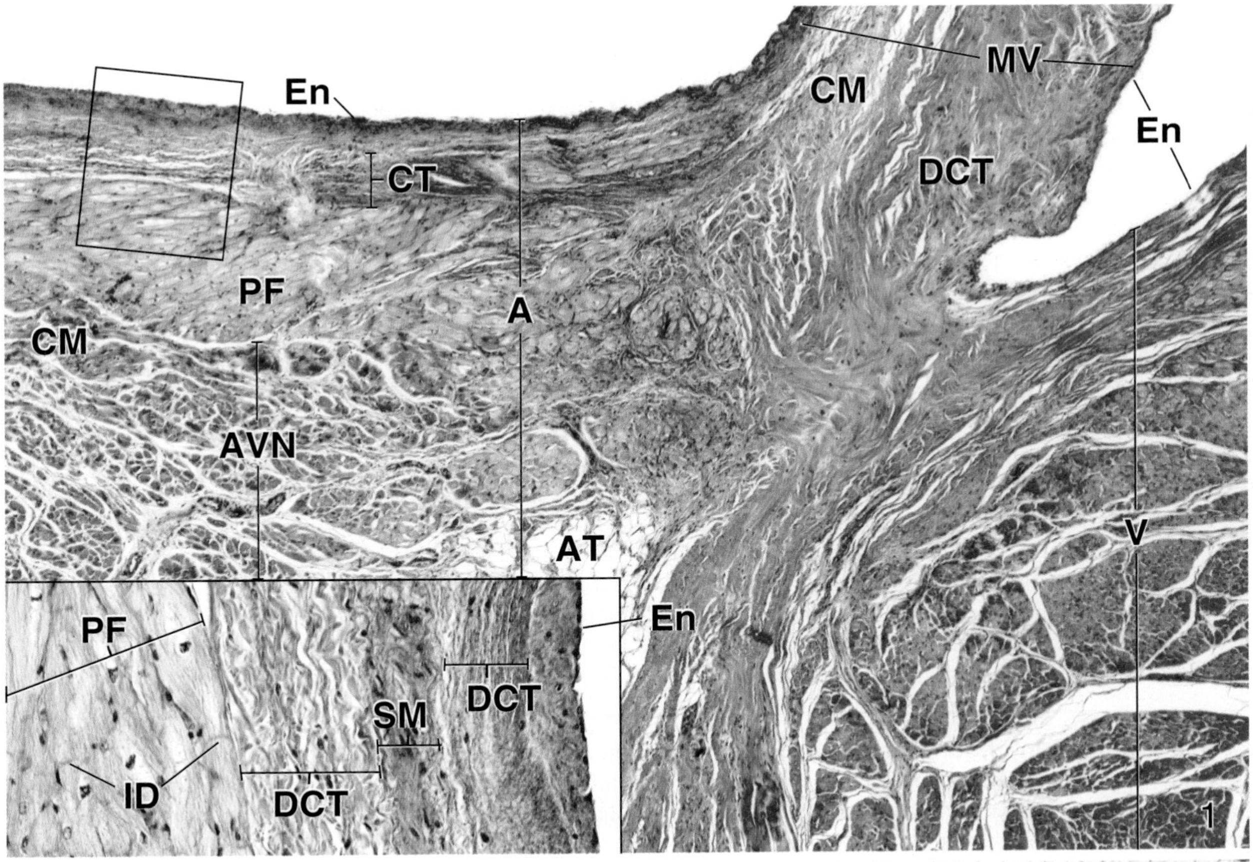
MV
En
CM
DCT
En
CT
A
PF
CM
AVN
AT
V
PF
En
DCT
SM
ID
DCT
1

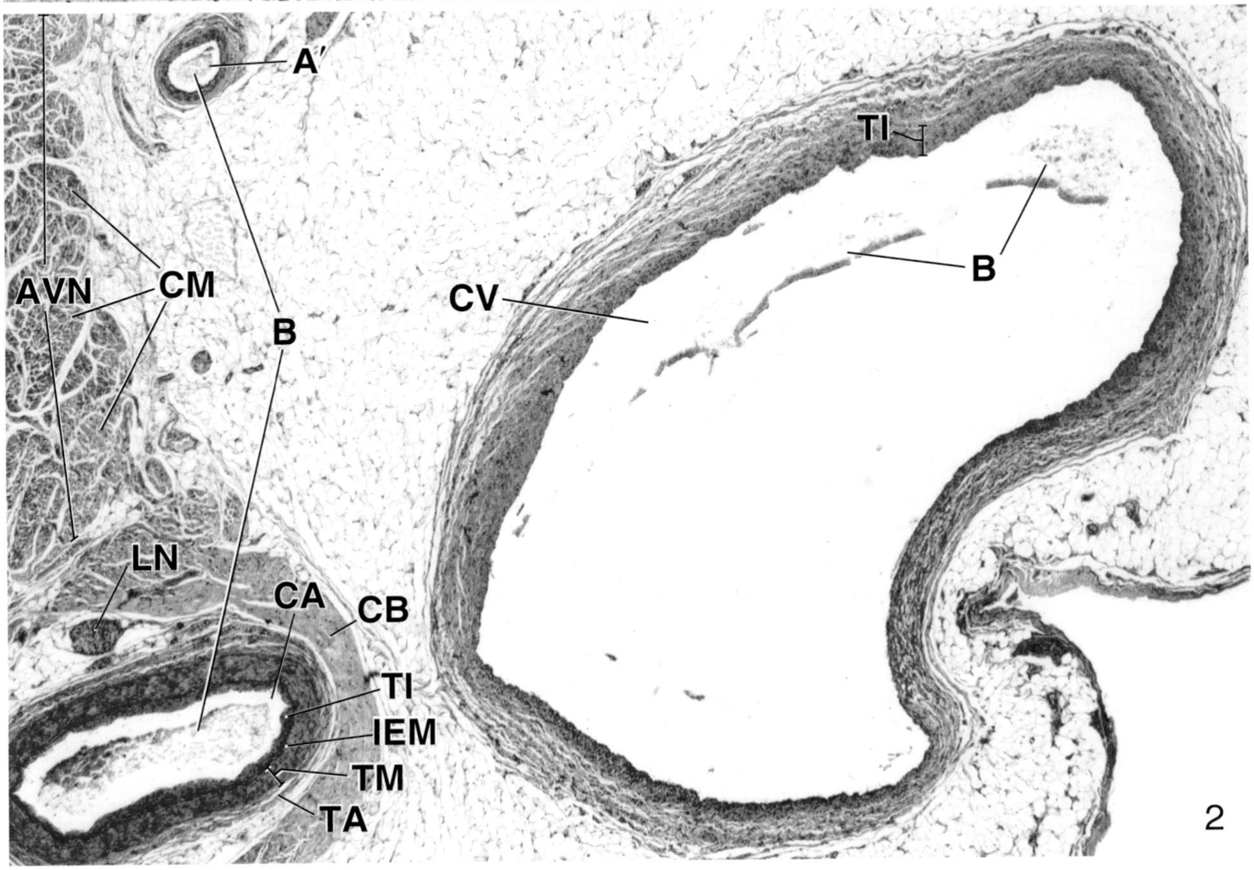
A
TI
B
AVN
CM
CV
B
LN
CA
CB
TI
IEM
TM
TA
2

PLATE 29. AORTA

Arteries are the blood vessels that carry blood from the heart to the capillaries in the tissues. Arteries are classified by their diameter and by the characteristics of the tunica media. The aorta is the artery that carries blood away from the left ventricle. It is called an *elastic artery* because of the large amount of elastic material, arranged as fenestrated lamellae, interspersed with the smooth muscle cells of the tunica media. The elastic lamellae in the aorta allow it to resist the pressure variations caused by the beating of the ventricle and to produce a relatively steady flow of blood into the arterial system. The elastic material may be seen because of its refractivity but is most easily demonstrated with special stains. Elastic arteries, also called conducting arteries, include the brachiocephalic, the subclavian, the beginning of the common carotid, and the pulmonary arteries.

Figure 1, aorta, human, H&E ×65.
The layers that make up the wall of the aorta are shown in this figure. This is a longitudinal section through the entire thickness of the arterial wall. Three layers can usually be recognized: the tunica intima *(TI)*, tunica media *(TM)*, and tunica adventitia *(TA)*. The tunica adventitia is the outermost part. It consists mainly of connective tissue and contains the blood vessels (vasa vasorum) and nerves (nervi vascularis) that supply the arterial wall.

Figure 2, aorta, human, H&E ×160.
The tunica intima *(TI)* is shown here at higher magnification. The boundary between it and the tissue below, the tunica media, is not sharply defined. Largely because of staining characteristics and degree of cellularity, the two tunics are more easily distinguished at low magnification (Fig. 1). The tunica intima consists of a lining of endothelial cells that rest on a layer of connective tissue. However, the endothelium is difficult to preserve in these vessels and is frequently lost. Both collagenous fibers and elastic lamellae are in the connective tissue. Smooth muscle cells are also present in the intima of the aorta *(arrows)*.

Figure 3, aorta, human, resorcin-fuchsin ×65.
The tunica media contains an abundance of smooth muscle; the more distinctive feature, however, is its large amount of elastic material. The elastic material is present not in the form of fibers but as fenestrated membranes. This figure and the higher magnification (Fig. 5) are from a specimen stained to demonstrate elastic material. This figure reveals elastic laminae present in the tunica media *(TM)* as well as the deep portion of the tunica intima *(TI)*. The tunica adventitia *(TA)*, however, essentially lacks these elastic laminae.

Figure 4, aorta, human, H&E ×160.
This figure shows a higher magnification of the tunica media of Figure 1. Here, the elastic lamellae are unstained, as is usually the case in H&E sections. (In some instances, the elastic material will stain lightly with eosin.) The *arrowheads* reveal the sites of some of the lamellae. Their presence is recognized by the apparent absence of structure, which, in turn, is due to the absence of staining of the elastic material. The smooth muscle cells of the media are arranged in a closely wound spiral between the elastic membranes. This arrangement, however, is difficult to recognize in sectioned material.

Figure 5, aorta, human, resorcin-fuchsin ×300.
Careful examination of the tunica media at higher magnification reveals what appear to be interruptions of some of the elastic lamellae. These are actually the fenestrations or openings in the elastic membranes.

Figure 6, aorta, human, H&E ×160.
The outermost layer of the aorta, the tunica adventitia, is shown here. The tunica adventitia *(TA)* consists mostly of collagenous fibers that course in longitudinal spirals. (Their course, like that of the smooth muscle fibers, however, is unrecognizable in tissue sections.) There are no elastic lamellae in the adventitia, but elastic fibers are present, though relatively few in number. The cells of the adventitia, represented by the nuclei seen in the adventitia, are fibroblasts. Occasionally, ganglion cells are present, as well as some scattered smooth muscle cells. The ganglion cells, when present, are quite conspicuous, whereas the smooth muscle cells may be overlooked.

KEY

TA, tunica adventitia
TI, tunica intima
TM, tunica media
arrows (Fig. 2), smooth muscle cell
arrowheads (Fig. 4), unstained elastic lamellae

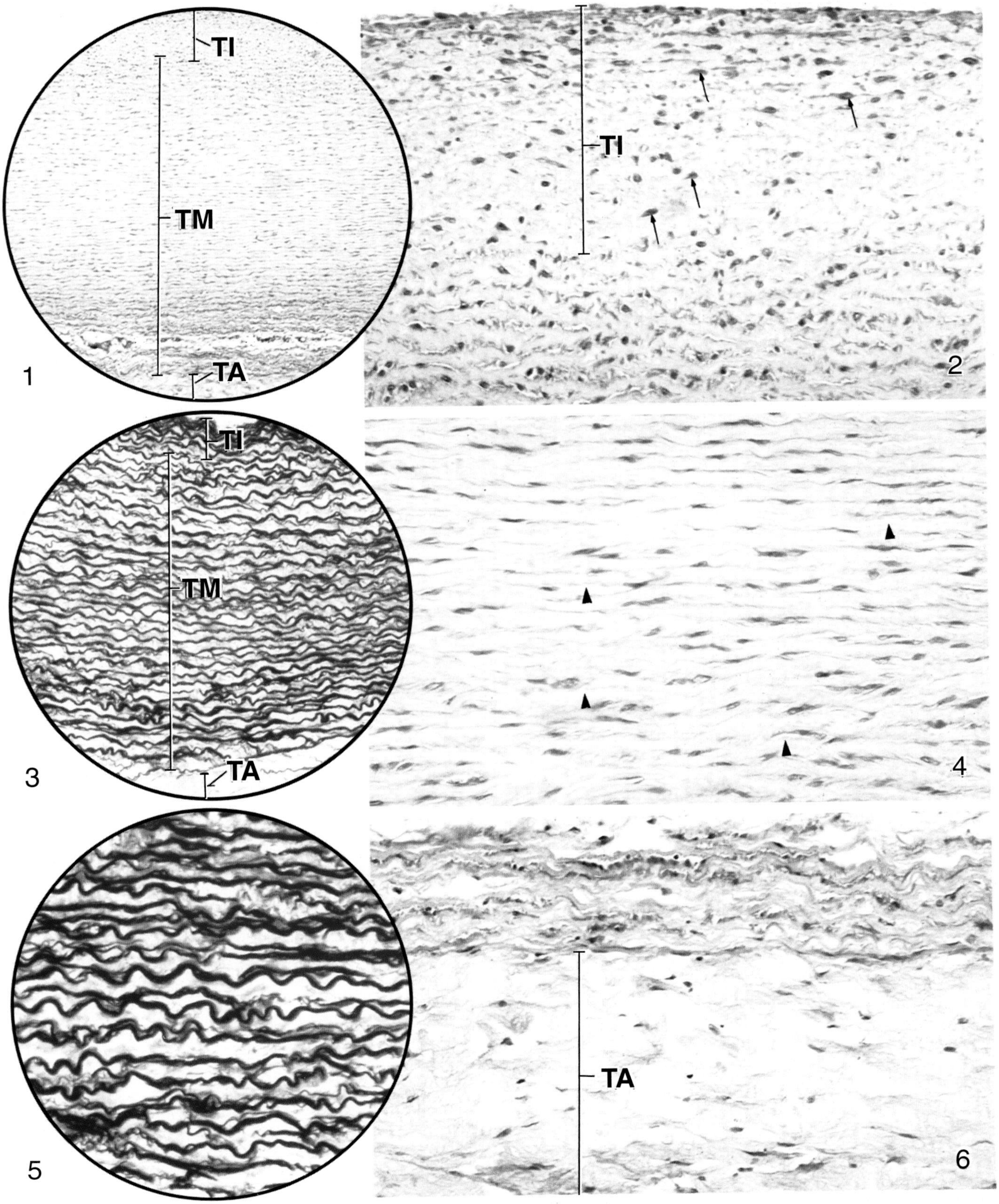
TI
TM
TA
1
TI
2
TI
TM
TA
3
4
5
TA
6

PLATE 30. MUSCULAR ARTERIES AND VEINS

Muscular arteries have more smooth muscle and less elastin in the tunica media than do elastic arteries. Thus, as the arterial tree is traced further from the heart, the elastic tissue is considerably reduced and smooth muscle becomes the predominant component of the tunica media. The muscular arteries are characterized, however, by a refractile *internal elastic lamina* separating the tunica intima from the tunica media and, usually, by an *external elastic lamina* separating the tunica media from the tunica adventitia. Muscular arteries, or arteries of medium caliber, constitute the majority of the named arteries in the body. Veins usually accompany arteries as they travel in the loose connective tissue. The veins have the same three layers in their walls, but the tunica media is thinner than in the accompanying artery, and the tunica adventitia is the predominant layer in the wall. The veins usually have the same name as the artery they accompany.

Figure 1, muscular artery and vein, monkey, H&E ×365.

In this photomicrograph, the lumen of the artery is at the right; the lumen of the vein is at the left. The arterial endothelium *(AEn)* is clearly seen on the corrugated surface of the tunica intima, whereas the venous endothelium *(VEn)* is somewhat harder to distinguish. The internal elastic lamina *(IEL)* is seen as a thin clear zone immediately beneath the endothelial layer, separating the tunica intima from the underlying smooth muscle *(SM)* of the tunica media *(TM)*. It is evident here that the tunica media is almost twice as thick as the tunica adventitia *(TA′)* even if the outer border of the latter is obscured by its blending almost imperceptibly with loose connective tissue separating it from the tunica adventitia of the accompanying vein *(TA)*. The arterial tunica adventitia is identified by the elastic fibers *(EF)* in it. In this specimen, only a few small smooth muscle cells *(SSm)* are visible in the tunica media of the vein. The tunica adventitia *(TA)* is much thicker than the tunica media and is characterized by a pale extracellular compartment containing a small number of cell nuclei *(N)*, most of which appear to be those of fibroblasts, and a sparsity of elastic fibers.

Figure 2, muscular artery, monkey, H&E ×545.

This is a higher-magnification micrograph of the portion of the figure above outlined by the *rectangle* turned 90°. At this magnification, it is evident that the flattened endothelial cells *(EN)* follow the contours of the refractile, corrugated internal elastic lamina *(IEL)*, which rests directly on the most luminal layer of smooth muscle cells *(SM)* of the thick tunica media *(TM)*. The thinner tunica adventitia *(TA′)* is recognized by the presence of numerous elastic fibers *(EF)* separating collagen bundles *(C)*. Nuclei *(N)* in this layer are those of fibroblasts.

Figure 3, medium vein, monkey, H&E ×600.

In this higher-magnification view of a portion of the wall of the vein in the figure above, the endothelial cells *(EN)* are more easily recognized and are seen to be plumper than those of the arterial endothelium. The margin between the tunica intima *(TI)* and the thin tunica media *(TM)* is difficult to discern, but the smooth muscle cells *(SM)* in the thin media are more easily recognized than in the figure above because of the shape of their nuclei and the slight basophilia of their cytoplasm. The tunica adventitia *(TA)* is about twice as thick as the tunica media and appears to contain only bundles of collagen fibers and fibroblasts, with the latter recognizable by their nuclei *(N)*. The collagen bundles of the loose connective tissue beneath the tunica adventitia are larger than those of the adventitia, and there are fewer cells in this portion of the specimen.

KEY

AEn, arterial endothelium
C, collagen bundles
EF, elastic fibers
EN, endothelial cells
IEL, internal elastic lamina
N, nuclei
SM, smooth muscle
SSm, small smooth muscle
TA′, tunica adventitia of artery
TA, tunica adventitia of accompanying vein
TI, tunica intima
TM, tunica media
VEn, venous endothelium

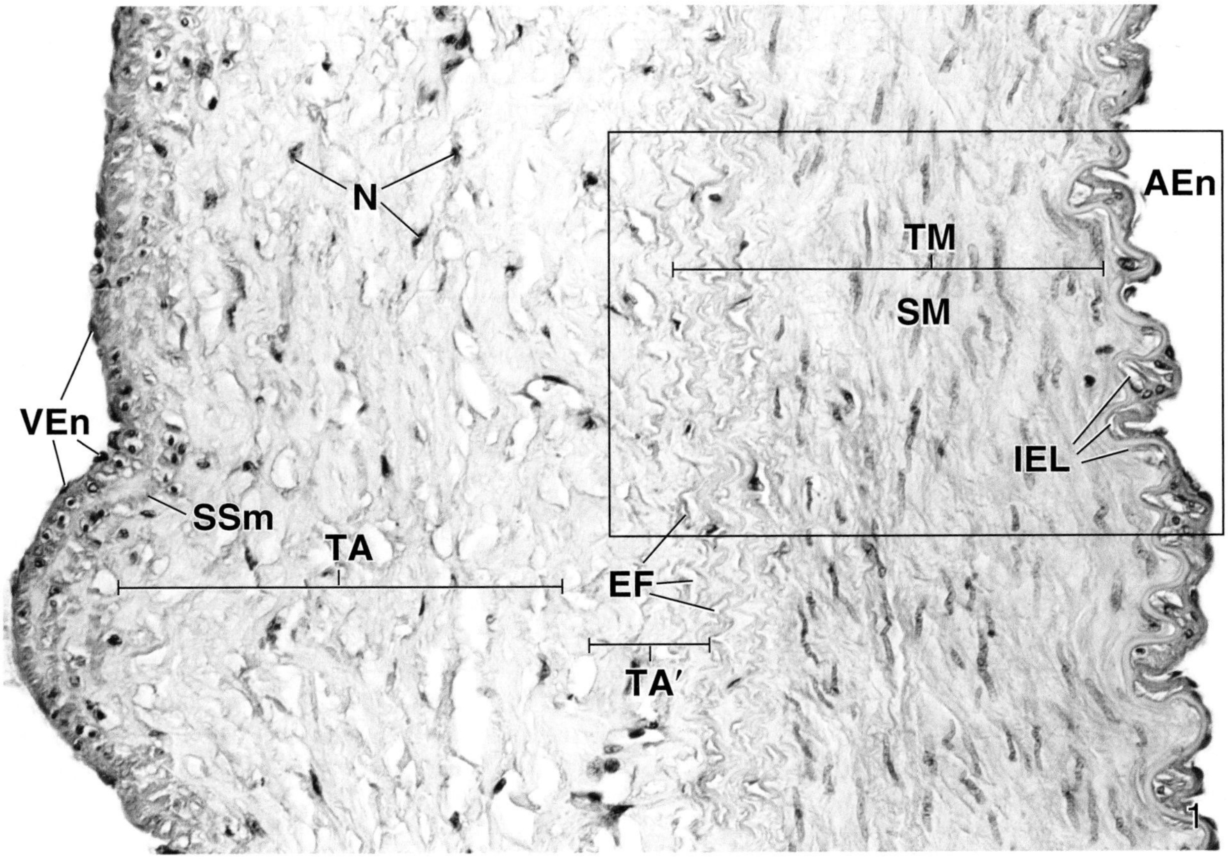
N
AEn
TM
SM
VEn
IEL
SSm
TA
EF
TA′
1

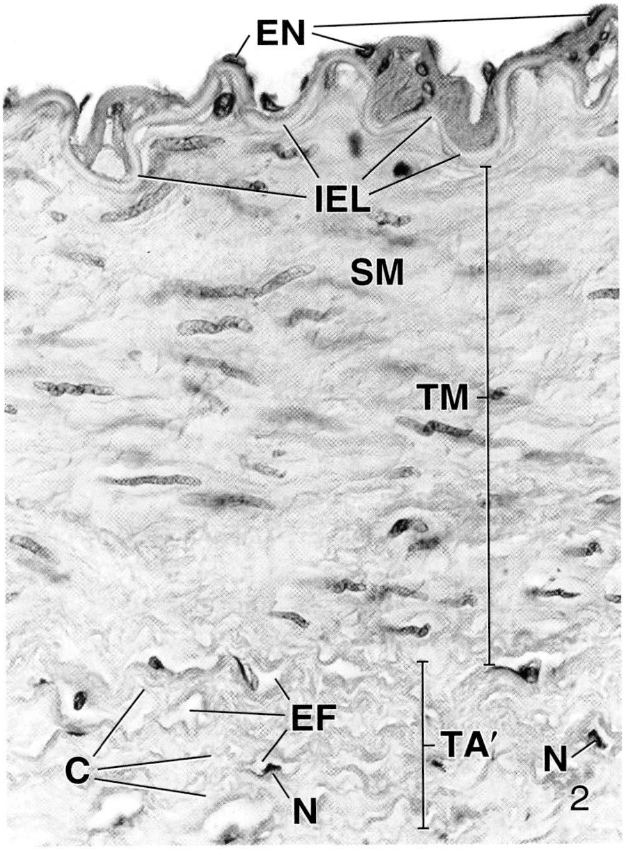
EN
IEL
SM
TM
EF
C
TA′
N
N
2

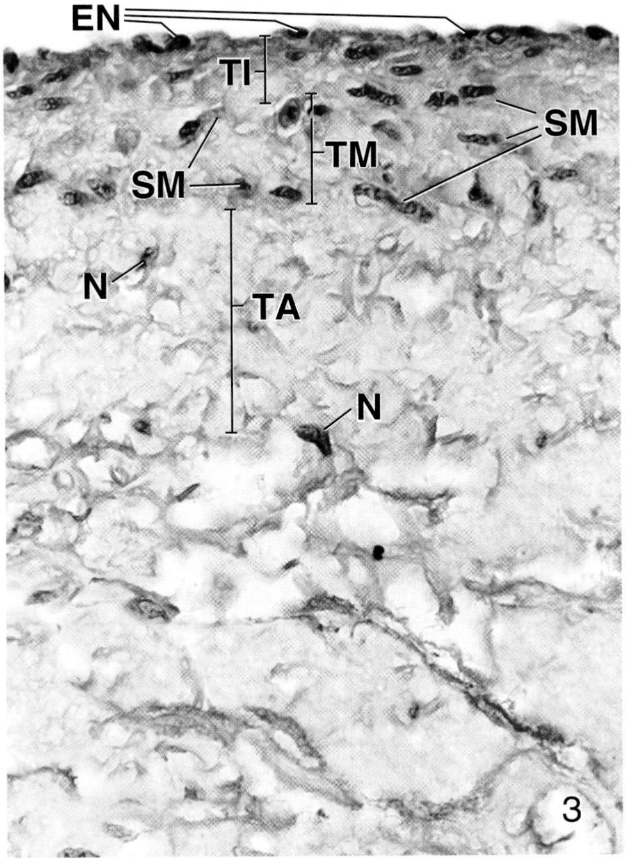
EN
TI
SM
TM
SM
N
TA
N
3

PLATE 31. ARTERIOLES AND LYMPHATIC VESSELS

The terminal components of the arterial tree just before a capillary bed or an arteriovenous shunt are the *arterioles.* Arterioles have an endothelial lining and smooth muscle in the wall but the smooth muscle is limited in thickness to one or two cells. There may or may not be an internal elastic membrane, according to the size of the vessel. Arterioles control blood flow into capillary networks. In the normal relationship between an arteriole and a capillary network, contraction of the smooth muscle of the arteriole wall reduces or shuts off the blood going to the capillaries. A *precapillary sphincter* is formed by a slight thickening of the smooth muscle at the origin of a capillary bed from an arteriole. Nerve impulses and hormonal stimulation can cause the muscle cells to contract, directing blood into capillary beds where it is most needed.

Figure 1, arteriole, venule, and small nerve, human, H&E ×600.

This micrograph shows two cross-sectioned arterioles *(A)* and a venule *(V).* The arteriole on the left is identified as a large arteriole, based on the presence of two discrete layers of smooth muscle cells that form the tunica media of the vessel. The nuclei of the muscle cells appear in longitudinal profile as a result of the circumferential arrangement of the cells. The endothelial cell nuclei of the vessel appear as small round profiles surrounding the lumen. These cells are elongate and oriented with their long axis in the direction of flow. Thus, their nuclei are seen here as cross-sectioned profiles. The arteriole on the right is a very small arteriole, having only a single layer of smooth muscle. Again, the muscle cell nuclei are seen in longitudinal profile. The endothelial cell nuclei appear as the small round profiles at the luminal surface. A venule is seen in proximity to the larger arteriole, and a cross section of peripheral nerve *(N)* is seen in proximity to the smaller arteriole. Compare the wall of the venule, consisting only of endothelium and a thin layer of connective tissue, with the arterioles. Also, note the relatively large lumen of the venule.

Figure 2, arteriole, human, H&E ×350.

This micrograph shows a longitudinal section of an arteriole. Because of its twisting path through the section, its wall has been cut such that the single layer of muscle cells of the tunica media is seen in different planes along its length. In the segment numbered *1,* at the left, the vessel wall has been cut tangentially. Thus, the vessel lumen is not included in the plane of section, but the smooth muscle cell nuclei of the tunica media are seen in longitudinal profile. After the arteriole makes an acute turn (segment numbered *2*), the vessel wall is cut to reveal the lumen. Here, the smooth muscle nuclei appear as round profiles and the nuclei of the endothelial cells lining the lumen appear in longitudinal profile. In the segment numbered *3,* the vessel wall is again only grazed. In the segment numbered *4,* the cut is deeper, again showing the lumen and some of the endothelial cells in face view *(arrowheads).* The structure below the vessel is a Pacinian corpuscle *(P).*

Figure 3, lymphatic vessel, human, H&E ×175.

The lymphatic vessel shown in this figure shows a region where the vessel is making a U-shaped turn in the plane of the section, thus disappearing at the top and bottom of the micrograph. The call of the vessel consists of an endothelial lining and a small amount of connective tissue, with one being indistinguishable from the other. A valve *(Val),* which is characteristic of lymphatic vessels, is seen within the vessel. It is formed of a miniscule layer of connective tissue that is covered on both sides by endothelium. The *arrows* indicate nuclei that are just barely visible at this magnification; most of them belong to endothelial cells. Typically, the lumen contains precipitated lymph material *(L);* sometimes, lymphocytes may be present. Adjacent to the vessel, on the right, is adipose tissue *(AT)* and on the upper left is dense connective tissue *(DCT).*

Figure 4, lymphatic vessel, human, Mallory ×375.

The lymphatic vessel shown here is contained within dense connective tissue *(DCT).* The lumen is irregular, appearing relatively narrow below the valve *(Val).* A few endothelial cell nuclei are evident *(arrows).* A thin layer of connective tissue that is present outside of the endothelium blends with the dense connective tissue beyond the wall of the vessel. A venule *(V)* is also present; it can readily be distinguished from the lymphatic vessel by the presence of red blood cells in the lumen.

KEY

A, arteriole
Ad, adipocyte
AT, adipose tissue
DCT, dense connective tissue
L, lymph material
N, nerve
P, Pacinian corpuscle
V, venule
Val, valve
arrowheads, endothelial cells
arrows, endothelial cell nuclei

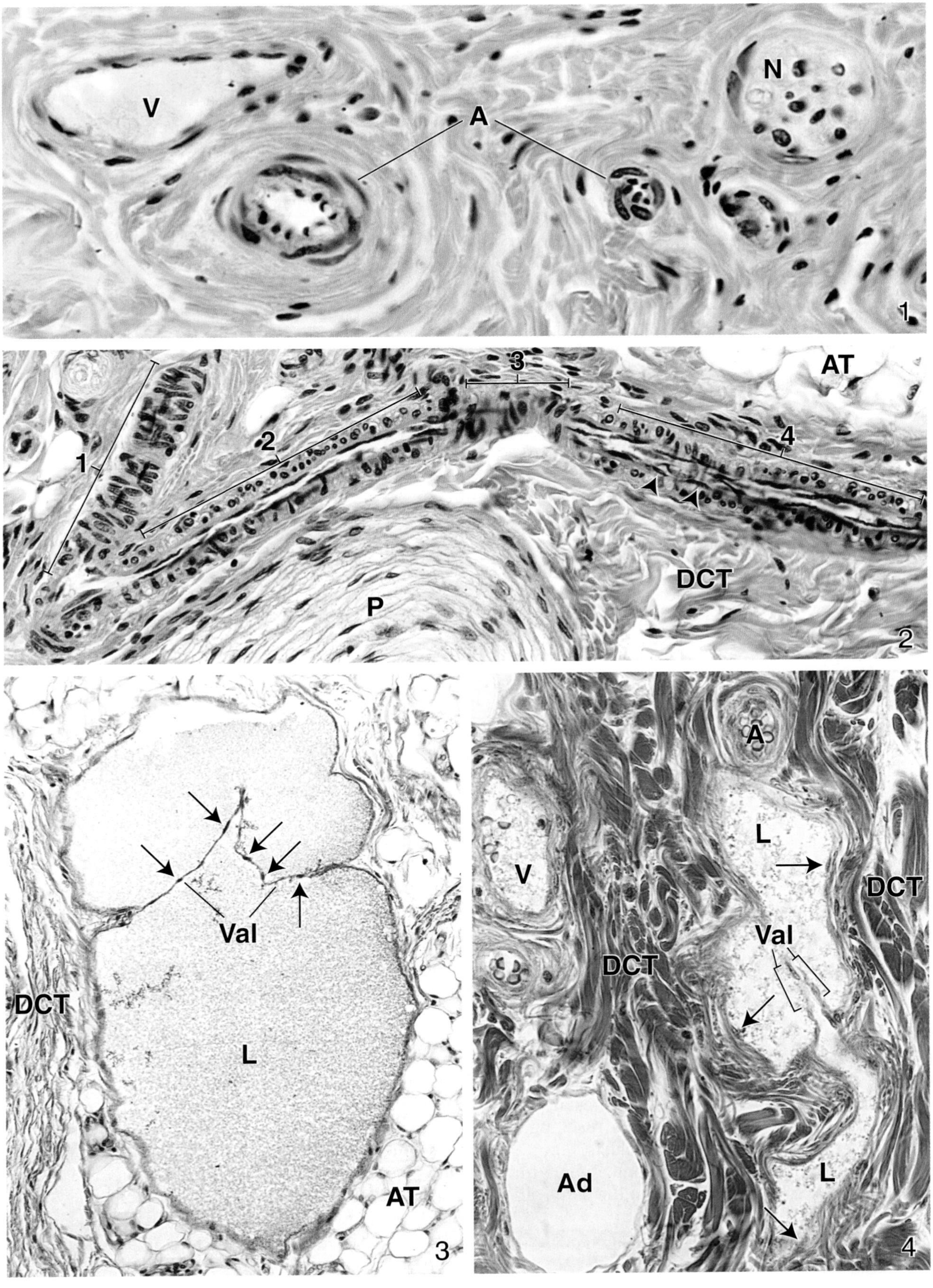
V
A
N
1
1
2
3
4
AT
P
DCT
2
Val
DCT
L
AT
3
A
L
V
DCT
Val
DCT
Ad
L
4

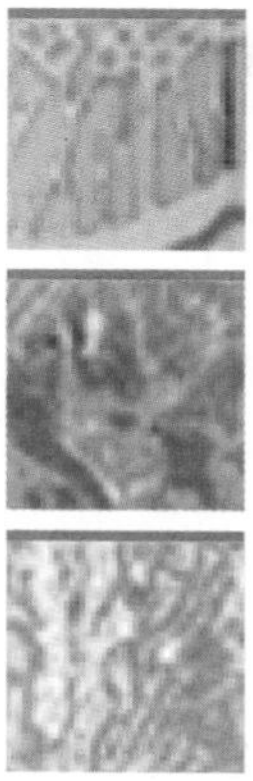

13

Lymphatic System

▼ OVERVIEW OF THE LYMPHATIC SYSTEM

Throughout history, it has been noted that people who recover from certain diseases, such as chickenpox, measles, or mumps, become resistant to the same disease, i.e., immune. Another longstanding observation is that immunity is specific, i.e., immunity to chickenpox does not prevent infection with measles. It has also been recognized that the immune system can react against itself, causing autoimmune diseases such as lupus erythematosus, autoimmune hemolytic anemia, some forms of diabetes mellitus, and autoimmune thyroiditis (Hashimoto's thyroiditis).

The *lymphatic system* consists of groups of cells, tissues, and organs that monitor body surfaces and internal fluid compartments and react to the presence of potentially harmful substances. ***Lymphocytes*** are the definitive cell type of the lymphatic system and are the effector cells in the response of the immune system to harmful substances. Included in this system are the ***diffuse lymphatic tissue, lymphatic nodules, lymph nodes, spleen, bone marrow,*** and ***thymus*** (Fig. 13.1). The various ***lymphatic organs*** and ***lymphatic tissues*** are often collectively referred to as the ***immune system. Lymphatic vessels*** connect parts of the system to the blood vascular system.

Lymphatic tissues serve as sites where lymphocytes proliferate, differentiate, and mature. In addition, in the ***thymus, bone marrow,*** and ***gut-associated lymphatic tissue (GALT),*** lymphocytes are "educated" to recognize and destroy specific antigens. These now ***immunocompetent cells*** can distinguish between ***"self"*** (molecules normally present

within an organism) and ***"nonself"*** (foreign molecules, i.e., those not normally present).

An antigen is any substance that can induce a specific immune response

The body is constantly exposed to pathogenic (disease-causing) organisms and hazardous substances from the external environment (infectious microorganisms, toxins, and foreign cells and tissues). In addition, changes may occur in cells (such as transformation of normal cells into cancerous cells) that give them characteristics of foreign cells. An immune response is generated against a specific ***antigen,*** which can be a soluble substance (e.g., a foreign protein, polysaccharide, or toxin) or an infectious organism, foreign tissue, or transformed tissue. Most antigens must be "processed" by cells of the immune system before other cells can mount the immune response.

The immune response can be divided into nonspecific and specific defenses

The body has two lines of immune defenses against foreign invaders and transformed cells. **Nonspecific defenses** consist of physical barriers (e.g., the skin and mucous membranes) that prevent foreign cells from invading the tissues, as well as various chemicals that neutralize foreign cells. If these nonspecific defenses fail, the immune system provides **specific defenses** that target individual invaders. Two types of specific defenses have been identified: the **antibody, or humoral, response,** which results in the production of proteins that mark invaders for destruction by other immune cells, and the **cellular immune response,** which targets transformed and virus-infected cells for destruction by lymphocytes.

▼ LYMPHATIC CELLS

Overview

Cells of the immune system include lymphocytes and various supporting cells

Lymphocytes and a variety of supporting cells make up the cells of the immune system. Three types of lymphocytes are recognized: B cells, T cells, and natural killer (NK) cells. Sup-

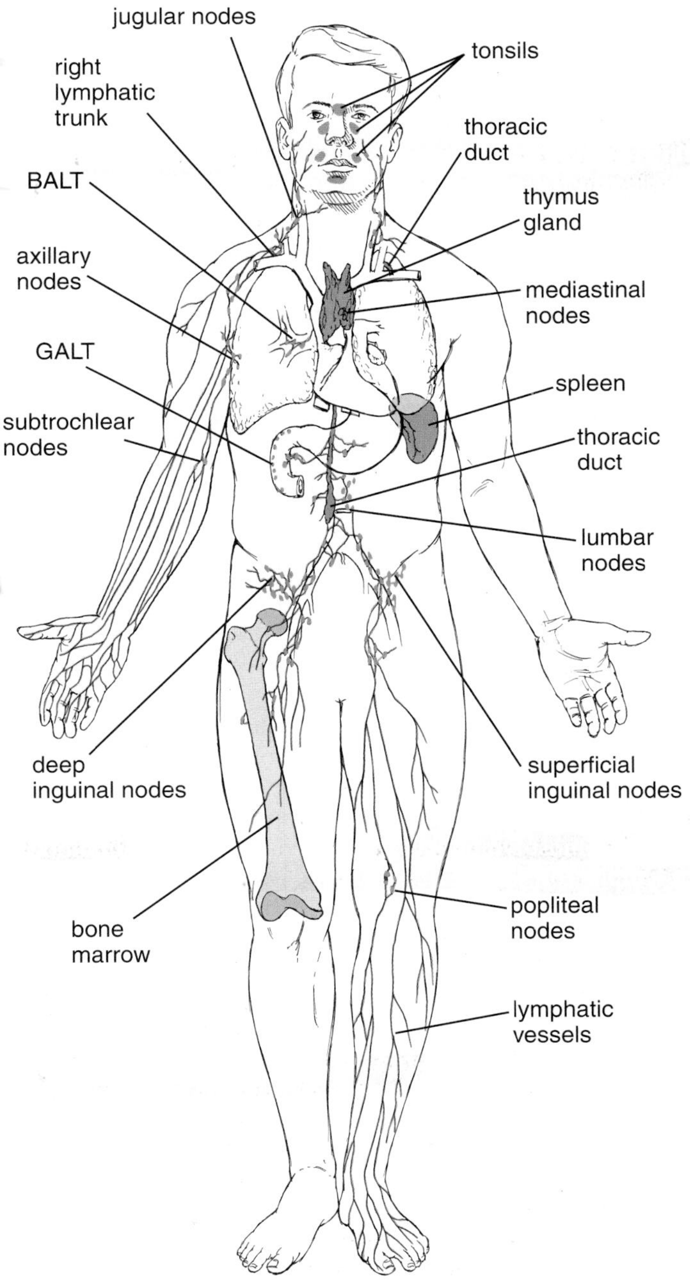

FIGURE 13.1
Overview of the structures constituting the lymphatic system. Because lymphatic tissue is the main component of some organs, they are regarded as organs of the lymphatic system (spleen, thymus, lymph nodes). Lymphatic tissue is present as part of other organs, such as red bone marrow, lymphatic nodules of the alimentary canal (tonsils, vermiform appendix, gut-associated lymphatic tissue [GALT]) and of the respiratory system (bronchus-associated lymphatic tissue [BALT]), and, not shown in the illustration, diffuse lymphatic tissue of mucous membranes (mucus-associated lymphatic tissue [MALT]). The lymph nodes are interspersed along the superficial lymphatic vessels (associated with the skin and superficial fascia) and deep lymphatic vessels (associated with main arteries); ultimately, the lymphatic vessels empty into the bloodstream by joining the large veins at the base of the neck. The thoracic duct is the largest lymphatic vessel.

porting cells include ***reticular cells, macrophages, follicular dendritic cells, Langerhans' cells,*** and ***epithelioreticular cells.***

Supporting cells in the lymphatic organs are organized into loose meshworks

In lymph nodules, lymph nodes, and the spleen, ***reticular cells*** and the ***reticular fibers*** produced by these cells form elaborate meshworks. Lymphocytes, macrophages, follicular dendritic cells and other cells of the immune system reside in these meshworks and in the loose connective tissue of the body; Langerhans' cells are found only in the middle layers of epidermis. At these sites, they carry out their mission of surveillance and defense. In the thymus, epithelioreticular cells form the structural meshwork within the tissue. Despite their name, these cells neither produce nor are related to reticular fibers.

Different types of cells in lymphatic tissue are identified by specific cluster of differentiation (CD) markers on their surface

Different lymphatic and hematopoietic tissue cells possess unique cell surface molecules. These specific markers, called ***cluster of differentiation (CD) molecules,*** are designated by numbers according to an international system that relates them to antigens expressed at different stages of their differentiation. CD molecules can be visualized by immunohistochemical methods using monoclonal antibodies and are useful in identifying specific subtypes of lymphatic or hematopoietic cells. Some CD markers are expressed by a cell line throughout its entire life; others are expressed only during one phase of differentiation or during cell activation. Table 13.1 lists the most clinically useful markers.

Lymphocytes

Circulating lymphocytes are the chief cellular constituent of lymphatic tissue

To understand the function of lymphocytes, one must realize that most lymphocytes (approximately 70%) in blood or lymph represent a ***circulating pool*** of immunocompetent cells. These cells participate in a cycle during which they exit the systemic circulation to enter the lymphatic tissue. While there, they are responsible for immunologic surveillance of surrounding tissues. The cells then return to the systemic circulation. This population of cells is represented mainly by long-lived, mature lymphocytes (mainly T cells). Mature lymphocytes have developed the capacity to recognize and respond to foreign antigens and are in transit from one site of lymphatic tissue to another.

The remaining 30% of lymphocytes in the blood vessels do not circulate between the lymphatic tissues and the systemic circulation. This population comprises mainly short-lived, immature cells or activated cells destined for a specific tissue. These cells leave the capillaries and migrate directly to the tissues, especially into the connective tissue that underlies the lining epithelium of the respiratory, gastrointestinal, and urogenital tracts as well as into the intercellular spaces of these epithelia.

Functionally, three types of lymphocytes are present in the body: T lymphocytes, B lymphocytes, and NK cells

The functional classification of lymphocytes is independent of their morphologic (size) characteristics. Functionally, three types of lymphocytes are recognized:

- ***T lymphocytes (T cells)*** are named for the thymus, where they differentiate. They have a long lifespan and are involved in ***cell-mediated immunity.*** They account for 60 to 80% of circulating lymphocytes. T cells express CD2, CD3, and CD7 markers; however, they are subclassified according to the presence or absence of two other important surface markers, CD4 and CD8. T cells that also express CD4 markers are called ***helper CD4⁺ T lymphocytes.*** T cells that also express CD8 markers are called ***cytotoxic CD8⁺ T lymphocytes.***
- ***B lymphocytes (B cells)*** are so named because they were first recognized as a separate population in the bursa of Fabricius in birds (page 361) or bursa-equivalent organs such as bone marrow and GALT in mammals. They have variable lifespans and are involved in the production and secretion of the various circulating ***antibodies,*** also called ***immunoglobulins,*** the immune proteins associated with ***humoral immunity*** (Fig. 13.2 and Table 13.2). B cells account for 20 to 30% of the circulating lymphocytes. In addition to secreting circulating immunoglobulins, B cells express immunoglobulin M (IgM) and immunoglobulin D (IgD) as well as the major histocompatibility complex II (MHC II) molecules on the cell surface. Their CD markers are CD9, CD19, CD20, and CD24.
- ***NK cells,*** which develop from the same precursor cell as B and T cells, are named for their ability to kill certain types of transformed cells. They constitute about 5 to 10% of circulating lymphocytes. During their development, they are genetically programmed to recognize transformed cells (i.e., cells infected with a virus or tumor cells). Following recognition of a transformed cell, they release ***perforins*** and ***fragmentins,*** substances that create channels in the cell's plasma membrane and cytoplasm, which induces them to self-destruct (a process known as **apoptosis**) and lyse. Their specific markers include CD16, CD56, and CD94.

LYMPHOCYTE DEVELOPMENT AND DIFFERENTIATION

Lymphocytes undergo antigen-independent differentiation in the primary lymphatic organs

In humans and other mammals, the bone marrow and ***GALT*** (together called the ***bursa-equivalent organ***) and the thymus have been identified as ***primary*** or ***central lym-***

TABLE 13.1. **Most Common CD Markers Used in Clinical Practice**

Marker	Main Cellular Expression	Function/Identity	Molecular Weight (kDa)
CD1	T cells in the midstage of development	Developmental marker for T cells and Langerhans' cells of the skin	49
CD2	T cells	Clinical marker for T cells	50
CD3	T cells	Forms complex with T cell receptor (TCR)	100
CD4	Helper T cells	Interacts with MHC II molecules	56
CD5	T cells, some B cells	High levels in chronic lymphocytic leukemia	67
CD7	T cells	Useful clinical marker for T cell leukemia	40
CD8	Cytotoxic T cells	Interacts with MHC I molecules	34
CD9	B cells	Facilitates aggregation of platelets	24
CD10	Pre-B cells	Common marker for acute lymphoblastic leukemia	100
CD16	Granulocytes, monocytes, NK cells	F_c receptor for aggregated IgG, mediates phagocytosis, clinical marker for NK cells	27
CD19	B cells	Clinical marker for all stages of B cell development	90
CD20	B cells	Marker for late stage of B cell development	37
CD21	B cells	Receptor for C3d complement protein and for Epstein-Barr virus	145
CD22	B cells	Participates in B cell adhesion	140
CD24	B cells	Expressed in late stage of B cell differentiation	41
CD34	Pluripotential stem cells (PPSCs) in bone marrow	Clinical marker for PPSCs and ligand for CD62L	120
CD35	B cells, monocytes	Promotes phagocytosis of complement-coated particles, binds C36 and C46 complement protein	250
CD38	Activated T cells	Marker for T cell activation	45
CD40	B cells	Active in proliferating B cells, receptor for CD40L	48
CD40L	Activated $CD4^+$ T cells	Facilitates interaction between T and B cells, ligand for CD40	39
CD45	All human leukocytes	Leukocyte common antigen	220
CD45RA	Suppressor/cytotoxic $CD8^+$ T cells	Facilitates TCR signaling	205
CD56	NK cells	Clinical marker for NK cells, isoform of neural adhesion molecules (N-CAM)	135
CD62L	Leukocytes	Represent selectins, leukocyte adhesion molecules	150
CD94	NK cells	Clinical marker for NK cells	43

phatic organs. Lymphocytes differentiate into immunocompetent cells in these organs. Initially, lymphocytes are genetically programmed to recognize a single antigen out of virtually an infinite number of possible antigens, a process called ***antigen-independent proliferation and differentiation.*** These immunocompetent cells then enter the blood or lymph and are transported throughout the body, where they are dispersed in the connective tissue.

Lymphocytes undergo antigen-dependent activation in the secondary lymphatic organs

Immunocompetent lymphocytes (together with plasma cells derived from B lymphocytes and with macrophages) organize around reticular cells and their reticular fibers to form the adult ***effector lymphatic tissues*** and organs, i.e., lymphatic nodules, lymph nodes, tonsils, and spleen. Within these ***secondary*** or ***peripheral lymphatic organs,*** T and B lymphocytes undergo ***antigen-dependent activation*** into ***effector lymphocytes*** and ***memory cells.***

IMMUNE RESPONSES TO ANTIGENS

Inflammation is the initial response to an antigen

The initial reaction of the body to invasion by an antigen, either a foreign molecule or a pathogenic organism, is the

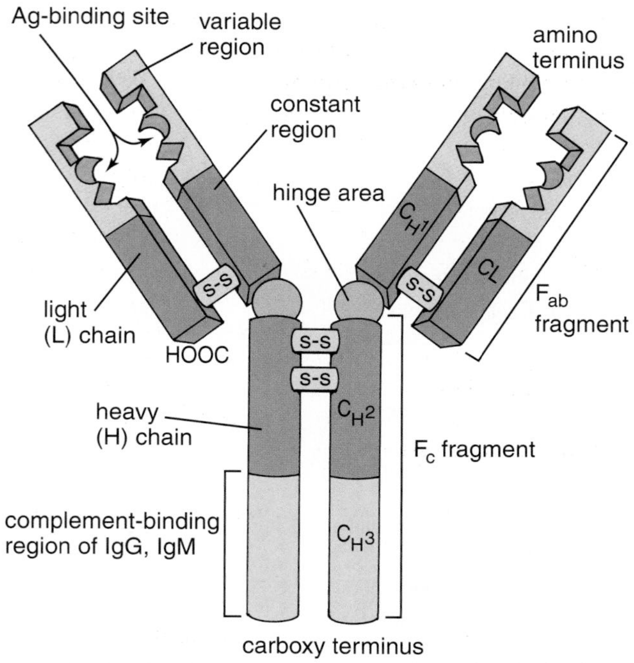

FIGURE 13.2
Schematic diagram of an antibody molecule. Antibodies are Y-shaped molecules produced by plasma cells. They consist of two heavy (H) and two light (L) polypeptide chains connected by disulfide bonds (S–S). Both H and L chains are composed of domains of amino acids that are constant (at the carboxy terminus) or variable (at the amino terminus) in their sequence. The five different immunoglobulin (Ig) isotypes (see Table 13.2) are determined by the type of heavy chain present. An antibody molecule binds an antigen (Ag) at the two sites of the amino terminus, where the heavy and light chains are associated with each other. Digestion of an antibody molecule by the proteolytic enzyme papain cleaves the antibody into two F_{ab} fragments and one crystallizable F_c fragment. The F_c fragment is composed of two carboxy-teminus heavy-chain segments (C_H2 and C_H3)

TABLE 13.2. **Characteristics of Human Immunoglobulins**

Isotype	Molecular Weight (kDa)	Serum Level (mg/mL)	Percentage of all Ig in the Adult Blood	Cells to Which Bound via F_c Region	Major Functions
IgG	145	12	85	Macrophages, B cells, NK cells, neutrophils, eosinophils,	Principal Ig in secondary immune response; the longest half-life (23 days) of all five Igs; activates complement; stimulates chemotaxis; crosses placenta, providing the newborn with passive immunity
IgM	190 (950)[A]	1	5–10	B cells	Principal Ig produced during primary immune response; the most efficient Ig in fixing complement; activates macrophages; serves as Ag receptor of B lymphocytes.
IgA	160 (385)[B]	2	5–15	B cells	Ig present in body secretions, including tears, colostrum, saliva, and vaginal fluid, and in the secretions of the nasal cavity, bronchi, intestine, and prostate; provides protection against the proliferation of microorganisms in these fluids and aids in the defense against microbes and foreign molecules penetrating the body via the cells lining these cavities
IgD	185	0.03	<1	B cells	Acts as an antigen receptor (together with IgM) on the surface of mature B lymphocytes (only traces in serum)
IgE	190	0.0003	<1	Mast cells, basophils	Stimulates mast cells to release histamine, heparin, leukotrienes, SRS-A[C], and eosinophil chemotactic factor of anaphylaxis; is responsible for anaphylactic hypersensitivity reactions; increased levels in parasitic infections

[A]IgM found in serum as a pentameric molecule.
[B]IgA found in serum as dimeric molecule.
[C]Slow-reacting substance of anaphylaxis.

BOX 13.1

Functional Considerations: Origin of the Names *T Lymphocyte* and *B Lymphocyte*

In the early 1960s, investigators using chicken embryos demonstrated that the ***bursa of Fabricius,*** a mass of lymphatic tissue associated with the cloaca of birds, was one of the anatomic sites of lymphocyte differentiation. When this tissue was destroyed in the chicken embryos (by either surgical removal or administration of high doses of testosterone), the adult chickens were unable to produce antibodies, leading to impaired humoral immunity. The chickens also demonstrated a marked reduction in the number of lymphocytes found in specific bursa-dependent areas of the spleen and lymph nodes. These affected lymphocytes were therefore named *B lymphocytes* or *B cells.* The **bursa-equivalent organs** in mammals (including humans) are the GALT and the bone marrow, where B lymphocytes differentiate into immunocompetent cells. Thus, the "B" refers to the bursa of birds or the "bursa-equivalent organs" of mammals.

Investigators studying newborn mice found that removal of the thymus results in profound deficiencies in cell-mediated immune responses. The rejection of transplanted skin from a heterologous donor is an example of cell-mediated immune response. Thymectomized mice demonstrate a marked reduction in the number of lymphocytes found in specific regions of the spleen and the lymph nodes (thymus-dependent areas). The areas of depletion differ from those identified after removal of the bursa of Fabricius in the chicken. These affected lymphocytes were therefore named *T lymphocytes* or *T cells;* the "T" refers to the thymus.

nonspecific defense known as the ***inflammatory response.*** The inflammatory response may either sequester the antigen, physically digest the antigen with enzymes secreted by neutrophils, or phagocytose and degrade the antigen in the cytoplasm of macrophages. Degradation of antigens by macrophages may lead to subsequent presentation of a portion of the antigen to immunocompetent lymphocytes to elicit a specific immune response.

Specific immune responses are either primary or secondary

When immunocompetent cells encounter a foreign antigen (e.g., antigen associated with pathogenic microorganisms, tissue transplants, or toxins), a ***specific immune response*** to the antigen is generated.

A ***primary immune response*** refers to the body's first encounter with an antigen. This response is characterized by a lag period of several days before antibodies (mostly IgM) or specific lymphocytes directed against the invading antigen can be detected in the blood. The initial response to an antigen is initiated by only one or a few B lymphocytes that have been genetically programmed to respond to that specific antigen. Following this initial immune response, a few antigen-specific B lymphocytes remain in circulation as ***memory cells.***

The ***secondary immune response*** is usually more rapid and more intense (characterized by higher levels of secreted antibodies, usually of the IgG class) than the primary response, because of the presence of specific memory B lymphocytes already programmed to respond to that specific antigen. The secondary response is the basis of most immunizations for common bacterial and viral diseases. Some antigens, such as penicillin and insect venoms, may trigger an intense secondary immune response that produces a ***hypersensitivity reaction*** or even anaphylaxis (see page 365). However, antibodies themselves do not kill or destroy invading antigens; they simply mark them for destruction by cells of the immune system.

The two types of specific immune responses are the humoral and cell-mediated responses

In general, an encounter with a given antigen triggers a response characterized as either a humoral immune response (antibody production) or a cell-mediated immune response. Typically, however, both cellular and humoral immune systems are involved, although one system generally predominates, depending on the stimulus.

- ***Humoral immunity*** is mediated by antibodies that act directly on an invading agent. These antibodies are produced by B lymphocytes and by plasma cells derived from B lymphocytes. In some diseases, e.g., tetanus, a nonimmune person can be rendered immune by receiving an injection of antibody purified from the blood of an immune person or animal. The effectiveness of this passive transfer proves that it is the antibody that is responsible for the protection.
- ***Cell-mediated immunity*** is mediated by specific T lymphocytes that attack and destroy virus-infected host cells or foreign cells. Cell-mediated immunity is important in the defense against viral, fungal, and mycobacterial infections, as well as tumor cells. Cell-mediated immunity is also responsible for transplant rejection.

Helper T and cytotoxic lymphocytes recognize and bind to antigens that are bound to MHC molecules

To understand how the specific immune responses (humoral and cell-mediated responses) are initiated, one must grasp the central role played by the helper and cytotoxic T lymphocytes. Helper T and cytotoxic lymphocytes act as the immune system "patrols." Both kinds of lymphocytes have a ***T cell receptor (TCR),*** a transmembrane protein whose exposed portion is on the T cell membrane in close proximity to the CD3 marker (Fig. 13.3). The TCR recognizes antigen only when it is attached to "identification molecules," the ***MHC molecules.*** In addition, helper T

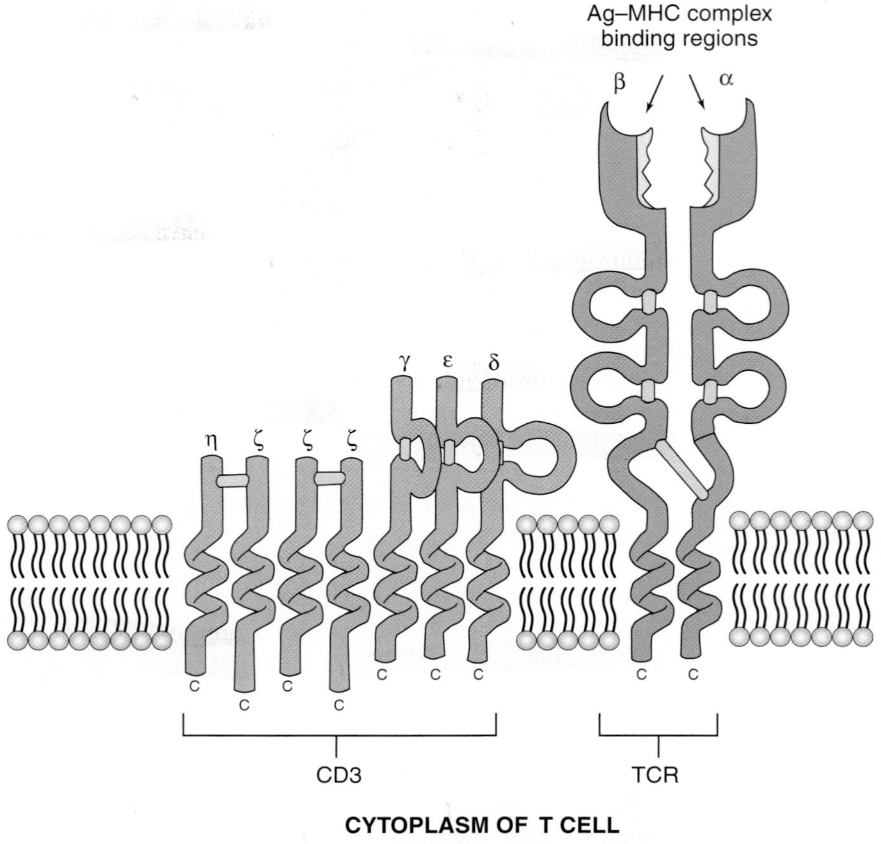

FIGURE 13.3
Schematic diagram of the molecular structure of the CD3–TCR complex. The CD3 molecule consists of five different polypeptide chains with molecular weights ranging from 16 to 28 kDa. This molecule is closely associated with the T cell receptor (TCR), which has two polypeptide chains (α and β). The T cell may be activated following the interaction of the TCR with antigen displayed on the surface of a MHC molecule. This interaction transmits the signals to the interior of the cell through the CD3 molecule. This signal stimulates the T cell to secrete interleukins, which in turn stimulate T cells to divide and differentiate.

lymphocytes can only recognize an antigen when it is "presented" to them by cells called ***antigen-presenting cells (APCs)***. Cytotoxic T lymphocytes can only recognize antigen on other body cells, such as cells transformed by cancer or infected with a virus.

When a helper T lymphocyte recognizes an antigen bound to a MHC molecule, the TCR attaches to the antigen–MHC complex. The binding of the TCR to the antigen–MHC complex then triggers the helper T lymphocyte to release immune chemicals, or ***cytokines***, immune substances (proteins) that are biologic modulators of immune responses. The specific cytokines produced by helper $CD4^+$ T lymphocytes are called ***interleukins***. Interleukins stimulate other T cells, B cells, and NK cells to differentiate and proliferate.

When a cytotoxic T lymphocyte recognizes an antigen–MHC complex and the TCR attaches to it, the cytotoxic T lymphocyte also releases cytokines that stimulate the cell to proliferate. These new cytotoxic T cells then seek out and destroy the abnormal host cells.

The two classes of MHC molecules display peptides on the surface of cells

MHC molecules display small fragments of digested foreign proteins on the surface of cells. These proteins bind to MHC molecules inside the cell and are then transported to the cell surface. MHC I and MHC II molecules are products of a "supergene" located on chromosome 6 in humans, known as the ***major histocompatability gene complex***. The expression of this gene complex produces molecules that are specific not only to the individual cell that produces them, but also to the tissue type and degree of cellular differentiation.

MHC I is expressed on the surface of all nucleated cells and platelets. MHC I molecules act as a target to allow the elimination of abnormal host cells (e.g., virus-infected or transformed cancer cells). *MHC I molecules perform this function by displaying on their surface all of the peptides that are actively synthesized by the cell.* Therefore, all endogenous "self" peptides are displayed on the surface of every cell in the body, but viral or cancer-specific peptides are displayed only on the surface of infected or transformed cells (Fig. 13.4).

MHC II is limited in its distribution (see Fig. 13.4). It is expressed on the surface of all APCs and is critical in immune interactions. *The MHC II molecules present partially digested, endocytosed foreign peptides to helper $CD4^+$ T lymphocytes.*

$CD8^+$ T lymphocytes are MHC I restricted, and $CD4^+$ T lymphocytes are MHC II restricted

MHC molecules are recognized by helper $CD4^+$ T lymphocytes or cytotoxic $CD8^+$ lymphocytes, depending on

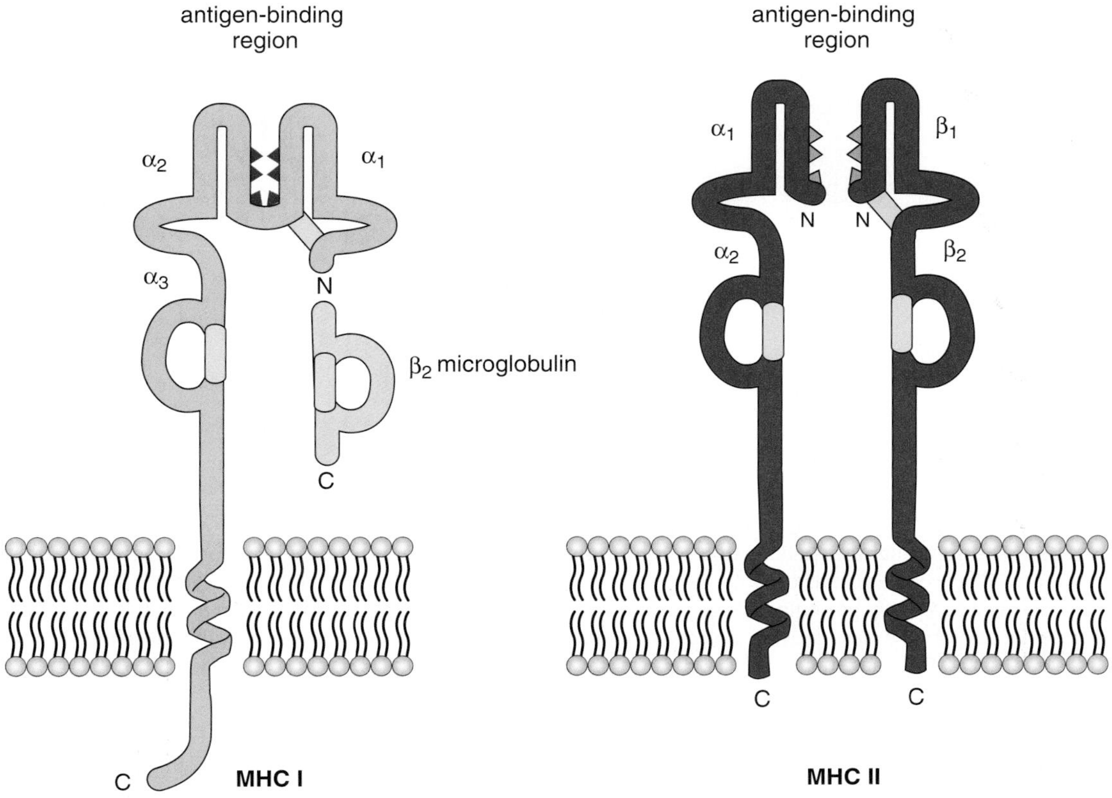

FIGURE 13.4
Schematic diagram of the molecular structure of MHC I and MHC II molecules. The MHC I molecule is a glycoprotein that is expressed on the surface of all nucleated cells of the body and on platelets. MHC I molecules present endogenously synthesized peptides for recognition by cytotoxic CD8$^+$ T lymphocytes. Therefore, the MHC I molecule acts as the target for the elimination of abnormal host cells producing abnormal proteins (e.g., cells infected by an intracellular agent, such as a virus, or cells that have been transformed, such as cancer cells). MHC I consists of an α heavy chain (45 kDa) and a smaller, noncovalently attached β_2 microglobulin polypeptide (12 kDa). The β_2 microglobulin promotes maturation of T cells and acts as a chemotactic factor. The MHC II molecule is also a glycoprotein but is expressed only on a restricted population of cells known as antigen-presenting cells (APCs). MHC II molecules present exogenous (foreign) peptides to helper CD4$^+$ T lymphocytes. They consist of two chains: an α chain (33 kDa) and a β chain (29 kDa), each of which possesses oligosaccharide groups.

the class of the MHC molecule engaged. This restricted presentation of foreign antigens by MHC molecules to either cytotoxic or helper T lymphocytes is a key component of immune surveillance.

The MHC I molecule with the peptide antigen displayed on its surface interacts only with the TCR and CD8$^+$ molecule expressed on cytotoxic CD8$^+$ T lymphocytes; these cells are therefore described as ***MHC I restricted.*** This interaction allows cytotoxic T lymphocytes to recognize infected or transformed target cells (Fig. 13.5a).

In contrast, the MHC II molecule with the peptide antigen displayed on its surface interacts only with the TCR and CD4 molecule expressed on helper CD4$^+$ T lymphocytes (Fig. 13.5b); these cells are therefore described as ***MHC II restricted.*** MHC II molecules are found on APCs, such as macrophages, whose main function is to present antigen to T lymphocytes.

The humoral immune response: Activated B lymphocytes differentiate into plasma cells that produce antibodies or into B memory cells

Each B lymphocyte reacts only with a single antigen or type of antigenic site that it has been genetically programmed to recognize. The reaction of a B lymphocyte with a TCR–MHC II–antigen complex activates the cell. Details of B cell activation are illustrated in Fig. 13.6. Activated B lymphocytes are transformed into ***immunoblasts (plasmablasts)*** that proliferate and then differentiate into

- ***Plasma cells,*** which synthesize and secrete a specific antibody
- ***Memory B cells,*** which respond more quickly to the next encounter with the same antigen

The specific antibody produced by the plasma cell binds to the stimulating antigen, forming an ***antigen–antibody***

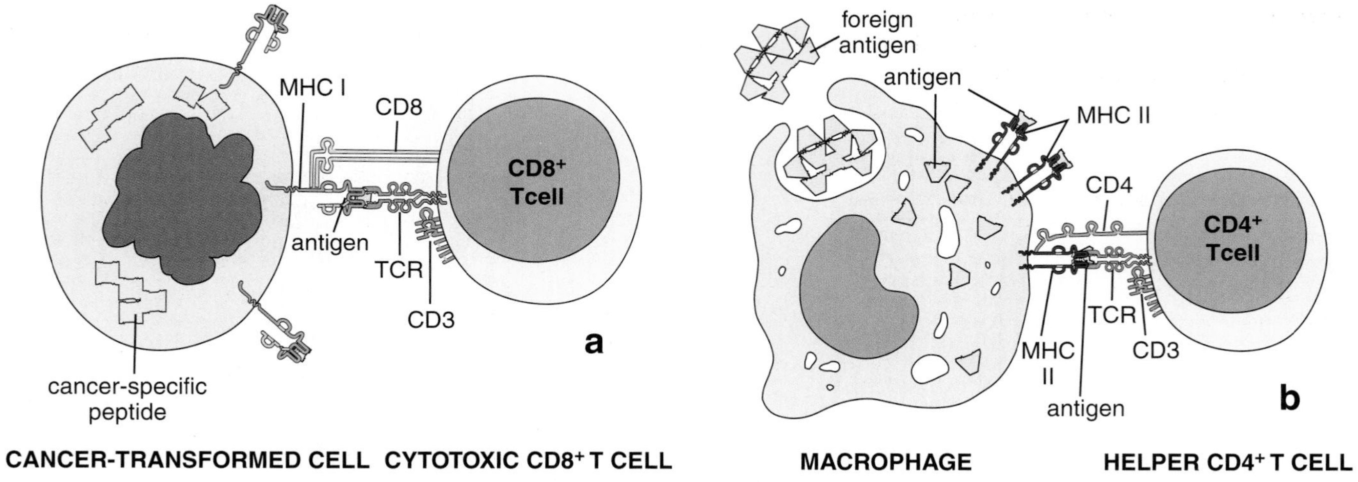

FIGURE 13.5

Schematic diagram of the molecular interactions that occur during antigen presentation. To become activated, both cytotoxic and helper T lymphocytes need to identify presented antigen as "nonself" as well as recognize the appropriate class of MHC molecules. **a.** In all nucleated cells of the body, viral antigen or cancer (tumor-specific) proteins are displayed in the context of MHC I molecules to interact with cytotoxic $CD8^+$ T lymphocytes. **b.** On antigen-presenting cells (e.g., macrophages), the foreign antigen is displayed in the context of MHC II molecules to interact with a helper $CD4^+$ T lymphocyte.

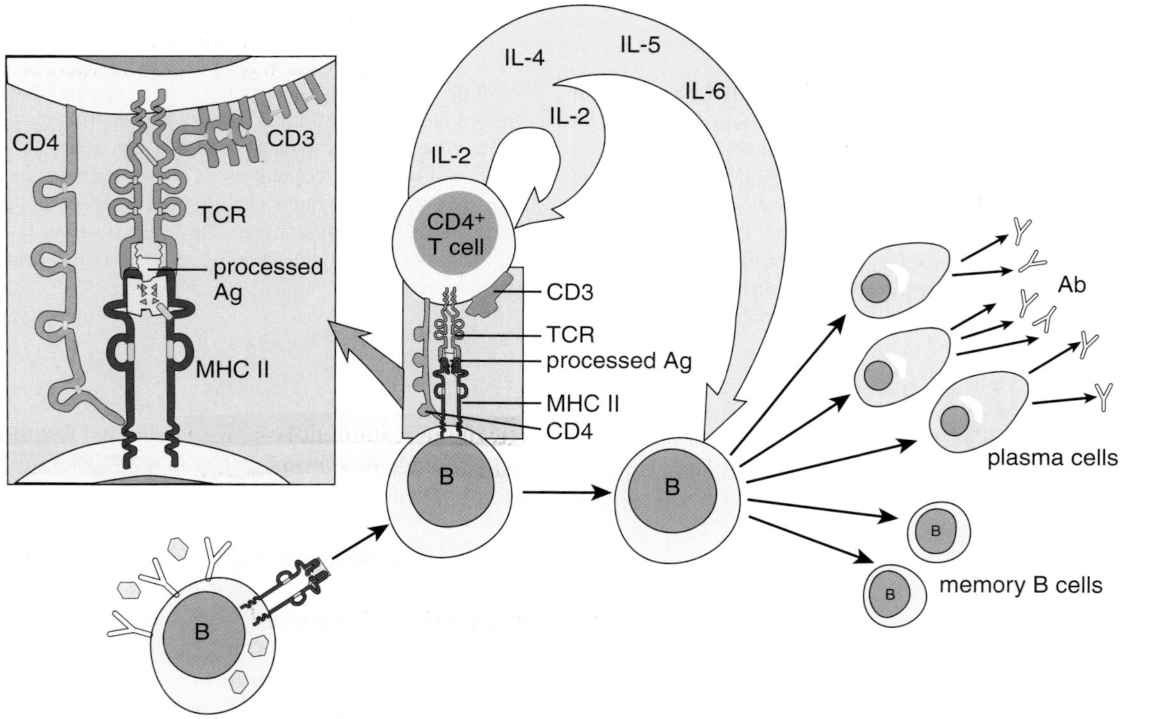

FIGURE 13.6

Schematic diagram of B lymphocyte activation leading to plasma cell and B memory cell formation. B cells are activated by the binding of antigen to antibodies expressed on their surface. As an antigen-presenting cell, a B cell internalizes the antibody–antigen complex, partially digests the antigen, and then displays parts of it on the surface of its own MHC II molecules. The T cell receptor *(TCR)* on a helper $CD4^+$ T lymphocyte recognizes both the antigen and the MHC II molecule, activating the helper $CD4^+$ T lymphocyte. The activated helper $CD4^+$ T lymphocyte releases interleukins IL-2, IL-4, IL-5, and IL-6, which promote division and differentiation of the B lymphocyte into plasma cells and memory B cells. *Ab,* antibody; *Ag,* antigen.

complex. These complexes are eliminated in a variety of ways, including destruction by NK cells and phagocytosis by macrophages and eosinophils. NK cells recognize the F_c region of antibodies and preferentially attack and destroy target cells, usually those coated with IgG antibodies (Fig. 13.7). NK cells act in concert with ***killer (K) cells*** and ***antibody-dependent cell-mediated cytotoxicity (ADCC) cells*** to induce the lysis of target cells, most commonly through the action of tumor-specific antibodies. ADCC reactions involve binding of an antibody or antibody and complement-coated target cell to an effector cell (NK, K, ADCC) bearing a receptor for the F_c portion of the antibody (see Fig. 13.2). This binding (through the F_c region) results in the lysis of the target cell.

If the antigen is a bacterium, the antigen–antibody complex may also activate a system of plasma proteins called the ***complement system*** and cause one of its components, usually C3, to bind to the bacterium and act as a ligand for its phagocytosis by macrophages. Complement binding induced by the antigen–antibody complex may also cause foreign cells to lyse.

The cell-mediated immune response: Cytotoxic T lymphocytes target and destroy transformed and virus-infected cells

When the TCR of a cytotoxic T lymphocyte recognizes and binds to an antigen–MHC I complex on the surface of a transformed or virus-infected cell, cytokines are released from the cell that cause it to proliferate. The cytotoxic T cells then secrete other cytokines (e.g., lymphokines, perforins, and fragmentins) that induce the cell to undergo apoptosis or to lyse (Fig. 13.8).

> **BOX 13.2**
>
> **Clinical Correlations: Hypersensitivity Reactions**
>
> When an individual has been immunologically sensitized by exposure to antigen, subsequent exposure may lead not only to secondary response but also to tissue-damaging reactions called ***hypersensitivity reactions.*** Such reactions are observed in sensitized humans, following insect bites or injections of penicillin. One common type of hypersensitivity reaction is the allergic reaction. Certain aspects of a hypersensitivity reaction are caused by the antibody-induced discharge of mast cell granules. These granules contain histamine that accounts for the distressing features of hypersensitivity reactions. Eosinophils are attracted to the site of mast cell degranulation, where they neutralize the effects of histamine. Thus, eosinophils are frequently seen in connective tissue at allergic or other hypersensitivity reaction sites.

Suppressor/cytotoxic T lymphocytes turn off the immune response

Suppressor/cytotoxic $CD8^+$, ***$CD45RA^+$ T lymphocytes*** diminish or suppress antibody formation by B cells. They also downregulate the ability of cytotoxic T lymphocytes to provide a cell-mediated immune response and participate in delayed hypersensitivity reactions (allergic reactions). Suppressor/cytotoxic T lymphocytes may also function in the regulation of erythroid cell maturation in bone marrow.

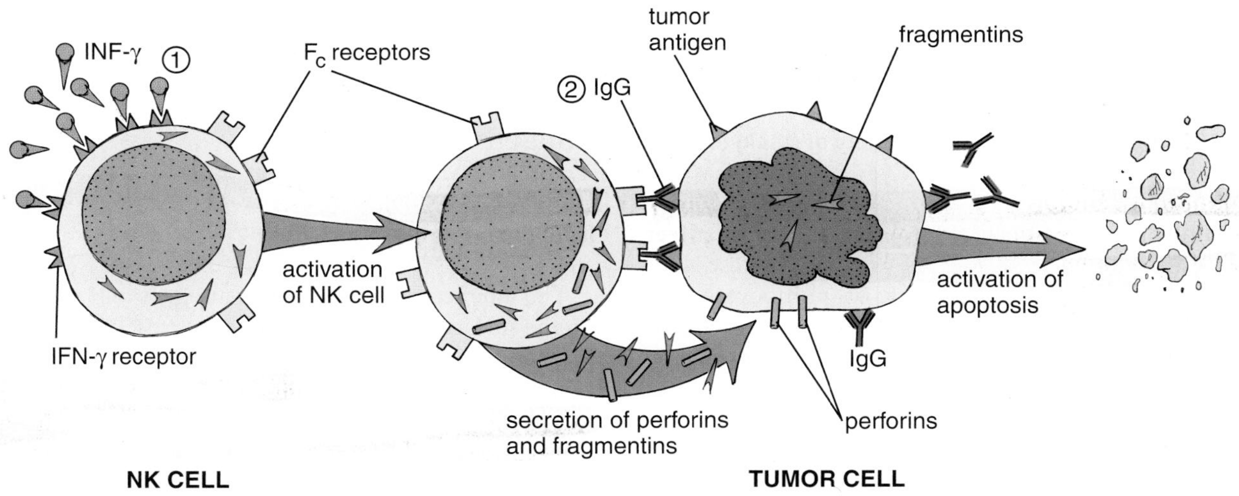

FIGURE 13.7
Schematic diagram of activation of NK cells leading to destruction of a transformed tumor cell by antibody-dependent, cell-mediated cytotoxicity (ADCC). The ADCC reaction involves activation of NK cells by ① the binding of interferon γ *(IFN-γ)*, the powerful NK cell activator, to its cell surface receptor *(IFN-γ receptor)* and ② the binding of an antibody- or an antibody- and complement-coated target cell to a NK cell bearing F_c receptors. These reactions induce apoptosis, or lysis of the target cell, usually through the action of tumor-specific antibodies or the action of perforins and fragmentins secreted by activated NK cells.

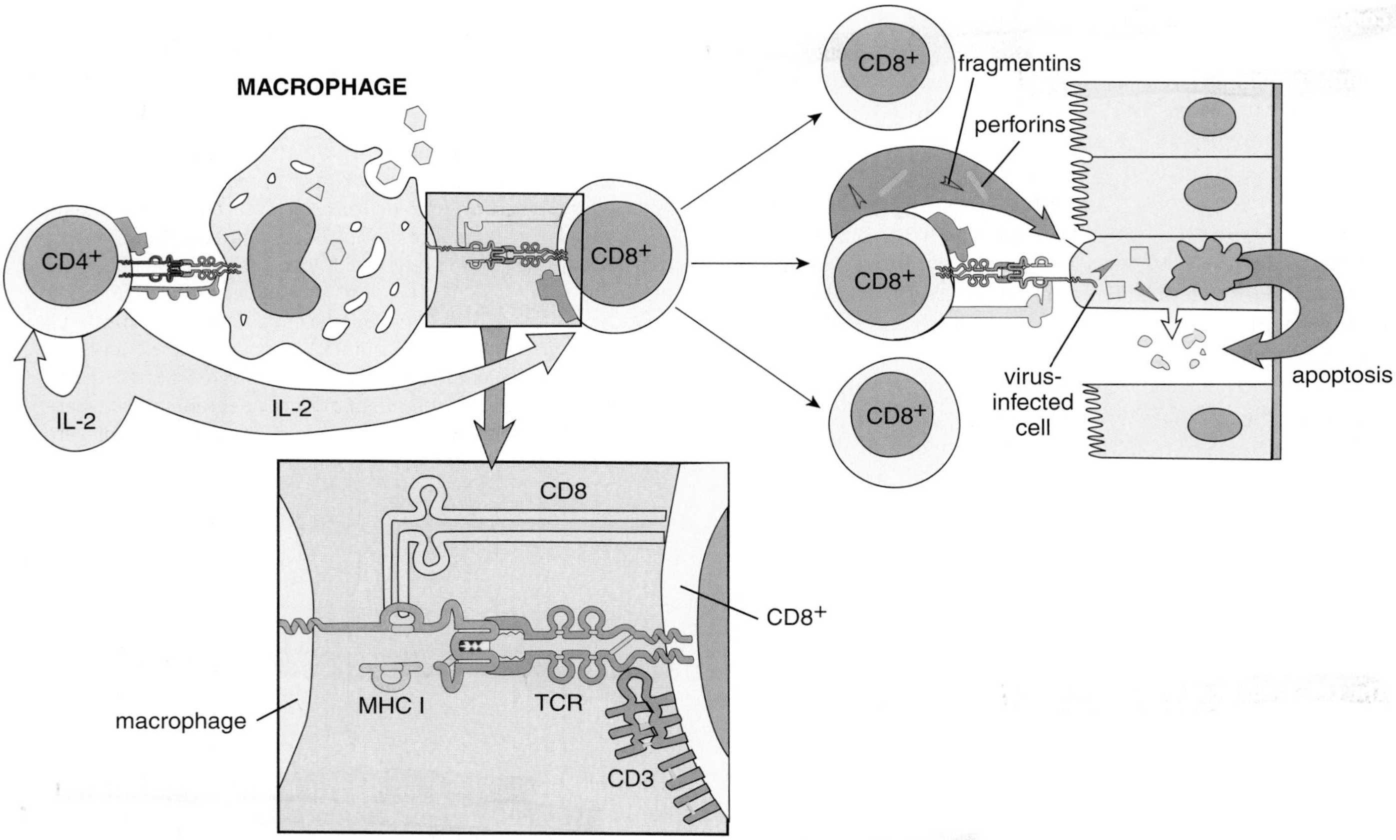

FIGURE 13.8

Schematic diagram of T cell activation leading to elimination of a virus-infected host cell. The TCR–CD3 complex on a helper $CD4^+$ T lymphocyte recognizes foreign antigen displayed on a MHC II molecule on the surface of a macrophage. This recognition triggers a rapid response from B lymphocytes and release of interleukin-2 (IL-2). The same macrophage also expresses MHC I molecules (like every other cell in the body) that interact with the appropriate TCR on the surface of a cytotoxic $CD8^+$ T lymphocyte. The cytotoxic $CD8^+$ T lymphocyte also possesses IL-2 receptors. IL-2 binding to these receptors stimulates the cell to divide and differentiate. The newly formed cytotoxic $CD8^+$ T lymphocytes migrate to the site of viral infection. There the TCRs recognize the viral antigens displayed on the surface of MHC I molecules of infected cells. After successfully recognizing these "nonself" proteins, the cytotoxic $CD8^+$ T lymphocytes secrete perforins and fragmentins, killing the infected cells.

Activated T lymphocytes synthesize a variety of cytokines

Cytokines are soluble polypeptide substances, synthesized mainly by activated T lymphocytes, which affect the function of other immune system cells. These substances also stimulate the activity of monocytes and macrophages in cell-mediated immunity. Included among these substances are chemotactic and mitogenic agents, migration inhibitory factors, interferon, and interleukins.

Interleukins are synthesized mainly by helper $CD4^+$ T lymphocytes and to a lesser extent by monocytes, macrophages, and endothelial cells. Interleukins promote growth and differentiation of T cells, B cells, and hematopoietic cells. Presently, more than 17 interleukins have been identified. Interleukin-2 was the first cytokine to be discovered and characterized. The major functions of known interleukins are summarized in Table 13.3.

Antigen-Presenting Cells

APCs interact with helper CD41 T lymphocytes to facilitate immune responses

The interaction between most antigens and the antibodies on the surface of B cells is insufficient to stimulate B cell proliferation, differentiation, and secretion of antibodies. For B cell stimulation to occur, the antigen must be broken into small peptides and presented in conjunction with MHC II molecules by APCs to the appropriate helper $CD4^+$ T lymphocytes. Most APCs belong to the mononuclear phagocytotic system (MPS) (described in Chapter 5, page 144). APCs include macrophages, ***perisinusoidal macrophages (Kupffer cells)*** of the liver, Langerhans' cells in the epidermis, and reticular dendritic cells of spleen and lymph nodes. Two APCs that do not belong to the MPS are B lymphocytes and ***type II and type III epithelioreticular cells*** of the thymus.

BOX 13.3

Clinical Correlations: Human Immunodeficiency Virus (HIV) and Acquired Immunodeficiency Syndrome (AIDS)

Human immunodeficiency virus (HIV) is a RNA retrovirus; it contains an enzyme called reverse transcriptase. HIV is the virus that causes **acquired immunodeficiency syndrome (AIDS)**. HIV has an incubation period that may be as long as 11 years before symptoms of clinical AIDS occur. The great majority of HIV-infected individuals eventually develop AIDS. HIV gains entry to helper T cells by binding to CD4 molecules. The virus then injects its own genetic information into the cell cytoplasm (Fig. 13.9). This injected genetic information consists of single-stranded RNA. The viral RNA is incorporated into the infected T cell genome through reverse transcription of the RNA into DNA. The transcribed DNA is then incorporated into the host DNA. The T cell then makes copies of the virus, which are extruded from the T cell through exocytosis. These HIV particles then infect other helper T cells, greatly reducing their number. The helper CD4$^+$ T cell count is used as a clinical indicator of the progress of HIV infection. Infected individuals eventually become incapable of generating an immune response against bacterial or viral infections. They usually die of secondary infections caused by opportunistic microorganisms or of malignancies.

Anti-HIV treatment is the major strategy against HIV infection and AIDS. Currently, the most effective is multiple drug therapy known as highly active antiretroviral therapy (HAART), which uses a combination of several chemotherapeutic agents. These include nucleoside and nonnucleoside reverse transcriptase inhibitors and HIV protease inhibitors. HAART offers several advantages over monotherapy such as synergistic dosage effects and reduced side effects as well as reduced drug resistance.

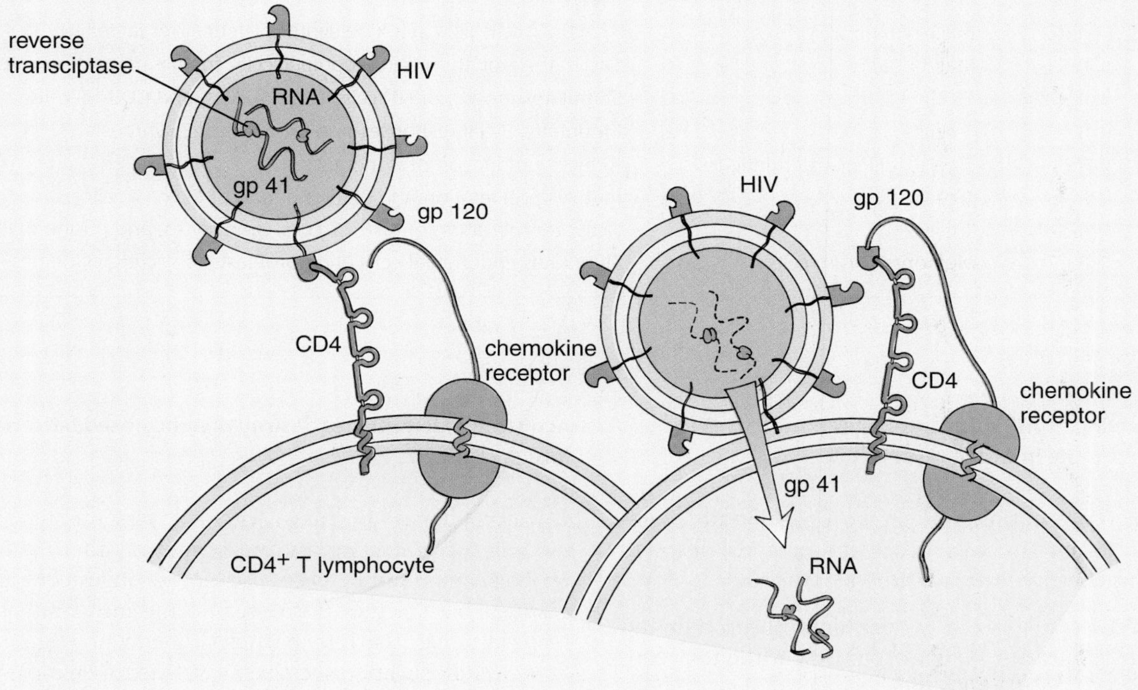

FIGURE 13.9
Schematic diagram of the interaction between HIV and the helper CD4$^+$ T cell. Human immunodeficiency virus (HIV) is the RNA virus that causes AIDS. It contains reverse transcriptase. HIV gains entry into the helper CD4$^+$ T lymphocyte by binding to the CD4 molecule and injecting its genetic information into the cell cytoplasm. Accessory cell surface molecules such as gp 120 assist in viral entry into the cell. These proteins interact with CD4 molecules. The injected genetic information is incorporated into the host cell genome through reverse transcription of RNA into DNA. This DNA containing viral information is then incorporated into host DNA.

To present an antigen to a helper T cell, the APC first processes the antigen intracellularly and then displays antigen peptides on its surface. Antigen processing begins when the APC endocytoses the antigen and breaks it down into 8 to 10 amino acid peptides. In the endosomal compartment of the APC, the peptides bind to MHC II molecules. The MHC II–antigen complex is then translocated to the plasma membrane of the APC and displayed on the cell surface (Fig. 13.10).

TABLE 13.3. **Characteristics of Interleukins**

Name	Symbol	Source	Major Functions
Interleukin-1	IL-1	Neutrophils, monocytes, macrophages, endothelial cells	Stimulates various cells in inflammatory response; induces fever; facilitates proliferation of $CD4^+$ T cells and proliferation and differentiation of B cells
Interleukin-2	IL-2	$CD4^+$ T cells	Induces proliferation and differentiation of $CD4^+$ T cells and to a lesser degree $CD8^+$ T cells, B cells, and NK cells
Interleukin-3	IL-3	$CD4^+$ T cells	Induces proliferation of hematopoietic stem cells
Interleukin-4	IL-4	$CD4^+$ T cells, mast cells	Induces proliferation and differentiation of B cells, $CD4^+$ T cells; activates macrophages
Interleukin-5	IL-5	$CD4^+$ T cells	Induces proliferation and differentiation of eosinophils; stimulates B cells to secrete IgA
Interleukin-6	IL-6	Endothelial cells, neutrophils, macrophages, T cells	Stimulates differentiation of hematopoietic cells; induces growth of activated B cells
Interleukin-7	IL-7	Adventitial cells of bone marrow	Stimulates growth and differentiation of progenitor B and T cells
Interleukin-8	IL-8	Macrophages, endothelial cells	Acts as a chemotactic factor on T lymphocytes and neutrophils
Interleukin-9	IL-9	$CD4^+$ T cells	Facilitates growth of $CD4^+$ T cell (but not $CD8^+$ T cells); stimulates growth of hematopoietic cells
Interleukin-10	IL-10	Macrophages, T cells	Acts on T cells as a cytokine synthesis inhibitory factor
Interleukin-11	IL-11	Macrophages	Facilitates growth of hematopoietic cells, mainly megakaryocytes
Interleukin-12	IL-12	T cells	Stimulates growth of NK cells, $CD4^+$ T cells, and $CD8^+$ T cells
Interleukin-13	IL-13	T cells	Modulates B cell responses and promotes IgE synthesis
Interleukin-14	IL-14	T cells, follicular dendritic cells	Induces production of B memory cells
Interleukin-15	IL-15	T cells	Induces proliferation and differentiation of $CD8^+$ T cells
Interleukin-16	IL-16	T cells	Activates migration of $CD8^+$ T cells, monocytes, and eosinophils
Interleukin-17	IL-17	Memory $CD4^+$ T cells	Stimulates endothelial cells and fibroblasts to secrete cytokines

In addition to acting as APCs, macrophages perform other crucial functions in the immune response

In addition to presenting antigens to both T and B lymphocytes, macrophages have other important, although nonspecific, functions in the immune response:

- They endocytose and partially degrade both protein and polysaccharide antigens before they present them in conjunction with MHC II molecules to helper $CD4^+$ T lymphocytes.
- They digest pathogenic microorganisms through lysosomal action in combination with the helper $CD4^+$ T lymphocytes.
- They secrete multiple cytokines including lymphokines, complement components, and interleukins, as well as acid hydrolases, proteases, and lipases.

Following contact with an antigen, macrophages undergo an activation process characterized by multiple functional and morphologic changes. The macrophage increases in size, as do the number of lysosomes and cytoplasmic vacuoles. The activated macrophage becomes avidly phagocytotic with a greater ability to lyse ingested pathogenic microorganisms (Fig. 13.11).

Activated macrophages destroy phagocytosed bacteria and foreign antigens

Macrophages also play a vital role in sequestering and removing foreign materials and organisms that either do not provoke an immune response or are ingested but not digested. These include both organic and inorganic particulate materials (e.g., carbon particles), pigment (e.g., from tattoos), cellulose, and asbestos, as well as tuberculosis and leprosy bacilli and the organisms that cause malaria and other diseases. In these instances, macrophages often fuse to form multinucleate, foreign body giant cells called ***Langhans' giant cells,*** which isolate these pathogens from the body.

▼ LYMPHATIC TISSUES AND ORGANS

Lymphatic Vessels

Lymphatic vessels are the route by which cells and large molecules pass from the tissue spaces back to the blood

Lymphatic vessels begin as networks of blind capillaries in loose connective tissue. They are most numerous beneath

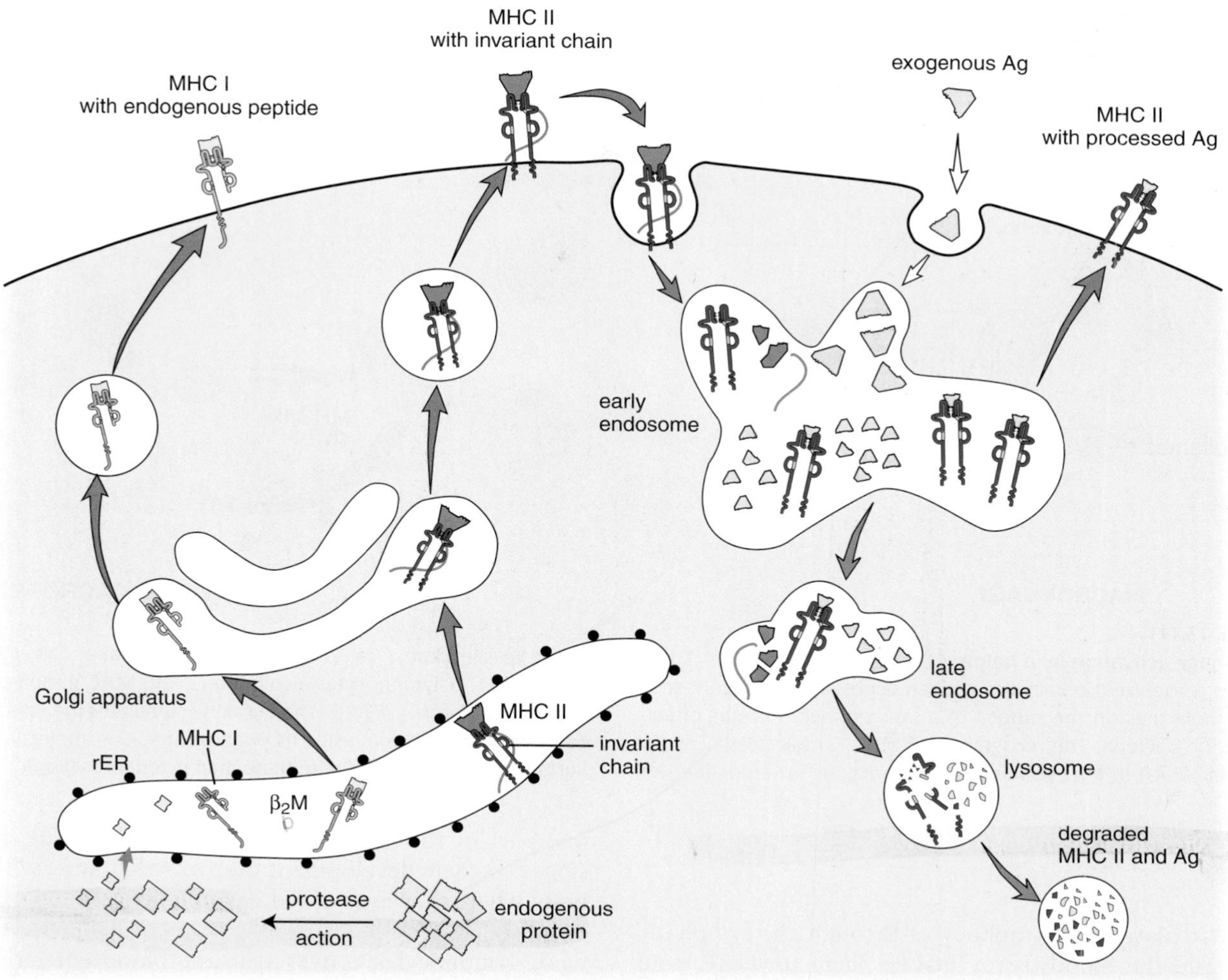

FIGURE 13.10

Schematic diagram of processing pathways for MHC I and MHC II synthesis and antigen presentation. During the processing and presentation of cytoplasmic antigen (Ag) for MHC I molecules *(red pathway),* cytoplasmic protein antigens are degraded by protease into 8 to 10 amino acid fragments, which then enter the rER. In the rER, newly synthesized α chains of MHC I molecules interact with both the processed antigen and β_2 microglobulin *(β_2M)* and form a stable complex. This complex leaves the rER via the typical secretory pathway through the Golgi apparatus. The antigen–MHC I complex is displayed on the cell surface, where it is available for recognition by cytotoxic CD8+ T lymphocytes. MHC II molecules are assembled in the rER and then bind to an invariant chain, which blocks the antigen-binding side. At this point the MHC II molecule and the invariant chain are secreted to the cell surface *(blue pathway).* After a brief stay on the cell surface, the MHC II molecule and invariant chain are endocytosed, and in an early endosome, the invariant chain is degraded. The foreign (exogenous) antigen is endocytosed and partially digested by proteolytic degradation in endosomes *(white pathway).* The MHC II molecule can now bind the processed foreign antigen and return with it to the cell surface. On the cell surface, the antigen–MHC II complex is recognized by helper CD4+ T lymphocytes, which initiates the immune response. If the MHC II molecule fails to capture the antigen, it will be degraded in the lysosomal compartment *(green pathway).*

the epithelium of skin and mucous membranes. These vessels remove substances and fluid from the extracellular spaces of the connective tissues, thus producing lymph. Because the walls of the lymphatic capillaries are more permeable than the walls of blood capillaries, large molecules, including antigens and cells, gain entry more readily into the lymphatic capillaries than into blood capillaries.

As lymph circulates through the lymphatic vessels, it passes through lymph nodes. Within the lymph nodes, foreign substances (antigens) conveyed in the lymph are trapped by the follicular dendritic cells and concentrated. These APCs process the antigens and present them to lymphocytes, which leads to an immune response that eliminates the antigens from the body.

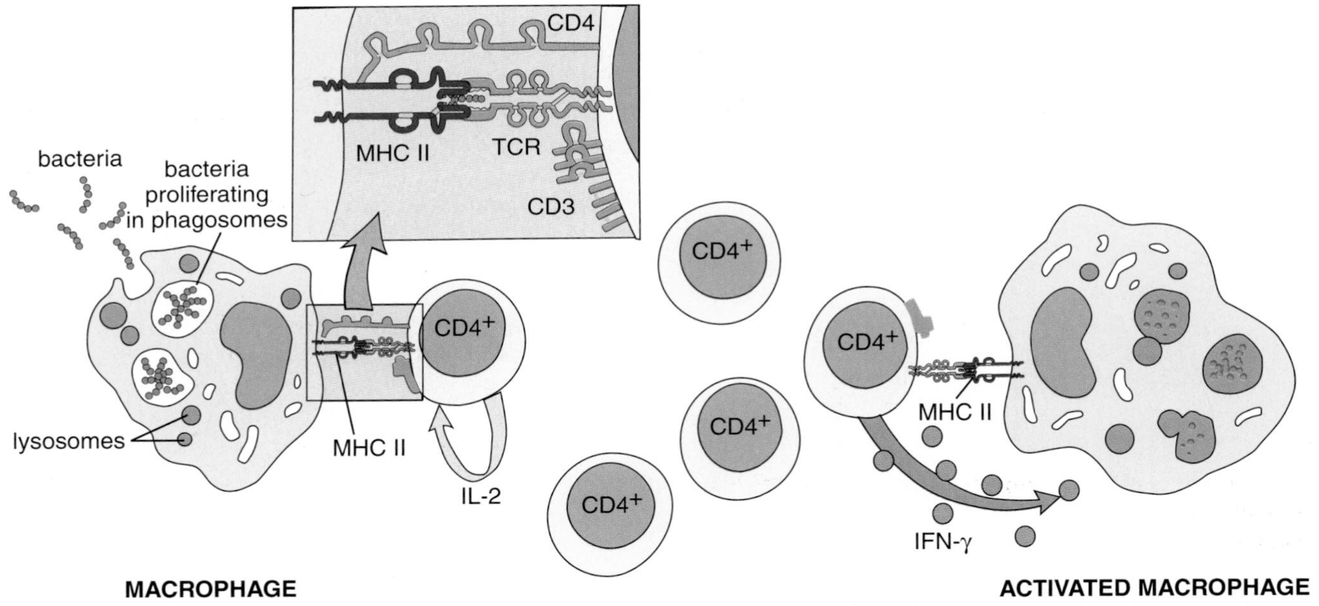

FIGURE 13.11
Macrophage activation by a helper CD4$^+$ T cell. Helper CD4$^+$ T lymphocytes recognize the bacterial antigen expressed in the context of MHC II molecules on the surface of a macrophage that has phagocytosed the bacteria. The recognition of MHC II molecules activates the T cell, which in turn secretes IL-2. IL-2 acts as an autocrine hormone to stimulate T cell division and differentiation. Newly formed helper CD4$^+$ T lymphocytes also interact with MHC II molecules and release interferon γ *(IFN-γ)*. This cytokine stimulates the macrophage to destroy the bacteria inside its phagosomes. CD4 molecules on the surface of the T cell also potentiate antibacterial reactions.

Lymphocytes circulate through both lymphatic and blood vessels

The circulation of lymphocytes through the lymphatic vessels and the bloodstream enables them to move from one part of the lymphatic system to another at different stages in their development and to reach sites within the body where they are needed. Lymphocytes conveyed in the lymph enter lymph nodes via ***afferent lymphatic vessels,*** while lymphocytes conveyed in the blood enter the node

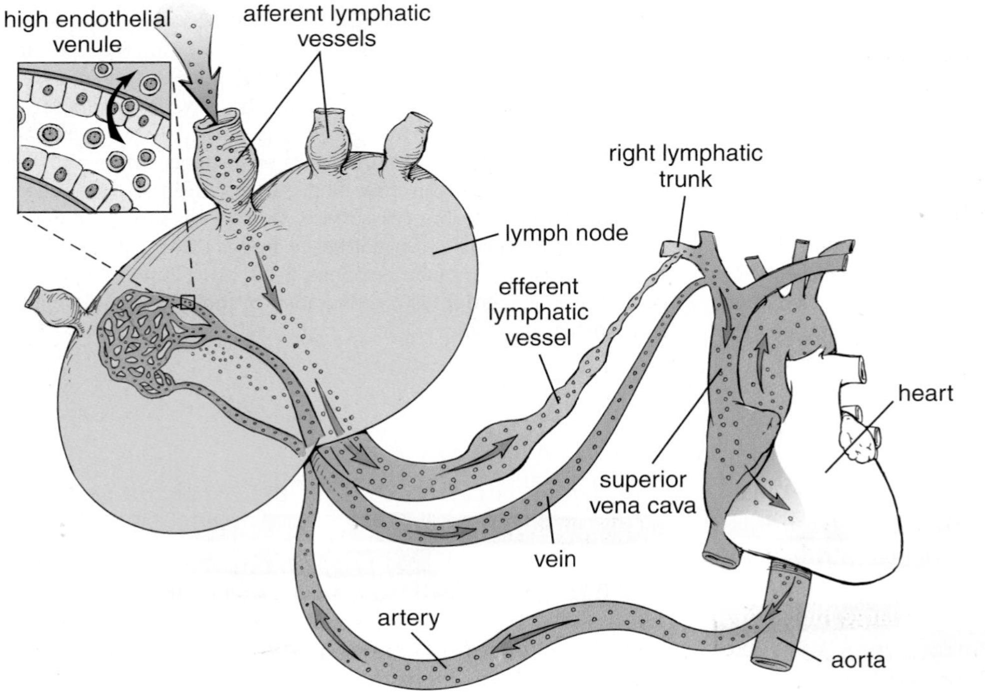

FIGURE 13.12
Diagram depicting circulation of lymphocytes in the body. Lymphocytes enter lymph nodes by two routes: afferent lymphatic vessels and through the wall of high endothelial venules (HEVs) in the deep cortex. Some lymphocytes move to the T and B domains of the lymph node; others pass through the parenchyma of the node and leave via an efferent lymphatic vessel. Ultimately, the lymphocytes enter a major lymphatic vessel—in this case the right lymphatic trunk—that opens into the junction of the right internal jugular and right subclavian vein. The lymphocytes continue to the arterial side of the circulation and, via the arteries, to the lymphatic tissues of the body or to tissues where they participate in immune reactions. From the lymphatic tissues, lymphocytes again return to the lymph nodes to gain entry via the HEV.

through the walls of ***postcapillary (high endothelial) venules*** (Fig. 13.12.). B and T cells migrate to and populate different regions within the lymph node. Some lymphocytes pass through the substance of the node and leave via the ***efferent lymphatic vessels,*** which lead to the right lymphatic trunk or to the thoracic duct. In turn, both of these channels empty into the blood circulation at the junctions of the internal jugular and subclavian veins at the base of the neck. The lymphocytes are conveyed to and from the various lymphatic tissues via the blood vessels.

Diffuse Lymphatic Tissue and Lymphatic Nodules

Diffuse lymphatic tissue and lymphatic nodules guard the body against pathogenic substances and are the site of the initial immune response

The alimentary canal, respiratory passages, and genitourinary tract are guarded by accumulations of lymphatic tissue that are not enclosed by a capsule. Lymphocytes and other free cells of this tissue are found in the ***lamina propria*** (subepithelial tissue) of these tracts. This form of lymphatic tissue is called ***diffuse lymphatic tissue*** or ***mucus-associated lymphatic tissue (MALT)*** because of its association with mucous membranes (Fig. 13.13). These cells are strategically located to intercept antigens and initiate an immune response. Following contact with antigen, they travel to regional lymph nodes, where they undergo proliferation and differentiation. Progeny of these cells then return to the lamina propria as effector B and T lymphocytes.

The importance of diffuse lymphatic tissue in protecting the body from antigens is indicated by

- The regular presence of large numbers of plasma cells, especially in the lamina propria of the gastrointestinal tract, a morphologic indication of local antibody secretion
- The presence of large numbers of eosinophils, also frequently observed in the lamina propria of the intestinal and respiratory tracts, an indication of chronic inflammation and hypersensitivity reactions

Lymphatic nodules are discrete concentrations of lymphocytes contained in a meshwork of reticular cells

In addition to diffuse lymphatic tissue, localized concentrations of lymphocytes are commonly found in the walls of the alimentary canal, respiratory passages, and genitourinary tract. These concentrations, called ***lymphatic nodules*** or ***lymphatic follicles,*** are sharply defined but not encapsulated (Fig. 13.14). A lymphatic nodule consisting chiefly of small lymphocytes is called a ***primary nodule.*** However, most nodules are ***secondary nodules*** and have distinctive features that include

- A ***germinal center*** located in the central region of the nodule (Fig. 13.15), which in histologic sections appears lightly stained. The germinal center develops when a lymphocyte that has recognized an antigen returns to a primary nodule and undergoes proliferation. The lighter staining is due to the large lymphocytes ***(lymphoblasts and plasmablasts)*** that it contains. These lymphocytes have large amounts of dispersed euchromatin in their nuclei rather than the dense heterochromatin of small lymphocytes. The germinal center is a morphologic indication of lymphatic tissue response to antigen. The presence of a germinal center represents a cascade of events that includes proliferation of lymphocytes, differentiation of plasma cells, and antibody production. Mitotic figures are frequently observed in the germinal center, reflecting the proliferation of new lymphocytes at this site. The number of macrophages in the germinal center often increases dramatically following a period of intense response to an antigen.

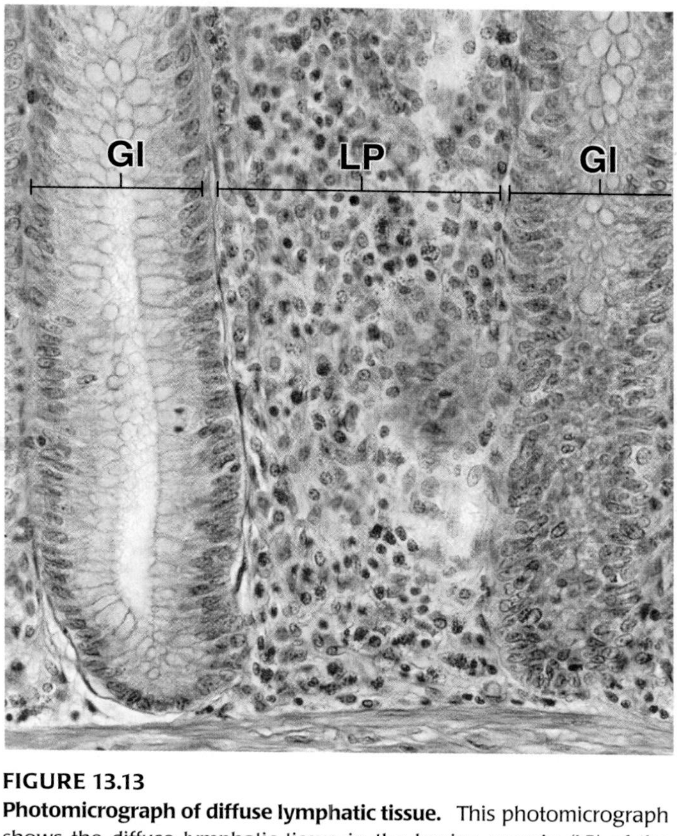

FIGURE 13.13
Photomicrograph of diffuse lymphatic tissue. This photomicrograph shows the diffuse lymphatic tissue in the lamina propria *(LP)* of the large intestine. The lower portion of two intestinal glands *(GI)* is also evident. The highly cellular, diffuse lymphatic tissue includes fibroblasts, plasma cells, and eosinophils. However, the most abundant cell component, whose presence characterizes diffuse lymphatic tissue, is the lymphocyte, which can be identified by its small, round, dark-staining nucleus. ×320.

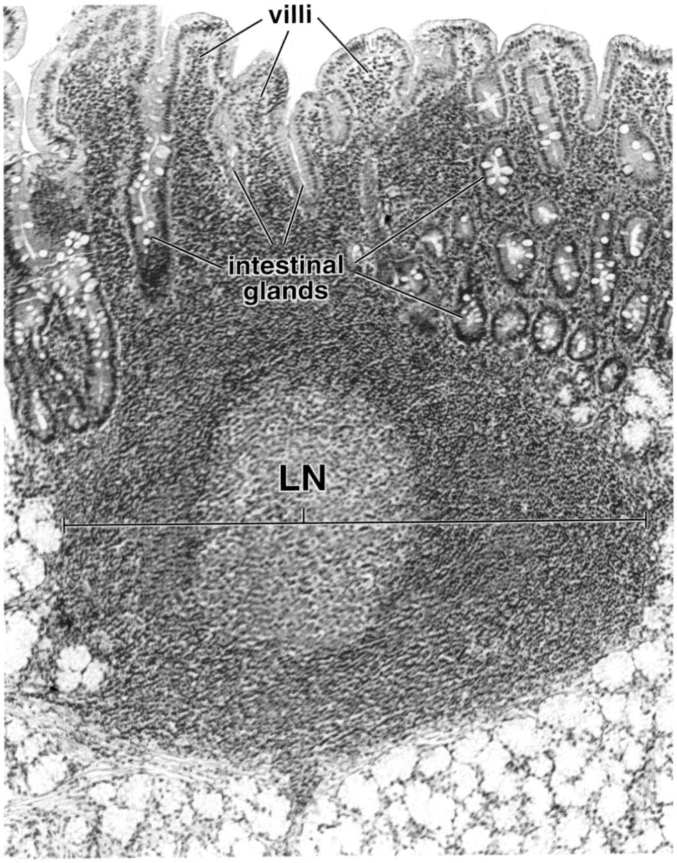

FIGURE 13.14
Photomicrograph of a lymphatic nodule. This photomicrograph shows a section of the wall of the small intestine (duodenum). Short villi and intestinal glands are present in the upper part of the micrograph. A lymphatic nodule *(LN)* occupies most of the remainder of the micrograph. The lighter central region of the nodule is the germinal center. The lymphocytes in the germinal center are larger than those in the more dense region of the nodule. They have more cytoplasm; consequently, their nuclei are more dispersed, giving the appearance of a less compact cellular mass. ×120.

- A *mantle zone* or *corona,* which represents an outer ring of small lymphocytes that encircles the germinal center.

Lymphatic nodules are usually found in structures associated with the alimentary canal such as the tonsils, ileum, and vermiform appendix

Generally, nodules are dispersed singly in a random manner. In the alimentary canal, however, some aggrega-

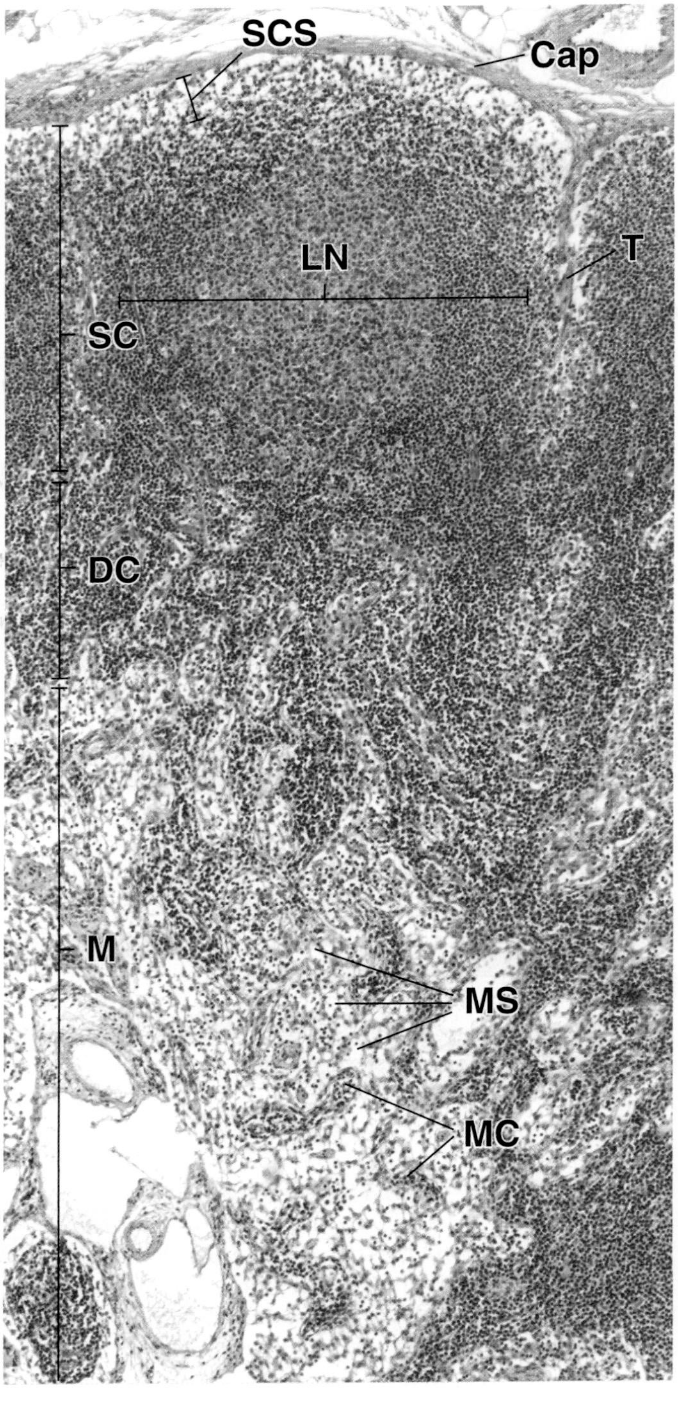

FIGURE 13.15
Photomicrograph of a lymph node. This photomicrograph shows the superficial cortex *(SC),* deep cortex *(DC),* and medulla *(M)* of the lymph node in a routine H&E preparation. The capsule *(Cap)* is composed of dense connective tissue from which trabeculae *(T)* penetrate into the organ. Below the capsule is the subcapsular sinus *(SCS).* It receives lymph from afferent lymphatic vessels that penetrate the capsule. The subcapsular sinus is continuous with the trabecular sinuses that course along the trabeculae. The superficial cortex contains the lymphatic nodules *(LN).* The deep cortex is nodule free. It consists of densely packed lymphocytes and contains the unique high endothelial venules (not visible at this magnification). The medulla consists of narrow strands of anastomosing lymphatic tissue called medullary cords *(MC),* separated by light-appearing spaces, the medullary sinuses *(MS).* The medullary sinuses receive lymph from the trabecular sinuses as well as lymph that has filtered through the cortical tissue. ×140.

tions of nodules are found in specific locations. These include

- ***Tonsils,*** which form a ring of lymphatic tissue at the entrance of the oropharynx. The ***pharyngeal tonsils,*** or ***adenoids,*** located in the roof of the pharynx; the ***palatine tonsils,*** or simply the tonsils, on either side of the pharynx, between the palatopharyngeal and palatoglossal arches; and the ***lingual tonsils,*** at the base of the tongue, all contain aggregates of lymphatic nodules. The palatine tonsils consist of dense accumulations of lymphatic tissue located in the mucous membrane. The squamous epithelium that forms the surface of the tonsil dips into the underlying connective tissue in numerous places, forming ***tonsillar crypts*** (Fig. 13.16). The walls of these crypts usually possess numerous lymphatic nodules. Like other aggregations of lymph nodules, tonsils do not possess afferent lymphatic vessels; however lymph drains from the lymphatic tissue of the tonsil via efferent lymphatic vessels.
- ***Peyer's patches,*** which are located in the ileum (distal portion of the small intestine). They consist of numerous aggregations of lymphatic nodules containing T and B lymphocytes (Fig. 13.17). In addition, numerous, isolated ***single (solitary) lymph nodules*** are located along both large and small intestines.
- ***Vermiform appendix,*** which arises from the cecum. The lamina propria is heavily infiltrated with lymphocytes and contains numerous lymphatic nodules. Although the appendix is often described as a vestigial organ, the abundant lymphatic tissue that it contains during early life suggests that it is functionally associated with bursa-equivalent organs. With age, the amount of lymphatic tissue within the organ regresses and is difficult to recognize.

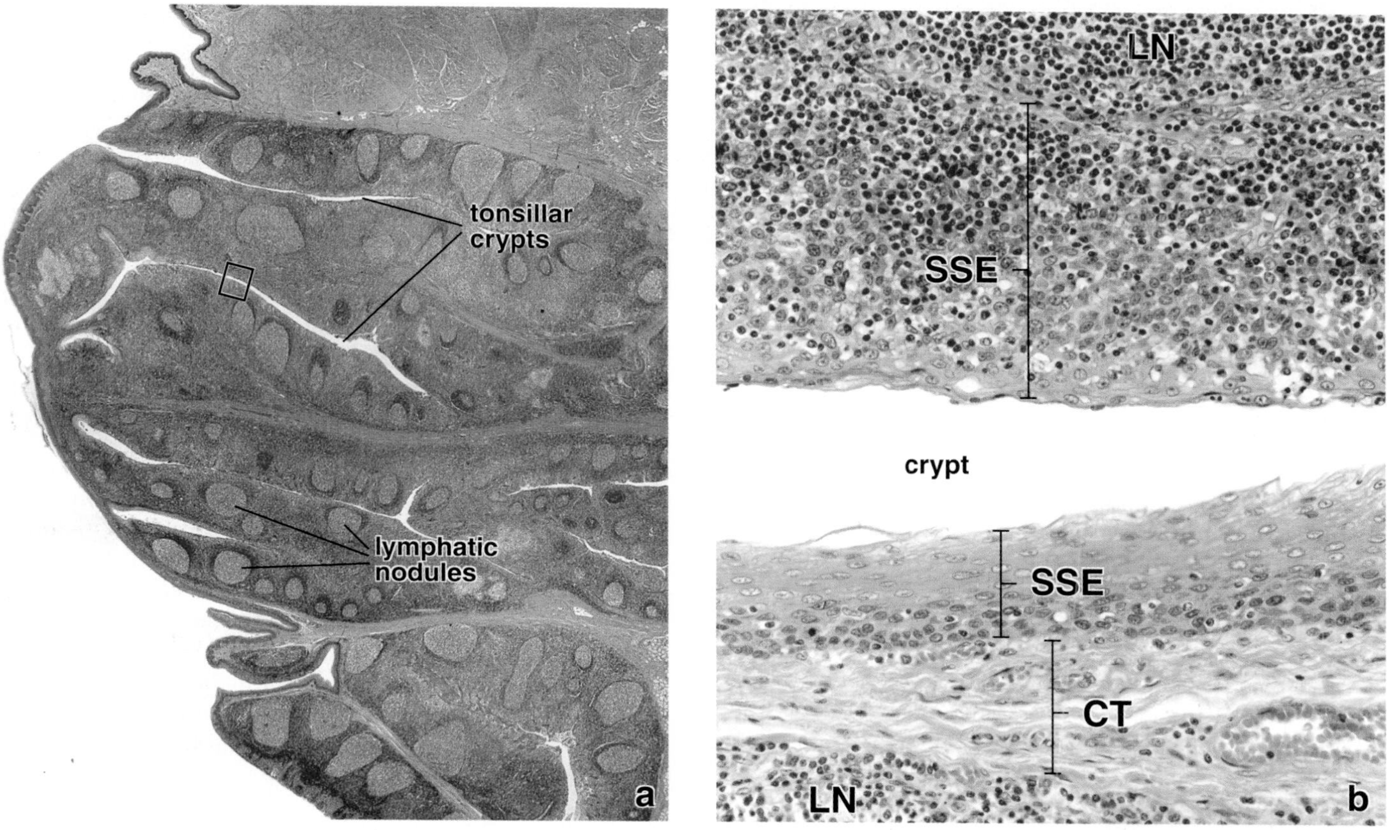

FIGURE 13.16
Photomicrograph of a palatine tonsil. a. This low-magnification photomicrograph shows a H&E–stained palatine tonsil. The stratified squamous epithelium that forms the surface of the tonsil dips into the underlying connective tissue in numerous places, forming tonsillar crypts. ×25. **b.** This higher-magnification photomicrograph of the *rectangular area* in *a* shows the stratified squamous epithelium *(SSE)* lining the tonsillar crypt. In the portion of the photomicrograph below the lumen of the crypt, SSE is well defined and separated by a connective tissue layer *(CT)* from the lymphatic nodule *(LN)*. In the upper portion of the photomicrograph, the SSE is just barely recognized because of the heavy infiltration of lymphocytes; the epithelial cells are present, however, although they are difficult to identify. In effect, the lymphatic nodule has literally grown into the epithelium, distorting it and resulting in the disappearance of the more typical, well-defined epithelial–connective tissue boundary. ×450.

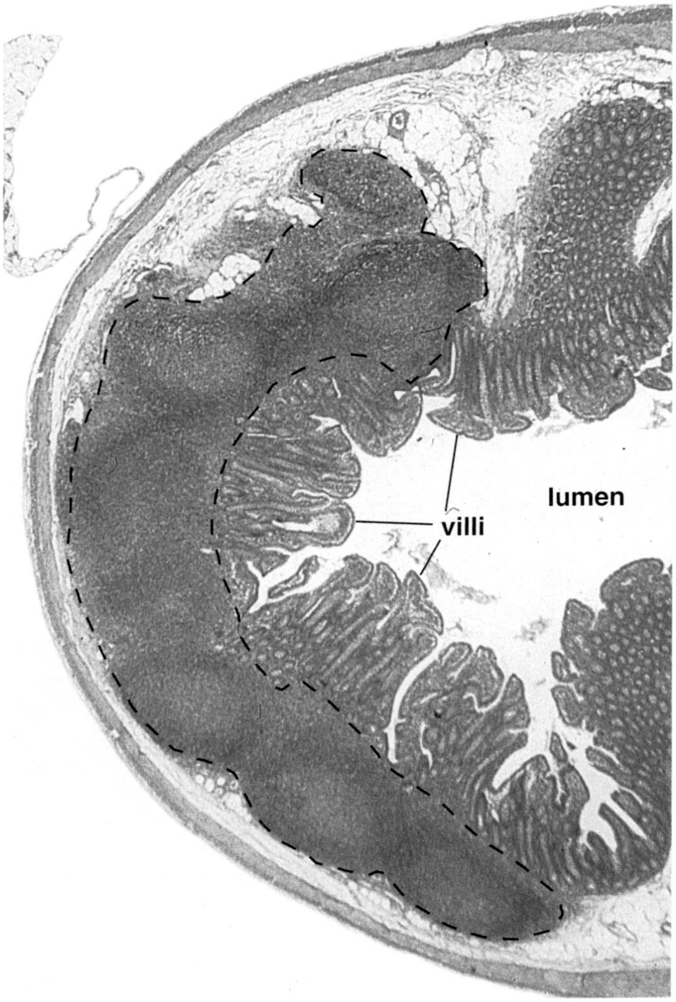

FIGURE 13.17
Photomicrograph of aggregated nodules in the wall of the ileum. This low-magnification photomicrograph provides an example of aggregated nodules. The multiple lymphatic nodules (indicated by a *dashed line*) with visible germinal centers are typically found in the ileum. This accumulation of lymphatic tissue is known as a Peyer's patch. The nodules originate in the lamina propria and extend into the submucosa of the ileum. ×5.

As noted, diffuse lymphatic tissue and lymphatic nodules are named according to the region or organ in which they appear. In the alimentary canal they are collectively referred to as GALT; in the bronchial tree they are known as ***bronchus-associated lymphatic tissue (BALT)***. The term ***mucus-associated lymphatic tissue (MALT)*** includes GALT and BALT. Diffuse lymphatic tissue and lymphatic nodules of MALT are present in many other regions of the body (e.g., female reproductive tract) where the mucosa is exposed to the external environment. All lymphatic nodules become enlarged as a consequence of encounters with antigen.

Lymph Nodes

Lymph nodes are small encapsulated organs located along the pathway of lymphatic vessels

Lymph nodes are small, bean-shaped, encapsulated lymphatic organs. They range in size from about 1 mm (barely visible with the unaided eye) to about 1 to 2 cm in their longest dimension. Lymph nodes are interposed along lymphatic vessels (Fig. 13.18) and serve as filters through which lymph percolates on its way to the blood vascular system. Although widely distributed throughout the body, they are concentrated in certain regions such as the axilla, groin, and mesenteries.

Two types of lymphatic vessels serve the lymph node:

- ***Afferent lymphatic vessels*** convey lymph toward the node and enter it at various points on the convex surface of the capsule.
- ***Efferent lymphatic vessels*** convey lymph away from the node and leave at the hilum, a depression on the concave surface of the node that also serves as the entrance and exit for blood vessels and nerves.

Note that activated lymphocytes, which remain in the lymph node to proliferate and differentiate, are carried to the node primarily by blood vessels.

The supporting elements of the lymph node are

- ***Capsule,*** composed of dense connective tissue that surrounds the node
- ***Trabeculae,*** also composed of dense connective tissue, which extend from the capsule into the substance of the node, forming a gross framework
- ***Reticular tissue,*** composed of reticular cells and reticular fibers that form a fine supporting meshwork throughout the remainder of the organ (Fig. 13.19)

The reticular meshwork of lymphatic tissues and organs (except the thymus) consists of cells of mesenchymal origin and reticular fibers and ground substance produced by those cells. The cells of the reticular meshwork appear as stellate or elongated cells with an oval euchromatic nucleus and a small amount of acidophilic cytoplasm. These cells can take up dyes and colloidal materials. Transmission electron microscopy, immunocytochemistry, and autoradiography indicate two populations of these cells:

- ***Reticular cells,*** indistinguishable from typical fibroblasts. These cells synthesize and secrete collagen (reticular fibers) and the associated ground substance that forms the stroma observed with the light microscope. Elongated cytoplasmic processes of these cells wrap around the bundles of reticular fibers, effectively isolating these structural components from the parenchyma of the lymphatic tissue and organs (Fig. 13.20).

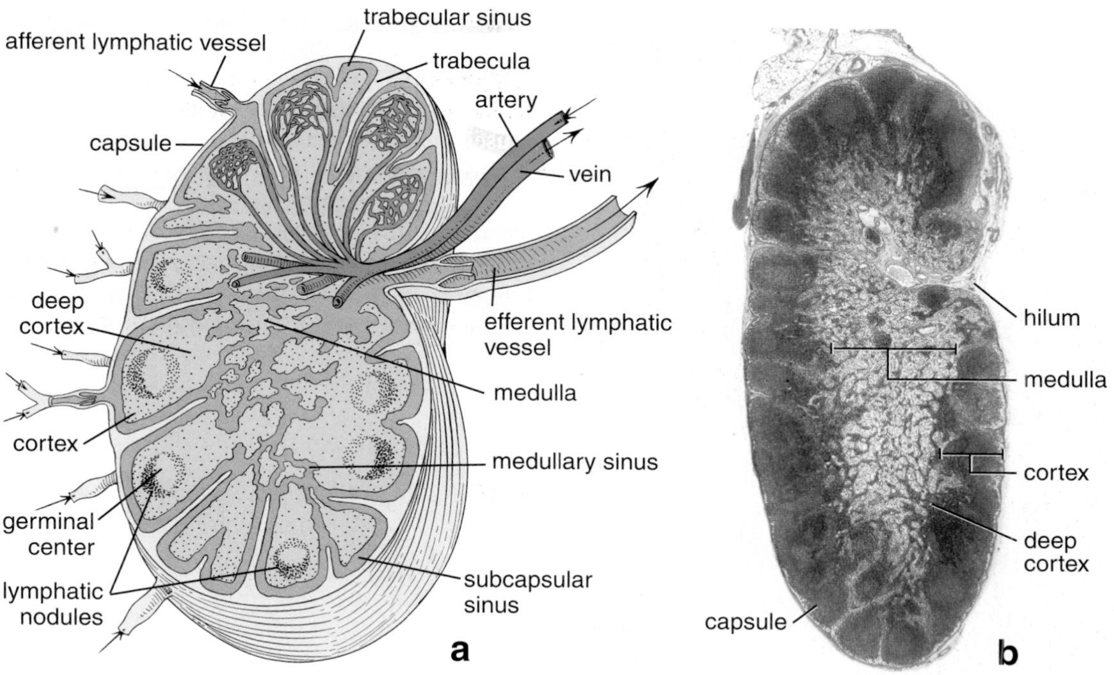

FIGURE 13.18

Structure of a lymph node. a. This diagram depicts the general features of a lymph node as seen in a section. The substance of the lymph node is divided into a cortex, including a deep cortex, and a medulla. The cortex, the outermost portion, contains spherical or oval aggregates of lymphocytes, called lymphatic nodules. In an active lymph node, nodules contain a lighter center, called the germinal center. The medulla, the innermost region of the lymph node, consists of lymphatic tissue that appears as irregular cords separated by lymphatic medullary sinuses. The dense population of lymphocytes between the superficial cortex and the medulla constitutes the deep cortex. It contains the high endothelial venules. Surrounding the lymph node is a capsule of dense connective tissue from which trabeculae extend into the substance of the node. Under the capsule and adjacent to the trabeculae are, respectively, the subcapsular sinus and the trabecular lymphatic sinuses. Afferent lymphatic vessels *(arrows)* penetrate the capsule and empty into the subcapsular sinus. The subcapsular sinus and trabecular sinuses communicate with the medullary sinuses. The upper portion of the lymph node shows an artery and a vein and the location of the high endothelial venules of the lymph node. **b.** Photomicrograph of a lymph node in a routine H&E preparation. The dense outer portion of the lymph node is the cortex. It consists of aggregations of lymphocytes organized as nodules and a nodule-free deep cortex. The innermost portion of the lymph node, the medulla, extends to the surface at the hilum, where blood vessels enter or leave and where efferent lymphatic vessels leave the node. Surrounding the lymph node is the capsule, and immediately beneath it is the subcapsular sinus. ×18.

- ***Follicular dendritic cells*** with multiple, thin, hair-like branching cytoplasmic processes that interdigitate between B lymphocytes in the germinal centers (Fig. 13.21). Antigen–antibody complexes adhere to the dendritic cytoplasmic processes by means of the antibody's F_c receptors, and the cell can retain antigen on its surface for weeks or months. Although this mechanism is similar to the adhesion of antigen–antibody complexes to macrophages, the antigen is not generally endocytosed, as it is by the macrophage. Follicular dendritic cells are not APCs, because they lack MHC II molecules.

The parenchyma of the lymph node is divided into a ***cortex*** and ***medulla*** (Fig. 13.22). The cortex forms the outer portion of the node except at the hilum. It consists of a dense mass of lymphatic tissue (reticular framework, follicular dendritic cells, lymphocytes, macrophages, and plasma cells) and lymphatic sinuses, the lymph channels. The medulla is the inner part of the lymph node.

Lymphocytes in the superficial cortex are organized into nodules

As elsewhere, the lymphatic nodules of the cortex are designated primary nodules if they consist chiefly of small lymphocytes and secondary nodules if they possess a germinal center. Lymphatic nodules are found in the outer part of the cortex, called the ***superficial*** or ***nodular cortex***. The portion of the cortex between the medulla and superficial cortex is free of nodules; it is called the ***deep cortex*** or ***paracortex***. This region contains most of the T cells in the lymph node. Because of its dependence

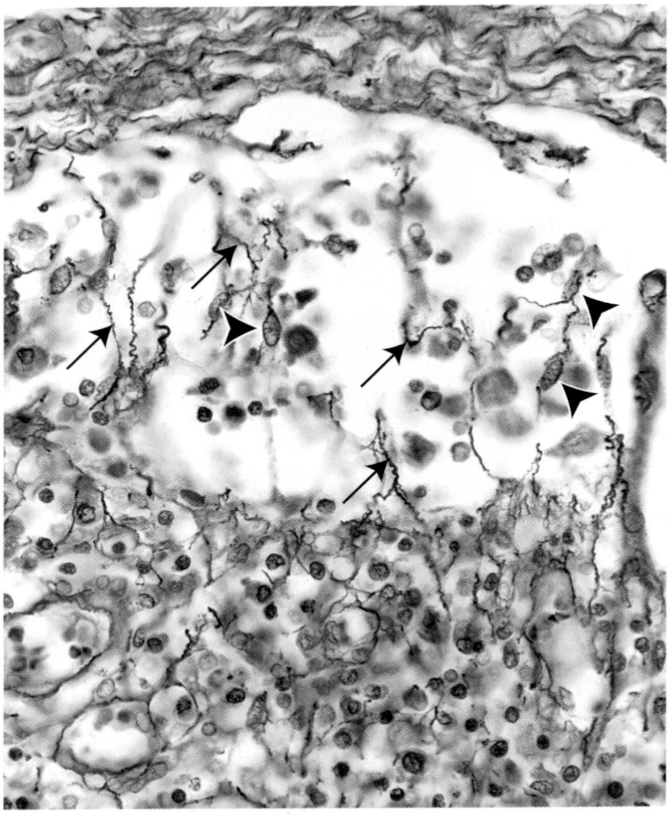

FIGURE 13.19
Photomicrograph of a lymph node. This silver preparation shows the connective tissue capsule (at the top), subcapsular sinus, and the superficial cortex of the lymph node (at the bottom). The reticular fibers *(arrows)* form an irregular anastomosing network throughout the stroma of the lymph node. Note elongated oval nuclei of reticular cells *(arrowheads)*, which are in intimate contact with reticular fibers in the sinus. ×640.

on the thymus, perinatal thymectomy in animals results in a poorly developed deep cortex. On the basis of this observation, the deep cortex is also called the ***thymus-dependent cortex.***

The medulla of the lymph node consists of the medullary cords and medullary sinuses

The medulla, the inner part of the lymph node, consists of cords of lymphatic tissue separated by lymphatic sinuses called medullary sinuses. As described above, a network of reticular cells and fibers traverses the medullary cords and medullary sinuses and serves as the framework of the parenchyma. In addition to reticular cells, the medullary cords contain lymphocytes (mostly B lymphocytes), macrophages, and plasma cells. The medullary sinuses converge near the hilum, where they drain into efferent lymphatic vessels.

Filtration of lymph in the lymph node occurs within a network of interconnected lymphatic channels called sinuses

There are three types of lymphatic channels called sinuses in the lymph node. Just beneath the capsule of the lymph node is a sinus interposed between the capsule and the cortical lymphocytes called the ***subcapsular sinus*** or ***cortical sinus.*** Afferent lymphatic vessels drain lymph into this sinus. ***Trabecular sinuses*** that originate from the subcapsular sinuses extend through the cortex along the trabeculae and drain into ***medullary sinuses.*** Lymphocytes and macrophages or their processes readily pass back and forth between the lymphatic sinuses and the parenchyma

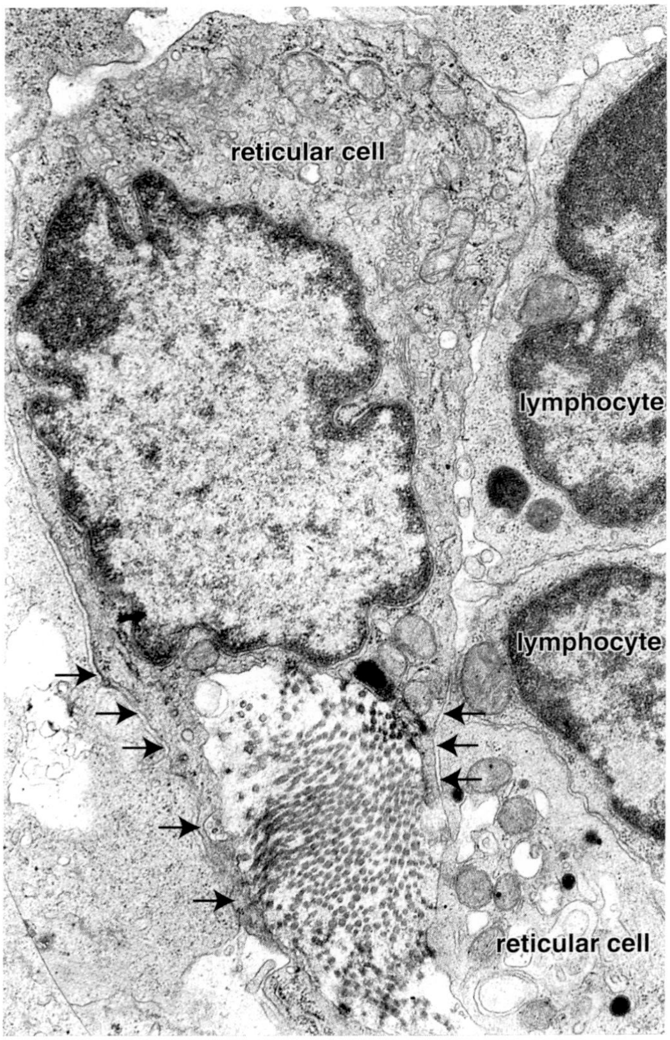

FIGURE 13.20
Electron micrograph of a reticular cell. The body of a reticular cell and its processes *(arrows)* are evident. The arrangement of the reticular cells contains and isolates the collagen fibrils from exposure to the lymphocytes. Note the adjacent lymphocytes on the right. In the light microscope and using a silver staining method, these collagen fibrils are recognized as a reticular fiber. ×12,600.

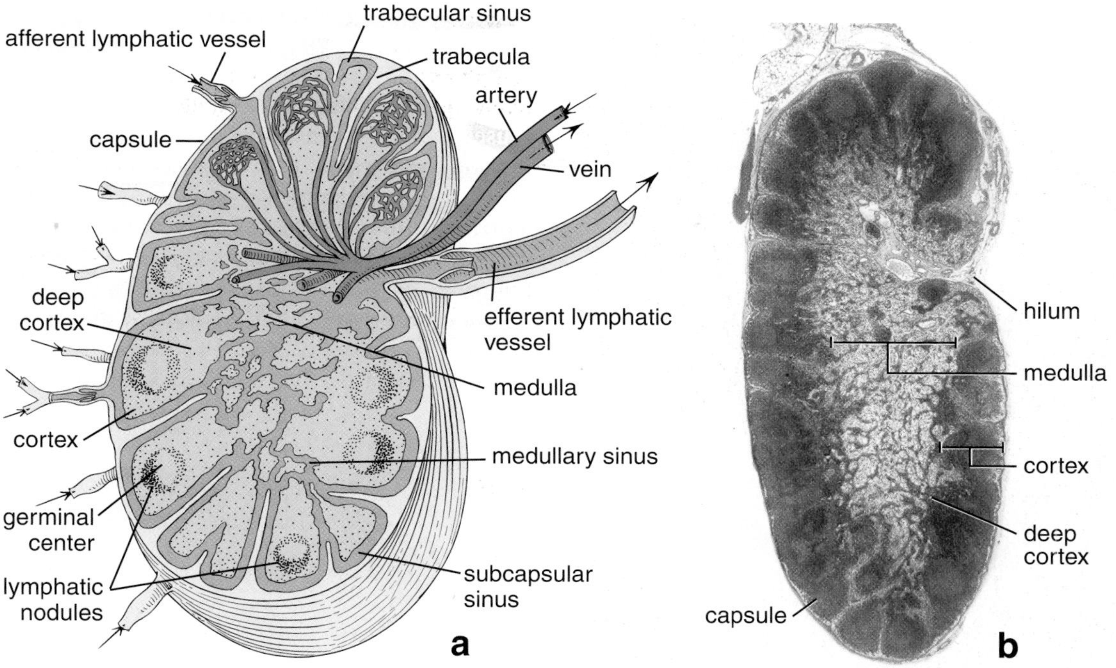

FIGURE 13.18
Structure of a lymph node. a. This diagram depicts the general features of a lymph node as seen in a section. The substance of the lymph node is divided into a cortex, including a deep cortex, and a medulla. The cortex, the outermost portion, contains spherical or oval aggregates of lymphocytes, called lymphatic nodules. In an active lymph node, nodules contain a lighter center, called the germinal center. The medulla, the innermost region of the lymph node, consists of lymphatic tissue that appears as irregular cords separated by lymphatic medullary sinuses. The dense population of lymphocytes between the superficial cortex and the medulla constitutes the deep cortex. It contains the high endothelial venules. Surrounding the lymph node is a capsule of dense connective tissue from which trabeculae extend into the substance of the node. Under the capsule and adjacent to the trabeculae are, respectively, the subcapsular sinus and the trabecular lymphatic sinuses. Afferent lymphatic vessels *(arrows)* penetrate the capsule and empty into the subcapsular sinus. The subcapsular sinus and trabecular sinuses communicate with the medullary sinuses. The upper portion of the lymph node shows an artery and a vein and the location of the high endothelial venules of the lymph node. **b.** Photomicrograph of a lymph node in a routine H&E preparation. The dense outer portion of the lymph node is the cortex. It consists of aggregations of lymphocytes organized as nodules and a nodule-free deep cortex. The innermost portion of the lymph node, the medulla, extends to the surface at the hilum, where blood vessels enter or leave and where efferent lymphatic vessels leave the node. Surrounding the lymph node is the capsule, and immediately beneath it is the subcapsular sinus. ×18.

- ***Follicular dendritic cells*** with multiple, thin, hair-like branching cytoplasmic processes that interdigitate between B lymphocytes in the germinal centers (Fig. 13.21). Antigen–antibody complexes adhere to the dendritic cytoplasmic processes by means of the antibody's F_c receptors, and the cell can retain antigen on its surface for weeks or months. Although this mechanism is similar to the adhesion of antigen–antibody complexes to macrophages, the antigen is not generally endocytosed, as it is by the macrophage. Follicular dendritic cells are not APCs, because they lack MHC II molecules.

The parenchyma of the lymph node is divided into a ***cortex*** and ***medulla*** (Fig. 13.22). The cortex forms the outer portion of the node except at the hilum. It consists of a dense mass of lymphatic tissue (reticular framework, follicular dendritic cells, lymphocytes, macrophages, and plasma cells) and lymphatic sinuses, the lymph channels. The medulla is the inner part of the lymph node.

Lymphocytes in the superficial cortex are organized into nodules

As elsewhere, the lymphatic nodules of the cortex are designated primary nodules if they consist chiefly of small lymphocytes and secondary nodules if they possess a germinal center. Lymphatic nodules are found in the outer part of the cortex, called the ***superficial*** or ***nodular cortex.*** The portion of the cortex between the medulla and superficial cortex is free of nodules; it is called the ***deep cortex*** or ***paracortex.*** This region contains most of the T cells in the lymph node. Because of its dependence

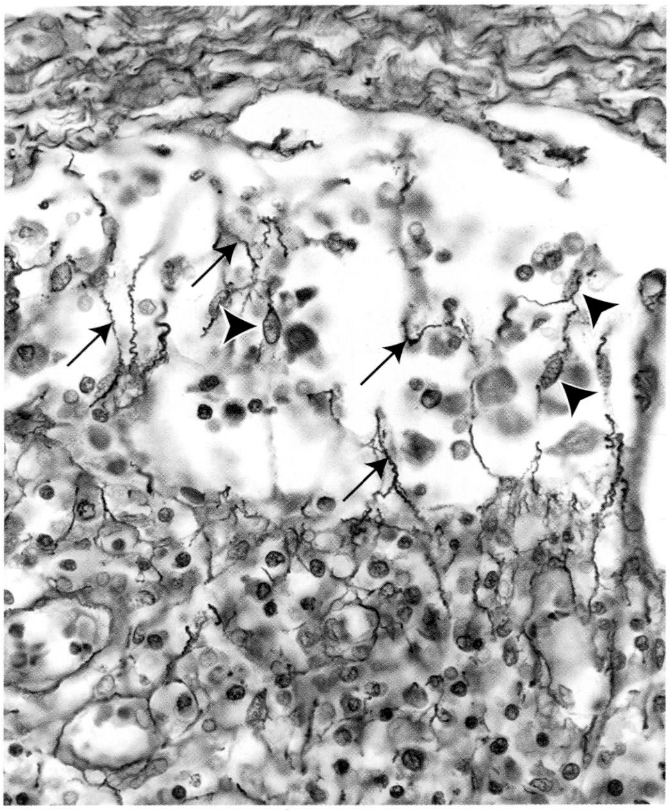

FIGURE 13.19
Photomicrograph of a lymph node. This silver preparation shows the connective tissue capsule (at the top), subcapsular sinus, and the superficial cortex of the lymph node (at the bottom). The reticular fibers *(arrows)* form an irregular anastomosing network throughout the stroma of the lymph node. Note elongated oval nuclei of reticular cells *(arrowheads),* which are in intimate contact with reticular fibers in the sinus. ×640.

on the thymus, perinatal thymectomy in animals results in a poorly developed deep cortex. On the basis of this observation, the deep cortex is also called the ***thymus-dependent cortex.***

The medulla of the lymph node consists of the medullary cords and medullary sinuses

The medulla, the inner part of the lymph node, consists of cords of lymphatic tissue separated by lymphatic sinuses called medullary sinuses. As described above, a network of reticular cells and fibers traverses the medullary cords and medullary sinuses and serves as the framework of the parenchyma. In addition to reticular cells, the medullary cords contain lymphocytes (mostly B lymphocytes), macrophages, and plasma cells. The medullary sinuses converge near the hilum, where they drain into efferent lymphatic vessels.

Filtration of lymph in the lymph node occurs within a network of interconnected lymphatic channels called sinuses

There are three types of lymphatic channels called sinuses in the lymph node. Just beneath the capsule of the lymph node is a sinus interposed between the capsule and the cortical lymphocytes called the ***subcapsular sinus*** or ***cortical sinus.*** Afferent lymphatic vessels drain lymph into this sinus. ***Trabecular sinuses*** that originate from the subcapsular sinuses extend through the cortex along the trabeculae and drain into ***medullary sinuses.*** Lymphocytes and macrophages or their processes readily pass back and forth between the lymphatic sinuses and the parenchyma

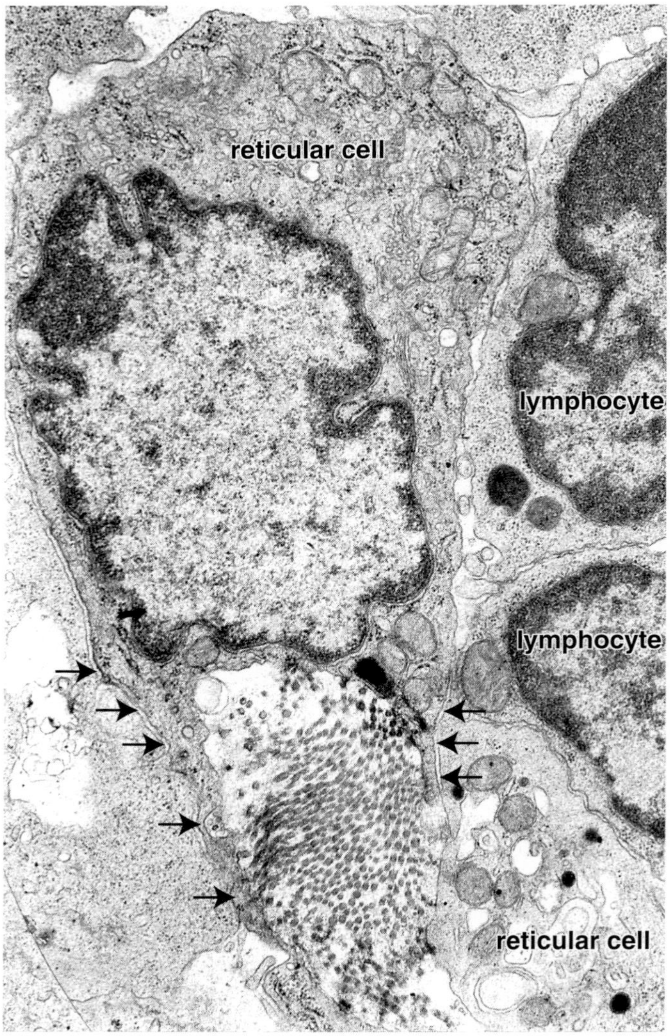

FIGURE 13.20
Electron micrograph of a reticular cell. The body of a reticular cell and its processes *(arrows)* are evident. The arrangement of the reticular cells contains and isolates the collagen fibrils from exposure to the lymphocytes. Note the adjacent lymphocytes on the right. In the light microscope and using a silver staining method, these collagen fibrils are recognized as a reticular fiber. ×12,600.

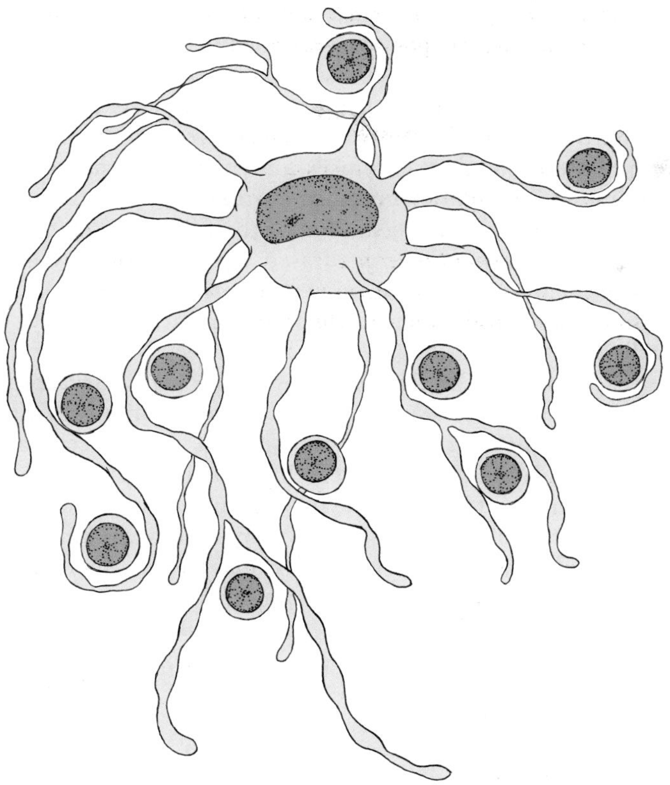

FIGURE 13.21
Diagram of a follicular dendritic cell. This cell, usually found in germinal centers, has multiple, thin, hair-like cytoplasmic processes that interdigitate between B lymphocytes. Antigen–antibody complexes adhere to the dendritic cytoplasmic processes by means of F_c receptors. Follicular dendritic cells are not antigen-presenting cells because they lack MHC II molecules.

of the node. The sinuses have a lining of endothelium that is continuous where it is directly adjacent to the connective tissue of the capsule or trabeculae but discontinuous where it faces the lymphatic parenchyma. Although a macrophage may reside in the lymphatic parenchyma, it often sends pseudopods (long cytoplasmic processes) into the sinus through these endothelial discontinuities. These pseudopods monitor the lymph as it percolates through the sinus.

Lymphatic sinuses are not open spaces, as are blood sinuses. Particularly in the medulla, macrophage processes, along with the reticular fibers surrounded by reticular cell processes, span the lumen of the sinus and form a crisscrossing meshwork that retards the free flow of lymph and enhances its filtration. Antigenic material and transformed cells of metastatic cancer are trapped by this mechanical filter and then phagocytosed by macrophages. In metastatic cancer, the system can be overwhelmed by an excessive number of cancer cells flowing through the lymphatic sinuses; as a result, the cells may establish a new metastatic site in the lymph node.

Specialized high endothelial venules (HEVs) are the site of entry for circulating lymphocytes into the lymph node

In addition to lymph, lymphocytes also circulate through the lymph nodes. Although some lymphocytes enter nodes through afferent lymphatic vessels as components of lymph, most enter the node through the wall of ***postcapillary venules*** located in the deep cortex (see Fig. 13.22). Because the postcapillary venules are lined by cuboidal or columnar endothelial cells, they are referred to as ***high endothelial venules (HEVs)*** (Fig. 13.23). These specialized endothelial cells possess receptors for antigen-primed lymphocytes. They signal lymphocytes to leave the circulation and migrate into the lymph node. Both B and T cells leave the bloodstream through HEVs, crossing the endothelium

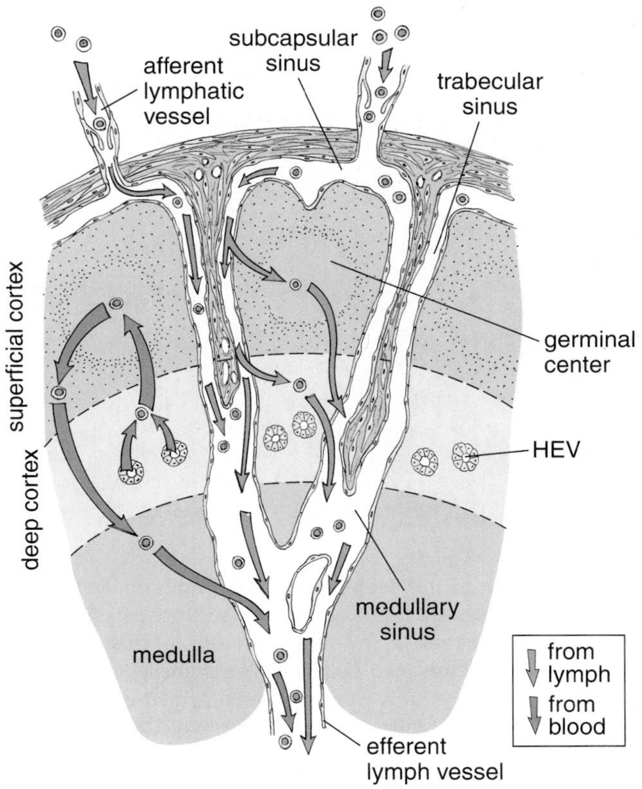

FIGURE 13.22
Schematic diagram of lymphocyte circulation within a lymph node. The *green arrows* indicate the circulation pathway of lymphocytes that enter the lymph node with the flow of lymph. Afferent lymphatic vessels carry lymph from the surrounding tissues and neighboring lymph nodes into the elaborate network of lymphatic sinuses. The wall of the sinuses allows lymph to percolate freely into the superficial and deep cortex, allowing lymphocytes to engage in immunosurveillance. The lymphocytes that enter the tissue next migrate back to the sinuses and leave the lymph node with the flow of the lymph. Lymphocytes that migrate to the lymph node from the blood *(blue arrows)* enter the deep cortex via high endothelial venules *(HEVs)* and also migrate to the superficial cortex. Here, lymphocytes perform the same functions as lymphocytes that enter via lymphatic vessels. They also leave the lymph node by the efferent lymph vessels.

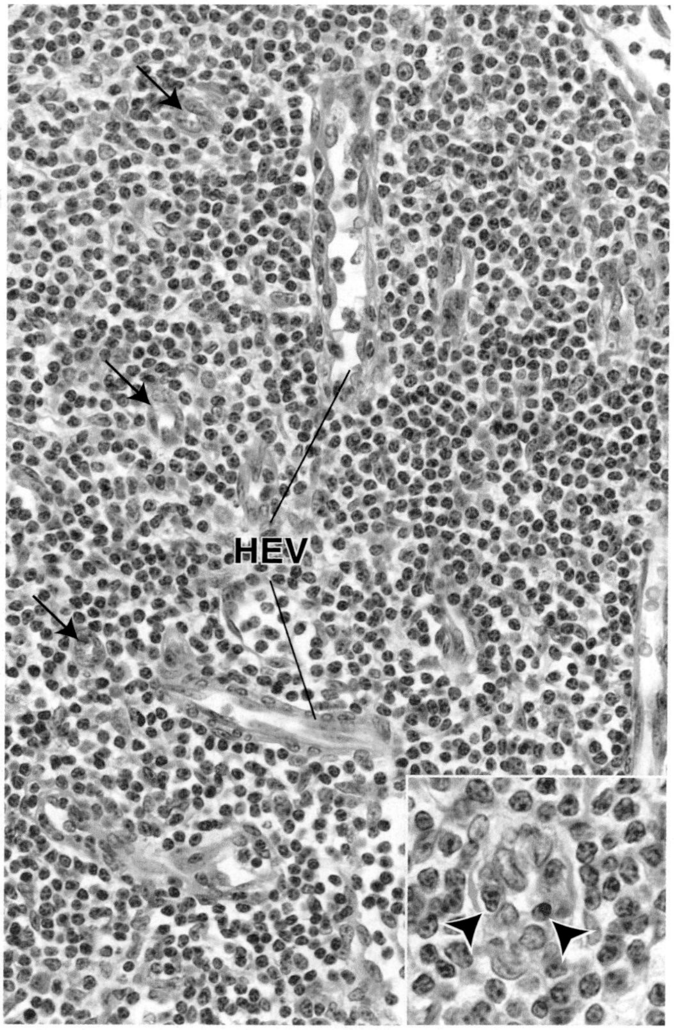

FIGURE 13.23
Photomicrograph of the deep cortex of a lymph node. This photomicrograph shows several longitudinally sectioned high endothelial venules *(HEVs)* as well as several that are seen in cross section (*arrows*). These vessels are lined by cuboidal endothelial cells. In some preparations, the walls of a HEV may be infiltrated with migrating lymphocytes, making it difficult to recognize. ×400. **Inset.** The cross section of a HEV shown here at higher magnification reveals several lymphocytes *(arrowheads)* in the process of migrating from the HEV into the parenchyma of the lymph node. ×640

by diapedesis, i.e., by migrating between the endothelial cells, in a manner similar to that described for neutrophils (see page 222). The T cells remain in the thymus-dependent deep cortex; the B cells migrate to the nodular cortex. Most lymphocytes leave the lymph node by entering lymphatic sinuses from which they flow to an efferent lymphatic vessel.

The lymph node is an important site for phagocytosis and initiation of immune responses

Phagocytosis of particulate material by phagocytotic cells within the lymph nodes is an important step in initiating an immune response. The physical accumulation of microorganisms and particulate substances conveyed in the lymph and phagocytosis of the particulate material help to concentrate antigen, thus enhancing its presentation to lymphocytes. Antigens conveyed in the lymph percolate through the sinuses and penetrate the lymph nodules to initiate an immune response. Some antigens become trapped on the surface of the follicular dendritic cells, while others are processed by macrophages and B cells, leading to activation and differentiation of B cells into antibody-producing plasma cells and memory B cells.

The plasma cells then migrate to the medullary cords where they synthesize and release specific antibodies into the lymph flowing through the sinuses. Plasma cells account for 1 to 3% of the cells in resting lymph nodules. Their number increases dramatically during an immune response, thereby increasing the amount of circulating immunoglobulins. Memory B cells may leave the lymph nodes and circulate to various regions through the body, where they can proliferate in response to subsequent exposure to their specific antigen. The presence of memory cells in various sites throughout the body ensures a more rapid response to an antigen, the secondary response.

Lymph nodes in which lymphocytes are responding to antigens often enlarge, reflecting formation of germinal centers and proliferation of lymphocytes. This phenomenon is most often seen in the lymph nodes of the neck in response to nasal or oropharyngeal infection. These enlarged lymph nodes are commonly referred to as "swollen glands."

Thymus

The thymus is a lymphoepithelial organ located in the superior mediastinum

The thymus is a bilobed organ located in the superior mediastinum, anterior to the heart and great vessels. It develops bilaterally from the third (and sometimes also the fourth) branchial (oropharyngeal) pouch. During development, the epithelium invaginates, and the thymic rudiment grows caudally as a tubular projection of the endodermal epithelium into the mediastinum of the chest. The advancing tip proliferates and ultimately becomes disconnected from the branchial epithelium. ***Multipotential lymphoid stem cells (CFU-Ls)*** from the bone marrow that are destined to develop into immunocompetent T cells invade the epithelial rudiment and occupy spaces between the epithelial cells so that the thymus develops into a lymphoepithelial organ.

The thymus is fully formed and functional at birth. It persists as a large organ until about the time of puberty, when T cell differentiation and proliferation are reduced and most of the lymphatic tissue is replaced by adipose tissue (involution). The organ can be restimulated under conditions that demand rapid T cell proliferation.

Connective tissue surrounds the thymus and subdivides it into thymic lobules

The thymus possesses a thin connective tissue ***capsule*** from which ***trabeculae*** extend into the parenchyma of the organ. The capsule and trabeculae contain blood vessels, efferent (but not afferent) lymphatic vessels, and nerves. In addition to collagen fibers and fibroblasts, the connective tissue of the thymus contains variable numbers of plasma cells, granulocytes, lymphocytes, mast cells, adipose cells, and macrophages.

The trabeculae establish domains in the thymus called ***thymic lobules.*** They are not true lobules, but cortical caps over portions of the highly convoluted but continuous inner medullary tissue (Fig. 13.24). In some planes of section, the "lobular" arrangement of the cortical cap and medullary tissue superficially resembles a lymphatic nodule with a germinal center, which often confuses students. Other morphologic characteristics (described below) allow positive identification of the thymus in histologic sections.

The thymic parenchyma contains developing T cells in an extensive meshwork formed by epithelioreticular cells

The outer portion of the parenchyma, the ***thymic cortex,*** is markedly basophilic in H&E preparations because of the closely packed developing T lymphocytes with their intensely staining nuclei. These T lymphocytes, also called ***thymocytes,*** occupy spaces within an extensive meshwork of ***epithelioreticular cells*** (Fig. 13.25). Macrophages are also dispersed among the cortical cells. The developing T cells arise from CFU-Ls, which originate in bone marrow. As development proceeds in the thymus, the cells derived from CFU-Ls pass through a series of developmental stages that are reflected by their expression of different CD molecules.

As their name implies, epithelioreticular cells have features of both epithelial and reticular cells. They provide a framework for the developing T cells; thus, they correspond to the reticular cells and their associated reticular fibers in other lymphatic tissues and organs. Reticular connective tissue cells and their fibers, however, are not present in the thymic parenchyma. Epithelioreticular cells exhibit certain features characteristic of epithelium, such as intercellular junctions and intermediate filaments.

Six types of epithelioreticular cells are recognized on the basis of function: three types in the cortex and three types in the medulla. Each type is designated by roman numerals. In the cortex the following cell types are recognized:

- ***Type I epithelioreticular cells*** are located at the boundary of the cortex and the connective tissue capsule as well as between the cortical parenchyma and the trabeculae. They also surround the adventitia of the cortical blood vessels. In essence, type I epithelioreticular cells serve to separate the thymic parenchyma from the connective tissue of the organ. The occluding junctions between these cells reflect their function as a barrier that isolates developing T cells from the connective tissue of the organ, i.e., capsule, trabeculae, and perivascular connective tissue.
- ***Type II epithelioreticular cells*** are located within the cortex. The transmission electron microscope (TEM) reveals maculae adherentes (desmosomes) that join long cytoplasmic processes of adjacent cells. The cell body and cytoplasmic processes contain abundant intermediate filaments. Because of their processes, these cells are stellate. They have a large nucleus that stains lightly with H&E because of its abundant euchromatin. This nuclear feature allows the cell to be easily identified in the light microscope. Type II cells compartmentalize the cortex

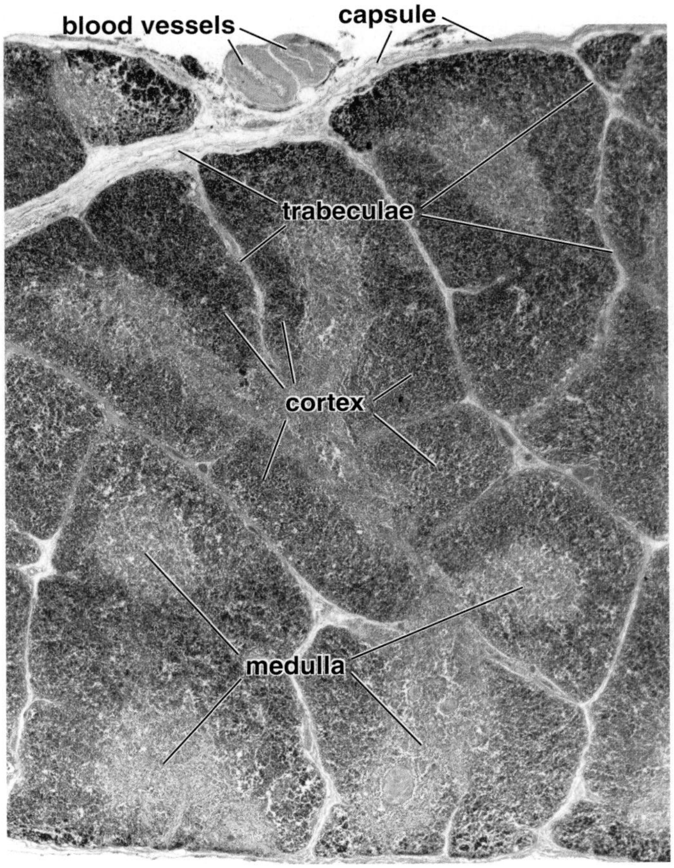

FIGURE 13.24
Photomicrograph of an infant human thymus. This H&E preparation reveals multiple lobules separated by connective tissue trabeculae that extend into the organ from the surrounding capsule. Each lobule is composed of a dark-staining basophilic cortex and a lighter-staining and relatively eosinophilic medulla. The medulla is actually a continuous branching mass surrounded by the cortex. The cortex contains numerous densely packed lymphocytes, whereas the medulla contains fewer lymphocytes. Note that in some instances the medulla may bear a resemblance to germinal centers of lymphatic nodules (upper right and center left). Such isolated medullary profiles are continuous with the overall medullary tissue, but this continuity may not be seen within the plane of section. ×25.

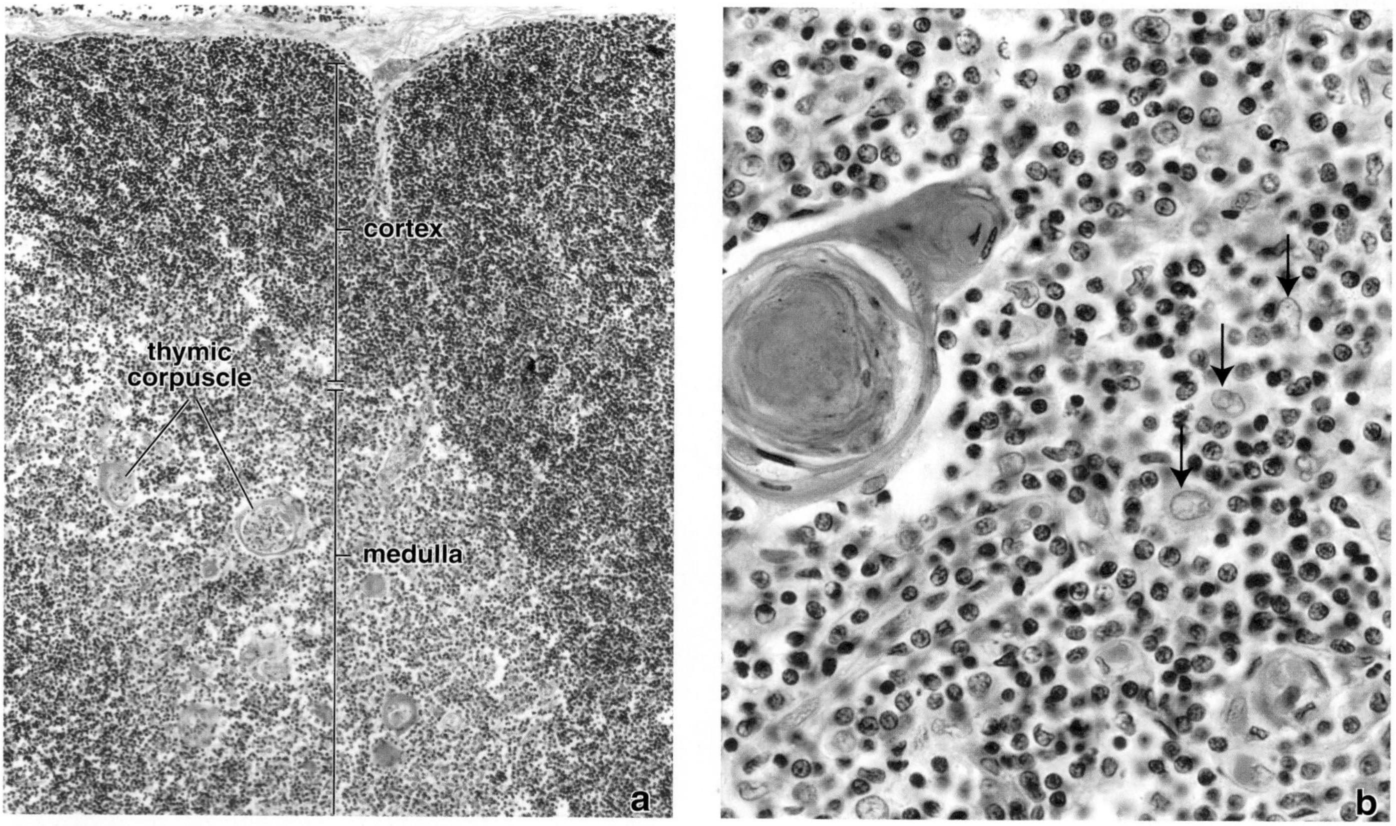

FIGURE 13.25
Photomicrograph of a human thymus. a. The cortex contains a dense population of small, maturing T cells that creates the dark staining of this region of the thymus. The medulla, in contrast, appears lighter. The medulla also contains the thymic corpuscles that stain with eosin and give it a further distinction. ×120. **b.** This higher-magnification photomicrograph shows the medulla with a thymic corpuscle (left) and surrounding cells. Thymic corpuscles are isolated masses of closely packed, concentrically arranged type VI epithelioreticular cells; these cells exhibit flattened nuclei. The more central mass of the corpuscle contains fully keratinized cells. In addition to numerous lymphocytes, the micrograph also shows type V epithelioreticular cells *(arrows)*, with their eosinophilic cytoplasm and large, pale-staining nuclei. ×600.

into isolated areas for the developing T cells. Unlike type I cells, type II cells express MHC I and MHC II molecules, which are involved in thymic cell education.

- *Type III epithelioreticular* cells are located at the boundary of the cortex and medulla. The TEM reveals occluding junctions between sheet-like cytoplasmic processes of adjacent cells. Like type I cells, type III epithelioreticular cells create a functional barrier, in this case between the cortex and medulla. Like type II cells, they possess MHC I and MHC II molecules.
- *Macrophages* reside within the thymic cortex and are responsible for phagocytosis of T cells that do not fulfill thymic education requirements. These T cells are programmed to die before leaving the cortex. Approximately 98% of the T cells undergo this apoptosis and are then phagocytosed by the macrophages. The macrophages in the cortex are difficult to identify in H&E preparations. However, the periodic acid–Schiff (PAS) reaction readily defines them because of the staining of their numerous large lysosomes. Accordingly, these macrophages are called ***PAS cells.***

While the epithelioreticular cells of the thymic cortex play an important role in the development of immunocompetent T cells, recent evidence shows that T cells at the different stages of differentiation control the microarchitecture of the thymic epithelioreticular cells, a phenomenon called "crosstalk." The developing lymphocytes and epithelioreticular cells thus influence each other during T cell development.

Thymic or Hassall's corpuscles (derived from type VI epithelioreticular cells) are a distinguishing feature of the thymic medulla

The ***thymic medulla,*** the inner portion of the parenchyma, contains a large number of epithelioreticular cells and loosely packed T cells (Fig. 13.25). The medulla

stains less intensely than the cortex because, like the germinal centers of lymph nodules, it contains mostly large lymphocytes. These lymphocytes have pale-staining nuclei and quantitatively more cytoplasm than small lymphocytes. Like the cortex, the medulla also contains three types of epithelioreticular cells:

- ***Type IV epithelioreticular cells*** are located between the cortex and the medulla close to type III cells. They possess sheet-like processes with occluding junctions between adjacent cells as well as between them and type III cells. In cooperation with type III cells, they create the barrier at the corticomedullary junction.
- ***Type V epithelioreticular cells*** are located throughout the medulla. Like the type II cells located in the cortex, processes of adjacent cells are joined by desmosomes to provide the cellular framework of the medulla and to compartmentalize groups of lymphocytes. These nuclei contrast markedly with the densely staining lymphocyte nuclei.
- ***Type VI epithelioreticular*** cells form the most characteristic feature of the thymic medulla, the ***thymic*** or ***Hassall's corpuscles*** (Fig. 13.26). Thymic corpuscles are isolated masses of closely packed, concentrically arranged type VI epithelioreticular cells that exhibit flattened nuclei. TEM studies of these cells reveal keratohyalin granules, bundles of cytoplasmic intermediate filaments, and lipid droplets. The cells are joined by desmosomes. The center of a thymic corpuscle may display evidence of keratinization, not a surprising feature for cells developed from oropharyngeal epithelium. Thymic corpuscles are unique, antigenically distinct, and functionally active multicellular components of the medulla. Although the function of thymic corpuscles is not fully understood, histochemical studies show that they produce thymic hormones (e.g., thymosin and thymopoietin).

Blood vessels pass from the trabeculae to enter the parenchyma of the thymus. Typically, the blood vessels enter the medulla from the deeper parts of the trabeculae and carry a sheath of connective tissue along with them. This perivascular connective tissue sheath varies in thickness. It is thicker around larger vessels and gradually becomes thinner around smaller vessels. Where it is thick, it contains reticular fibers, fibroblasts, macrophages, plasma cells, and other cells found in loose connective tissue; where it is thin, it may contain only reticular fibers and occasional fibroblasts.

The blood–thymus barrier protects developing lymphocytes in the thymus from exposure to antigens

Lymphocytes reaching the thymic cortex are prevented from contact with antigen by a physical barrier called the ***blood–thymus barrier*** (Fig. 13.27). The components that

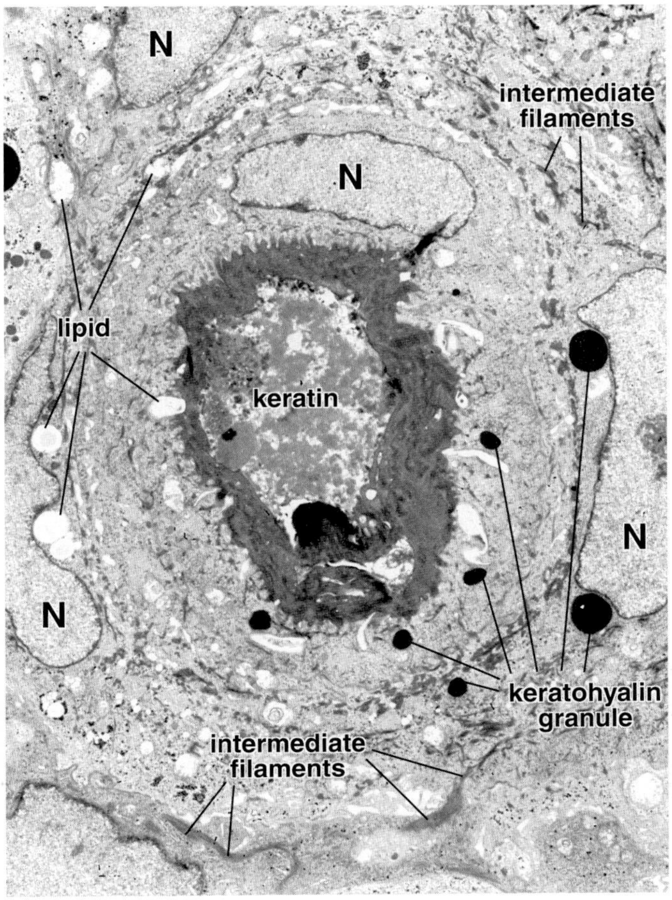

FIGURE 13.26
Electron micrograph of a thymic (Hassall's) corpuscle. This relatively low magnification electron micrograph shows some of the nuclei *(N)* and cytoplasm of the concentrically arranged epithelioreticular cells of a thymic (Hassall's) corpuscle. Bundles of intermediate filaments, keratohyalin granules, and lipid droplets are also evident within the cytoplasm of the epithelioreticular cells. Fully keratinized cells *(black layer)* are present in the center of the thymic corpuscle. ×5,000. (Courtesy of Dr. Johannes A. G. Rhodin.)

constitute the blood–thymus barrier between the T cells and the lumen of cortical blood vessels from the lumen outward, are

- Lining ***endothelium*** of the capillary wall. The endothelium is of the continuous type with occluding junctions. It is highly impermeable to macromolecules and is considered a major structural component of the barrier within the cortical parenchyma. The underlying ***basal lamina*** of endothelial cells and occasional ***pericytes*** are also part of the capillary wall.
- ***Macrophages*** in the surrounding perivascular connective tissue. Antigenic molecules that escape from the capillary lumen into the cortical parenchyma may be phagocytosed by macrophages residing in this tissue.

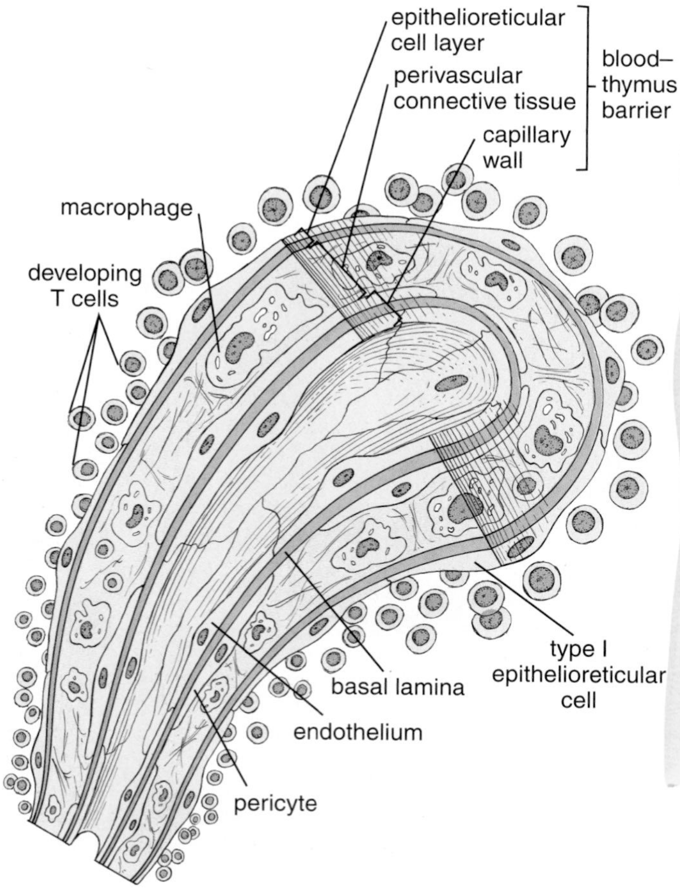

FIGURE 13.27
Schematic diagram of the blood–thymus barrier. The blood–thymus barrier consists of three major elements: (1) capillary endothelium and its basal lamina, (2) perivascular connective tissue space occupied by macrophages, and (3) type I epithelioreticular cells with their basal lamina. The perivascular connective tissue is enclosed between the basal lamina of the epithelioreticular cells and the endothelial cell basal lamina. These layers provide the necessary protection to the developing immature T cells and separate them from mature immunocompetent lymphocytes circulating in the bloodstream.

- *Type I epithelioreticular cells* with their occluding junctions. These cells provide further protection to the developing T cells. The epithelioreticular cells surround the capillary wall in the cortex and with their basal lamina represent another major structural component of the blood–thymus barrier.

The thymus is the site of T cell education

During fetal life, the thymus is populated by multipotential lymphoid stem cells that originate from the bone marrow and are destined to develop into immunocompetent T cells. Stem cell maturation and differentiation into immunocompetent T cells is called ***thymic cell education*** (Fig. 13.28). This process is characterized by the expression and deletion of specific surface CD antigens.

The expression of CD2 and CD7 molecules on the cell surface indicates an early ***(double negative)*** stage of differentiation. This early stage is followed by the expression of the CD1 molecule, which indicates the middle stage of T cell differentiation. As maturation progresses, the cells express TCRs, CD3, and both CD4 and CD8 molecules ***(double-positive stage)***. These cells are then presented with self and foreign antigens by type II and III epithelioreticular cells. If the lymphocyte recognizes "self" MHC molecules and "self" or foreign antigen, it will survive ***(positive selection)***. If not, the cell will die. Cells that pass the positive selection test leave the cortex and enter the medulla. Here, they undergo another selection process in which cells that recognize "self" antigen displayed by self MHC are eliminated ***(negative selection)***. The cells that survive become either cytotoxic $CD8^+$ T lymphocytes (by losing CD4 and retaining CD8) or helper $CD4^+$ T lymphocytes (by losing CD8 and retaining CD4). This stage is called the ***single-positive stage***. Now the cells leave the thymus by passing from the medulla into the blood circulation. The process of thymic cell education is promoted by substances secreted by the epithelioreticular cells, including interleukins, colony stimulating factors, interferon γ, ***thymosin***, and ***thymopoietin***.

Spleen

The spleen is about the size of a clenched fist and is the largest lymphatic organ. It is located in the upper left quadrant of the abdominal cavity and has a rich blood supply.

The spleen filters blood and reacts immunologically to blood-borne antigens

The spleen has both morphologic and immunologic filtering functions. In addition to large numbers of lymphocytes, it contains specialized vascular spaces or channels, a meshwork of reticular cells and reticular fibers, and a rich supply of macrophages. These contents allow the spleen to monitor the blood immunologically, much as the macrophages of the lymph nodes monitor the lymph.

Most of the spleen consists of splenic pulp. Splenic pulp, in turn, is divided into two functionally and morphologically different regions: ***white pulp*** and ***red pulp***, based on the color of fresh sections. White pulp appears as circular or elongated whitish gray areas surrounded by red pulp.

The spleen is enclosed by a dense connective tissue ***capsule*** from which ***trabeculae*** extend into the parenchyma of the organ (Fig. 13.29). The connective tissue of the capsule and trabeculae contains ***myofibroblasts***. These contractile cells also produce extracellular connective tissue fibers. In

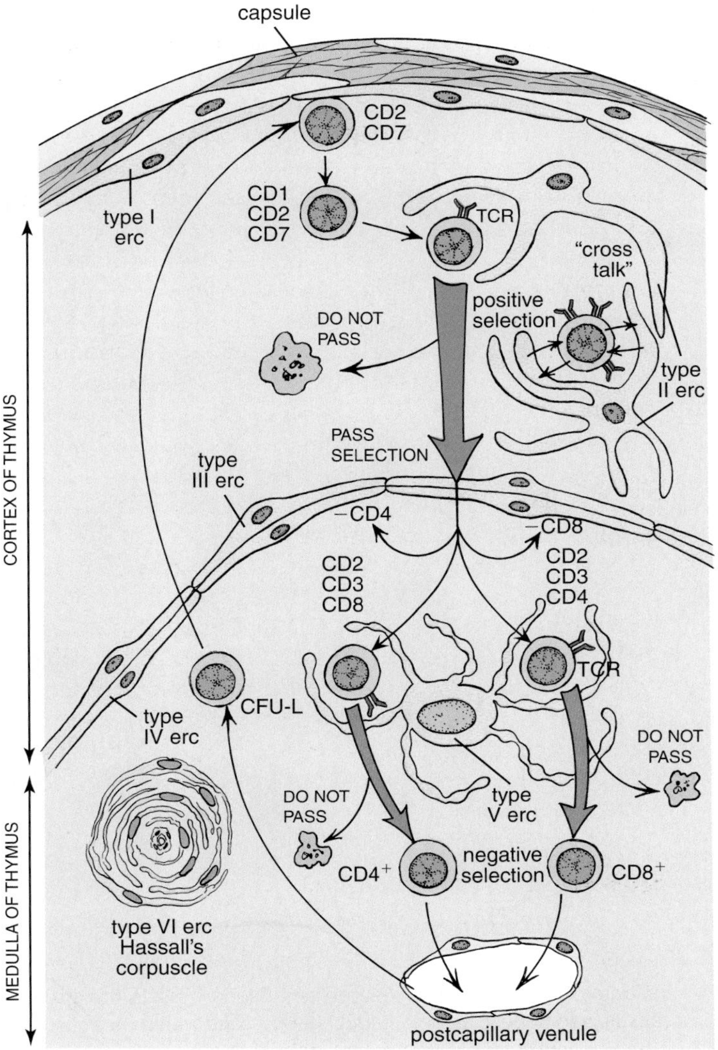

FIGURE 13.28
Schematic drawing of the major steps in thymic education. The process of multipotential lymphatic stem cell (CFU-L) maturation and differentiation into immunocompetent T cells is accomplished by the expression and deletion of specific surface CD antigens. The CFU-L stem cells enter the medulla of the thymus via a postcapillary venule and then migrate to the periphery of the thymic lobule. The presence of CD2 and CD7 molecules on the cell surface indicates an early stage of differentiation. This is followed by expression of the CD1 molecule, indicating the midstage of T cell differentiation. As maturation progresses, the cells express TCRs, CD3, CD4, and CD8 molecules. These cells are then presented with self and foreign antigens by type II and III epithelioreticular *(erc)* cells. If the lymphocyte recognizes self MHC and self or foreign antigen, it will survive the selection (positive selection); if not, death of the cell will occur. Cells that pass the positive selection test leave the cortex and enter the medulla. Here they undergo another selection process in which cells directed to self-antigen displayed by self MHC are eliminated (negative selection). Cells that survive that selection then become either cytotoxic $CD8^+$ T lymphocytes or helper $CD4^+$ T lymphocytes. These cells are now ready for the immune response; they leave the thymus from the medulla and enter the blood circulation. Hormonal substances secreted by type VI epithelioreticular cells within the thymic (Hassall's) corpuscle promote the process of thymic cell education. Note the distribution of all six types of epithelioreticular cells.

many mammals the spleen holds large volumes of red blood cells in reserve. In these species, contraction in the capsule and trabeculae helps discharge stored red blood cells into the systemic circulation. The human spleen normally retains relatively little blood, but it has the capacity for contraction by means of the contractile cells in the capsule and trabeculae.

The ***hilum***, located on the medial surface of the spleen, is the site for the passage of the splenic artery and vein, nerves, and lymphatic vessels. The lymphatic vessels originate in the white pulp near the trabeculae and constitute a route for lymphocytes leaving the spleen.

White pulp consists of a thick accumulation of lymphocytes surrounding an artery

The white pulp consists of lymphatic tissue, mostly lymphocytes. In H&E–stained sections, white pulp appears basophilic because of the dense heterochromatin in the nuclei of the numerous lymphocytes. Branches of the splenic artery course through the capsule and trabeculae of the spleen and then enter the white pulp. Within the white pulp, the branch of the splenic artery is called the ***central artery.*** Lymphocytes that aggregate around the central artery constitute the ***periarterial lymphatic sheath (PALS).*** The PALS has a roughly cylindrical configuration that conforms to the course of the central artery. In cross sections, the PALS appears circular and may resemble a lymphatic nodule. The presence of the central artery, however, distinguishes the PALS from typical lymphatic nodules found in other sites. Nodules appear as localized expansions of the PALS and displace the central artery, so that it occupies an eccentric rather than a central position.

The nodules are the territory of B lymphocytes; other lymphocytes of the PALS are chiefly T lymphocytes that

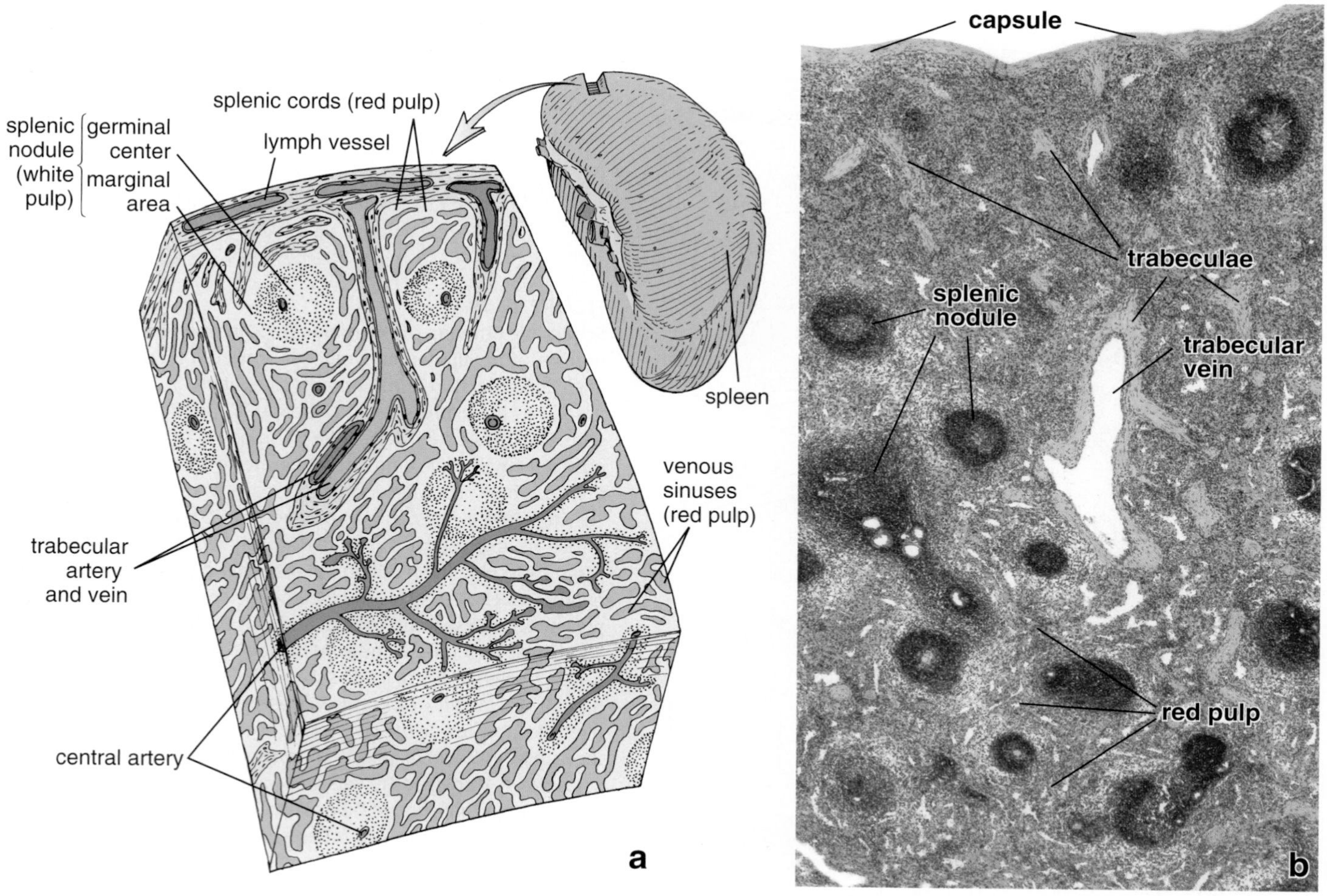

FIGURE 13.29

Schematic diagram and photomicrograph of splenic structure. a. The substance of the spleen is divided into white pulp and red pulp. White pulp consists of a cylindrical mass of lymphocytes arranged around a central artery that constitutes the periarterial lymphatic sheath (PALS). Splenic nodules occur along the length of the PALS. When observed in cross section through part of the sheath that contains a nodule, the central artery appears eccentrically located with respect to the lymphatic mass. The red pulp consists of splenic sinuses surrounded by splenic cords (cords of Billroth). A capsule surrounds the spleen and from it trabeculae project into the substance of the spleen. Both capsule and trabeculae give the appearance of dense connective tissue infiltrated by numerous myofibroblasts. Blood vessels traverse the capsule and trabeculae before and after passage within the substance of the spleen. Lymphatic vessels originate in the white pulp near the trabeculae. **b.** This low-magnification photomicrograph of the spleen reveals the same components shown in the previous drawing. Note the capsule with several trabeculae projecting into the substance of the spleen. In the center, there is a trabecula containing a trabecular vein through which blood leaves the organ. The red pulp constitutes the greater bulk of the splenic tissue. The white pulp contains lymphatic tissue that follows and ensheathes the central artery. Expansion of the white pulp creates the splenic nodules. $\times 45$.

surround the nodules. Thus, the PALS may be considered a thymus-dependent zone similar to the deep cortex of a lymph node. The nodules usually contain germinal centers, which, as in other lymphatic tissues, develop as B cells proliferate following their activation. In humans, germinal centers develop within 24 hours after antigen exposure and may become extremely large and visible with the naked eye. These enlarged nodules are called ***splenic nodules*** or Malpighian corpuscles (not to be confused with the renal corpuscles that have the same name).

Red pulp contains large numbers of red blood cells that it filters and degrades

Red pulp has a red appearance in the fresh state as well as in histologic sections because it contains large numbers of red blood cells. Essentially, red pulp consists of ***splenic sinuses*** separated by ***splenic cords*** (cords of Billroth). Splenic cords consist of the now-familiar loose meshwork of reticular cells and reticular fibers that contain large numbers of erythrocytes, macrophages,

lymphocytes, plasma cells, and granulocytes. Splenic macrophages phagocytose damaged red blood cells. The iron from destroyed red blood cells is used in the formation of new red blood cells; splenic macrophages begin the process of hemoglobin breakdown and iron reclamation. Megakaryocytes are also present in certain species, such as rodents and the cat, but not in humans except during fetal life.

The splenic or venous sinuses are special sinusoidal vessels lined by rod-shaped endothelial cells

The endothelial cells that line the splenic sinuses are extremely long. Their longitudinal axis runs parallel to the direction of the vessel (Fig. 13.30). There are few contact points between adjacent cells, thus producing prominent intercellular spaces. These spaces allow blood cells to pass readily into and out of the sinuses. Processes of macrophages extend between the endothelial cells and into the lumen of the sinuses to monitor the passing blood for foreign antigens.

The sinuses do not possess a continuous basal lamina. Strands of basal lamina loop around the outside of the sinus much like the hoops that loop around the staves of a barrel. These strands are at right angles to the long axes of the endothelial cells. This material stains with silver-containing reagents or with the PAS reaction. Neither smooth muscle nor pericytes are present in the wall of splenic sinuses. Reticular cell processes may extend to the basal side of the endothelial cells and are probably associated with the reticular fibers that appear to merge with the perisinusoidal loops of basal lamina. Blood fills both the sinuses and cords of the red pulp, often obscuring the underlying structures and making it difficult to distinguish between the cords and the sinuses in histologic sections.

Circulation within red pulp allows macrophages to screen antigens in the blood

Branches of the splenic artery enter the white pulp from the trabeculae. The central artery sends branches to the white pulp itself and to the sinuses at the perimeter of the white pulp, called ***marginal sinuses*** (see Fig. 13.29). The central artery continues into the red pulp, where it branches into several relatively straight arterioles called ***penicillar arterioles. The penicillar arterioles then continue as*** arterial capillaries. Some arterial capillaries are surrounded by aggregations of macrophages and are thus called ***sheathed capillaries.*** Sheathed capillaries then empty directly into the reticular meshwork of the splenic cords rather than connecting to the endothelium-lined splenic sinuses. Blood entering the red pulp in this manner percolates through the cords and is exposed to the macrophages of the cords before returning to the circulation by squeezing through the walls of the splenic sinuses (Fig. 13.31). This type of circulation is referred to as ***open circulation,*** and it is the only route by which blood returns to the venous circulation in humans. In other species such as the rat and dog, some of the blood from the sheathed capillaries passes directly to the splenic sinuses of the red pulp. This type of circulation is referred to as ***closed circulation.***

Open circulation exposes the blood more efficiently to the macrophages of the red pulp. Both transmission and scanning electron micrographs often show blood cells in transit across the endothelium of the sinus, presumably reentering the vascular system from the red pulp cords. The blood collected in the sinuses drains to tributaries of the trabecular veins that converge into larger veins and eventually leaves the spleen by the splenic vein. The splenic vein in turn joins the drainage from the intestine in the hepatic portal vein (see page 535).

The spleen performs both immune and hemopoietic functions

Because the spleen filters blood as the lymph nodes filter lymph, it functions in both the immune and the hemopoietic systems.

Immune system functions of the spleen include

- Antigen presentation by APCs and initiation of immune response
- Activation and proliferation of B and T lymphocytes
- Production of antibodies against antigen present in circulating blood
- Removal of macromolecular antigens from the blood
- Proliferation of lymphocytes and differentiation of B cells and plasma cells, as well as secretion of antibodies, occur in the white pulp of the spleen; in this regard, the white pulp is the equivalent of other lymphatic organs

Hemopoietic functions of the spleen include

- Removal and destruction of senescent, damaged, and abnormal erythrocytes and platelets
- Retrieval of iron from erythrocyte hemoglobin
- Formation of erythrocytes during early fetal life
- Storage of blood, especially red blood cells, in some species

The role of the red pulp is primarily ***blood filtration,*** i.e., removal of particulate material; macromolecular antigens; and aged, abnormal, or damaged blood cells and platelets from the circulating blood. These functions are accomplished by the macrophages embedded in the reticular meshwork of the red pulp. Senescent, damaged, or abnormal red cells are broken down by the lysosomes of the macrophages; the iron of the hemoglobin is retrieved and stored as ferritin or hemosiderin for future recycling. The heme portion of the molecule is broken down to bilirubin, which is transported to the liver via the portal system and there conjugated to glucuronic acid. Conjugated bilirubin is secreted into the bile, giving it a characteristic color.

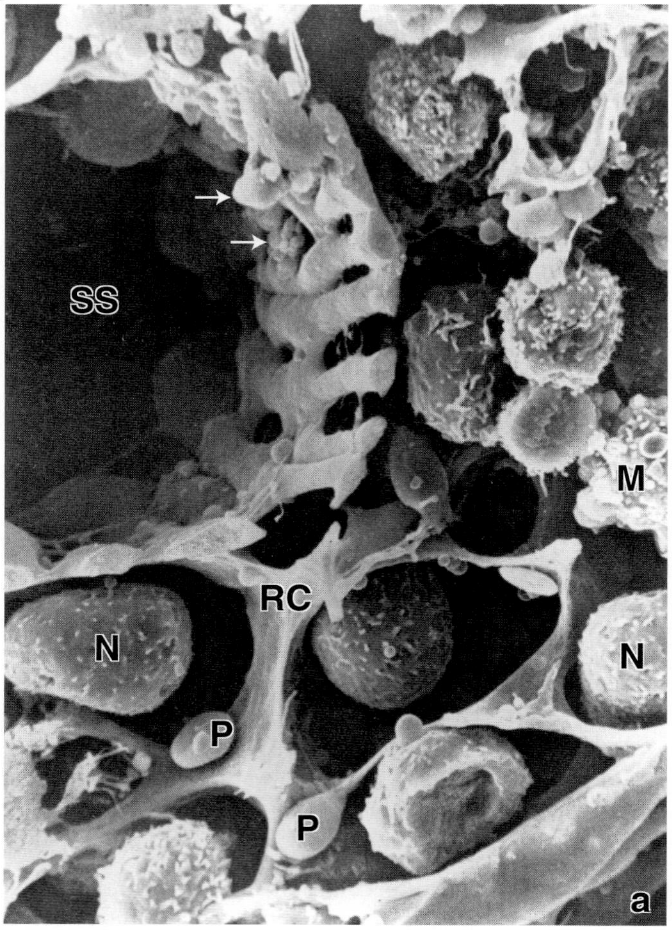

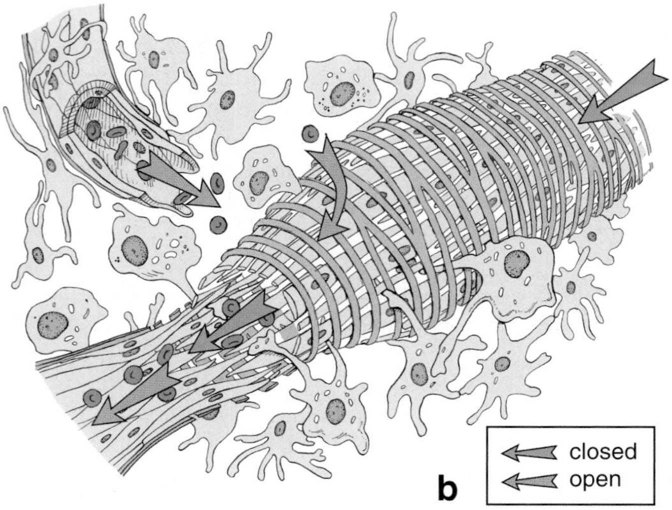

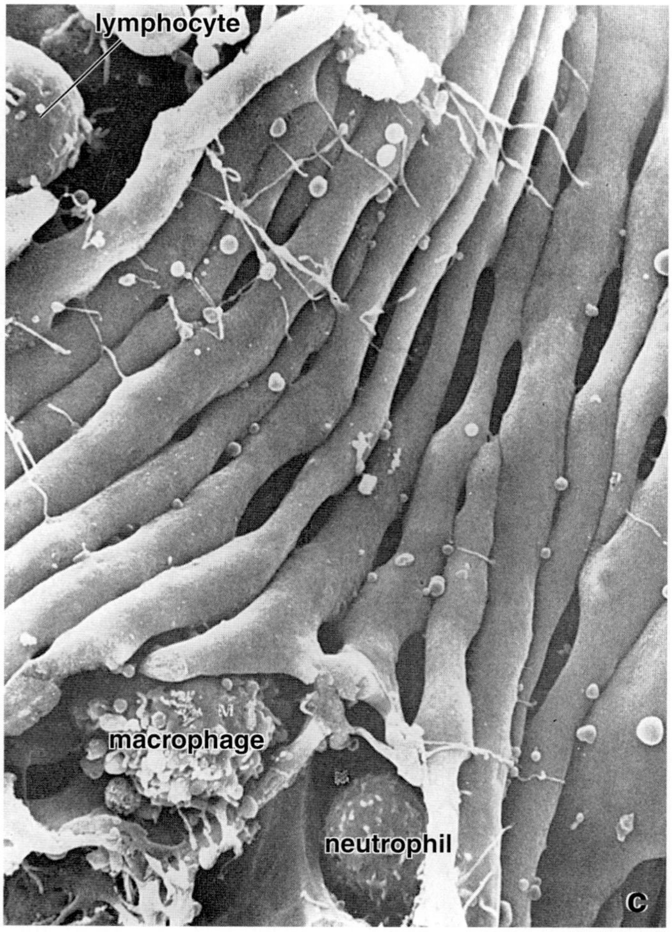

FIGURE 13.30
Splenic sinus and splenic cord structure. a. This scanning electron micrograph shows a cross section of a splenic sinus *(SS),* revealing the lattice structure of its wall. Through the multiple openings in the wall, processes of macrophages *(arrows)* are inserted into the sinus lumen. The remainder of the micrograph shows characteristically smooth-surfaced processes of reticular cells *(RC).* The spaces of the reticular cell framework contain neutrophils *(N),* macrophages *(M),* and blood platelets *(P).* ×4,400. **b.** Schematic diagram of the reconstructed structure of splenic sinus. Note the direction of blood flow in open and closed circulation. **c.** Scanning electron micrograph of the splenic sinus, showing the architecture of the sinus wall as seen from its luminal side. Rod-like endothelial cells run in parallel and are intermittently connected to each other by side processes. A nuclear swelling is shown at lower right. The tapered ends of a few of the rod cells are seen. The macrophage *(M),* neutrophil *(N),* and lymphocyte *(L)* are outside the sinus. ×5,300. (From Fujita T, Tanaka K, Tokunga J. *SEM Atlas of Cells and Tissues.* Tokyo: Igaku-Shoin, 1981.)

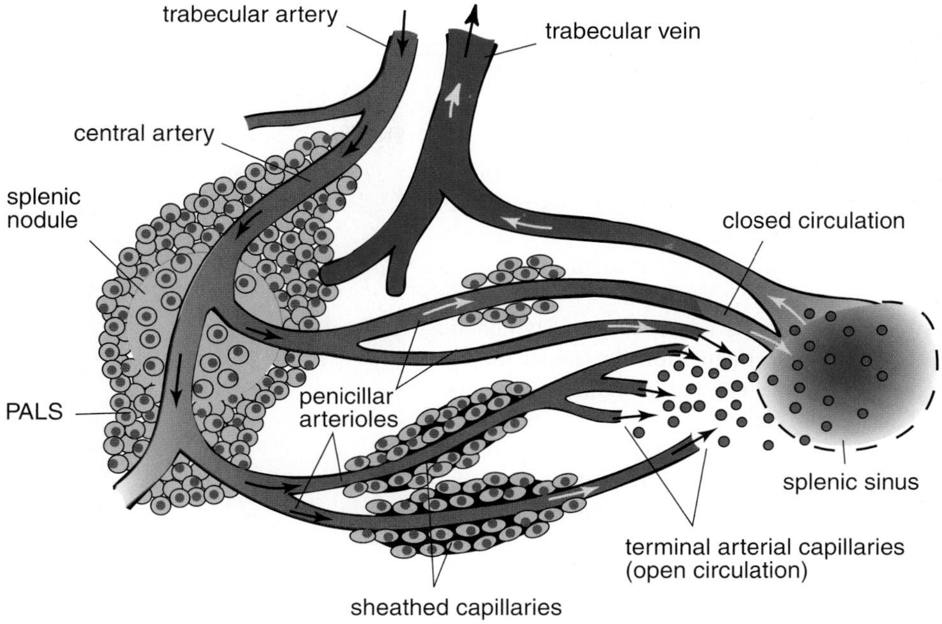

FIGURE 13.31
Schematic diagram of open and closed splenic circulation. In the open circulation, which occurs in humans, penicillar arterioles empty directly into the reticular meshwork of the cords rather than connecting to the endothelium-lined splenic sinuses. Blood entering the red pulp then percolates through the cords and is exposed to the macrophages residing there. In the closed circulation, which occurs in other species, the penicillar arterioles empty directly into the splenic sinuses of the red pulp.

Macrophages recognize senescent or abnormal blood cells by several different mechanisms:

- ***Nonspecific mechanisms*** involve morphologic and biochemical changes that occur in aged erythrocytes; they become more rigid and are thus more easily trapped in the mesh of the red pulp.
- ***Specific mechanisms*** include opsonization of the cell membrane with anti–band 3 IgG antibodies, which trigger F_c receptor–dependent phagocytosis of erythrocytes. In addition, specific changes in glycosylation of glycophorins (see page 217) in aging erythrocytes act as a recognition signal that triggers the elimination of senescent erythrocytes by macrophages.

Despite these important functions, the spleen is not essential for human life. It can be removed surgically, which is often done following trauma that causes intractable bleeding from the spleen. The removal and destruction of aging red blood cells then occurs in the bone marrow and liver.

PLATE 32. TONSIL

The palatine tonsils (faucial tonsils) are paired, ovoid structures that consist of dense accumulations of lymphatic tissue located in the mucous membrane of the fauces (the junction of the oropharynx and oral cavity). This low-magnification (×30) survey micrograph shows the general structural features of part of the human tonsil. The epithelium that forms the surface of the tonsil dips into the underlying connective tissue in numerous places, forming crypts known as *tonsillar crypts.* One of these crypts is seen in the survey micrograph (*arrows*). Numerous lymphatic nodules are evident in the walls of the crypts.

In addition to the palatine tonsils illustrated here, similar aggregations of lymphatic tissue are present beneath the epithelium of the tongue (lingual tonsils), under the epithelium of the roof of the nasopharynx (pharyngeal tonsils), and in smaller accumulations around the openings of the auditory (Eustachian) tubes.

The tonsils guard the opening of the pharynx, the common entry to the respiratory and digestive tracts. They can become inflamed because of repeated infection in the oropharynx and nasopharynx and can even harbor bacteria that cause repeated infections if they are overwhelmed. When this occurs, the inflamed palatine tonsils and pharyngeal tonsils (also called adenoids) are removed surgically (tonsillectomy and adenoidectomy).

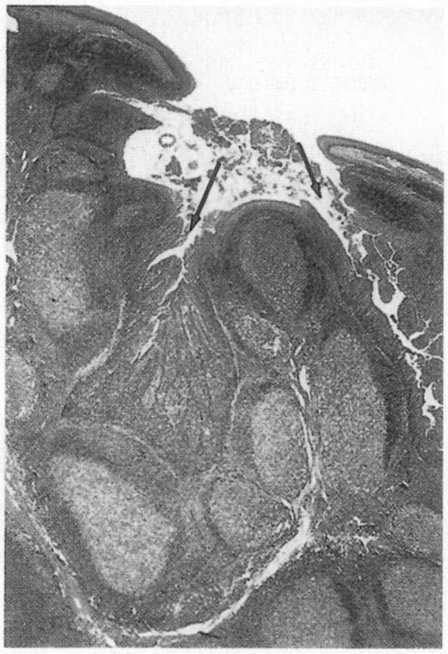

Figure 1, tonsil, human, H&E ×180.
This shows, at a higher magnification, part of the same crypt as in the survey micrograph, as well as the adjacent epithelium *(Ep)* and one of the lymphatic nodules *(LN).* The crypt contains some cellular debris, a frequent occurrence. The lymphatic nodule exhibits a germinal center, the lighter central region of the nodule. The darker-staining peripheral portion of the nodule contains numerous, closely packed small lymphocytes intimately related to the epithelium; they have actually become incorporated in the epithelium. Portions of the germinal center have also become incorporated into the epithelium.

Figure 2, tonsil, human, H&E ×400; inset ×800.
The *rectangular area* in Figure 1 is shown here at higher magnification, rotated 90° counterclockwise. The stratified squamous epithelium *(Ep)* is just barely recognized because of the heavy infiltration of lymphocytes, with the deepest portion of the epithelium totally obscured, hence the *question mark* on the lead line. Epithelial cells are present, though difficult to identify, in the germinal center as well as in the periphery of the nodule *(small arrows).* The **inset** shows the *oval inscribed area* at higher magnification and the epithelial cells *(arrows)* more clearly. In effect, this nodule has literally grown into the epithelium, distorting it and resulting in the disappearance of the well-defined epithelial–connective tissue boundary.

KEY

Ep, epithelium
LN, lymphatic nodule
LP, lamina propria

arrow (survey micrograph), tonsillar crypt
large arrow (Fig. 1), crypt
rectangular area (Fig. 1), shown at higher magnification in Fig. 2

small arrows (Fig. 2), strands of epithelial cells in nodule

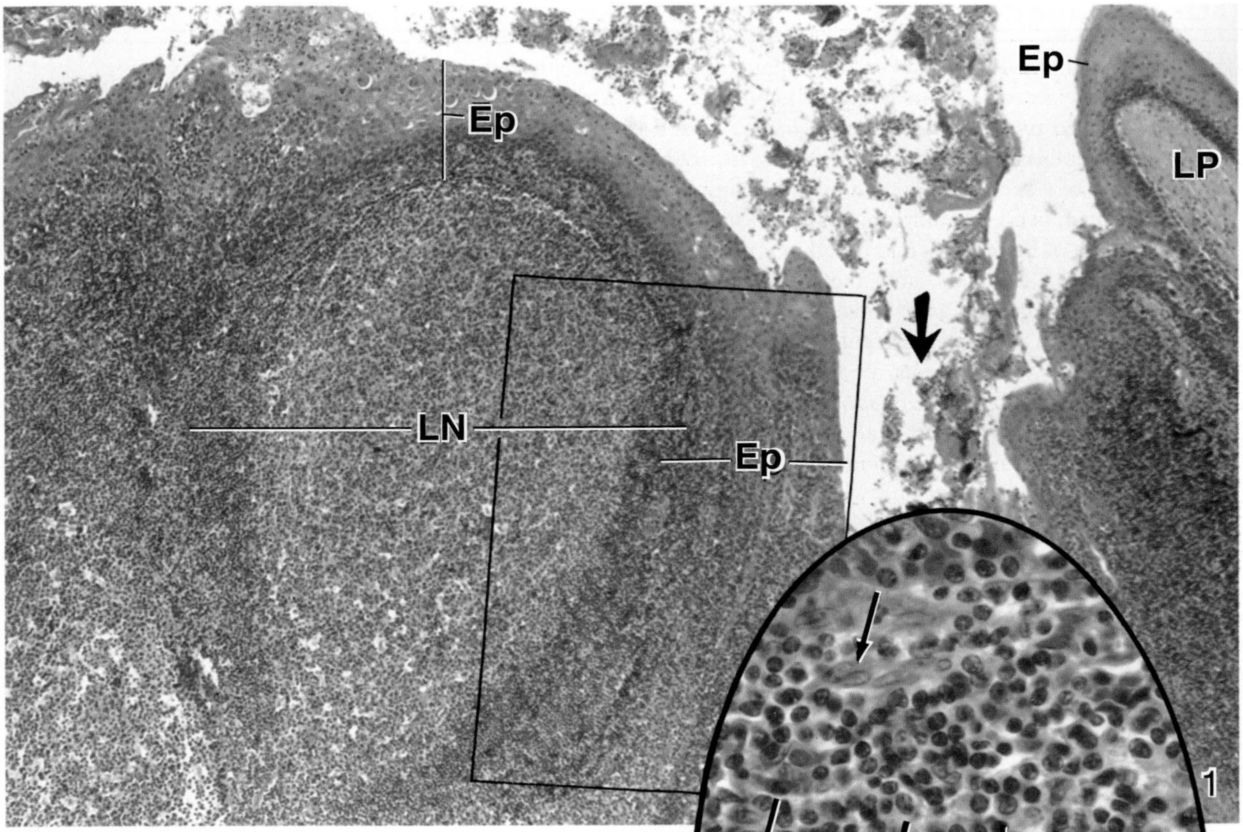
Ep
Ep
LP
LN
Ep
1

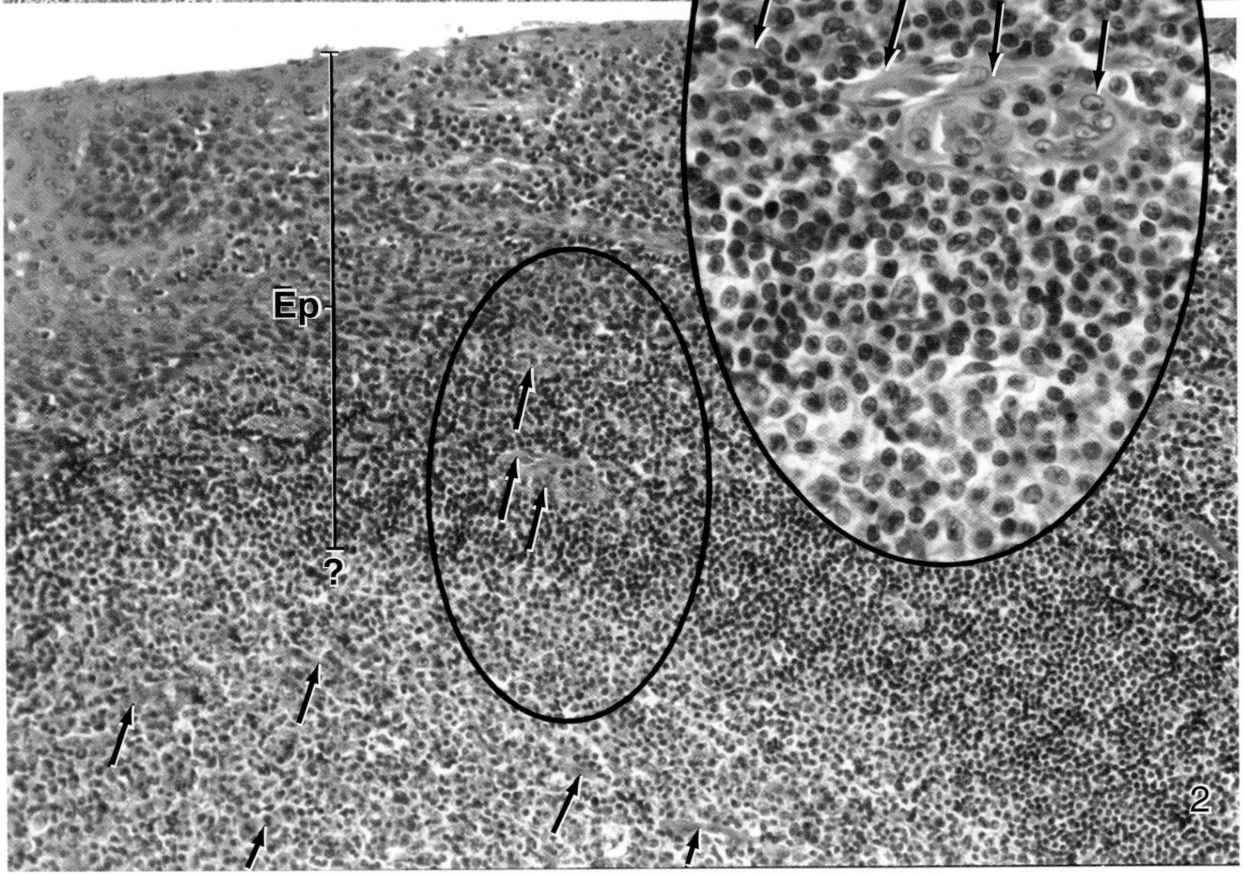
Ep
?
2

PLATE 33. LYMPH NODE I

Lymph nodes are small, encapsulated lymphatic organs that are located in the path of the lymph vessels. They serve as filters of the lymph and as the principal site in which T and B lymphocytes undergo *antigen-dependent proliferation* and differentiation into *effector lymphocytes* (plasma cells and T cells) and *memory B cells* and *T cells.* A low-magnification (×14) micrograph of a section through a human lymph node is shown on this page for orientation. The capsule appears as a thin connective tissue covering.

The parenchyma of the node is composed of a mass of lymphatic tissue, arranged as a cortex *(C)* that surrounds a less dense area, the medulla *(M).* The cortex is interrupted at the *hilum* of the organ *(H),* where there is a recognizable concavity. It is at this site that blood vessels enter and leave the lymph node; the efferent lymphatic vessels also leave the node at the hilum.

Afferent lymphatic vessels penetrate the capsule at multiple sites to empty into an endothelium-lined space, the *cortical* or *subcapsular sinus.* This sinus drains into the trabecular sinuses that extend through the cortex alongside the trabeculae and then supply the *medullary sinuses.* These, in turn, drain to the *efferent lymphatics* that leave the node at the hilum.

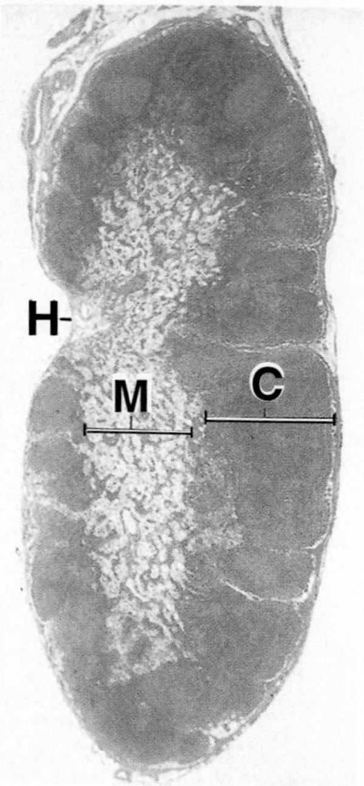

Figure 1, lymph node, human, H&E ×120.

An area from the cortex is shown here at higher magnification. The capsule *(Cap)* is composed of dense connective tissue from which trabeculae *(T)* penetrate into the organ. Immediately below the capsule is the cortical or subcapsular sinus *(CS),* which receives lymph from the afferent lymphatic vessels after they penetrate the capsule. The cortical sinus is continuous with the trabecular sinuses *(TS)* that course along the trabeculae.

The cortex contains the lymphatic nodules *(LN)* and a deeper component that lacks nodules, known as the deep cortex. Whereas lymph nodules and their lighter-staining germinal centers characterize the outer cortex, a more dense mass of lymphocytes, which impart a distinct basophilia, characterize the deep cortex. In contrast to these areas, the medulla is characterized by narrow strands of anastomosing lymphatic tissue containing numerous lymphocytes, the medullary cords *(MC),* separated by light-appearing areas known as the medullary sinuses *(MS).* The medullary sinuses receive lymph from the trabecular sinuses and lymph filtered through the cortical tissue.

Figure 2, lymph node, human, H&E ×400; inset ×640.

This higher-magnification micrograph of a lymphatic nodule from Figure 1 illustrates the germinal center *(GC)* containing medium and large lymphocytes. Germinal centers also contain plasma cells. Dividing lymphocytes are shown at slightly higher magnification in the **inset** *(arrows),* which corresponds to the area in the *circle* in Figure 2. The **inset** also reveals nuclei of the reticular cells *(RC)* that form the connective tissue stroma throughout the organ. The ovoid reticular cell has a large pale-staining nucleus, and its cytoplasm forms long processes that surround the reticular fibers. In H&E preparations, the reticular fibers and the surrounding cytoplasm are difficult to identify. Reticular cells are best seen in the sinuses, where they extend across the lymphatic space and are relatively unobscured by other cells.

A unique vessel, the postcapillary venule *(PCV),* is found in relation to the lymphatic nodules, particularly in the deep cortex. These vessels have an endothelium composed of tall cells between which lymphocytes migrate from the vessel lumen into the parenchyma.

KEY

C, cortex
Cap, capsule
CS, cortical or subcapsular sinus
GC, germinal center
H, hilum
LN, lymphatic nodule
M, medulla
MC, medullary cords
MS, medullary sinus
PCV, postcapillary venule
RC, reticular cells
T, trabecula
TS, trabecular sinus
arrows, dividing lymphocytes

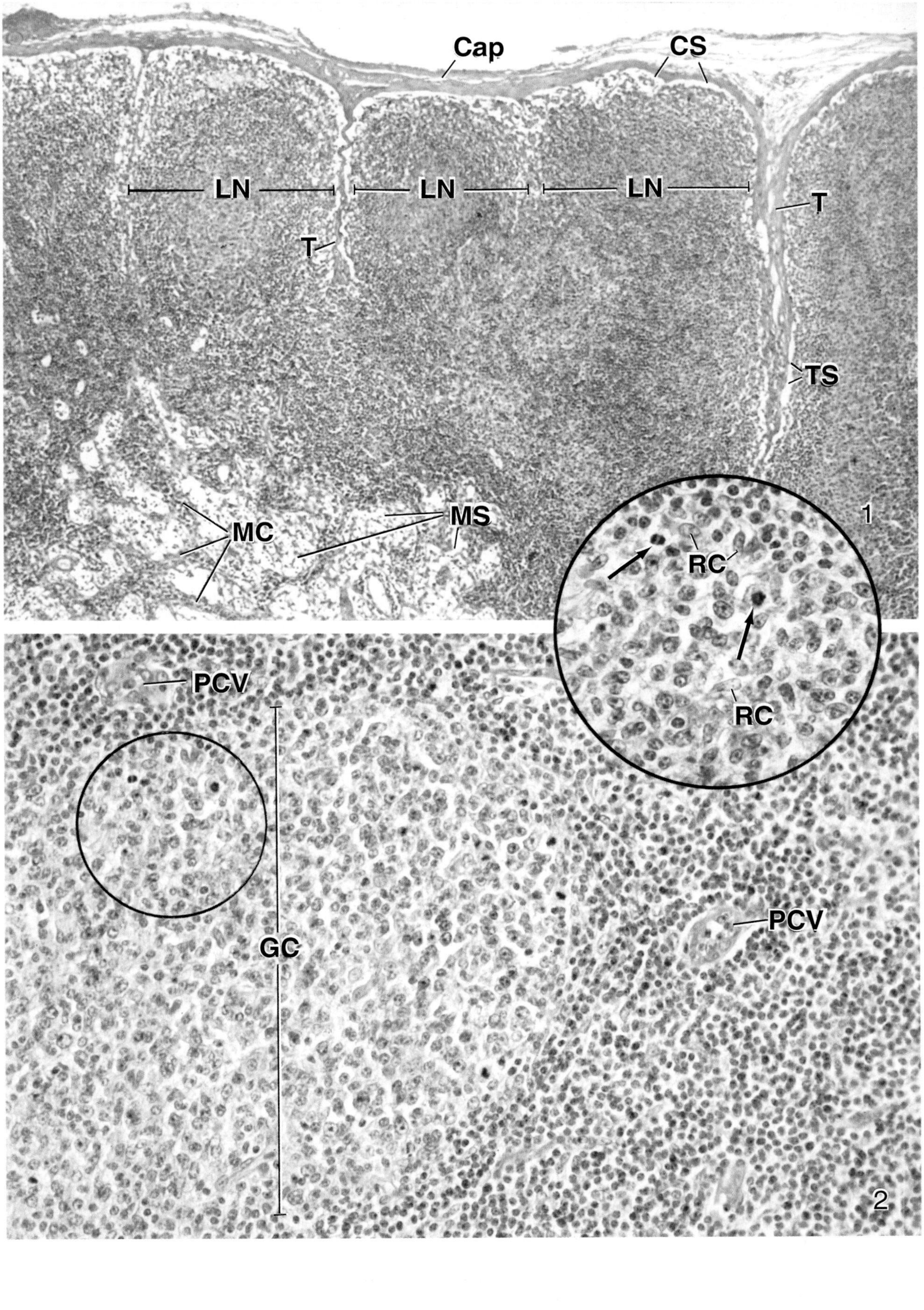
Cap
CS
LN
LN
LN
T
T
TS
MC
MS
RC
RC
1
PCV
GC
PCV
2

PLATE 34. LYMPH NODE II

Immunocompetent B cells that have been exposed to an antigen that they can recognize and bind migrate to a lymph node, where they undergo *blastic transformation* and begin a series of mitotic divisions that produce large numbers of immature immunoblasts. The immunoblasts proliferate further and then differentiate into a clone of lymphocytes that differentiate into antibody-secreting plasma cells and memory cells. Immunocompetent T lymphocytes behave in a similar manner but differentiate into several types of T cells (rather than plasma cells) and memory cells. B cell proliferation and differentiation take place in *germinal centers* in the cortex of the lymph node. T cell proliferation and differentiation take place in the *juxtamedullary cortex*. Newly differentiated plasma cells migrate to the medulla, where they release antibodies into the lymph leaving the node. They may also leave the node, enter the blood vascular system at the thoracic duct, and travel to localized sites in the connective tissue where they may continue to produce antibodies or may remain as memory cells.

Figure 1, lymph node, human, H&E ×365.
This micrograph shows the lymph node deep cortex. As noted in the previous plate, it lies below the region containing the lymph nodules and consists of closely packed lymphocytes. A number of blood vessels can be seen in this region. Whereas typical small blood vessels such as capillaries (*Cap*) and venules are present, the more unusual postcapillary venule (*PCV*) is also found in this region. A small vessel that can be identified as a venule (*Ven*), based on lumen size and wall thickness, is seen at a point of transition to become a postcapillary venule (*arrowheads*). The endothelial cell nuclei at this point of juncture have become cuboidal. The postcapillary venule is identified by its endothelium, which is composed of cells that are cuboidal. A cross-sectioned profile of a postcapillary venule is shown in the **inset** at higher magnification (×700). The endothelial cell nuclei are round and are lightly stained, in contrast to the nuclei of the surrounding lymphocytes, which are of similar size and shape but are densely stained. This vessel also shows three lymphocytes (*arrows*) that are in the process of migrating through the wall of the vessel. The lower right corner of Figure 1 reveals a region where there is a considerably lesser concentration of lymphocytes. This area, part of the medulla, contains spaces that represent medullary sinuses (*MS*).

Figure 2, lymph node, human, H&E ×250.
The area shown here, near the hilar region of the node, shows part of a lymph nodule (*LN*), the cortical sinus (*CS*) just below the capsule (*Cap*), and some of the medullary sinus (*MS*). Both the cortical sinus and the medullary sinus are spanned by reticular cells (*RC*). These cells wrap around the collagen bundles that form the supporting trabecular framework of the node. The **inset** reveals the *boxed area* at higher magnification (×530). The nuclei of the reticular cells (*RC*) are larger and less densely staining than the lymphocyte nuclei, which are round and densely stained. In H&E preparations, these characteristics allow for the distinction between the reticular cell and the lymphocyte.

Figure 3, lymph node, monkey, H&E ×530.
This micrograph shows an area in the region of the hilum of the node. Two of the vessels here are efferent lymphatics; both contain a valve (*Val*). The upper lymphatic vessel exhibits what appears to be an incomplete wall. The openings in the vessel wall (*arrows*) are sites in which the medullary sinuses are emptying their contents into the lymphatic vessel. Also present are a small artery (*A*) and a vein (*V*).

KEY

A, artery
Cap, capillary
CS, cortical sinus
LN, lymph nodule
MS, medullary sinus
PCV, postcapillary venule
RC, reticular cells
V, vein
Val, valve
Ven, venule
arrowheads, endothelial cells of postcapillary venule
arrows, Fig. 1, endothelial cells; Fig. 3, opening of medullary sinus to lymph vessel

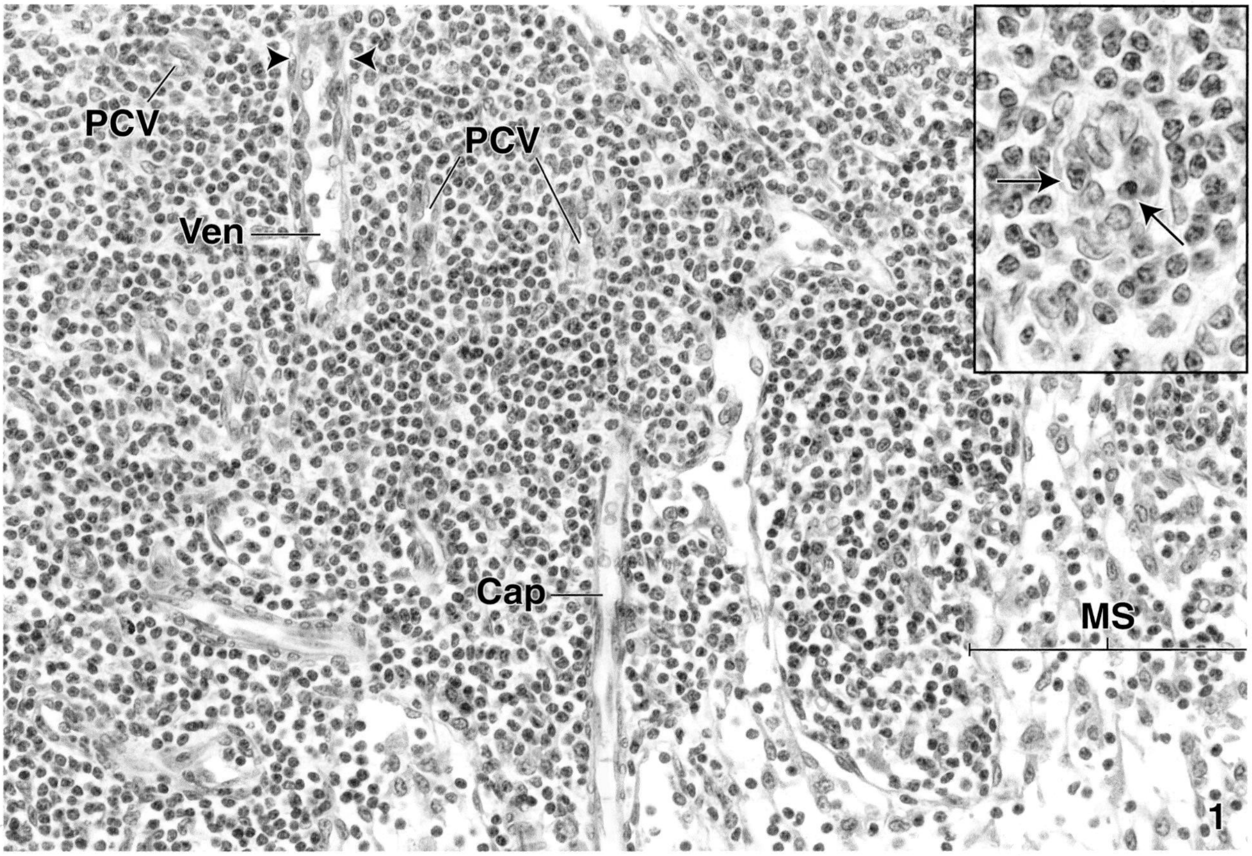
PCV
PCV
Ven
Cap
MS
1

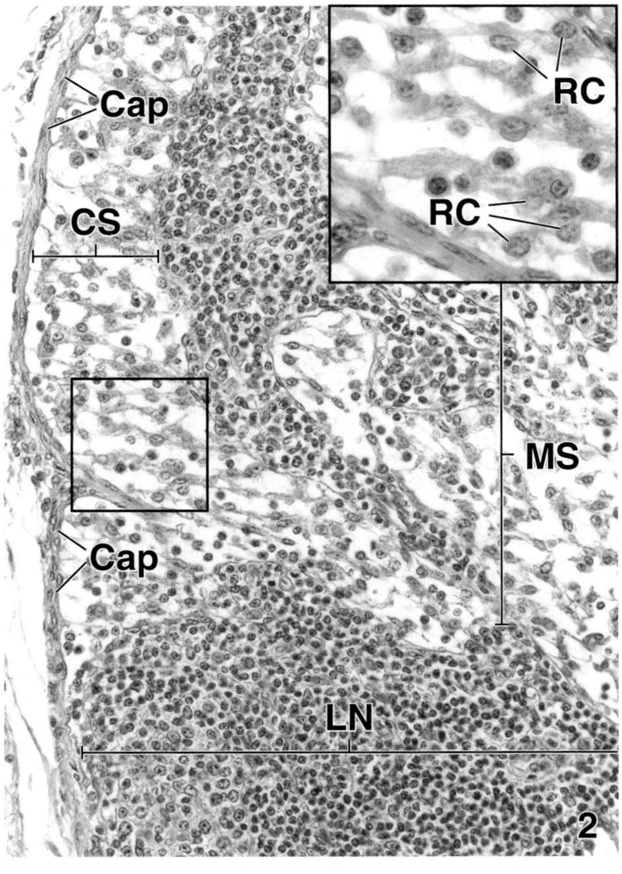
Cap
CS
RC
RC
MS
Cap
LN
2

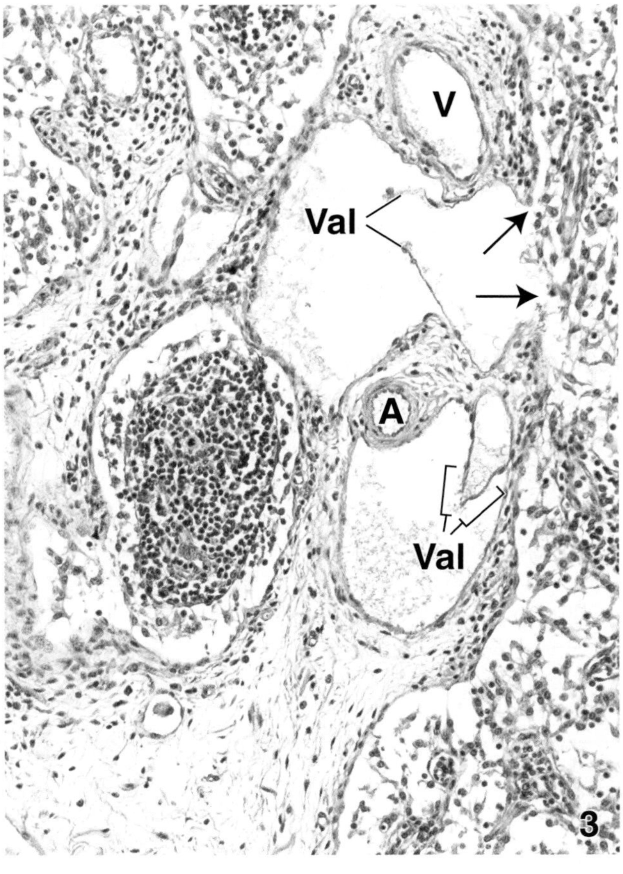
V
Val
A
Val
3

PLATE 35. SPLEEN I

The spleen is the largest lymphatic organ; it is surrounded by a capsule and located in the path of the bloodstream (splenic artery and vein). The spleen filters the blood and reacts immunologically to blood-borne antigens. It has both morphologic and immunologic filtering functions. The substance of the spleen, the splenic pulp, consists of *red pulp* and *white pulp,* so named because of their appearance in fresh tissue. The white pulp is rich in lymphocytes that form a *periarterial lymphatic sheath (PALS)* around branches of the splenic artery that penetrate the white pulp. The red pulp contains large numbers of red blood cells that it filters and degrades. Aged, damaged, or abnormal red blood cells are trapped by macrophages associated with unusual vascular sinuses in the red pulp. These macrophages break down the red cells, begin the metabolic breakdown of hemoglobin, and retrieve and store the iron from the heme for reutilization in the formation of new red blood cells in the bone marrow.

Figure 1, spleen, human, H&E ×65.
This low-magnification micrograph of the spleen reveals its two major components, the red pulp *(RP)* and white pulp *(WP).* In the center of the figure, there is a trabecula containing a blood vessel, a trabecular vein *(TV)* through which blood leaves the organ. The red pulp constitutes the greater bulk of the splenic tissue. In life, the red pulp has pulp-like texture; it is red as a result of the natural coloration of the numerous red blood cells present, hence its name.

The white pulp, on the other hand, is so named because its content of lymphocytes appears in life as whitish areas. In tissue sections, however, the nuclei of the closely packed lymphocytes impart an overall blue-staining response. The lymphatic tissue that constitutes the white pulp differs from nodules seen elsewhere in that it follows and ensheathes a blood vessel, the central artery. The lymphatic tissue surrounding the artery exhibits periodic expansion, thus forming the nodules. When this occurs, the central artery *(CA)* is displaced peripherally within the nodule.

In those regions where the lymphatic tissue is not in nodular form, it is present as a thin cuff around the central artery and is referred to as the periarterial lymphatic sheath. If the plane of section does not include the artery, the sheath may appear only as a localized and irregular aggregation of lymphocytes.

Figure 2, spleen, human, H&E ×160.
This figure reveals, at a higher magnification, the red pulp and a portion of the trabecular vein from the area enclosed in the *uppermost rectangle* in Figure 1. The red pulp is composed of two elements: venous sinuses *(VS)* and the splenic cords (of Billroth), the tissue that lies between the sinuses. In this specimen, the venous sinuses can be seen to advantage because the red blood cells in the sinuses have lysed and appear as unstained "ghosts"; only the nuclei of the white cells are readily seen. (This is better shown in Plate 36.) The paler, unstained areas thus represent the sinus lumina.

Near the top of the micrograph, two venous sinuses *(arrows)* empty into the trabecular vein *(TV),* thus showing the continuity between venous sinuses and the trabecular veins. The wall of the vein is thin, but the trabecula *(T)* containing the vessel gives the appearance of being part of the vessel wall. In humans as well as in other mammals, the capsule and the trabeculae that extend from the capsule contain myofibroblasts. Under conditions of increasing physical stress, contraction of these cells will occur and cause rapid expulsion of blood from the venous sinuses into the trabecular veins and, thus, into the general circulation.

Figure 3, spleen, human, H&E ×240.
This figure reveals, at higher magnification, the splenic nodule in the *rectangle* in the right portion of Figure 1. Present are a germinal center *(GC)* and a cross section through the thick-walled central artery *(CA).* As noted above, the central artery is eccentrically placed in the nodule. The marginal zone *(MZ)* is the area that separates white pulp and red pulp *(RP).* Small arterial vessels and capillaries, branches of the central artery, supply the white pulp, and some pass into the reticular network of the marginal zone, terminating in a funnel-shaped orifice. Venous sinuses are also found in the marginal zone, and occasionally, arterial vessels may open into the sinuses. The details of the vascular supply are, at best, difficult to resolve in typical H&E preparations. The penicillar arterioles, the terminal branches of the central artery, supply the red pulp but are likewise difficult to resolve.

KEY

CA, central artery
GC, germinal center
MZ, marginal zone
RP, red pulp
T, trabecula
TV, trabecular vein
VS, venous sinus
WP, white pulp
arrows (Fig. 2), venous sinuses emptying into the trabecular vein

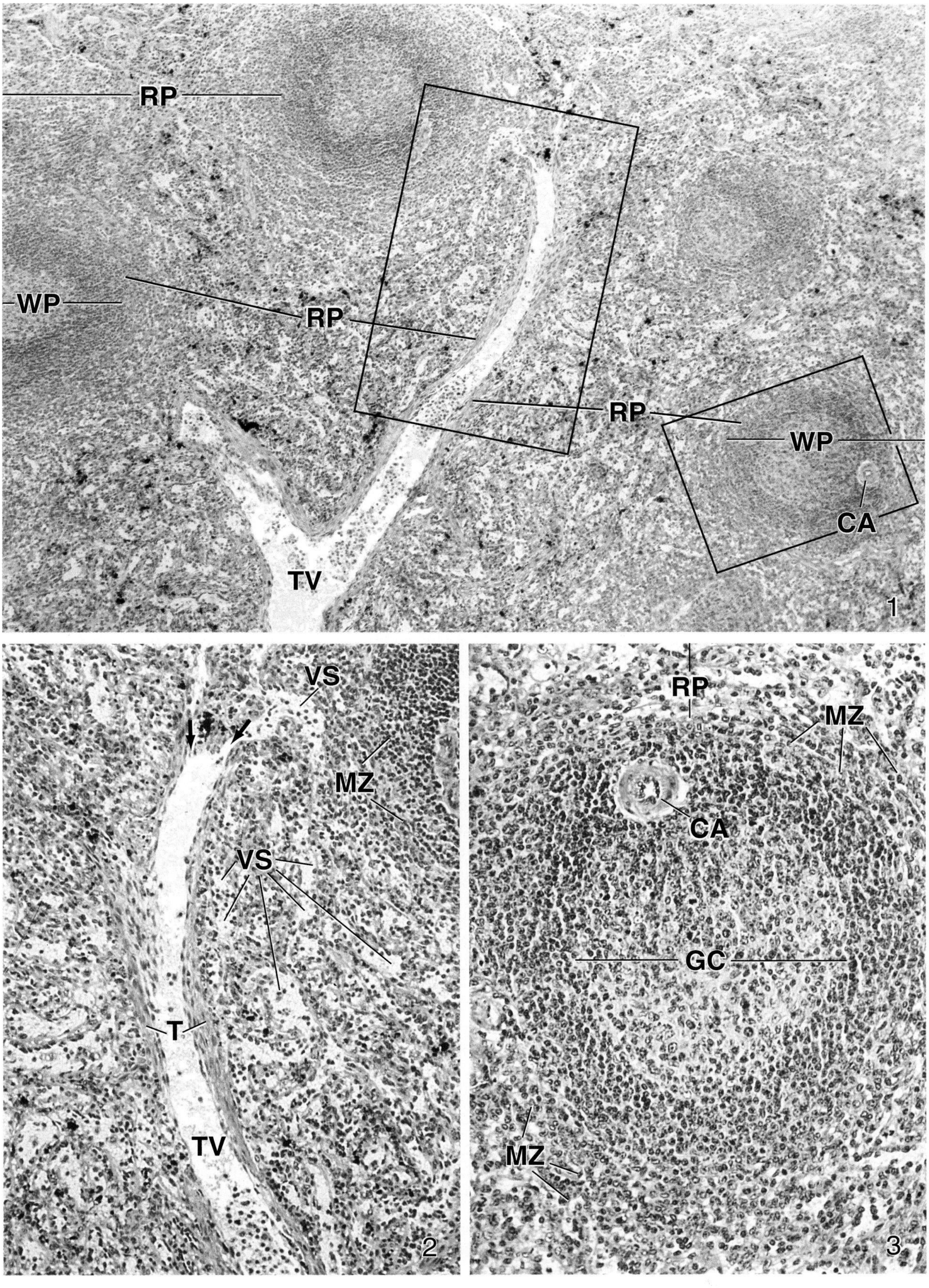
RP
WP
RP
RP
WP
CA
TV
1
VS
MZ
VS
T
TV
2
RP
MZ
CA
GC
MZ
3

PLATE 36. SPLEEN II

Figure 1, spleen, human, H&E ×360.

The red pulp, as noted in the previous plate, has two components: venous sinuses and the splenic cords (of Billroth). The venous sinuses *(VS)* can be recognized by their circumscribing endothelial wall. The red cells within the lumina of the vessels are apparent only by virtue of their outline, with the contents of the cells having been lost during the preparation of the tissue (lysed), leaving only a ghost image. The cords are filled with a variety of cell types, among which are numerous lysed red blood cells. These red cells have left the vascular channels; i.e., they are extravascular. Macrophages can be identified in this specimen by the pigment that they have sequestered *(arrows),* specifically, the breakdown products of old red blood cells.

Figure 2, spleen, human, H&E ×1200.

This figure reveals, at higher magnification, one of the venous sinuses and the surrounding splenic (Billroth's) cord *(BC)* from the preceding figure. The wall of the sinus consists of elongated rod-like endothelial cells that are oriented parallel to each other in the long axis of the sinus. A narrow, but clearly visible, intercellular space is usually present between adjacent cells. (The space seen in light microscopic preparations is an exaggeration due to shrinkage during routine preparation.) When a venous sinus is cut in cross section, as in this figure, the rod-shaped endothelial lining cells are also cut in cross section, and the cut edges of the adjoining cells are seen in the form of a ring. The narrow intercellular spaces then appear as slits between the cross-sectioned cells. Occasionally, the wall of a sinus is tangentially sectioned, and the cytoplasm of the endothelial cells appears as a series of narrow stripes, as can be seen in the lower left of Figure 1 *(asterisks).* Each linear component here is a single endothelial cell.

The endothelial cell nuclei *(En)* project into the sinus lumen. In effect, the nuclei form a bleb-like structure that then appears to sit within the lumen of the vessel. Unless examined carefully, they may give the impression that they are nuclei of white blood cells. This is especially true if the white blood cells *(WBC)* within the lumen of the sinus are numerous.

Figure 3, spleen, human, silver preparation ×120; inset ×300.

The framework of the spleen consists of a capsule, trabeculae that extend from the capsule into the substance of the spleen, and a reticular stroma. The silver-stained reticular stroma is illustrated in this figure. In the white pulp, the germinal centers *(GC)* can be recognized by the circular arrangement and, to some degree, the paucity of the reticular fibers. The central arteries *(CA)* are surrounded by a relative abundance of reticular fibers, hence the dense outline of these vessels. The arrangement of the fibers in the red pulp is more variable in appearance. A special arrangement of blackened fibers is seen in relation to the venous sinus *(VS)* of the red pulp. These fibers often appear as an organized lattice that circumscribes the vessel.

The **inset** in Figure 3 is a higher magnification of the area immediately above it. One of the vessels seen in the **inset** has been sectioned tangentially along its wall, and its circumscribing fibers can be seen lying parallel to one another like the rungs of a ladder *(arrows).* The vessel above and in very close proximity (with the label *VS* in its lumen) has also been sectioned longitudinally, but the section passes deeper into the vessel; thus, the cut ends of the fibers are seen in cross-sectional profile *(arrowheads)* and give the appearance of a series of dots outlining the wall of the vessel. These fibers are actually composed of basal lamina material. The basal lamina is not a thin sheath in this instance but, rather, forms a cord-like structure that facilitates the passage of cells across the endothelium. The true reticular fibers (composed of collagen fibrils) are darker staining and thicker. They can be seen between the closely apposed vessels.

KEY

BC, Billroth's cord (splenic cord)
CA, central artery
En, endothelial cell nucleus
GC, germinal center
VS, venous sinus
WBC, white blood cells
arrowheads (Fig. 3, inset), silver-positive fibers (basal lamina material) circumscribing the venous sinus endothelium seen in cross-sectional profile
arrows: Fig. 1, pigment (contained in macrophages); Fig. 3 (inset), silver-positive fibers (basal lamina material) circumscribing the venous sinus endothelium
asterisks (Fig. 1), wall of venous sinus seen in tangential section

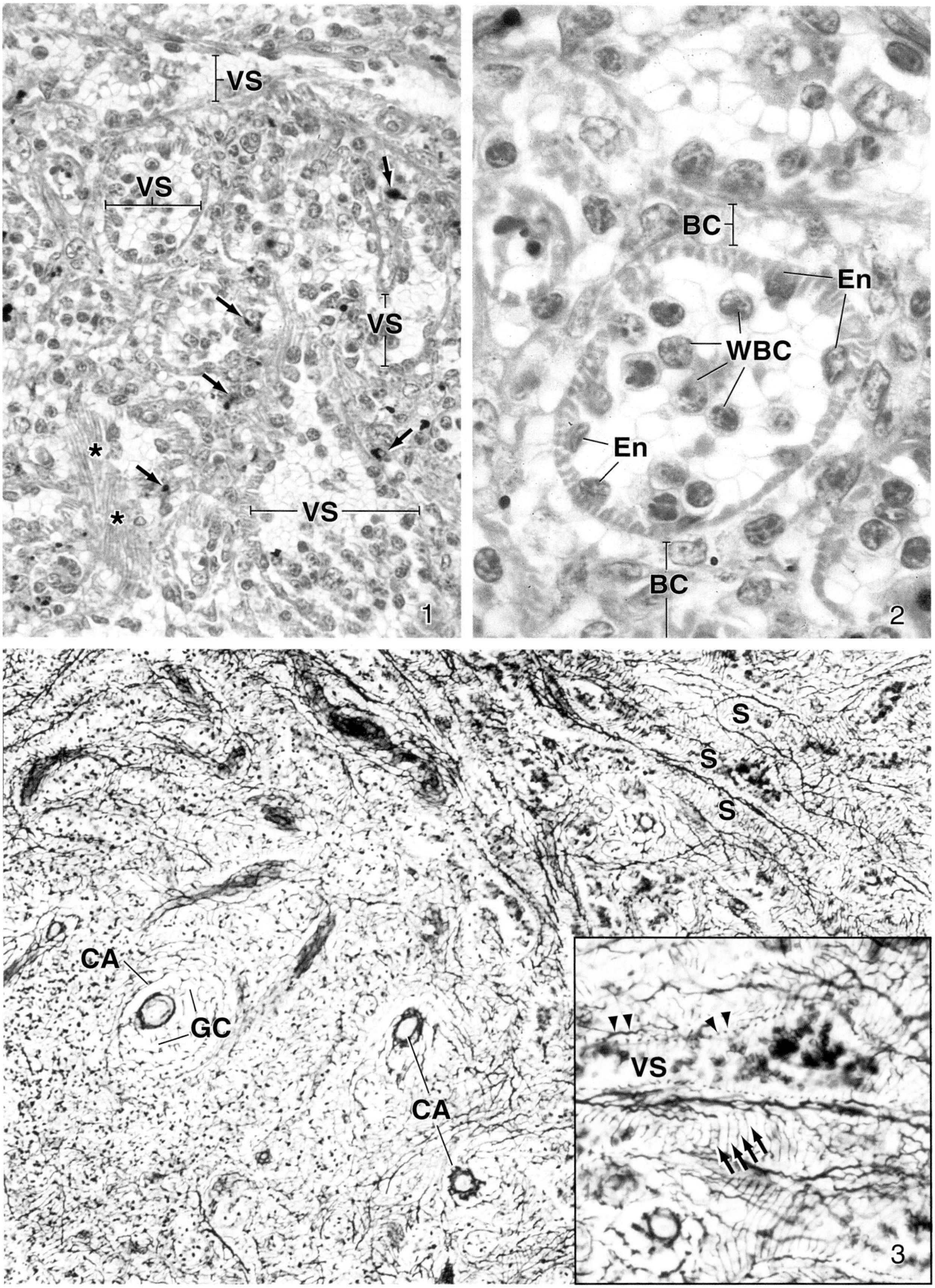
VS
VS
VS
*
*
VS
1
BC
En
WBC
En
BC
2
S
S
S
CA
GC
CA
VS
3

PLATE 37. THYMUS

The thymus is a lymphatic organ that exhibits certain unique structural features. The supporting reticular stroma arises from endodermal epithelium and produces a cellular reticulum. There are no reticular fibers associated with these cells; instead, the cells, designated *epithelioreticular cells,* serve as the stroma. Lymphocytes come to lie in the interstices of the cellular reticulum, and these two cellular elements, the lymphocytes and the epithelioreticular cells, comprise the bulk of the organ. The stem lymphocytes that migrate into the endodermal rudiment in the embryo derive from the yolk sac and, later, from the red bone marrow. These lymphocytes proliferate and become immunologically competent in the thymus, differentiating into the *thymus-dependent lymphocytes* (i.e., T lymphocytes). Some of these lymphocytes migrate to other tissues to populate the thymus-dependent portions of lymph nodes and spleen as well as to reside in the loose connective tissue. Many lymphocytes die or are destroyed in the thymus because in the random process by which they acquire the ability to recognize and react to antigens they become programmed against "self" antigens. Numerous macrophages are present to phagocytize these destroyed lymphocytes. A blood–thymus barrier is formed by the sheathing of the perivascular connective tissue of the thymus by the epithelioreticular cells. In addition, there are no afferent lymphatic vessels to the thymus. Thus, it cannot react to circulating antigens. The thymus involutes during adolescence and is often difficult to recognize in the adult.

A connective tissue capsule *(Cap)* surrounds each lobe of the two lobes of the thymus and sends trabeculae *(T)* into the parenchyma to form lobules. The lobules are not completely separate units; rather, they interconnect because of the discontinuous nature of the trabeculae.

Figure 1, thymus, human, H&E ×40.
Examination of the thymus at low magnification reveals the lobules *(L)* composed of a dark-staining basophilic cortex *(C)* and a lighter-staining and relatively eosinophilic medulla *(M).* The cortex contains numerous densely packed lymphocytes, whereas the medulla contains fewer lymphocytes and is consequently less densely packed.

Figure 2, thymus, human, H&E ×140.
It is the relative difference in the lymphocyte population (per unit area) and, in particular, the staining of their nuclei with hematoxylin that creates the difference in appearance between cortex *(C)* and medulla *(M).* Note that some of the medullary areas bear a resemblance to germinal centers of other lymphatic organs because of the medulla appearing as isolated circular areas (upper left of Fig. 1). The medullary component, however, is actually a continuous branching mass surrounded by cortical tissue. Thus, the "isolated" medullary profiles are actually united with one another, although not within the plane of section. A suggestion of such continuity can be seen on the right in Figure 1, where the medulla appears to extend across several lobules.

The main cellular constituents of the thymus are lymphocytes (thymocytes), with characteristic small, round, dark-staining nuclei, and epithelioreticular supporting cells, with large pale-staining nuclei. Both of the cell types can be distinguished in Figure 3, which provides a high-magnification view of the medulla. Because there are fewer lymphocytes in the medulla, it is the area of choice to examine the epithelioreticular cells. The thymus also contains macrophages; however, they are difficult to distinguish from the epithelioreticular cells.

Figure 3, thymus, human, H&E ×600.
The medulla usually possesses varying numbers of circular bodies called Hassall's, or thymic, corpuscles *(HC).* The corpuscles are large concentric layers of flattened epithelioreticular cells *(Ep).* They stain readily with eosin and can be distinguished easily with low magnification, as in Figures 1 and 2 *(arrows).* The center of a corpuscle, particularly a large one, may show evidence of keratinization and appear somewhat amorphous.

The thymus gland remains as a large structure until the time of puberty. At that time, regressive changes occur that result in a significant reduction in the amount of thymic tissue. The young thymus is highly cellular and contains a minimum of adipose tissue. On the other hand, in the older thymus, much adipose tissue is present between the lobules. With continued involution, adipose cells are found even within the thymic tissue itself. Occasional plasma cells may be present in the periphery of the thymic cortex of the involuting thymus gland.

KEY

BV, blood vessels
C, cortex
Cap, capsule
Ep, epithelioreticular cells
HC, Hassall's corpuscles
L, lobule
M, medulla
T, trabeculae
arrowheads, nuclei of epithelioreticular cells of Hassall's corpuscles
arrows (Figs. 1 and 2), Hassall's corpuscles

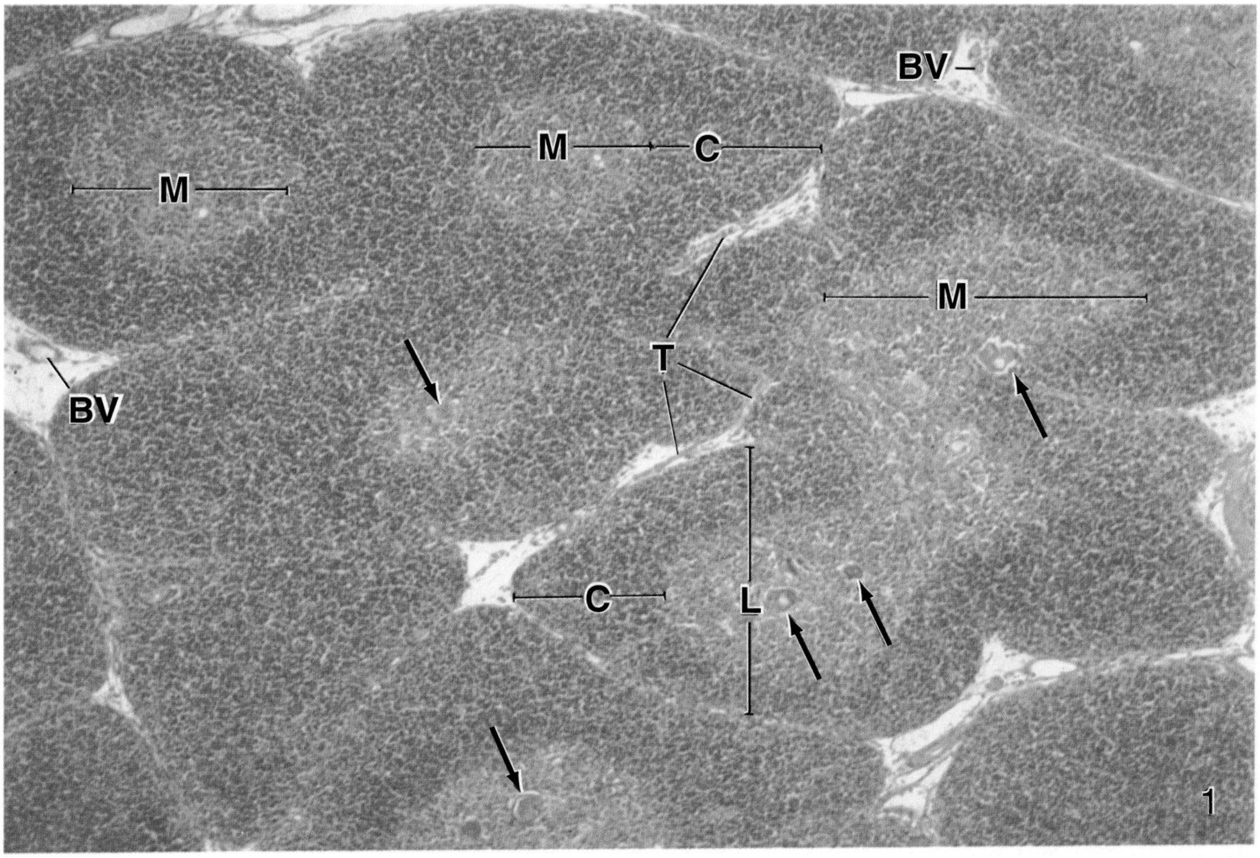
BV
M
C
M
T
M
BV
C
L
1

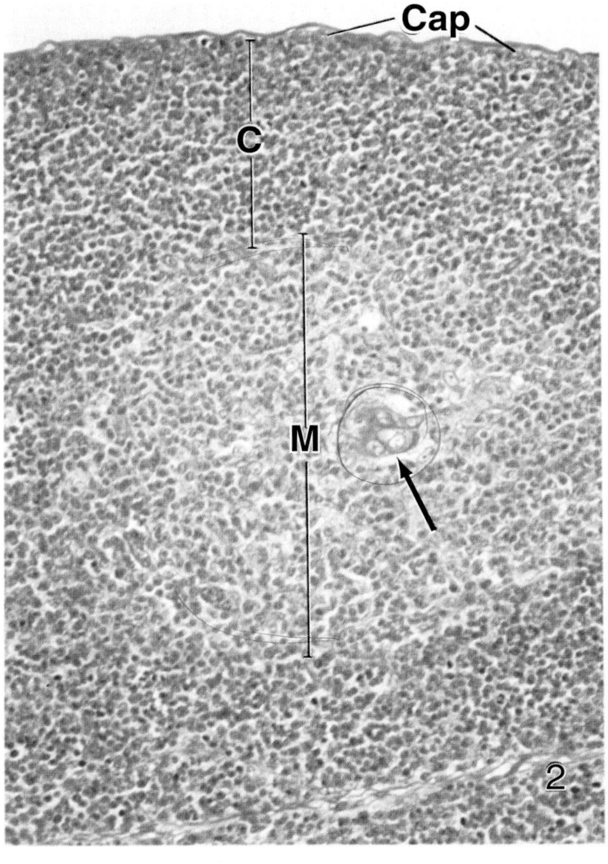
Cap
C
M
2

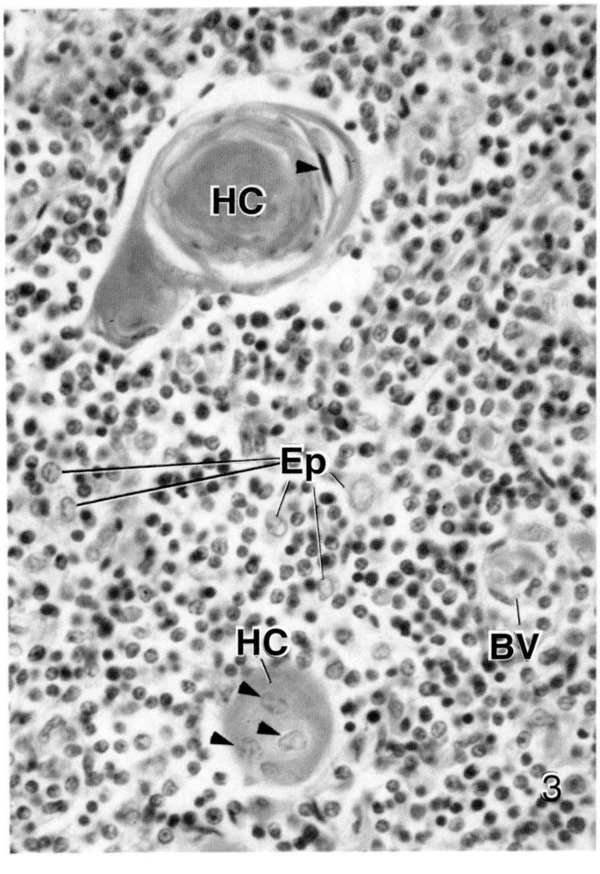
HC
Ep
HC
BV
3

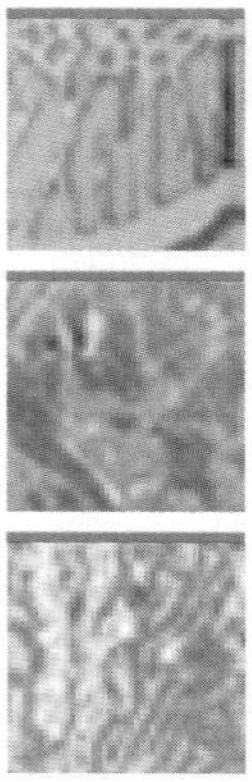

14

Integumentary System

OVERVIEW OF THE INTEGUMENTARY SYSTEM

The skin *(cutis, integument)* and its derivatives constitute the ***integumentary system.*** The skin forms the external covering of the body and is its largest organ, constituting 15 to 20% of its total mass. The skin consists of two main layers:

- ***Epidermis,*** composed of a keratinized stratified squamous epithelium that grows continuously but maintains its normal thickness by the process of desquamation. Epidermis is derived from ectoderm.
- ***Dermis,*** composed of a dense connective tissue that imparts mechanical support, strength, and thickness to the skin. Dermis is derived from mesoderm.

The ***hypodermis*** contains variable amounts of adipose tissue arranged into lobules separated by connective tissue septa. It lies deep to the dermis and is equivalent to the ***subcutaneous fascia*** described in gross anatomy. In well-

nourished individuals and in individuals living in cold climates, the adipose tissue can be quite thick.

The ***epidermal derivatives of the skin (epithelial skin appendages)*** include the following structures and integumentary products:

- ***Hair follicles*** and ***hair***
- ***Sweat (sudoriferous) glands***
- ***Sebaceous glands***
- ***Nails***
- ***Mammary glands***

The integumentary system performs essential functions related to its external surface location

Skin and its derivatives constitute a complex organ composed of many different cell types. The diversity of these cells and their ability to work together provide a number of functions that allow the individual to cope with the external environment. Major functions of the skin include

- It acts as a ***barrier*** that protects against physical, chemical, and biologic agents in the external environment (i.e., mechanical barrier, permeability barrier, ultraviolet barrier).
- It provides ***immunologic*** information obtained during antigen processing to the appropriate effector cells in the lymphatic tissue.
- It participates in ***homeostasis*** by regulating body temperature and water loss.
- It conveys ***sensory*** information about the external environment to the nervous system.
- It performs ***endocrine*** functions by secreting hormones, cytokines, and growth factors and converting precursor molecules into hormonally active molecules (vitamin D).
- It functions in ***excretion*** through exocrine secretion of sweat, sebaceous, and apocrine glands.

In addition, certain lipid-soluble substances may be absorbed through the skin. Although not a function of skin, this property is frequently used in delivery of therapeutic agents.

Skin is categorized as thick or thin, a reflection of thickness and location

The thickness of the skin varies over the surface of the body, from less than 1 mm to more than 5 mm. However, the skin is obviously both grossly and histologically different at two locations, the palms of the hands and the soles of the feet; these areas are subject to the most abrasion, are hairless, and have a much thicker epidermal layer than skin in any other location. This hairless skin is referred to as ***thick skin.*** Elsewhere, the skin possesses a much thinner epidermis and is called ***thin skin.*** It contains hair follicles in all but a few locations.

The terms *thick skin* and *thin skin,* as used in histologic description, are misnomers and refer only to the thickness of the epidermal layer. Anatomically, the thickest skin is found on the upper portion of the back where the dermis is exceedingly thick. The epidermis of the upper back, however, is comparable to that of thin skin found elsewhere on the body. In contrast, in certain other sites such as the eyelid, the skin is extremely thin.

▽ LAYERS OF THE SKIN

Epidermis

The ***epidermis*** is composed of stratified squamous epithelium in which four distinct layers can be identified. In the case of thick skin, a fifth layer is observed (Figs. 14.1 and 14.2). Beginning with the deepest layer, these are

- ***Stratum basale,*** also called the ***stratum germinativum*** because of the presence of mitotically active cells, the stem cells of the epidermis
- ***Stratum spinosum,*** also called the ***spinous*** or ***prickle cell layer*** because of the characteristic light microscopic appearance of short processes extending from cell to cell
- ***Stratum granulosum,*** which contains numerous intensely staining granules
- ***Stratum lucidum,*** limited to thick skin and considered a subdivision of the stratum corneum
- ***Stratum corneum,*** composed of keratinized cells

Differentiation of epithelial cells constitutes a specialized form of apoptosis

Terminal differentiation of the epidermal cells, which begins with the cell divisions in the stratum basale, is considered a specialized form of apoptosis. Cells in the stratum granulosum exhibit typical apoptotic nuclear morphology, including fragmentation of their DNA. However, the cellular fragmentation associated with normal apoptosis does not occur; instead, the cells become filled with filaments of the intracellular protein ***keratin*** and are later sloughed from the skin surface.

The stratum basale provides for epidermal cell renewal

The ***stratum basale*** is represented by a single layer of cells that rests on the basal lamina. It contains the ***stem cells*** from which new cells, the ***keratinocytes,*** arise by mitotic division. For this reason, the stratum basale is also called the ***stratum germinativum.*** The cells are small and

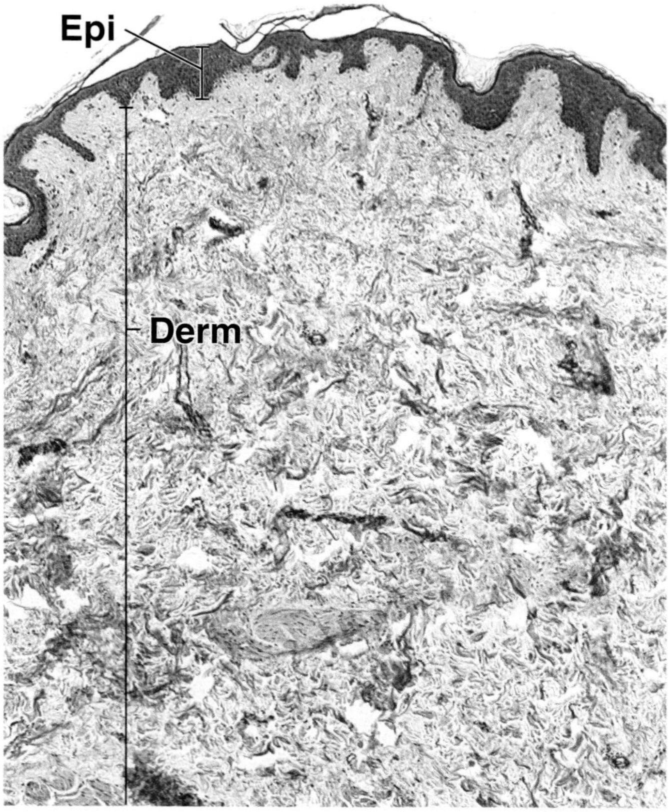

FIGURE 14.1
Photomicrograph showing the layers of thin skin. This H&E–stained specimen from human skin shows the two chief layers of the skin, the epidermis *(Epi)* and dermis *(Derm)*. The epidermis forms the surface; it consists of stratified squamous epithelium that is keratinized. The dermis consists of two layers: the papillary layer, which is the most superficial layer and is adjacent to the epidermis, and the more deeply positioned reticular layer. The boundary between these two layers is not conspicuous; the papillary layer is, however, more cellular than the reticular layer. In addition, the collagen fibers of the reticular layer are thick (clearly visible in the lower part of the figure); those of the papillary layer are thin. ×45.

are cuboidal to low columnar. They have less cytoplasm than the cells in the layer above; consequently, their nuclei are more closely spaced. The closely spaced nuclei, in combination with the basophilic cytoplasm of these cells, imparts a noticeable basophilia to the stratum basale. The basal cells also contain various amounts of melanin (described later) in their cytoplasm that is transferred from neighboring melanocytes interspersed in this layer. Basal cells exhibit extensive cell junctions; they are connected to each other and to keratinocytes by desmosomes and to the underlying basal lamina by hemidesmosomes. As new keratinocytes arise in this layer by mitotic division, they move into the next layer, thus beginning their process of upward migration. This process terminates when the cell becomes a mature keratinized cell, which is eventually sloughed off at the skin surface.

The cells of the stratum spinosum characteristically exhibit spinous processes

The ***stratum spinosum*** is at least several cells thick. The cells are larger than those of the stratum basale. They exhibit numerous cytoplasmic processes or spines, which gives this layer its name (Fig. 14.3). The processes are attached to similar processes of adjacent cells by desmosomes. In the light microscope, the site of the desmosome appears as a slight thickening called the ***node of Bizzozero.*** The processes are usually very conspicuous, in part because the cells shrink during preparation and a resultant expanded intercellular space develops between the spines. Be-

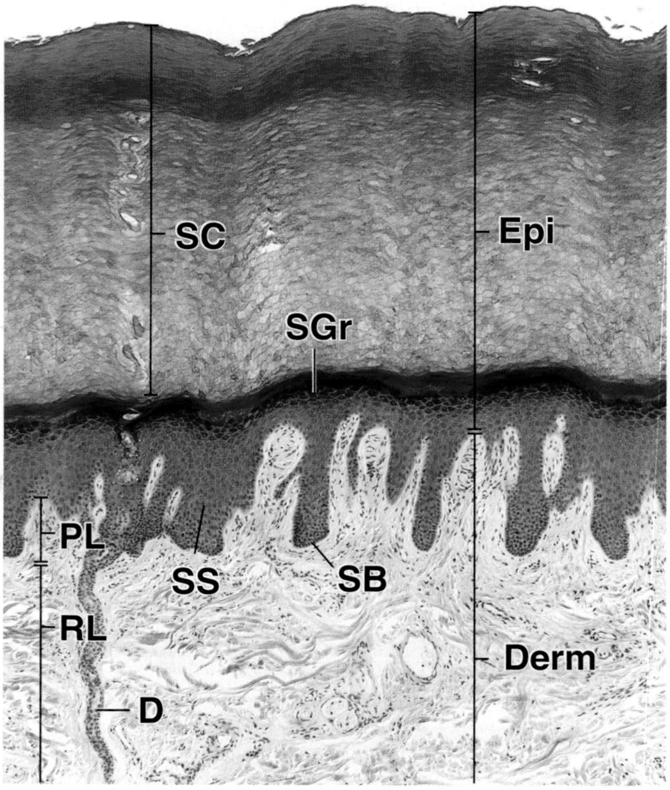

FIGURE 14.2
Photomicrograph showing the layers of thick skin. Specimen obtained from the skin of the sole of the foot (human) shows epidermis *(Epi)* containing the extremely thick stratum corneum *(SC)*. Remaining layers of the epidermis (except for the stratum lucidum, which is not present on this slide), i.e., the stratum basale *(SB)*, the stratum spinosum *(SS)*, and the stratum granulosum *(SGr)*, are clearly visible in this routine H&E preparation. The duct of a sweat gland *(D)* can be seen on the left as it traverses the dermis (*Derm*) and further spirals through the epidermis. At the sites where the ducts of the sweat gland enter the epidermis, note the epidermal downgrowths known as interpapillary pegs. The dermis contains papillae, protrusions of connective tissue that lie between the interpapillary pegs. Note also the greater cellularity of the papillary layer *(PL)* and that the collagen fibers of the reticular layer *(RL)* are thicker than those of the papillary layer. ×65.

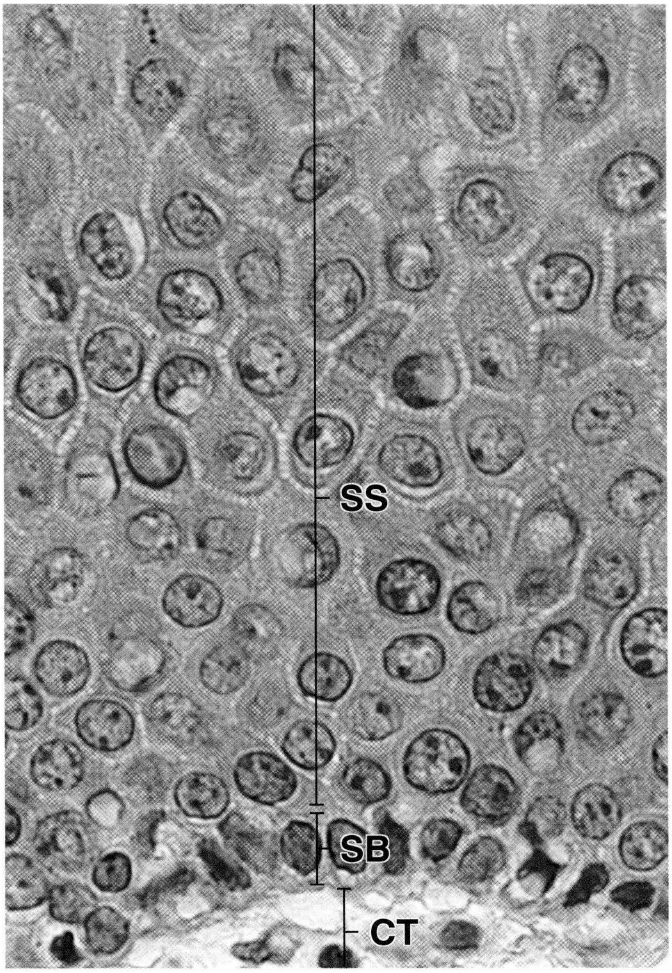

FIGURE 14.3
Photomicrograph of the stratum spinosum and stratum basale. The epidermis of thin skin is shown here at higher magnification. The one-cell-deep layer at the base of the epidermis just above the connective tissue *(CT)* of the dermis is the stratum basale *(SB).* The cells of this layer rest on the basement membrane. A layer referred to as the stratum spinosum *(SS)* is located just above the stratum basale. It consists of cells with spinous processes on their surfaces. These processes are attached to spinous processes of neighboring cells by desmosomes and together appear as intercellular bridges. ×640.

cause of their appearance, the cells that constitute this layer are often referred to as ***prickle cells.*** As the cells mature and move to the surface, they increase in size and become flattened in a plane parallel to the surface. This arrangement is particularly notable in the most superficial spinous cells, where the nuclei also become elongate instead of ovoid, matching the acquired squamous shape of the cells.

The cells of the stratum granulosum contain conspicuous keratohyalin granules

The ***stratum granulosum*** is the most superficial layer of the nonkeratinized portion of the epidermis. This layer varies from one to three cells thick. The cells contain numerous ***keratohyalin granules,*** hence the name of the layer. These granules contain cystine-rich and histidine-rich proteins, which are the precursors of the protein ***filaggrin*** that aggregates the keratin filaments present within the cornified cells of the stratum corneum. Keratohyalin granules are irregular in shape and variable in size. Because of their intense basophilic staining, they are readily seen in routine histologic sections.

The stratum corneum consists of anucleate squamous cells largely filled with keratin filaments

Usually, an abrupt transition occurs between the nucleated cells of the stratum granulosum and the flattened, desiccated, anucleate cells of the ***stratum corneum.*** The cells in the stratum corneum are the most differentiated cells in the skin. They lose their nucleus and cytoplasmic organelles and become filled almost entirely with keratin filaments. The thick plasma membrane of these cornified, keratinized cells is coated from the outside, in the deeper portion of this layer, with an extracellular layer of lipids that form the major constituent of the ***water barrier*** in the epidermis (see page 406).

The stratum corneum is the layer that varies most in thickness, being thickest in thick skin. The thickness of this layer constitutes the principal difference between the epidermis of thick and thin skin. This cornified layer will become even thicker at sites subjected to unusual amounts of friction, as in the formation of calluses on the palms of the hand and on the fingertips.

The ***stratum lucidum,*** considered a subdivision of the stratum corneum by some histologists, is found only in thick skin. In the light microscope, it often has a refractile appearance and may stain poorly. This highly refractile layer contains eosinophilic cells in which the process of keratinization is well advanced. The nucleus and cytoplasmic organelles become disrupted and disappear as the cell gradually fills with keratin.

Dermis

Attachment of epidermis to dermis is enhanced by an increased interface between the two tissues

The junction between the dermis and epidermis is seen in the light microscope as an uneven boundary except in the thinnest skin. Sections of skin cut perpendicular to the surface reveal numerous finger-like connective tissue protrusions, ***dermal papillae,*** that project into the undersurface of the epidermis (see Figs. 14.1 and 14.2). The papillae are complemented by what appear to be similar epidermal protrusions, called ***epidermal ridges*** or ***rete ridges,*** that project into the dermis. If the plane of section is parallel to the surface of the epidermis and passes at a level that includes the

dermal papillae, however, the epidermal tissue appears as a continuous sheet of epithelium, containing circular islands of connective tissue within it. The islands are cross sections of true finger-like dermal papillae that project into the epidermis. At sites where increased mechanical stress is placed on the skin, the epidermal ridges are much deeper (the epithelium is thicker), and the dermal papillae are much longer and more closely spaced, creating a more extensive interface between the dermis and epidermis. This phenomenon is particularly well demonstrated in histologic sections that show both palmar and dorsal surfaces of the hand, as in a section of a finger.

True dermal ridges are present in thick skin in addition to dermal papillae

Dermal ridges tend to have a parallel arrangement, with the dermal papillae located between them. These ridges form a distinctive pattern that is genetically unique to each individual and is reflected in the appearance of epidermal grooves and ridges on the surface of the skin. These patterns are the basis of the science of ***dermatoglyphics,*** or fingerprint and footprint identification.

The dermal ridges and papillae are most prominent in the thick skin of the palmar and plantar surfaces. Here, the basal surface of the epidermis greatly exceeds its free surface. The germinal layer is thus spread over a large area, and assuming a near-constant rate of mitosis in the stratum germinativum, more cells per unit time enter the stratum corneum in thick skin than in thin skin. These additional cells are thought to account for the greater thickness of the cornified layer in thick skin.

Hemidesmosomes strengthen the attachment of the epidermis to the underlying connective tissue

When studied with the transmission electron microscope (TEM), the basal surface of the basal epidermal cells exhibits a pattern of irregular cytoplasmic protrusions that increase the attachment surface between the epithelial cell and its subjacent basal lamina. A series of ***hemidesmosomes*** link the intermediate filaments of the cytoskeleton into the basal lamina. In addition, ***focal adhesions*** that anchor actin filaments into the basal lamina are also present. These specialized anchoring junctions are discussed on page 109.

The dermis is composed of two layers: the papillary layer and the reticular layer

Examination of the full thickness of the dermis at the light microscope level reveals two structurally distinct layers:

- The ***papillary layer,*** the more superficial layer, consists of loose connective tissue immediately beneath the epidermis. The collagen fibers located in this part of the dermis are not as thick as those in the deeper portion. This delicate collagen network contains predominately type I and type III collagen molecules. Similarly, the elastic fibers are thread-like and form an irregular network. The papillary layer is relatively thin and includes the substance of the dermal papillae and dermal ridges. It contains blood vessels that serve but do not enter the epidermis. It also contains nerve processes that either terminate in the dermis or penetrate the basal lamina to enter the epithelial compartment. Because the blood vessels and sensory nerve endings are concentrated in this layer, they are particularly apparent in the dermal papillae.
- The ***reticular layer*** lies deep to the papillary layer. Although its thickness varies in different parts of the body, it is always considerably thicker and less cellular than the papillary layer. It is characterized by thick, irregular bundles of mostly type I collagen and by coarser elastic fibers. The collagen and elastic fibers are not randomly oriented but form regular lines of tension in the skin, called ***Langer's lines.*** Skin incisions made parallel to Langer's lines heal with the least scarring.

In the skin of the areolae, penis, scrotum, and perineum, smooth muscle cells form a loose plexus in the deepest parts of the reticular layer. This arrangement accounts for the puckering of the skin at these sites, particularly in erectile organs.

Layers of adipose tissue, smooth muscle, and, in some sites, striated muscle may be found just beneath the reticular layer

Deep to the reticular layer is a layer of adipose tissue, the ***panniculus adiposus,*** which varies in thickness. This layer serves as a major energy storage site and also provides insulation. It is particularly thick in individuals who live in cold climates. This layer and its associated loose connective tissue constitute the ***hypodermis*** or ***subcutaneous layer.***

Individual smooth muscle cells or small bundles of smooth muscle cells that originate in this layer form the ***arrector pili muscles*** that connect the deep part of hair follicles to the more superficial dermis. Contraction of these muscles in humans produces the erection of hairs and puckering of skin called "goose flesh." In animals, the erection of hairs serves in both thermal regulation and fright reactions.

A thin layer of striated muscle, the ***panniculus carnosus,*** lies deep to the panniculus adiposus in many animals. Although largely vestigial in humans, it remains well defined in the skin of the neck, face, and scalp, where it constitutes the ***platysma*** muscle and the other muscles of facial expression.

CELLS OF THE EPIDERMIS

The cells of the epidermis consist of four different cell types:

- Keratinocytes
- Melanocytes
- Langerhans' cells
- Merkel's cells

Keratinocytes

The keratinocyte is the predominate cell type of the epidermis. These cells originate in the basal epidermal layer. On leaving this layer, keratinocytes assume two essential activities:

- They produce keratin, the major structural protein of the epidermis. Keratin constitutes almost 85% of fully differentiated keratinocytes.
- They participate in the formation of the epidermal water barrier.

The keratinocytes in the basal layer contain numerous free ribosomes, scattered 7- to 9-nm intermediate (keratin) filaments, a small Golgi apparatus, mitochondria, and rough endoplasmic reticulum (rER). The cytoplasm of immature keratinocytes appears basophilic in histologic sections because of the large number of free ribosomes, most of which are engaged in the synthesis of keratin, which will later be assembled into ***keratin filaments.*** These filaments are classified as intermediate filaments although they are more commonly called ***tonofilaments.***

As the cells enter and are moved through the stratum spinosum, the synthesis of keratin filaments continues, and the filaments become grouped into bundles sufficiently thick to be visualized in the light microscope. These bundles are called ***tonofibrils.*** The cytoplasm becomes eosinophilic because of the staining reaction of the tonofibrils that fill more and more of the cytoplasm.

Keratohyalin granules contain intermediate filament–associated proteins that aid in aggregation of keratin filaments

In the upper part of the stratum spinosum (Fig. 14.4), the free ribosomes within the keratinocytes begin to synthesize ***keratohyalin granules*** that become the distinctive feature of the cells in the stratum granulosum. Keratohyalin granules contain the two major intermediate filament–associated proteins, ***filaggrin*** and ***trichohyalin.*** The appearance of the granules and expression of filaggrin in the keratinocytes is often used as a clinical marker for the initiation of the final stage of apoptosis. As the number of granules increases, the contents of the granules are released into the keratinocyte cytoplasm. Filaggrin and trichohyalin function as promoters in the aggregation of keratin filaments into tonofibrils, thus initiating the conversion of granular cells into cornified cells. This process is called ***keratinization*** and occurs in 2 to 6 hours, the time it takes for the cells to leave the stratum granulosum and enter the stratum corneum. The keratin fibril formed in this process is called ***soft keratin*** in contrast to the hard keratin of hair and nails (see below).

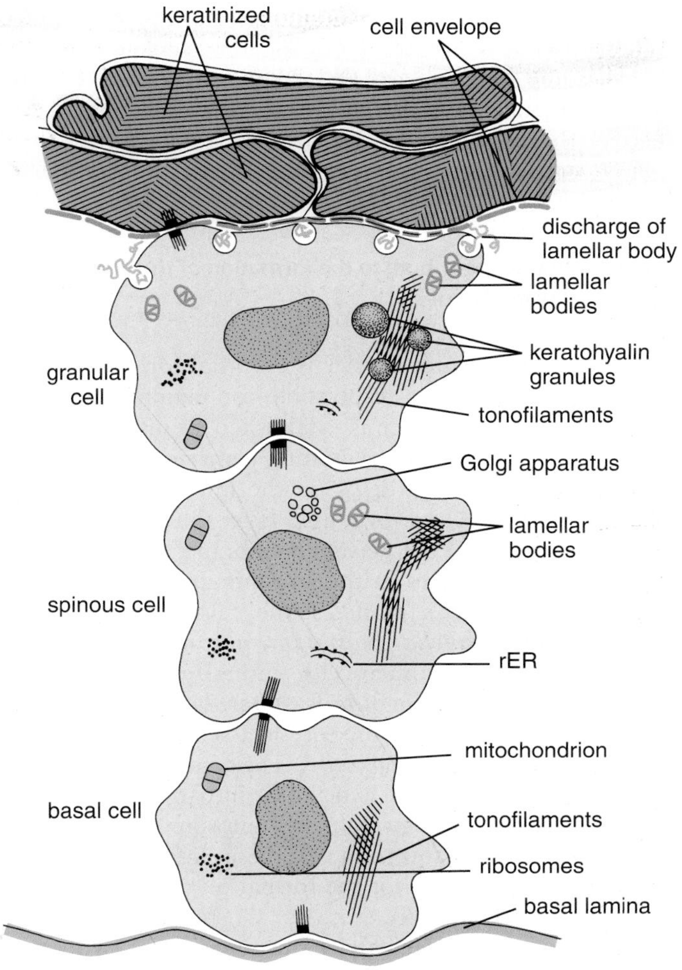

FIGURE 14.4
Schematic diagram of keratinocytes in the epidermis. The keratinocytes in this figure reflect different stages in the life cycle of the cell as it passes from the basal layer through the spinous and granular layers to the surface keratinized layer. The basal cell begins to synthesize tonofilaments (intermediate [keratin] filaments); these are grouped into bundles and seen in the light microscope as tonofibrils. The cell enters the spinous layer, where the synthesis of tonofilaments continues. In the upper part of the spinous layer, the cells begin to produce keratohyalin granules containing intermediate filament–associated proteins and glycolipid-containing lamellar bodies. Within the granular layer, the cell discharges lamellar bodies; the remainder of the cell cytoplasm contains numerous keratohyalin granules in close association with tonofilaments. The surface cells are keratinized; they contain a thickened plasma membrane and bundles of tonofilaments in a specialized matrix. (From Matoltsy AG, Parrakal PF. In: Zelickson AS, eds. *Ultrastructure of Normal and Abnormal Skin.* Philadelphia: Lea & Febiger, 1967.)

The transformation of a granular cell into a cornified cell also involves breakdown of the nucleus and other organelles and thickening of the plasma membrane. Finally, cells are regularly exfoliated (desquamated) from the surface of the stratum corneum. The cells that will desquamate accumulate acid phosphatase, which is thought to participate in the exfoliation of these keratinized cells.

Lamellar bodies contribute to the formation of the intercellular epidermal water barrier

An epidermal water barrier is essential for mammalian "dry" epithelia and is responsible for maintaining body homeostasis. The barrier is established primarily by two factors in terminally differentiating keratinocytes: *(a)* deposition of insoluble proteins on the inner surface of the plasma membrane and *(b)* a lipid layer that is attached to the outer surface of the plasma membrane.

As the keratinocytes in the stratum spinosum begin to produce keratohyalin granules, they also produce membrane-bounded ***lamellar bodies (membrane-coating granules).*** Spinous and granular cells synthesize a heterogenous mixture of ***glycosphingolipids, phospholipids,*** and ***ceramides*** (Fig. 14.5); this mixture is assembled into lamellar bodies in the Golgi apparatus. The contents of the granules is then secreted by exocytosis into the intercellular spaces between the stratum granulosum and stratum corneum. The organization of these intercellular lipid lamellae is responsible for the formation of the epidermal water barrier (Fig. 14.6).

The epidermal water barrier thus consists of two structural elements:

- The ***cell envelope (CE),*** a 15-nm-thick layer of insoluble proteins deposited on the inner surface of the plasma membrane that contributes to the strong mechanical properties of the barrier. The thickness of the CE increases in epithelia that are subject to considerable mechanical stress (e.g., lip, palm of the hand, sole of the foot). The CE is formed by cross-linking ***small proline-rich (SPR) proteins*** and larger structural proteins. The structural proteins include ***cystatin, desmosomal proteins (desmoplakin), elafin, envoplakin, filaggrin, involucrin,*** five different ***keratin*** chains, and ***loricrin.*** Loricrin is the major structural protein and accounts for almost 80% of the total CE protein mass. This 26-kDa insoluble protein has the highest glycine content of any known protein in the body.
- The ***lipid envelope,*** a 5-nm-thick layer of lipids attached to the cell surface by ester bonds. The major lipid components of the lipid envelope are ceramides, which belong to the class of sphingolipids; ***cholesterol;*** and ***free fatty acids.*** However, the most important component is the monomolecular layer of ***acylglucosylceramide,*** which provides a "Teflon-like" coating on the cell surface. Ceramides also play an important role in cell signaling and are partially responsible for inducing cell differentiation, triggering apoptosis, and reducing cell proliferation. As the cells continue to move toward the free surface, the barrier is constantly maintained by keratinocytes entering the process of terminal differentiation. Lamellae may remain as recognizable disks in the intercellular space or may fuse into broad sheets or layers.

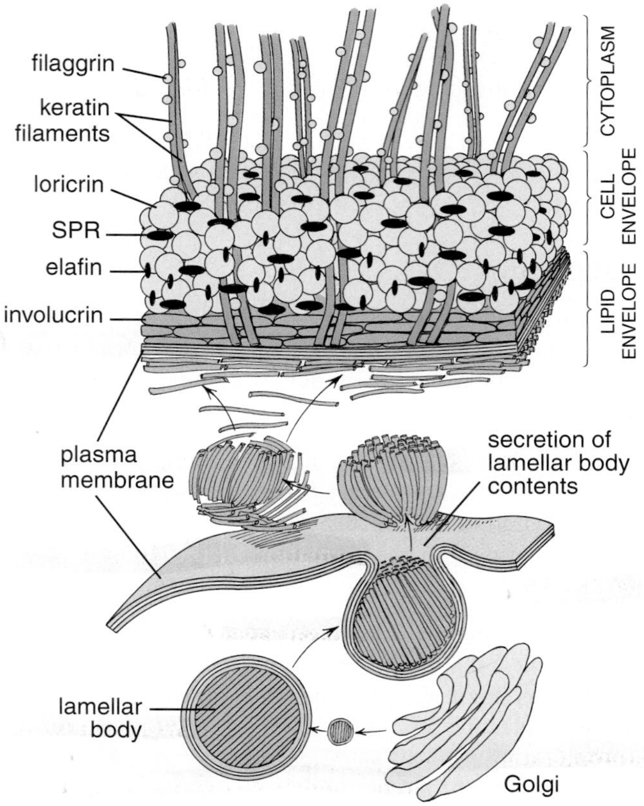

FIGURE 14.5
Schematic diagram of the epidermal water barrier. The heterogeneous mixture of glycosphingolipids, phospholipids, and ceramides makes up the lamellae of the lamellar bodies. The lamellar bodies, produced within the Golgi apparatus, are secreted by exocytosis into the intercellular spaces between the stratum granulosum and stratum corneum, where they form the lipid envelope. The lamellar arrangement of lipid molecules is depicted in the intercellular space just below the thickened plasma membrane and forms the cell envelope of the keratinized keratinocyte. The innermost part of the cell envelope consists primarily of loricrin molecules *(pink spheres)* that are cross-linked by small proline-rich (SPR) proteins and elafin. The layer adjacent to the cytoplasmic surface of the plasma membrane consists of the two tightly packed proteins involucrin and cystatin α. Keratin filaments (tonofilaments) bound by filaggrin are anchored into the cell envelope.

Experiments have shown that the epidermis of animals with induced essential fatty acid deficiency (EFAD) is more permeable than normal to water. The membrane-coating granules also have fewer lamellae than normal. Destruc-

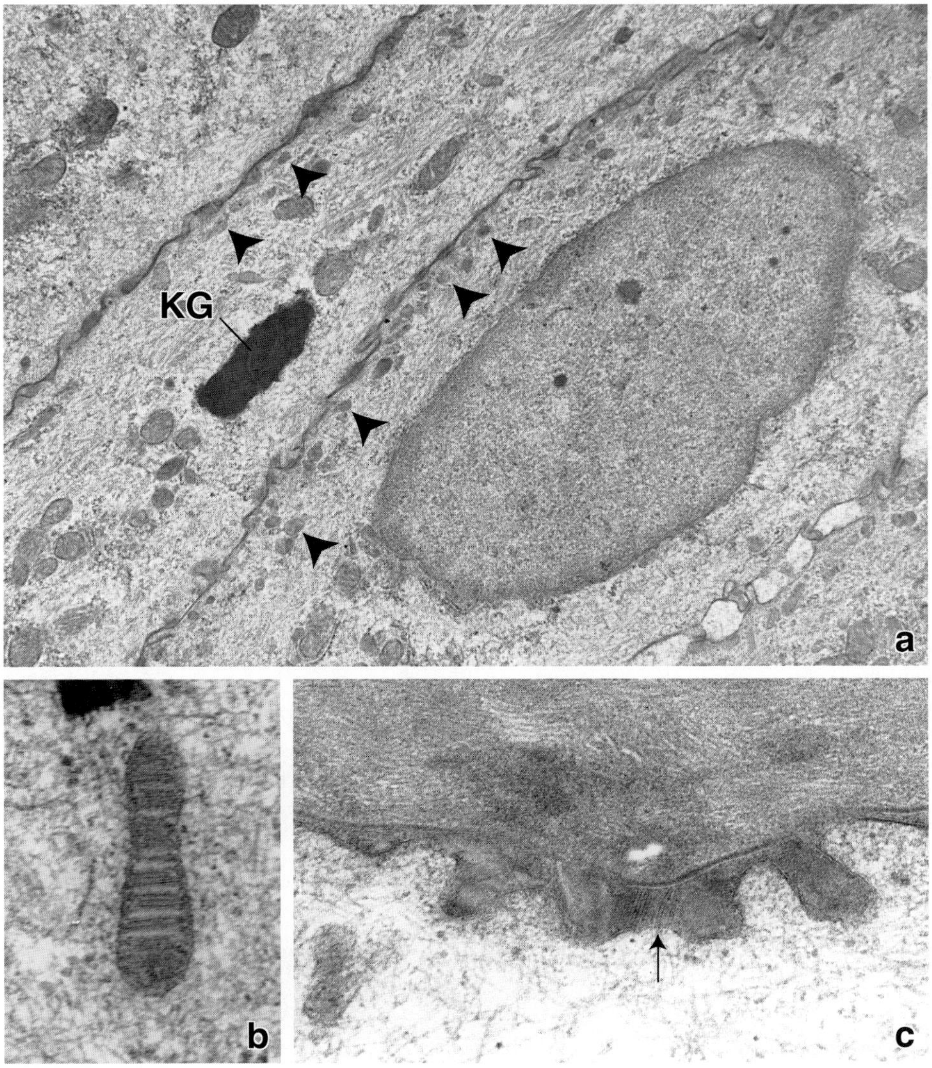

FIGURE 14.6
Electron micrographs of keratinocytes. **a.** Much of the keratinocyte cytoplasm is filled with tonofilaments. One keratinocyte exhibits a keratohyalin granule *(KG).* Near the plasma membrane closest to the surface (upper left), two keratinocytes display lamellar bodies *(arrowheads).* ×8,500. **b.** A lamellar body at higher magnification. ×135,000. **c.** Part of a keratinized cell and the underlying keratinocyte. Located between the cells are the contents of the lamellar bodies, which have been discharged into the intercellular space *(arrow)* to form the lipid envelope. ×90,000. (Courtesy of Dr. Albert I. Farbman.)

tion of the epidermal barrier over large areas, as in severe burns, can lead to life-threatening loss of fluid from the body.

Melanocytes

Neural crest–derived melanocytes are scattered among the basal cells of the stratum basale

During embryonic life, melanocyte precursor cells migrate from the neural crest and enter the developing epidermis. A specific functional association is then established, the ***epidermal-melanin unit,*** in which one melanocyte maintains an association with a given number of keratinocytes. This ratio varies in different parts of the body.

The epidermal ***melanocyte*** is a dendritic cell that is scattered among the basal cells of the stratum basale (Fig. 14.7). They are called dendritic cells because the rounded cell body resides in the basal layer and extends long processes between the keratinocytes of the stratum spinosum. Neither the processes nor the cell body forms desmosomal attachments with neighboring keratinocytes. However, melanocytes that reside close to the basal lamina have structures that resemble hemidesmosomes. The ratio of melanocytes to keratinocytes or their precursors in the basal layer ranges from 1:4 to 1:10 in different parts of the body and is constant in all races. In routine hematoxylin and eosin (H&E) preparations melanocytes are seen in the stratum basale with elongated nuclei surrounded by a clear cytoplasm. With the TEM, however, they are readily identified by the developing and mature melanin granules in the cytoplasm (Fig. 14.8). Melanocytes maintain the capacity to replicate throughout their life, although at a much slower rate than keratinocytes, thus maintaining the epidermal-melanin unit.

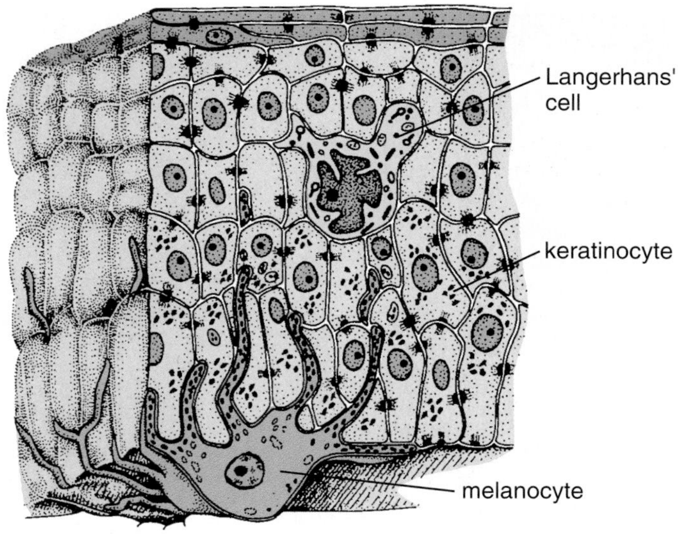

FIGURE 14.7
Diagram of the epidermis. This diagram shows a melanocyte interacting with several cells of the stratum basale and the stratum spinosum. The melanocyte has long dendritic processes that contain accumulated melanosomes and extend between the cells of the epidermis. The Langerhans' cell is a dendritic cell often confused with a melanocyte. It is actually part of the mononuclear phagocytotic system and functions as an antigen-presenting cell of the immune system in the initiation of cutaneous hypersensitivity reactions (contact allergic dermatitis). (Modified from Weiss L, ed. *Cell and Tissue Biology: A Textbook of Histology.* 6th ed. Baltimore: Urban & Schwarzenberg, 1988.)

Melanocytes produce and distribute melanin into keratinocytes

The epidermal melanocytes produce and secrete the pigment ***melanin.*** The most important function of melanin is to protect the organism against the damaging effects of nonionizing ultraviolet irradiation. Melanin is produced by the oxidation of ***tyrosine*** to ***3,4-dihydroxyphenylalanine (DOPA)*** by ***tyrosinase*** and the subsequent transformation of DOPA into melanin. These reactions initially occur in membrane-bounded structures, called ***premelanosomes,*** that are derived from the Golgi apparatus (Fig. 14.9). Premelanosomes and the ***early melanosomes,*** which have a low melanin content, exhibit a finely ordered internal structure with the TEM, reflecting their content of tyrosinase molecules. As more melanin is produced by oxidation of tyrosine, the internal structure of the premelanosome becomes obscured until the mature melanin granule, the ***melanosome,*** is formed and then appears as an electron-opaque granule. Premelanosomes are concentrated near the Golgi apparatus; nearly mature melanosomes at the bases of the cell processes; and mature melanosomes most commonly in and at the ends of the processes (see Fig. 14.9). Developing melanosomes and their melanin contents are transferred to neighboring keratinocytes by ***pigment donation.*** This process, which involves the phagocytosis of the tips of the melanocyte processes by keratinocytes, is a type of ***cytocrine secretion*** because a small amount of cytoplasm surrounding the melanosome is also phagocytosed.

Langerhans' Cells

Langerhans' cells are antigen-presenting cells in the epidermis

Langerhans' cells are dendritic-appearing, antigen-presenting cells in the epidermis. They encounter and present antigens entering through the skin. Langerhans' cells cannot be distinguished with certainty in routine H&E–stained paraffin sections. Like melanocytes, Langerhans' cells do not form desmosomes with neigh-

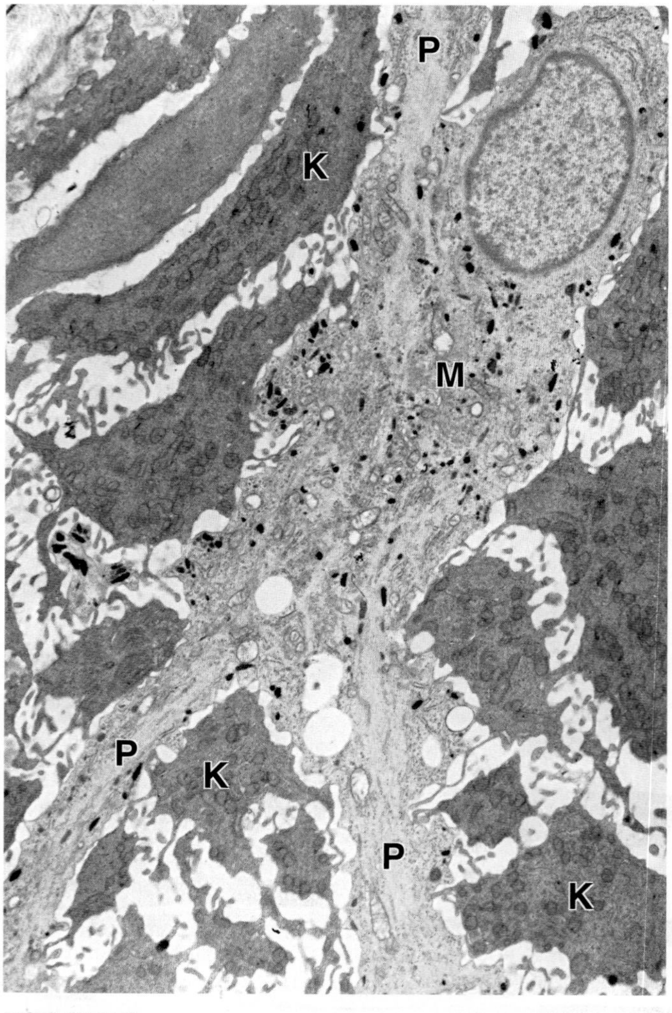

FIGURE 14.8
Electron micrograph of a melanocyte. The melanocyte *(M)* reveals several processes *(P)* extending between neighboring keratinocytes *(K)*. The small dark bodies are melanosomes. ×8,500. (Courtesy of Dr. Bryce L. Munger.)

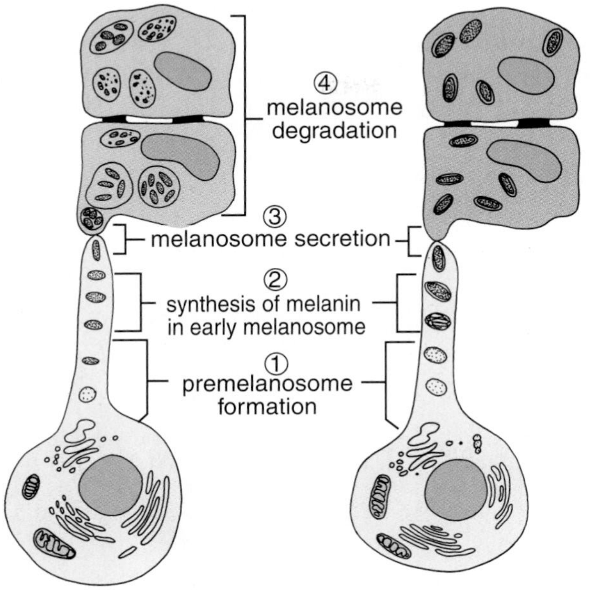

FIGURE 14.9
Formation of melanin pigment and secretion of pigment granules into keratinocytes. Melanocytes produce membrane-bounded structures that originate in the Golgi apparatus as premelanosomes ①. Within the early melanosomes, as maturation proceeds, melanin is produced from tyrosine by a series of enzymatic reactions ②. Mature melanosomes and their melanin contents are transferred to neighboring keratinocytes by pigment donation, which involves the phagocytosis of the tips of the melanocyte ③. In darker skin (on the right), the melanin is degraded slowly, and melanosomes remain discrete; in lighter skin (on the left), the melanin is degraded more rapidlly ④ through the process of macroautophagy. (Based on Weiss L, Greep RO. *Histology.* New York: McGraw-Hill, 1977.)

boring keratinocytes. The nucleus stains heavily with hematoxylin, and the cytoplasm is clear. With special techniques, such as gold chloride impregnation or immunostaining with antibody against CD1a molecules, Langerhans' cells can be readily seen in the stratum spinosum. They possess dendritic processes resembling those of the melanocyte. The TEM reveals several distinctive features of a Langerhans' cell (Fig. 14.10). Its nucleus is characteristically indented in many places, so the nuclear profile is uneven. Also, it possesses characteristic, tennis racket–shaped ***Birbeck granules.*** They represent relatively small vesicles, which appear as rods with a bulbous expansion at their end.

Like macrophages, Langerhans' cells express both MHC I and MHC II molecules, as well as F_c receptors for immunoglobulin G (IgG). Langerhans' cells also express complement C3b receptors as well as fluctuating quantities of CD1a molecules. As an antigen-presenting cell, the Langerhans' cell is involved in ***delayed-type hypersensitivity reactions*** (e.g., contact allergic dermatitis and other cell-mediated immune responses in the skin) through the uptake of antigen in the skin and its transport to the lymph nodes. Skin biopsy specimens from individuals with AIDS or AIDS-related complex reveal that Langerhans' cells contain HIV in their cytoplasm. Langerhans' cells appear to be more resistant than T cells to the deadly effects of the HIV and may, therefore, serve as a reservoir for the virus. Langerhans' cells are of mesenchymal origin and are derived from the $CD34^+$ stem cell in the bone marrow.

BOX 14.1
Functional Considerations: Skin Color

The color of an individual's skin is due to a number of factors. The most significant is melanin content. Although the number of melanocytes is essentially the same in all races, the nature of the melanin that is produced by the melanocytes differs. For example, due to the lysosomal activity of the keratinocytes, melanin is degraded more rapidly in individuals with light skin than in individuals with dark skin. In the former, melanosomes are more concentrated in the keratinocytes nearest the basal layer and are relatively sparse in the midregion of the stratum granulosum. In contrast, dark skin may exhibit melanosomes throughout the epidermis, including the stratum corneum.

In addition, melanin pigment comprises two distinct forms. One form, ***eumelanin,*** is a brownish black pigment. The other form, ***pheomelanin,*** is a reddish yellow pigment. Each is genetically determined. Coloration is most apparent in hair because of the concentration of melanin pigment granules, but it is also reflected in skin coloration.

Exposure to ultraviolet light, particularly the sun's rays, accelerates the rate of melanin production and thus protects against further radiation effects. Increased pigmentation of the skin may also result from hormonal imbalance, as, for example, in Addison's disease. Lack of pigmentation occurs in a condition known as ***albinism.*** In this condition, premelanosomes are produced by melanocytes, but because of the absence of tyrosinase, the transformation of tyrosine into DOPA and the subsequent transformation of DOPA into melanin fail to occur. Thus, there is no pigmentation in the skin or hair of these individuals.

The number of melanocytes decreases with age, resulting in decreasing availability of pigment donation to keratinocytes. Therefore, in older age the skin becomes lighter and the incidence of skin cancer increases. Other normal factors that affect skin coloration include the presence of oxyhemoglobin in the dermal vascular bed, which imparts a red hue; the presence of carotenes, an exogenous orange pigment taken up from foods and concentrated in tissues containing fat; and the presence of certain endogenous pigments. The latter include degradation products of hemoglobin, iron-containing hemosiderin and iron-free bilirubin, all of which impart color to the skin. Hemosiderin is a golden brown pigment, whereas bilirubin is a yellowish brown pigment. Bilirubin is normally removed from the bloodstream by the liver and eliminated via the bile. A yellowish skin color due to abnormal accumulation of bilirubin reflects liver dysfunction and is evidenced as ***jaundice.***

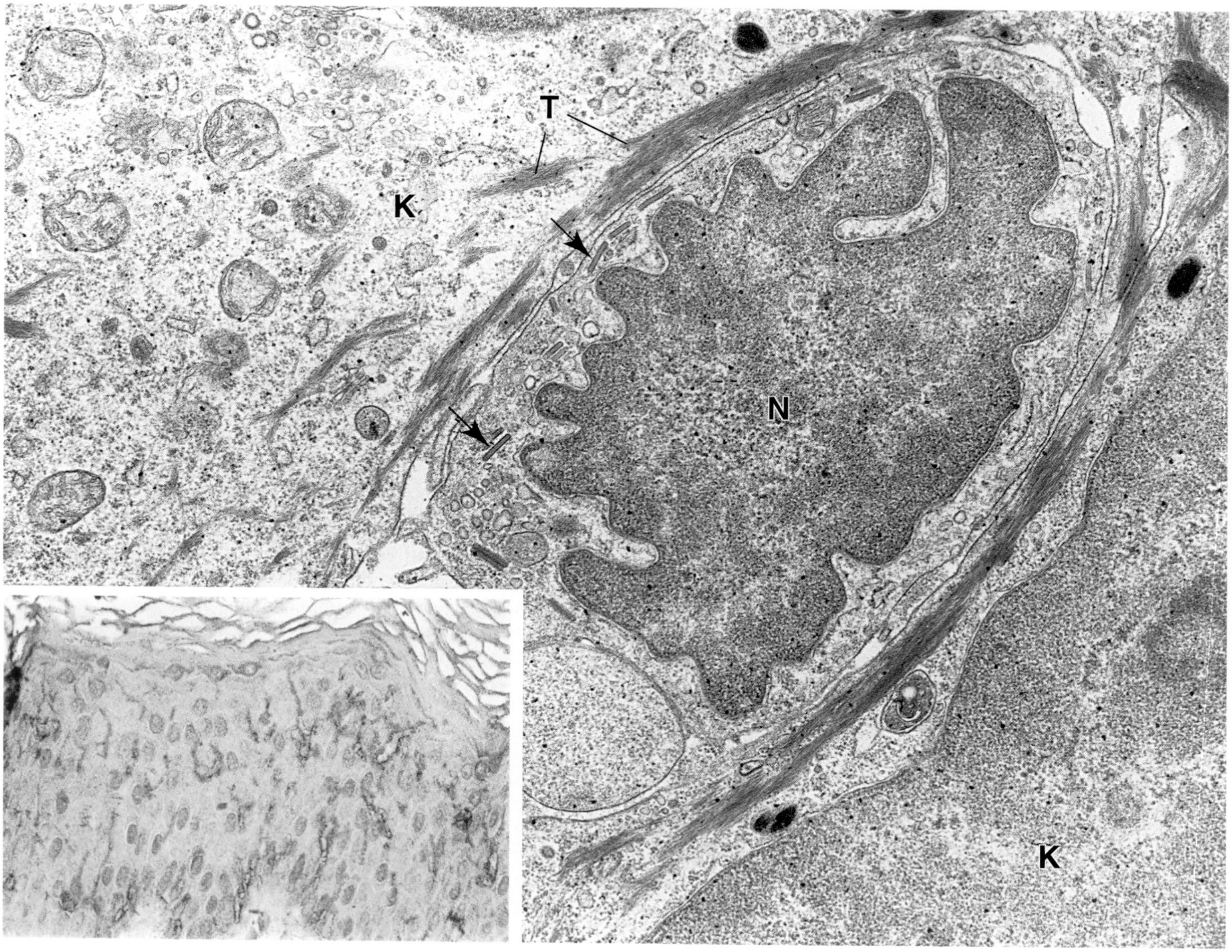

FIGURE 14.10
Electron micrograph of a Langerhans' cell. The nucleus *(N)* of a Langerhans' cell is characteristically indented in many places, and the cytoplasm contains distinctive rod-shaped bodies *(arrows).* Note the presence of tonofilaments *(T)* in adjacent keratinocytes *(K)* but the absence of these filaments in the Langerhans' cell. ×19,000. **Inset.** Photomicrograph of the epidermis shows the distribution and dendritic nature of the Langerhans' cells that were stained via immunostaining techniques with antibodies against CD1a surface antigen. ×300. (From Urmacher CD. In: Sternberg SS, ed. *Histology for Pathologists.* Philadelphia: Lippincott-Raven, 1997.)

Therefore, they constitute part of the mononuclear phagocytotic system (MPS) (page 144).

Merkel's Cells

Merkel's cells are epidermal cells that function in cutaneous sensation

Merkel's cells are modified epidermal cells located in the stratum basale. They are most abundant in skin where sensory perception is acute, such as the fingertips. Merkel's cells are bound to adjoining keratinocytes by desmosomes and contain intermediate (keratin) filaments in their cytoplasm. The nucleus is lobed, and the cytoplasm is somewhat denser than that of melanocytes and Langerhans' cells. They may contain some melanosomes in their cytoplasm, but they are best characterized by the presence of ***80-nm dense-cored neurosecretory granules*** that resemble those found in the adrenal medulla and carotid body (Fig. 14.11). Merkel's cells are closely associated with the expanded terminal bulb of afferent myelinated nerve fibers. The neuron terminal loses its Schwann cell covering and immediately penetrates the basal lamina, where it expands into a disk or plate-like ending that lies in close apposition to the base of the Merkel's cell. The combination of the neuron and

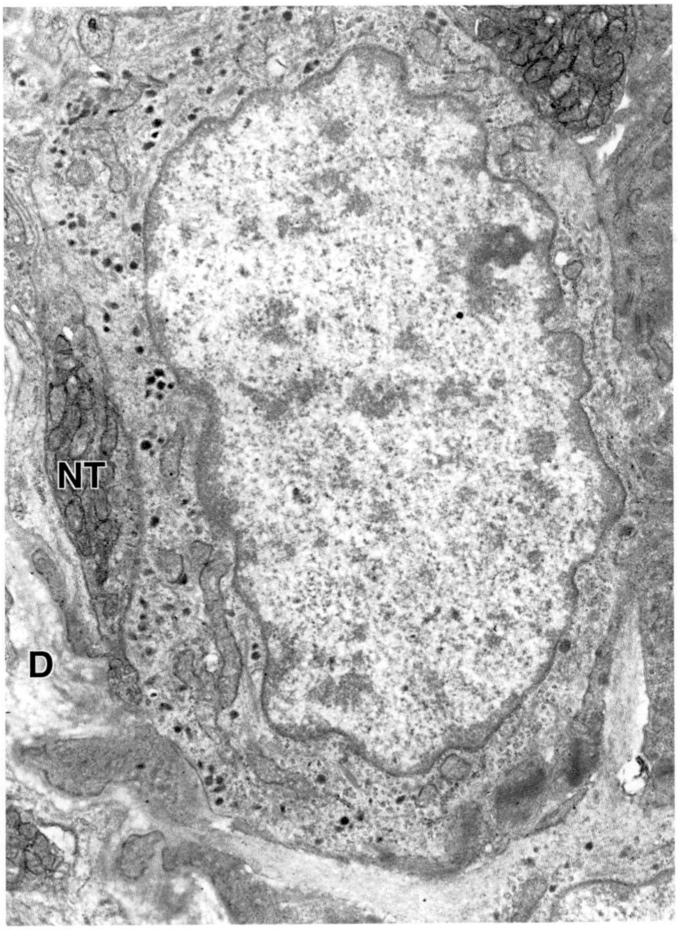

FIGURE 14.11
Electron micrograph of a Merkel's cell. The cell has small neurosecretory granules in the cytoplasm and makes contact with a peripheral terminal *(NT)* of a neuron. The dermis *(D)* is in the lower part of the micrograph. ×14,450. (Courtesy of Dr. Bryce L. Munger.)

epidermal cell, called a *Merkel's corpuscle,* is a sensitive *mechanoreceptor.*

STRUCTURES OF SKIN

Nerve Supply

The skin is endowed with sensory receptors of various types that are peripheral terminals of sensory nerves (Fig. 14.12). It is also well supplied with motor nerve endings to the blood vessels, arrector pili muscles, and sweat glands.

Free nerve endings are the most numerous neuronal receptors in the epidermis

Free nerve endings in the epidermis terminate in the stratum granulosum. The endings are "free" in that they lack a connective tissue or Schwann cell investment. Such neuronal endings subserve multiple sensory modalities including fine touch, heat, and cold, without apparent morphologic distinction. Networks of free dermal endings surround most hair follicles and attach to their outer root sheath (Fig. 14.13). In this position they are particularly sensitive to hair movement and serve as mechanoreceptors. This relationship imparts a sophisticated degree of specialization in the receptors that surround tactile hairs (vibrissae), such as the whiskers of a cat or rodent, in which each vibrissa has a specific representation in the cerebral cortex.

Other nerve endings in the skin are enclosed in a connective tissue capsule. ***Encapsulated nerve endings*** include

- *Pacinian corpuscles*
- *Meissner's corpuscles*
- *Ruffini's corpuscles*

Pacinian corpuscles are deep pressure receptors for mechanical and vibratory pressure

Pacinian corpuscles are large ovoid structures found in the deeper dermis and hypodermis (especially in the fingertips), in connective tissue in general, and in association with joints, periosteum, and internal organs. Pacinian corpuscles usually have macroscopic dimensions, measuring more than 1 mm along their long axis. They are composed of a myelinated nerve ending surrounded by a capsule structure (see Figs. 14.12 and 14.13a). The nerve enters the capsule at one pole with its myelin sheath intact. The myelin is retained for one or two nodes and is then lost. The unmyelinated portion of the axon extends toward the opposite pole from which it entered, and its length is covered by a series of tightly packed, flattened Schwann cell lamellae that form the ***inner core*** of the corpuscle. The remainder or bulk of the capsule, the outer core, is formed by a series of concentric lamellae; each lamella is separated from its neighbor by a narrow space containing lymph-like fluid. The appearance of the concentric lamellae as observed in the light microscope is reminiscent of the cut surface of a hemisected onion. Each lamella is composed of flattened cells that correspond to the cells of the endoneurium outside the capsule. In addition to fluid between the lamellae, collagen fibrils are present, although sparse, as well as occasional capillaries.

Pacinian corpuscles respond to pressure and vibration through the displacement of the capsule lamellae. This displacement effectively causes depolarization of the axon.

Meissner's corpuscles are localized within dermal papillae and serve as touch receptors

Meissner's corpuscles (see Figs. 14.12 and 14.13b) are touch receptors that are particularly responsive to low-frequency stimuli in the papillary layer of hairless skin,

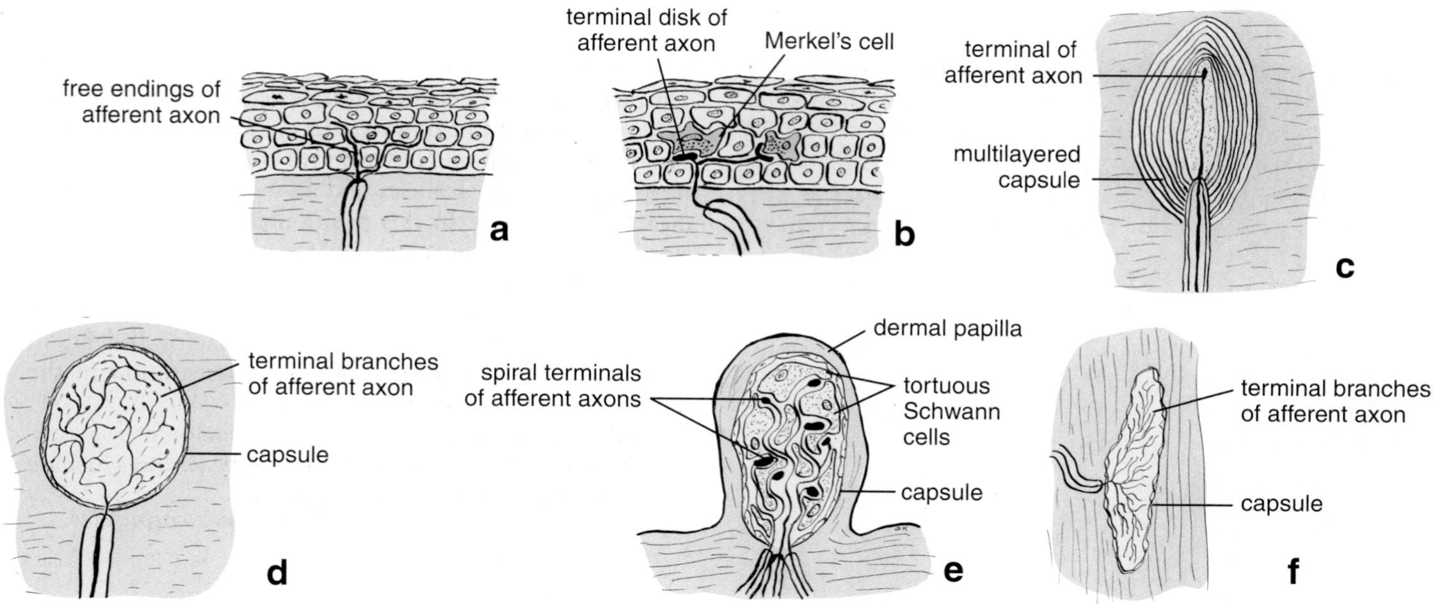

FIGURE 14.12

Diagram of the sensory receptors in skin. a. Epidermal free ending. **b.** Merkel's ending. **c.** Pacinian corpuscle. **d.** Krause's end bulb. **e.** Meissner's corpuscle. **f.** Ruffini's corpuscle. Note that axons *c* to *f* are encapsulated, i.e., surrounded by a capsule of connective tissue.

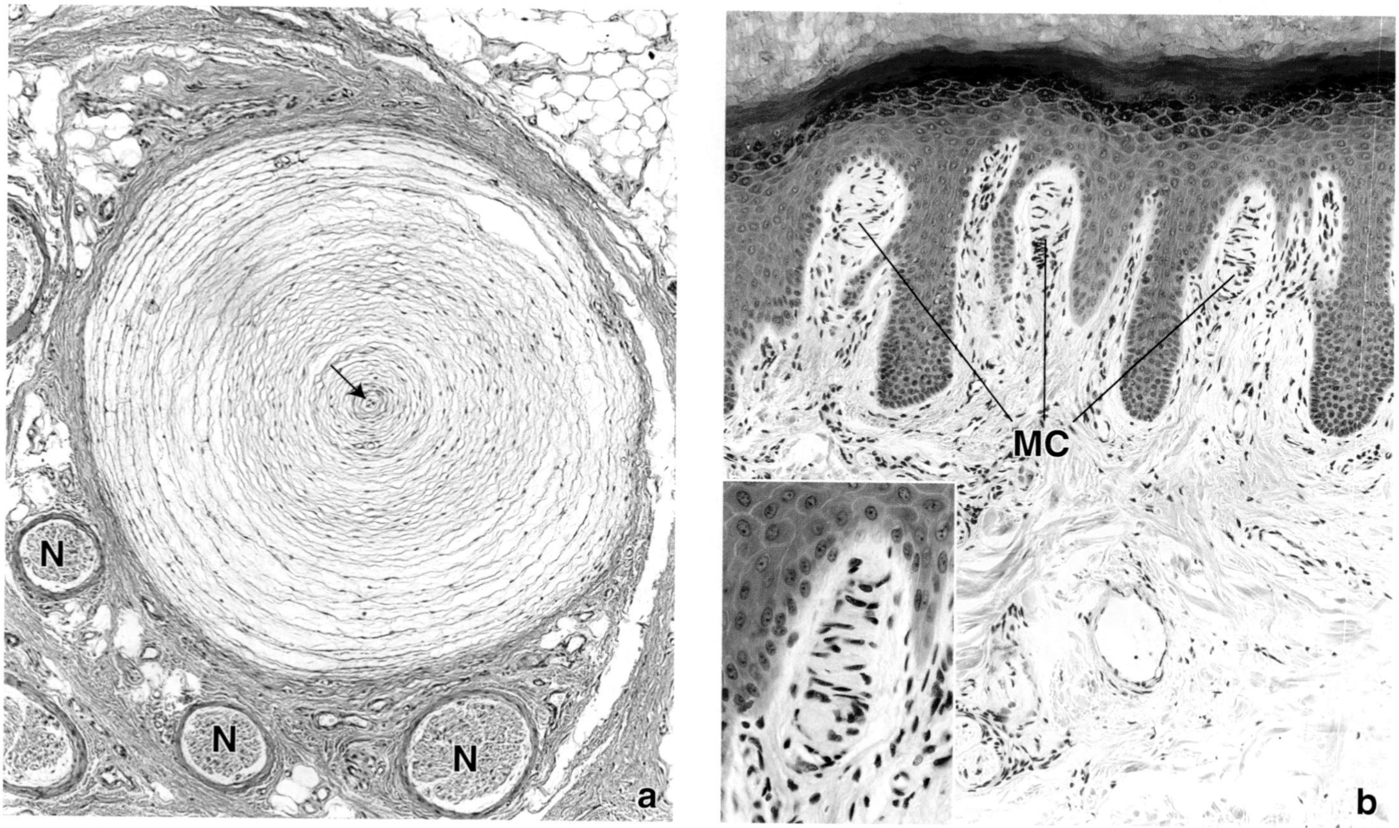

FIGURE 14.13

Pacinian and Meissner's corpuscles in H&E preparations. a. In this photomicrograph, the concentric cellular lamellae of the Pacinian corpuscle are visible because of flat, fibroblast-like supportive cells. Although not evident within the tissue section, these cells are continuous with the endoneurium of the nerve fiber. The spaces between lamellae contain mostly fluid. The neural portion of the Pacinian corpuscle travels longitudinally through the center of the structure *(arrow)*. Several nerves *(N)* are present adjacent to the corpuscle. ×85. **b.** Three Meissner's corpuscles *(MC)* are shown residing within the dermal papillae. Note the direct proximity of the corpuscle to the undersurface of the epidermis. ×150. **Inset.** A higher magnification of a Meissner's corpuscle. The nerve fiber terminates at the superficial pole of the corpuscle. Note that supporting cells are oriented approximately at right angles to the long axis of the corpuscle. ×320.

e.g., the lips and the palmar and volar surfaces, particularly those of the fingers and toes. Generally, they are tapered cylinders that measure about 150 μm along their long axis and are oriented perpendicular to the skin surface. Meissner's corpuscles are present in the dermal papillae just beneath the epidermal basal lamina. Within these receptors, one or two unmyelinated endings of myelinated nerve fibers follow spiral paths in the corpuscle. The cellular component consists of flattened Schwann cells that form several irregular lamellae through which the axons course to the pole of the corpuscle. In H&E–stained slides of sagittal sections, this structure resembles a loose, twisted skein of wool. It is the Schwann cells that give this impression.

Ruffini's corpuscles respond to mechanical displacement of adjacent collagen fibers

Ruffini's corpuscles are the simplest encapsulated mechanoreceptors. They have an elongated fusiform shape and measure 1 to 2 μm in length (see Fig. 14.12f). Structurally, they consist of a thin connective tissue capsule that encloses a fluid-filled space. Collagen fibers from the surrounding connective tissue pass through the capsule. The neural element consists of a single myelinated fiber that enters the capsule, where it loses its myelin sheath and branches to form a dense arborization of fine axonal endings, each terminating in a small knob-like bulb. The axonal endings are dispersed and intertwined inside the capsule. The axonal endings respond to displacement of the collagen fibers induced by sustained or continuous mechanical stress.

Epidermal Skin Appendages

Skin appendages are derived from downgrowths of epidermal epithelium during development. They include

- ***Hair follicles*** and their product, ***hair***
- ***Sebaceous glands*** and their product, ***sebum***
- ***Eccrine sweat glands*** and their product, ***sweat***
- ***Apocrine sweat glands*** and their mixed product

Both hairs and sweat glands play specific roles in regulation of body temperature. Sebaceous glands secrete an oily substance that may have protective functions. Apocrine glands produce a serous secretion containing pheromones that act as a sex attractant in animals and possibly humans. The epithelium of the skin appendages can serve as a source of new epithelial cells for skin wound repair.

HAIR FOLLICLES AND HAIR

Each hair follicle represents an invagination of the epidermis in which a hair is formed

Hair follicles and *hairs* are present over almost the entire body; they are absent only from the sides and palmar surfaces of the hands, sides and plantar surfaces of the feet, the lips, and the region around the urogenital orifices. Hair distribution is influenced to a considerable degree by sex hormones; these include, in the male, the thick, pigmented facial hairs that begin to grow at puberty and the pubic and axillary hair that develops at puberty in both genders. In the male, the hairline tends to recede with age, and in both genders, the scalp hair thins with age because of reduced secretion of estrogen and estrogen-like hormones.

The hair follicle is responsible for the production and growth of a hair. Coloration of the hair is due to the content and type of melanin (see page 409) that the hair contains. The follicle varies in histologic appearance, depending on whether it is in a growing or a resting phase. The growing follicle shows the most elaborate structure; thus, it is described here.

The hair follicle is divided into three segments:

- ***Infundibulum,*** which extends from the surface opening of the follicle to the level of the opening of its sebaceous gland. The infundibulum is a part of the ***pilosebaceous canal*** that is used as a route for the discharge of sebum.
- ***Isthmus,*** which extends from the infundibulum to the level of insertion of the arrector pili muscle.
- ***Inferior segment,*** which in the growing follicle (Fig. 14.14) is of nearly uniform diameter except at its base, where it expands to form the ***bulb.*** The base of the bulb is invaginated by a tuft of vascularized loose connective tissue called, not surprisingly, a ***dermal papilla.***

Other cells forming the bulb, including those that surround the connective tissue papilla, are collectively referred to as the matrix, which consists simply of ***matrix cells.*** Matrix cells immediately adjacent to the dermal papilla represent the germinative layer of the follicle. Division and proliferation of these cells accounts for the growth of the hair. Scattered melanocytes are also present in this germinative layer. They contribute melanosomes to the developing hair cells in a manner analogous to that in the stratum germinativum of the epidermis. The dividing matrix cells in the germinative layer differentiate into the keratin-producing cells of the hair and the ***internal root sheath.*** The internal root sheath is a multilayered cellular covering that surrounds the deep part of the hair. The internal root sheath has three layers:

- The ***cuticle,*** which consists of squamous cells whose outer free surface faces the hair shaft.
- ***Huxley's layer,*** which consists of a single or double layer of flattened cells that form the middle plate of the internal root sheath.
- ***Henle's layer,*** which consists of an outer single layer of cuboidal cells. These cells are in direct contact with the outermost part of the hair follicle, which represents a downgrowth of the epidermis and is designated the ***external (outer) root sheath.***

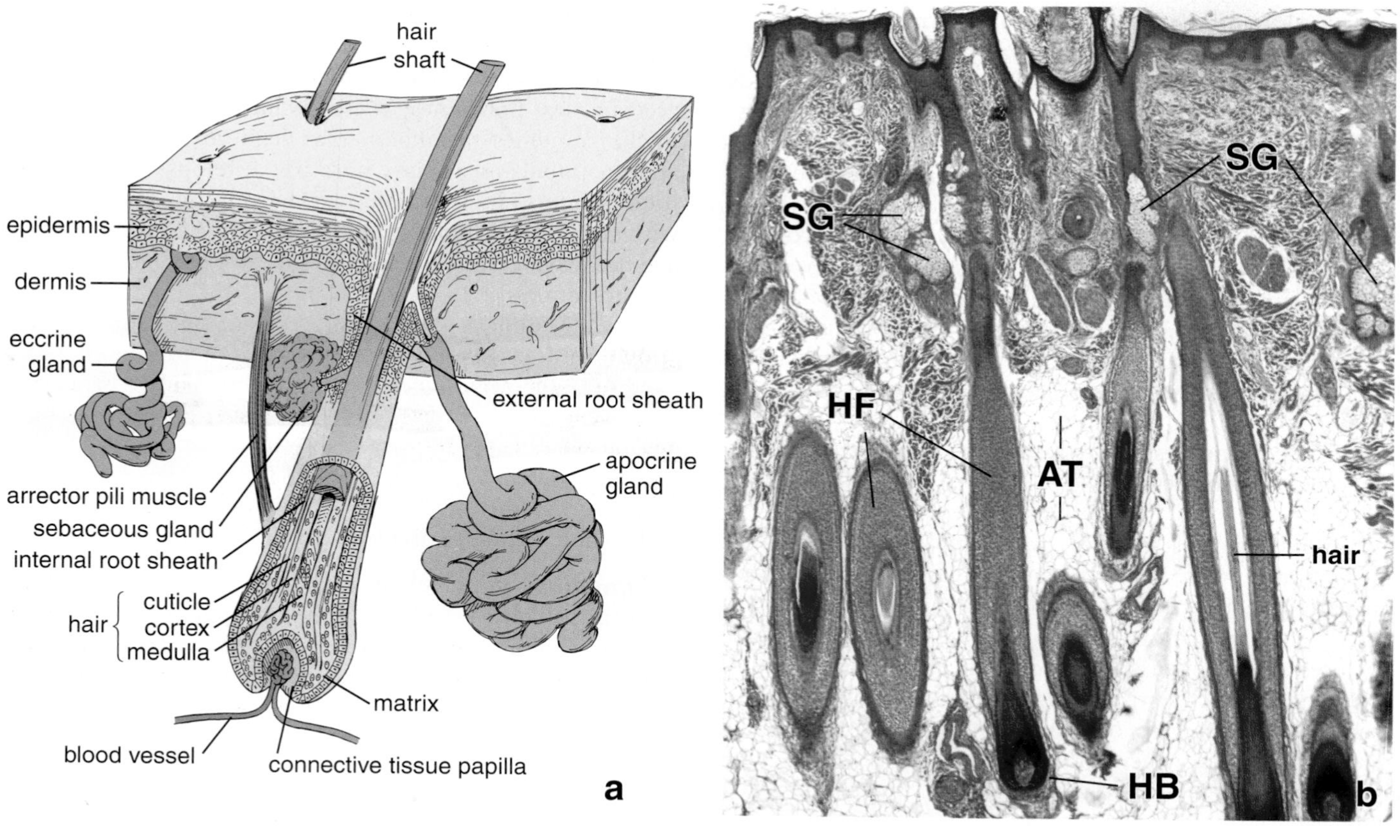

FIGURE 14.14
Hair follicle and other skin appendages. a. Diagram showing a hair follicle. Note the cell layers that form the hair shaft and the surrounding external and internal root sheaths. The sebaceous gland consists of the secretory portion and a short duct that empties into the infundibulum. The arrector pili muscle accompanies the sebaceous gland; its contraction assists in gland secretion and discharge into the infundibulum. The apocrine gland also empties into the infundibulum of the hair follicle. Note that eccrine sweat glands are independent structures and are not associated directly with the hair follicle. **b.** Photomicrograph of H&E–stained section of thin skin from human scalp. The growing end of a hair follicle consists of an expanded hair bulb *(HB)* of epithelial cells that is invaginated by a papilla of connective tissue. The epithelial cells form the unspecialized matrix surrounding the papilla; as the cells leave the matrix, they form cell layers that differentiate into the shaft of the hair and the inner and outer root sheaths of the hair follicle *(HF)*. Note that several oblique and longitudinal sections of the hair follicles are embedded in the adipose tissue *(AT)* of the hypodermis. Some of them reveal a section of the hair. Sebaceous glands *(SG)* are visible in conjunction with the upper part of the hair follicle. ×60.

Hairs are composed of keratinized cells that develop from hair follicles

Keratinization of the hair and internal root sheath occurs shortly after the cells leave the matrix, in a region called the ***keratogenous zone.*** By the time the hair emerges from the follicle, it is entirely keratinized as ***hard keratin.*** The internal root sheath, consisting of soft keratin, does not emerge from the follicle with the hair but is broken down at about the isthmus level where sebaceous secretions enter the follicle. A thick basal lamina, called the ***glassy membrane,*** separates the hair follicle from the dermis. Surrounding the follicle is a dense irregular connective tissue sheath to which the ***arrector pili muscle*** is attached.

Hairs are elongated filamentous structures that project from the hair follicles. They also consist of three layers (see Fig. 14.14):

- ***Medulla,*** which forms the central part of the shaft and contains large vacuolated cells. The medulla is present only in thick hairs.
- ***Cortex,*** which is located peripheral to the medulla and contains cuboidal cells. These cells undergo differentiation into keratin-filled cells.
- ***Cuticle of the hair shaft,*** which contains squamous cells that form the outermost layer of the hair.

In addition, the hair shaft contains melanin pigment produced by melanocytes present in the germinative layer of the hair bulb.

BOX 14.2

Functional Considerations: Hair Growth and Hair Characteristics

Unlike the renewal of the surface epidermis, hair growth is not a continuous process. A period of growth ***(anagen)*** in which a new hair develops is followed by a brief period in which growth stops ***(catagen).*** Catagen is followed by a long rest period in which the follicle atrophies ***(telogen),*** and the hair is eventually lost. More than 80% of the hair present in the normal scalp is in the anagen phase. In catagen, the germinative zone is reduced to an epithelial strand still attached to a remnant of the dermal papilla. In the telogen phase, the atrophied follicle may contract to one half or less of its original length. The hair may remain attached to the follicle for several months during this stage and is called a ***club hair*** because of the shape of its proximal end.

Hairs vary in size from long, coarse ***terminal hairs*** that may reach a meter or more in length (scalp hair and beard hair in males) to short, fine ***vellus hairs*** that may be visible only with the aid of a magnifying lens (vellus hairs of the forehead and anterior surface of the forearm). Terminal hairs are produced by large-diameter, long follicles; vellus hairs are produced by relatively small follicles. Terminal hair follicles may spend up to several *years* in anagen and only a few *months* in telogen. In the balding individual, large terminal follicles are gradually converted into small vellus follicles after several growth cycles. The ratio of vellus follicles to terminal follicles increases as baldness progresses. The "completely bald" scalp is not hairless but is populated by vellus follicles that produce fine hairs and remain in telogen for relatively long periods.

SEBACEOUS GLANDS

Sebaceous glands secrete sebum that coats the hair and skin surface

Sebaceous glands develop as outgrowths of the external root sheath of the hair follicle, usually producing several glands per follicle (see Fig. 14.14). The oily substance produced in the gland, ***sebum,*** is the product of holocrine secretion. The entire cell produces and becomes filled with the fatty product while it simultaneously undergoes programmed cell death (apoptosis) as the product fills the cell. Ultimately, both the secretory product and cell debris are discharged from the gland as sebum into the infundibulum of a hair follicle, which with the short duct of the sebaceous gland forms the ***pilosebaceous canal.*** New cells are produced by mitosis of the basal cells at the periphery of the gland, and the cells of the gland remain linked to one another by desmosomes. The basal lamina of these cells is continuous with that of the epidermis and the hair follicle. The process of sebum production from the time of basal cell mitosis to the secretion of the sebum takes about 8 days.

The basal cells of the sebaceous gland contain smooth endoplasmic reticulum (sER), rER, free ribosomes, mitochondria, glycogen, and a well-developed Golgi apparatus (Fig. 14.15). As the cells move away from the basal layer and begin to produce the lipid secretory product, the amount of sER increases, reflecting the role of the sER in lipid synthesis and secretion. The cells gradually become filled with numerous lipid droplets separated by thin strands of cytoplasm (see Fig. 14.15).

SWEAT GLANDS

Sweat glands are classified on the bases of their structure and the nature of their secretion. Two types of sweat glands are recognized:

- *Eccrine sweat glands,* which are distributed over the entire body surface except for the lips and part of the external genitalia.
- *Apocrine sweat glands,* which are limited to the axilla, areola and nipple of the mammary gland, skin around the anus, and the external genitalia. The ***ceruminous glands*** of the external acoustic meatus canal and the apocrine glands of eyelashes (**glands of Moll**) are also apocrine-type glands.

Eccrine Sweat Glands

Eccrine sweat glands are simple coiled glands that regulate body temperature

Eccrine sweat glands are independent structures, not associated with the hair follicle that arises as a downgrowth from the fetal epidermis. Each eccrine gland is arranged as a blind-ended, simple, coiled tubular structure. It consists of two segments: a *secretory segment* located deep in the dermis or in the upper part of the hypodermis and a di-

BOX 14.3

Functional Considerations: The Role of Sebum

The role of sebum is not clearly defined. Various investigators have ascribed bacteriostatic, emollient, barrier, and pheromone functions to sebum. Sebum does appear to play a critical role in the development of acne. The amount of sebum secreted increases significantly at puberty in both males and females. Triglycerides contained in sebum are broken down to fatty acids by bacteria on the skin surface, and the free fatty acids liberated may be an irritant in the formation of ***acne lesions.*** On histologic examination, acne is characterized by retention of the sebum in the isthmus of the hair follicle, with variable lymphocytic infiltration. In severe cases, dermal abscesses may form in association with inflamed hair follicles.

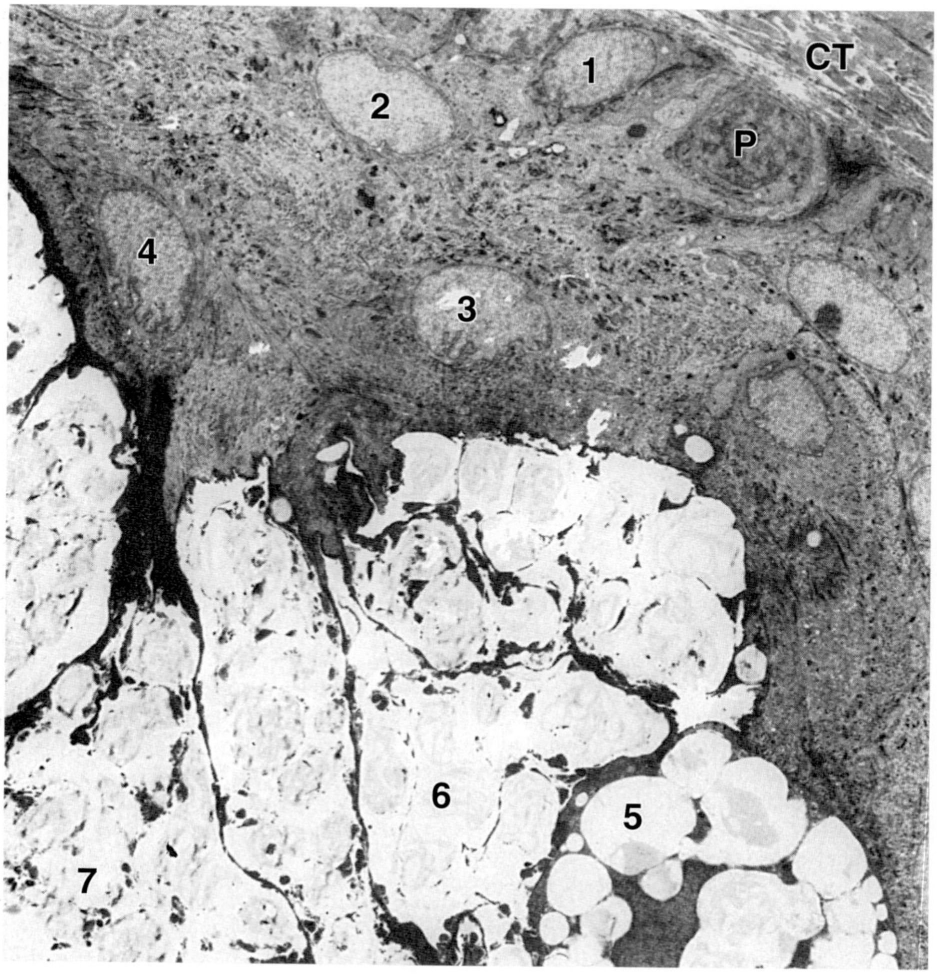

FIGURE 14.15
Electron micrograph of a sebaceous gland. Basal cells *(1)* close to the connective tissue *(CT)* are small and undifferentiated. Among these cells are dividing cells, one of which *(P)* appears to be in early prophase. From this peripheral position the cells move toward the opening of the gland *(2 to 4)* and produce a fatty secretory product. This oily product is first seen in the cytoplasm as small lipid droplets *(5)* that gradually fuse *(6)*. The cells perish *(7)* during the secretion of the secretory product, producing sebum. ×6,800. (Courtesy of Dr. Bryce L. Munger.)

rectly continuous, less coiled ***duct segment*** that leads to the epidermal surface (Fig.14.16).

Eccrine sweat glands play a major role in temperature regulation through the cooling that results from evaporation of water from sweat on the body surface. The secretory portion of the glands produces a secretion similar in composition to an ultrafiltrate of blood. Resorption of some of the sodium and water in the duct results in the release of a hypotonic sweat at the skin surface. This hypotonic watery solution is low in protein and contains varying amounts of sodium chloride, urea, uric acid, and ammonia. Thus, the eccrine sweat gland also serves, in part, as an excretory organ.

Excessive sweating can lead to loss of other electrolytes, such as potassium and magnesium, and to significant water loss. Normally, the body loses about 600 mL of water a day through evaporation from the lungs and skin. Under conditions of high ambient temperature, water loss can be increased in a regulated manner by an increased rate of sweating. This ***thermoregulatory sweating*** first occurs on the forehead and scalp, extends to the face and to the rest of the body, and occurs last on the palms and soles. Under conditions of emotional stress, however, the palms, soles, and axillae are the first surfaces to sweat. Control of thermoregulatory sweating is cholinergic, while ***emotional sweating*** may be stimulated by adrenergic portions of the sympathetic division of the autonomic nervous system.

The secretory segment of the eccrine sweat gland contains three cell types

Three cell types are present in the secretory segment of the gland: ***clear cells*** and ***dark cells***, both of which are secretory epithelial cells, and ***myoepithelial cells***, which are contractile epithelial cells (Fig. 14.17). All of the cells rest on the basal lamina; their arrangement is that of a pseudostratified epithelium.

- ***Clear cells*** are characterized by abundant glycogen. The glycogen is conspicuous in Fig. 14.17a because of its amount it would stain intensely with the periodic

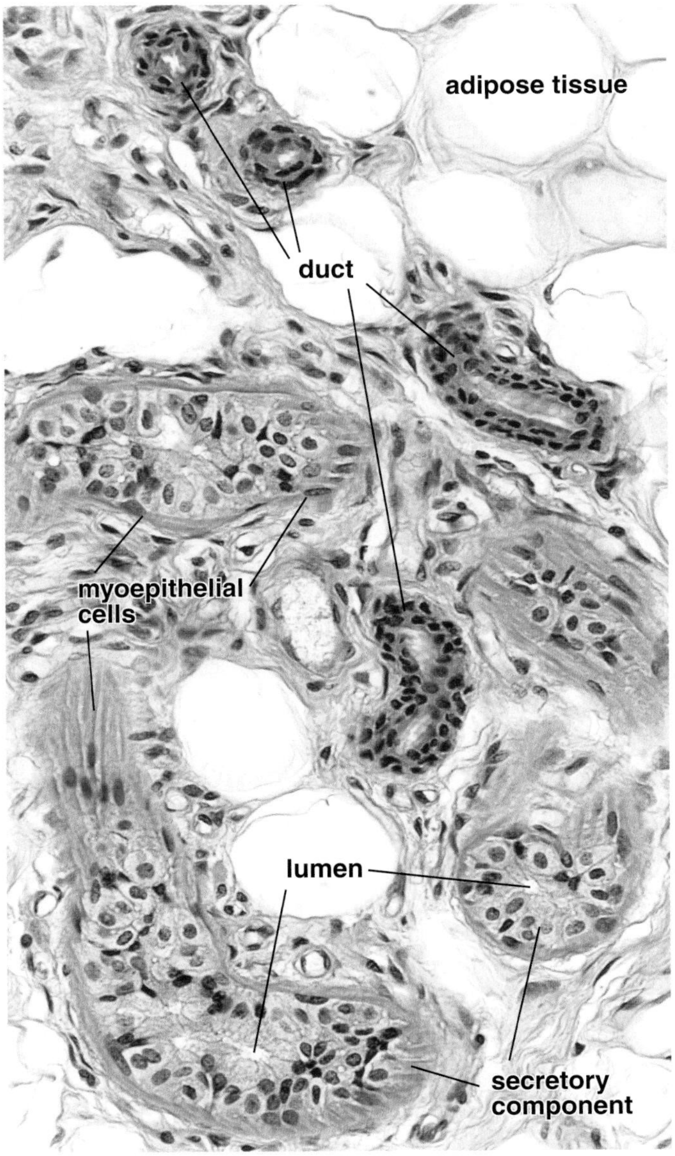

FIGURE 14.16
Photomicrograph of an eccrine sweat gland. This photomicrograph of a H&E–stained section of human skin shows profiles of both the secretory component and the duct of an eccrine sweat gland. The secretory component appears as a double layer of cuboidal epithelial cells and peripherally, within the basal lamina, a layer of myoepithelial cells. The duct portion of the gland has a narrower outside diameter and lumen than the secretory portion of the gland. It consists of a double layer of small cuboidal cells without the myoepithelial cells. ×320.

acid–Schiff (PAS) method. In routine H&E preparations, the cytoplasm of clear cells stains poorly. Membranous organelles include numerous mitochondria, profiles of sER, and a relatively small Golgi apparatus. The plasma membrane is remarkably amplified at the lateral and apical surfaces by extensive cytoplasmic folds. In addition, the basal surface of the cell possesses infoldings, although they are considerably less complex than the cytoplasmic folds. The morphology of these cells indicates that they produce the watery component of sweat.

- ***Dark cells*** are characterized by abundant rER and secretory granules (see Fig. 14.17). The Golgi apparatus is relatively large, a feature consistent with the glycoprotein secretion of these cells. The apical cytoplasm contains mature secretory granules and occupies most of the luminal surface (see Fig. 14.17a). Clear cells have considerably less cytoplasmic exposure to the lumen; their secretion is largely via the lateral surfaces of the cell, which are in contact with intercellular canaliculi that allow the watery secretion to reach the lumen. Here, it mixes with the proteinaceous secretion of the dark cells.
- ***Myoepithelial cells*** are limited to the basal aspect of the secretory segment. They lie between the secretory cells, with their processes oriented transversally to the tubule. The cytoplasm contains numerous contractile filaments (actin) that stain deeply with eosin, thus making them readily identifiable in routine H&E specimens. Contraction of these cells is responsible for rapid expression of sweat from the gland.

The duct segment of eccrine glands is lined by stratified cuboidal epithelium and lacks myoepithelial cells

The duct segment of the gland continues from the secretory portion with coiling. In histologic sections, multiple duct profiles typically appear among the secretory profiles. As the duct passes upward through the dermis, it takes a gentle spiral course until it reaches the epidermis, where it then continues in a tighter spiral to the surface. When the duct enters the epidermis, however, the duct cells end and the epidermal cells form the wall of the duct. The duct is composed of stratified cuboidal epithelium, consisting of a basal cell layer and a luminal cell layer. The duct cells are smaller and appear darker than the cells of the secretory portion of the gland. Also, the duct has a smaller diameter than the secretory portion. In contrast to the secretory portion of the eccrine gland, the duct portion does not possess myoepithelial cells. These features are useful in distinguishing the duct from the secretory portion in a histologic section (see Fig. 14.16).

The basal or peripheral cells of the duct have a rounded or ovoid nucleus and contain a prominent nucleolus. The cytoplasm is filled with mitochondria and ribosomes. The apical or luminal cells are smaller than the basal cells, but their nuclei are similar in appearance. The most conspicuous feature of the luminal cells is the deeply stained, glassy (hyalinized) appearance of the apical cytoplasm. The glassy appearance is due to the presence of large numbers of aggregated tonofilaments in the apical cytoplasm.

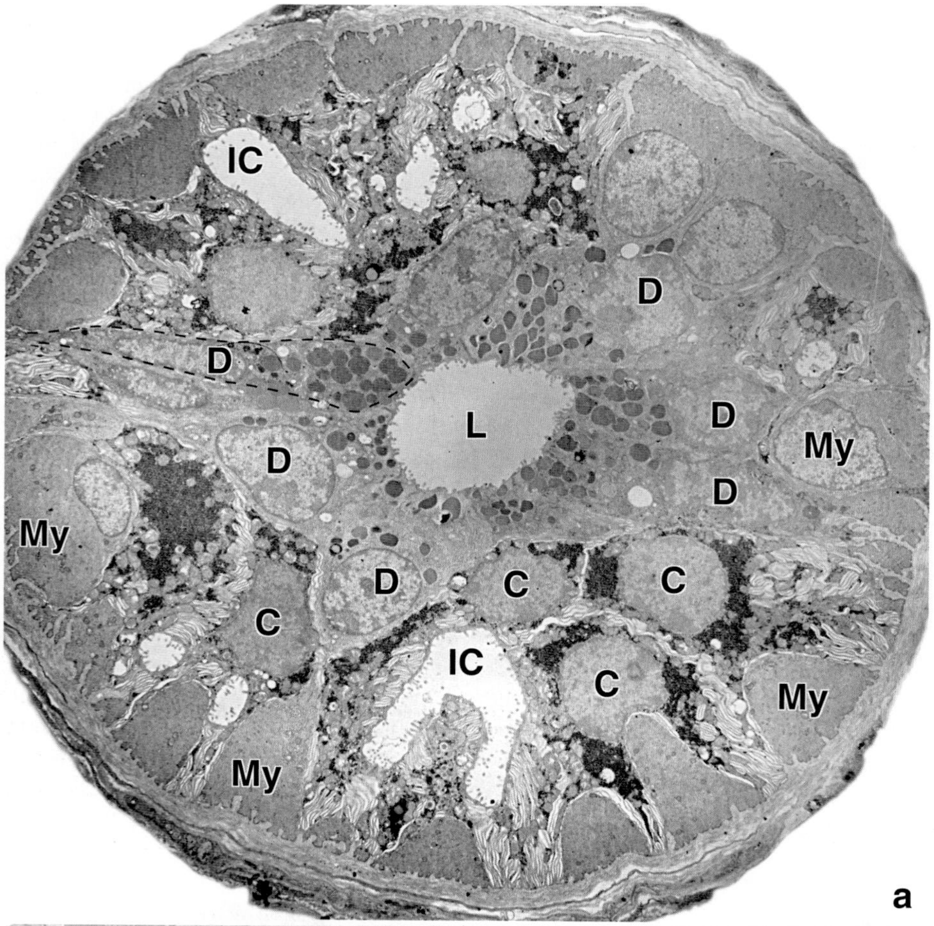

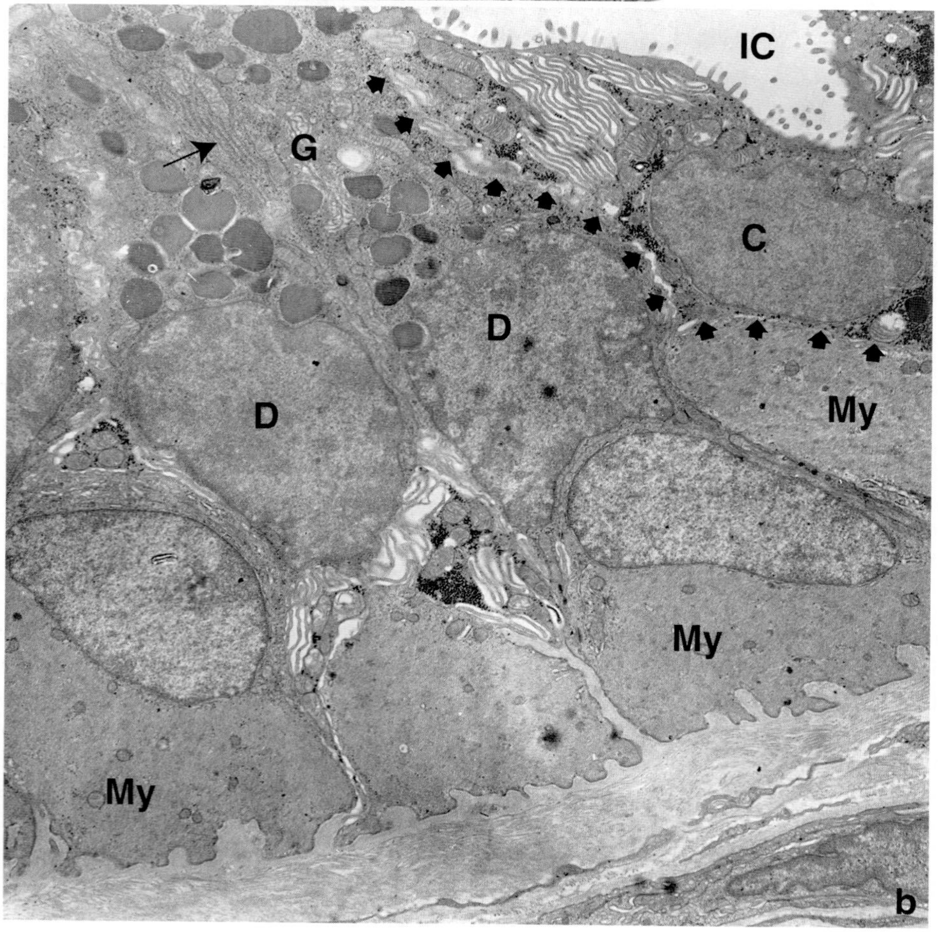

FIGURE 14.17
Electron micrographs of an eccrine sweat gland. a. This micrograph shows myoepithelial cells *(My)* and two distinctive gland cell types, dark cells *(D)* and clear cells *(C)*. The apical portion of the dark cell is broad; it faces the lumen *(L)* of the gland and contains numerous secretory granules. The *dashed line* marks the boundary of one dark cell. The clear cell is more removed from the lumen of the gland. Its base rests on the myoepithelial cells or directly on the basal lamina. Most of the free surface of the clear cell faces an intercellular canaliculus *(IC)*. Clear cells contain numerous mitochondria, extensive infoldings of the plasma membrane, and large numbers of electron-dense glycogen inclusions. ×5,600. (Courtesy of Dr. John A. Terzakis.) **b.** At higher magnification, dark cells display rER *(arrow)* and a Golgi apparatus *(G)* in addition to secretory granules. Clear cells show large amounts of folded membrane, mitochondria, and glycogen. The myoepithelial cells *(My)* contain large numbers of contractile actin filaments. *Short stubby arrows* (upper right) mark the boundary of a clear cell. ×17,500. (Courtesy of Dr. John A. Terzakis.)

Apocrine Sweat Glands

Apocrine glands are large-lumen tubular glands associated with hair follicles

Apocrine sweat glands develop from the same downgrowths of epidermis that give rise to hair follicles. The connection to the follicle is retained, allowing the secretion of the gland to enter the follicle, typically at a level just above the entry of the sebaceous duct. From here, the secretion makes its way to the surface.

Like eccrine glands, apocrine glands are coiled tubular glands. They are sometimes branched. The secretory portion of the gland is located deep in the dermis or, more commonly, in the upper region of the hypodermis.

The secretory portion of apocrine glands has a wider lumen than that of eccrine glands and is composed of a single cell type

The secretory portion of apocrine glands differs in several respects from that of eccrine glands. The most obvious difference, readily noted in the light microscope, is its very wide lumen (Fig. 14.18). Unlike eccrine glands, apocrine glands store their secretory product in the lumen. The secretory portion of the gland is composed of simple epithelium. Only one cell type is present, and the cytoplasm of the cell is eosinophilic. The apical part of the cell often exhibits a bleb-like protrusion. It was once thought that this part of the cell pinched off and was discharged into the lumen as an apocrine secretion, thus the name of the gland. However, TEM studies confirm that the secretion is a merocrine type. The apical cytoplasm contains numerous small granules, the secretory component within the cell, which are discharged by exocytosis. Other features of the cell include numerous lysosomes and lipofuscin pigment granules. The latter represent secondary and tertiary lysosomes. Mitochondria are also numerous. During the refractory phase, after expulsion of the secretion, the Golgi apparatus enlarges, in preparation for a new secretory phase.

Myoepithelial cells are also present in the secretory portion of the gland and are situated between the secretory cells and the adjacent basal lamina. As in eccrine glands, contraction of the processes of myoid cells facilitates expulsion of the secretory product from the gland.

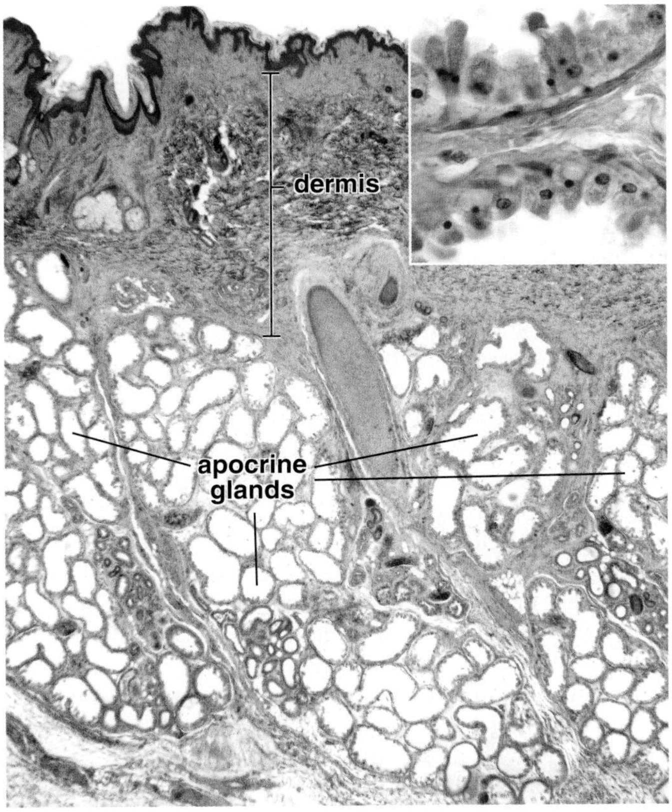

FIGURE 14.18
Photomicrograph of an apocrine sweat gland. This section of adult skin from the area around the anus shows several apocrine (anal) sweat glands, which are easily identified by the large lumen of their secretory components. This apocrine sweat gland is close to a hair follicle (center of photomicrograph) and deep to the dense, irregular connective tissue of the dermis. ×45. **Inset.** Higher magnification of secretory component shows the cell types of the apocrine gland. The gland consists of a simple epithelium whose cells are either cuboidal or columnar and myoepithelial cells located in the basal portion of the epithelial cell layer. ×230.

The duct portion of apocrine glands is lined by stratified cuboidal epithelium and lacks myoepithelial cells

The duct of the apocrine gland is similar to that of the eccrine duct; it has a narrow lumen. However, it continues from the secretory portion of the gland in a relatively straight path to empty into the follicle canal. Because of its straight course, the probability of viewing both the duct and the secretory portion of an apocrine gland in the same histologic section is reduced. Also in contrast to the eccrine duct, resorption does not take place in the apocrine duct. The secretory product is not altered in its passage through the duct.

BOX 14.4

Clinical Correlations: Sweating and Disease

Although many neural and emotional factors can alter the composition of sweat, altered sweat composition can also be a sign of disease. For example, elevated sodium levels in sweat can serve as an indicator of cystic fibrosis. In pronounced uremia, when the kidneys are unable to rid the body of urea, the concentration of urea in sweat increases. In this condition, after the water evaporates, crystals may be discerned on the skin, especially on the upper lip. These include urea crystals and are called ***urea frost***.

The duct epithelium is stratified cuboidal, usually two but sometimes three cell layers thick. The apical cytoplasm of the luminal cells appears hyalinized, a consequence of the aggregated tonofilaments in the apical cytoplasm. In this aspect they resemble the luminal cells of the eccrine duct.

Apocrine glands produce a protein-rich secretion containing pheromones

Apocrine glands produce a secretion that contains protein, carbohydrate, ammonia, lipid, and certain organic compounds that may color the secretion. However, the secretions vary with the anatomic location. In the axilla, the secretion is milky and slightly viscous. When secreted, the fluid is odorless, but through bacterial action on the skin surface it develops an acrid odor.

Apocrine glands become functional at puberty; as with axillary and pubic hair, their development depends on sex hormones. In the female, both axillary and areolar apocrine glands undergo morphologic and secretory changes that parallel the menstrual cycle.

In many mammals, similar glands secrete pheromones, chemical signals used in marking territory, in courtship behavior, and in certain maternal and social behaviors. It is generally believed that apocrine secretions may function as pheromones in humans. Male pheromones (androstenol/androstenone) in the secretion of apocrine glands have a direct impact on the female menstruation cycle. Furthermore, female pheromones (copulins) influence male perception of females and may also induce hormonal changes in males.

Innervation of Sweat Glands

Both eccrine and apocrine sweat glands are innervated by the sympathetic portion of the autonomic nervous system. Eccrine sweat glands are stimulated by cholinergic transmitters (usually identified with the parasympathetic component of the autonomic system), whereas apocrine glands are stimulated by adrenergic transmitters. As described above, eccrine glands respond to heat and stress. Apocrine glands respond to emotional and sensory stimuli but not to heat.

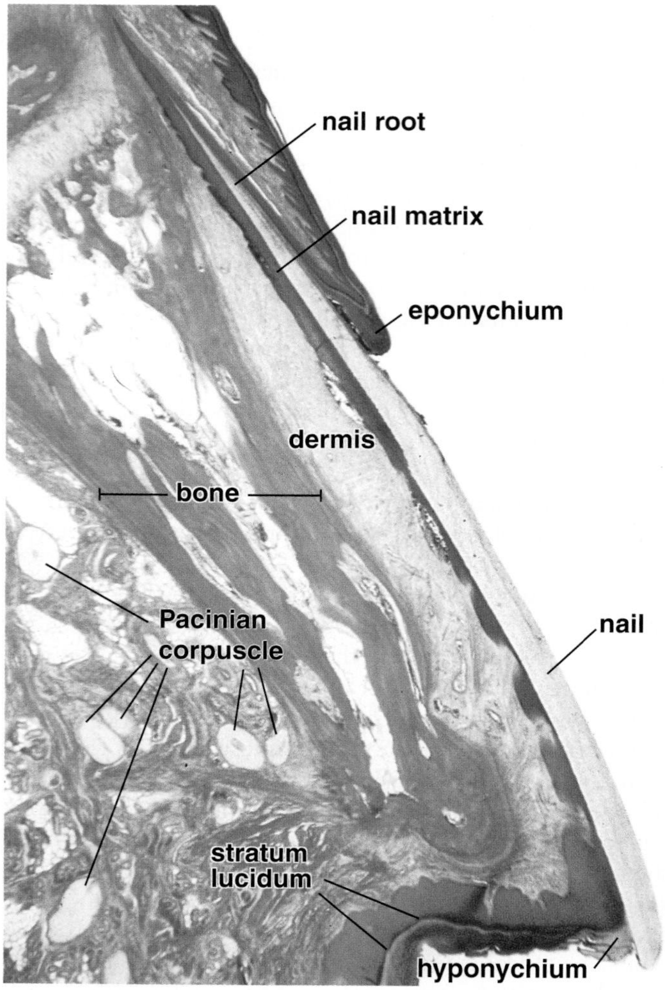

FIGURE 14.19
Photomicrograph of a sagittal section of distal phalanx with a nail. A nail is a keratinized plate located on the dorsal aspect of the distal phalanges. Under the free edge of the nail is a boundary layer, the hyponychium, which is continuous with the stratum corneum of the adjacent epidermis. The proximal end, the root of the nail, is overlapped by skin, the eponychium, which is also continuous with the stratum corneum of the adjacent epidermis. Deep to the nail is a layer of epithelium with underlying dermis. The proximal portion of this epithelium is referred to as the nail matrix. The bone in this section represents a distal phalanx. Numerous Pacinian corpuscles are present in the connective tissue of the palmar side of the finger. Note that even at this low magnification, the stratum lucidum in visible in the epidermis of the fingertip. ×10.

NAILS

Nails are plates of keratinized cells containing hard keratin

The slightly arched ***fingernails*** and ***toenails,*** more properly referred to as ***nail plates,*** rest on ***nail beds.*** The nail bed consists of epithelial cells that are continuous with the stratum basale and stratum spinosum of the epidermis (Fig. 14.19).

The proximal part of the nail, the ***nail root,*** is buried in a fold of epidermis and covers the cells of the germinative zone, or ***matrix.*** The matrix contains a variety of cells including stem cells, epithelial cells, melanocytes, Merkel's cells, and Langerhans' cells. The stem cells of the matrix regularly divide, migrate toward the root of the nail, and there differentiate and produce the keratin of the nail. Nail keratin is a hard keratin, like that of the hair cortex. Unlike the soft keratin of the epidermis, it does not desqua-

BOX 14.5

Clinical Correlations: Skin Repair

Epidermal repair is effected by basal cell proliferation or, in extensive trauma, by hair follicle and sweat gland epithelia. The repair of an incision or laceration of the skin requires stimulated growth of both the dermis and the epidermis. Dermal repair involves *(a)* removal of damaged collagen fibers in the wound site, primarily through the effort of macrophage activity; and *(b)* proliferation of fibroblasts and subsequent production of new collagen and other extracellular matrix components. Application of sutures reduces the extent of the repair area through maximal closure of a wound, minimizing scar formation. Surgical incisions are typically made along cleavage lines; the cut tends to parallel the collagen fibers, thus minimizing the need for excess collagen production and the inherent scarring that may occur.

Repair of the epidermis involves the proliferation of the basal keratinocytes in the stratum germinativum in the undamaged site surrounding the wound (Fig. 14.20). Mitotic activity is markedly increased within the first 24 hours. In a short time, the wound site is covered by a scab. The proliferating basal cells of the stratum germinativum begin migrating beneath the scab and across the wound surface. The migration rate may be up to 0.5 mm/day, starting within 8 to 18 hours after wounding. Further proliferation and differentiation occur behind the migration front, leading to restoration of the multilayered epidermis. As new cells ultimately keratinize and desquamate, the overlying scab is freed with the desquamating cells, which explains why a scab detaches from its periphery inward.

In cases in which the full thickness of the epidermal layer is removed either by trauma or in surgery, the deepest parts of hair follicles and glands that remain as islands of epithelial cells in the dermis will divide and produce cells that migrate over the exposed surface to reestablish a complete epithelial (epidermal) layer. Massive destruction of all of the epithelial structures of the skin, as in a third-degree burn or extensive full-thickness abrasion, prevents reepithelialization. Such wounds can be healed only by grafting epidermis to cover the wounded area. In the absence of a graft, the wound would, at best, reepithelialize slowly and imperfectly by ingrowth of cells from the margins of the wound.

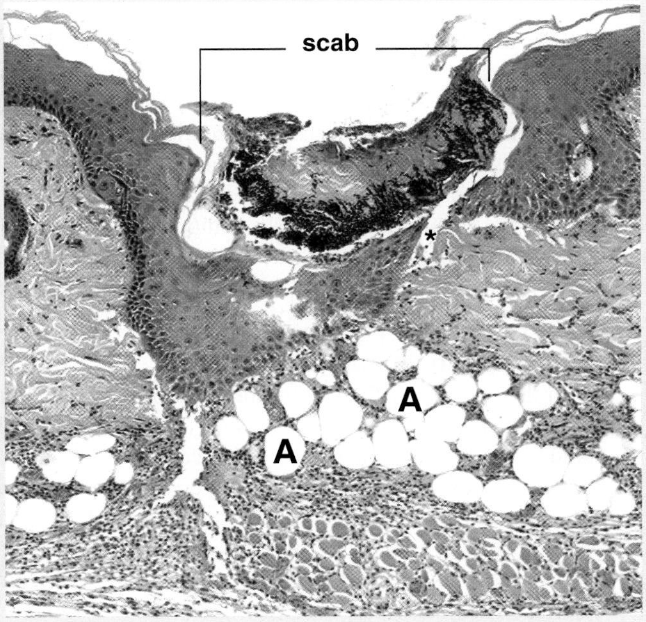

FIGURE 14.20
Photomicrograph showing a late stage in the epidermal repair of a skin wound. The initial injury was caused by an incision through the full thickness of the skin and partially into the hypodermis, which contains adipose cells *(A)*. The epidermis has re-formed beneath the scab. The *asterisk* marks an artifact where epithelium separated during specimen preparation. The scab, which contains numerous dead neutrophils in its inferior aspect, is close to the point of release. The dermis at this stage shows little change during the repair process but will ultimately reestablish itself to form a continuous layer. ×110.

mate. It consists of densely packed keratin filaments embedded in a matrix of amorphous keratin with a high sulfur content, which is responsible for the hardness of the nail. The process of hard keratin formation, as with the hair cortex, does not involve keratohyalin granules. In addition, a cornified cell envelope contains proteins similar to those found in the epidermis.

The constant addition of new cells at the root and their keratinization account for nail growth. As the nail plate grows, it moves over the nail bed. On the microscopic level, the nail plate contains closely packed interdigitating ***corneocytes*** lacking nuclei and organelles.

The crescent-shaped white area near the root of the nail, the ***lunula,*** derives its color from the thick, opaque layer of partially keratinized matrix cells in this region. When the nail plate becomes fully keratinized, it is more transparent and takes on the coloring of the underlying vascular bed. The edge of the skin fold covering the root of the nail is the ***eponychium,*** or cuticle. The cuticle is also composed of hard keratin, and for this reason it does not desquamate. Because of its thinness it tends to break off or, as with many individuals, it is trimmed and pushed back. A thickened epidermal layer, the ***hyponychium,*** secures the free edge of the nail plate at the fingertip.

PLATE 38. SKIN I

The skin, or integument, consists of two main layers: the *epidermis,* composed of stratified squamous epithelium that is keratinized, and the *dermis,* composed of connective tissue. Under the dermis is a layer of loose connective tissue called the *hypodermis,* which is also generally referred to as the subcutaneous tissue or, by gross anatomists, as the superficial fascia. Typically, the hypodermis contains large amounts of adipose tissue, particularly in an adequately nourished individual.

The epidermis gives rise to nails, hairs, sebaceous glands, and sweat glands. On the palms of the hands and soles of the feet, the epidermis has an outer keratinized layer that is substantially thicker than that over the other parts of the body. Accordingly, the skin over the palms and soles is referred to as *thick skin,* in contrast to the skin over other parts of the body, which is referred to as *thin skin.*

There are no hairs in thick skin. In addition, the interface between the epidermis and the dermis is more complex in thick skin than in thin skin. The finger-like projections of the dermis into the base of the epidermis, the *dermal papillae,* are much longer and more closely spaced in thick skin. This provides greater resistance to frictional forces acting on this skin.

Figure 1, skin, human, H&E ×45.

In this sample of thick skin, the epidermis *(Ep)* is at the top; the remainder of the field consists of dermis, in which a large number of sweat glands *(SW)* can be observed. Although the layers of the epidermis are examined more advantageously at higher magnification (e.g., Fig. 3), it is easy to see, even at this relatively low magnification, that about half of the thickness of the epidermis consists of a distinctive surface layer that stains more lightly than the remainder of the epidermis. This is the keratinized layer. The dome-shaped surface contours represent a cross section through the minute ridges on the surface of thick skin that produce the characteristic fingerprints of an individual.

In addition to sweat glands, the dermis displays blood vessels *(BV)* and adipose tissue *(AT).* The ducts of the sweat glands *(D)* extend from the glands to the epidermis. One of the ducts is shown as it enters the epidermis at the bottom of an epithelial ridge. It will pass through the epidermis in a spiral course to open onto the skin surface.

Figure 2, skin, human, H&E ×60.

A sample of thin skin is shown here to compare with the thick skin in Figure 1. In addition to sweat glands, thin skin contains hair follicles *(HF)* and their associated sebaceous glands *(SGl).* Each sebaceous gland opens into a hair follicle. Often, as in this tissue sample, the hair follicles and the glands, both sebaceous and sweat, extend beyond the dermis *(De)* and into the hypodermis. Note the blood vessels *(BV)* and adipose tissue *(AT)* in the hypodermis.

Figure 3, skin, human, H&E ×320; inset ×640.

The layers of the epidermis of thin skin are shown here at higher magnification. The cell layer that occupies the deepest location is the stratum basale *(SB).* This is one cell deep. Just above this is a layer several cells in thickness, the stratum spinosum *(SS).* It consists of cells that have spinous processes on their surface. These processes meet with spinous processes of neighboring cells and, together, appear as intercellular bridges (*arrows,* **inset**). The next layer is the stratum granulosum *(SGr),* whose cells contain keratohyalin granules (*arrowhead,* **inset**). On the surface is the stratum corneum *(SC).* This consists of keratinized cells, i.e., cells that no longer possess nuclei. The keratinized cells are flat and generally adhere to other cells above and below without evidence of cell boundaries. In thick skin, a fifth layer, the stratum lucidum, is seen between the stratum granulosum and the stratum corneum. The pigment in the cells of the stratum basale is melanin; some of this pigment *(P)* is also present in connective tissue cells of the dermis.

KEY

AT, adipose tissue
BV, blood vessels
D, duct of sweat glands
De, dermis
Ep, epidermis
HF, hair follicle
P, pigment
SB, stratum basale
SC, stratum corneum
SGl, sebaceous gland
SGr, stratum granulosum
SS, stratum spinosum
SW, sweat gland
arrowhead (inset), granules in cell of stratum granulosum
arrows (inset), "intercellular bridges"

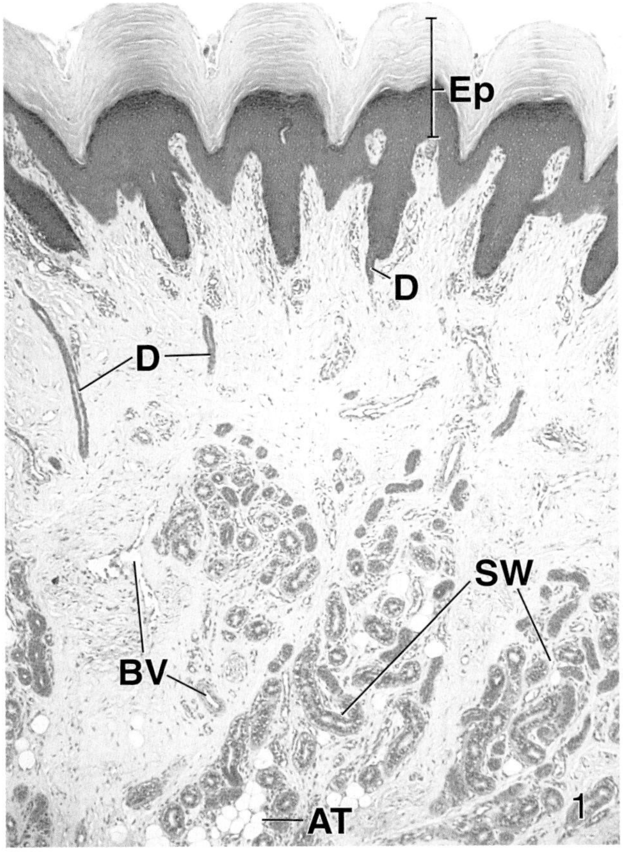
Ep
D
D
SW
BV
AT
1

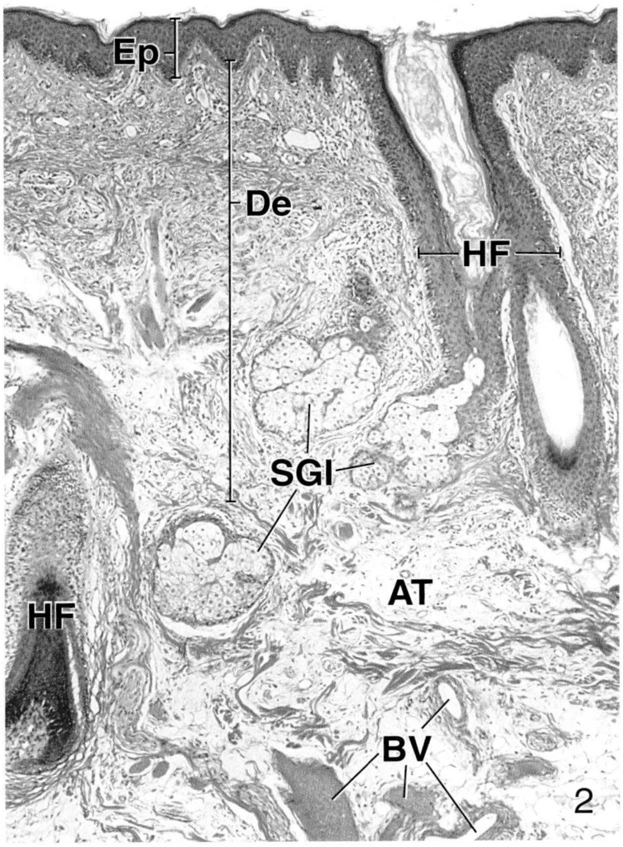
Ep
De
HF
SGl
HF
AT
BV
2

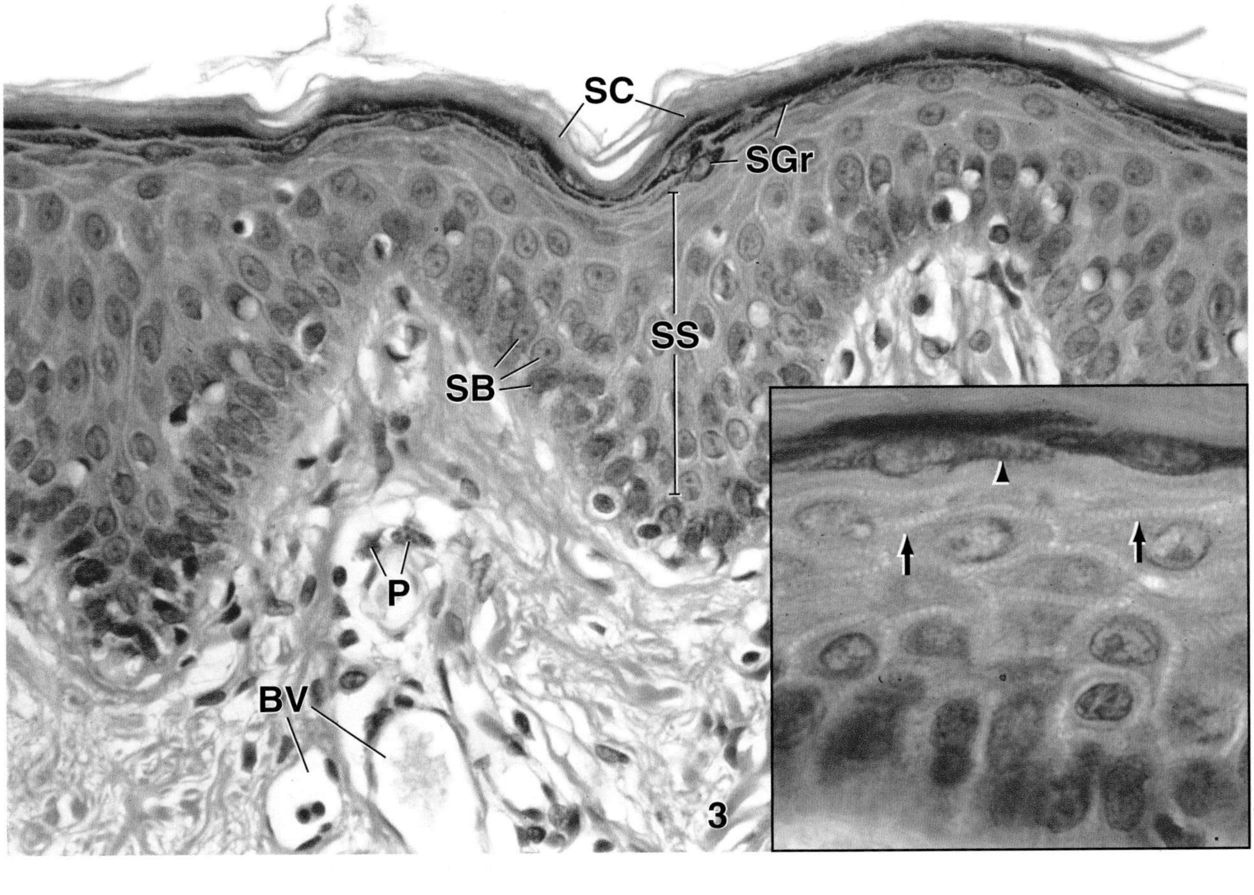
SC
SGr
SS
SB
P
BV
3

PLATE 39. SKIN II

The epidermis contains four distinctive cell types: *keratinocytes, melanocytes, Langerhans' cells,* and *Merkel's cells.* Keratinocytes are the most numerous of these cells; they are generated in the *stratum basale* and move toward the surface. As they do so, they produce the intracellular protein *keratin* and the special extracellular lipid that serves as a water barrier in the upper layers of the epidermis. Histologically, the keratinocytes are the cells that show spinous processes in the *stratum spinosum.* The other three cell types are not readily identified in H&E–stained paraffin sections. The product of the melanocyte is, however, evident in H&E sections, and this is considered in the first two figures of this plate.

The skin contains a pigment, *melanin,* which protects the tissue against the harmful effects of ultraviolet light. It is formed by the melanocytes that then pass the pigment to the keratinocytes. More pigment is present in dark skin than in light skin; this can be seen by comparing light skin (Fig. 1) and dark skin (Fig. 2.). The epidermis and a small amount of the dermis are shown in each figure. Whereas the deep part of the dark skin contains considerable pigment, the amount of pigment in light skin is insufficient to be noticeable at this magnification. Cells for producing the pigment are present in both skin types and *in approximately equal numbers.* The difference is due to more rapid digestion of the pigment by lysosomes of keratinocytes in light skin. After prolonged exposure to sunlight, pigment is also produced in sufficient amounts to be seen in light skin.

Figure 1, light skin, human, H&E ×300.

In routine H&E–stained paraffin sections of light skin, such as this sample, the melanocytes are among the cells that appear as small, rounded, clear cells *(CC)* mixed with the other cells of the stratum basale. However, not all clear cells of the epidermis are melanocytes. For example, Langerhans' cells may also appear as clear cells, but they are located more superficially in the stratum spinosum. Merkel's cells may also appear as clear cells, thus making it difficult to identify these three cell types with certainty.

Figure 2, dark skin, human, H&E ×300.

In dark skin, most of the pigment is in the basal portion of the epidermis, but it is also present in cells progressing toward the surface and within the nonnucleated cells of the keratinized layer. The *arrows* indicate the melanin pigment in keratinocytes of the stratum spinosum and in the stratum corneum. In light skin, the melanin is broken down before it leaves the upper part of the stratum spinosum. Thus, pigment is not seen in the upper layers of the epidermis.

Figure 3, skin, human, H&E and elastin stain ×200; inset ×450.

This figure is included because it shows certain features of the dermis, the connective tissue layer of the skin. The dermis is divided into two layers: the papillary layer *(PL)* of loose connective tissue and the reticular layer *(RL)* of more dense connective tissue. The papillary layer is immediately under the epidermis. It includes the connective tissue papillae that project into the undersurface of the epidermis. The reticular layer is deep to the papillary layer. The boundary between these two layers is not demarcated by any specific structural feature except for the change in the histologic composition of the two layers.

This specimen was stained with H&E and also with a procedure to display elastic fibers *(EF).* They are relatively thick and conspicuous in the reticular layer (see also **inset**), where they appear as the dark-blue profiles, some of which are elongate, whereas others are short. In the papillary layer, the elastic fibers are thinner and relatively sparse *(arrows).* The **inset** shows the typical eosinophilic staining of the thick collagenous fibers in the reticular layer. Although the collagenous fibers at the lower magnification of this figure are not as prominent, it is nevertheless possible to note that they are thicker in the reticular layer than in the papillary layer. The papillary layer is evidently more cellular than the reticular layer. Many of the small dark-blue profiles in the reticular layer represent oblique and cross sections through elastic fibers (see **inset**) and not nuclei of cells.

KEY

CC, clear cells
EF, elastic fibers
PL, papillary layer
RL, reticular layer
arrows, Figure 2, pigment in different layers of epidermis; Figure 3, delicate elastic fibers

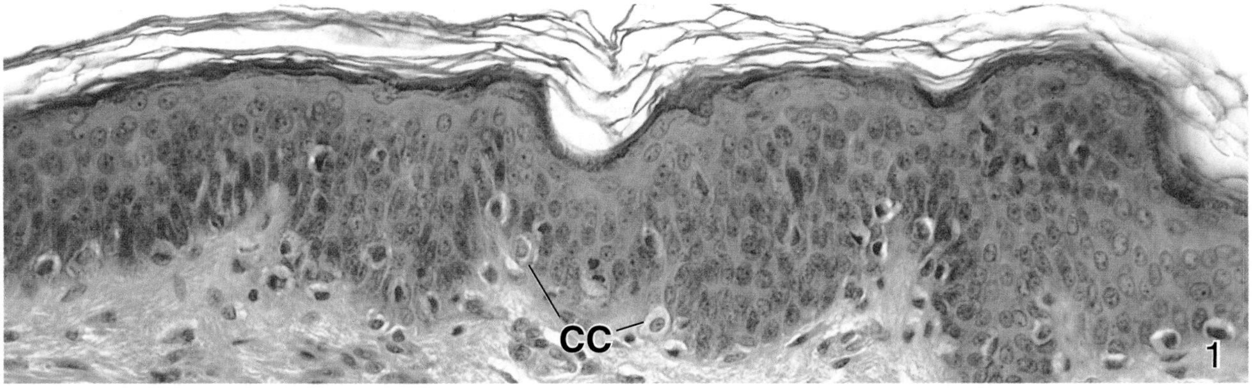
CC
1

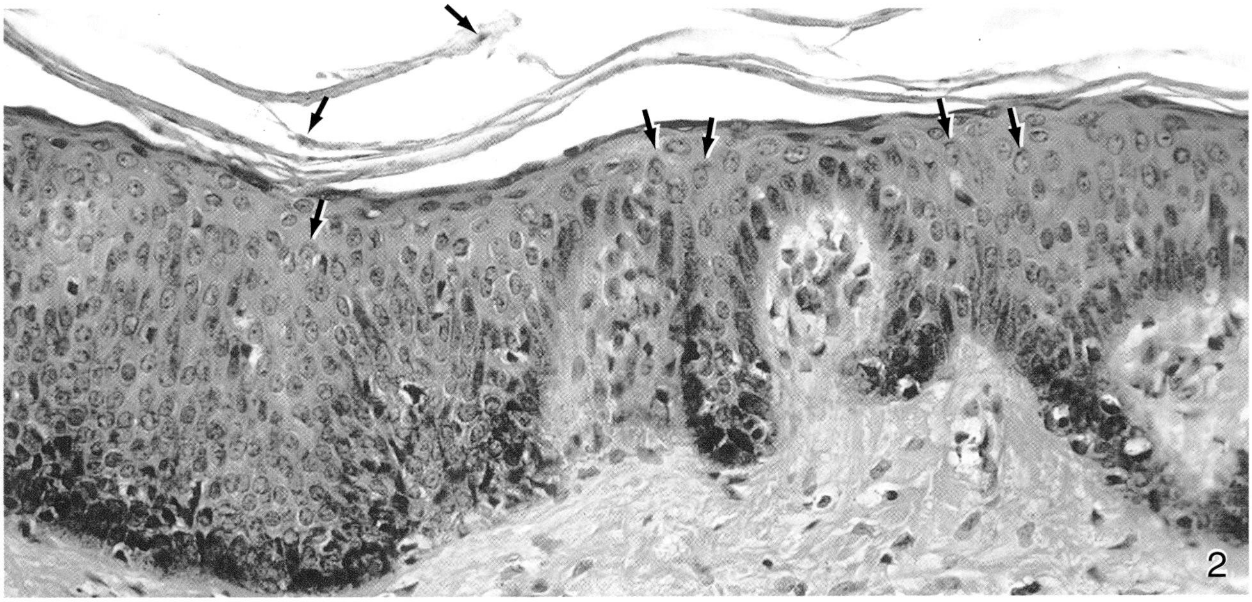
2

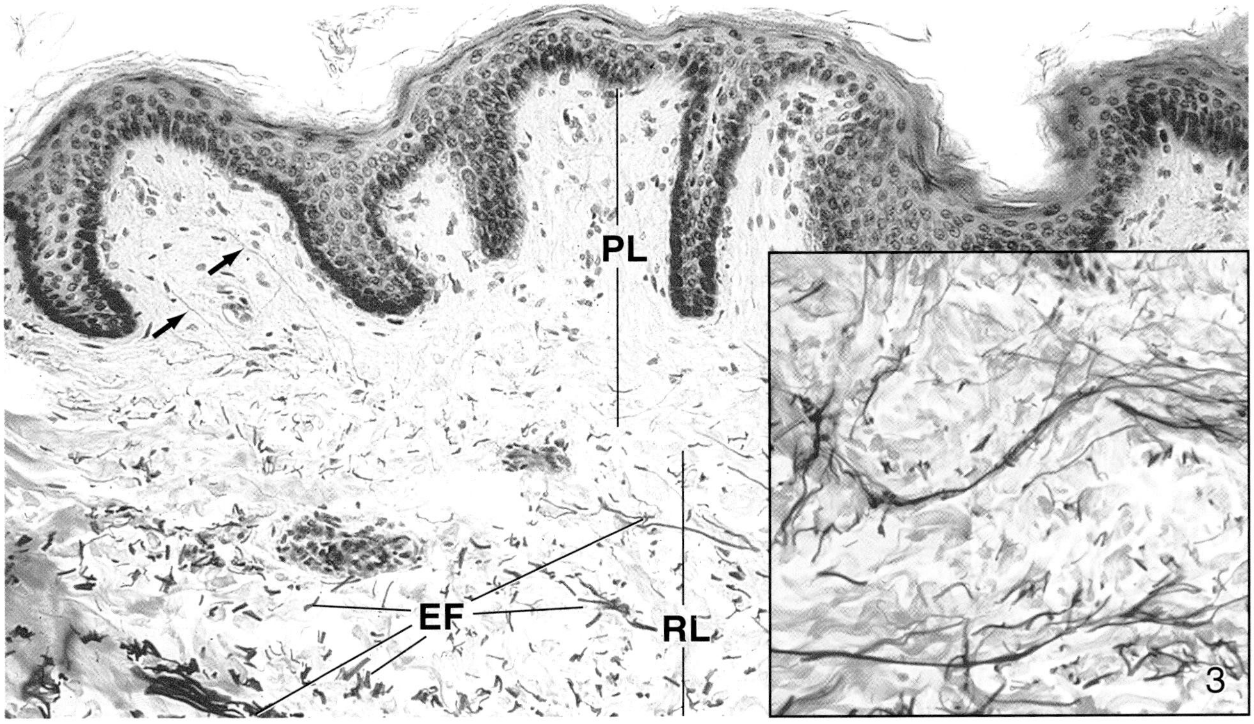
PL
EF
RL
3

PLATE 40. ECCRINE AND APOCRINE SWEAT GLANDS

Sweat glands are of two types: *apocrine* and *eccrine.* Apocrine glands have a limited distribution; in the human, they are found in the axilla, anogenital region, and mammary areola. Apocrine sweat glands are large tubular structures that are sometimes branched. They empty into the upper portion of the hair follicle and produce a product that becomes odoriferous after being secreted. The product of the apocrine sweat gland is important in other mammals, serving as a sex attractant and a marker of territory. Apocrine glands develop at puberty under the influence of sex hormones. They respond to nerve stimulation but not to elevated ambient temperature. In addition to the apocrine glands that are obviously sweat glands, two other types of glands, namely, the ceruminous glands of the external ear and the glands of Moll in the eyelids, are also classified as apocrine glands.

Eccrine sweat glands in the human are distributed over the entire body surface except for the lips, glans penis, inner surface of the prepuce, clitoris, and labia minora. They are simple coiled tubular structures located in the deep dermis or upper hypodermis and are directly continuous with a duct segment that leads to the epidermal surface. Eccrine sweat glands principally function in regulating body temperature through the cooling that results from evaporation of water from the hypotonic sweat secreted onto the body surface. Excessive sweating can lead to significant loss of water and electrolytes from the body. Eccrine sweat glands are particularly numerous in the thick skin of the hands and feet.

Figure 1, skin, human, H&E ×120; insets ×1200.

This section of adult skin shows both apocrine and eccrine sweat glands. The apocrine sweat glands *(aSG)* are easily identified by virtue of the large lumen of their secretory portion. This histologic feature is in striking contrast to the small lumen displayed by the secretory portion of the eccrine sweat gland *(SG).* Coincidentally, the apocrine sweat gland is close to a hair follicle *(HF).* As mentioned, the apocrine gland opens into the upper portion of a hair follicle. The two *small rectangular areas* are enlarged in the **rectangular insets** to show the cell types of the apocrine gland at higher magnification. Note that the *upper small rectangular area* includes a tangential section through one of the glandular units.

The secretory portion of the apocrine sweat gland consists of a single secretory cell type and myoepithelial cells. These can be seen in the **upper rectangular inset.** The epithelial cells are either cuboidal or columnar, and if columnar, they typically display granules *(G)* in their apical cytoplasm. The myoepithelial cells are in the basal portion of the epithelial cell layer. Nuclei of myoepithelial cells are elongate and, when cut in cross section, appear as rounded nuclear profiles in the base of the epithelial cell layer (*arrows,* **upper rectangular inset**). On the other hand, when seen in different planes of section, the profiles of myoepithelial cell nuclei may appear more elongate, as they are in the **lower rectangular inset** *(arrows).* This **inset** also shows the cytoplasmic portion of the myoepithelial cells, cut in cross section *(arrowheads),* in an adjacent glandular unit.

Figure 2, skin, human, H&E ×400; inset ×800.

This figure shows eccrine sweat glands at higher magnification. Typically, a section includes profiles of both the secretory portion *(SG)* and the duct portion *(D)* of the gland. The secretory portion of the gland consists of a double layer of cuboidal epithelial cells and, peripherally, along the basal lamina, a conspicuous layer of myoepithelial cells. The duct portion of the gland has a narrower outside diameter than the secretory portion, and the lumen of the duct portion is typically narrower than that of the gland. Occasionally, the duct may be distended *(asterisk).* The **inset** shows where a secretory unit *(SG)* continues into the ductal unit *(D).* The duct has been cut as it turns, so that in the upper part of the **inset** the duct is seen essentially in cross section, whereas in the middle part of the **inset** it has been cut in a more or less longitudinal plane. Moreover, where the duct has been cut longitudinally, the lumen is not in the plane of section. The duct consists of a double layer of small cuboidal cells and no myoepithelial cells. In addition, there is acidophilic staining associated with the apical portion of the duct cells that are adjacent to the lumen. This is evident in the duct seen in the **inset** and can be contrasted readily with the absence of such staining in the apical region of the secretory cells *(SG),* also seen in the **inset.**

KEY

aSG, apocrine sweat gland
BV, blood vessel
C, capillary
D, duct of eccrine sweat gland
G, granules in apocrine secretory cells
HF, hair follicle
SG, eccrine sweat gland, secretory portion
arrowheads, myoepithelial cell cytoplasm
arrows, myoepithelial cell, nuclei
asterisk, lumen of eccrine duct

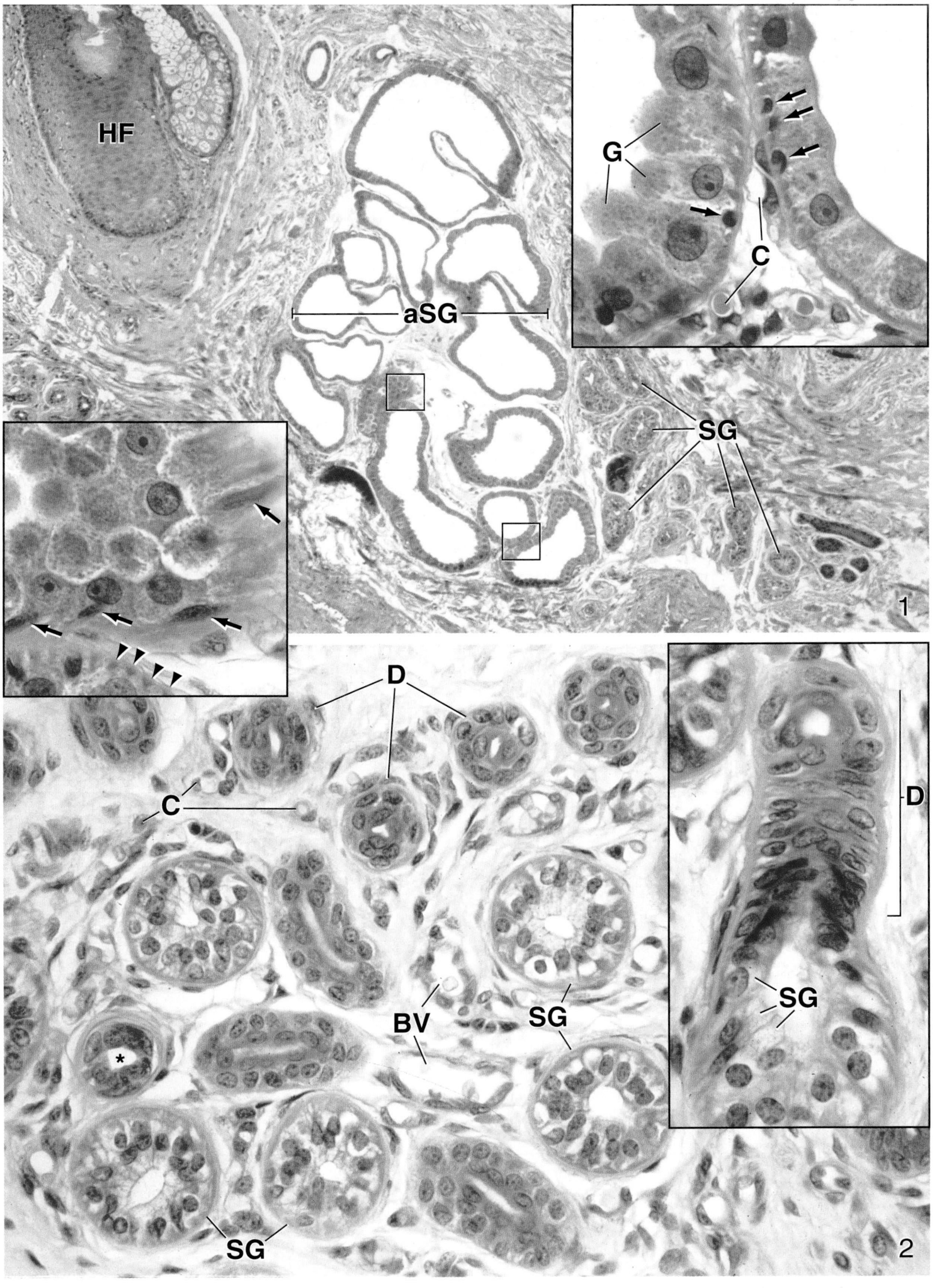
HF
G
C
aSG
SG
1
D
C
D
BV
SG
SG
*
SG
2

PLATE 41. SWEAT AND SEBACEOUS GLANDS

Normally, the body loses ~600 mL of water a day through evaporation from the lungs and skin. Under conditions of high ambient temperature, water loss is increased by an increased rate of sweating. This *thermoregulatory sweating* first occurs on the forehead and scalp, extends to the face and the rest of the body, and occurs last on the palms and soles. *Emotional sweating,* however, occurs first on the palms and soles and in the axillae. Sweating is under both nervous control through the autonomic nervous system and hormonal control.

Sebaceous glands secrete *sebum,* an oily substance that coats the hair and skin surface. Sebaceous secretion is a *holocrine* secretion; the entire cell produces, and becomes filled with, the fatty secretory product while it simultaneously undergoes progressive disruption, followed by necrosis, as the product fills the cell. Both secretory product and cell debris are discharged into the *pilosebaceous canal.*

Figure 1, skin, human, H&E ×1000.

This section through a sweat gland shows five profiles of the ductal portion *(D)* and two profiles of the secretory portion *(SG).* The larger secretory segment is through a region either just below or above where a U turn was made; therefore, it shows two luminal profiles. The lumina of both the ductal and the secretory units are marked by *asterisks.*

The glandular unit of the eccrine sweat gland contains two epithelial cell types and myoepithelial cells *(M). Arrowheads* show small cross sections of myoepithelial cell cytoplasm; *large arrows* show where more elongate profiles of myoepithelial cytoplasm are evident. The epithelial cells are of two types, designated dark cells and clear cells. Unfortunately, the characteristic dark cytoplasmic staining of the dark cells is not evident unless special precautions are taken to preserve the secretory granules in their apical cytoplasm. Nevertheless, note that the dark cells are closer to the lumen, whereas the clear cells are closer to the base of the epithelial layer, making contact with either the basal lamina or, more frequently, the myoepithelial cells. In addition, the clear cells are in contact with intercellular canaliculi. Several such intercellular canaliculi are shown in the secretory units *(small arrows).* This figure also shows that the duct consists of two layers of small cuboidal cells.

Figure 2, skin, human, H&E ×160.

Sebaceous glands develop from the epithelial cells of the hair follicle and discharge their secretion into the follicle, from where it reaches the skin surface. The sebaceous secretion is rich in lipid, and this is reflected in the cells of the sebaceous gland. A section of a sebaceous gland and its related hair follicle is shown in this figure. At this level, the hair follicle consists of the external root sheath *(RS)* surrounding the hair shaft. The sebaceous gland *(Seb)* appears as a cluster of cells, most of which display a washed-out or finely reticulated cytoplasm. This is because these cells contain numerous lipid droplets and the lipid is lost by dissolution in fat solvents during the routine preparation of the H&E–stained paraffin section. The opening of the sebaceous gland through the external root sheath *(eRS)* and into the hair follicle is shown in the lower right.

Figure 3, skin, human, H&E ×320.

The same sebaceous gland as in Figure 2 is shown here at higher magnification. *Numbers 1 to 4* show a series of cells filled with an increasingly greater amount of lipid and progressively closer to the opening of the gland into the hair follicle. The sebaceous secretion includes the entire cell, and therefore, cells need to be replaced constantly in the functional gland. Cells at the periphery of the gland are basal cells *(BC).* Dividing cells in the basal layer replace those that are lost with the secretion.

KEY

BC, basal cells
CT, connective tissue
D, duct of eccrine sweat gland
eRS, junction between sebaceous gland and external root sheath
M, myoepithelial cell
RS, external root sheath of hair follicle
Seb, sebaceous gland
SG, secretory component of eccrine sweat gland
arrowheads, myoepithelial cell cytoplasm (cross section)
asterisks, lumina of glands
large arrows, myoepithelial cell cytoplasm (longitudinal section)
numbers 1 to 4 (Fig. 3), see text
small arrows, intercellular canaliculi

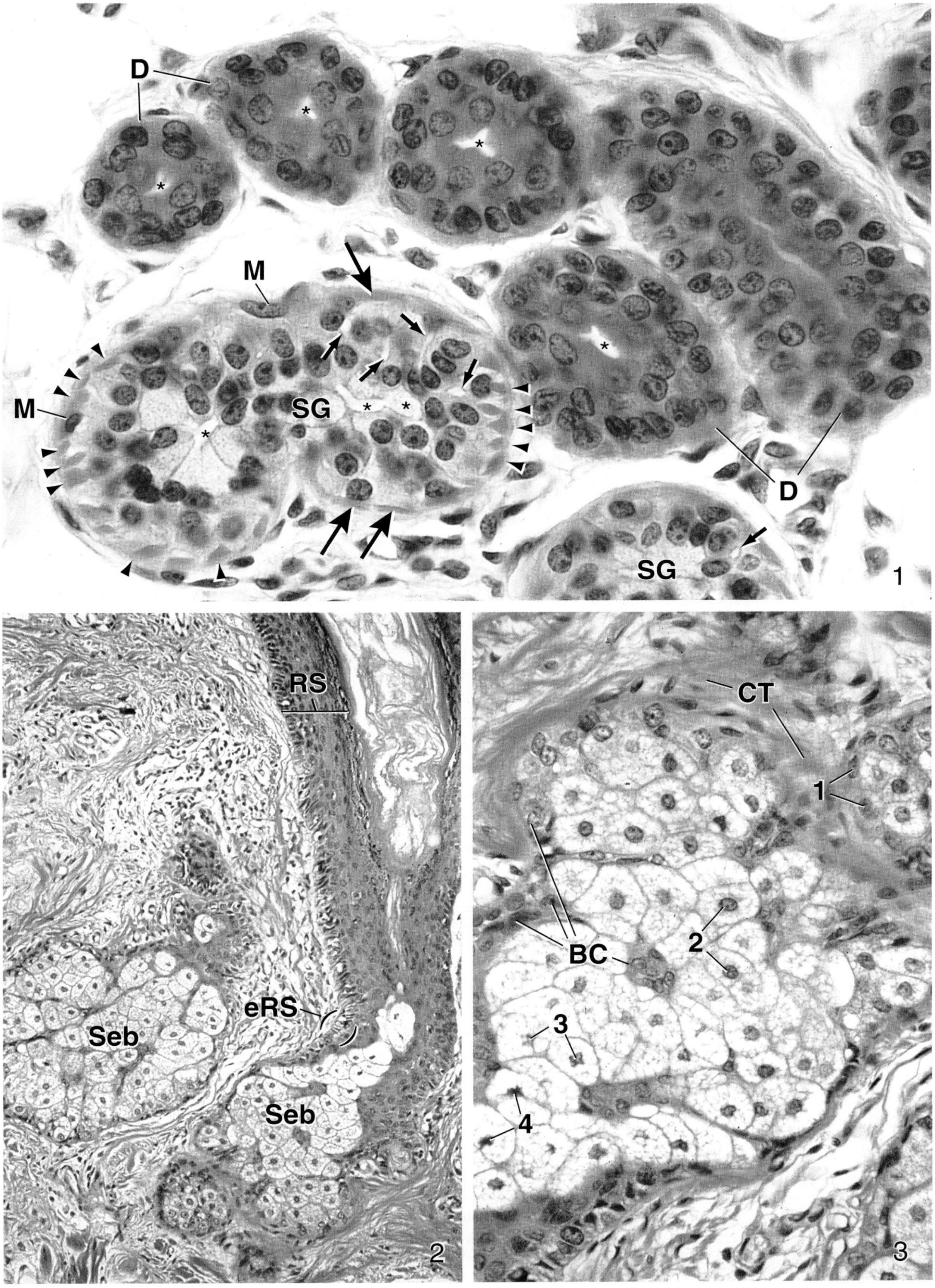
D
D
M
M
SG
SG
D
1
RS
eRS
Seb
Seb
2
CT
1
BC
2
3
4
3

PLATE 42. INTEGUMENT AND SENSORY ORGANS

The skin is endowed with numerous sensory receptors of various types. These are the peripheral terminals of sensory nerves whose cell bodies are in the dorsal root ganglia. The receptors in the skin are described as *free nerve endings* and *encapsulated nerve endings.* Free nerve endings are the most numerous. They subserve fine touch, heat, and cold and are found in the basal layers of the epidermis and as a network around the root sheath of hair follicles. Encapsulated nerve endings include *Pacinian corpuscles* (deep pressure), *Meissner's corpuscles* (touch, especially in the lips and thick skin of fingers and toes), and *Ruffini endings* (sustained mechanical stress on the dermis).

Motor endings of the autonomic nervous system supply the blood vessels, the arrector pili muscles, and the apocrine and eccrine sweat glands.

Figure 1, skin, human, H&E ×20.

This specimen is a section of thick skin from the finger tip, showing the epidermis *(Ep)* and the dermis *(De)* and, under the skin, a portion of the hypodermis *(Hy).* The thickness of the epidermis is largely due to the thickness of the stratum corneum. This layer is more lightly stained than the deeper portions of the epidermis. Note, even at this low magnification, the thick collagenous fibers in the reticular layer of the dermis. Sweat glands *(SG)* are present in the upper part of the hypodermis, and several sweat ducts *(D)* are seen passing through the epidermis.

A feature of this specimen is that it depicts those sensory receptors that can be recognized in a routine low-power H&E–stained paraffin section. They are Meissner's corpuscles and Pacinian corpuscles *(PC).* Several nerve bundles *(N)* are seen in proximity to the Pacinian corpuscles. Meissner's corpuscles are in the upper part of the dermis, in the dermal papillae immediately under the epidermis. These corpuscles are small and difficult to identify at this low magnification; however, their location is characteristic. Knowing where they are located is a major step in finding Meissner's corpuscles in a tissue section; they are shown at higher magnification in Figure 3.

Pacinian corpuscles are seen in the lower part of the hypodermis. These corpuscles are large, slightly oval structures, and even at low magnification, a layered or lamellated pattern can be discerned.

Figure 2, skin, human, H&E ×320.

At this higher magnification, the concentric layers or lamellae of the Pacinian corpuscle can be seen to be due to flat cells. These are fibroblast-like cells, and although not evident within the tissue section, these cells are continuous with the endoneurium of the nerve fiber. The space between the cellular lamellae contains mostly fluid. The neural portion of the Pacinian corpuscle travels longitudinally through the center of the corpuscle. In this specimen, the corpuscle has been cross-sectioned; an *arrowhead* points to the centrally located nerve fiber.

Figure 3, skin, human, H&E ×190.

This high-magnification micrograph shows portions of the upper left field of Figure 1 in which two Meissner's corpuscles *(MC)* are in direct proximity to the undersurface of the epidermis in adjacent dermal papillae. The section shows the long axis of the corpuscles. A Meissner's corpuscle consists of an axon (sometimes two) taking a zigzag or flat spiral course from one pole of the corpuscle to the other. The nerve fiber terminates at the superficial pole of the corpuscle. Consequently, as seen here, the nerve fibers and supporting cells are oriented approximately at right angles to the long axis of the corpuscle. Meissner's corpuscles are particularly numerous near the tips of the fingers and toes.

Figure 4, skin, human, H&E ×550.

At the even higher magnification of this figure, the close apposition of Meissner's corpuscle to the undersurface of the epidermis is well demonstrated throughout the entire area of the dermal papilla. The flat spiral path of the neuron (not seen) and its supporting cells is evident here, as is the fibrous capsule *(FC)* that surrounds the ending.

KEY

D, ducts of sweat glands
De, dermis
Ep, epidermis
FC, fibrous capsule
Hy, hypodermis
MC, Meissner's corpuscles
N, nerve bundles
PC, Pacinian corpuscles
SG, sweat glands
arrowhead, nerve fiber in center of Pacinian corpuscle

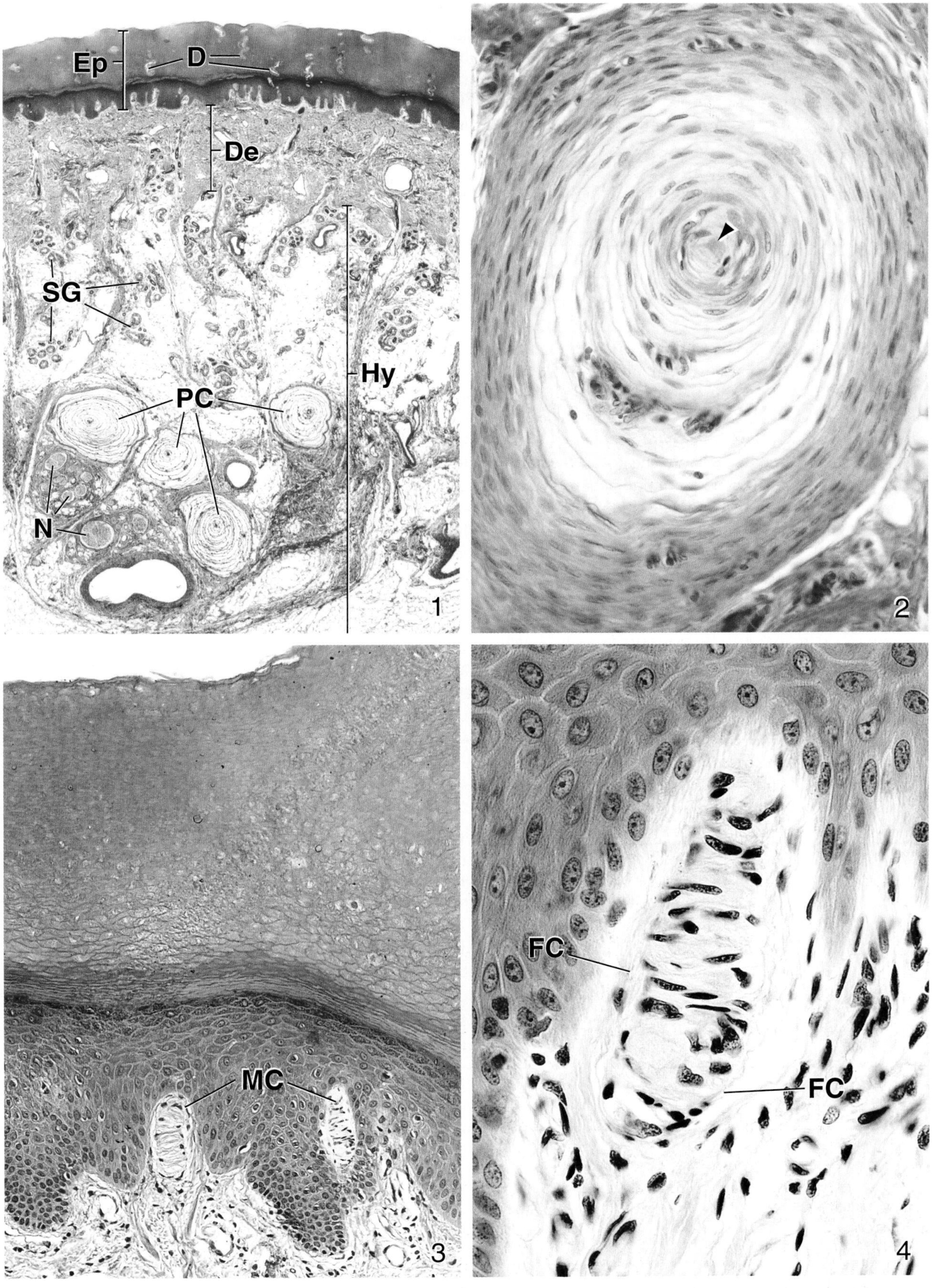
Ep
D
De
SG
Hy
PC
N
1
2
MC
3
FC
FC
4

PLATE 43. HAIR FOLLICLE AND NAIL

Hairs are composed of keratinized cells that develop from hair follicles. Hairs are present over almost the entire body, being conspicuously absent only from the sides and palmar surfaces of the hands, from the sides and plantar surfaces of the feet, from the lips, and from the skin around the urogenital orifices. Coloration of the hair is due to the content and type of melanin that it contains. The follicle varies in appearance, depending on whether it is in a growing or a resting phase; the growing follicle is the more elaborate.

The skin appendages (adnexa), especially hair follicles and sweat glands, are particularly important in healing of skin wounds. They serve as the source of new epithelial cells when there is extensive loss of epidermis, as in deep abrasions and second-degree burns.

Figure 1, skin, human, H&E ×300; inset ×440.

The growing end of a hair follicle consists of an expanded bulb of epithelial cells that is invaginated by a papilla *(HP)* of connective tissue. The epithelial cells surrounding the papilla at the very tip of the follicle are not yet specialized; they constitute the matrix, the region of the hair follicle where cell division occurs. As the cells leave the matrix, they form cell layers that will become the shaft of the hair and the inner and outer root sheaths of the hair follicle.

The cells that will develop into the shaft of the hair are seen just to the right of the expanded bulb. They constitute the cortex *(C)*, medulla *(M)*, and cuticle *(asterisks)* of the hair. The cells of the cortex become keratinized. This layer will come to constitute most of the hair shaft as a thick cylinder. The medulla forms the centrally located axis of the hair shaft; it does not always extend through the entire length of the hair and is absent from some hairs. The cuticle consists of overlapping cells that ultimately lose their nuclei and become filled with keratin. The cuticle covers the hair shaft like a layer of overlapping shingles.

The root sheath *(RS)* has two parts: the outer root sheath, which is continuous with the epidermis of the skin, and the inner root sheath, which extends only as far as the level at which sebaceous glands enter the hair follicle. The inner root sheath is further divided into three layers: Henle's layer, Huxley's layer, and the cuticle of the inner root sheath. These layers are seen in the growing hair follicle and are shown at higher magnification in the **inset** with *numbers 1 to 5: 1,* cells of the outer root sheath; *2,* Henle's layer; *3,* Huxley's layer; *4,* cuticle of the inner root sheath; and *5,* future cuticle of the hair.

Many of the cells of the growing hair follicle contain pigment that contributes to the color of the hair. Most of this pigment is inside the cell **(inset)**; however, in very dark hair some pigment is also extracellular.

The connective tissue surrounding the hair follicle forms a distinct layer referred to as the *sheath,* or *dermal sheath (DS),* of the hair follicle.

Figure 2, skin, human, H&E ×12.

A nail is a keratinized plate located on the dorsal aspect of the distal phalanges. A section through a nail plate is shown here. The nail itself *(N)* is difficult to stain. Under the free edge of the nail is a boundary layer, the *hyponychium (Hypon),* which is continuous with the stratum corneum of the adjacent epidermis. The proximal end of the nail is overlapped by skin; here, the junctional region is called the *eponychium (Epon)* and is also continuous with the stratum corneum of the adjacent epidermis. Under the nail is a layer of epithelium, the posterior portion of which is referred to as the *nail matrix (NM).* The cells of the nail matrix function in the growth of the nail. Together, the epithelium under the nail and the underlying dermis *(D)* constitute the nail bed. The posterior portion of the nail, covered by the fold of the skin, is the root of the nail *(NR).*

The relationship of the nail to other structures in the fingertip is also shown in this figure. The bone *(B)* in the specimen represents a distal phalanx. Note that in this bone there is an epiphyseal growth plate *(EP)* at the proximal extremity of the bone but not at the distal extremity. Numerous Pacinian corpuscles *(PC)* are present in the connective tissue of the palmar side of the finger. Also seen to advantage in this section is the stratum lucidum *(SL)* in the epidermis of the thick skin of the fingertip.

KEY

B, bone
C, cortex
D, dermis
DS, dermal sheath
EP, epiphyseal plate
Epon, eponychium
HP, dermal papilla of hair follicle
Hypon, hyponychium
M, medulla
N, nail or nail plate
NM, nail matrix
NR, nail root
PC, Pacinian corpuscles
RS, root sheath
SL, stratum lucidum
asterisks, cuticle of hair
numbers: *1,* external root sheath; *2,* Henle's layer; *3,* Huxley's layer; *4,* cuticle of inner root sheath; *5,* future cuticle of the hair

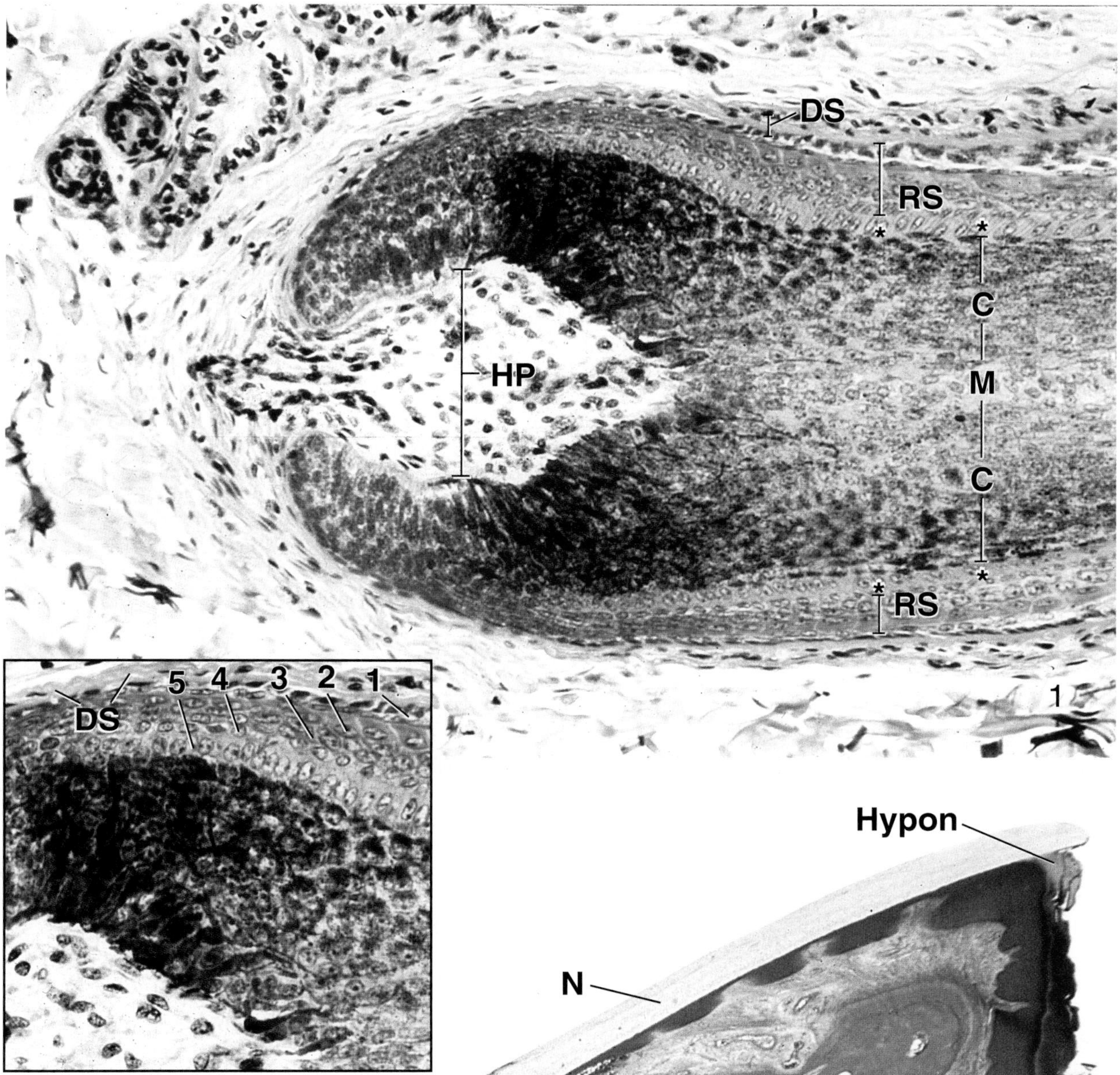
DS
RS
HP
C
M
C
RS
DS
5
4
3
2
1
1

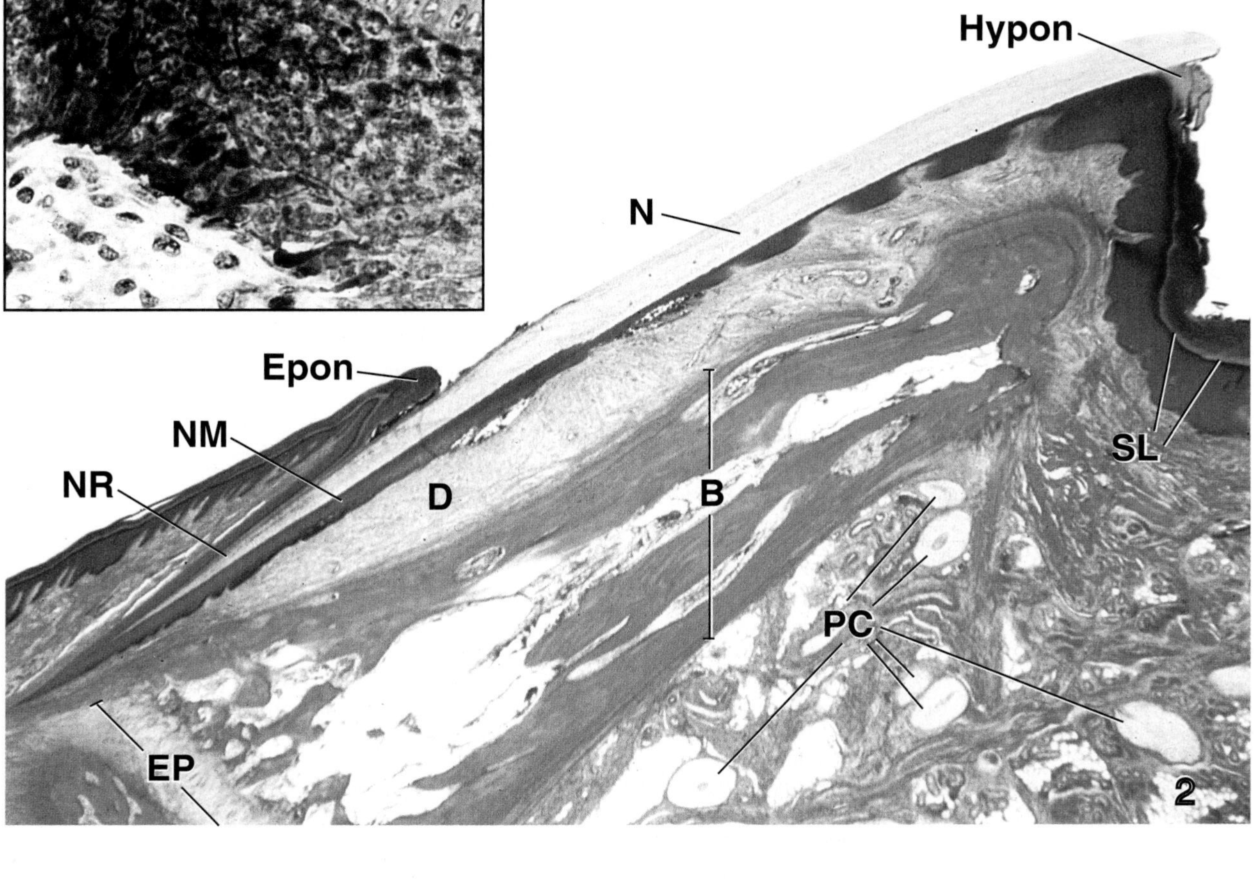
Hypon
N
Epon
NM
NR
D
B
SL
PC
EP
2

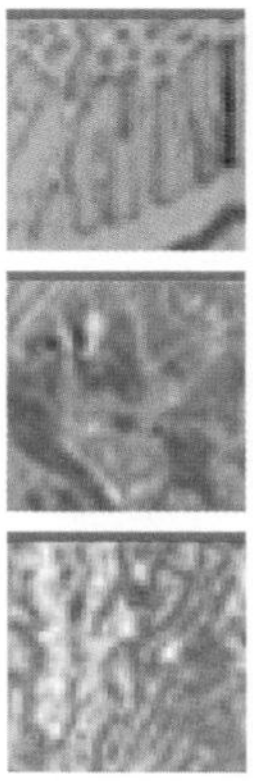

15

Digestive System I: Oral Cavity and Associated Structures

BOXES

OVERVIEW OF THE DIGESTIVE SYSTEM

The digestive system consists of the ***alimentary canal*** and its principal associated organs, namely, the ***tongue, teeth, salivary glands, pancreas, liver,*** and ***gallbladder.***

The lumen of the alimentary canal is physically and functionally external to the body

As it passes through the alimentary canal, food is broken down physically and chemically so that the degraded products can be absorbed into the body. The various segments

of the alimentary canal are morphologically specialized for specific aspects of digestion and absorption.

After preliminary maceration, moistening, and formation into a ***bolus*** by the actions of the structures of the oral cavity and salivary glands, food passes rapidly through the pharynx to the esophagus. The rapid passage of food through the pharynx keeps it clear for the passage of air. The food passes more slowly through the gastrointestinal tract, and during its transit through the stomach and small intestine, the major alterations associated with digestion, solubilization, and absorption occur. Absorption occurs chiefly through the wall of the small intestine. Undigested food and other substances within the alimentary canal, such as mucus, bacteria, desquamated cells, and bile pigments, are excreted as *feces*.

The alimentary mucosa is the surface across which most substances enter the body

The alimentary ***mucosa*** performs numerous functions in its role as an interface between the body and the environment. These include

- ***Secretion.*** The lining of the alimentary canal secretes, at specific sites, digestive enzymes, hydrochloric acid, mucin, and antibodies.
- ***Absorption.*** The epithelium of the mucosa absorbs metabolic substrates, e.g., the breakdown products of digestion, as well as vitamins, water, electrolytes, recyclable materials such as bile components and cholesterol, and other substances essential to the functions of the body.
- ***Barrier.*** The mucosa serves as a barrier to prevent the entry of noxious substances, antigens, and pathogenic organisms.
- ***Immunologic protection.*** Lymphatic tissue within the mucosa serves as the body's first line of immune defense.

The functions listed above are discussed at the beginning of the next chapter. The digestive system is considered in three chapters that deal, respectively, with the oral cavity and pharynx (this chapter), the esophagus and gastrointestinal tract (Chapter 16), and the liver, gallbladder, and pancreas (Chapter 17).

▽ ORAL CAVITY

The oral cavity consists of the mouth and its structures, which include the tongue, teeth and their supporting structures (peridontium), major and minor salivary glands, and tonsils

The *oral cavity* is divided into a ***vestibule*** and the ***oral cavity proper.*** The ***vestibule*** is the space between the lips, cheeks, and teeth. The ***oral cavity proper*** lies behind the teeth and is bounded by the hard and soft palates superiorly, the tongue and the floor of the mouth inferiorly, and the entrance to the oropharynx posteriorly.

Each of the three ***major salivary glands*** are paired structures; they include the

- ***Parotid gland,*** the largest of the three glands, located in the temporal region of the head. Its excretory duct, the ***parotid (Stensen's) duct,*** opens at the ***parotid papilla,*** a small elevation on the mucosal surface of the cheek opposite the second upper molar tooth.
- ***Submandibular gland,*** located in the submandibular triangle of the neck. Its excretory duct, the ***submandibular (Wharton's) duct*** opens at a small fleshy prominence (the ***sublingual caruncle***) on each side of the lingual frenulum on the floor of the oral cavity.
- ***Sublingual gland,*** lying inferior to the tongue within the sublingual folds at the floor of the oral cavity. It has a number of small excretory ducts; some enter the submandibular duct, and others enter individually into the oral cavity.

The parotid and submandibular glands have relatively long ducts that extend from the secretory portion of the gland to the oral cavity. The sublingual ducts are relatively short.

The ***minor salivary glands*** are located in the submucosa of the oral cavity. They empty directly into the cavity via short ducts and are named for their location i.e., buccal, labial, lingual, and palatine.

The tonsils consist of aggregations of lymphatic nodules that are clustered around the posterior opening of the oral and nasal cavities

Lymphatic tissue is organized into a ***tonsillar ring (Waldeyer's ring)*** of immunologic protection located at the shared entrance to the digestive and respiratory tracts. This lymphatic tissue surrounds the posterior orifice of the oral and nasal cavities and contains aggregates of lymphatic nodules that include

- ***Palatine tonsils,*** or simply the ***tonsils,*** which are located at either side of the entrance to the oropharynx between the palatopharyngeal and palatoglossal arches
- ***Tubal tonsils,*** which are located in the lateral walls of the nasopharynx posterior to the opening of the auditory tube
- ***Pharyngeal tonsil,*** or ***adenoid,*** which is located in the roof of the nasopharynx
- ***Lingual tonsil,*** which is located at the base of the tongue on its superior surface

The oral cavity is lined by a masticatory mucosa, a lining mucosa, and a specialized mucosa

The ***masticatory mucosa*** is found on the gingiva (gums) and the hard palate (Fig. 15.1). It has a ***keratinized*** and, in some areas, a ***parakeratinized*** stratified squamous epithelium (see Fig. 15.2). Parakeratinized epithelium is similar to keratinized epithelium except that the superficial cells do not lose their nuclei and their cytoplasm does not stain intensely with eosin. The nuclei of the parakeratinized cells are pyknotic (highly condensed) and remain until the cell is exfoliated (see Fig. 15.2). The keratinized epithelium of the masticatory mucosa resembles that of the skin but lacks a stratum lucidum. The underlying lamina propria consists of a thick papillary layer of loose connective tissue that contains blood vessels and nerves, some of which send bare axon endings into the epithelium as sensory receptors, and some of which end in Meissner's corpuscles. Deep to the lamina propria is a reticular layer of more dense connective tissue.

As in the skin, the depth and number of connective tissue papillae contribute to the relative immobility of the masticatory mucosa, thus protecting it from frictional and shearing stress. At the midline of the hard palate, in the ***palatine raphe,*** the mucosa adheres firmly to the underlying bone. The reticular layer of the lamina propria blends with the periosteum, and thus there is no submucosa. The same is true of the gingiva. Where there is a submucosa underlying the lamina propria on the hard palate (see Fig. 15.1), it contains adipose tissue anteriorly (fatty zone) and mucous glands posteriorly (glandular zone) that are continuous with those of the soft palate. In the submucosal regions, thick collagenous bands extend from the mucosa to the bone.

Lining mucosa is found on the lips, cheeks, alveolar mucosal surface, floor of the mouth, inferior surfaces of the tongue, and soft palate. At these sites it covers striated muscle (lips, cheeks, and tongue), bone (alveolar mucosa), and glands (soft palate, cheeks, inferior surface of the tongue). The lining mucosa has fewer and shorter papillae so that it can adjust to the movement of its underlying muscles.

Generally, the epithelium of the lining mucosa is nonkeratinized, although in some places it may be parakeratinized. The epithelium of the vermilion border of the lip (the reddish portion between the moist inner surface and the facial skin) is keratinized. The nonkeratinized lining epithelium is thicker than keratinized epithelium. It consists of only three layers:

- ***Stratum basale,*** a single layer of cells resting on the basal lamina
- ***Stratum spinosum,*** which is several cells thick
- ***Stratum superficiale,*** the most superficial layer of cells, also referred as the ***surface layer*** of the mucosa

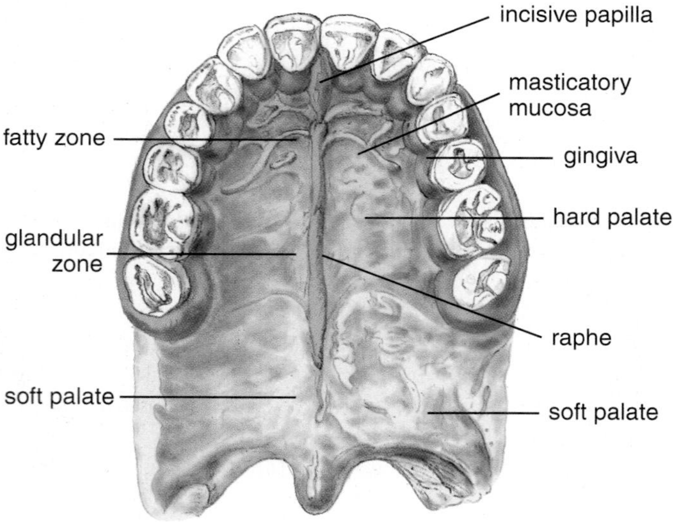

FIGURE 15.1
Roof of oral cavity. The hard palate, which contains bone, is bisected into right and left halves by a raphe. Anteriorly, in the fatty zone, the submucosa of the hard palate contains adipose tissue; posteriorly, in the glandular zone, there are mucous glands within the submucosa. Neither the raphe nor the gingiva contains a submucosa; instead, the mucosa is attached directly to the bone. The soft palate has muscle instead of bone, and its glands are continuous with those of the hard palate in the submucosa. (Based on Bhaskar SN, ed. *Orban's Oral Histology and Embryology.* St. Louis: CV Mosby, 1991.)

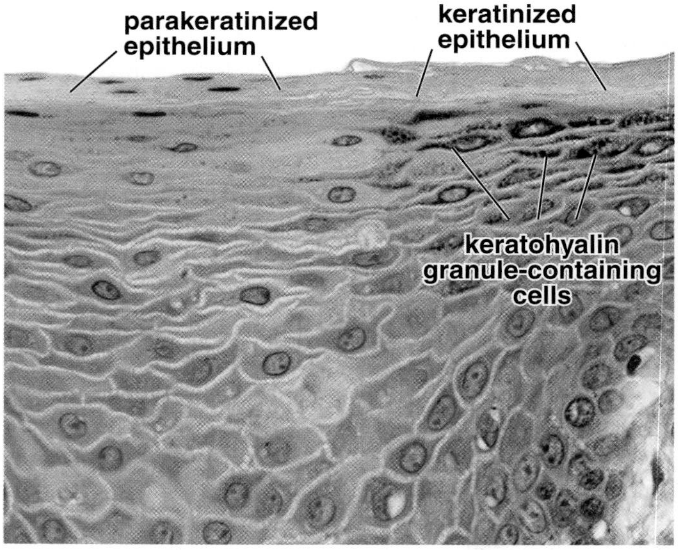

FIGURE 15.2
Stratified squamous epithelium of the hard palate. This photomicrograph shows a transition in the oral mucosa from a stratified squamous epithelium (on the right) to a stratified squamous parakeratinized epithelium (on the left). The flattened surface cells of the keratinized epithelium are devoid of nuclei. The layer of keratohyalin granule–containing cells is clearly visible in this type of epithelium. The flattened surface cells of the parakeratinized epithelium display the same characteristics as the keratinized cells, except they retain their nuclei; i.e., they are parakeratinized. In addition, note the paucity of keratohyalin granules present in the subsurface cells. ×380.

The cells of the mucosal epithelium are similar to those of the epidermis of the skin and include keratinocytes, Langerhans' cells, melanocytes, and Merkel's cells.

The lamina propria contains blood vessels, nerves that send bare axon endings into the basal layers of the epithelium, and encapsulated sensory endings in some papillae. The sharp contrast between the numerous deep papillae of the alveolar mucosa and the shallow papillae in the rest of the lining mucosa allows easy identification of the two different regions in a histologic section.

A distinct submucosa underlies the lining mucosa except on the inferior surface of the tongue. This layer contains large bands of collagen and elastic fibers that bind the mucosa to the underlying muscle; it also contains the many minor salivary glands of the lips, tongue, and cheeks. Occasionally, sebaceous glands not associated with a hair follicle are found in the submucosa just lateral to the corner of the mouth and in the cheeks opposite the molar teeth. They are visible to the eye and are called ***Fordyce spots.*** The submucosa contains the larger blood vessels, nerves, and lymphatic vessels that supply the subepithelial neurovascular networks in the lamina propria throughout the oral cavity.

Specialized mucosa is restricted to the dorsal surface of the tongue, where it contains papillae and taste buds.

▼ TONGUE

The ***tongue*** is a muscular organ projecting into the oral cavity from its inferior surface. ***Lingual*** (i.e., pertaining to the tongue) ***muscles*** are both extrinsic (having one attachment outside of the tongue) and intrinsic (confined entirely to the tongue, without external attachment). The striated muscle of the tongue is arranged in bundles that generally run in three planes, with each arranged at right angles to the other two. This arrangement of muscle fibers allows enormous flexibility and precision in the movements of the tongue, which are essential to human speech as well as to its role in digestion and swallowing. This form of muscle organization is found only in the tongue, which allows easy identification of this tissue as lingual muscle. Variable amounts of adipose tissue are found among the muscle fiber groups.

Grossly, the dorsal surface of the tongue is divided into an anterior two thirds and a posterior one third by a V-shaped depression, the ***sulcus terminalis*** (Fig. 15.3). The apex of the V points posteriorly and is the location of the ***foramen cecum,*** the remnant of the site from which an evagination of the floor of the embryonic pharynx occurred to form the thyroid gland.

Papillae cover the dorsal surface of the tongue

Numerous mucosal irregularities and elevations called ***lingual papillae*** cover the dorsal surface of the tongue anterior to the sulcus terminalis. The lingual papillae and their associated taste buds constitute the ***specialized mucosa*** of the oral cavity. Four types of papillae are described: ***filiform, fungiform, circumvallate,*** and ***foliate.***

- ***Filiform papillae*** are the smallest and most numerous in humans. They are conical, elongated projections of connective tissue that are covered with highly keratinized stratified squamous epithelium (Fig. 15.4a). This epithelium does not contain taste buds. The papillae serve only a mechanical role. Filiform papillae are distributed over the entire anterior dorsal surface of the tongue, with their tips pointing backward. They appear to form rows that diverge to the left and right from the midline and that parallel the arms of the sulcus terminalis.
- ***Fungiform papillae,*** as the name implies, are mushroom-shaped projections located on the dorsal surface

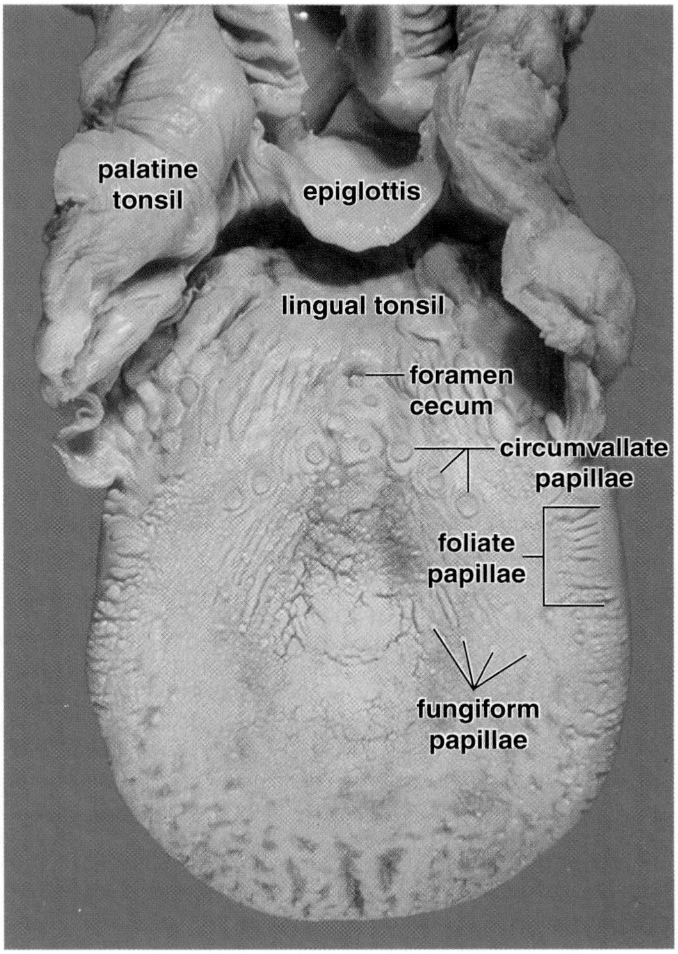

FIGURE 15.3
Human tongue. Circumvallate papillae are positioned in a V configuration, separating the anterior two thirds of the tongue from the posterior third. Fungiform and filiform papillae are on the anterior portion of the dorsal tongue surface. The uneven contour of the posterior tongue surface is due to the lingual tonsils. The palatine tonsil is at the junction between the oral cavity and the pharynx. (Specimen Courtesy of Dr. Gunther von Hagen.)

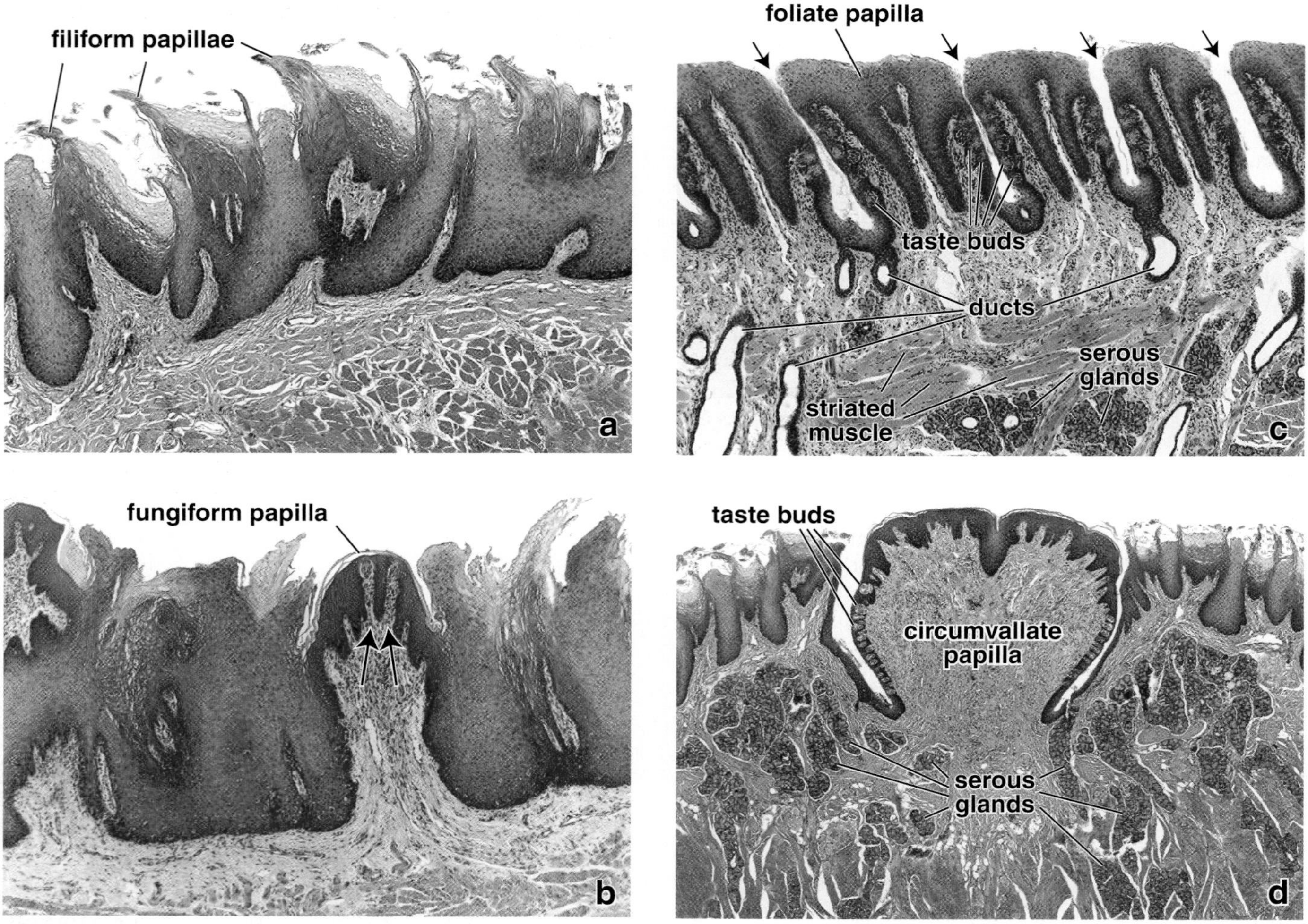

FIGURE 15.4

a. Structurally, the filiform papillae are posteriorly bent conical projections of the epithelium. These papillae do not possess taste buds and are composed of stratified squamous keratinized epithelium. ×45. **b.** Fungiform papillae are slightly rounded, elevated structures situated among the filiform papillae. A highly vascularized connective tissue core forms the center of the fungiform papilla and projects into the base of the surface epithelium. Because of the deep penetration of connective tissue into the epithelium *(arrows)*, combined with a very thin keratinized surface, the fungiform papillae appear as small red dots when the dorsal surface of the tongue is examined by gross inspection. ×45. **c.** In a section, foliate papillae can be distinguished from fungiform papillae because they appear in rows separated by deep clefts *(arrows)*. The foliate papillae are covered by stratified squamous nonkeratinized epithelium containing numerous taste buds on their lateral surfaces. The free surface epithelium of each papilla is thick and has a number of secondary connective tissue papillae projecting into its undersurface. The connective tissue within and under the foliate papillae contains serous glands (von Ebner's glands) that open via ducts into the cleft between neighboring papillae. ×45. **d.** Circumvallate papillae are covered by stratified squamous epithelium that may be slightly keratinized. Each circumvallate papilla is surrounded by a trench or cleft. Numerous taste buds are on the lateral walls of the papillae. The dorsal surface of the papilla is smooth. The deep trench surrounding the circumvallate papillae and the presence of taste buds on the sides rather than on the free surface are features that distinguish circumvallate from fungiform papillae. The connective tissue near the circumvallate papillae also contains many serous-type glands that open via ducts into the bottom of the trench. ×25.

of the tongue (Fig. 15.4b). They project above the filiform papillae, among which they are scattered, and are just visible to the unaided eye as small spots (see Fig. 15.3). They tend to be more numerous near the tip of the tongue. ***Taste buds*** are present in the stratified squamous epithelium on the dorsal surface of these papillae.

- ***Circumvallate papillae*** are the large, dome-shaped structures that reside in the mucosa just anterior to the sulcus terminalis (see Fig. 15.3). The human tongue has 8 to 12 of these papillae. Each papilla is surrounded by a moat-like invagination lined with stratified squamous epithelium that contains numerous taste buds (Fig. 15.4d). Ducts of ***lingual salivary glands (von Ebner's glands)*** empty

their serous secretion into the base of the moats. This secretion presumably flushes material from the moat to enable the taste buds to respond rapidly to changing stimuli.

- ***Foliate papillae*** consist of parallel low ridges separated by deep mucosal clefts (see Fig. 15.4c), which are aligned at right angles to the long axis of the tongue. They occur on the lateral edge of the tongue. In aged individuals, the foliate papillae may not be recognized; in younger individuals, they are easily found on the posterior lateral surface of the tongue and contain many taste buds in the epithelium of the facing walls of neighboring papillae (Fig. 15.3e). Small serous glands empty into the clefts. In some animals, such as the rabbit, foliate papillae constitute the principal site of aggregation of taste buds.

The dorsal surface of the base of the tongue exhibits smooth bulges that reflect the presence of the lingual tonsil in the lamina propria (see Fig. 15.3).

Taste buds are present on fungiform, foliate, and circumvallate papillae

In histologic sections, taste buds appear as oval, pale-staining bodies that extend through the thickness of the epithelium (Fig. 15.5). A small opening onto the epithelial surface at the apex of the taste bud is called the ***taste pore.***

Three principal cell types are found in taste buds:

- ***Neuroepithelial (sensory) cells*** are the most numerous cells in the taste bud. These elongated cells extend from the basal lamina of the epithelium to the taste pore, through which the tapered apical surface of each cell extends microvilli (see Fig. 15.5). Near their apical surface they are connected to neighboring neuroepithelial or supporting cells by tight junctions. At their base they form a synapse with the processes of afferent sensory neurons of the ***facial*** (cranial nerve VII), ***glossopharyn-***

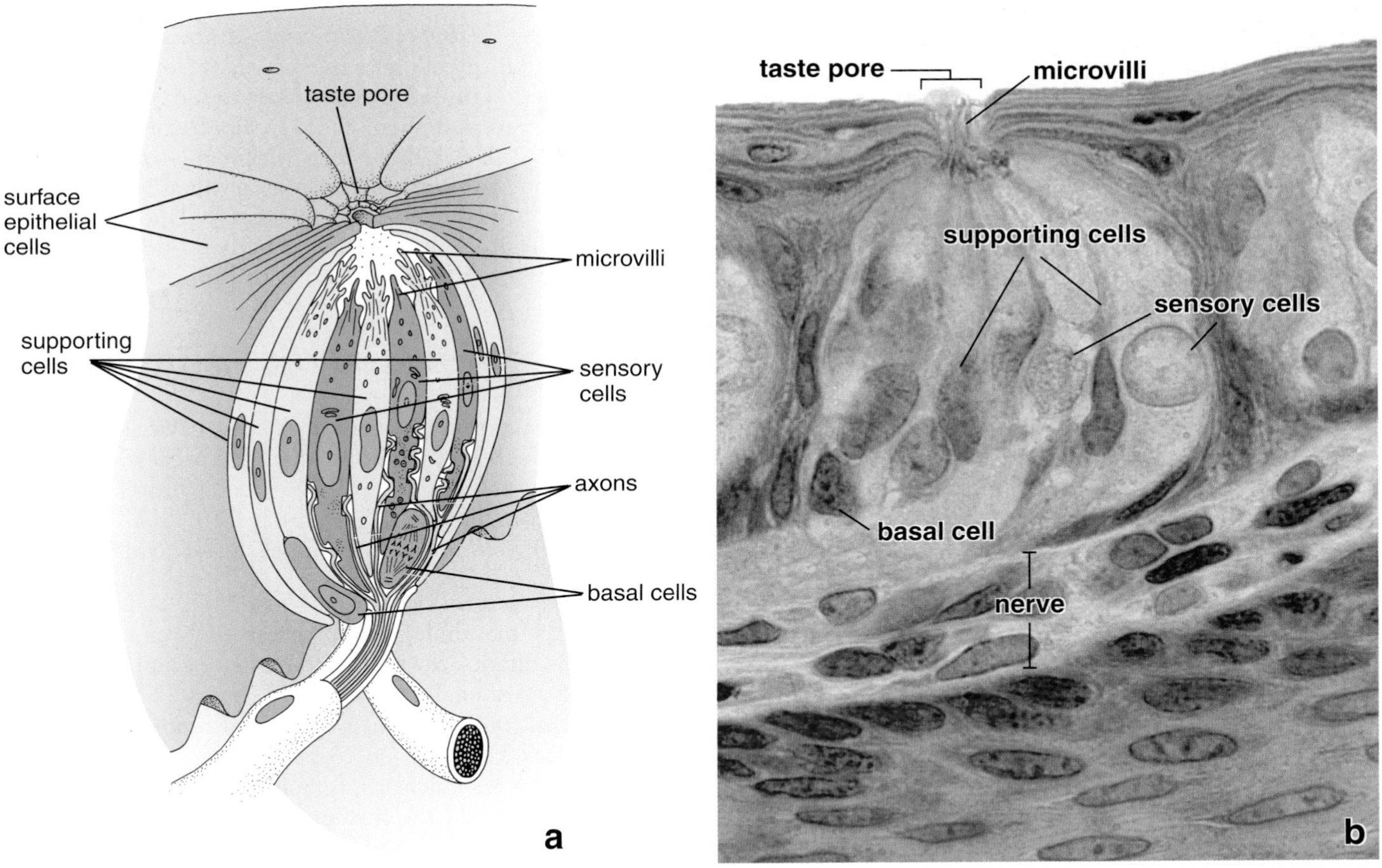

FIGURE 15.5
Diagram and photomicrograph of a taste bud. a. This diagram of a taste bud shows the neuroepithelial (sensory), supporting, and basal cells. One of the basal cells is shown in the process of dividing. Nerve fibers have synapses with the neuroepithelial cells. (Based on Warwick R, Williams PL, eds. *Gray's Anatomy.* 35th ed. Edinburgh: Churchill Livingstone, 1973.) **b.** This high-magnification photomicrograph shows the organization of the cells within the taste bud. The sensory and supporting cells extend through the full length of the taste bud. The apical surface of these cells contains microvilli. The basal cells are located at the bottom of the taste bud. Note that the taste bud opens at the surface by means of a taste pore. ×640.

BOX 15.1

Clinical Correlations: Inherited Absence of Taste

The general ability to taste as well as the ability to sense specific tastes is genetically determined. At one extreme are those rare individuals, such as wine tasters and tea tasters, who have prodigious taste discrimination and taste memory. At the other extreme are individuals who are totally unable to taste. In one rare inherited condition, ***familial dysautonomia,*** taste buds and fungiform papillae are absent. The disease may be diagnosed easily in the newborn, where the absence of these papillae is particularly clear.

A common test used to identify "tasters" and "nontasters" is to place a drop of a solution containing phenylthiocarbamide (PTC) on the tip of the tongue. Tasters report a bitter taste; nontasters are unaware of any taste.

geal (cranial nerve IX), or ***vagus*** (cranial nerve X) nerves. The turnover time of neuroepithelial cells is about 10 days.

- ***Supporting cells*** are less numerous. They are also elongated cells that extend from the basal lamina to the taste pore. Like neuroepithelial cells, they contain microvilli on their apical surface and possess tight junctions, but they do not synapse with the nerve cells. The turnover time of supporting cells is also about 10 days.
- ***Basal cells*** are small cells located in the basal portion of the taste bud, near the basal lamina. They are the stem cells for the two other cell types.

In addition to those associated with the papillae, taste buds are also present on the glossopalatine arch, the soft palate, the posterior surface of the epiglottis, and the posterior wall of the pharynx down to the level of the cricoid cartilage.

Taste buds react to only four stimuli: sweet, salty, bitter, and acid. In general, taste buds at the tip of the tongue detect sweet stimuli, those immediately posterolateral to the tip detect salty stimuli, and those more posterolateral detect acid or sour testing stimuli. Taste buds on the circumvallate papillae detect bitter stimuli.

Lingual tonsil consists of accumulations of lymphatic tissue at the base of the tongue

The ***lingual tonsil*** is located in the lamina propria of the root or base of the tongue. It is found posterior to the sulcus terminalis (see Fig. 15.3). The lingual tonsil contains diffuse lymphatic tissue with lymphatic nodules containing germinal centers. These structures are discussed in Chapter 13.

Epithelial crypts usually invaginate into the lingual tonsil. However, the structure of the epithelium may be difficult to distinguish because of the extremely large number of lymphocytes that normally invade it. Between nodules, the lingual epithelium has the characteristics of lining epithelium. Mucous lingual salivary glands may be seen within the lingual tonsil and may extend into the muscle of the base of the tongue.

The complex nerve supply of the tongue is provided by cranial nerves and the autonomic nervous system

- General sensation for the anterior two thirds of the tongue (anterior to the sulcus terminalis) is carried in the ***mandibular division trigeminal nerve*** (cranial nerve V). General sensation for the posterior one third of the tongue is carried in the glossopharyngeal (cranial nerve IX) and the vagus nerve (cranial nerve X).
- Taste sensation is carried by the ***chorda tympani,*** a branch of the facial nerve (cranial nerve VII) anterior to the sulcus terminalis and by the glossopharyngeal (cranial nerve IX) and vagus nerves (cranial nerve X) posterior to the sulcus.
- Motor innervation for the musculature of the tongue is supplied by the ***hypoglossal nerve*** (cranial nerve XII).
- Vascular and glandular innervation is provided by the ***sympathetic*** and ***parasympathetic nerves.*** They supply blood vessels and small salivary glands of the tongue. Ganglion cells are often seen within the tongue. These cells belong to postganglionic parasympathetic neurons and are destined for the minor salivary glands within the tongue. The cell bodies of sympathetic postganglionic neurons are located in the superior cervical ganglion.

▽ TEETH AND SUPPORTING TISSUES

Teeth are a major component of the oral cavity and are essential for the beginning of the digestive process. Teeth are embedded in and attached to the alveolar processes of the maxilla and mandible. Children have 10 ***deciduous (primary, milk) teeth*** in each jaw, on each side, consisting of

- A ***medial (central) incisor,*** the first tooth to erupt (usually in the mandible) at approximately 6 months of age (in some infants, the first teeth may not erupt until 12 to 13 months of age)
- A ***lateral incisor,*** which erupts at approximately 8 months
- A ***canine tooth,*** which erupts at approximately 15 months
- Two **molar teeth,** the first of which erupts at 10 to 19 months and the second of which erupts at 20 to 31 months

Over a period of years, usually beginning at about age 6 and finishing at about age 12 to 13, deciduous teeth are gradually replaced by 16 ***permanent (secondary) teeth*** in each jaw. Each side of both upper and lower jaws consists of

- A ***medial (central) incisor,*** which erupts at age 7 to 8
- A ***lateral incisor,*** which erupts at age 8 to 9

BOX 15.2

Clinical Correlations: Classification of Permanent (Secondary) and Deciduous (Primary) Dentition

Three systems are currently used to classify permanent and deciduous teeth (Fig. 15.6):

- ***Palmer system,*** which was the most commonly used notation worldwide. In this system, uppercase letters are used for the deciduous teeth, and arabic numerals are used for the permanent teeth. Each quadrant in this system is designated by angled lines: ┘ for upper right (UR), └ for upper left (UL), ┐ for lower right (LR), and ┌ for lower left (LL). For example, permanent canines are called number 3 in each quadrant, and the quadrant is designated by its angled line.
- ***International system,*** which uses two arabic numerals to designate the individual tooth. In this system, the first numeral indicates the location of the tooth in a specific quadrant. The permanent quadrants are designated UR = 1, UL = 2, LL =3, and LR = 4; the deciduous quadrants are designated UR = 5, UL = 6, LL = 7, and LR = 8. The second numeral designates the individual tooth, which is numbered beginning from the dental midline. For example, in this system, the permanent canines are named 13, 23, 33, and 43, and the deciduous canines would be 53, 63, 73, and 83.
- ***American (Universal) system,*** which is the most commonly used notation in North America. In this system, the permanent dentition is designated by arabic numerals, and the deciduous dentition is designated with uppercase letters. For permanent dentition, numbering begins in the UR quadrant, with the UR third molar designated number 1. Numbering continues across the maxillary arch to the UL third molar, designated tooth number 16. Tooth number 17 is the third molar located in the LL quadrant inferior and opposite to tooth number 16. Then, the numbering progresses across the mandibular arch and terminates with tooth number 32, the LR third molar. ***In this system, the sum of the numbers of opposing teeth adds up to 33.*** For the deciduous dentition, the same pattern is followed, but the letters A to T are used to designate the individual teeth. Thus, in this system, the permanent canines are designated 6, 11, 22, and 27, and the deciduous canines, C, H, M, and R.

Also note that in Figure 15.6 the color outline demonstrates the relationship of the deciduous and permanent dentitions. Examination of the table reveals that deciduous molars are replaced with permanent premolars after exfoliation and that the permanent molars have no deciduous precursors.

- A ***canine,*** which erupts at age 10 to 12
- Two ***premolar teeth,*** which erupt between ages 10 and 12
- Three ***molar teeth,*** which erupt at different times; the first molar usually erupts at age 6, the second molar in the early teens, and the third molar ***(wisdom teeth)*** during the late teens or early twenties

Incisors, canines, and premolars have one root each, except for the first premolar of the maxilla, which has two roots. Molars have three and, on rare occasions, four roots. All teeth have the same basic structure, however.

Teeth consist of several layers of specialized tissues

Teeth are made up of three specialized tissues:

- enamel
- dentin
- cementum

Enamel is an acellular mineralized tissue that covers the crown of the tooth. Once formed it cannot be replaced. Enamel is a unique tissue because unlike bone, which is formed from connective tissue, it is a ***mineralized material*** derived from epithelium. Enamel is more highly mineralized and harder than any other mineralized tissue in the body. The enamel that is exposed and visible above the gum line is called the ***clinical crown;*** the ***anatomic crown*** describes all of the tooth that is covered by enamel, some of which is below the gum line. Enamel varies in thickness over the crown and may be as thick as 2.5 mm on the ***cusps*** (biting and grinding surfaces) of some teeth. The enamel layer ends at the ***neck*** or ***cervix*** of the tooth at the ***cementoenamel junction*** (Fig. 15.7); the ***root*** of the tooth is then covered by ***cementum,*** a bone-like material. ***Dentin*** lies deep to the enamel and cementum.

Enamel

Enamel is the hardest substance in the body; it consists of 96% to 98% hydroxyapatite

The nonstoichiometric carbonated calcium hydroxyapatite enamel crystals that form the enamel are arranged as ***rods*** that measure 4 μm wide and 8 μm high. Each enamel rod spans the full thickness of the enamel layer from the dentinoenamel junction to the enamel surface. When examined in cross section at higher magnification, the rods reveal a keyhole shape (Fig. 15.8; the ballooned part or head is oriented superiorly and the tail is directed inferiorly toward the root of the tooth. The enamel crystals are primarily oriented parallel to the long axis of the rod within the head, and in the tail they are oriented more obliquely (Figs. 15.8 and 15.9). The limited spaces between the rods are also filled with enamel crystals. Striations observed on enamel rods (contour lines of Retzius) may represent evidence of rhythmic growth of the enamel in the developing tooth. A wider line of hypomineralization is observed in the enamel of the deciduous teeth. This line, called the neonatal line, marks the nutritional changes that take place between prenatal and postnatal life.

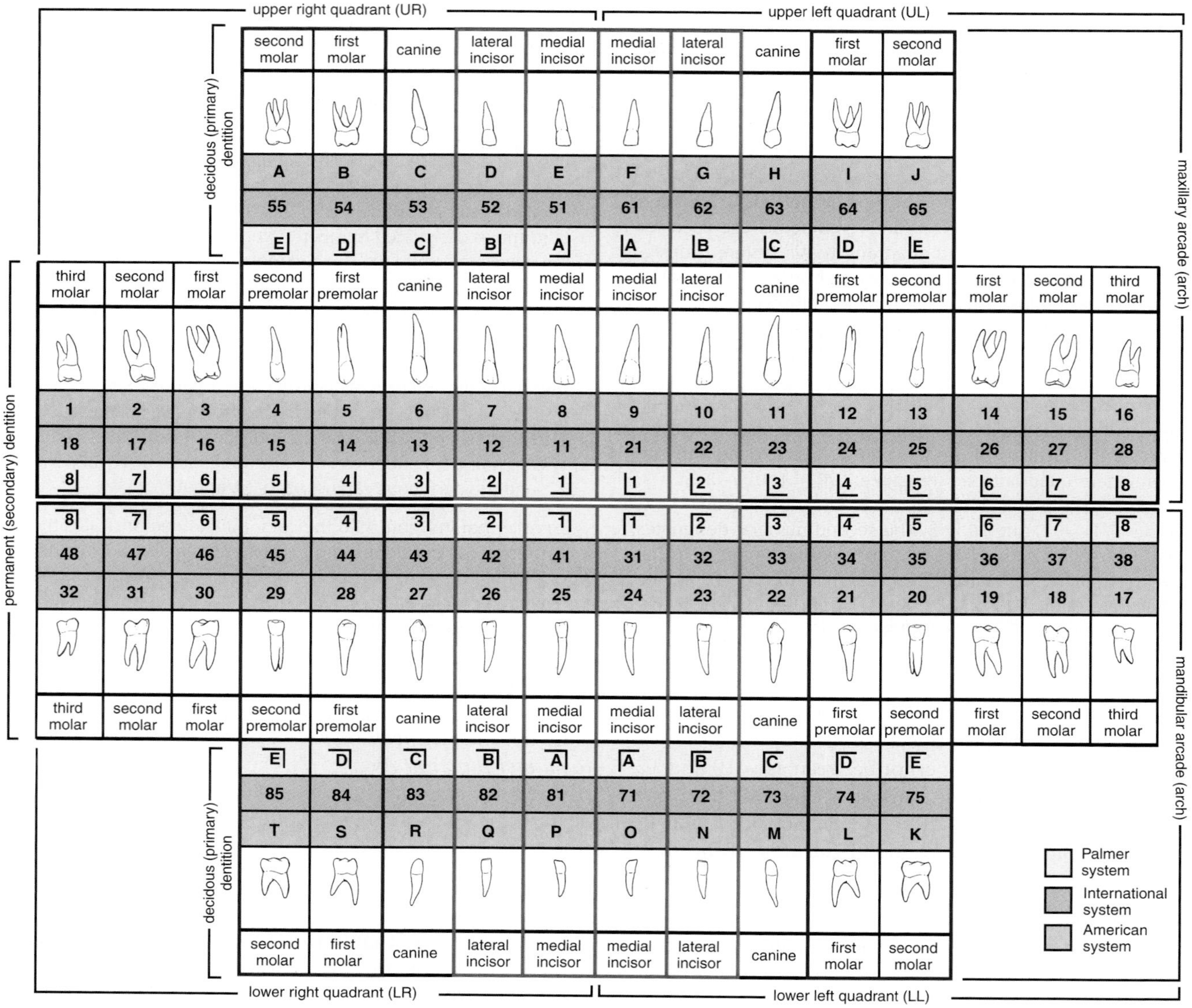

FIGURE 15.6

Classification of permanent and deciduous teeth. Three systems of tooth classification are used. The *central panel* of the diagram shows the permanent teeth, while the *upper and lower panels* show the deciduous teeth. Dentition is divided into four quadrants: upper left (UL), upper right (UR), lower left (LL), and lower right (LR). Each quadrant includes 8 permanent teeth and/or 5 deciduous teeth. In the American (Universal) system *(blue)*, permanent teeth are designated with Arabic numerals. The numbering begins from the wisdom tooth in the upper right quadrant designated as tooth number 1 and continues along all the teeth in the maxilla to tooth number 16 that designates the third upper left molar. The numbering progresses to the mandible, beginning at the third left lower molar designated as number 17 to the third lower right molar designated as number 32. In the American system, deciduous teeth are marked with capital letters designated for each tooth. The pattern is the same as that for permanent teeth, so the numbering begins from the second upper right molar and finishes with the second lower right molar. In the International system *(red)*, also referred to as the Two Digit System, each tooth is designated with two numbers: The first number indicates the dentition quadrant, which is marked from 1 to 4 and from 5 to 8 in clockwise direction beginning from the upper right quadrant for permanent and deciduous teeth, respectively. The second number specifies individual teeth in each quadrant beginning from the midline where the medial incisors are designated as number 1 and third molars are designated as number 8. In the Palmer system *(yellow)*, the dentition is divided into four quadrants with a right-angle bracket. The vertical line of the bracket divides the dentition into a right and a left side beginning at the midline. The horizontal line of the bracket divides the dentition into the upper and lower parts to designate teeth in the maxilla and mandible. In the Palmer system permanent teeth are numbered with Arabic numerals beginning from the midline. The deciduous teeth are marked with capital letters also starting from the midline. To mark a particular tooth with the Palmer system, two lines (vertical and horizontal) and the correct number or letter of the tooth are needed. (Table design courtesy of Dr. Wade T. Schultz.)

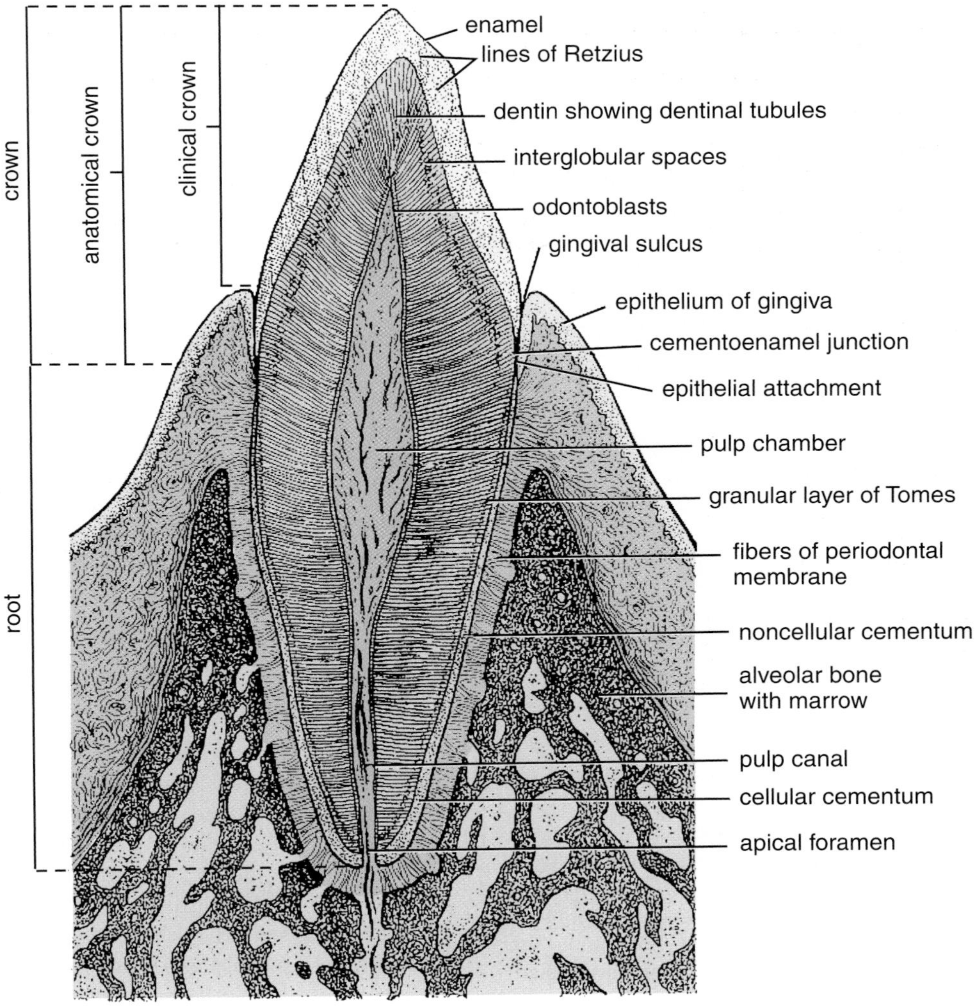

FIGURE 15.7

Diagram of a section of an incisor tooth and surrounding bony and mucosal structures. The three mineralized components of the tooth are dentin, enamel, and cementum. The central soft core of the tooth is the pulp. The periodontal ligament (membrane) contains bundles of collagenous fibers that bind the tooth to the surrounding alveolar bone. The clinical crown of the tooth is the portion that projects into the oral cavity. The anatomical crown is the entire portion of the tooth covered by enamel. (Modified from Copenhaver WM, ed. *Bailey's Textbook of Histology.* Baltimore: Williams & Wilkins, 1964.)

Although the enamel of an erupted tooth lacks cells and cell processes, it is not a static tissue. It is influenced by substances in saliva, the secretion of the salivary glands, which are essential to its maintenance. The substances in saliva that affect teeth include

- Digestive enzymes
- Antibacterial enzymes
- Antibodies
- Inorganic (mineral) components

Mature enamel contains very little organic material. Despite its hardness, enamel can be decalcified by acid-producing bacteria acting on food products trapped on the enamel surface. This is the basis of the initiation of ***dental caries.*** Fluoride added to the hydroxyapatite complex makes the enamel more resistant to acid demineralization. The widespread use of fluoride in drinking water, toothpaste, pediatric vitamin supplements, and mouthwashes significantly reduces the incidence of dental caries.

Enamel is produced by ameloblasts of the enamel organ, and dentin by odontoblasts of the adjacent mesenchyme

The ***enamel organ*** is an epithelial formation that is derived from ectodermal epithelial cells of the oral cavity. The onset of tooth development is marked by proliferation of oral epithelium to form a horseshoe-shaped cellular band of tissue, the dental lamina, in the adjacent mes-

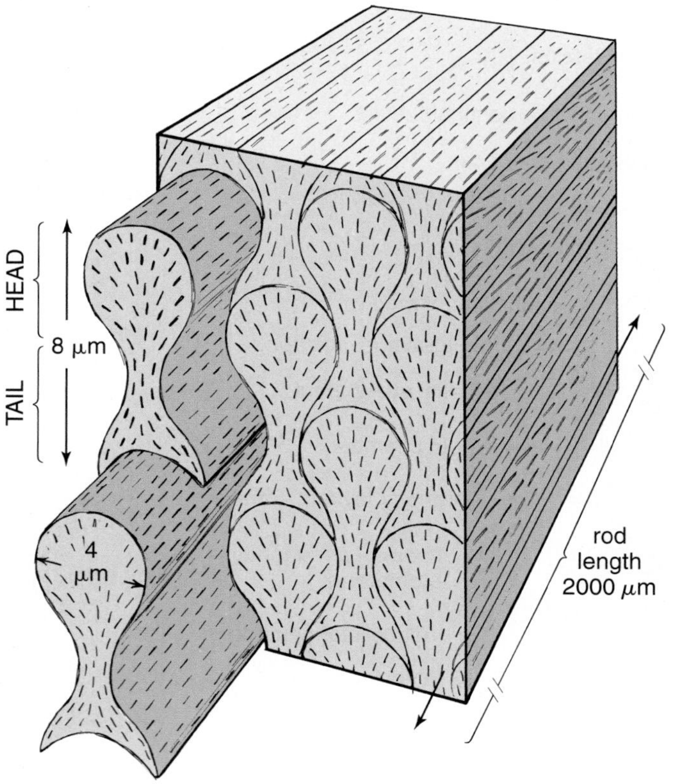

FIGURE 15.8
Diagram showing the basic organization and structure of enamel rods. The enamel rod is a thin structure extending from the dentinoenamel junction to the surface of the enamel. Where the enamel is thickest, at the tip of the crown, the rods are longest, measuring up to 2,000 μm. On cross section, the rods reveal a keyhole shape. The upper ballooned part of the rod, called the head, is oriented superiorly, and the lower part of the rod, called the tail, is directed inferiorly. Within the head, most of the enamel crystals are oriented parallel to the long axis of each rod. Within the tail, the crystals are oriented more obliquely.

enchyme where the upper and lower jaws will develop. At the site of each future tooth, there is a further proliferation of cells that arise from the dental lamina, resulting in a rounded, cellular, bud-like outgrowth, one for each tooth, that projects into the underlying mesenchymal tissue. This outgrowth, referred to as the ***bud stage,*** represents the early enamel organ (Fig. 15.10a). Gradually, the rounded cell mass enlarges and then develops a concavity at the site opposite where it arose from the dental lamina. The enamel organ is now referred to as being in the *cap stage* (Fig. 15.10b). Further growth and development of the enamel organ results in the ***bell stage*** (Fig. 15.10, c and d). At this stage the enamel organ consists of four recognizable cellular components:

- ***Outer enamel epithelium,*** made up of a cell layer that forms the convex surface
- ***Inner enamel epithelium,*** made up of a cell layer that forms the concave surface
- ***Stratum intermedium,*** a cell layer that develops internal to the inner enamel epithelium
- ***Stellate reticulum,*** made up of cells that have a stellate appearance and occupy the inner portion of the enamel organ

The mesenchymal cells within the "bell" adjacent to the inner enamel epithelial cells become columnar and have an epithelial type appearance. They will become ***odontoblasts*** and form the dentin of the tooth. The inner enamel epithelial cells of the enamel organ will become ***ameloblasts.*** Along with the cells of the stratum intermedium, they will be responsible for enamel production. At the early stage, just prior to dentinogenesis and amelogenesis, the dental lamina degenerates, leaving the developing tooth primordium detached from its site of origin.

Dental enamel is formed by a matrix-mediated biomineralization process known as ***amelogenesis.*** The major stages of amelogenesis are

- ***Matrix production,*** or ***secretory stage.*** In the formation of mineralized tissues of the tooth, dentin is produced first. Then, partially mineralized enamel matrix (Fig. 15.11) is deposited directly on the surface of the previously formed dentin. The cells producing this partially mineralized organic matrix are called ***secretory-stage ameloblasts.*** As do osteoblasts in bone, these cells produce an organic proteinaceous matrix by activity of the rough endoplasmic reticulum (rER), Golgi apparatus, and secretory granules. The secretory-stage ameloblasts continue to produce enamel matrix until the full thickness of the future enamel is achieved.
- ***Matrix maturation.*** Maturation of the partially mineralized enamel matrix involves the removal of organic material as well as continued influx of calcium and phosphate into the maturing enamel. Cells involved in this second stage of enamel formation are called ***maturation-stage ameloblasts.*** Maturation-stage ameloblasts differentiate from secretory-stage ameloblasts and function primarily as a transport epithelium, moving substances into and out of the maturing enamel. Maturation-stage ameloblasts undergo cyclical alterations in their morphology that correspond to cyclical entry of calcium into the enamel.

Secretory-stage ameloblasts are polarized columnar cells that produce enamel

The secretory-stage ameloblast lies directly adjacent to the developing enamel. At the apical pole of each ameloblast is a process, ***Tomes' process,*** which is surrounded by the developing enamel (Fig. 15.12). A cluster of mitochondria in the base of the cell accounts for the

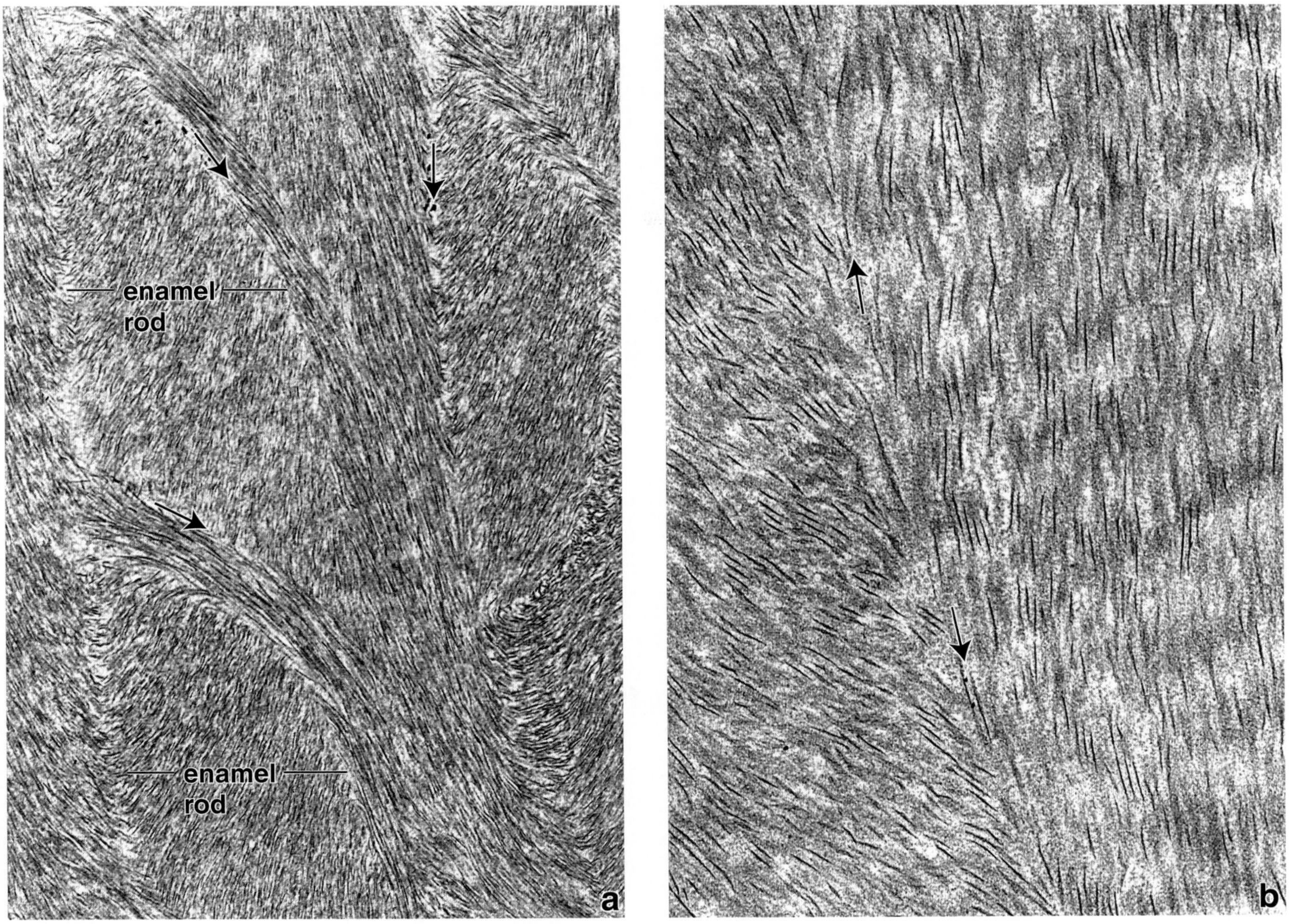

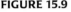

FIGURE 15.9
Structure of young enamel. a. This electron micrograph shows enamel rods cut obliquely. *Arrows* indicate the boundaries between adjacent rods. ×14,700. **b.** Parts of two adjacent rods are seen at higher magnification. *Arrows* mark the boundary between the two rods. The dark needle-like objects are young hydroxyapatite crystals; the substance between the hydroxyapatite crystals is the organic matrix of the developing enamel. As the enamel matures, the hydroxyapatite crystals grow, and the bulk of the organic matrix is removed. ×60,000.

eosinophilic staining of this region in hematoxylin and eosin (H&E)–stained paraffin sections (Fig. 15.13). Adjacent to the mitochondria is the nucleus; in the main column of cytoplasm are the rER, Golgi, secretory granules, and other cell elements. Junctional complexes are present at both apical and basal parts of the cell. They maintain the integrity and orientation of the ameloblasts as they move away from the dentoenamel junction. Actin filaments joined to these junctional complexes are involved in moving the secretory-stage ameloblast over the developing enamel. The rod produced by the ameloblast follows in the wake of the cell. Thus, in mature enamel, the direction of the enamel rod is a record of the path taken earlier by the secretory-stage ameloblast.

At their base, the secretory-stage ameloblasts are adjacent to a layer of enamel organ cells called the ***stratum intermedium*** (see Fig. 15.10, b, c, and g). The plasma membrane of these cells, especially at the base of the ameloblasts, contains alkaline phosphatase, an enzyme active in calcification. Stellate enamel organ cells are external to the stratum intermedium and are separated from the adjacent blood vessels by a basal lamina.

Maturation-stage ameloblasts transport substances needed for enamel maturation

The histologic feature that marks the cycles of maturation-stage ameloblasts is a striated or ruffled border (Fig.

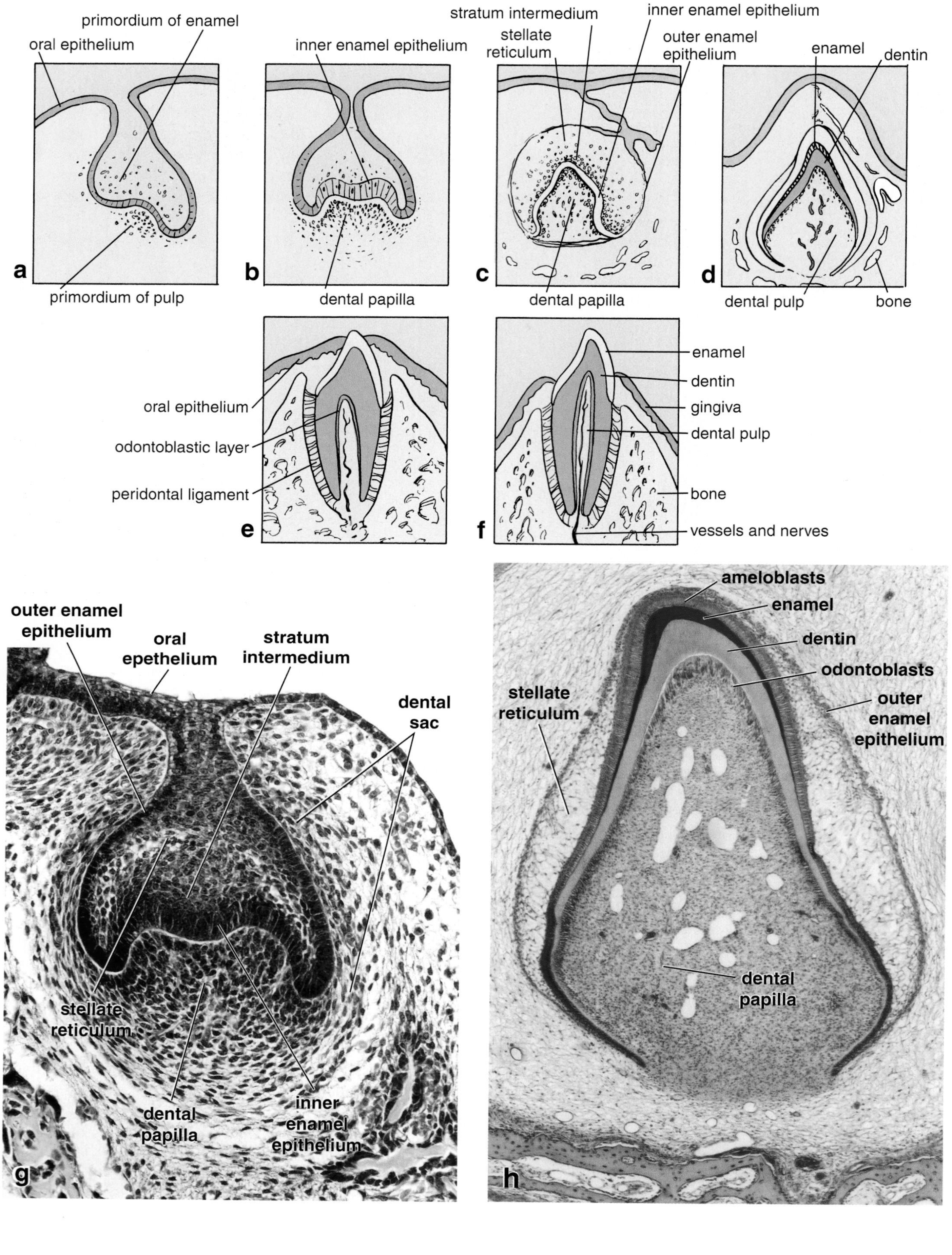
oral epithelium
primordium of enamel
primordium of pulp
a
inner enamel epithelium
dental papilla
b
stratum intermedium
stellate reticulum
inner enamel epithelium
outer enamel epithelium
dental papilla
c
enamel
dentin
dental pulp
bone
d
oral epithelium
odontoblastic layer
peridontal ligament
e
enamel
dentin
gingiva
dental pulp
bone
vessels and nerves
f
outer enamel epithelium
oral epethelium
stratum intermedium
dental sac
stellate reticulum
dental papilla
inner enamel epithelium
g
ameloblasts
enamel
dentin
odontoblasts
stellate reticulum
outer enamel epithelium
dental papilla
h

FIGURE 15.10
Diagrams and photomicrographs of a developing tooth. a. In this bud stage, the oral epithelium invaginates into the underlying mesenchyme, giving origin to the enamel organ (primordium of enamel). Mesenchymal cells adjacent to the tooth bud begin to differentiate, forming the dental papilla that protrudes into the tooth bud. **b.** Tooth bud in cap stage. In this stage, cells located in the concavity of the cap differentiate into tall, columnar cells (ameloblasts) forming the inner enamel epithelium. The condensed mesenchyme invaginates into the inner enamel epithelium, forming the dental papilla, which gives rise to the dentin and the pulp. **c.** In this bell stage, the connection with the oral epithelium is almost cut off. The enamel organ consists of a narrow line of outer enamel epithelium, an inner enamel epithelium formed by ameloblasts, several condensed layers of cells that form the stratum intermedium, and the widely spaced stellate reticulum. The dental papilla is deeply invaginated against the enamel organ. **d.** In this appositional dentin and enamel stage, the tooth bud is completely differentiated and independent from the oral epithelium. The relationship of the two mineralized tissues of the dental crown, enamel and dentin, is clearly visible. The surrounding mesenchyme has developed into bony tissue. **e.** In this stage of tooth eruption, the apex of the tooth emerges through the surface of the oral epithelium. The odontoblastic layer lines the pulp cavity. Note the developed periodontal ligaments that fasten the root of the tooth to the surrounding bone. The apex of the root is still open, but after eruption occurs, it becomes narrower. **f.** Functional tooth stage. Note the distribution of enamel and dentin. The tooth is embedded in surrounding bone and gingiva. **g.** This photomicrograph of the developing tooth in the cap stage (comparable to *b*) shows its connection with the oral epithelium. The enamel organ consists of a single layer of cuboidal cells forming the outer enamel epithelium; the inner enamel epithelium has differentiated into columnar ameloblasts; and the layer of cells adjacent to the inner enamel epithelium has formed the stratum intermedium. The remainder of the structure is occupied by the stellate reticulum. The mesenchyme of the dental papilla has proliferated and pushed into the enamel organ. At this stage, the forming tooth is surrounded by condensed mesenchyme, called the dental sac, which gives rise to periodontal structures. ×300. **h.** This photomicrograph shows the developing crown of an incisor, which is surrounded by the outer enamel epithelium and remnants of the stellate reticulum. It is comparable to *d*. The underlying lighter-stained layer of dentin is a product of the odontoblasts. These tall columnar odontoblasts have differentiated from cells of the dental papilla. The pulp cavity is filled with dental pulp, and blood vessels permeate the pulp tissue. ×40.

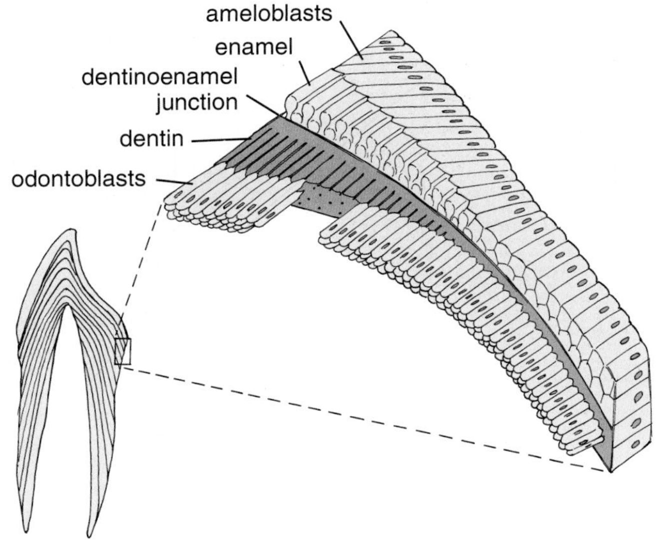

FIGURE 15.11
Diagram showing the cellular relationships during enamel formation. In the initial secretory stage, dentin is produced first by odontoblasts. Enamel matrix is then deposited directly on the surface of the previously formed dentin by secretory-stage ameloblasts. The secretory-stage ameloblasts continue to produce enamel matrix until the full thickness of the future enamel is achieved. (Adapted from Schour I. The neonatal line in the enamel and dentin of the human deciduous teeth and first permanent molar. *J Am Dent Assoc* 1936;23:1946. Fig 2. Copyright © 2002 American Dental Association. Adapted 2002 with permission of ADA Publishing, a Division of ADA Business Enterprises, Inc.)

15.14). Maturation-stage ameloblasts with a striated border occupy approximately 70% of a specific cycle, and those that are smooth-ended, approximately 30% of a specific cycle. There is no stratum intermedium in the enamel organ during enamel maturation; stellate ***papillary cells*** are adjacent to the maturation-stage ameloblasts.

The maturation-stage ameloblasts and the adjacent papillary cells are characterized by numerous mitochondria. Their presence indicates cellular activity that requires large amounts of energy and reflects the function of maturation-stage ameloblasts and adjacent papillary cells as a transporting epithelium.

Recent advances in the molecular biology of ameloblast gene products have revealed the enamel matrix to be highly heterogenous. It contains proteins encoded by a number of different genes. The principal proteins in the extracellular matrix of the developing enamel are

- ***Amelogenins,*** important proteins in establishing and maintaining the spacing between enamel rods in early stages of enamel development
- ***Ameloblastins,*** proteins produced by ameloblasts from the early secretory to late maturation stages. Their function is not well understood; however, their developmental pattern suggests that ameloblastins play a much broader role in amelogenesis than the other proteins, and they are believed to guide the enamel mineralization process by controlling elongation of the enamel crystals.
- ***Enamelins,*** proteins distributed throughout the enamel layer. These enamel proteinases (ameloproteases-I) are responsible for degradation of amelogenins in maturing enamel.
- ***Tuftelins,*** acidic enamel proteins located near the dentinoenamel junction that participate in the nucleation of enamel crystal. Tuftelins are present in ***enamel tufts*** and account for hypomineralization; i.e., enamel tufts have a higher percentage of organic material than the remainder of the mature enamel.

The maturation of the developing enamel results in its continued mineralization, so that it becomes the hardest

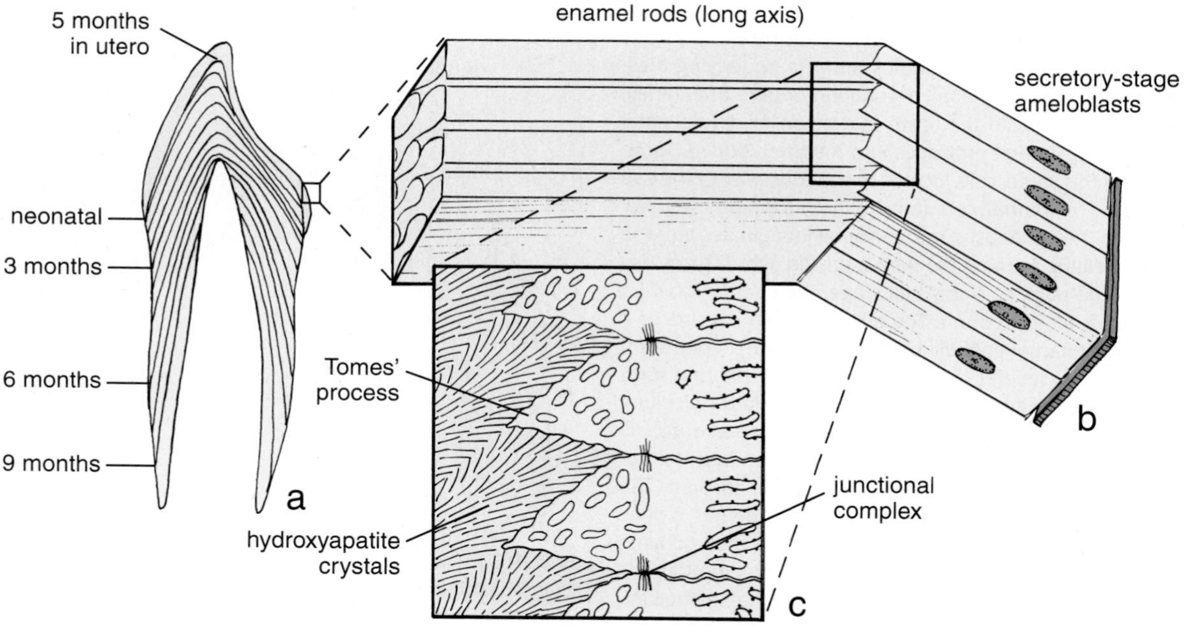

FIGURE 15.12
Schematic diagrams of a partially formed tooth showing details of amelogenesis. a. The enamel is drawn to show the enamel rods extending from the dentinoenamel junction to the surface of the tooth. Although the full thickness of the enamel is formed, the full thickness of the dentin has not yet been established. The contour lines within the dentin show the extent to which the dentin has developed at a particular time, as labeled in the illustration. Note that the pulp cavity in the center of the tooth becomes smaller as the dentin develops. (Based on Schour I, Massler M. *J Am Dent Assoc* 1936;23:1948.) **b.** During amelogenesis, enamel formation is influenced by the path of the ameloblasts. The rod produced by the ameloblast forms in the wake of the cell. Thus, in mature enamel, the direction of the enamel rod is a record of the path taken earlier by the secretory-stage ameloblast. **c.** At the apical pole of the secretory-stage ameloblasts are Tomes' processes, surrounded by the developing enamel. Junctional complexes at the apical pole are also shown. Note the numerous matrix-containing secretory vesicles in the cytoplasm of the processes.

substance in the body. Amelogenins and ameloblastins are removed during enamel maturation. Thus, mature enamel contains only enamelins and tuftelins. The ameloblasts degenerate after the enamel is fully formed, at about the time of tooth eruption through the gum.

Cementum

Cementum covers the root of the tooth

The root is the part of the tooth that fits into its ***socket*** or ***alveolus*** in the maxilla or mandible. ***Cementum*** is a thin layer of bone-like material that is secreted by ***cementocytes,*** cells that closely resemble osteocytes. Like bone, cementum is 65% mineral. The lacunae and canaliculi in the cementum contain the cementocytes and their processes, respectively. They resemble those structures in bone that contain osteocytes and osteocyte processes.

Unlike bone, cementum is avascular. Also, the canaliculi in cementum do not form an interconnecting network. A layer of ***cementoblasts*** (cells that resemble the osteoblasts of the surface of growing bone) is seen on the outer surface of the cementum, adjacent to the ***periodontal ligament.***

Collagen fibers that project out of the matrix of the cementum and embed in the bony matrix of the socket wall form the bulk of the periodontal ligament. These fibers are another example of ***Sharpey's fibers*** (Fig. 15.15). In addition, elastic fibers are also a component of the periodontal ligament. This mode of attachment of the tooth in its socket allows slight movement of the tooth to occur naturally. It also forms the basis of orthodontic procedures used to straighten teeth and reduce malocclusion of the biting and grinding surfaces of the maxillary and mandibular teeth. During corrective tooth movements, the alveolar bone of the socket is resorbed and resynthesized, but the cementum is not.

Dentin

Dentin is a calcified material that forms most of the tooth substance

Dentin lies deep to the enamel and cementum. It contains less hydroxyapatite than enamel, about 70%, but more than is found in bone and cementum. Dentin is secreted by ***odontoblasts*** that form an epithelial layer over the inner surface of the dentin, i.e., the surface that is in

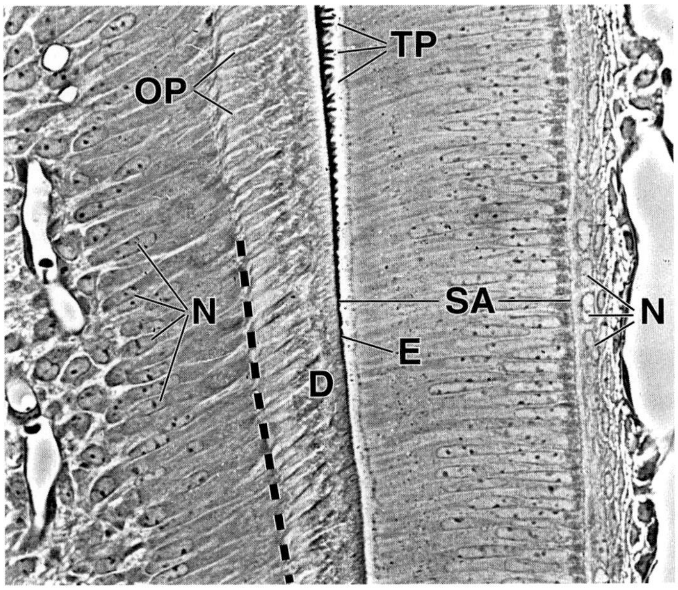

FIGURE 15.13
Enamel organ cells and odontoblasts in a developing tooth. This photomicrograph of an unstained plastic thick section viewed with the phase contrast microscope shows enamel organ cells and odontoblasts as they begin to produce enamel *(E)* and dentin *(D)*, respectively. Young enamel is deposited by secretory-stage ameloblasts *(SA)* onto the previously formed dentin. The enamel appears dark in the illustration. At the top, the enamel surface displays a characteristic picket-fence pattern because of the sharp contrast between the lightly stained Tomes' processes *(TP)* of the secretory-stage ameloblasts and the darkly stained young enamel product that partly surrounds the cell processes. The nuclei *(N)* at the right belong to cells of the stratum intermedium. The nuclei *(N)* on the left belong to odontoblasts located in the basal part of the cells. The odontoblast cytoplasm extends to the *dashed line.* At this point, cytoplasmic processes *(OP)* extend into the dentin. ×85.

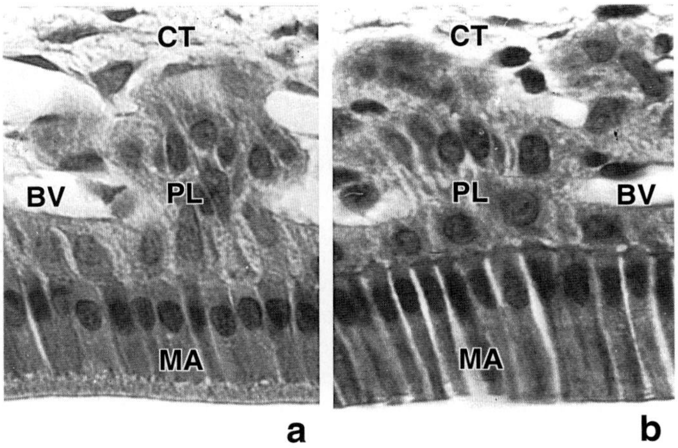

FIGURE 15.14
Ameloblasts in different stages of maturation. a. This black and white microphotograph of an H&E–stained specimen shows maturation-stage ameloblasts *(MA)* in demineralized tissue. The maturing enamel has been lost during slide preparation, and the space below the ameloblasts previously occupied by the enamel appears empty. Maturation-stage ameloblasts with a striated border account for 80% of the cell population in the maturation zone. *BV,* blood vessels; *CT,* connective tissue; *PL,* papillary layer. ×650. **b.** This photomicrograph shows smooth-ended maturation-stage ameloblasts *(MA),* which account for 20% of the cell population in the mature zone. At the basal pole of the ameloblasts are the cells of the papillary layer *(PL).* A layer of stratum intermedium is no longer present during this stage of ameloblast maturation. ×650.

BOX 15.3

Functional Considerations: Histologic Preparation of Tooth Tissues

Because most parts of the tooth are highly mineralized, teeth are prepared for histologic study by methods similar to those used for bone, namely, by means of ground sections and stained demineralized sections. Ground sections are most often used to study an extracted or exfoliated tooth. As in the preparation of bone, the ground section displays mineralized tissue but destroys soft tissue; demineralization removes mineral and retains soft tissue. Demineralized sections have the advantage that they can be used to view a section of a tooth to study its relationship to the adjacent supporting structures. In routinely demineralized sections of a mature tooth, however, the enamel is dissolved and lost. Therefore, diagrams of a tooth showing features of both enamel and soft tissues are composite diagrams that combine data derived from both ground and demineralized sections (see Fig. 15.7).

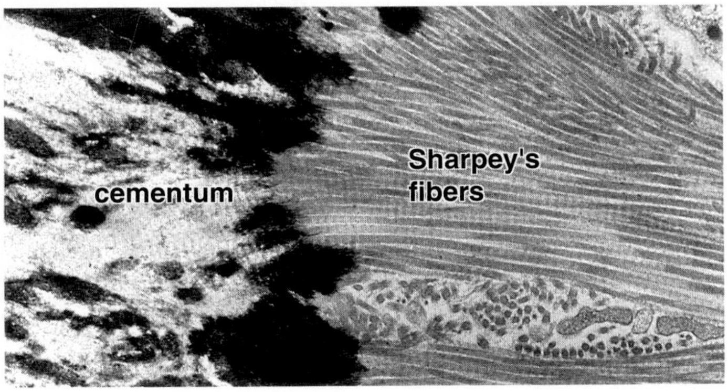

FIGURE 15.15
Electron micrograph of Sharpey's fibers. Sharpey's fibers extend from the periodontal ligament (right) into the cementum. They consist of collagen fibrils. Sharpey's fibers within the cementum are mineralized; those within the periodontal ligament are not mineralized. ×13,000.

contact with the pulp (Fig. 15.16). Like ameloblasts, odontoblasts are columnar cells that contain a well-developed rER, a large Golgi apparatus, and other organelles associated with the synthesis and secretion of large amounts of protein (Fig. 15.17). The apical surface of the odontoblast is in contact with the forming dentin; junctional complexes between the odontoblasts at that level separate the dentinal compartment from the pulp compartment.

The layer of odontoblasts retreats as the dentin is laid down, leaving odontoblast processes embedded in the dentin in narrow channels called ***dentinal tubules*** (see Fig. 15.15). The tubules and processes continue to elongate as the dentin continues to thicken by rhythmic growth. The rhythmic growth of dentin produces certain "growth lines" in the dentin (incremental lines of von Ebner and thicker lines of Owen) that mark significant developmental times such as birth ***(neonatal line)*** and when unusual substances such as lead are incorporated into the growing tooth. Study of growth lines has proved useful in forensic medicine.

Predentin is the newly secreted organic matrix, closest to the cell body of the odontoblast, which has yet to be mineralized. Although most of the proteins in the organic matrix are similar to those of bone, predentin contains two unique proteins:

- ***Dentin phosphoprotein (DPP),*** which is rich in aspartic acid and phosphoserine and binds large amounts of calcium. DPP is involved in initiation of mineralization and in control of mineral size and shape.
- ***Dentin sialoprotein (DSP),*** which is rich in aspartic acid, serine, glutamic acid, and glycine and is also involved in the mineralization process.

An unusual feature of the secretion of collagen and hydroxyapatite by odontoblasts is the presence, in Golgi vesicles, of arrays of a formed filamentous collagen precursor. Granules believed to contain calcium attach to these precursors, giving rise to structures called ***abacus bodies*** (Figs. 15.17 and 15.18). Abacus bodies become more condensed as they mature into secretory granules.

Dentin is produced by odontoblasts

Dentin is the first mineralized component of the tooth to be deposited. The outermost dentin, which is referred to as mantle dentin, is formed by subodontoblastic cells that produce small bundles of collagen fibers (von Korff's

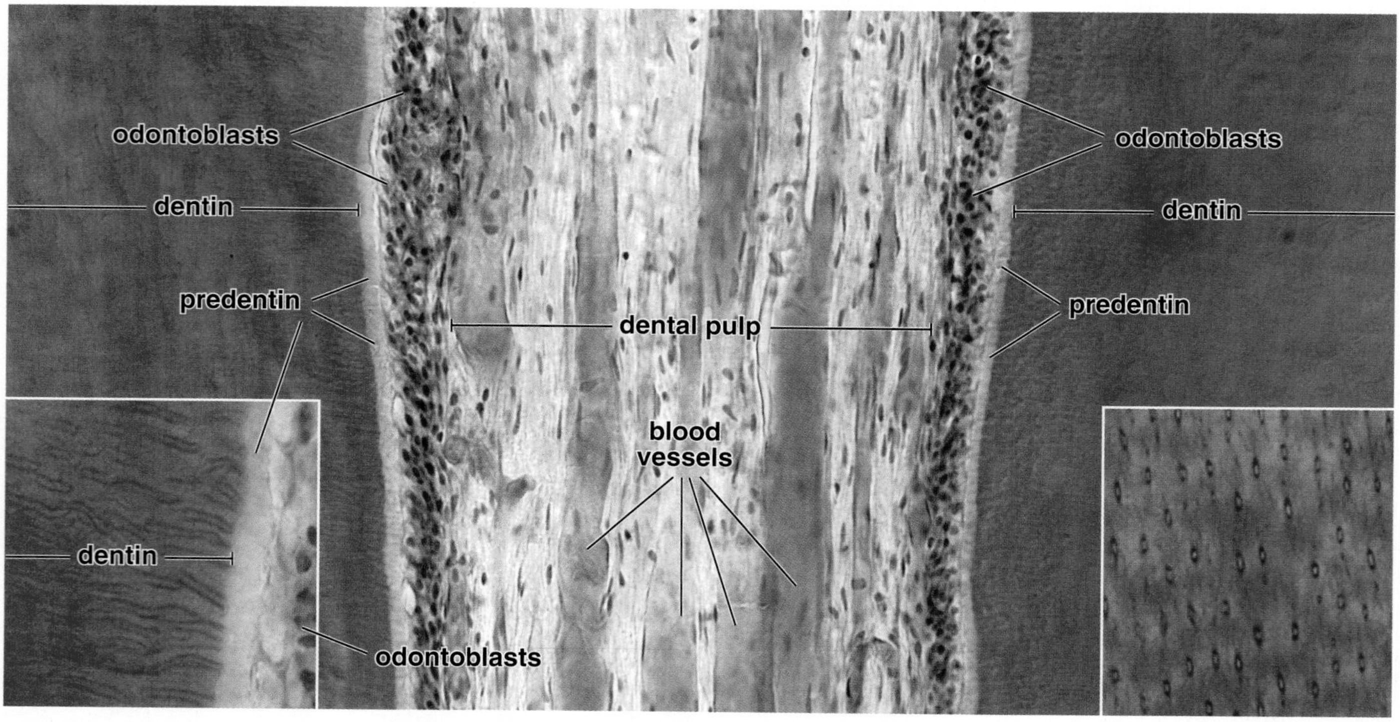

FIGURE 15.16

Dental pulp and structure of dentin. This photomicrograph of a decalcified tooth shows the centrally located dental pulp, surrounded by dentin on both sides. The dental pulp is a soft tissue core of the tooth that resembles embryonic connective tissue, even in the adult. It contains blood vessels and nerves. Dentin contains the cytoplasmic processes of the odontoblasts within dentinal tubules. They extend into the dentinoenamel junction. The cell bodies of the odontoblasts are adjacent to the unmineralized dentin called the predentin. ×120. **Left inset.** Longitudinal profiles of the dentinal tubules. ×240. **Right inset.** Cross-sectional profiles of dentinal tubules. The dark outline of the dentinal tubules, as seen in both *insets,* represents the peritubular dentin, which is the more mineralized part of the dentin. ×240.

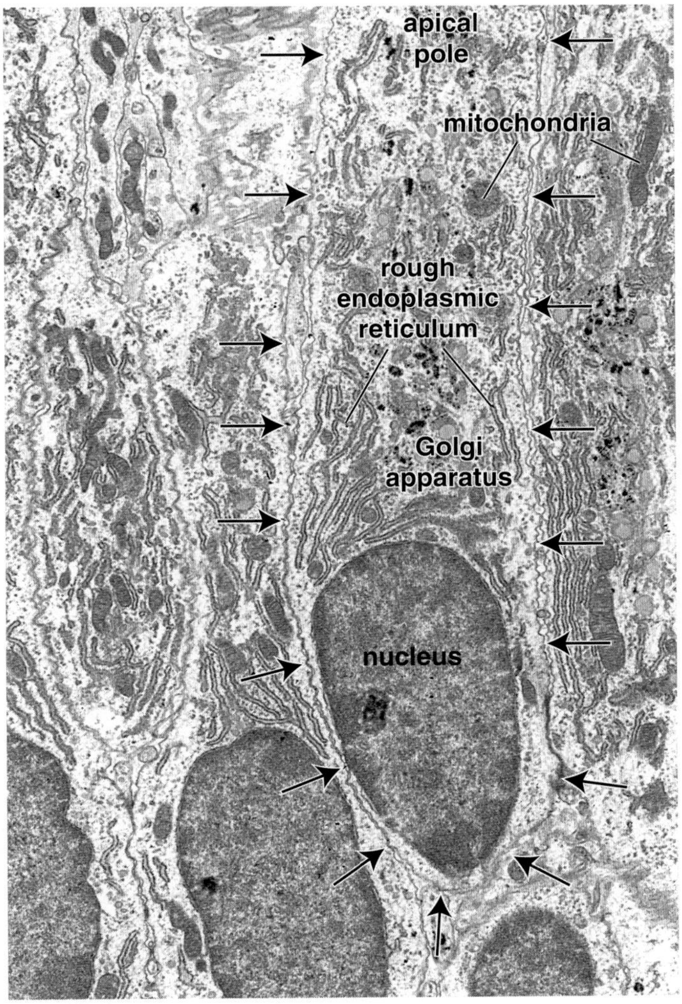

FIGURE 15.17
Electron micrograph of odontoblasts. The plasma membrane of one odontoblast has been marked with *arrows.* The cell contains a large amount of rough endoplasmic reticulum and a large Golgi apparatus. The odontoblast processes are not included in this image; one process would extend from the apical pole of each cell (top). The black objects in the Golgi region are abacus bodies. The tissue has been treated with pyroantimonate, which forms a black precipitate with calcium. ×12,000.

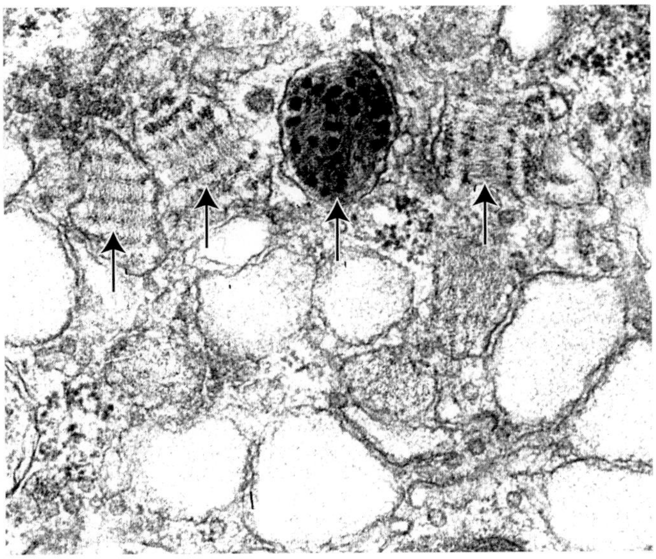

FIGURE 15.18
Golgi apparatus in an odontoblast. This electron micrograph shows a region of the Golgi apparatus containing numerous large vesicles. Note the abacus bodies *(arrows)* that contain parallel arrays of filaments studded with granules. ×52,000.

fibers). The odontoblasts differentiate from cells at the periphery of the dental papilla. The progenitor cells have the appearance of typical mesenchymal cells; i.e., they contain little cytoplasm. During their differentiation into odontoblasts, the cytoplasmic volume and organelles characteristic of collagen-producing cells increase. The cells form a layer at the periphery of the dental papilla, and they secrete the organic matrix of dentin, or predentin, at their apical end (away from the dental papilla) (Fig. 15.19). As the predentin thickens, the odontoblasts move or are displaced centrally (see Fig. 15.12). A wave of mineralization follows the receding odontoblasts; this mineralized product is the dentin. As the cells move centrally, the odontoblastic processes elongate; the longest are surrounded by the mineralized dentin. In newly formed dentin, the wall of the dentinal tubule is simply the edge of the mineralized dentin. With time, the dentin immediately surrounding the dentinal tubule becomes more highly mineralized; this more mineralized sheath of dentin is referred to as the ***peritubular dentin.*** The remainder of the dentin is called the ***intertubular dentin.***

Dental Pulp and Central Pulp Cavity (Pulp Chamber)

The dental pulp cavity is a connective tissue compartment bounded by the tooth dentin

The ***central pulp cavity*** is the space within a tooth that is occupied by ***dental pulp,*** a loose connective tissue that is richly vascularized and supplied by abundant nerves. The pulp cavity takes the general shape of the tooth. The blood vessels and nerves enter the pulp cavity at the tip (apex) of the root, at a site called the ***apical foramen.*** (The designations *apex* and *apical* in this context refer only to the narrowed tip of the root of the tooth rather than to a luminal (apical) surface, as used in describing secretory and absorptive epithelia.)

The blood vessels and nerves extend to the crown of the tooth where they form vascular and neural networks beneath and within the layer of odontoblasts. Some bare nerve fibers also enter the proximal portions of the denti-

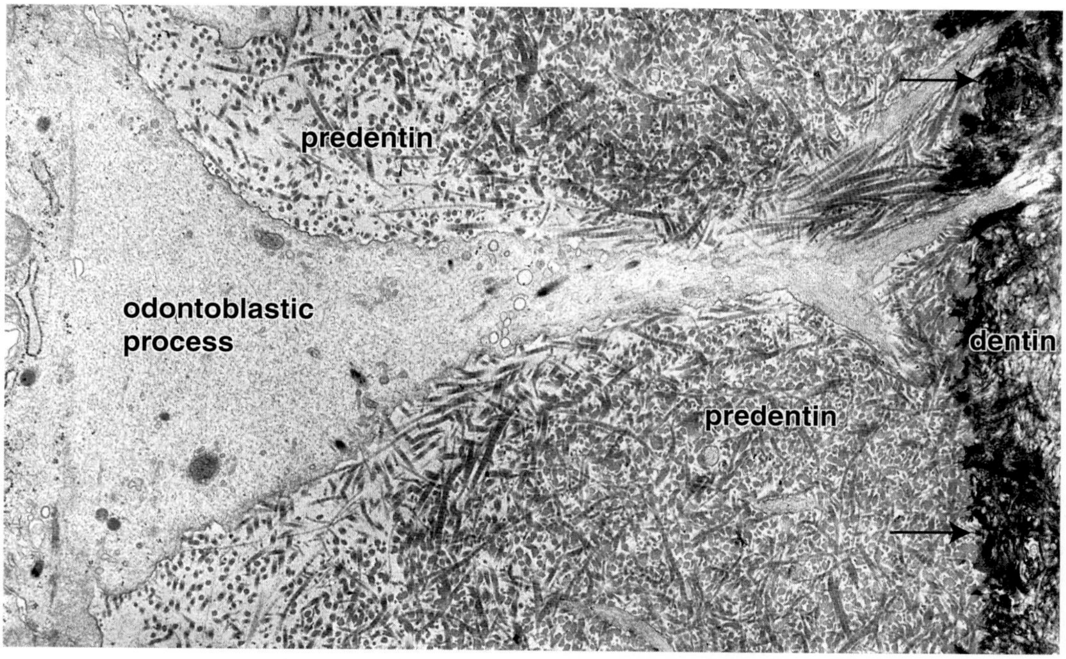

FIGURE 15.19
Odontoblast process of a young odontoblast. This electron micrograph shows a process of the odontoblast entering a dentinal tubule. The process extends into the predentin and, after passing the mineralization front *(arrows)*, lies within the dentin. The collagen fibrils in the predentin are finer than the more mature, courser fibrils of the mineralization front and beyond. ×34,000.

nal tubules and contact odontoblast processes. The odontoblast processes are believed to serve a transducer function in transmitting stimuli from the tooth surface to the nerves in the dental pulp. In teeth with more than one cusp, ***pulpal horns*** extend into the cusps and contain large numbers of nerve fibers. More of these fibers extend into the dentinal tubules than at other sites. Because dentin continues to be secreted throughout life, the pulp cavity decreases in volume with age.

Supporting Tissues of the Teeth

Supporting tissues of the teeth include the alveolar bone of the alveolar processes of the maxilla and mandible, periodontal ligaments, and gingiva.

The alveolar processes of the maxilla and mandible contain the sockets or alveoli for the roots of the teeth

The ***alveolar bone proper,*** a thin layer of compact bone, forms the wall of the alveolus (see Fig. 15.7) and is the bone to which the periodontal ligament is attached. The rest of the alveolar process consists of supporting bone.

The surface of the alveolar bone proper usually shows regions of bone resorption and bone deposition, particularly when a tooth is being moved (Fig. 15.20). Periodontal disease usually leads to loss of alveolar bone, as does the absence of functional occlusion of a tooth with its normal opposing tooth.

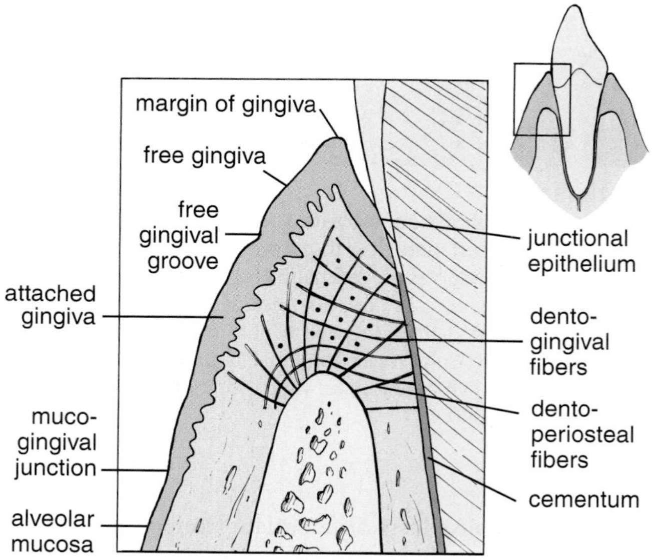

FIGURE 15.20
Schematic diagram of gingiva. This schematic diagram of gingiva corresponds to the *rectangular area* of the orientation diagram. The gingival epithelium is attached to the enamel of the tooth. Here, the junction between epithelium and connective tissue is smooth. Elsewhere, the gingival epithelium is deeply indented by connective tissue papillae, and the junction between the two is irregular. The *black lines* represent collagen fibers from the cementum of the tooth and from the crest of the alveolar bone that extend toward the gingival epithelium. Note the shallow papillae in the lining mucosa (alveolar mucosa) that contrast sharply with those of the gingiva.

The periodontal ligament secures the attachment of the tooth to the surrounding bone

The ***periodontal ligament*** is the fibrous connective tissue joining the tooth to its surrounding bone. This ligament is also called the ***periodontal membrane,*** but neither term describes its structure and function adequately. The periodontal ligament provides for

- Tooth attachment (fixation)
- Tooth support
- Bone remodeling (during movement of a tooth)
- Proprioception
- Tooth eruption

A histologic section of the periodontal ligament shows that it contains areas of both dense and loose connective tissue. The dense connective tissue contains collagen fibers and fibroblasts that are elongated parallel to the long axis of the collagen fibers. The fibroblasts are believed to move back and forth, leaving behind a trail of collagen fibers. Periodontal fibroblasts also contain internalized collagen fibrils that are digested by the hydrolytic enzymes of the cytoplasmic lysosomes. These observations indicate that the fibroblasts not only produce collagen fibrils but also resorb collagen fibrils, thereby adjusting continuously to the demands of tooth stress and movement.

The loose connective tissue in the periodontal ligament contains blood vessels and nerve endings. In addition to fibroblasts and thin collagenous fibers, the periodontal ligament also contains thin, longitudinally disposed ***oxytalan fibers.*** They are attached to bone or cementum at each end. Some appear to be associated with the adventitia of blood vessels.

The gingiva is the part of the mucous membrane commonly called the gums

The ***gingiva*** is a specialized part of the oral mucosa located around the neck of the tooth. It is firmly attached to the teeth and to underlying alveolar bony tissue. An idealized diagram of the gingiva is presented in Figure 15.20. The gingiva is composed of two parts:

- ***Gingival mucosa,*** which is synonymous with the masticatory mucosa described above (page 436)
- ***Junctional epithelium*** or ***attachment epithelium,*** which adheres firmly to the tooth. A basal lamina-like material is secreted by the junctional epithelium and adheres firmly to the tooth surface. The cells then attach to this material via hemidesmosomes. The basal lamina and the hemidesmosomes are together referred to as the ***epithelial attachment.*** In young individuals, this attachment is to the enamel; in older individuals, where passive tooth eruption and gingival recession expose the roots, the attachment is to the cementum.

BOX 15.4

Clinical Correlations: Dental Caries

Dental caries is an infectious microbial disease of teeth that results in the destruction of affected calcified tissues; i.e., enamel, dentin, and cementum. Carious lesions generally occur under masses of bacterial colonies referred to as "dental plaque." The onset of dental caries is primarily associated with bacterial colonies of *Streptococcus mutans,* while lactobacilli are associated with active progression of the disease. These bacterial colonies metabolize carbohydrates, producing an acidic environment that demineralizes the underlying tooth structure. Frequent sucrose ingestion is strongly associated with the development of these acidogenic bacterial colonies.

Trace amounts of fluoride, from sources such as water supplies (0.5 to 1.0 ppm is optimal), toothpaste, and even diet, can improve resistance to the effects of cariogenic bacteria. Fluoride improves the acid resistance of the tooth structure, acts as an antimicrobial agent, and promotes remineralization of small carious lesions. Resistance to acid breakdown of enamel is facilitated by the substitution of fluoride ion for the hydroxyl ion in the hydroxyapatite crystal. This decreases enamel crystal solubility in acid.

Treatment of cavitated lesions, or "tooth cavities" (Fig. 15.21), includes excavation of the infected tooth tissue and replacement with dental materials such as amalgam, composite, and glass ionomer cements. Microbial invasion of tooth structure can reach the "pulp" of the tooth and elicit an inflammatory response. In this case, endodontic treatment, or a "root canal," is generally recommended, with subsequent placement of a crown to add strength to the compromised coronal tooth structure.

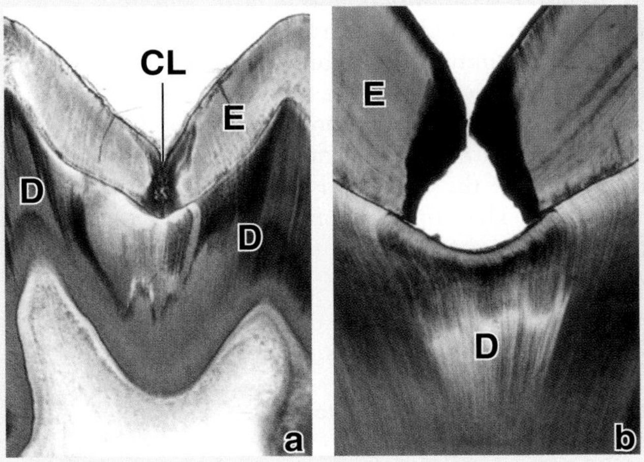

FIGURE 15.21
Photomicrographs of carious lesions. a. Photomicrograph of an unstained ground section of a tooth showing a carious lesion *(CL)* that has penetrated the entire thickness of the enamel *(E)* and spread laterally at the amelodentinal junction. *D,* dentin. **b.** The lesion here is more advanced. The enamel *(E)* has been undermined and weakened, causing fracture and a resulting cavity. At this point, bacteria can invade and penetrate down the exposed dental tubules, resulting in destructive liquefaction foci in the dentin *(D)* and, ultimately, exposure of the pulp. ×15. (From Eveson JW, Scully C. *Color Atlas of Oral Pathology.* London: Times Mirror International Publishers, 1995.)

Above the attachment of the epithelium to the tooth, a shallow crevice called the ***gingival sulcus,*** is lined with ***crevicular epithelium*** that is continuous with the attachment epithelium. The term ***periodontium*** refers to all the tissues involved in the attachment of a tooth to the mandible and maxilla. These include the crevicular and junctional epithelium, the cementum, the periodontal ligament, and the alveolar bone.

SALIVARY GLANDS

The major salivary glands are paired glands with long ducts that empty into the oral cavity

The major salivary glands, as noted above, consist of the paired parotid, submandibular, and sublingual glands. The parotid and the submandibular glands are actually located outside the oral cavity; their secretions reach the cavity by ducts. The parotid gland is located subcutaneously, below and in front of the ear in the temporal region of the head, and the submandibular gland is located under the floor of the mouth, in the submandibular triangle of the neck. The sublingual gland is located in the floor of the mouth anterior to the submandibular gland.

The minor salivary glands are located in the submucosa of different parts of the oral cavity. They include the ***lingual, labial, buccal, molar,*** and ***palatine glands.***

Each salivary gland arises from the developing oral cavity epithelium. Initially, the gland takes the form of a solid cord of cells that enters the mesenchyme. The proliferation of epithelial cells eventually produces highly branched epithelial cords with bulbous ends. Degeneration of the innermost cells of the cords and bulbous ends leads to their canalization. The cords become ducts, and the bulbous ends become ***secretory acini.***

Secretory Gland Acini

Secretory acini are organized into lobules

The major salivary glands are surrounded by a capsule of moderately dense connective tissue from which septa divide the secretory portions of the gland into lobes and lobules. The septa contain the larger blood vessels and excretory ducts. The connective tissue associated with the groups of secretory acini blends imperceptibly into the surrounding loose connective tissue. The minor salivary glands do not have a capsule.

Numerous lymphocytes and plasma cells populate the connective tissue surrounding the acini in both the major and minor salivary glands. Their significance in the secretion of salivary antibodies is described below.

Acini are of three types: serous, mucous, or mixed

The basic secretory unit of salivary glands, the ***salivon,*** consists of the acinus, intercalated duct, and excretory duct (Fig. 15.22). The ***acinus*** is a blind sac composed of secretory cells. The term *acinus [L., berry or grape]* refers to the secretory unit of the salivary glands. The acini of salivary glands contain either ***serous cells*** (protein secreting), ***mucous cells*** (mucin secreting), or both. The relative frequencies of the three types of acini is a prime characteristic by which the major salivary glands are distinguished. Thus, three types of acini are described:

- ***Serous acini,*** which contain only serous cells and are generally spherical
- ***Mucous acini,*** which contain only mucous cells and are usually more tubular
- ***Mixed acini,*** which contain both serous and mucous cells. In routine H&E preparations, mucous acini have a cap of serous cells that are thought to secrete into the highly convoluted intercellular space between the mucous cells. Because of their appearance in histologic sections, such caps are called ***serous demilunes*** *[Fr., half-moon].*

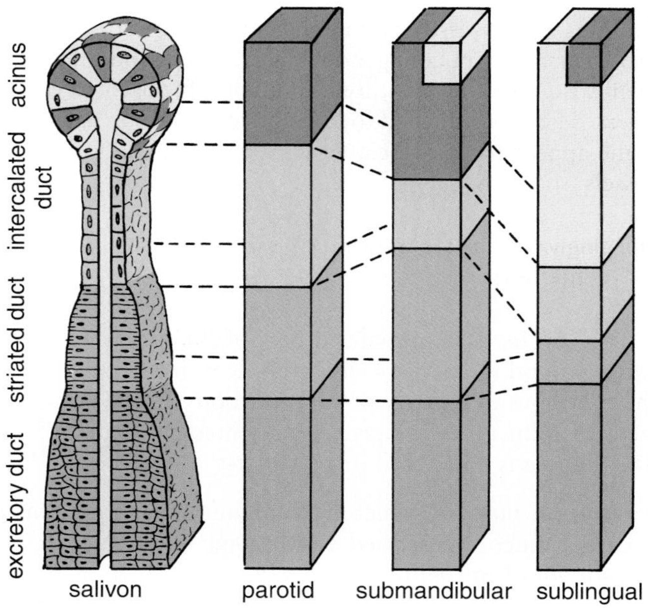

FIGURE 15.22
Diagram comparing the components of the salivon in the three major salivary glands. The four major parts of the salivon, the acinus, intercalated duct, striated duct, and excretory duct, are color coded. The three columns on the right of the salivon compare the length of the different ducts in the three salivary glands. The *red-colored cells* of the acinus represent serous-secreting cells, and the *yellow-colored cells* represent mucous-secreting cells. The ratio of serous-secreting cells to mucous-secreting cells is depicted in the acini of the various glands.

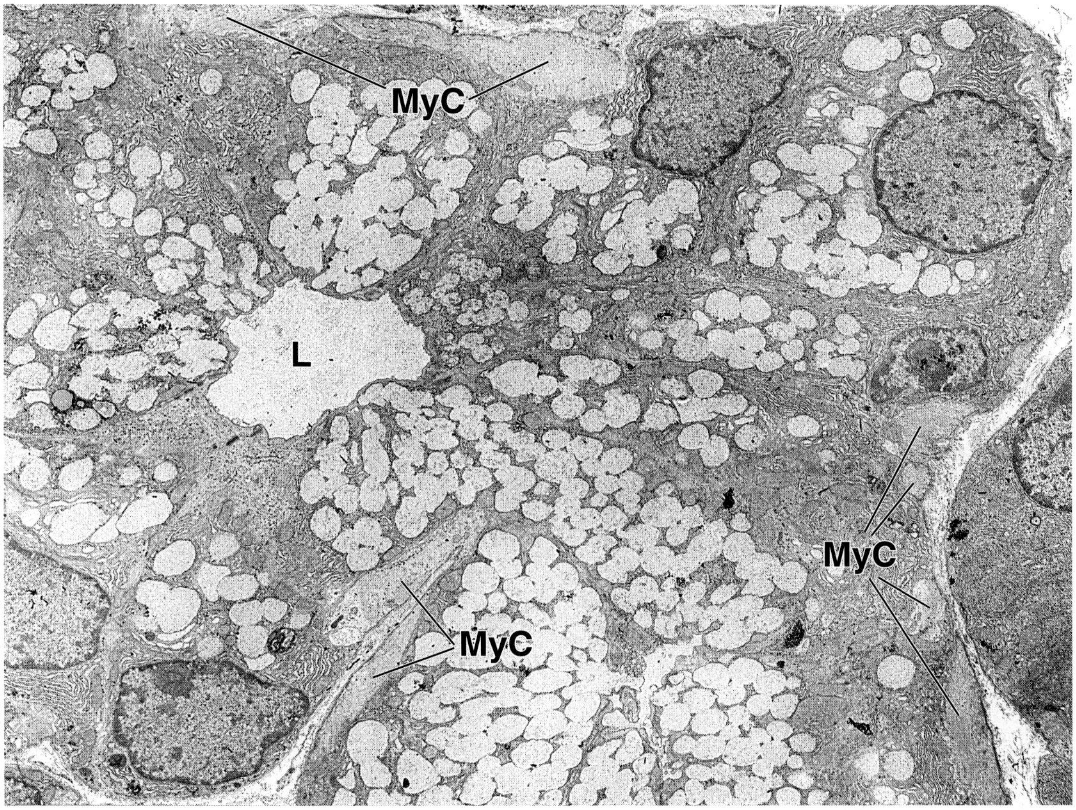

FIGURE 15.25

Low-magnification electron micrograph of a mucous acinus. The mucous cells contain numerous mucinogen granules. Many of the granules have coalesced to form larger irregular masses that will ultimately discharge into the lumen *(L)* of the acinus. Myoepithelial cell processes *(MyC)* are evident at the periphery of the acinus. ×5,000.

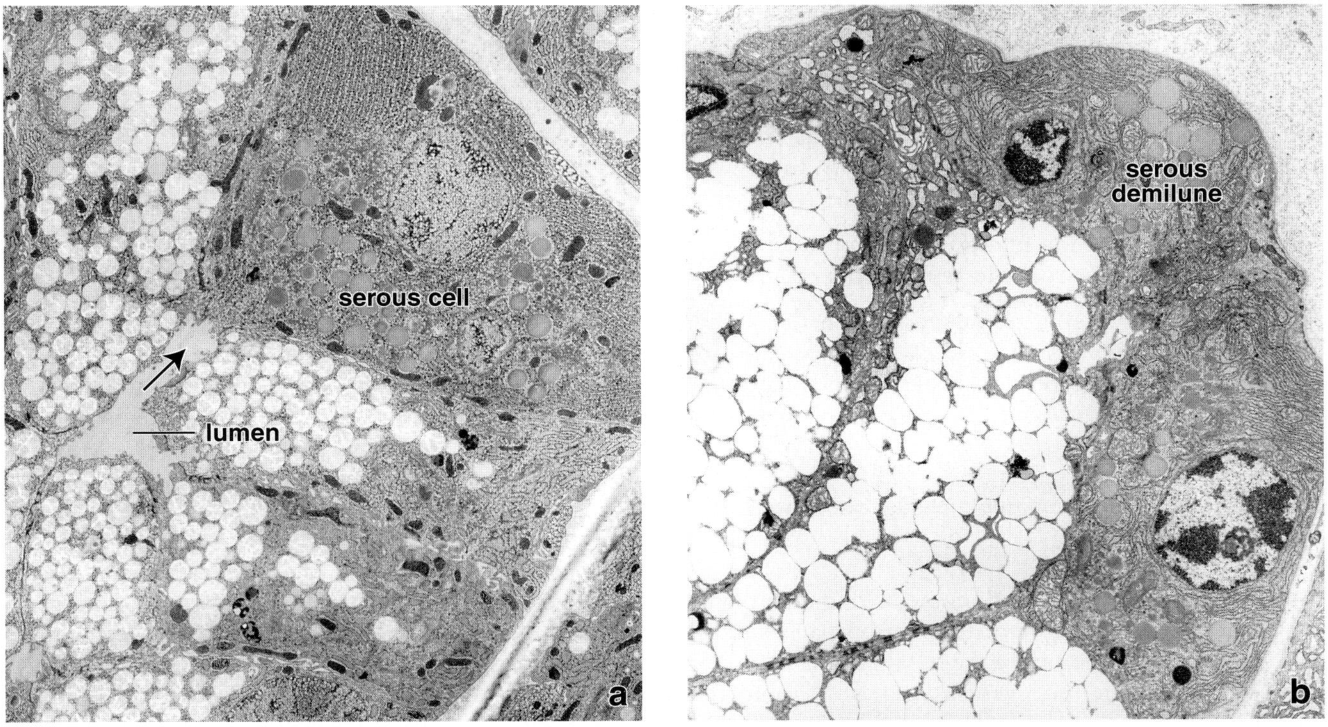

FIGURE 15.26

Electron micrographs of mixed acini. a. Low-magnification electron micrograph of the sublingual gland, prepared by the rapid freezing and freeze-substitution method, shows the arrangement of the cells within a single acinus. The mucous cells have well-preserved round mucinogen granules. The mucous and serous cells are aligned to surround the acinus lumen. Serous demilunes are not evident. ×6,000. **b.** Electron micrograph of the sublingual gland prepared by traditional fixation in formaldehyde. Note the considerable expansion and coalescence of the mucinogen granules and the formation of a serous demilune. ×15,000. (Courtesy of Dr. Shohei Yamashina.)

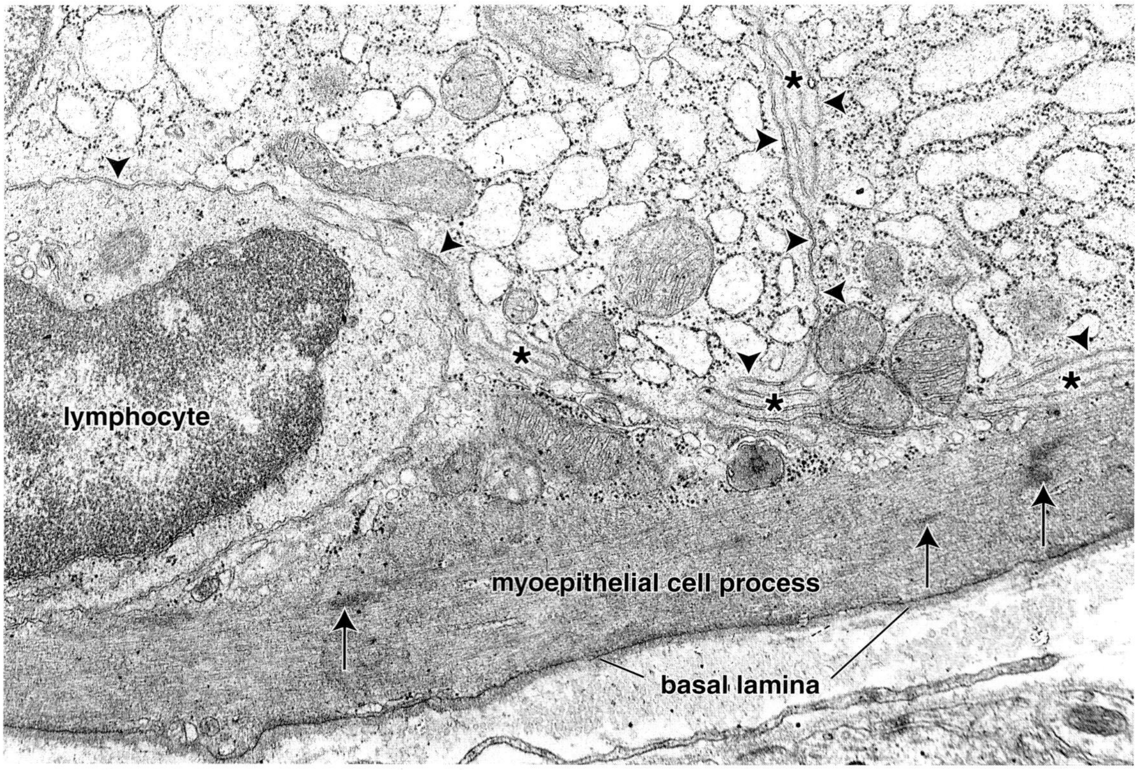

FIGURE 15.27
Electron micrograph of the basal portion of an acinus. This electron micrograph shows the basal portion of two secretory cells from a submandibular gland. A myoepithelial cell process is also evident. Note the location of the myoepithelial cell process on the epithelial side of the basal lamina. The cytoplasm of the myoepithelial cell contains contractile filaments and densities *(arrows)* similar to those seen in smooth muscle cells. The cell on the left with the small nucleus is a lymphocyte. Having migrated through the basal lamina, it is also within the epithelial compartment. *Arrowheads,* cell boundries; *asterisks,* basal-lateral folds. ×15,000.

other than that of a conduit. However, the cells of intercalated ducts possess carbonic anhydrase activity. In serous secreting glands and mixed glands, they have been shown to

- ***Secrete bicarbonate*** ion into the acinar product
- ***Absorb chloride*** ion from the acinar product

As noted above, intercalated ducts are most prominent in those salivary glands that produce a watery serous secretion. In mucus-secreting salivary glands, the intercalated ducts, when present, are short and difficult to identify.

Striated duct cells have numerous infoldings of the basal plasma membrane

Striated ducts are lined by a simple cuboidal epithelium that gradually becomes columnar as it approaches the excretory duct. The infoldings of the basal plasma membrane are seen in histologic sections as "striations." Longitudinally oriented, elongated mitochondria are enclosed in the infoldings. Basal infoldings associated with elongated mitochondria are a morphologic specialization associated with reabsorption of fluid and electrolytes. The striated duct cells also have numerous basal-lateral folds that are interdigitated with those of adjacent cells. The nucleus typically occupies a central (rather than basal) location in the cell. Striated ducts are the sites of

- ***Reabsorption of*** Na^+ from the primary secretion
- ***Secretion of*** K^+ and HCO_3^- into the secretion

More Na^+ is resorbed than K^+ is secreted, so the secretion becomes hypotonic. When secretion is very rapid, more Na^+ and less K^+ appear in the final saliva because the reabsorption and secondary secretion systems cannot keep up with the rate of primary secretion. Thus, the saliva may become isotonic to hypertonic.

The diameter of striated ducts often exceeds that of the secretory acinus. Striated ducts are located in the parenchyma of the glands (they are ***intralobular ducts***) but may be surrounded by small amounts of connective tissue in which blood vessels and nerves can be seen running in parallel with the duct.

Excretory ducts travel in the interlobular and interlobar connective tissue

Excretory ducts constitute the principal ducts of each of the major glands. They ultimately connect to the oral cav-

ity. The epithelium of small excretory ducts is simple cuboidal. It gradually changes to pseudostratified columnar or stratified cuboidal. As the diameter of the duct increases, stratified columnar epithelium is often seen, and as the ducts approach the oral epithelium, stratified squamous epithelium may be present. The parotid duct (Stensen's duct) and the submandibular duct (Wharton's duct) travel in the connective tissue of the face and neck, respectively, for some distance from the gland before penetrating the oral mucosa.

Major Salivary Glands

PAROTID GLAND

The parotid glands are completely serous

The paired serous parotid glands are the largest of the major salivary glands. The parotid duct travels from the gland, which is located below and in front of the ear, to enter the oral cavity opposite the second upper molar tooth. The secretory units in the parotid are serous and surround numerous, long, narrow intercalated ducts. Striated ducts are large and conspicuous (Fig. 15.28a).

Large amounts of adipose tissue often occur in the parotid gland; this is one of its distinguishing features. The facial nerve (cranial nerve VII) passes through the parotid gland; large cross sections of this nerve may be encountered in routine H&E sections of the gland and are useful in identifying the parotid. Mumps, a viral infection of the parotid gland, can damage the facial nerve.

SUBMANDIBULAR GLAND

The submandibular glands are mixed glands that are mostly serous in humans

The large, paired, mixed submandibular glands are located under either side of the floor of the mouth, close to the mandible. A duct from each of the two glands runs forward and medially to a papilla located on the floor of the mouth just lateral to the *frenulum* of the tongue. Some mucous acini capped by serous demilunes are generally found among the predominant serous acini. Intercalated ducts are less extensive than in the parotid gland (Fig. 15.28b).

SUBLINGUAL GLAND

The small sublingual glands are mixed glands that are mostly mucus-secreting in humans

The sublingual glands, the smallest of the paired major salivary glands, are located in the floor of the mouth anterior to the submandibular glands. Their multiple small sublingual ducts empty into the submandibular duct as well as directly onto the floor of the mouth. Some of the predominant mucous acini exhibit serous demilunes, but purely serous acini are rarely present (Fig. 15.28c). Intercalated ducts and striated ducts are short, difficult to locate, or sometimes absent. The mucous secretory units may be more tubular than purely acinar.

Saliva

Saliva includes the combined secretions of all the major and minor salivary glands

Most saliva is produced by the salivary glands. A smaller amount is derived from the gingival sulcus, tonsillar crypts, and general transudation from the epithelial lining of the oral cavity. One of the unique features of saliva is the large and variable volume produced. The volume (per weight of gland tissue) of saliva exceeds that of other digestive secretions by as much as 40 times. The large volume of saliva produced is undoubtedly related to its many functions, only some of which are concerned with digestion.

Saliva performs both protective and digestive functions

The salivary glands produce about 1200 mL of saliva a day. Saliva has numerous functions relating to metabolic and nonmetabolic activities. These include

- Moistening the oral mucosa
- Moistening dry foods to aid swallowing
- Providing a medium for dissolved and suspended food materials that chemically stimulate taste buds
- Buffering the contents of the oral cavity, because of its high concentration of bicarbonate ions
- Digesting carbohydrates with the digestive enzyme ***α-amylase*** that breaks 1-4 glycosidic bonds and continues to act in the esophagus and stomach
- Controlling the bacterial flora of the oral cavity by use of ***lysozyme (muramidase),*** an enzyme that lyses the muramic acid in certain bacteria (e.g., staphylococci).

The unique composition of saliva is summarized in Table 15.1.

Saliva is a source of calcium and phosphate ions essential for normal tooth development and maintenance

Calcium and phosphate in the saliva are essential for the mineralization of newly erupted teeth and for repair of precarious lesions of the enamel in erupted teeth. In addition, saliva serves several other roles in protecting the teeth. Proteins in saliva cover the teeth with a protective coat called the ***acquired pellicle.*** Antibodies and other antibacterial agents retard bacterial action that would otherwise lead to tooth decay. Patients whose salivary glands are irradiated, as in the treatment of salivary gland tumors, fail to produce normal amounts of saliva; these patients typically develop rampant caries. Anticholinergic drugs used

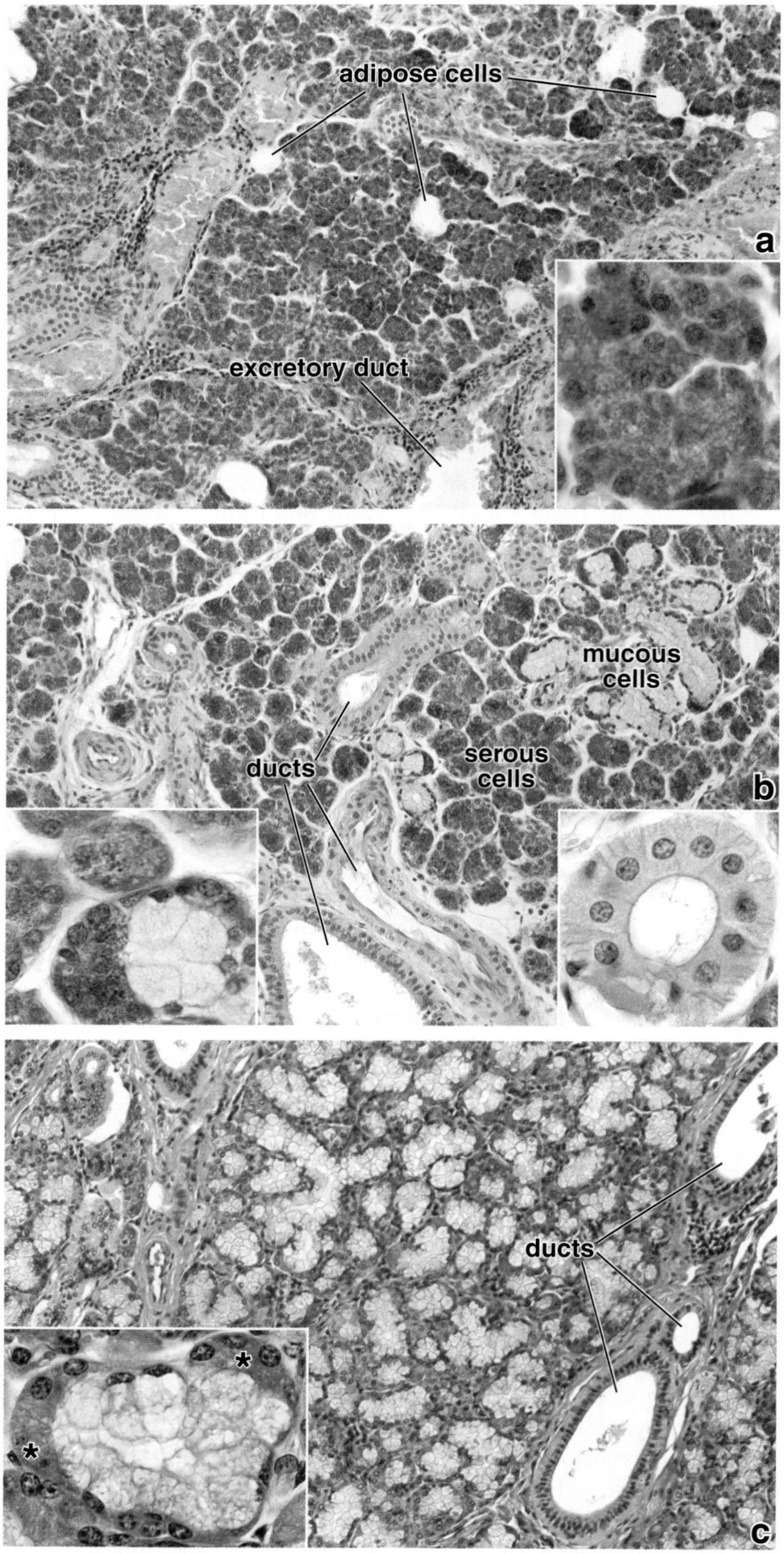

FIGURE 15.28

Photomicrographs of the three major salivary glands. **a.** The parotid gland in the human is composed entirely of serous acini and their ducts. Typically, adipose cells are also distributed throughout the gland. The lower portion of the figure reveals an excretory duct within a connective tissue septum. ×120. **Inset.** Higher magnification of the serous acinar cells. ×320. **b.** The submandibular glands contain both serous and mucous acini. In humans, the serous components predominate. The mucus-secreting acini are readily discernable at this low magnification because of their light staining. The remainder of the field is composed largely of serous acini. Various ducts—excretory, striated, and intercalated—are evident in the field. ×120. **Left inset.** Higher magnification of an acinus revealing a serous demilune surrounding mucus-secreting cells. ×360. **Right inset.** Higher magnification of a striated duct. These ducts have columnar epithelium with visible basal striations. ×320. **c.** The sublingual gland also contains both serous and mucous elements. Here, the mucous acini predominate. The mucous acini are conspicuous because of their light staining. Critical examination of the mucous acini at this relatively low magnification reveals that they are not spherical structures but, rather, elongate or tubular structures with branching outpockets. Thus, the acinus is rather large, and much of it is usually not seen within the plane of a single section. The ducts of the sublingual gland that are observed with the greatest frequency in a section are the interlobular ducts. ×120. **Inset.** The serous component of the gland is composed largely of demilunes *(asterisks)*, artifacts of conventional fixation. ×320.

TABLE 15.1. **Composition of Unstimulated Saliva**

	Mean (mg/mL)
Organic constituents	
Protein	220.0
Amylase	38.0
Mucin	2.7
Muramidase (lysozyme)	22.0
Lactoferrin	0.03
ABO group substances	0.005
EGF	3.4
sIgA	19.0
IgG	1.4
IgM	0.2
Glucose	1.0
Urea	20.0
Uric acid	1.5
Creatinine	0.1
Cholesterol	8.0
cAMP	7.0
Inorganic constituents	
Sodium	15.0
Potassium	80.0
Thiocyanate	
Smokers	9.0
Nonsmokers	2.0
Calcium	5.8
Phosphate	16.8
Chloride	50.0
Fluoride	Traces (according to intake)

Modified from Jenkins GN. *The Physiology and Biochemistry of the Mouth.* 4th ed. Oxford: Blackwell Scientific Publications, 1978.

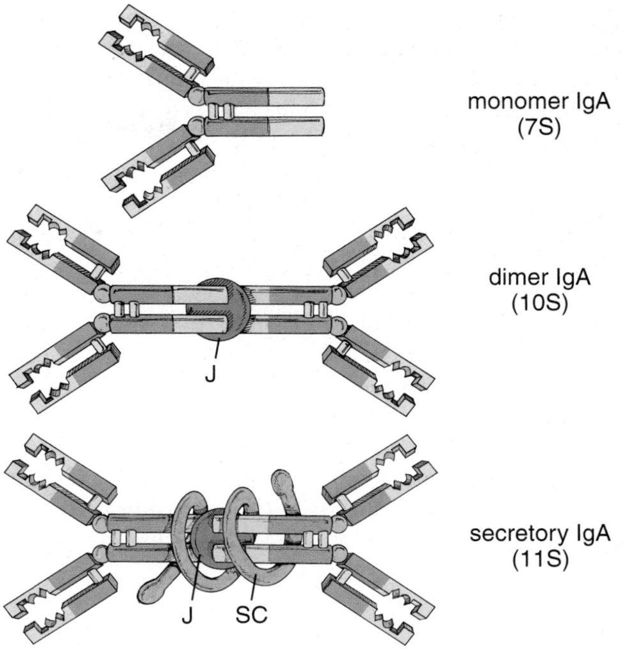

FIGURE 15.29
Diagram of different forms of immunoglobulin A (IgA). This drawing shows the monomer of IgA *(top).* The dimer of IgA is a product of the plasma cell and contains a J chain *(J)* connecting two monomers *(middle).* The secretory component *(SC),* a product of the epithelial cells, is added to the dimer to form secretory IgA (sIgA, *bottom*).

to treat some forms of heart disease also significantly reduce salivary secretion, leading to dental caries.

Saliva performs immunologic functions

As noted, saliva contains antibodies, salivary ***immunoglobulin A (IgA).*** IgA is synthesized by plasma cells in the connective tissue surrounding the secretory acini of the salivary glands, and both dimeric and monomeric forms are released into the connective tissue matrix (Fig. 15.29). A secretory glycoprotein is synthesized by the salivary gland cells and inserted into the basal plasma membrane, where it serves as a receptor for dimeric IgA.

When the dimeric IgA binds to the receptor, the ***secretory IgA complex*** thus formed is internalized by receptor-mediated endocytosis and carried through the acinar cell to the apical plasma membrane, where it is released into the lumen as secretory IgA (sIgA). This process of synthesis and secretion of IgA is essentially identical to that which occurs in the more distal parts of the gastrointestinal tract, where sIgA is transported across the absorptive columnar epithelium of the small intestine and colon.

Saliva contains water, various proteins, and electrolytes

Saliva contains chiefly water, proteins and glycoproteins (enzymes and antibodies), and electrolytes. It has a high potassium concentration that is approximately 7 times that of blood, a sodium concentration approximately one tenth that of blood, a bicarbonate concentration approximately 3 times that of blood, and significant amounts of calcium, phosphorus, chloride, thiocyanate, and urea. Lysozyme and α-amylase are the principal enzymes present (see Table 15.1).

PLATE 44. LIP, A MUCOCUTANEOUS JUNCTION

The lips are the entry point of the alimentary canal. Here, the thin keratinized epidermis of face skin changes to the thick parakeratinized epithelium of the oral mucosa. The transition zone, the red portion of the lips, is characterized by deep penetration of connective tissue papillae into the base of the stratified squamous keratinized epithelium. The blood vessels and nerve endings in these papillae are responsible for both the color and the exquisite touch sensitivity of the lips.

A H&E–stained sagittal section through the lip in this low-power orientation photomicrograph to the right (×8) reveals the skin of the face, the red margin of the lip, and the transition to the oral mucosa. The *numbered rectangles* indicate representative areas of each of these sites, shown at higher magnifications in Figures 1, 3, and 5, respectively, on the adjacent plate. Note the change in thickness of the epithelium from the exterior or facial portion of the lip (the vertical surface on the right) to the interior surface of the oral cavity (the surface beginning with *rectangle 5* and continuing down the left surface of the lip) in this micrograph.

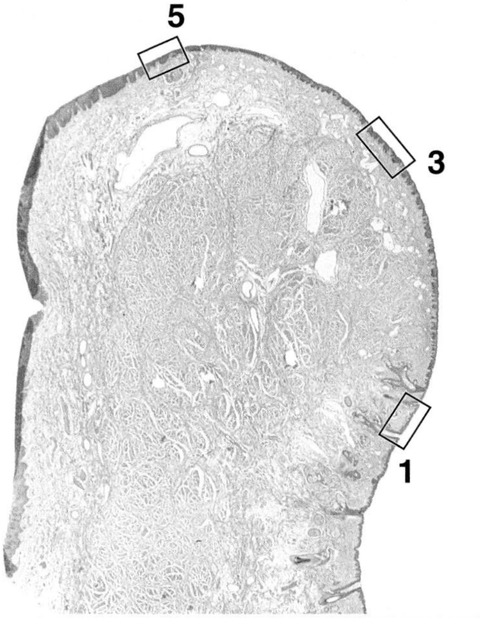

Figure 1, lip, human, H&E ×120.
The epithelium *(EP)* of the face is relatively thin and has the general features of thin skin found in other sites. Associated with it are hair follicles *(HF)* and sebaceous glands *(SGl).*

Figure 2, lip, human, H&E ×380.
The *circled area* in Figure 1 is shown at higher magnification here. The reddish brown material in the basal cells is the pigment melanin *(M),* and the dark blue near the surface is the stratum granulosum *(SG)* with its deep-blue–stained keratohyalin granules.

Figure 3, lip, human, H&E×120.
The epithelium of the red margin of the lip is much thicker than that of the face. The stratum granulosum is still present (see Fig. 4); thus, the epithelium is keratinized. The feature that accounts for the coloration of the red margin is the deep penetration of the connective tissue papillae into the epithelium *(arrowheads).* The thinness of the epithelium combined with the extensive vascularity of the underlying connective tissue, particularly the extensive venous blood vessels *(BV),* allows the color of the blood to show through.

Figure 4, lip, human, H&E×380.
The sensitivity of the red margin to stimuli such as light touch is due to the presence of an increased number of sensory receptors. In fact, each of the two deep papillae seen in Figure 3 contains a Meissner's corpuscle, one of which *(MC)* is more clearly seen in this figure.

Figure 5, lip, human, H&E×120.
The transition from the keratinized red margin to the fairly thick stratified squamous parakeratinized epithelium of the oral mucosa is evident in this figure. Note how the stratum granulosum suddenly ends. This is more clearly shown at higher magnification in Figure 6.

Figure 6, lip, human, H&E×380.
Beyond the site where the stratum granulosum cells disappear, nuclei are seen in the superficial cells up to the surface *(arrows).* The epithelium is also much thicker at this point and remains so throughout the oral cavity.

KEY

BV, venous blood vessels
EP, epithelium
HF, hair follicle
M, melanin pigment
MC, Meissner's corpuscle
SG, stratum granulosum
SGl, sebaceous gland
arrowheads, connective tissue papillae
arrows, nuclei of superficial cells up to surface

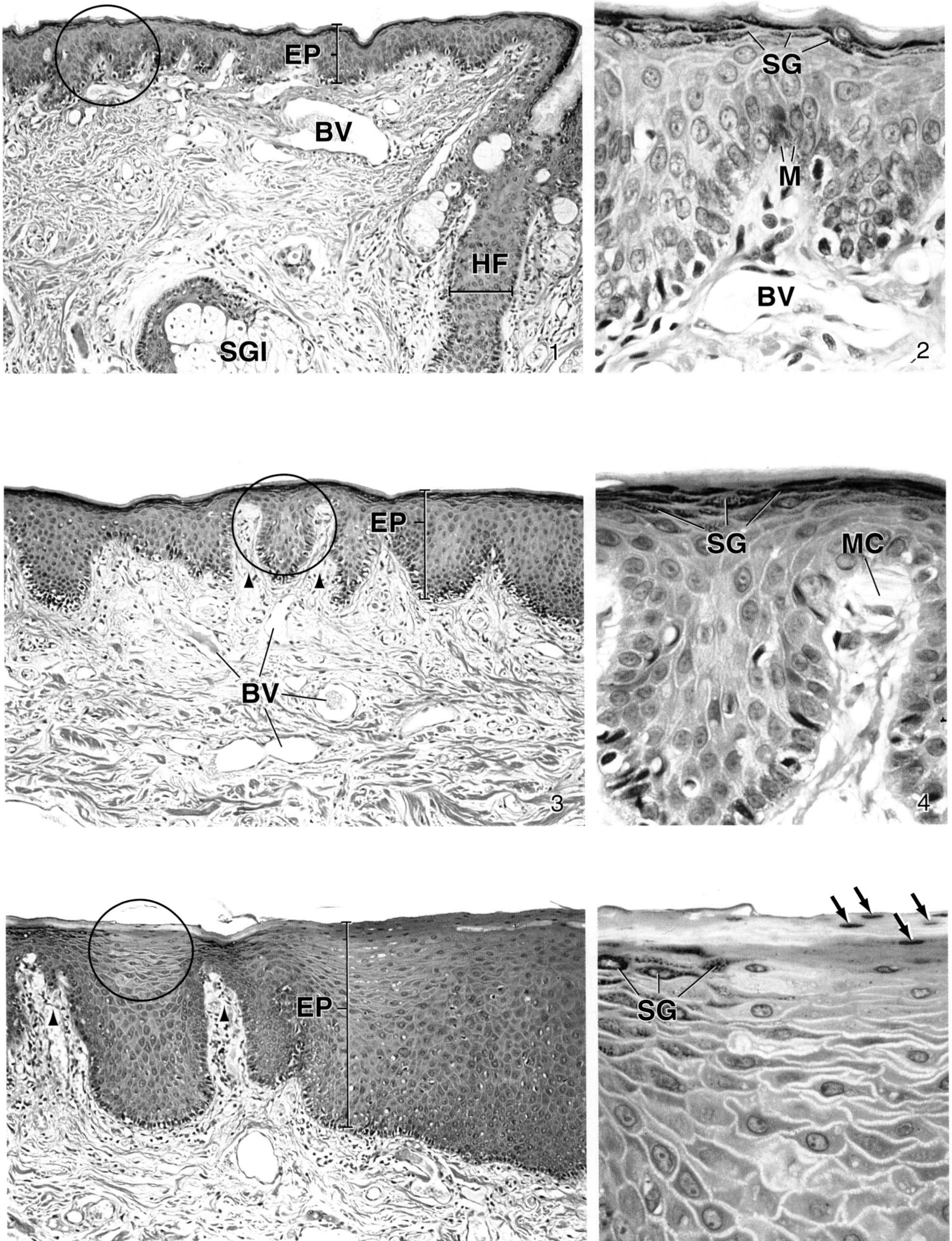
EP
BV
HF
SGl
1
SG
M
BV
2
EP
BV
3
SG
MC
4
EP
5
SG
6

PLATE 45. TONGUE I

The tongue is a muscular organ projecting into the oral cavity from its inferior surface. It is covered with a mucous membrane that consists of stratified squamous epithelium, keratinized in parts, resting on a loose connective tissue. The undersurface of the tongue is relatively uncomplicated. The mucosa of the dorsal surface, however, is modified to form three types of papillae: *filiform, fungiform,* and *circumvallate.* The circumvallate papillae form a V-shaped row that divides the tongue into a body and a root; the dorsal surface of the body, i.e., the portion anterior to the circumvallate papillae, contains filiform and fungiform papillae. Parallel ridges bearing taste buds are found on the sides of the tongue and are particularly evident in infants. When sectioned at right angles to their long axis, they appear as papillae and, although not true papillae, are called *foliate papillae.*

The tongue contains both intrinsic and extrinsic voluntary striated muscle. The striated muscles of the tongue are arranged in three interweaving planes, with each arrayed at right angles to the other two. This arrangement is unique to the tongue. It provides enormous flexibility and precision in the movements of the tongue that are essential to human speech as well as to its role in digestion and swallowing. The arrangement also allows easy identification as lingual muscle.

Figure 1, tongue, monkey, H&E ×65; inset ×130.
This figure shows the dorsal surface of the tongue with the filiform papillae *(Fil P).* They are the most numerous of the three types of papillae. Structurally, they are bent, conical projections of the epithelium, with the point of the projection directed posteriorly. These papillae do not possess taste buds and are composed of stratified squamous keratinized epithelium.

The fungiform papillae are scattered about as isolated, slightly rounded, elevated structures situated among the filiform papillae. A fungiform papilla is shown in the **inset.** A large connective tissue core (primary connective tissue papilla) forms the center of the fungiform papilla, and smaller connective tissue papillae (secondary connective tissue papillae) project into the base of the surface epithelium *(arrowhead).* The connective tissue of the papillae is highly vascularized. Because of the deep penetration of connective tissue into the epithelium, combined with a very thin keratinized surface, the fungiform papillae appear as small red dots when the dorsal surface of the tongue is examined by gross inspection.

Figure 2, tongue, monkey, H&E ×65.
The undersurface of the tongue is shown in this figure. The smooth surface of the stratified squamous epithelium *(Ep)* contrasts with the irregular surface of the dorsum of the tongue. Moreover, the epithelial surface on the underside of the tongue is usually not keratinized. The connective tissue *(CT)* is immediately deep to the epithelium; deeper still is the striated muscle *(M).*

The numerous connective tissue papillae that project into the base of the epithelium of both ventral and dorsal surfaces give the epithelial–connective tissue junction an irregular profile. Often, these connective tissue papillae are cut obliquely and then appear as small islands of connective tissue within the epithelial layer (see Fig. 1).

The connective tissue extends as far as the muscle without changing character, and no submucosa is recognized. The muscle *(M)* is striated and is unique in its organization; i.e., the fibers travel in three planes. Therefore, most sections will show bundles of muscle fibers cut longitudinally, at right angles to each other, and in cross section. Nerves *(N)* that innervate the muscle are also frequently observed in the connective tissue septa between the muscle bundles.

The surface of the tongue behind the vallate papillae (the root of the tongue) contains lingual tonsils (not shown). These are similar in structure and appearance to the palatine tonsils illustrated in Plate 32.

KEY

CT, connective tissue
Ep, epithelium
Fil P, filiform papillae
M, striated muscle bundles
N, nerves
arrowhead (Fig. 1, inset), secondary connective tissue papilla

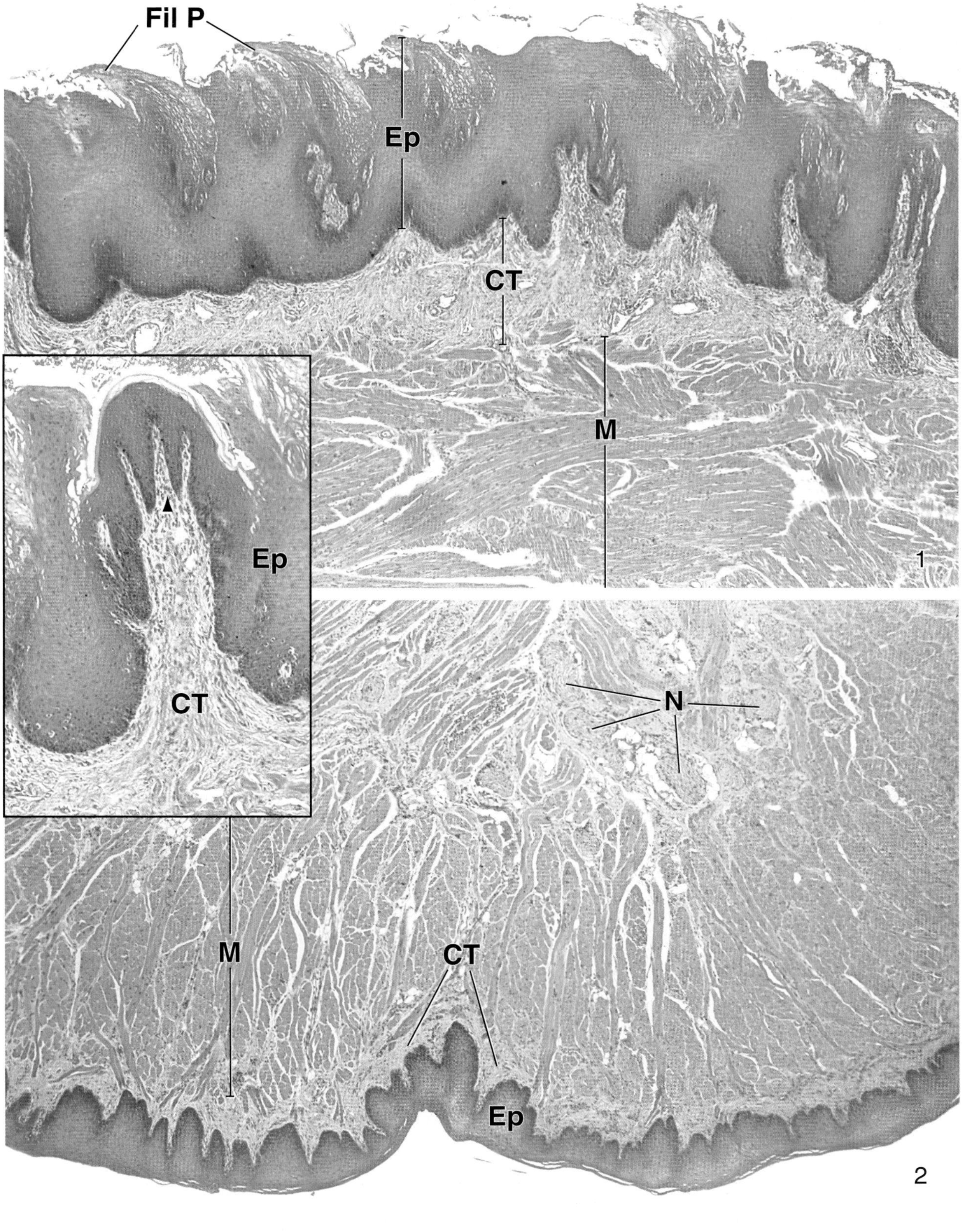
Fil P
Ep
CT
M
Ep
CT
1
N
M
CT
Ep
2

PLATE 46. TONGUE II

The papillae and their associated *taste buds* constitute the *specialized mucosa* of the oral cavity. Although filiform papillae do not have taste buds, the other three types, viz., fungiform, circumvallate, and foliate, contain taste buds in their epithelium. The fungiform (i.e., mushroom-shaped) papillae (see Plate 45) are most numerous near the tip of the tongue. Taste buds are present in the epithelium on their dorsal surface. The taste buds in the epithelium covering the circumvallate and foliate papillae are located in deep clefts that separate the papillae from adjacent mucosa or from each other, respectively. Ducts of lingual salivary glands (von Ebner's glands; a component of the *minor salivary glands*) empty their serous secretions into the moat surrounding each circumvallate papilla. The secretions flush material from the moat to allow the taste buds to respond to new stimuli. Similarly, ducts of small serous glands empty into the clefts between foliate papillae.

Taste buds in section appear as oval, pale-staining bodies that extend through the thickness of the epithelium. A small opening at the epithelial surface is called the *taste pore.* Taste buds react to only four stimuli: sweet, salty, bitter, and sour. These modalities appear to be spatially separated; taste buds at the tip of the tongue detect sweet stimuli, those immediately posterolateral to the tip detect salty stimuli, those on the circumvallate papillae detect bitter stimuli.

Figure 1, tongue, monkey, H&E ×55.

The sides of the tongue contain a series of vertical ridges that bear taste buds. When these ridges are cut at right angles to their long axis, they appear as a row of papillae. These ridges are called ***foliate papillae.*** Foliate papillae are not always conspicuous in the adult human tongue but are quite evident in the infant tongue. They can be distinguished immediately from fungiform papillae in a section because they appear in rows, whereas fungiform papillae (not illustrated) appear alone. Moreover, numerous taste buds *(TB)* are present on adjacent walls of neighboring foliate papillae. In contrast, fungiform papillae have taste buds on the dorsal surface. The foliate papillae are covered by stratified squamous epithelium that is usually not keratinized or is only slightly keratinized. The part of the epithelium *(EP)* that is on the free surface of the foliate papillae is thick and has a number of secondary connective tissue papillae projecting into its undersurface.

The connective tissue within and under the foliate papillae contains serous-type glands *(Gl),* called ***von Ebner's glands,*** which open via ducts *(D)* into the cleft between neighboring papillae. In addition to von Ebner's glands, which are entirely of the serous type, the tongue contains mixed (serous and mucous) glands near the apex and mucous glands in the root (not illustrated).

The dense patches *(arrows)* within the connective tissue consist of accumulations of lymphocytes in the form of diffuse lymphatic tissue. They are typically seen just below the clefts of the papillae.

Figure 2, tongue, monkey, H&E ×55; inset ×640.

Of the true papillae found on the dorsal surface of the tongue—filiform, fungiform, and circumvallate (vallate)—the circumvallate are the largest. About 7 to 11 of these form a "V" between the body and root of the tongue. ***Circumvallate papillae*** are covered by stratified squamous epithelium that may be slightly keratinized. Each circumvallate papilla is surrounded by a trench or cleft. Numerous taste buds *(TB)* are on the lateral walls of the papillae; moreover, the tongue epithelium *(EP)* facing the papilla within the cleft may contain some taste buds. The dorsal surface of the papilla is rather smooth; however, numerous secondary connective tissue *(CT)* papillae project into the underside of the epithelium. The deep trench surrounding the circumvallate papillae and the presence of taste buds on the sides rather than on the surface are features that distinguish circumvallate from fungiform papillae.

The connective tissue near the circumvallate papillae also contains many serous-type glands *(Gl),* von Ebner's glands, which open via ducts *(D)* into the bottom of the trench.

The taste buds extend through the full thickness of the stratified squamous epithelium **(inset)** and open at the surface at a small pore *(arrowheads).* The cells of the taste bud are chiefly spindle shaped and oriented at a right angle to the surface. The nuclei of the cells are elongated and mainly in the basal two-thirds of the bud. At least three cell types are present in the taste bud; one is a special receptor cell, the sensory or neuroepithelial cell. Nerve fibers enter the epithelium and terminate in close contact with the sensory cells of the taste bud, but they cannot be identified in routine H&E preparations. Other cell types in the taste bud include the supporting cells and the basal cells. The latter sometimes exhibit mitotic figures *(asterisk)* and give rise to the other cell types.

KEY

CT, connective tissue
D, ducts
EP, epithelium
Gl, serous (von Ebner's) glands
M, striated muscle bundles
TB, taste buds
arrowheads (inset), taste bud pore
arrows (Fig. 1), lymphocytes
asterisk (inset), mitotic figure

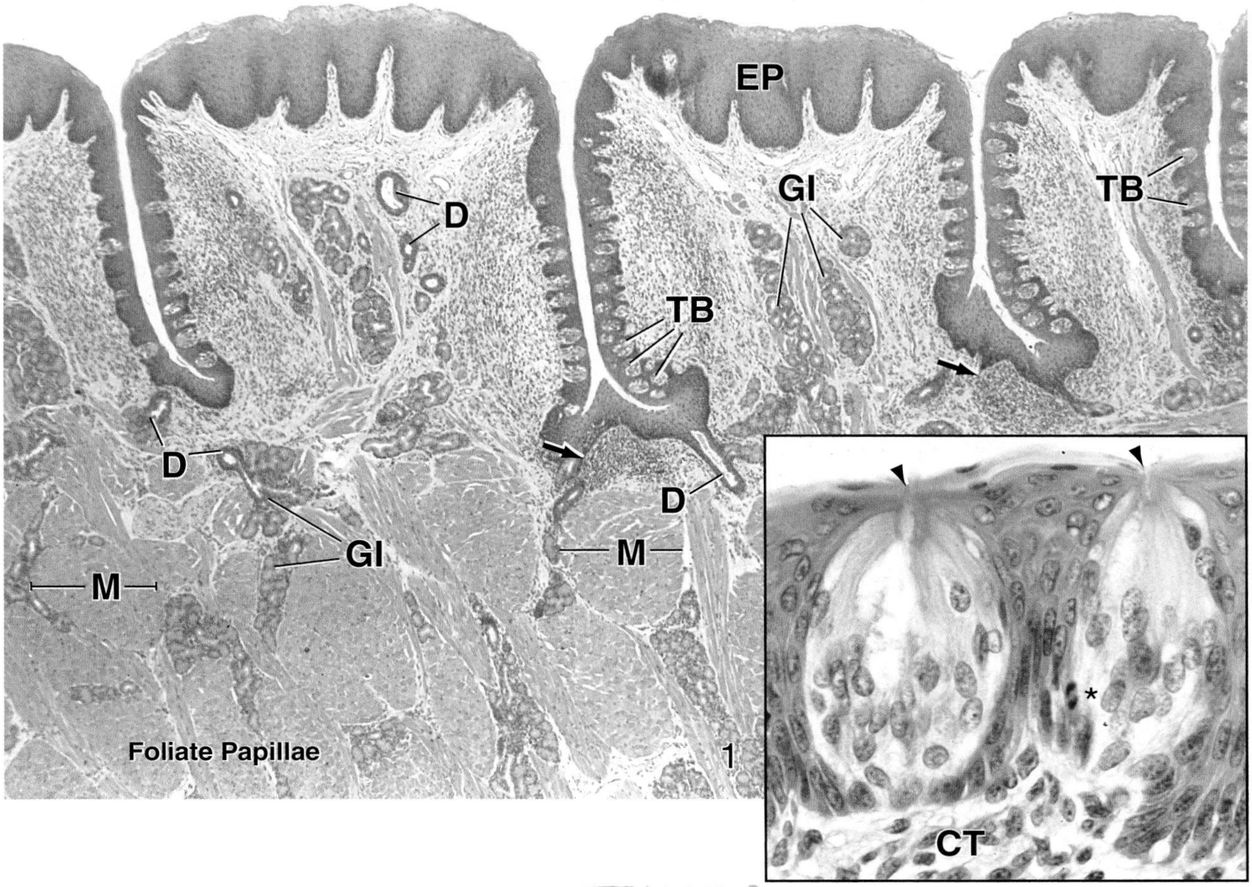
EP
D
GI
TB
TB
D
D
GI
M
M
CT
Foliate Papillae
1

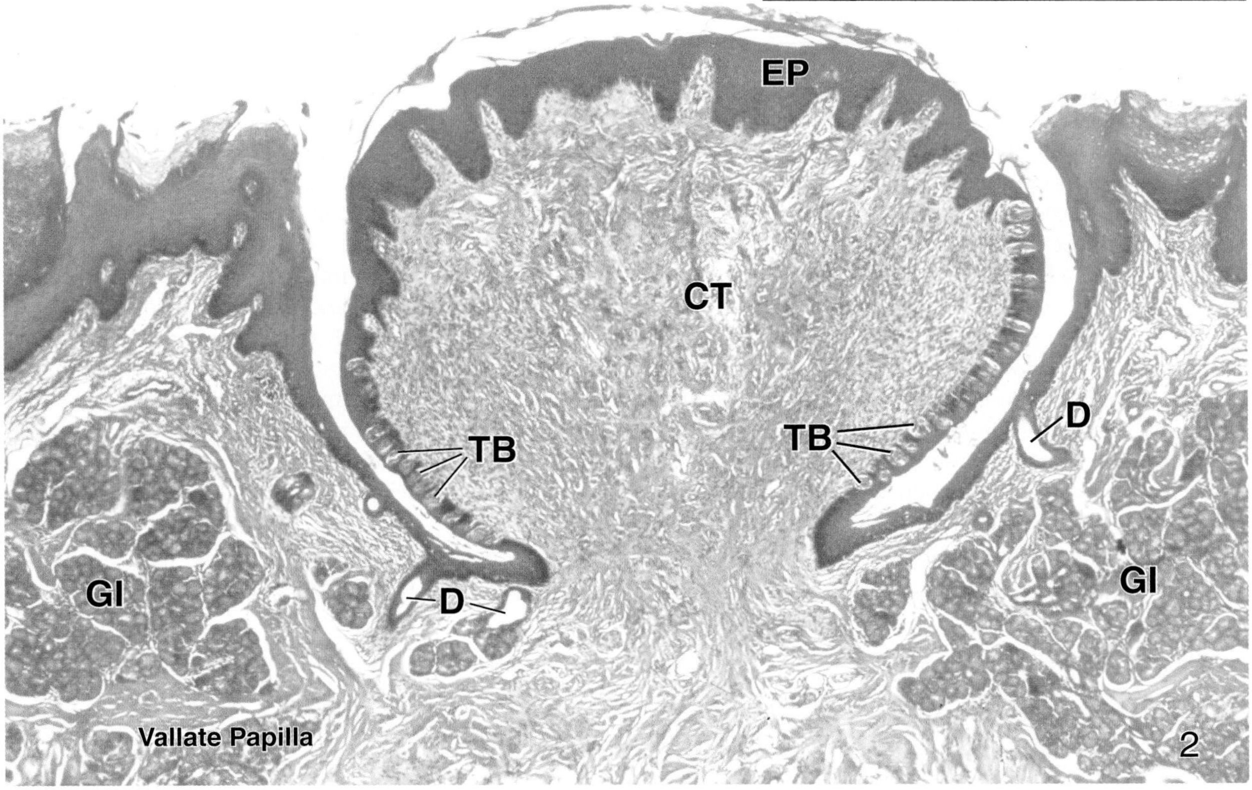
EP
CT
TB
TB
D
GI
D
GI
Vallate Papilla
2

PLATE 47. SUBMANDIBULAR GLAND

The major salivary glands, the *parotid, submandibular,* and *sublingual* glands, are paired glands with long ducts. The parotid and submandibular glands are actually located outside the oral cavity. The parotid gland is located subcutaneously, below and in front of the ear. The submandibular gland is located under the floor of the mouth, close to the mandible. The sublingual gland is located in the floor of the mouth, anterior to the submandibular gland.

The salivary glands are *compound* (branched) *tubuloacinar glands.* They are surrounded by a moderately dense connective tissue from which septa divide the secretory portion of the gland into lobes and lobules. The secretory unit is the *acinus,* which is made up of either *serous cells* (serous acini), *mucous cells* (mucous acini), or both cell types (mixed acini). Generally, in H&E preparations, serous cells can readily be distinguished from mucous cells by the deep staining of the cytoplasm of the serous cell in contrast to the empty or washed-out appearance of the mucous cell—a characteristic feature due to loss of the stored mucinogen granules from the cell during tissue preparation. A second distinguishing feature relates to nuclear shape. The nuclei of mucous cells are typically flattened against the base of the cell, whereas the nuclei of serous cells are spherical.

Numerous lymphocytes and plasma cells populate the connective tissue surrounding the acini in both major and minor salivary glands. The plasma cells synthesize the antibodies that are secreted by the salivary cells as *secretory immunoglobulin A.*

Myoepithelial cells are contractile cells that embrace the basal aspect of the acinar secretory cells. They lie between the basal plasma membrane of the epithelial cells and the basal lamina of the epithelium and may extend onto the proximal portion of the duct system. In both locations, myoepithelial cells are instrumental in moving secretory products toward the excretory duct.

Figure 1, submandibular gland, human, H&E ×160.

The submandibular glands contain both serous and mucous acini. In humans, the serous components predominate. The *rectangle* reveals a cluster of mucous acini *(MA).* The mucus-secreting cells of the acini are readily discernable at this low magnification because of their light staining. The remainder of the field is composed largely of serous acini *(SA).* A few adipose cells *(A)* and various ducts—excretory *(ED),* striated *(StD),* and intercalated *(ID)*—are also evident in the field.

The nature of the duct system of the submandibular gland is shown to advantage in this figure. The initial ducts leading from the acinus, the intercalated ducts, are very small. They possess a flattened to cuboidal epithelium and exhibit a distinct lumen. Intercalated ducts in the submandibular gland (and the parotid gland) tend to be relatively long; thus, they are frequently encountered in a section. They merge *(arrows)* to form the larger striated ducts *(StD).* These ducts have an epithelium of low to tall columnar cells and, at high magnification, show basal striations (see Plate 48).

Figure 2, submandibular gland, human H&E ×400.

When examined at higher magnification, as in this figure, the individual mucous cells exhibit distinct cell boundaries. Their nuclei are flattened (except those that are tangentially sectioned). In contrast, the cytoplasm of the serous cells stains deeply, and the nuclei appear ovoid or round.

Serous cells are also found forming a cap known as a serous demilune *(SD)* on the periphery of many of the mucous acini *(MA).* Recent evidence indicates this is an artifact of fixation in which the serous cells are squeezed out of their normal position by swelling of the mucous cells. Some acini that appear to be of the serous type *(SA)* and particularly the acini that appear as small spherical profiles may actually be demilunes of mucous acinus that have been cut in a plane that excludes the mucous cells from the section.

Associated with the acinar epithelium are myoepithelial cells. They are located between the basal aspect of the secretory cells and the basal lamina. However, myoepithelial cells are difficult to identify in H&E–stained preparations of salivary glands, and none can be identified with assurance here.

This figure also provides a comparison between an intercalated duct *(ID)* and a small striated duct *(StD)* from the *rectangle* in Figure 1. Outside the lobule, the striated duct joins the excretory duct *(ED)* (Fig. 1, upper left). The excretory duct is characterized by a wider lumen and a taller columnar epithelium. As the excretory ducts increase in size, the epithelium becomes pseudostratified and, finally, stratified in the main excretory ducts.

KEY

A, adipose cell
ED, excretory duct
ID, intercalated duct
MA, mucous acini
SA, serous acini
SD, serous demilune
StD, striated duct
arrows (Fig. 1), intercalated ducts joining to form a striated duct
asterisks, lumina of mucous acini
rectangle (Fig. 1), cluster of mucous acini

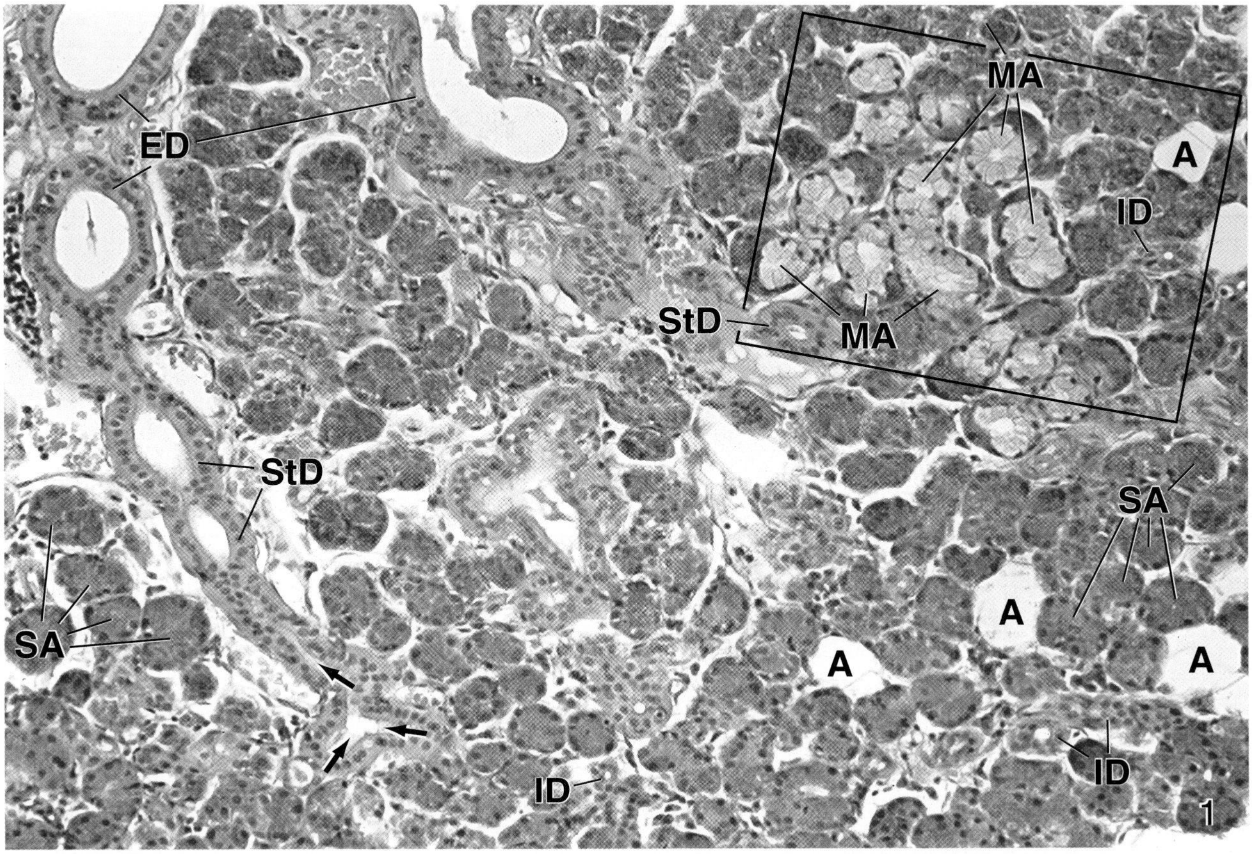
ED
MA
A
ID
StD
MA
StD
SA
SA
A
A
A
ID
ID
1

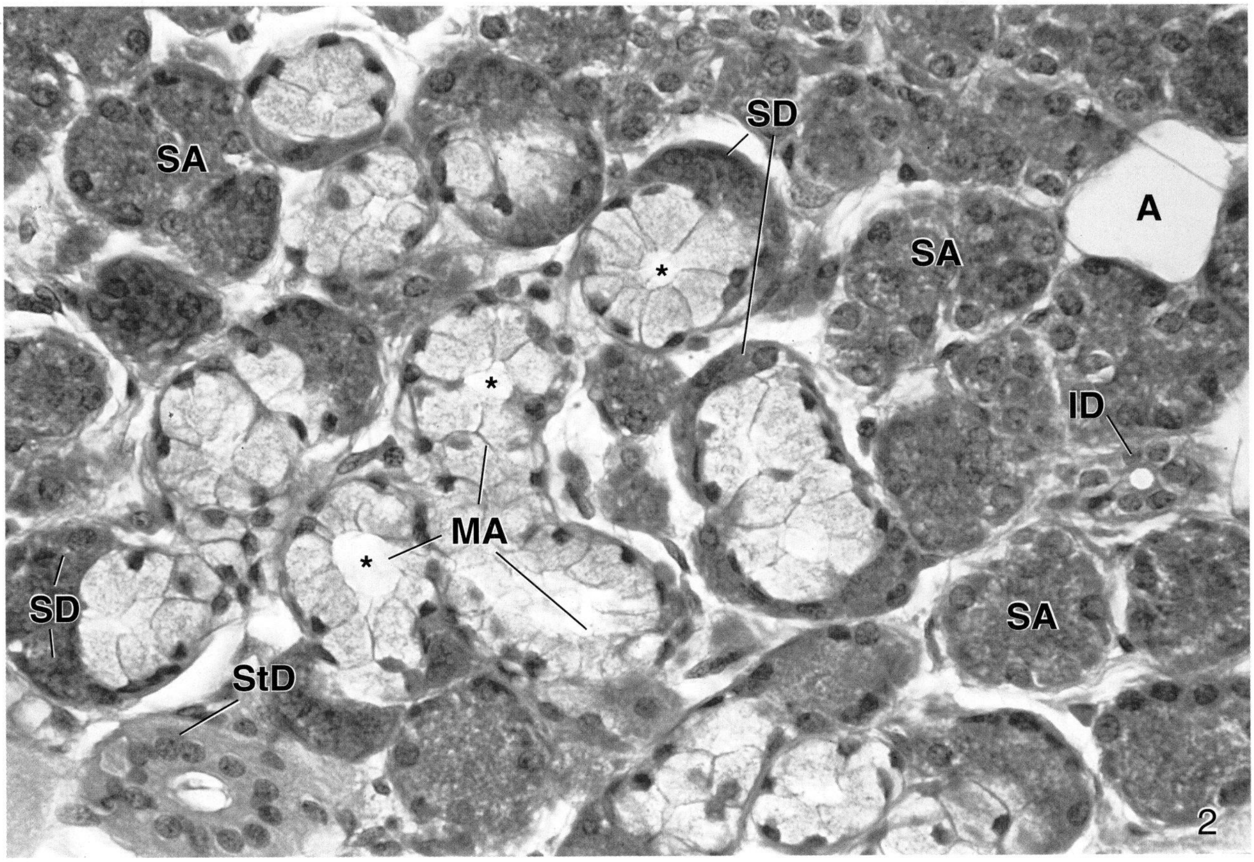
SD
SA
A
SA
*
*
ID
MA
*
SD
SA
StD
2

PLATE 48. PAROTID GLAND

The parotid glands are the largest of the major salivary glands. They are composed of alveoli containing only serous secretory cells. Adipose tissue often occurs in the parotid gland and may be one of its distinguishing features. The facial nerve (cranial nerve VII) passes through the parotid gland; large cross sections of this nerve, often found in routine H&E sections of the gland, may also be of help in identifying the parotid. Mumps, a viral infection of the parotid gland, can damage the facial nerve.

Figure 1, parotid gland, human, H&E ×160.

The parotid gland in the human is composed entirely of serous acini *(A)* and their ducts. However, numerous adipose cells *(AC)* are usually distributed throughout the gland. Both the serous acini and their duct system in the parotid gland are comparable in structure and arrangement to the same components in the submandibular gland. Within the lobule, the striated ducts *(StD)* are readily observed. They exhibit a simple columnar epithelium. The intercalated ducts are smaller; at the low magnification of this figure, they are difficult to recognize. A few intercalated ducts *(ID)* are indicated. The lower portion of the figure reveals an excretory duct *(ED)* within a connective tissue septum *(CT)*. The epithelium of this excretory duct exhibits two layers of nuclei and is either pseudostratified or, possibly, already true stratified epithelium.

Figure 2, parotid gland, monkey, glutaraldehyde–osmium tetroxide fixed, H&E ×640.

The serous cells are optimally preserved in this specimen and reveal their secretory (zymogen) granules. The granules appear as fine dot-like objects within the cytoplasm. The acinus in the upper right of the figure has been cut in cross section and reveals the acinar lumen *(AL)*. The *small rectangle* drawn in the acinus represents an area comparable to the electron micrograph shown as Figure 15.24. The large acinar profile to the left of the striated duct *(StD)* shows that the acini are not simple spheres but, rather, irregular elongate structures. Because of the small size of the acinar lumen and the variability in sectioning an acinus, the lumen is seen infrequently.

A cross-sectional profile of an intercalated duct *(ID)* appears on the left of the micrograph; note its simple cuboidal epithelium. A single flattened nucleus is present at the top of the duct and may represent one of the myoepithelial cells that are associated with the beginning of the duct system as well as with the acini *(A)*. The large duct occupying the center of the micrograph is a striated duct *(StD)*. It is composed of columnar epithelium. The striations *(S)* that give the duct its name are evident. Also of significance is the presence of plasma cells *(PC)* within the connective tissue surrounding the duct. These cells produce the immunoglobulins taken up and resecreted by the acinar cells, particularly secretory IgA (sIgA).

KEY

A, acinus
AC, adipose cell
AL, acinar lumen
CT, connective tissue
ED, excretory duct
ID, intercalated duct
PC, plasma cells
S, striations of duct cells
StD, striated duct

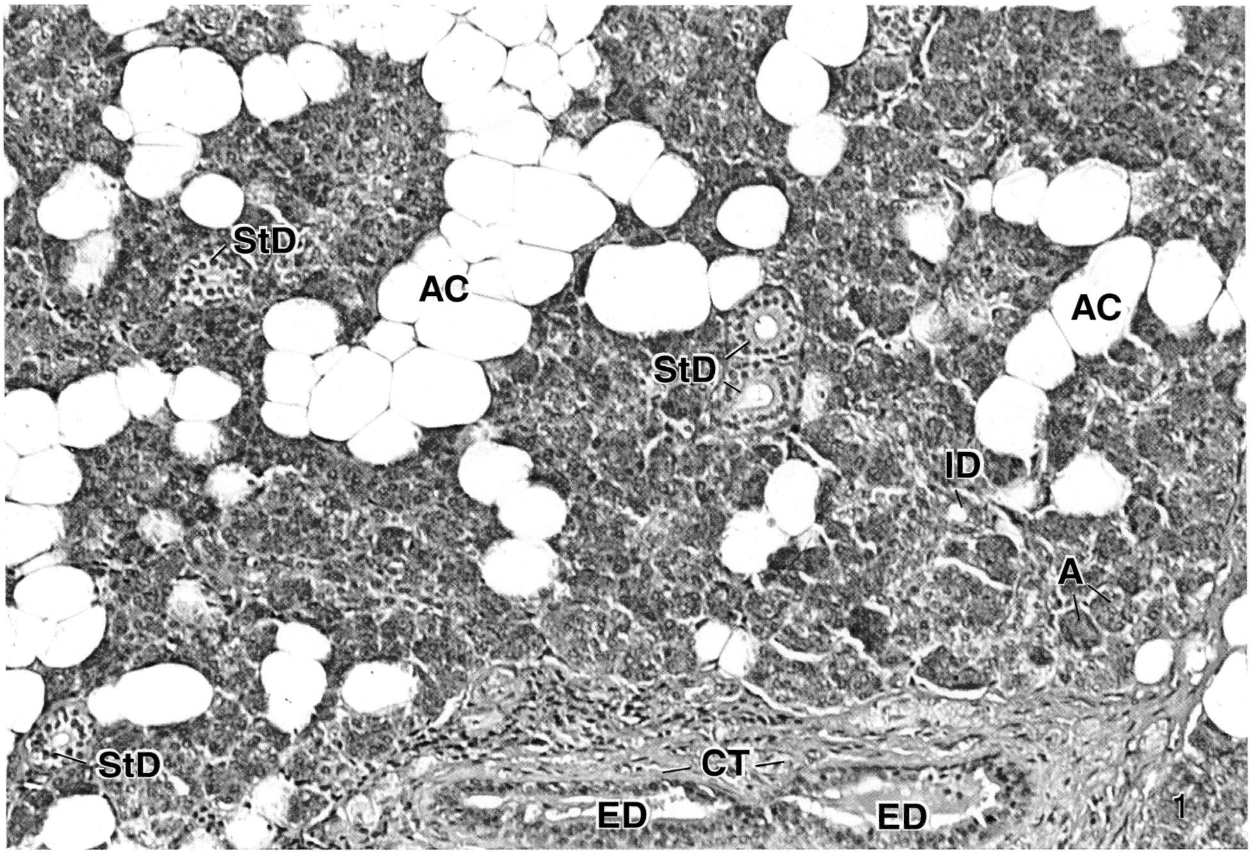
StD
AC
StD
AC
ID
A
StD
CT
ED
ED
1

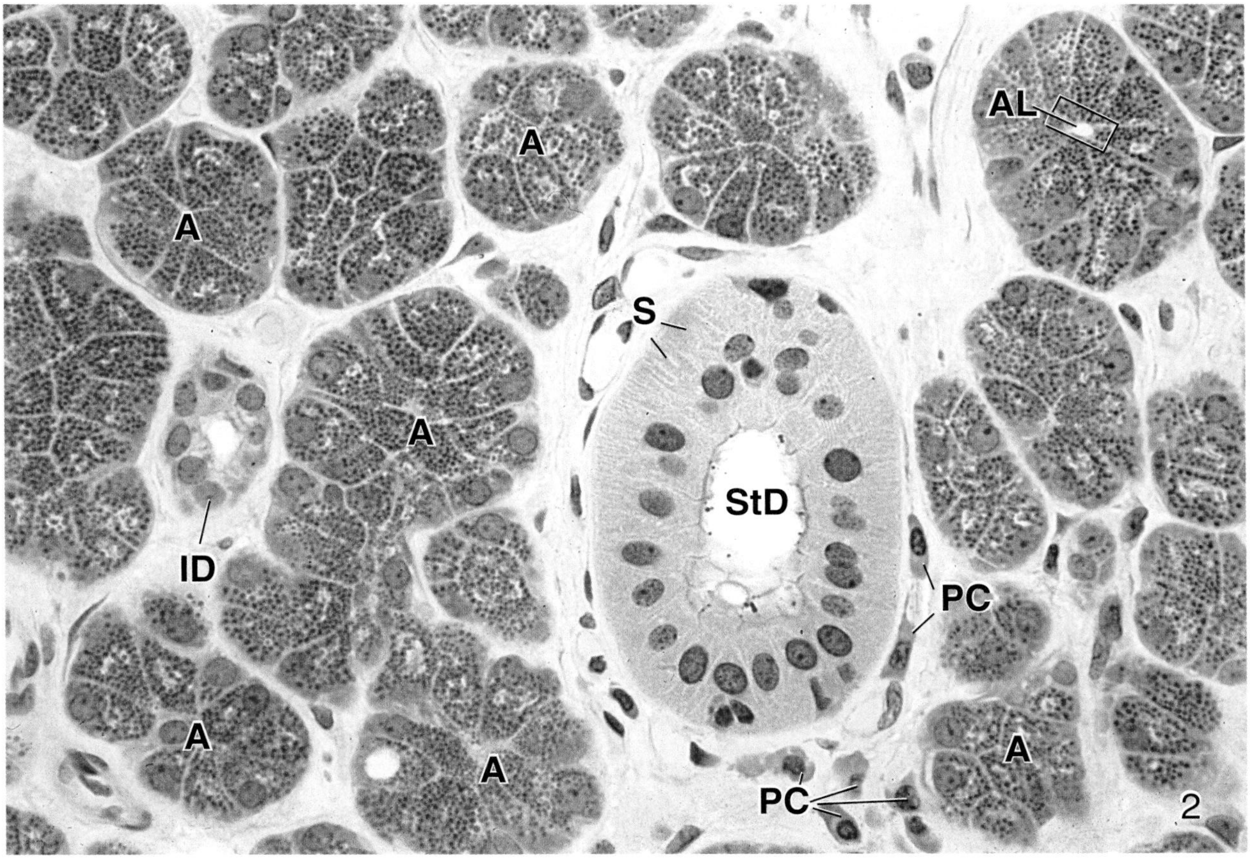
AL
A
A
S
A
StD
ID
PC
A
A
A
PC
2

PLATE 49. SUBLINGUAL GLAND

The sublingual glands are the smallest of the paired major salivary glands. Their multiple small ducts empty into the submandibular ducts as well as directly onto the floor of the mouth. The sublingual gland resembles the submandibular gland, in that it contains both serous and mucous elements. In the sublingual gland, however, the mucous acini predominate. Some of the predominant mucous acini have serous demilunes, but purely serous acini are rarely present.

Saliva includes the combined secretions of all the major and minor salivary glands. The functions of saliva include *moistening* dry foods to aid swallowing, *dissolving* and *suspending* food materials that chemically stimulate taste buds, *buffering* the contents of the oral cavity through its high concentration of bicarbonate ion, *digestion* of carbohydrates by the digestive enzyme α-amylase (which breaks the 1-4 glycoside bonds and continues to act in the esophagus and stomach), and *controlling* the bacterial *flora* of the oral cavity because of the presence of the antibacterial enzyme *lysozyme.*

Saliva is a source of calcium and phosphate ions essential for normal tooth development and maintenance. It also contains antibodies, notably salivary sIgA. Salivation is part of a reflex arc that is normally stimulated by the ingestion of food, although sight, smell, or even thoughts of food can also stimulate salivation.

Figure 1, sublingual gland, human, H&E ×160.

This figure shows a sublingual gland at low power. The mucous acini *(MA)* are conspicuous because of their light staining. Critical examination of the mucous acini at this relatively low magnification reveals that they are not spherical structures but, rather, elongate or tubular structures with branching outpockets. Thus, the acinus is rather large, and much of it is usually not seen within the plane of a single section.

The serous component of the gland is composed largely of demilunes, but occasional serous acini are present. As noted earlier, some of the serous demilunes may be sectioned in a plane that does not include the mucous component of the acinus, thus giving the appearance of a serous acinus.

The ducts of the sublingual gland that are observed most frequently in a section are the intralobular ducts. They are the equivalent of the striated duct of the submandibular and parotid glands but lack the extensive basal infoldings and mitochondrial array that creates the striations. One of the intralobular ducts *(InD)* is evident in this figure (upper right). The area within the *rectangle* includes part of this duct and is shown at higher magnification in Figure 2.

Figure 2, sublingual gland, human, H&E ×400.

Note that through a fortuitous plane of section the lumen of a mucous acinus *(MA)* (upper right) is seen joining an intercalated duct *(ID)*. The juncture between the acinus and the beginning of the intercalated duct is marked by an *arrowhead.* The intercalated duct is composed of a flattened or low columnar epithelium similar to that seen in the other salivary glands. The intercalated ducts of the sublingual gland are extremely short, however, and thus are usually difficult to find. The intercalated duct seen in this micrograph joins with one or more other intercalated ducts to become the intralobular duct *(InD),* which is identified by its columnar epithelium and relatively large lumen. The point of transition from intercalated to intralobular duct is not recognizable in the micrograph, however, because the duct wall has only been grazed and the shape of the cells cannot be determined.

Examination of the acini at this higher magnification also reveals the serous demilunes *(SD)*. Note how they form a cap-like addition to the mucous end pieces. The cytologic appearance of the mucous cells *(MC)* and serous cells is essentially the same as that described for the submandibular gland. The area selected for this higher magnification also reveals isolated cell clusters that bear some resemblance to serous acini. It is likely, however, that these cells are actually mucous cells that either have been cut in a plane parallel to their base and do not include the mucinogen-containing portions of the cell or are in a state of activity in which, after depletion of their granules, the production of new mucinogen granules does not yet suffice to give the characteristic "empty" mucous cell appearance.

An additional important feature of the connective tissue stroma is the presence of numerous lymphocytes and plasma cells. Some of the plasma cells are indicated by the *arrows.* The plasma cells are associated with the production of salivary IgA and are also present in the other salivary glands.

KEY

MA, mucous acinus
MC, mucous cells
ID, intercalated duct
InD, intralobular duct
SD, serous demilune
arrowhead, mucous acinus joining intercalated duct
arrows, plasma cells

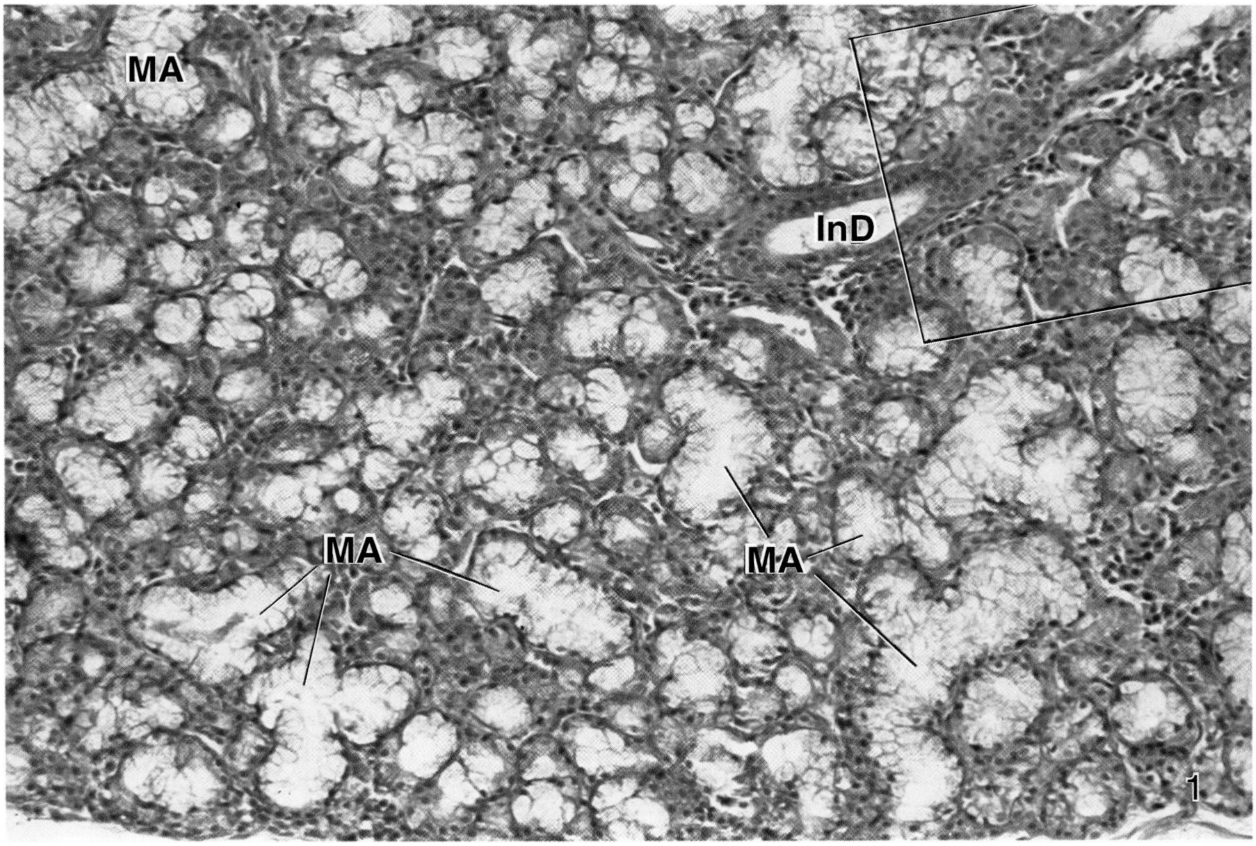
MA
InD
MA
MA
1

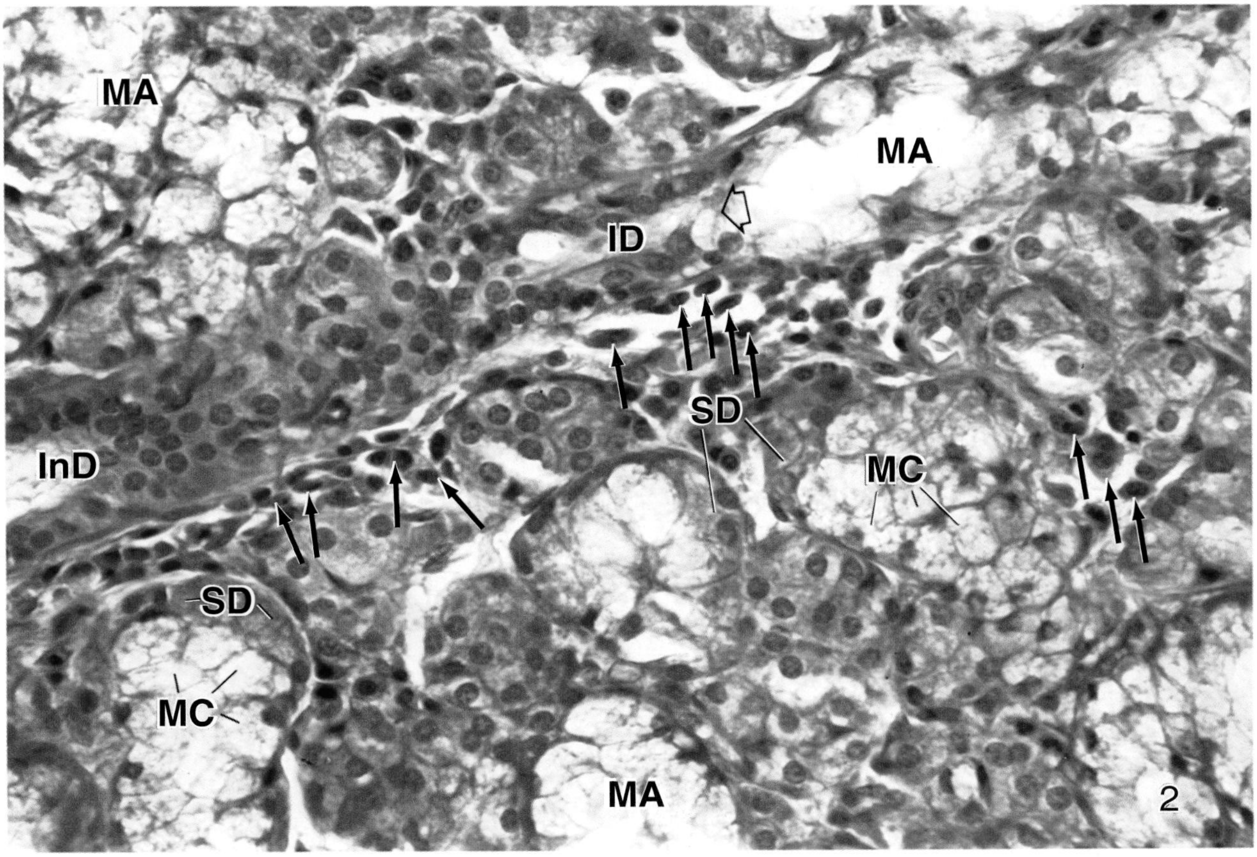
MA
MA
ID
SD
InD
MC
SD
MC
MA
2

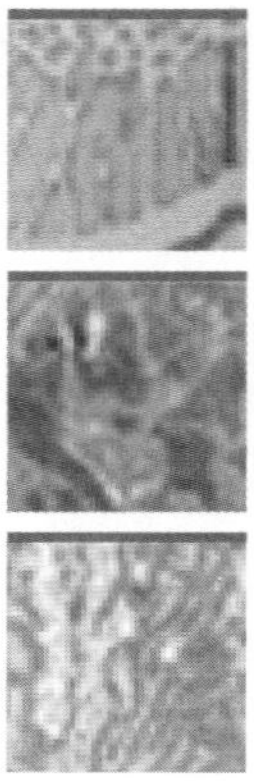

16

Digestive System II: Esophagus and Gastrointestinal Tract

OVERVIEW OF THE ESOPHAGUS AND GASTROINTESTINAL TRACT

The portion of the alimentary canal that extends from the proximal part of the esophagus to the distal part of the anal canal is a hollow tube of varying diameter. This tube has the same basic structural organization throughout its length. Its wall is formed by four distinctive layers. From the lumen outward (Fig. 16.1), they are

- *Mucosa,* consisting of a lining epithelium, an underlying connective tissue called the *lamina propria,* and the *muscularis mucosae,* composed of smooth muscle
- *Submucosa,* consisting of dense irregular connective tissue
- *Muscularis externa,* consisting in most parts of two layers of smooth muscle
- *Serosa,* a serous membrane consisting of a simple squamous epithelium, the mesothelium, and a small amount of underlying connective tissue. An *adventitia* consisting only of connective tissue is found where the wall of the tube is directly attached or fixed to adjoining structures (i.e., body wall and certain retroperitoneal organs).

Mucosa

The structure of the esophagus and gastrointestinal tract varies considerably from region to region; most of the variation occurs within the mucosa. The epithelium differs throughout the alimentary canal and is adapted to the specific function of each part of the tube. The histologic characteristics of these layers are described below in relation to specific regions of the digestive tube. The mucosa has three principal functions: ***protection, absorption,*** and ***secretion.***

The epithelium of the mucosa serves as a barrier that separates the lumen of the alimentary canal from the rest of the organism

The epithelial barrier separates the external luminal environment of the tube from the tissues and organs of the body. The barrier aids in protection of the individual from the entry of antigens, pathogens, and other noxious substances. In the esophagus, a stratified squamous epithelium provides protection from physical abrasion by ingested food. In the gastrointestinal portion of the alimentary tract, tight junctions between the simple columnar epithelial cells of the mucosa serve as a selectively permeable barrier. Most epithelial cells transport products of digestion and other essential substances such as water through the cell and into the extracellular space beneath the tight junctions.

The absorptive function of the mucosa allows the movement of digested nutrients, water, and electrolytes into the blood and lymph vessels

The absorption of digested nutrients, water, and electrolytes is possible because of projections of the mucosa and submucosa into the lumen of the digestive tract. These surface projections greatly increase the surface area available for absorption and vary in size and orientation. They consist of the following structural specializations (see Fig. 16.1)

- ***Plicae circulares*** are circumferentially oriented submucosal folds present along most of the length of the small intestine.
- ***Villi*** are mucosal projections that cover the entire surface of the small intestine, the principal site of absorption of the products of digestion.
- ***Microvilli*** are tightly packed, microscopic projections of the apical surface of intestinal absorptive cells. They further increase the surface available for absorption.

In addition, the ***glycocalyx*** consists of glycoproteins that project from the apical plasma membrane of epithelial absorptive cells. It provides additional surface for adsorption and includes enzymes secreted by the absorptive cells that are essential for the final steps of digestion of proteins and sugars. The epithelium selectively absorbs the products of digestion both for its own cells and for transport into the vascular system for distribution to other tissues.

The secretory function of the mucosa provides lubrication and delivers digestive enzymes, hormones, and antibodies into the lumen of the alimentary tube.

Secretion is carried out largely by glands distributed throughout the length of the digestive tube. The various se-

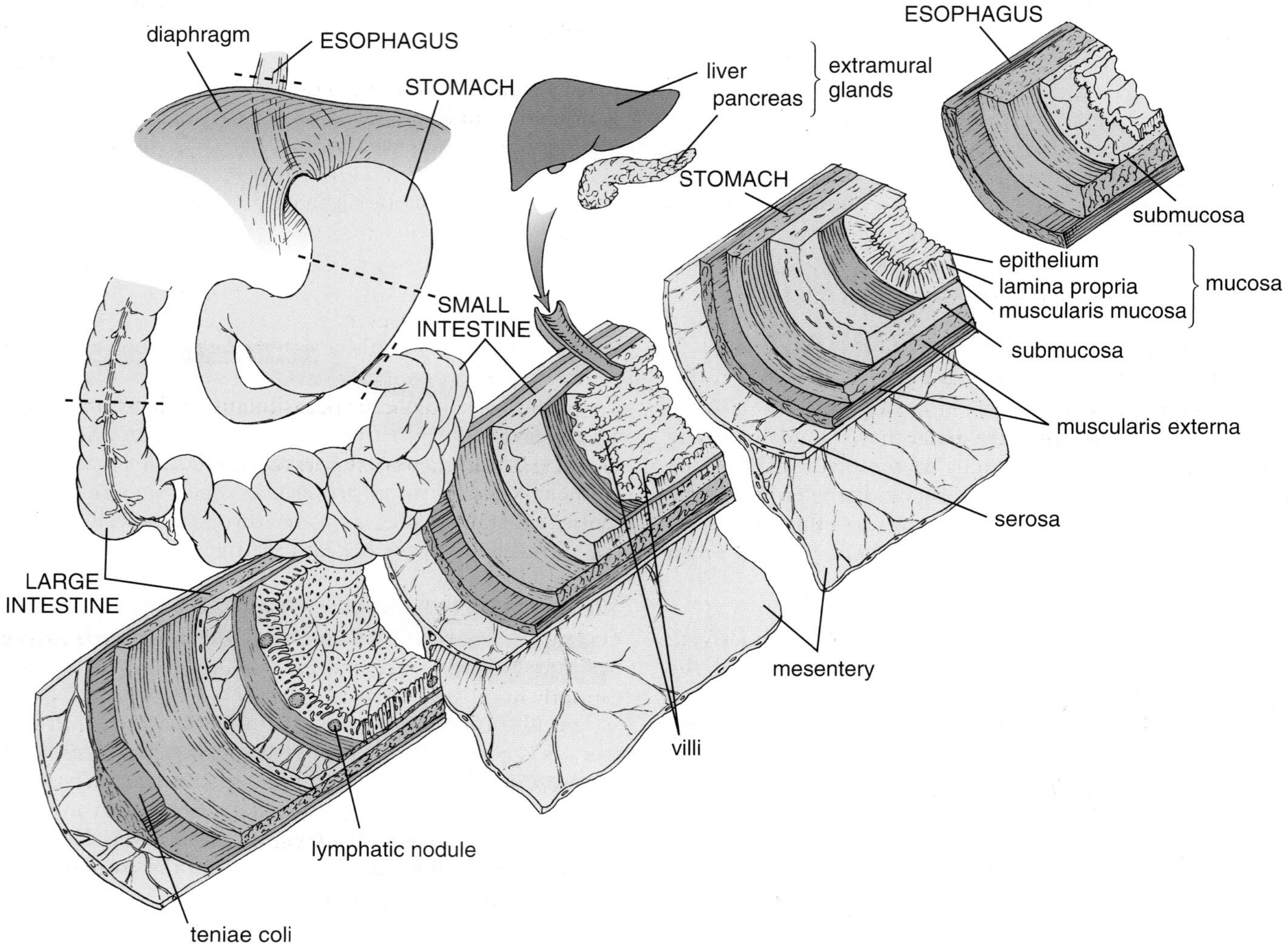

FIGURE 16.1

Diagram of general organization of the alimentary canal. This composite diagram shows the wall structure of the alimentary canal in four representative organs: esophagus, stomach, small intestine, and large intestine. Note that villi, a characteristic feature of the small intestine, are not present in other parts of the alimentary canal. Mucosal glands are present throughout the length of the alimentary canal but sparingly in the esophagus and oral cavity. Submucosal glands are present in the esophagus and duodenum. The extramural glands (liver and pancreas) empty into the duodenum. Diffuse lymphatic tissues and nodules are found in the lamina propria throughout the entire length of the alimentary canal (shown here only in the large intestine). Nerves, blood vessels, and lymphatic vessels reach the alimentary canal via the mesenteries or via the adjacent connective tissue (as in the retroperitoneal organs).

cretory products provide mucus for protective lubrication, as well as buffering of the tract lining and substances that assist in digestion, including enzymes, hydrochloric acid, peptide hormones, and water (see Fig. 16.1). The mucosal epithelium also secretes antibodies that it receives from the underlying connective tissue.

The glands of the alimentary tract (see Fig. 16.1) develop from invaginations of the luminal epithelium and include

- *Mucosal glands* that extend into the lamina propria.
- *Submucosal glands* that either deliver their secretions directly to the lumen of mucosal glands or via ducts that pass through the mucosa to the luminal surface.
- *Extramural glands* that lie outside the digestive tract and deliver their secretions via ducts that pass through the wall of the intestine to enter the lumen. The liver and the pancreas are extramural digestive glands (see Chapter 17) that greatly increase the secretory capacity of the digestive system. They deliver their secretions into the ***duodenum***, the first part of the small intestine

The lamina propria contains glands, vessels that transport absorbed substances, and components of the immune system

As noted, the mucosal glands extend into the lamina propria throughout the length of the alimentary canal. In ad-

dition, in several parts of the alimentary canal (e.g., the esophagus and anal canal), the lamina propria contains aggregations of mucus-secreting glands. In general they lubricate the epithelial surface to protect the mucosa from mechanical and chemical injury. These glands are described below in relation to specific regions of the digestive tube.

In segments of the digestive tract in which absorption occurs, principally the small and large intestines, the absorbed products of digestion diffuse into the blood and lymphatic vessels of the lamina propria for distribution. Typically, the blood capillaries are of the fenestrated type and collect most of the absorbed metabolites. In the small intestine, lymphatic capillaries are numerous and receive some absorbed lipids and proteins.

The lymphatic tissues in the lamina propria function as an integrated immunologic barrier that protects against pathogens and other antigenic substances that could potentially enter through the mucosa from the lumen of the alimentary canal. The lymphatic tissue is represented by

- ***Diffuse lymphatic tissue*** consisting of numerous lymphocytes and plasma cells, located in the lamina propria, and lymphocytes transiently residing in the intercellular spaces of the epithelium
- ***Lymphatic nodules*** with well-developed germinal centers
- ***Eosinophils***, ***macrophages***, and sometimes ***neutrophils***

The diffuse lymphatic tissue and the lymphatic nodules are referred to as ***gut-associated lymphatic tissue (GALT)***. In the distal small intestine, the ***ileum***, extensive aggregates of nodules, called ***Peyer's patches***, occupy much of the lamina propria and submucosa. They tend to be located on the side of the tube opposite the attachment of the mesentery. Aggregated lymphatic nodules are also present in the appendix.

The muscularis mucosae forms the boundary between mucosa and submucosa

The ***muscularis mucosae***, the deepest portion of the mucosa, consists of smooth muscle cells arranged in an inner circular and outer longitudinal layer. Contraction of this muscle produces movement of the mucosa, forming ridges and valleys that facilitate absorption and secretion. This localized movement of the mucosa is independent of the peristaltic movement of the entire wall of the digestive tract.

Submucosa

The submucosa consists of a dense, irregular connective tissue layer containing blood and lymphatic vessels, a nerve plexus, and occasional glands

The submucosa contains the larger blood vessels that send branches to the mucosa, muscularis externa, and serosa. The submucosa also contains lymphatic vessels and a nerve plexus. The extensive nerve network in the submucosa contains visceral sensory fibers mainly of sympathetic origin, parasympathetic (terminal) ganglia, and preganglionic and postganglionic parasympathetic nerve fibers. The nerve cell bodies of parasympathetic ganglia and their postganglionic nerve fibers represent the ***enteric nervous system***, the third division of the autonomic nervous system. This system is primarily responsible for innervating the smooth muscle layers of the alimentary canal and can function totally independent of the central nervous system. In the submucosa, the network of unmyelinated nerve fibers and ganglion cells constitute the ***submucosal plexus (Meissner's plexus)***.

As noted, glands occur occasionally in the submucosa in certain locations. For example, they are present in the esophagus and the initial portion of the duodenum. In histologic sections, the presence of these glands often aids in identifying the specific segment or region of the tract.

Muscularis Externa

In most parts of the digestive tract, the ***muscularis externa*** consists of two concentric and relatively thick layers of smooth muscle. The cells in the inner layer form a tight spiral, described as a ***circularly oriented layer;*** those in the outer layer form a loose spiral, described as a ***longitudinally oriented layer.*** Located between the two muscle layers is a thin connective tissue layer. Within this connective tissue lies the ***myenteric plexus (Auerbach's plexus)*** containing nerve cell bodies (ganglion cells) of postganglionic parasympathetic neurons and neurons of the enteric nervous system, as well as blood vessels and lymphatic vessels.

Contractions of the muscularis externa mix and propel the contents of the digestive tract

Contraction of the inner circular layer of the muscularis externa compresses and mixes the contents by constricting the lumen; contraction of the outer, longitudinal layer propels the contents by shortening the tube. The slow, rhythmic contraction of these muscle layers under the control of the enteric nervous system produces ***peristalsis***, i.e., waves of contraction. Peristalsis is marked by constriction and shortening of the tube, which moves the contents through the intestinal tract.

A few sites along the digestive tube exhibit variations in the muscularis externa. For example, in the wall of the proximal portion of the esophagus (pharyngoesophageal sphincter) and around the anal canal (external anal sphincter), striated muscle forms part of the muscularis externa. In the stomach, a third, obliquely oriented layer of smooth muscle is present deep to the circular layer. Finally, in the large intestine, part of the longitudinal smooth muscle layer is thickened to form three distinct, equally spaced longitudinal bands called ***teniae coli***. Dur-

ing contraction, the teniae facilitate shortening of the tube to move its contents.

The circular smooth muscle layer forms sphincters at specific locations along the digestive tract

At several points along the digestive tract the circular muscle layer is thickened to form *sphincters* or *valves.* From the oropharynx distally, these structures include

- *Pharyngoesophageal sphincter.* Actually, the lowest part of the cricopharyngeus muscle is physiologically referred to as the superior esophageal sphincter. It prevents the entry of air into the esophagus. The inferior esophageal sphincter creates a pressure difference between the esophagus and stomach that prevents reflux of gastric contents into the esophagus.
- *Pyloric sphincter.* Located at the junction of the pylorus of the stomach and duodenum (gastroduodenal sphincter), it controls the release of ***chyme,*** the partially digested contents of the stomach, into the duodenum.
- *Ileocecal valve.* Located at the junction of the small and large intestines, it prevents reflux of the contents of the colon with its high bacterial count into the distal ileum, which normally has a low bacterial count.
- *Internal anal sphincter.* This, the most distally located sphincter, surrounds the anal canal and prevents passage of the feces into the anal canal from the undistended rectum.

Serosa and Adventitia

Serosa or adventitia constitutes the outermost layer of the alimentary canal

The ***serosa*** is a serous membrane consisting of a layer of simple squamous epithelium, called the ***mesothelium,*** and a small amount of underlying connective tissue. It is equivalent to the visceral peritoneum described in gross anatomy. The serosa is the most superficial layer of those parts of the digestive tract that are suspended in the peritoneal cavity. As such, the serosa is continuous with both the ***mesentery*** and the lining of the abdominal cavity.

Large blood and lymphatic vessels and nerve trunks travel through the serosa (from and to the mesentery) to reach the wall of the digestive tract. Large amounts of adipose tissue can develop in the connective tissue of the serosa (and in the mesentery).

Parts of the digestive tract do not possess a serosa. These include the thoracic part of the esophagus and portions of structures in the abdominal and pelvic cavities that are fixed to the cavity wall—the duodenum, ascending and descending colon, rectum, and anal canal. These structures are attached to the abdominal and pelvic wall by connective tissue, the ***adventitia,*** which blends with the connective tissue of the wall.

▼ ESOPHAGUS

The esophagus is a fixed muscular tube that delivers food and liquid from the pharynx to the stomach

The esophagus courses through the neck and mediastinum where it is fixed to adjacent structures by connective tissue. As it enters the abdominal cavity, it is free for a short distance, approximately 1 to 2 cm. The overall length of the esophagus is about 25 cm. On cross section (Fig. 16.2), the lumen in its normally collapsed state has a branched appearance due to longitudinal folds. When a bolus of food passes through the esophagus the lumen expands without mucosal injury.

The ***mucosa*** that lines the length of the esophagus has a nonkeratinized stratified squamous epithelium (Fig. 16.3). In many animals, however, the epithelium is keratinized, reflecting a coarse food diet. In humans, the surface cells may exhibit some keratohyalin granules, but keratinization does not normally occur. The underlying lamina propria is similar to the lamina propria throughout the alimentary tract; diffuse lymphatic tissue is scattered throughout, and lymphatic nodules are present, often in proximity to ducts of the esophageal mucous glands (described below). The deep layer of the mucosa, the muscularis mucosae, is composed of longitudinally organized smooth muscle that begins near the level of the cricoid cartilage. It is unusually thick in the proximal portion of the esophagus and presumably functions as an aid in swallowing.

The ***submucosa*** consists of dense irregular connective tissue that contains the larger blood and lymphatic vessels, nerve fibers, and ganglion cells. The nerve fibers and ganglion cells make up the submucosal plexus (Meissner's plexus). Glands are also present (described below). In addition, diffuse lymphatic tissue and lymphatic nodules are present mostly in the upper and lower parts of the esophagus where submucosal glands are more prevalent.

The ***muscularis externa*** consists of two muscle layers, an inner circular layer and an outer longitudinal layer. It differs from the muscularis externa found in the rest of the digestive tract in that the upper one third is striated muscle, a continuation of the muscle of the pharynx. Striated muscle and smooth muscle bundles are mixed and interwoven in the muscularis externa of the middle third of the esophagus; the muscularis externa of the distal third consists only of smooth muscle, as in the rest of the digestive tract. A nerve plexus, the myenteric plexus (Auerbach's plexus), is present between the outer and inner muscle layers. As in the submucosal plexus (Meissner's plexus), nerves and ganglion cells are present here. This plexus innervates the muscularis externa and produces peristaltic activity.

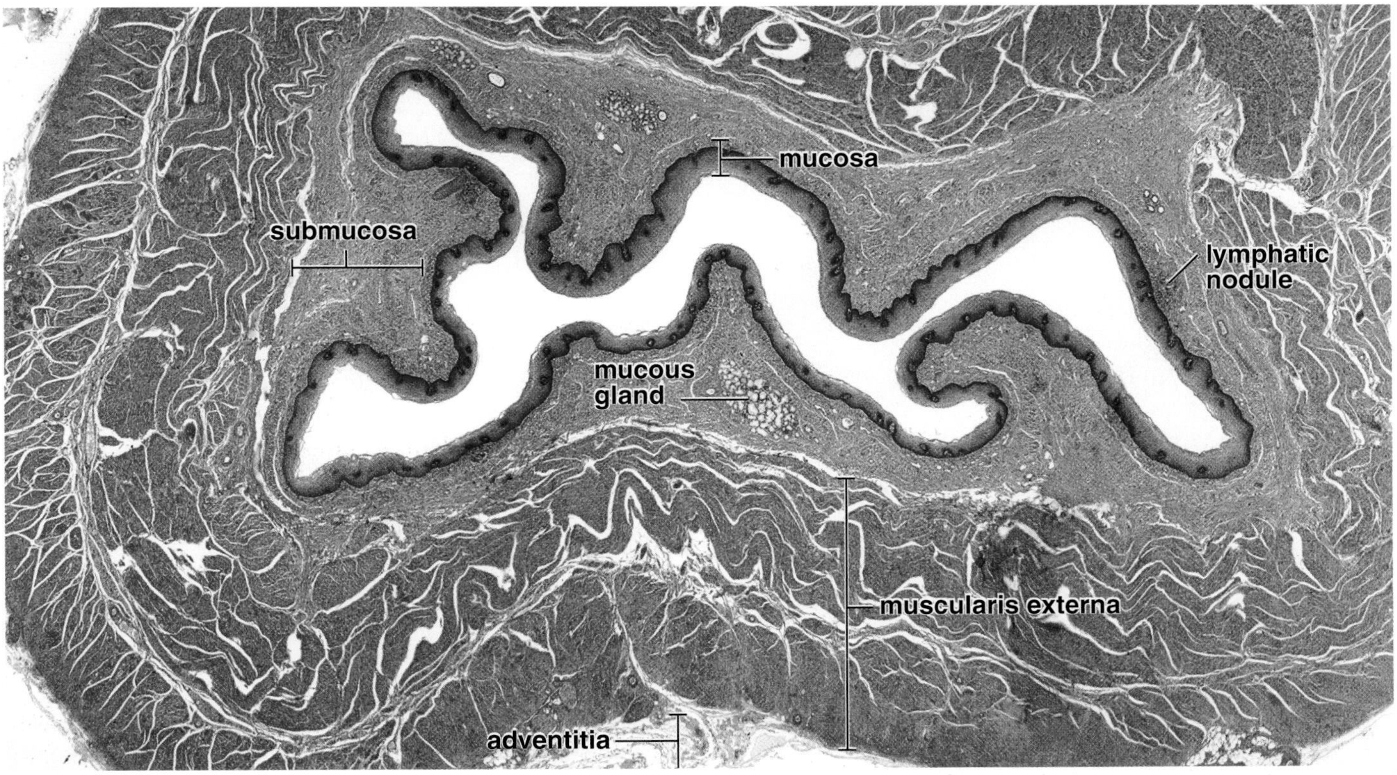

FIGURE 16.2
Photomicrograph of the esophagus. This low-magnification photomicrograph shows a H&E–stained section of the esophagus with its characteristically folded wall, giving the lumen an irregular appearance. The mucosa consists of a relatively thick stratified squamous epithelium, a thin layer of lamina propria containing occasional lymphatic nodules, and a muscularis mucosae. Mucous glands are present in the submucosa; their ducts, which empty into the lumen of the esophagus, are not evident in this section. External to the submucosa in this part of the esophagus there is a thick muscularis externa made up of an inner layer of circularly arranged smooth muscle and an outer layer of longitudinally arranged smooth muscle. The adventitia is seen just external to the muscularis externa. ×8.

As noted, the esophagus is fixed to adjoining structures throughout most of its length; thus its outer layer is composed of adventitia. After entering the abdominal cavity, the short remainder of the tube is covered by serosa, the visceral peritoneum.

Mucosal and submucosal glands of the esophagus secrete mucus to lubricate and protect the luminal wall

Glands are present in the wall of the esophagus and are of two types. Both secrete mucus, but their locations differ.

- *Esophageal glands proper* occur in the submucosa. These glands are scattered along the length of the esophagus but are somewhat more concentrated in the upper half. They are small, compound, tubuloalveolar glands (Fig. 16.4). The excretory duct is composed of stratified squamous epithelium and is usually conspicuous when present in a section, because of its dilated appearance.
- *Esophageal cardiac glands* are named for their similarity to the cardiac glands of the stomach and occur in the lamina propria of the mucosa. They are present in the terminal part of the esophagus and frequently, though not consistently, in the beginning portion of the esophagus.

The mucus produced by the esophageal glands proper is slightly acidic and serves to lubricate the luminal wall. Because the secretion is relatively viscous, transient cysts often occur in the ducts. The esophageal cardiac glands produce a neutral mucus. Those glands near the stomach tend to protect the esophagus from regurgitated gastric contents. Under certain conditions, however, they are not fully effective, and excessive reflux results in ***pyrosis***, a condition more commonly known as ***heartburn***.

The muscle of the esophageal wall is innervated by both autonomic and somatic nervous systems

The striated musculature in the upper part of the esophagus is innervated by somatic motor neurons of the ***vagus nerve***, cranial nerve X (from the nucleus ambiguus). The

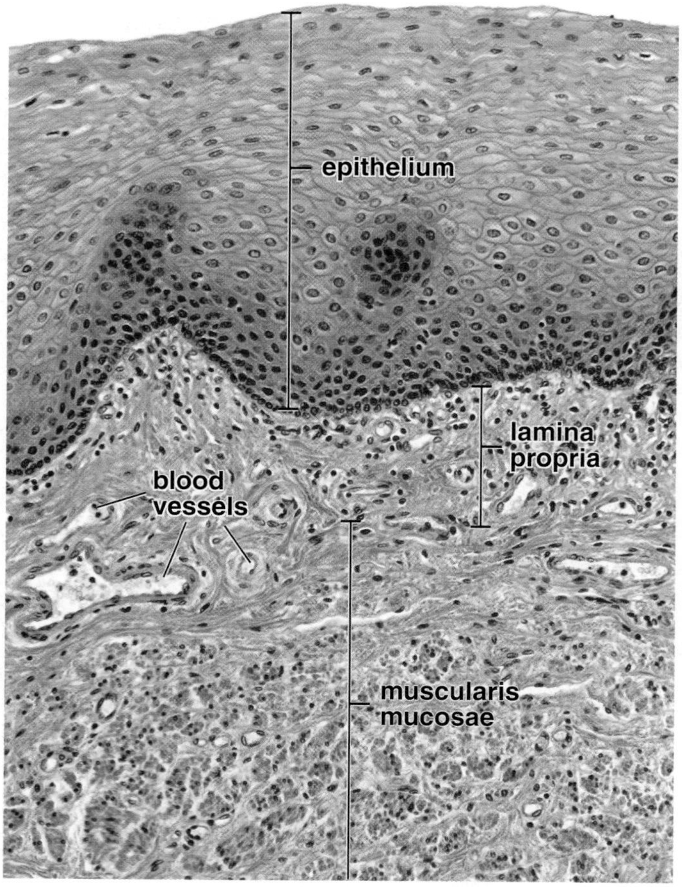

FIGURE 16.3
Photomicrograph of the esophageal mucosa. This higher-magnification photomicrograph shows the mucosa of the wall of the esophagus in a H&E preparation. It consists of a stratified squamous epithelium, lamina propria, and muscularis mucosae. The boundary between the epithelium and lamina propria is distinct, although uneven, because of the connective tissue papillae. The basal layer of the epithelium stains intensely, appearing as a dark band because the basal cells are smaller and have a high nucleus-to-cytoplasm ratio. Note that the loose connective tissue of the lamina propria is very cellular, containing many lymphocytes. The deepest part of the mucosa is the muscularis mucosae that is arranged in two layers (inner circular and outer longitudinal) similar in orientation to the muscularis externa. ×240.

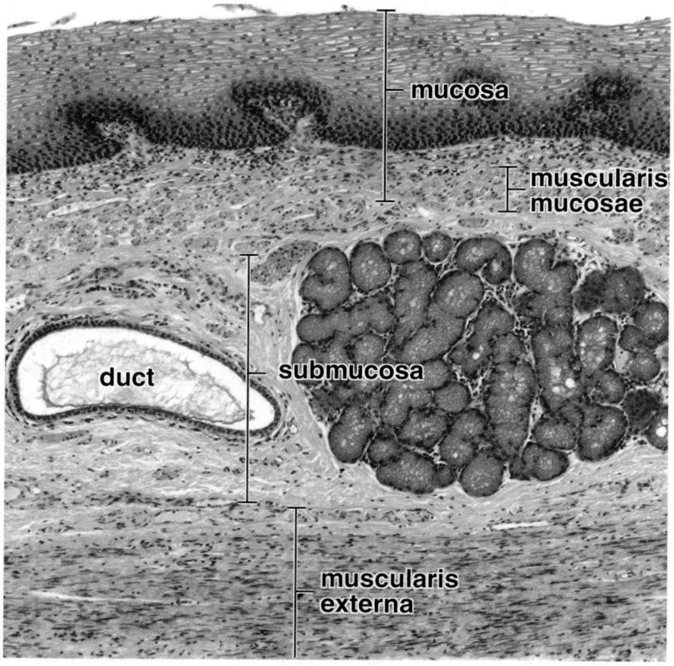

FIGURE 16.4
Photomicrograph of an esophageal submucosal gland. This photomicrograph shows a mucicarmine-stained section of the esophagus. An esophageal gland, deeply stained red by the carmine, and an adjacent excretory duct are seen in the submucosa. These small, compound, tubuloalveolar glands produce mucus that lubricates the epithelial surface of the esophagus. Note the stained mucus within the excretory duct. The remaining submucosa consists of irregular dense connective tissue. The inner layer of the muscularis externa *(bottom)* is composed of circularly arranged smooth muscle. ×110.

smooth muscle of the lower part of the esophagus is innervated by visceral motor neurons of the vagus (from the dorsal motor nucleus). These motor neurons synapse with postganglionic neurons whose cell bodies are located in the wall of the esophagus.

▼ STOMACH

The stomach is an expanded part of the digestive tube that lies beneath the diaphragm. It receives the bolus of macerated food from the esophagus. Mixing and partial digestion of the food in the stomach by its gastric secretions produces a pulpy fluid mix called chyme. The chyme then passes into the small intestine for further digestion and absorption.

The stomach is divided histologically into three regions on the basis of the type of gland that each contains

Gross anatomists subdivide the stomach into four regions. The ***cardia*** surrounds the esophageal orifice; the ***fundus*** lies above the level of a horizontal line drawn through the esophageal (cardiac) orifice; the ***body*** lies below this line; and the ***pyloric part*** is the funnel-shaped region that leads into the ***pylorus,*** the distal, narrow sphincteric region between the stomach and duodenum. Histologists also subdivide the stomach, but into only three regions (Fig. 16.5). These subdivisions are based not on location but on the types of glands that occur in the gastric mucosa. The histologic regions are the

- ***Cardiac region (cardia),*** the part near the esophageal orifice, which contains the ***cardiac glands*** (Fig. 16.6)
- ***Pyloric region (pylorus),*** the part proximal to the pyloric sphincter, which contains the ***pyloric glands***

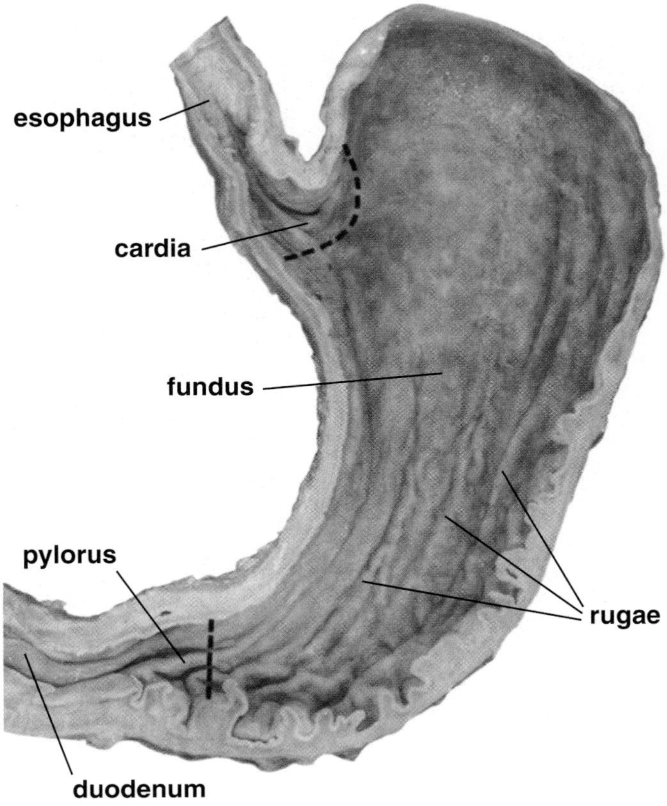

FIGURE 16.5
Photograph of a hemisected human stomach. This photograph shows the mucosal surface of the posterior wall of the stomach. Numerous longitudinal gastric folds are evident. These folds or rugae allow the stomach to distend as it fills. The histologic divisions of the stomach differ from the anatomic division. The former is based on the types of glands found in the mucosa. Histologically, the portion of the stomach adjacent to the entrance of the esophagus is the cardiac region *(cardia)* in which cardiac glands are located. A *dashed line* approximates its boundary. A slightly larger region leading toward the pyloric sphincter, the pyloric region *(pylorus)*, contains the pyloric glands. Another *dashed line* approximates its boundary. The remainder of the stomach, the fundic region *(fundus)*, is located between the two *dashed lines* and contains the fundic (gastric) glands.

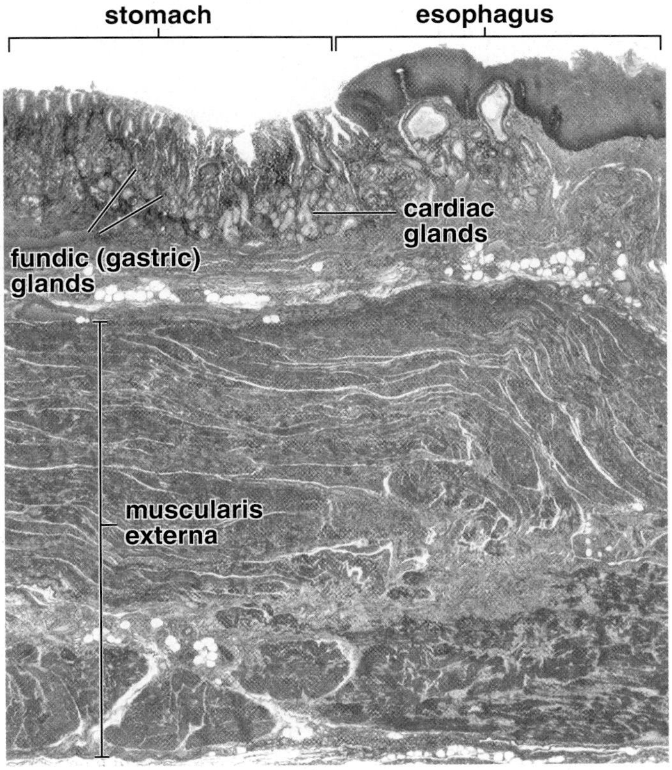

FIGURE 16.6
Photomicrograph of esophagogastric junction. This low-magnification photomicrograph shows the junction between the esophagus and stomach. At the esophagogastric junction, the stratified squamous epithelium of the esophagus ends abruptly, and the simple columnar epithelium of the stomach mucosa begins. The surface of the stomach contains numerous and relatively deep depressions called gastric pits that are formed by the surface epithelium. The glands in the vicinity of the esophagus, the cardiac glands, extend from the bottom of these pits. The fundic (gastric) glands similarly arise at the base of the gastric pits and are evident in the remaining part of the mucosa. Note the relatively thick muscularis externa. ×40.

- ***Fundic region (fundus)***, the largest part of the stomach, which is situated between the cardia and pylorus and contains the ***fundic*** or ***gastric glands*** (see Fig. 16.6)

Gastric Mucosa

Longitudinal submucosal folds, rugae, allow the stomach to distend when filled

The stomach has the same general structural plan throughout, consisting of a mucosa, submucosa, muscularis externa, and serosa. Examination of the inner surface of the empty stomach reveals a number of longitudinal folds or ridges called ***rugae.*** They are prominent in the narrower regions of the stomach but poorly developed in the upper portion (see Fig. 16.5). When the stomach is fully distended, the rugae, composed of the mucosa and underlying submucosa, virtually disappear. The rugae do not alter total surface area; rather, they serve to accommodate expansion and filling of the stomach.

A view of the stomach's surface with a hand lens shows that smaller regions of the mucosa are formed by grooves or shallow trenches that divide the stomach surface into bulging irregular areas called ***mamillated areas.*** These grooves provide a slightly increased surface area for secretion.

At higher magnification, numerous openings can be observed in the mucosal surface. These are the ***gastric pits,*** or ***foveolae.*** They can be readily demonstrated with the scanning electron microscope (Fig. 16.7). The gastric glands open into the bottom of the gastric pits.

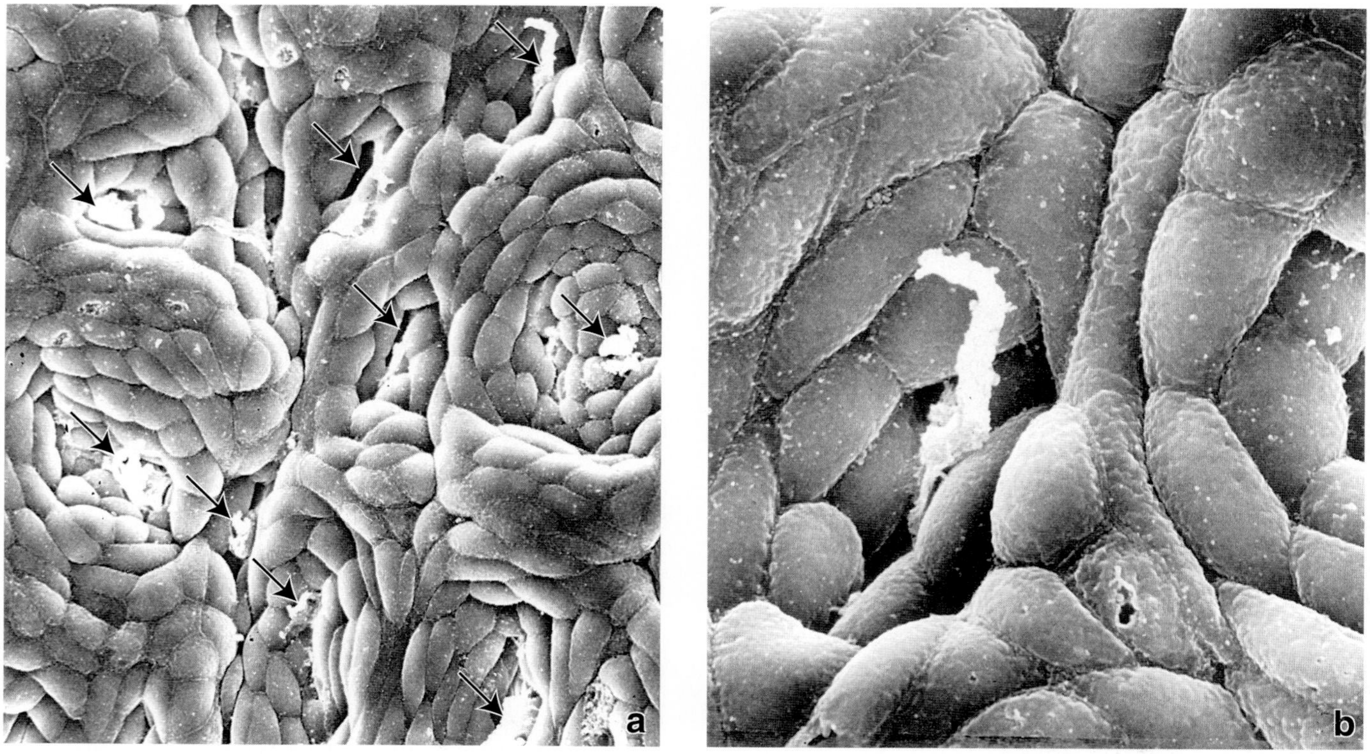

FIGURE 16.7
Mucosal surface of the stomach. a. Scanning electron micrograph showing the mucosal surface of the stomach. The gastric pits contain secretory material, mostly mucus *(arrows)*. The surface mucus has been washed away to reveal the surface mucous cells. ×1,000. **b.** Higher magnification showing the apical surface of the surface mucous cells that line the stomach and gastric pits. Note the elongate polygonal shape of the cells. ×3,000.

Surface mucous cells line the inner surface of the stomach and the gastric pits

The epithelium that lines the surface and the gastric pits of the stomach is simple columnar. The columnar cells are designated ***surface mucous cells.*** Each cell possesses a large, apical cup of ***mucinogen granules,*** creating a glandular sheet of cells (Fig. 16.8). The mucous cup occupies most of the volume of the cell. It typically appears empty in routine hematoxylin and eosin (H&E) sections because the mucinogen is lost in fixation and dehydration. When the mucinogen is preserved by appropriate fixation, however, the granules stain intensely with toluidine blue and with the periodic acid–Schiff (PAS) procedure. The toluidine blue staining reflects the presence of many strongly anionic groups in the glycoprotein of the mucin, among which is bicarbonate.

The nucleus and Golgi apparatus of the surface mucous cells are located below the mucous cup. The basal part of the cell contains small amounts of rough endoplasmic reticulum (rER) that may impart a light basophilia to the cytoplasm when observed in well-preserved specimens.

The mucous secretion from the surface mucous cells is described as ***visible mucus*** because of its cloudy appearance. It forms a thick, viscous, gel-like coat that adheres to the epithelial surface; thus, it protects against abrasion from rougher components of the chyme. Additionally, its high bicarbonate concentration protects the epithelium from the acidic content of the gastric juice. The bicarbonate that makes the mucus alkaline is secreted by the surface cells but is prevented from mixing rapidly with the contents of the gastric lumen by its containment within the mucus coat.

The lining of the stomach does not function in an absorptive capacity. However, some water, salts, and lipid-soluble drugs may be absorbed; alcohol and certain drugs, e.g., aspirin, enter the lamina propria by damaging the surface epithelium.

FUNDIC GLANDS OF THE GASTRIC MUCOSA

The fundic glands produce the gastric juice of the stomach

The ***fundic glands,*** also called ***gastric glands,*** are present throughout the entire gastric mucosa except for the relatively small regions occupied by cardiac and pyloric glands. The fundic glands are simple, branched, tubular glands that extend from the bottom of the gastric pits to the muscularis mucosae (see Fig. 16.8). Located between the gastric pit and the gland below is a short segment

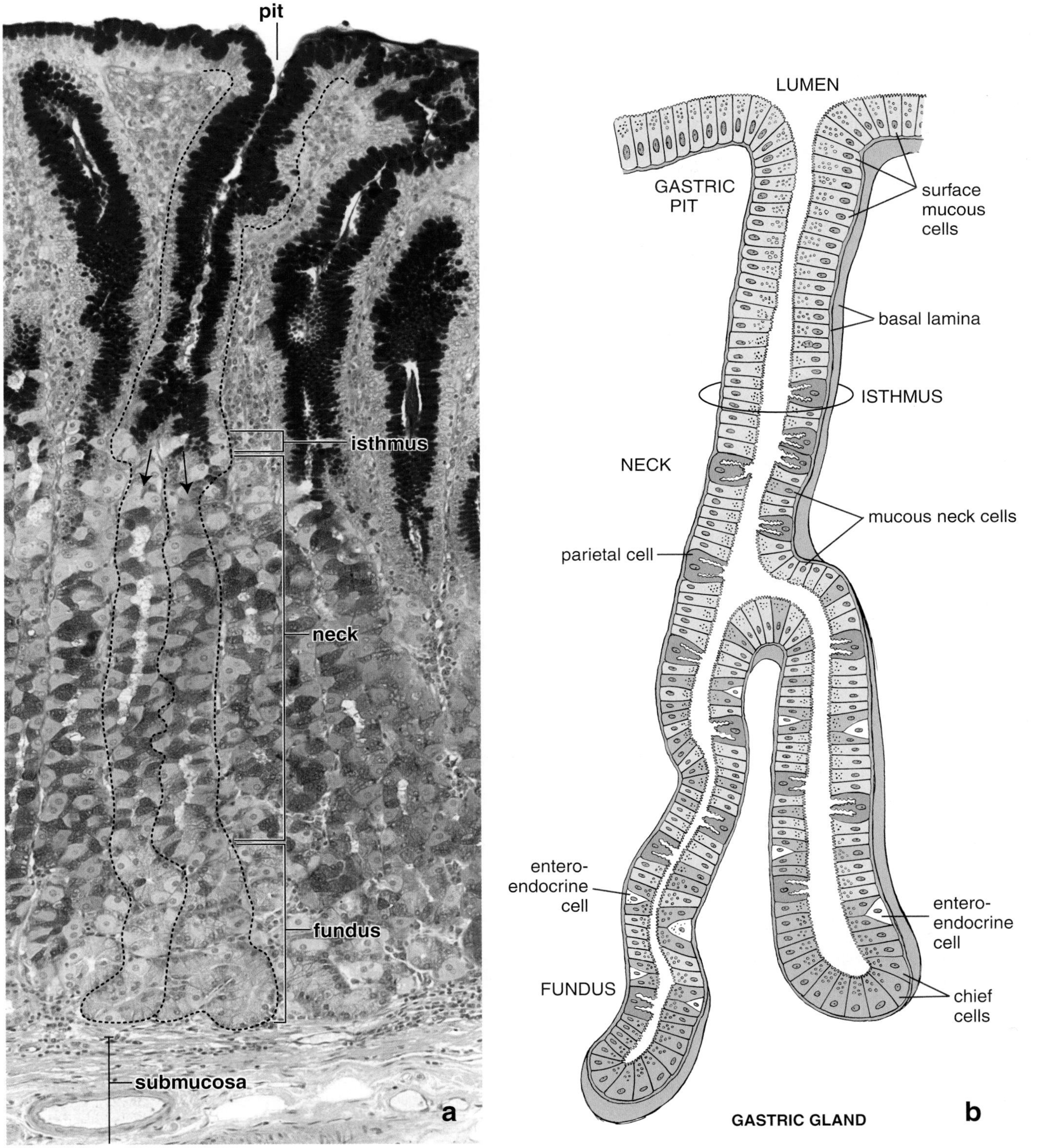

FIGURE 16.8

Gastric glands. a. This photomicrograph shows the fundic mucosa from an Alcian blue/PAS preparation to visualize mucus. Note that the surface epithelium invaginates to form the gastric pits. The surface mucous cells and the cells lining the gastric pits are readily identified in this preparation because the neutral mucus within these cells is stained intensely. One of the gastric pits and its associated fundic gland are depicted by the *dashed lines.* This gland represents a simple branched tubular gland *(arrows* indicate the branching pattern). It extends from the bottom of the gastric pit to the muscularis mucosae. Note the segments of the gland: the short isthmus, the site of cell divisions; the relatively long neck; and a shorter and wider fundus. The mucous secretion of mucous neck cells is different from that produced by the surface mucous cells as evidenced by the *lighter magenta* staining in this region of the gland. ×320. **b.** Schematic diagram of a gastric gland, illustrating the relationship of the gland to the gastric pit. Note that the isthmus region contains dividing cells and undifferentiated cells; the neck region contains mucous neck cells, parietal cells, and enteroendocrine cells, including amine precursor uptake and decarboxylation (APUD) cells. Parietal cells are large, pear-shaped acidophilic cells found throughout the gland. The fundus of the gland contains mainly chief cells, some parietal cells, and several types of enteroendocrine cells.

known as the ***isthmus,*** the site of cell replication. Cells destined to become mucous surface cells migrate upward in the gastric pits to the stomach surface. Other cells migrate downward, maintaining the population of the fundic gland epithelium. Typically, several glands open into a single gastric pit. Each gland has a narrow, relatively long ***neck segment*** and a shorter and wider ***base*** or ***fundic segment.*** The base of the gland usually divides into two and sometimes three branches that become slightly coiled near the muscularis mucosae. The cells of the gastric glands produce gastric juice (about 2 L/day), which contains a variety of substances. In addition to water and electrolytes, gastric juice contains four major components:

- ***Hydrochloric acid (HCl)*** in a concentration ranging from 150 to 160 mmol/L, which gives the gastric juice a low pH (<1.0 to 2.0). It is produced by ***parietal cells*** and initiates digestion of dietary protein (it promotes acid hydrolysis of substrates). It also converts inactive pepsinogen into the active enzyme pepsin. Because HCl is bacteriostatic, most of the bacteria entering the stomach with the ingested food are destroyed.
- ***Pepsin,*** a potent proteolytic enzyme. It is converted from ***pepsinogen*** produced by the ***chief cells*** by HCl at a pH lower than 5. Pepsin hydrolyzes proteins into small peptides by splitting interior peptide bonds. Peptides are further digested into amino acids by enzymes in the small intestine.
- ***Mucus,*** an acid-protective coating for the stomach secreted by several types of mucus-producing cells. The mucus and bicarbonates trapped within the mucous layer maintain a neutral pH and contribute to the so-called ***physiologic gastric mucosa barrier.*** In addition, mucus serves as a physical barrier between the cells of the gastric mucosa and the ingested material in the lumen of the stomach.
- ***Intrinsic factor,*** a glycoprotein that binds to vitamin B_{12}. It is essential for absorption of vitamin B_{12}, which occurs in the distal part of the ileum.

In addition, ***gastrin*** and other hormones and hormone-like secretions are produced by enteroendocrine cells in the fundic glands and secreted into the lamina propria where they enter the circulation or act locally on other gastric epithelial cells.

Fundic glands are composed of four functionally different cell types

The cells that constitute the fundic glands are of four functional types. Each has a distinctive appearance. In addition, undifferentiated cells that give rise to these cells are also present. The various cells that constitute the gland are

- ***Mucous neck cells***
- ***Chief cells***
- ***Parietal cells,*** also called ***oxyntic cells***
- ***Enteroendocrine cells***
- ***Undifferentiated cells***

Mucous neck cells are localized in the neck region of the gland and are interspersed with parietal cells

As the name implies, the ***mucous neck cells*** are located in the neck region of the fundic gland. Parietal cells are usually interspersed between groups of these cells. The mucous neck cell is much shorter than the surface mucous cell and contains considerably less mucinogen in the apical cytoplasm. Consequently, these cells do not exhibit a prominent mucous cup. Also, the nucleus tends to be spherical compared with the more prominent, elongate nucleus of the surface mucous cell.

The mucous neck cells secrete a ***soluble mucus*** compared with the ***insoluble*** or ***cloudy mucus*** produced by the surface mucous cell. Release of mucinogen granules is induced by vagal stimulation; thus, secretion from these cells does not occur in the resting stomach.

Chief cells are located in the deeper part of the fundic glands

Chief cells are typical protein-secreting cells (Fig. 16.9). The abundant rER in the basal cytoplasm gives this part of the cell a basophilic appearance, whereas the apical cytoplasm is eosinophilic due to the presence of the secretory granules, also called zymogen granules because they contain enzyme precursors. The basophilia, in particular, allows easy identification of these cells in H&E sections. The eosinophilia may be faint or absent when the secretory granules are not adequately preserved. Chief cells secrete ***pepsinogen*** and a weak lipase. On contact with the acid gastric juice, pepsinogen is converted to pepsin, a proteolytic enzyme.

Parietal cells secrete HCl and intrinsic factor

Parietal (oxyntic) cells are found in the neck of the fundic glands, among the mucous neck cells, and in the deeper part of the gland. They tend to be most numerous in the upper and middle portions of the neck. They are large cells, sometimes binucleate, and appear somewhat triangular in sections, with the apex directed toward the lumen of the gland and the base resting on the basal lamina. The nucleus is spherical, and the cytoplasm stains with eosin and other acidic dyes. Their size and distinctive staining characteristics allow them to be easily distinguished from other cells in the fundic glands.

When examined with the transmission electron microscope (TEM), parietal cells (Fig. 16.10) are seen to have an extensive ***intracellular canalicular system*** that communicates with the lumen of the gland. Numerous microvilli project from the surface of the canaliculi, and an elaborate ***tubulovesicular membrane system*** is present in the cytoplasm adjacent to the canaliculi. In an actively secreting

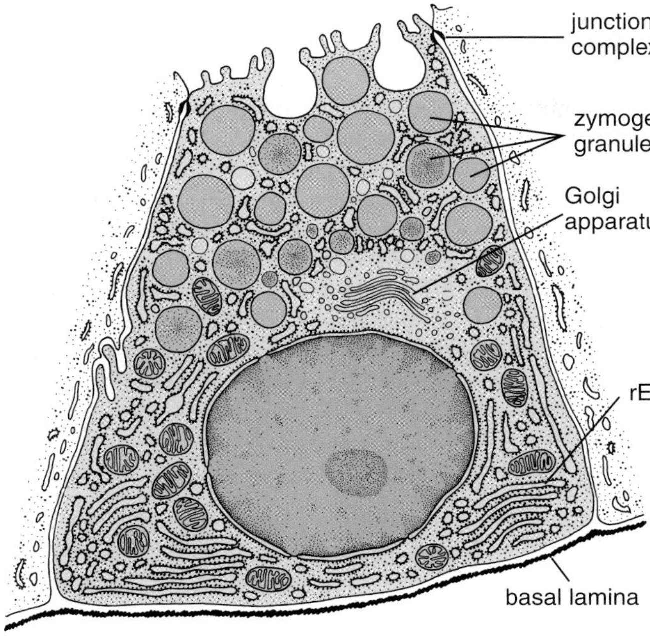

FIGURE 16.9
Diagram of a chief cell. The large amount of rER in the basal portion of the cell accounts for the intense basophilic staining seen in this region. Zymogen granules containing pepsinogen and a weak lipase are not always adequately preserved, and thus the staining in the apical region of the cell is somewhat variable. This cell produces and secretes the precursor enzyme of the gastric secretion. (Based on Lentz TL. *Cell Fine Structure: An Atlas of Drawings of Whole-Cell Structure.* Philadelphia: WB Saunders, 1971.)

cell, the number of microvilli in the canaliculi increases, and the tubulovesicular system is reduced significantly or disappears. The membranes of the tubulovesicular system serve as a reservoir of plasma membrane containing active proton pumps. This membrane material can be inserted into the plasma membrane of the canaliculi to increase their surface area and the number of proton pumps available for acid production. Numerous mitochondria with complex cristae and many matrix granules supply the high levels of energy necessary for acid secretion.

HCl is produced in the lumen of the intracellular canaliculi

Parietal cells have three different types of membrane receptors for substances that activate HCl secretion: ***gastrin, histamine*** H_2, and ***acetylcholine*** M_3 receptors. Activation of the gastrin receptor by ***gastrin,*** a gastrointestinal peptide hormone, is the major path for parietal cell stimulation. Following stimulation, several steps occur in the production of HCl (Fig. 16.11):

- ***Production of*** H^+ ***ions*** in the parietal cell cytoplasm by the enzyme carbonic anhydrase. This enzyme hydrolyzes carbonic acid (H_2CO_3) to H^+ and HCO_3^-. Carbon dioxide (CO_2) necessary for synthesis of carbonic acid diffuses across the basement membrane into the cell from the blood capillaries in the lamina propria.
- ***Transport of*** H^+ ***ions*** from the cytoplasm, across the membrane to the lumen of the canaliculus by the H^+/K^+-ATPase proton pump. Simultaneously, K^+ from the canaliculus is transported into the cell cytoplasm in exchange for the H^+ ions.
- ***Transport of*** K^+ ***and*** Cl^- from the parietal cell cytoplasm into the lumen of the canaliculus through activation of K^+ and Cl^- channels (uniporters) in the plasma membrane.
- ***Formation of HCl*** from the H^+ and Cl^- that were transported into the lumen of the canaliculus.

In humans, ***intrinsic factor*** is secreted by the parietal cells (chief cells do so in some other species). Its secretion is stimulated by the same receptors that stimulate gastric acid secretion. Intrinsic factor is a glycoprotein that com-

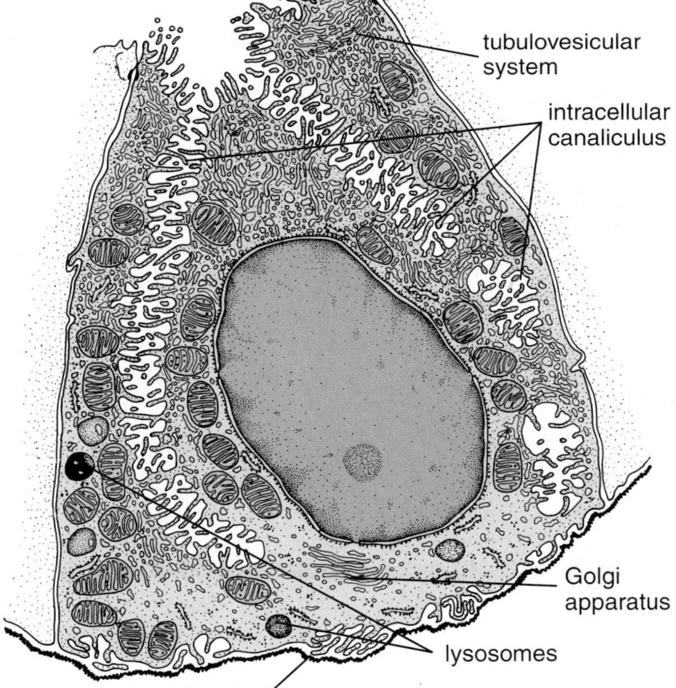

FIGURE 16.10
Diagram of a parietal cell. The cytoplasm of the parietal cell stains with eosin largely because of the extensive amount of membrane comprising the intracellular canaliculus, tubulovesicular system, mitochondria, and the relatively small number of ribosomes. This cell produces HCl and intrinsic factor. (Based on Lentz TL. *Cell Fine Structure: An Atlas of Drawings of Whole-Cell Structure.* Philadelphia: WB Saunders, 1971.)

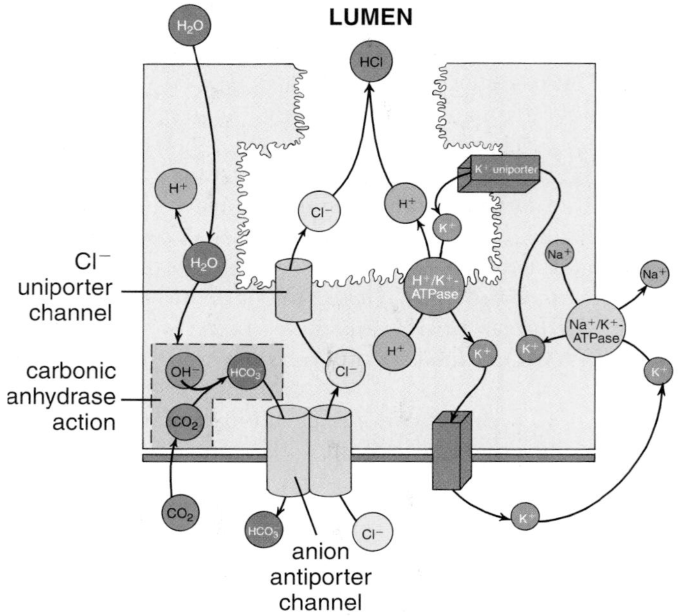

FIGURE 16.11
Diagram of parietal cell HCl synthesis. Following parietal cell stimulation, several steps occur leading to the production of HCl. Carbon dioxide (CO_2) from the blood diffuses across the basement membrane into the cell to form H_2CO_3. The H_2CO_3 dissociates into H^+ and HCO_3^-. The reaction is catalyzed by carbonic anhydrase, which leads to the production of H^+ ions in the cytoplasm, which are then transported across the membrane to the lumen of the intracellular canaliculus by a H^+/K^+-ATPase proton pump. Simultaneously, K^+ within the canaliculus is transported into the cell in exchange for the H^+ ions. Cl^- ions are also transported from the cytoplasm of the parietal cell into the lumen of the canaliculus by Cl^- channels in the membrane. HCl is then formed from H^+ and Cl^-. The HCO_3^-/Cl^- anion channels maintain the normal concentration of both ions in the cell, as well as Na^+/K^+-ATPase on the basolateral cell membrane.

plexes with vitamin B_{12} in the stomach and duodenum, a step necessary for subsequent absorption of the vitamin in the ileum.

Enteroendocrine cells secrete their products into the lamina propria

Enteroendocrine cells are found at every level of the fundic gland, although they tend to be somewhat more prevalent in the base. They are small cells that rest on the basal lamina and do not always reach the lumen (Fig. 16.12). Some, however, have a thin cytoplasmic extension bearing microvilli that are exposed to the gland lumen. It is thought that these cells sample the contents of the gland lumen and release hormones on the basis of the information from those samples.

Electron micrographs reveal small membrane-bounded secretory granules throughout the cytoplasm; however, the granules are typically lost in H&E preparations, and the cytoplasm appears clear because of the lack of sufficient stainable material. Although these cells are often difficult to identify because of their small size and lack of distinctive staining, the clear cytoplasm of the cell sometimes stands out in contrast to adjacent chief or parietal cells, thus allowing their easy recognition.

The names given to the enteroendocrine cells in the older literature were based on their staining with salts of silver and chromium, i.e., ***enterochromaffin cells, argentaffin cells,*** and ***argyrophil cells.*** Such cells are currently identified and characterized by immunochemical staining for the more than 20 peptide and polypeptide hormones and hormone-like regulating agents that they secrete (a list of many of these agents and their actions is given in Fig. 16.13 and in Tables 16.1 and 16.2). With the aid of the TEM, at least 17 different types of enteroendocrine cells

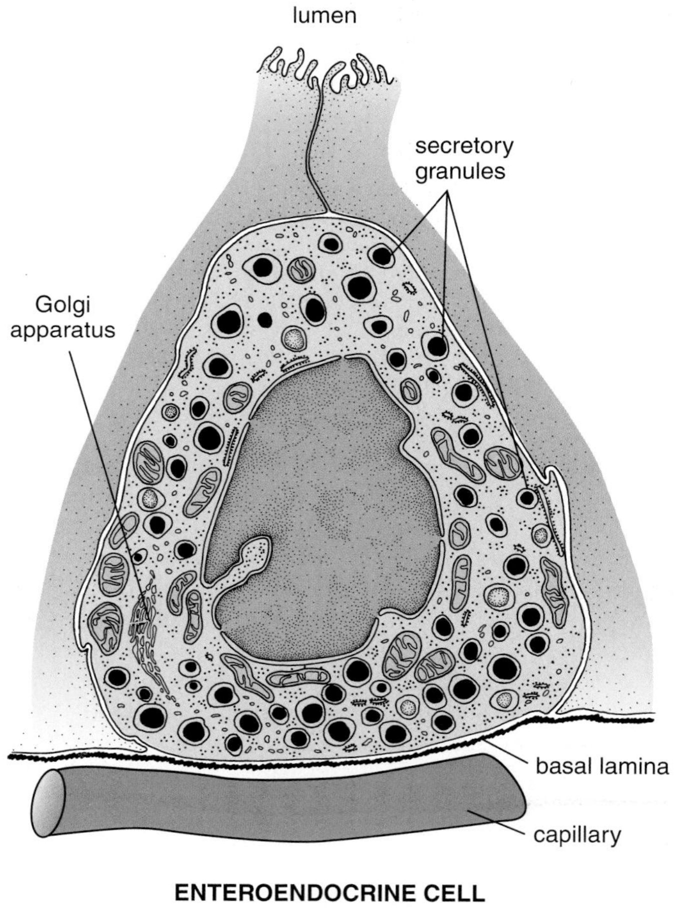

FIGURE 16.12
Diagram of an enteroendocrine cell. This cell is drawn to show that it does not reach the epithelial surface. The secretory granules are regularly lost during routine preparation. Because of the absence of other distinctive organelles, the nucleus appears to be surrounded by a small amount of clear cytoplasm in H & E–stained sections. (Based on Ito S, Winchester RJ. The fine structure of the gastric mucosa of the bat. *J Cell Biol* 1963;16:574.)

BOX 16.1

Clinical Correlations: Pernicious Anemia and Peptic Ulcer Disease

Achlorhydria is a condition characterized by the absence of parietal cells. Consequently, intrinsic factor is not secreted, thereby leading to ***pernicious anemia.*** Lack of intrinsic factor is the most common cause of vitamin B_{12} deficiency. However, other factors such as Gram-negative anaerobic bacterial overgrowth in the small intestine are associated with B_{12} deficiency. These bacteria bind to the vitamin B_{12}–intrinsic factor complex, preventing its absorption. Parasitic tapeworm infections also produce clinical symptoms of pernicious anemia. Because the liver has extensive reserve stores of vitamin B_{12}, the disease is often not recognized until long after significant changes in the gastric mucosa have taken place.

Another cause of reduced secretion of intrinsic factor and subsequent pernicious anemia is the loss of gastric epithelium because of chronic or recurrent ***peptic ulcer disease.*** Often, even healed ulcerated regions produce insufficient intrinsic factor. Repeated loss of epithelium and consequent scarring of the gastric mucosa can significantly reduce the amount of functional mucosa.

Histamine H_2 receptor antagonist drugs (e.g., Zantac and Tagamet), which block attachment of histamine to its receptors in the gastric mucosa, suppress both acid and intrinsic factor production and have been used extensively in the treatment of peptic ulcers. They prevent further mucosal erosion and promote healing of the previously eroded surface. However, long-term use can cause vitamin B_{12} deficiency. Recently, new proton pump inhibitors (e.g., Omeprazole and Lansoprazole) have been designed that inhibit the H^+/K^+-ATPase. They suppress acid production in the parietal cells and do not affect intrinsic factor secretion.

Although it was generally thought that the parietal cells are the direct target of the H_2 receptor antagonist drugs, recent evidence from a combination of in situ hybridization histochemistry and antibody staining has unexpectedly revealed that the immunoglobulin A (IgA)–secreting plasma cells and some of the macrophages in the lamina propria display a positive reaction for gastrin receptor mRNA, not the parietal cells. These findings indicate that the agents used to treat peptic ulcers may act directly on plasma cells and/or macrophages and that these cells then transmit their effects to the parietal cells to inhibit HCl secretion. The factor that mediates the interaction between the connective tissue cells and the epithelial cells has not been elucidated.

Recent evidence, however, suggests that most common peptic ulcers (95%) are actually caused by a chronic infection of the gastric mucosa by the bacterium ***Helicobacterium pylori.*** Lipopolysaccharide antigens are expressed on its surface that mimic those on human gastric epithelial cells. The mimicry appears to cause an initial immunologic tolerance to the pathogen by the host immune system, thus helping to enhance the infection and ultimately causing the production of antibodies. These antibodies against *H. pylori* bind to the gastric mucosa and cause damage to the mucosal cells. Treatment includes antibiotic eradication of the bacteria. These treatments for ulcerative disease have made the common surgical interventions of the past infrequent.

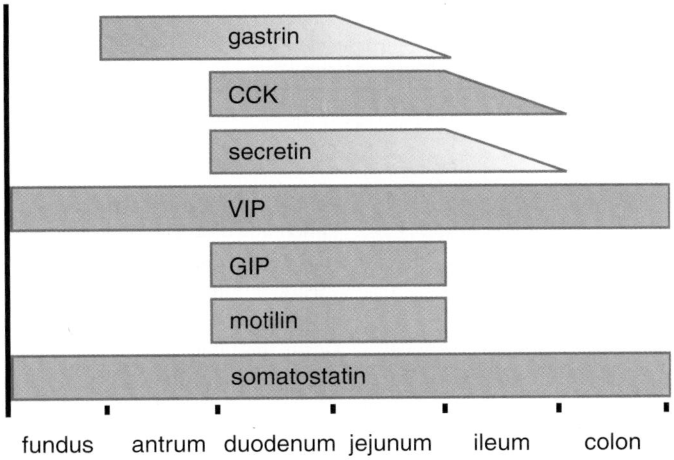

FIGURE 16.13
Gastrointestinal hormones. This schematic diagram shows the distribution of gastrointestinal peptide hormones produced by enteroendocrine cells in the alimentary canal. *CCK,* cholecystokinin; *VIP,* vasoactive intestinal peptide; *GIP,* gastric inhibitory peptide. (Modified from Johnson LR, ed. *Gastrointestinal Physiology.* St. Louis: Mosby-Year Book, 1997.)

have been described on the basis of size, shape, and density of their secretory granules.

CARDIAC GLANDS OF THE GASTRIC MUCOSA

Cardiac glands are composed of mucus-secreting cells

Cardiac glands are limited to a narrow region of the stomach (the cardia) that surrounds the esophageal orifice. Their secretion, in combination with that of the esophageal cardiac glands, contributes to the gastric juice and also helps protect the esophageal epithelium against gastric reflux. The glands are tubular, somewhat tortuous, and occasionally branched (Fig. 16.14). They are composed mainly of mucus-secreting cells, with occasional interspersed enteroendocrine cells. The mucus-secreting cells are similar in appearance to the cells of the esophageal cardiac glands. They have a flattened basal nucleus, and the apical cytoplasm is typically filled with mucin granules. A short duct segment containing columnar cells with elongate nuclei is interposed between the secretory portion of the gland and the shallow pits into which the glands secrete. The duct segment is the site at which the surface mucous cells and the gland cells are produced.

TABLE 16.1. **Physiologic Action of Gastrointestinal Hormones**

Hormone	Site of Synthesis	Major Action: Stimulates	Major Action: Inhibits
Gastrin	Stomach	Gastric acid secretion	
Cholecystokinin (CCK)	Duodenum Jejunum	Gallbladder contraction Pancreatic enzyme secretion Pancreatic bicarbonate ion secretion Pancreatic growth	Gastric emptying
Secretin	Duodenum	Pancreatic enzyme secretion Pancreatic bicarbonate ion secretion Pancreatic growth	Gastric acid secretion
Gastric inhibitory peptide (GIP)	Duodenum Jejunum	Insulin release	Gastric acid secretion
Motilin	Duodenum Jejunum	Gastric motility Intestinal motility	

Adapted from Johnson LR, ed. *Essential Medical Physiology.* Philadelphia: Lippincott-Raven, 1998.

PYLORIC GLANDS OF THE GASTRIC MUCOSA

Pyloric gland cells are similar to surface mucous cells and help protect the pyloric mucosa

Pyloric glands are located in the pyloric antrum (the part of the stomach between the fundus and the pylorus). They are branched, coiled, tubular glands. The lumen is relatively wide, and the secretory cells are similar in appearance to the surface mucous cells, suggesting a relatively viscous secretion. Enteroendocrine cells are found interspersed within the gland epithelium along with occasional parietal cells. The glands empty into deep gastric pits that occupy about half the thickness of the mucosa (Fig. 16.15).

Epithelial Cell Renewal in the Stomach

Surface mucous cells are renewed approximately every 3 to 5 days

The relatively short lifespan of the surface mucous cells, 3 to 5 days, is accommodated by mitotic activity in the isth-

TABLE 16.2. **Physiologic Action of Other Hormones in the Gastrointestinal Tract**

Hormone	Site of Synthesis	Major Action: Stimulates	Major Action: Inhibits
Candidate hormones			
Pancreatic polypeptide	Pancreas		Pancreatic enzyme secretion Pancreatic bicarbonate secretion
Peptide YY	Ileum Colon		Gastric acid secretion Gastric emptying
Glucagon-like peptide-1 (GLP-1)	Ileum Colon	Insulin release	Gastric acid secretion Gastric emptying
Paracrine hormones			
Somatostatin	Mucosa throughout GI tract		Gastrin release Gastric acid secretion Release of other GI hormones
Histamine	Mucosa throughout GI tract	Gastric acid secretion	
Neurocrine hormones			
Bombesin	Stomach	Gastric release	
Enkephalins	Mucosa and smooth muscle throughout GI tract	Smooth muscle contraction	Intestinal secretion
Vasoactive inhibitory peptide (VIP)	Mucosa and smooth muscle throughout GI tract	Pancreatic enzyme secretion Intestinal secretion	Smooth muscle contraction Sphincter contraction

Adapted from Johnson LR, ed. *Essential Medical Physiology.* Philadelphia: Lippincott-Raven, 1998.

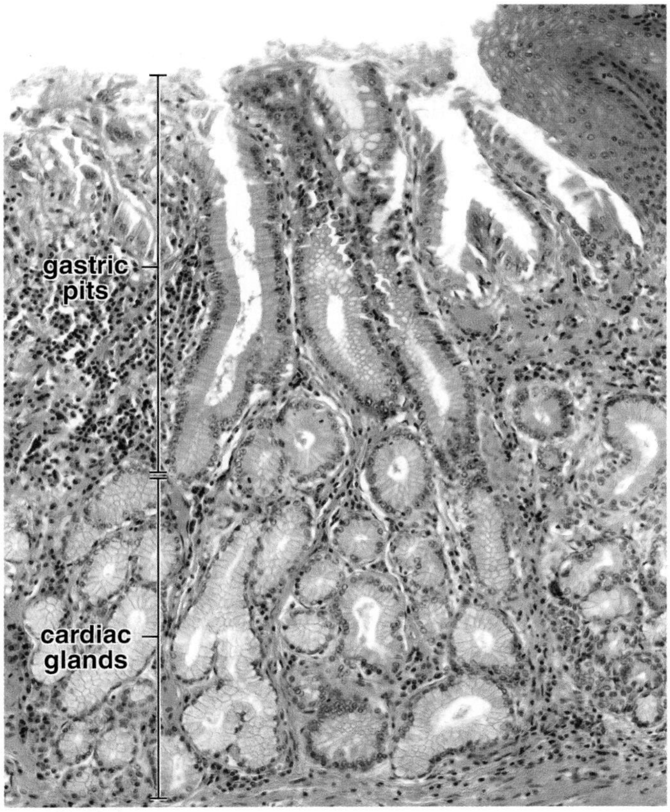

FIGURE 16.14
Photomicrograph of cardiac glands. This photomicrograph shows the esophagogastric junction. Note the presence of the stratified squamous epithelium of the esophagus in the upper right corner of the micrograph. The cardiac glands are tubular, somewhat tortuous, and occasionally branched. They are composed mainly of mucus-secreting cells similar in appearance to the cells of the esophageal glands. Mucous secretion reaches the lumen of the gastric pit via a short duct segment containing columnar cells. ×240.

mus, the narrow segment that lies between the gastric pit and the fundic gland (Fig. 16.16). This mitotic activity provides continuous cell renewal. Most of the newly produced cells at this site become surface mucous cells. They migrate upward along the wall of the pit to the luminal surface of the stomach and are ultimately shed into the stomach lumen.

The cells of the fundic glands have a relatively long lifespan

Other cells from the isthmus migrate down into the gastric glands to give rise to the parietal cells, chief cells, mucous gland cells, and enteroendocrine cells that constitute the gland epithelium. These cells have a relatively long lifespan. The parietal cells have the longest lifespan, approximately 150 to 200 days. Although parietal cells develop from the same undifferentiated stem cells, their lifespan is distinctly different. Recently, it has been hypothesized that parietal cells may have evolved from a bacterium called *Neurospora crassa* that previously ex-

BOX 16.2

Functional Considerations: Enteroendocrine Cells, APUD Cells, and Gastrointestinal Hormones

Enteroendocrine cells are present in most of the digestive tract, including the ducts of the pancreas and liver, and in the respiratory system, another endodermal derivative that originates by invagination of the epithelium of the embryonic foregut. The endocrine islets (of Langerhans) of the pancreas can be considered specialized accumulations of enteroendocrine cells derived from pancreatic buds that also arise from the embryonic foregut. It has been estimated that the enteroendocrine cells collectively would constitute the largest endocrine "organ" in the body. These cells have also been called ***gastroenteropancreatic (GEP) endocrine cells*** and closely resemble neurosecretory cells of the central nervous system that secrete many of the same hormones and regulatory agents. For that reason, they are also described as constituting part of a ***diffuse neuroendocrine system.*** These endocrine cells are not grouped as clusters in any specific part of the gastrointestinal tract. Rather, they are distributed singly throughout the gastrointestinal epithelium. Figure 16.13 shows the parts of the gastrointestinal tract from which the hormones are released into the blood.

Some enteroendocrine cells may be classifiable functionally as ***amine precursor uptake and decarboxylation (APUD) cells.*** They should not, however, be confused with the APUD cells that are derived from the embryonic neural crest and migrate to other sites in the body. Enteroendocrine cells, as discussed above, differentiate from the progeny of the same stem cells as all of the other epithelial cells of the digestive tract. The fact that two different cells may produce similar products should not imply that they have the same origin.

Enteroendocrine cells produce not only gastrointestinal hormones such as secretin, gastrin, cholecystokinin (CCK), gastric inhibitory peptide (GIP), and motilin but also ***paracrine substances (paracrines).*** A paracrine substance differs from a hormone in that it diffuses locally to its target cell instead of being carried by the bloodstream to a target cell. A well-known substance that appears to act as a paracrine substance within the gastrointestinal tract and pancreas is ***somatostatin,*** which inhibits other gastrointestinal and pancreatic islet endocrine cells. APUD cells secrete a variety of regulator substances in tissues and organs including the respiratory epithelium, adrenal medulla, islets of Langerhans, thyroid gland (parafollicular cells), and pituitary gland.

In addition to the established gastrointestinal hormones, several gastrointestinal peptides have not been definitely classified as hormones or paracrines. These peptides are designated ***candidate*** or ***putative hormones.***

Other locally active agents isolated from the gastrointestinal mucosa are ***neurotransmitters.*** These agents are released from nerve endings close to the target cell, usually the smooth muscle of the muscularis mucosae, the muscularis externa, or the tunica media of a blood vessel. In addition to acetylcholine (not a peptide), peptides found in nerve fibers of the gastrointestinal tract are vasoactive intestinal peptide (VIP), bombesin, and enkephalins. Thus, a particular peptide may be produced by endocrine and paracrine cells and also be localized in nerve fibers.

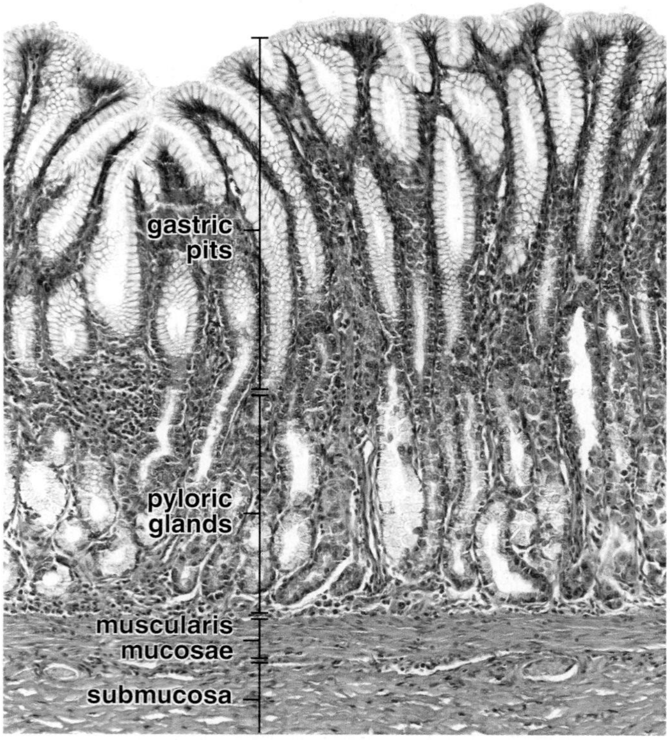

FIGURE 16.15
Photomicrograph of pyloric glands. This photomicrograph shows a section of the wall of the pylorus. The pyloric glands are relatively straight for most of their length but are slightly coiled near the muscularis mucosae. The lumen is relatively wide, and the secretory cells are similar in appearance to the surface mucous cells, suggesting a relatively viscous secretion. They are restricted to the mucosa and empty into the gastric pits. The boundary between the pits and glands is, however, hard to ascertain in routine H&E preparations. ×120.

BOX 16.3

Clinical Correlations: Zollinger-Ellison Syndrome

Excessive secretion of gastrin usually has its origin in a tumor of the gastrin-producing GEP endocrine cells located in the duodenum or in the pancreatic islet. This condition, known as the ***Zollinger-Ellison syndrome*** or ***gastrinomas***, is characterized by excessive secretion of hydrochloric acid by continuously stimulated parietal cells. The excess acid cannot be adequately neutralized in the duodenum, thereby leading to gastric and duodenal ulcers. Gastric ulcers are present in 95% of patients with this syndrome and are 6 times more prevalent than the duodenal ulcers. Treatment of Zollinger-Ellison syndrome in the past involved blockage of the parietal cell membrane receptors that stimulate HCl production. Recently, proton pump inhibitors have become the treatment of choice in managing HCl hypersecretion. In addition, surgical excision of the tumor, when possible, removes the source of gastrin production and alleviates symptoms.

isted in a symbiotic relationship with the cells of the human stomach. The basis for this hypothesis is that the human proton pump (H^+/K^+-ATPase) found in parietal cells bears a strong genetic similarity to proton pumps found in this bacterium. The bacterial DNA is thought to have been translocated and subsequently incorporated into the nucleus of the stem cells, probably with the help of a virus.

The chief and enteroendocrine cells are estimated to live for about 60 to 90 days before they are replaced by new cells migrating downward from the isthmus. The mucous neck cell, in contrast, has a much shorter lifespan, approximately 6 days.

Lamina Propria and Muscularis Mucosae

The ***lamina propria*** of the stomach is relatively scant and restricted to the limited spaces surrounding the gastric pits and glands. The stroma is composed largely of reticular

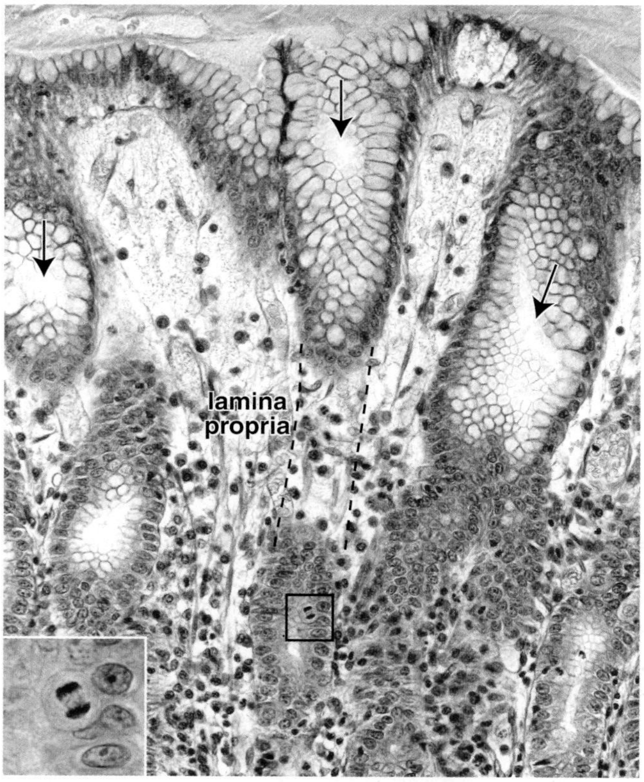

FIGURE 16.16
Photomicrograph of a dividing cell in the isthmus of a pyloric gland. The gastric pits in this photomicrograph were sectioned in a plane that is oblique to the axis of the pit. Note that on this section, gastric pits *(arrows)* can be recognized as invaginations of surface epithelium that are surrounded by lamina propria. The lamina propria is highly cellular because of the presence of large numbers of lymphocytes. ×240. **Inset.** This high magnification of the area indicated by the *rectangle* shows a dividing cell in the isthmus. ×580.

fibers with associated fibroblasts and smooth muscle cells. Other components include cells of the immune system, namely, lymphocytes, plasma cells, macrophages, and some eosinophils. When inflammation occurs, as is often the case, neutrophils may also be prominent. Occasional lymphatic nodules are also present, usually intruding partially into the muscularis mucosae.

The ***muscularis mucosae*** is composed of two relatively thin layers, usually arranged as an inner circular and outer longitudinal layer. In some regions a third layer may be present; its orientation tends to be in a circular pattern. Thin strands of smooth muscle cells extend toward the surface in the lamina propria from the inner layer of the muscularis mucosae. These smooth muscle cells in the lamina propria are thought to help outflow of the gastric gland secretions.

Gastric Submucosa

The ***submucosa*** is composed of a dense connective tissue containing variable amounts of adipose tissue and blood vessels, as well as the nerve fibers and ganglion cells that compose the ***submucosal (Meissner's) plexus.*** The latter innervates the vessels of the submucosa and the smooth muscle of the muscularis mucosae.

Gastric Muscularis Externa

The ***muscularis externa*** of the stomach is traditionally described as consisting of an outer longitudinal layer, a middle circular layer, and an inner oblique layer. This description is somewhat misleading, as distinct layers may be difficult to discern. As with other hollow, spheroidal organs (e.g., gallbladder, urinary bladder, and uterus), the smooth muscle of the muscularis externa of the stomach is somewhat more randomly oriented than the term "layer" implies. Moreover, the longitudinal layer is absent from much of the anterior and posterior stomach surfaces, and the circular layer is poorly developed in the periesophageal region. The arrangement of the muscle layers is functionally important, as it relates to its role in mixing chyme during the digestive process as well as to its ability to force the partially digested contents into the small intestine. Groups of ganglion cells and bundles of unmyelinated nerve fibers are present between the muscle layers. Collectively, they represent the ***myenteric (Auerbach's) plexus,*** which provides innervation of the muscle layers.

Gastric Serosa

The ***serosa*** of the stomach is as described above for the alimentary canal in general. It is continuous with the parietal peritoneum of the abdominal cavity via the greater omentum and with visceral peritoneum of the liver at the lesser omentum. Otherwise, it exhibits no special features.

▼ SMALL INTESTINE

The small intestine is the longest component of the digestive tract, measuring over 6 m, and is divided into three anatomic portions:

- ***Duodenum*** (~25 cm long) is the first, shortest, and widest part of the small intestine. It begins at the pylorus of the stomach and ends at the duodenojejunal junction.
- ***Jejunum*** (~2.5 m long) begins at the ***duodenojejunal junction*** and constitutes the upper two fifths of the small intestine. It gradually changes its morphologic characteristics to become the ileum.
- ***Ileum*** (~3.5 m long) is a continuation of the jejunum and constitutes the lower three fifths of the small intestine. It ends at the ***ileocecal junction,*** the union of the distal ileum and cecum.

The small intestine is the principal site for the digestion of food and absorption of the products of digestion

Chyme from the stomach enters the duodenum, where enzymes from the pancreas and bile from the liver are also delivered to continue the solubilization and digestion process. Enzymes, particularly disaccharidases and dipeptidases, are also located in the glycocalyx of the microvilli of the ***enterocytes,*** the ***intestinal absorptive cells.*** These enzymes contribute to the digestive process by completing the breakdown of most sugars and proteins to monosaccharides and amino acids, which are then absorbed. Water and electrolytes that reach the small intestine with the chyme and pancreatic and hepatic secretions are also reabsorbed in the small intestine, particularly in the distal portion.

Plicae circulares, villi, and microvilli increase the absorptive surface area of the small intestine

The absorptive surface area of the small intestine is amplified by tissue and cell specializations of the submucosa and mucosa.

- ***Plicae circulares (circular folds),*** also known as the valves of Kerckring, are permanent transverse folds that contain a core of submucosa. Each circular fold is circularly arranged and extends about one half to two thirds of the way around the circumference of the lumen (Fig. 16.17). The folds begin to appear about 5 to 6 cm beyond the pylorus. They are most numerous in the distal part of the duodenum and the beginning of the jejunum and become reduced in size and frequency in the middle of the ileum.
- ***Villi*** are unique, finger-like and leaf-like projections of the mucosa that extend from the theoretical mucosal surface for 0.5 to 1.5 mm into the lumen (Fig. 16.18). They completely cover the surface of the small intestine, giving it a velvety appearance when viewed with the unaided eye.

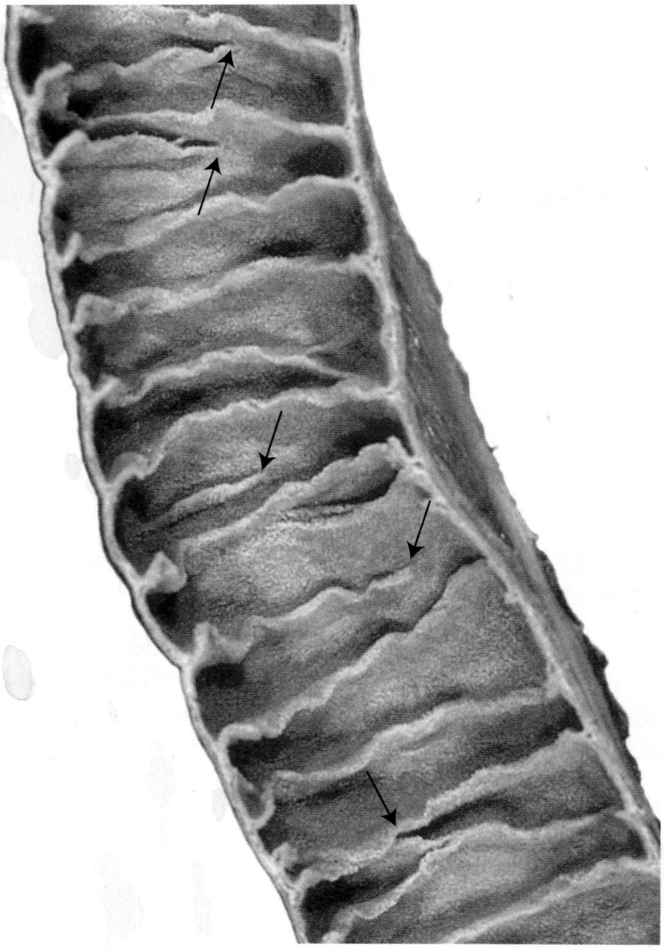

FIGURE 16.17
Photograph of the mucosal surface of the small intestine. This photograph of a segment of a human jejunum shows the mucosal surface. The circular folds (plica circulares) appear as a series of transversely oriented ridges that extend partially around the lumen. Consequently, some of the circular folds appear to end (or begin) at various sites along the luminal surface *(arrows)*. The entire mucosa has a velvety appearance because of the presence of villi.

- *Microvilli* of the enterocytes provide the major amplification of the luminal surface. Each cell possesses several thousand closely packed microvilli. They are visible in the light microscope and give the apical region of the cell a striated appearance, the so-called ***striated border***. Enterocytes and their microvilli are described below.

The villi, intestinal glands, along with the lamina propria, associated GALT, and muscularis mucosae, constitute the essential features of the small intestinal mucosa

Villi, as noted, are projections of the mucosa. They consist of a core of loose connective tissue covered by a simple columnar epithelium. The core of the villus is an extension of the lamina propria, which contains numerous fibroblasts, smooth muscle cells, lymphocytes, plasma cells, eosinophils, macrophages, and a network of fenestrated blood capillaries located just beneath the epithelial basal lamina. In addition, the lamina propria of the villus contains a central, blind-ending lymphatic capillary, the ***lacteal*** (Fig. 16.19). Smooth muscle cells derived from the muscularis mucosae extend into the villus and accompany the lacteal. These smooth muscle cells may account for reports that villi contract and shorten intermittently, an action that may force lymph from the lacteal into the lymphatic vessel network that surrounds the muscularis mucosae.

The ***intestinal glands,*** or ***crypts of Lieberkühn,*** are simple tubular structures that extend from the muscularis mucosae through the thickness of the lamina propria, where they open onto the luminal surface of the intestine at the base of the villi (see Fig. 16.18). The glands are composed of a simple columnar epithelium that is continuous with the epithelium of the villi.

As in the stomach, the lamina propria surrounds the intestinal glands and contains numerous cells of the immune system (lymphocytes, plasma cells, mast cells, macrophages, and eosinophils), particularly in the villi. The lamina propria also contains numerous nodules of lymphatic tissue that represent a major component of the GALT. The nodules are particularly large and numerous in the ileum, where they are preferentially located on the side of the intestine opposite the mesenteric attachment (Fig. 16.20). These nodular aggregations are known as ***aggregated nodules*** or ***Peyer's patches.*** In gross specimens, they appear as aggregates of white specks.

The muscularis mucosae consists of two thin layers of smooth muscle cells, an inner circular and an outer longitudinal layer. As noted above, strands of smooth muscle cells extend from the muscularis mucosae into the lamina propria of the villi.

At least five types of cells are found in intestinal mucosal epithelium

The mature cells of the intestinal epithelium are found both in the intestinal glands and on the surface of the villi. They include

- ***Enterocytes,*** whose primary function is absorption
- ***Goblet cells,*** unicellular mucin-secreting glands
- ***Paneth cells,*** whose primary function is to maintain mucosal innate immunity by secreting antimicrobial substances
- ***Enteroendocrine cells,*** which produce various paracrine and endocrine hormones
- ***M cells (microfold cells),*** modified enterocytes that cover enlarged lymphatic nodules in the lamina propria

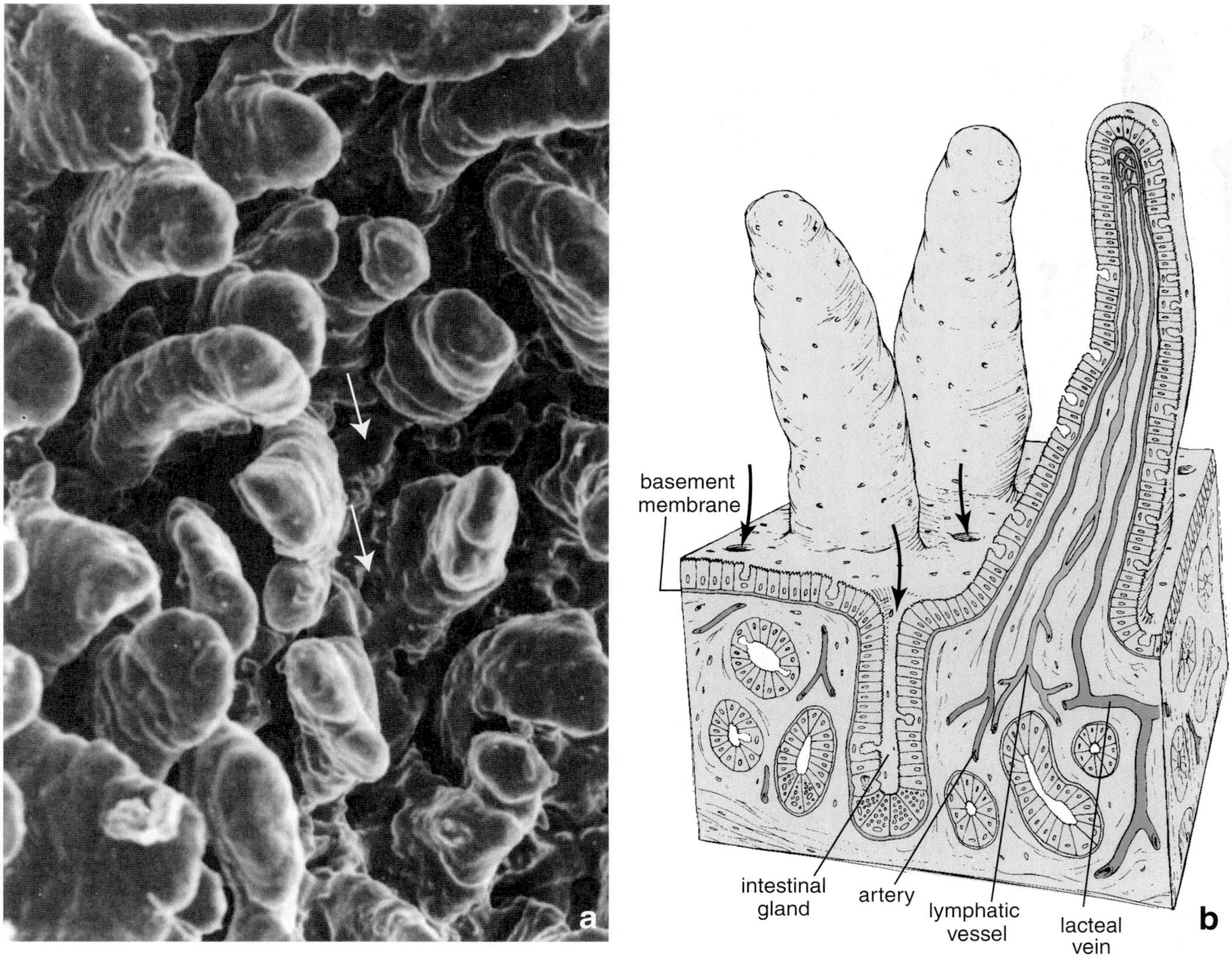

FIGURE 16.18
Intestinal villi in the small intestine. a. Scanning electron micrograph of the intestinal mucosa showing its villi. Note the openings *(arrows)* located between the bases of the villi that lead into the intestinal glands (crypts of Lieberkühn). ×800. **b.** This three-dimensional diagram of the intestinal villi shows the continuity of the epithelium covering the villi with the epithelium lining the intestinal glands. Note blood vessels and the blind-ending lymphatic capillary, called a lacteal, in the core of the villus. Between the bases of the villi, the openings of the intestinal glands can be seen *(arrows).* Also, the small openings on the surface of the villi indicate the location of discharged goblet cells.

Enterocytes are absorptive cells specialized for the transport of substances from the lumen of the intestine to the circulatory system

Enterocytes are tall columnar cells with a basally positioned nucleus (see Figs. 16.18 and 16.21). Microvilli increase the apical surface area as much as 600 times; they are recognized in the light microscope as forming a ***striated border*** on the luminal surface.

Each microvillus has a core of vertically oriented actin microfilaments that are anchored to villin located in the tip of the microvillus and that also attach to the microvillus plasma membrane by myosin I molecules. The actin microfilaments extend into the apical cytoplasm and insert into the ***terminal web,*** a network of horizontally oriented contractile microfilaments that form a layer in the most apical cytoplasm and attach to the intracellular density associated with the zonula adherens. Contraction of the terminal web causes the microvilli to spread apart, thus increasing the space between them to allow more surface area exposure for absorption to take place. In addition, contraction of the terminal web may aid in "closing" the holes left in the epithelial sheet by exfoliation of aging cells. Enterocytes are bound to one another and to the goblet, enteroendocrine, and other cells of the epithelium by junctional complexes.

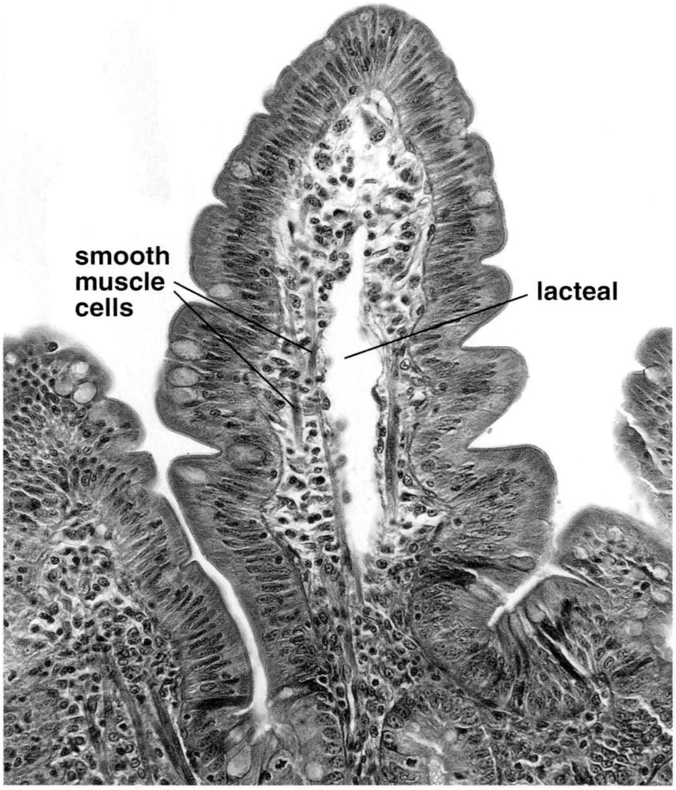

FIGURE 16.19
Photomicrograph of an intestinal villus. The surface of the villus consists of columnar epithelial cells, chiefly enterocytes with a striated border. Also evident are goblet cells that can be readily identified by the presence of the apical mucous cup. Located beneath the epithelium is the highly cellular loose connective tissue, the lamina propria. The lamina propria contains large numbers of round cells, mostly lymphocytes. In addition, smooth muscle cells can be identified. A lymphatic capillary called a lacteal occupies the center of the villus. When the lacteal is dilated, as it is in this specimen, it is easily identified. ×160.

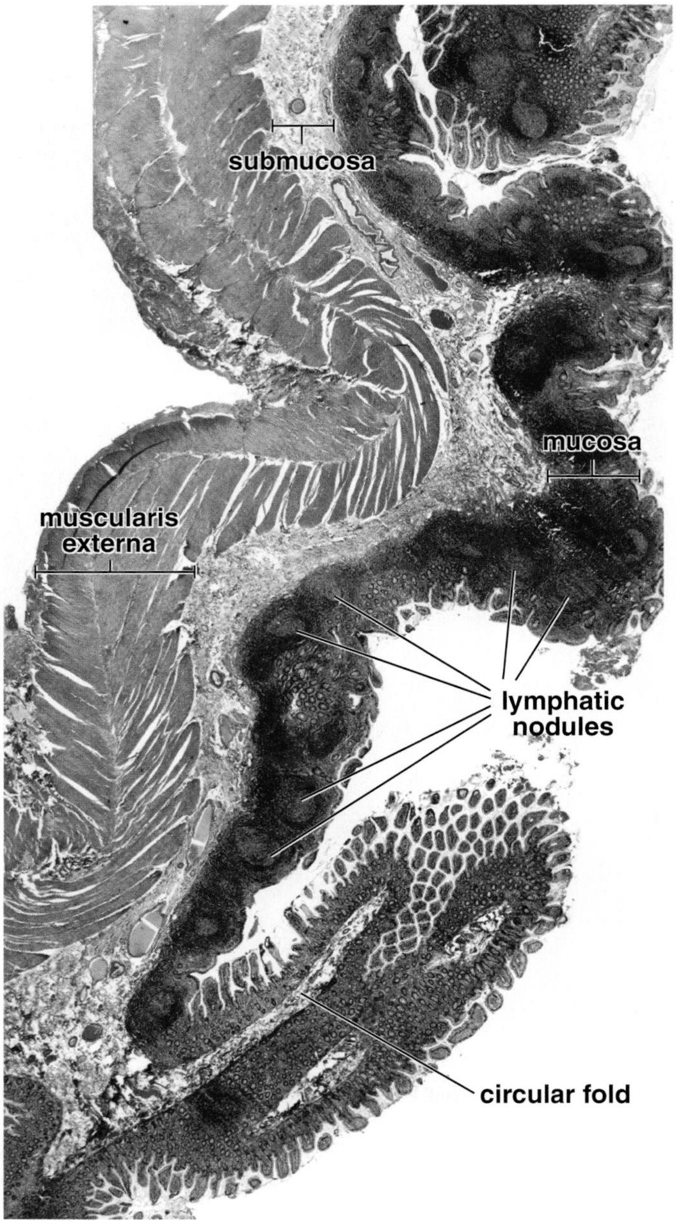

FIGURE 16.20
Photomicrograph of Peyer's patches. This photomicrograph shows a longitudinal section through the wall of a human ileum. Note the extensive lymphatic nodules located in the mucosa and the section of a circular fold projecting into the lumen of the ileum. Lymphatic nodules within the Peyer's patch are primarily located within the lamina propria, although many extend into the submucosa. They are covered by the intestinal epithelium, which contains enterocytes, occasional goblet cells, and specialized antigen-presenting M cells. ×40.

Tight junctions establish a barrier between the intestinal lumen and the epithelial intercellular compartment

The tight junctions between the intestinal lumen and the connective tissue compartment of the body allow selective retention of substances absorbed by the enterocytes. As noted in the section on occluding junctions (see page 97), the "tightness" of these junctions can vary.

In relatively impermeable tight junctions, as in the ileum and colon, active transport is required to move solutes across the barrier. In simplest terms, active transport systems, e.g. sodium pumps (Na^+/K^+-ATPase), located in the lateral plasma membrane transiently reduce the cytoplasmic concentration of Na^+ by transporting it across the lateral plasma membrane into the extracellular space below the tight junction. This transport of Na^+ creates a high intercellular Na^+ concentration, causing water from the cell to enter the intercellular space, reducing both the water and Na^+ concentrations in the cell. Consequently, water and Na^+ enter the cell at its apical surface, passing through the cell, and exiting at the lateral plasma membrane as long as the sodium pump continues to function. Increased osmolarity in the intercellular space draws water into this space, establishing a hydrostatic pressure

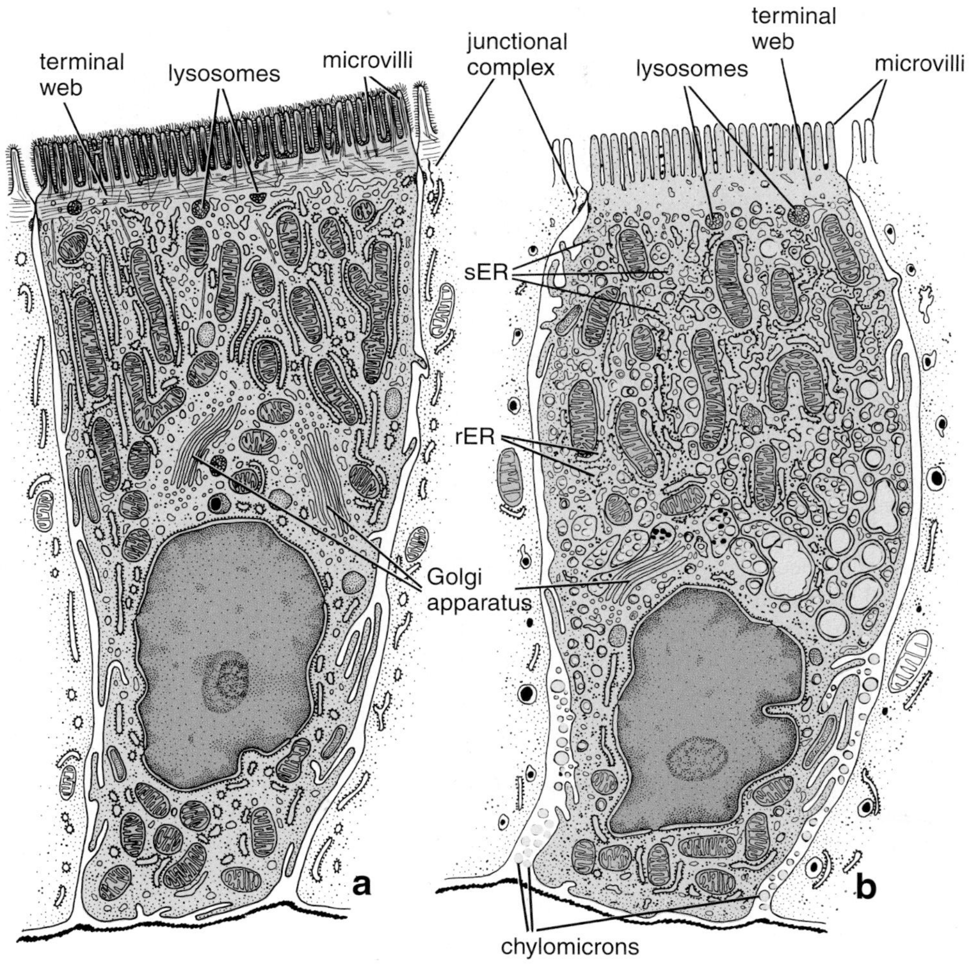

FIGURE 16.21
Diagrams of an enterocyte in different phases of absorption. a. This cell has a striated border on its apical surface and junctional complexes that seal the lumen of the intestine from the lateral intercellular space. The characteristic complement of organelles is depicted in the diagram. **b.** This cell shows the distribution of lipid during fat absorption as seen with the TEM. Initially, lipids are seen in association with the microvilli of the striated border. Lipids are internalized and seen in vesicles of the smooth endoplasmic reticulum (sER) in the apical portion of the cell. The membrane-bounded lipid can be traced to the center of the cell, where many of the lipid-containing vesicles fuse. The lipid is then discharged into the intercellular space. The extracellular lipids, recognized as chylomicrons, pass beyond the basal lamina for further transport. (Based on Lentz TL. *Cell Fine Structure: An Atlas of Drawings of Whole-Cell Structure.* Philadelphia: WB Saunders, 1971.)

that drives Na^+ and water across the basal lamina into the connective tissue.

In epithelia with more permeable tight junctions, such as those in the duodenum and jejunum, a sodium pump also creates low intracellular Na^+ concentration. When the contents that pass into the duodenum and jejunum are hypotonic, however, considerable absorption of water, along with additional Na^+ and other small solutes, takes place directly across the tight junctions of the enterocytes into the intercellular spaces. This mechanism of absorption is referred to as ***solvent drag.***

Other transport mechanisms also increase the concentrations of specific substances, such as sugars, amino acids, and other solutes in the intercellular space. These substances then diffuse or flow down their concentration gradients within the intercellular space to cross the epithelial basal lamina and enter the fenestrated capillaries in the lamina propria located immediately beneath the epithelium. Substances that are too large to enter the blood vessels, such as lipoprotein particles, enter the lymphatic lacteal.

The lateral cell surface of the enterocytes exhibits elaborate, flattened cytoplasmic processes (plicae) that interdigitate with those of adjacent cells (see Fig. 4.15). These folds increase the lateral surface area of the cell, thus increasing the amount of plasma membrane containing transport enzymes. During active absorption, especially of solutes, water, and lipids, these ***lateral plications*** separate, enlarging the intercellular compartment. The increased hydrostatic pressure from the accumulated solutes and solvents causes a directional flow through the basal lamina into the lamina propria (see Fig. 4.1).

In addition to the membrane specializations associated with absorption and transport, the enterocyte cytoplasm is also specialized for these functions. Elongated mitochondria that provide energy for transport are concentrated in the apical cytoplasm between the terminal web and the nucleus. Tubules and cisternae of the smooth endoplasmic reticulum (sER), which are involved in the absorption of fatty acids and glycerol and in the resynthesis of neutral fat, are found in the apical cytoplasm beneath the terminal web.

Enterocytes are also secretory cells, producing enzymes needed for terminal digestion and absorption as well as secretion of water and electrolytes

The secretory function of enterocytes, primarily the synthesis of glycoprotein enzymes that will be inserted into the apical plasma membrane, is represented morphologically by aligned stacks of Golgi cisternae in the immediate supranuclear region and by the presence of free ribosomes and rER lateral to the Golgi apparatus (see Fig. 16.21). Small secretory vesicles containing glycoproteins destined for the cell surface are located in the apical cytoplasm, just below the terminal web, and along the lateral plasma membrane. Histochemical or autoradiographic methods are needed, however, to distinguish these ***secretory vesicles*** from endocytotic vesicles or small lysosomes.

The small intestine also secretes water and electrolytes. This activity occurs mainly in the cells within the intestinal glands. The secretion that occurs in these glands is thought to assist the process of digestion and absorption by maintaining an appropriate liquid state of the intestinal chyme. Under normal conditions, the absorption of fluid by the villus enterocyte is balanced by the secretion of fluid by the gland enterocyte.

Goblet cells represent unicellular glands that are interspersed among the other cells of the intestinal epithelium

As in other epithelia, ***goblet cells*** produce mucus. In the small intestine, goblet cells increase in number from the duodenum to the terminal part of the ileum. Also, as in other epithelia, because water-soluble mucinogen is lost during preparation of routine H&E sections, the part of the cell that normally contains mucinogen granules appears empty. Examination with the TEM reveals a large accumulation of mucinogen granules in the apical cytoplasm that distends the apex of the cell and distorts the shape of neighboring cells (Fig. 16.22). With the apex of the cell containing a large accumulation of mucinogen granules, the basal portion of the cell resembles a narrow stem. This basal portion is intensely basophilic in histologic preparations because it is occupied by a heterochromatic nucleus, extensive rER, and free ribosomes. Mitochondria are also concentrated in the basal cytoplasm. The characteristic shape, with the apical accumulation of granules and the narrow basal stem, is responsible for the name of the cell, as in a glass "goblet." An extensive array of flattened Golgi cisternae forms a wide cup around the newly formed mucinogen granules adjacent to the basal part of the cell (Fig. 16.23). The microvilli of goblet cells are restricted to a thin rim of cytoplasm (the theca) that surrounds the apical-lateral portion of the mucinogen granules. Microvilli are more obvious on the immature goblet cells in the deep one half of the intestinal gland.

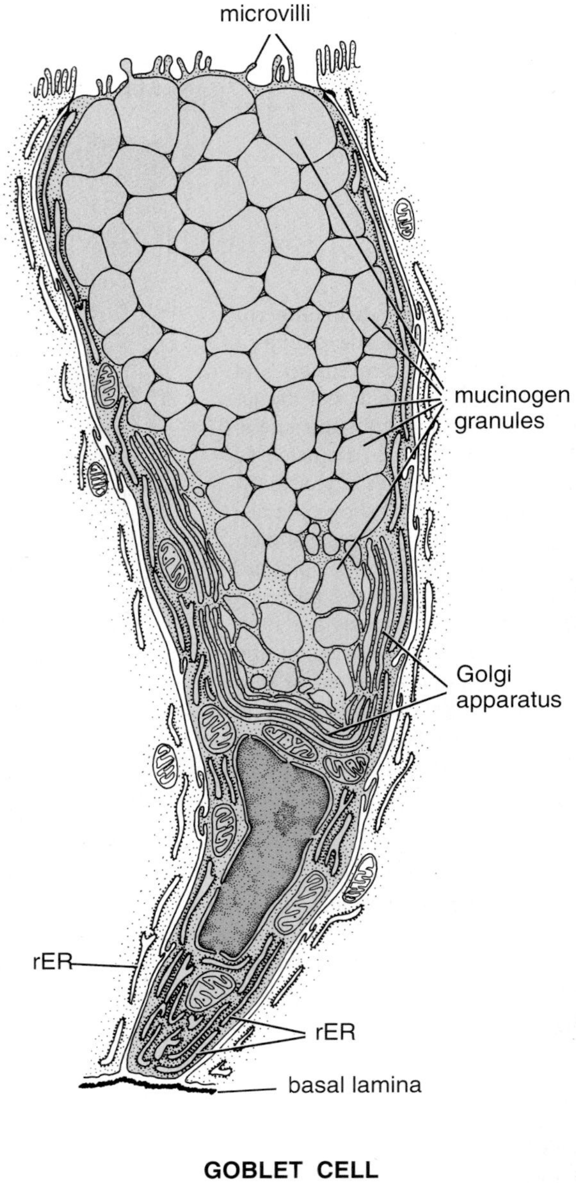

FIGURE 16.22
Diagram of a goblet cell. The nucleus is located at the basal portion of the cell. The major portion of the cell is filled with mucinogen granules forming the mucous cup that is evident in the light microscope. At the base and lower sides of the mucous cup are flattened saccules of the large Golgi apparatus. Other organelles are distributed throughout the remaining cytoplasm, especially in the perinuclear cytoplasm in the base of the cell. (Based on Neutra MR, Leblond CP. *J Cell Biol* 1966;30:119–136.)

Paneth cells play a role in regulation of normal bacterial flora of the small intestine

Paneth cells are found in the bases of the intestinal glands. (They are also occasionally found in the normal colon in small numbers; their number may increase in cer-

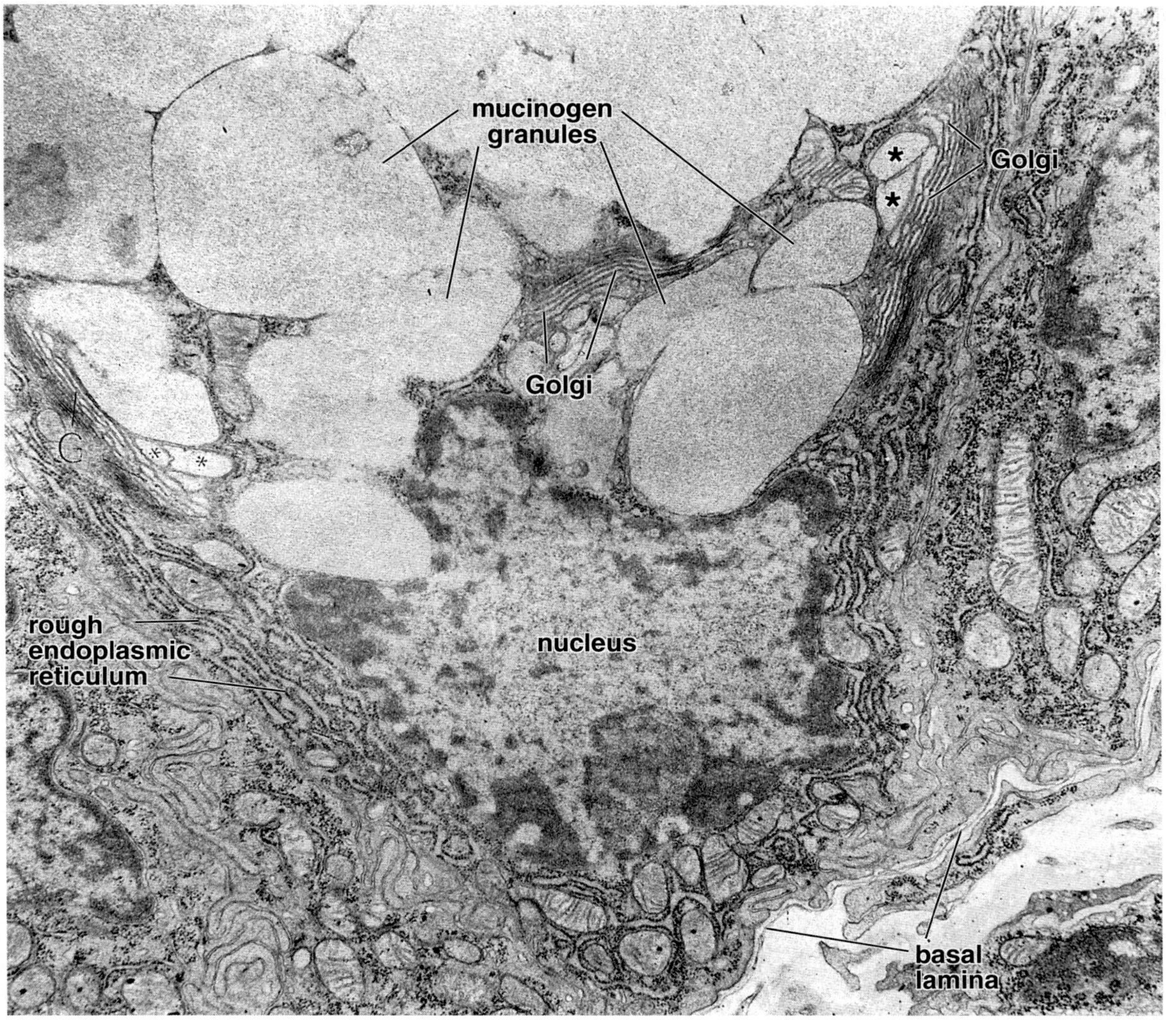

FIGURE 16.23
Electron micrograph of the basal portion of a goblet cell. The cell rests on the basal lamina. The basal portion of the cell contains the nucleus, rough endoplasmic reticulum, and mitochondria. Just apical to the nucleus are extensive profiles of Golgi apparatus. As the mucous product accumulates in the Golgi cisternae, they become enlarged *(asterisks).* The large mucinogen granules fill most of the apical portion of the cell and collectively constitute the "mucous cup" seen in the light microscope. ×15,000.

tain pathologic conditions.) They have a basophilic basal cytoplasm; a supranuclear Golgi apparatus; and large, intensely acidophilic, refractile apical secretory granules. These granules allow their easy identification in routine histologic sections (Fig. 16.24).

The secretory granules contain the antibacterial enzyme lysozyme, α-defensins, other glycoproteins, an arginine-rich protein (probably responsible for the intense acidophilia), and zinc. Lysozyme digests the cell walls of certain groups of bacteria. α-Defensins are homologues of peptides that function as mediators in cytotoxic $CD8^+$ T lymphocytes. This antibacterial action and their ability to phagocytose certain bacteria and protozoa suggest that Paneth cells play a role in regulating the normal bacterial flora of the small intestine.

Enteroendocrine cells in the small intestine produce nearly all of the same peptide hormones as they do in the stomach

Enteroendocrine cells in the small intestine resemble those that reside in the stomach. They are concentrated in the lower portion of the intestinal gland but migrate slowly and can be found at all levels of each villus (Fig. 16.25). Nearly all of the same peptide hormones identified in this cell type in the stomach can be demonstrated in the enteroendocrine cells of the intestine (see Table 16.1). ***CCK, secretin, GIP,*** and ***motilin*** are the most active regulators of gastrointestinal physiology that are released in this portion of the gut (see Fig. 16.13). CCK and secretin increase pancreatic and gallbladder activity and inhibit gastric secretory function and motility. GIP stimu-

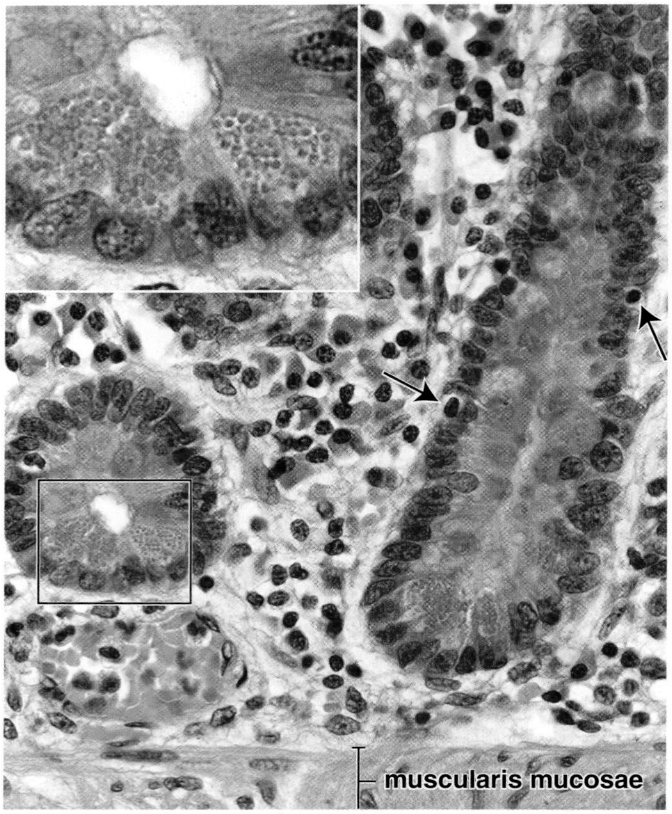

FIGURE 16.24
Photomicrograph of intestinal glands showing Paneth cells. This photomicrograph shows the base of intestinal (jejunal) glands in a H&E preparation. The gland on the right is sectioned longitudinally; the circular cross-sectional profile of another gland is seen on the left. Paneth cells are typically located in the base of the intestinal glands and are readily seen in the light microscope because of the intensive eosin staining of their granules. The lamina propria contains an abundance of plasma cells, lymphocytes, and other connective tissue cells. Note several lymphocytes in the epithelium of the gland *(arrows)*. ×240. **Inset.** This high magnification of the area indicated by the *rectangle* shows the characteristic basophilic cytoplasm in the basal portion of the cell and large accumulations of intensely staining, eosinophilic, refractile secretory granules in the apical portion of the cell. An arginine-rich protein found in the granules is probably responsible for the intense eosinophilic reaction. ×680.

lates insulin release in the pancreas, and motilin initiates gastric and intestinal motility. Although other peptides produced by enteroendocrine cells have been isolated, they are not considered hormones and are therefore called ***candidate hormones*** (page 488). Enteroendocrine cells also produce at least two hormones, somatostatin and histamine, which act as ***paracrine hormones*** (see page 488), i.e., hormones that have a local effect and do not circulate in the bloodstream. In addition, several peptides are secreted by the nerve cells located in the submucosa and muscularis externa. These peptides, called ***neurocrine hormones,*** are represented by VIP, bombesin, and the enkephalins. The functions of these peptides are listed in Table 16.2.

M cells convey microorganisms and other macromolecules from the intestinal lumen to Peyer's patches

M cells are epithelial cells that overlie Peyer's patches and other large lymphatic nodules; they differ significantly from the surrounding intestinal epithelial cells. M cells have ***microfolds*** rather than microvilli on their apical surface, and they take up microorganisms and macromolecules from the lumen in endocytotic vesicles. The vesicles are transported to the basolateral membrane where they discharge their contents into the epithelial intercellular space in the vicinity of $CD4^+$ T lymphocytes. Thus, substances that gain access to the body from the intestinal lumen via M cells come into contact with cells of the immune system as they reach the basolateral surface. Antigens that reach lymphocytes in this manner stimulate a response in the GALT that is described below.

Intermediate cells have characteristics of both immature absorptive cells and goblet cells

Intermediate cells constitute most of the cells in the lower half of the intestinal gland. These cells are still capable of cell division and usually undergo one or two divisions before they become committed to differentiation into either absorptive or goblet cells. These cells have short, irregular microvilli with long core filaments extending deep into the apical cytoplasm and numerous macular (desmosomal) junctions with adjacent cells. Small mucin-like secretory granules form a column in the center of the supranuclear cytoplasm. Intermediate cells that are committed to becoming goblet cells develop a small, rounded collection of secretory granules just beneath the apical plasma membrane; those that are committed to becoming absorptive cells lose the secretory granules and begin to show concentrations of mitochondria, rER, and ribosomes in the apical cytoplasm.

GALT is prominent in the lamina propria of the small intestine

As noted above, the lamina propria of the digestive tract is heavily populated with elements of the immune system; approximately one fourth of the mucosa consists of a loosely organized layer of lymphatic nodules, lymphocytes, macrophages, plasma cells, and eosinophils in the lamina propria. Lymphocytes are also located between epithelial cells. This GALT serves as an immunologic barrier throughout the length of the gastrointestinal tract. In cooperation with the overlying epithelial cells, particularly M cells, the lymphatic tissue samples the antigens in the epithelial intercellular spaces. Lymphocytes and other antigen-presenting cells process the antigens and migrate to lymphatic nodules in the lamina propria where they un-

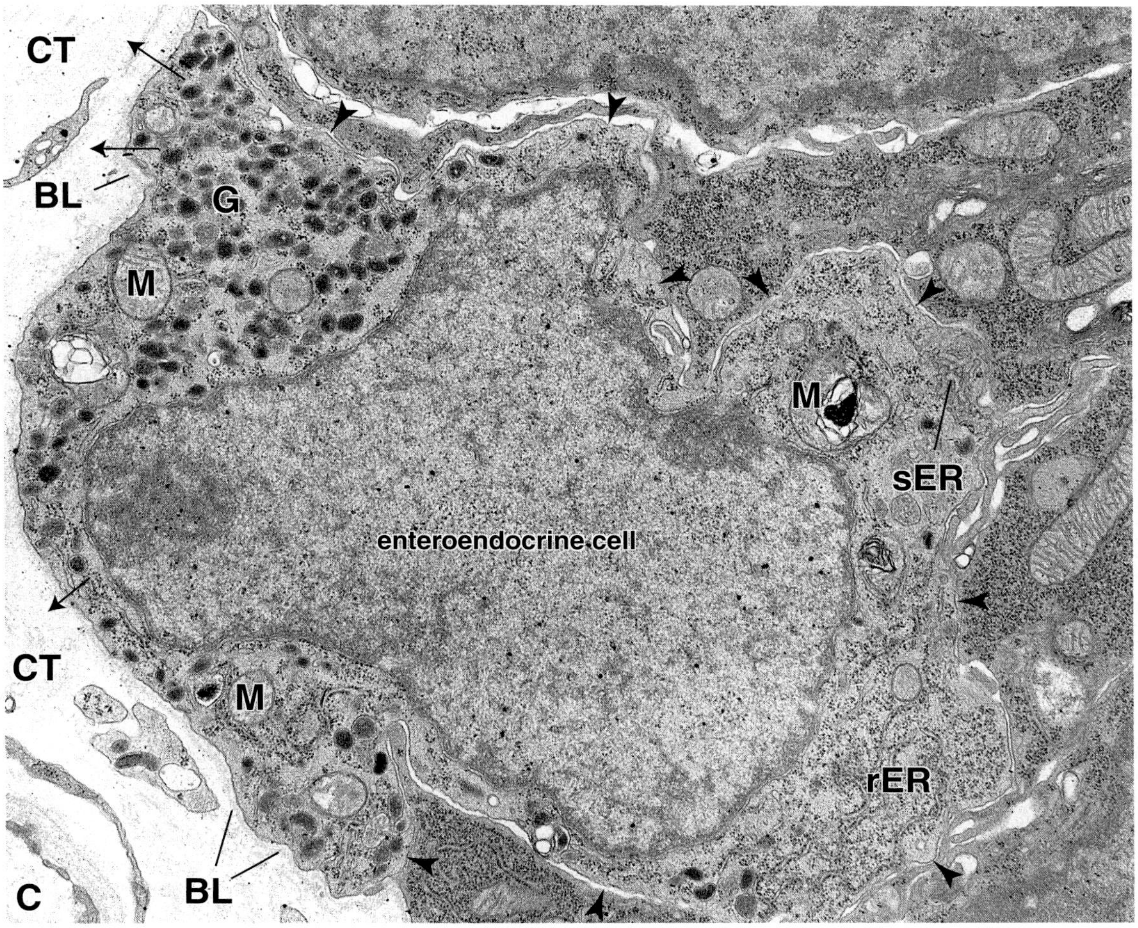

FIGURE 16.25
Electron micrograph of an enteroendocrine cell of the colon. *Arrowheads* mark the boundary between the enteroendocrine cell and the adjacent epithelial cells. At its base, the enteroendocrine cell rests on the basal lamina *(BL)*. This cell does not extend to the epithelial or luminal surface. Numerous secretory granules *(G)* in the base of the cell are secreted in the direction of the arrows across the basal lamina and into the connective tissue *(CT)*. C, capillary; *M*, mitochondria; *rER*, rough endoplasmic reticulum; and *sER*, smooth endoplasmic reticulum.

dergo activation (see page 358), leading to antibody secretion by newly differentiated plasma cells.

Most of the plasma cells in the lamina propria of the intestine secrete dimeric IgA rather than the more common IgG; other plasma cells produce IgM and IgE (see page 461). IgA is transported across the epithelium, linked to a secretory (75 kDa) glycoprotein component that is synthesized by enterocytes and inserted in the basal plasma membrane as a receptor for IgA. The complex of IgA and secretory component enters into the epithelial cell by endocytosis at the basal plasma membrane and is subsequently released from the cell into the gut lumen by exocytosis at the apical plasma membrane (Fig. 16.26). In the lumen IgA binds to antigens, toxins, and microorganisms. Secretory IgA (sIgA) is the principal molecule of mucosal immunity and is the only immunoglobulin isotype that can be selectively passed across the mucosal wall to reach the lumen of the gut. Some of the IgE binds to the plasma membranes of mast cells in the lamina propria (see page 144), selectively sensitizing them to specific antigens derived from the lumen.

Submucosa

A distinguishing characteristic of the duodenum is the presence of submucosal glands

The submucosa consists of a dense connective tissue and localized sites that contain aggregates of adipose cells. A conspicuous feature in the duodenum is the presence of ***submucosal glands,*** also called ***Brunner's glands.***

The branched, tubular submucosal glands of the duodenum have secretory cells with characteristics of both zymogen-secreting and mucus-secreting cells (Fig. 16.27). The secretion of these glands has a pH of 8.1 to 9.3 and contains neutral and alkaline glycoproteins and bicarbon-

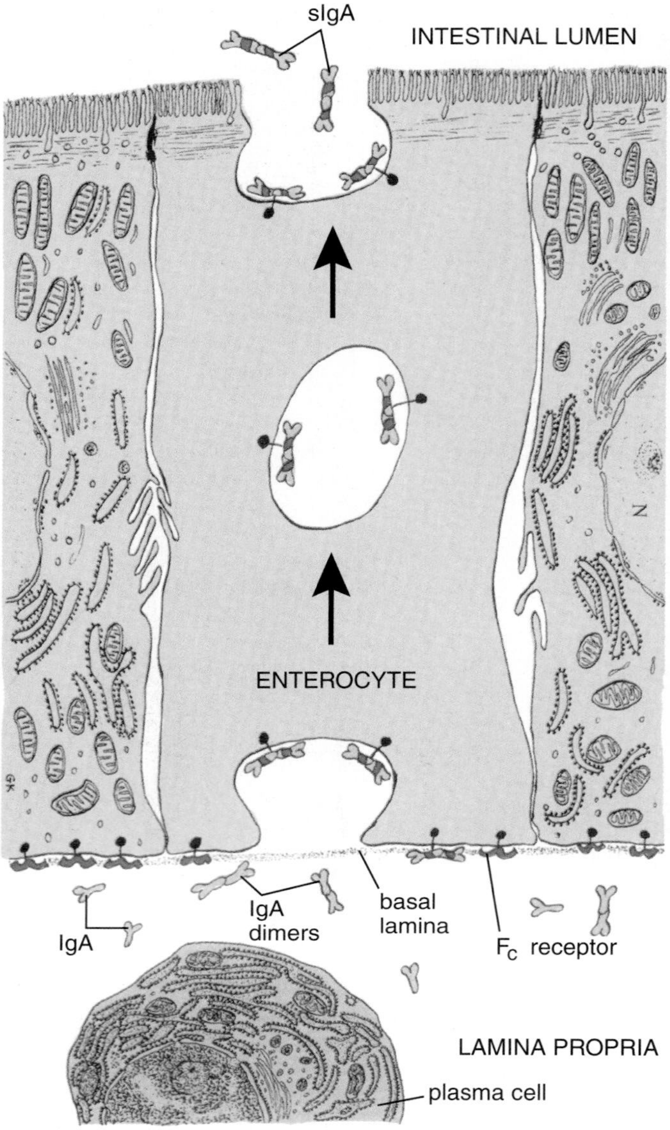

FIGURE 16.26
Diagram of immunoglobulin A (IgA) secretion and transport. Immunoglobulin A (IgA) is secreted by plasma cells into the lamina propria. Here, it dimerizes and then binds to a transmembrane F_c receptor on the membrane of the enterocyte. The extracellular portion of the membrane receptor will remain with the IgA dimer and will later become the secretory component of the IgA. The IgA–receptor complex enters the cell by endocytosis and is carried to the apical surface within the endocytotic vesicles (a process called transcytosis). The vesicle fuses with the apical plasma membrane, releasing the IgA–receptor complex as secretory IgA *(sIgA)*. The IgA monomers and dimers, the F_c receptors, and the endocytotic vesicles are greatly exaggerated in size for clarity. The actual sizes of the vesicles involved approximate those shown in the adjacent enterocytes.

ate ions. This highly alkaline secretion probably serves to protect the proximal small intestine by neutralizing the acid-containing chyme delivered to it. It also brings the intestinal contents close to the optimal pH for the pancreatic enzymes that are also delivered to the duodenum.

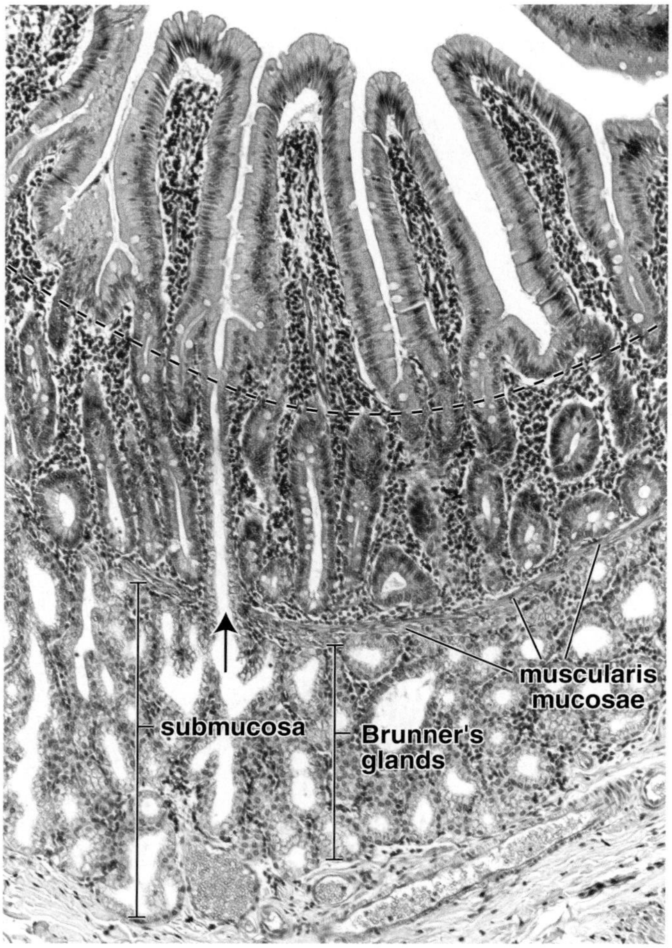

FIGURE 16.27
Photomicrograph of Brunner's glands in the duodenum. This photomicrograph shows part of the duodenal wall in a H&E preparation. A distinctive feature of the duodenum is the presence of Brunner's glands. The *dashed line* marks the boundary between the villi and the typical intestinal glands (crypts of Lieberkühn). The latter extend to the muscularis mucosae. Under the mucosa is the submucosa, which contains Brunner's glands. These are branched tubular glands whose secretory component consists of columnar cells. The duct of the Brunner's gland opens into the lumen of the intestinal gland *(arrow)*. ×120

Muscularis Externa

The ***muscularis externa*** consists of an inner layer of circularly arranged smooth muscle cells and an outer layer of longitudinally arranged smooth muscle cells. The main components of the myenteric plexus (Auerbach's plexus) are located between these two muscle layers (Fig. 16.28). Two kinds of muscular contraction occur in the small intestine. Local contractions displace intestinal contents both proximally and distally, this type of contraction is called ***segmentation.*** These contractions primarily involve the circular muscle layer. They serve to circulate the chyme locally, mixing it with digestive juices and moving it into contact with the mucosa for absorption. ***Peristal-***

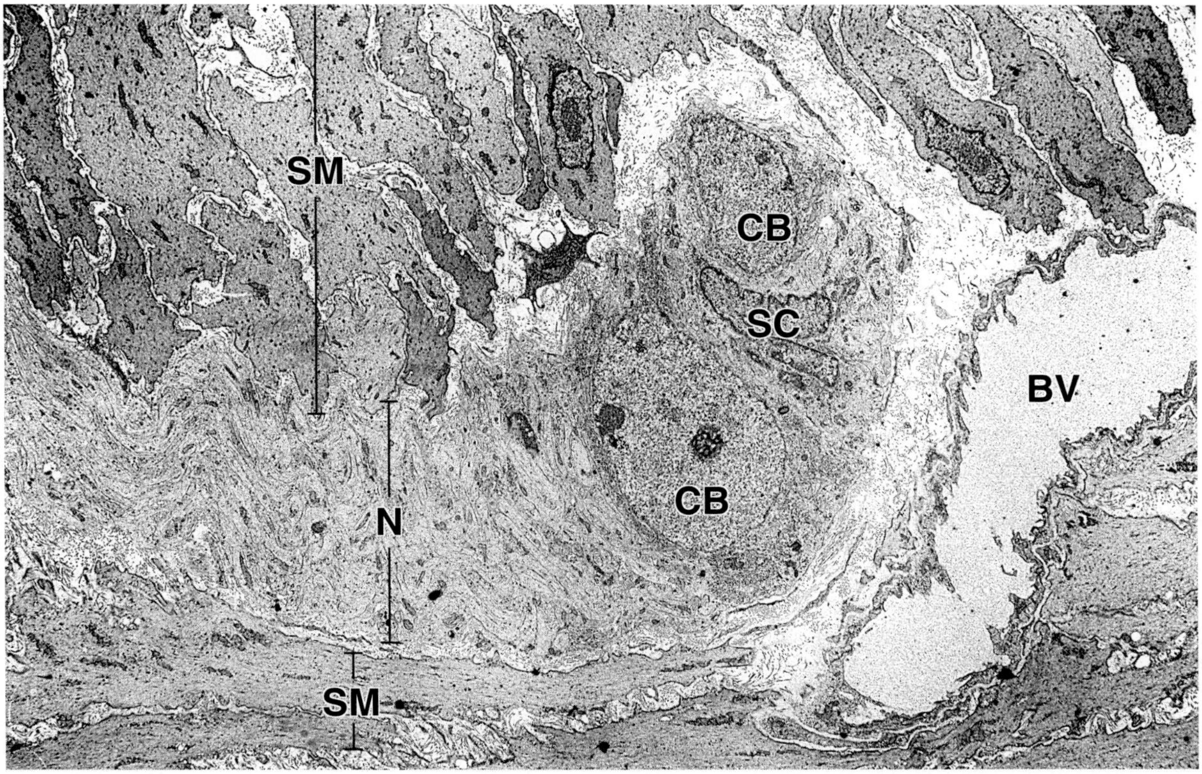

FIGURE 16.28
Electron micrograph of the myenteric (Auerbach's) plexus. The plexus is located between the two smooth muscle *(SM)* layers of the muscularis externa. It consists of nerve cell bodies *(CB)* and an extensive network of nerve fibers *(N)*. A satellite cell *(SC)*, also referred to as an enteric glial cell, is seen in proximity to the neuron cell bodies. These cells have structural and chemical features in common with glial cells of the CNS. BV, Blood vessel. ×3,800.

sis, the second type of contraction, largely involves the longitudinal muscle layer and moves the intestinal contents distally.

Serosa

The ***serosa*** of the parts of the small intestine that are located intraperitoneally in the abdominal cavity corresponds to the general description at the beginning of the chapter.

Epithelial Cell Renewal in the Small Intestine

All of the mature cells of the intestinal epithelium are derived from a single stem cell population

Stem cells are located in the base of the intestinal gland. The ***zone of cell replication*** is restricted to the lower one half of the gland. A cell destined to become a goblet cell or absorptive cell usually undergoes several additional divisions after it leaves the pool of stem cells. The epithelial cells migrate upward in the intestinal gland onto the villus and are shed at the tip of the villus. Autoradiographic studies have shown that the renewal time for absorptive and goblet cells in the human small intestine is 5 to 6 days (see Fig. 4.32).

Enteroendocrine cells and Paneth cells are also derived from the stem cells at the base of the intestinal gland. Enteroendocrine cells appear to divide only once before differentiating. They migrate with the absorptive and goblet cells but at a slower rate. Paneth cells do not migrate; they remain in the base of the intestinal gland near the stem cells from which they are derived. They live for approximately 4 weeks and are then replaced by differentiation of a nearby "committed" cell in the intestinal gland. Cells that are recognizable as Paneth cells no longer divide.

▼ LARGE INTESTINE

The large intestine comprises the ***cecum*** with its projecting ***vermiform appendix,*** the ***colon,*** the ***rectum*** and the ***anal canal.*** The colon is further subdivided on the basis of its anatomic location into ***ascending colon, transverse colon, descending colon,*** and ***sigmoid colon.*** The four layers characteristic of the alimentary canal are present throughout. However, several distinctive features exist at the gross level (Fig. 16.32):

- Except for the rectum, anal canal, and vermiform appendix, the outer longitudinal layer of the muscularis

BOX 16.4

Functional Considerations: Digestive and Absorptive Functions of Enterocytes

The plasma membrane of the microvilli of the enterocyte plays a role in digestion as well as absorption. Digestive enzymes are anchored in the plasma membrane, and their functional groups extend outward to become part of the glycocalyx. This arrangement brings the end products of digestion close to their site of absorption. Included among the enzymes are peptidases and disaccharidases. The plasma membrane of the apical microvilli also contains the enzyme *enteropeptidase (enterokinase),* which is particularly important in the duodenum, where it converts trypsinogen into trypsin. Trypsin can then continue to convert additional trypsinogen into trypsin, and trypsin converts several other pancreatic zymogens into active enzymes (Fig. 16.29). A summary of digestion and absorption of the three major nutrients is outlined in the following paragraphs.

Triglycerides are broken down into glycerol, monoglycerides, and long- and short-chain fatty acids. These substances are emulsified by bile salts and pass into the apical portion of the enterocyte. Here, the glycerol and long-chain fatty acids are resynthesized into triglycerides. The resynthesized triglycerides appear first in apical vesicles of the sER (see Fig. 16.21), then in the Golgi (where they are converted into ***chylomicrons,*** small droplets of neutral fat), and finally in vesicles that discharge the chylomicrons into the intercellular space. The chylomicrons are conveyed away from the intestine via both venous capillaries and lacteals. Short-chain fatty acids and glycerol leave the intestine exclusively via capillaries that lead to the portal vein and the liver.

Carbohydrate final digestion is brought about by enzymes bound to the microvilli of the enterocytes (Fig. 16.30). Galactose, glucose, and fructose are conveyed to the liver by the vessels of the hepatic portal system. Some infants and a larger percentage of adults cannot tolerate milk and unfermented milk products because of the absence of lactase, the disaccharidase that splits lactose into galactose and glucose. If given milk, these individuals become bloated because of the gas produced by bacterial digestion of the unprocessed lactose and suffer from diarrhea. The condition is completely alleviated if lactose (milk sugar) is eliminated from the diet. For some individuals, milk intolerance may be also partially or completely alleviated by using lactose-reduced milk products or tablets of lactase (enzyme that digests lactose), which are available as over-the-counter drugs.

Protein digestion and absorption is shown in Figure 16.31. The major end products of protein digestion are amino acids, which are absorbed by enterocytes. However, some peptides are also absorbed and are evidently broken down intracellularly. In one disorder of amino acid absorption (Hartnup's disease), free amino acids appear in the blood when dipeptides are fed to patients but not when free amino acids are fed. This supports the conclusion that dipeptides of certain amino acids are absorbed via a pathway different from that of the free amino acids.

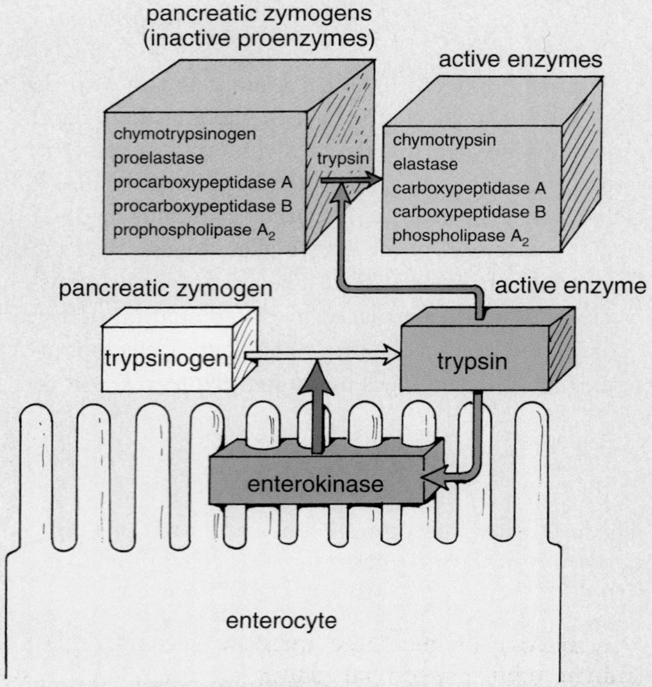

FIGURE 16.29
Diagram showing events in the activation of the proteolytic enzymes of the pancreas. The majority of pancreatic enzymes (proteases) are secreted as inactive proenzymes. Their activation is triggered by the arrival of chyme into the duodenum. This stimulates the mucosal cells to release and to activate the enterokinase *(blue box)* within the glycocalyx. The enterokinase activates trypsinogen, converting it into its active form, trypsin *(green box).* In turn, trypsin activates other pancreatic proenzymes *(red box)* into their active forms *(purple box).* The active proteases hydrolyze peptide bonds of proteins or polypeptides and reduce them to small peptides and amino acids.

BOX 16.4

Functional Considerations: Digestive and Absorptive Functions of Enterocytes (Continued)

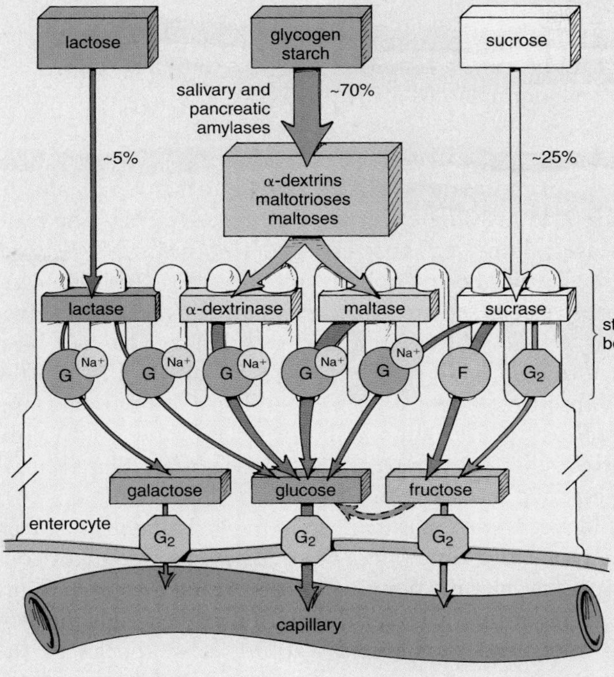

FIGURE 16.30
Diagram showing the digestion and absorption of carbohydrates by an enterocyte. Carbohydrates are delivered to the alimentary canal as monosaccharides (e.g., glucose, fructose, and galactose), disaccharides (e.g., sucrose, lactose, and maltose), and as polysaccharides (e.g., glycogen and starch). Enzymes evolved in digestion of carbohydrates are classified as salivary and pancreatic amylases. Further digestion is performed at the striated border of the enterocytes by enzymes breaking down oligosaccharides and polysaccharides into three basic monosaccharides (glucose, galactose, and fructose). Glucose and galactose are absorbed by the enterocyte via an active transport utilizing Na^+-dependent glucose transporters (SGLT1). These transporters are localized at the apical cell membrane *(brown circles with G and Na^+ labels).* Fructose enters the cell via facilitated Na^+-independent transport utilizing GLUT5 *(gray circle with F label)* and GLUT2 glucose transporters *(orange octagon with G_2 label).* The three absorbed monosaccharides then pass through the basal membrane of the enterocyte, utilizing GLUT2 glucose transporters, into the underlying capillaries of the portal circulation to reach their final destination in the liver.

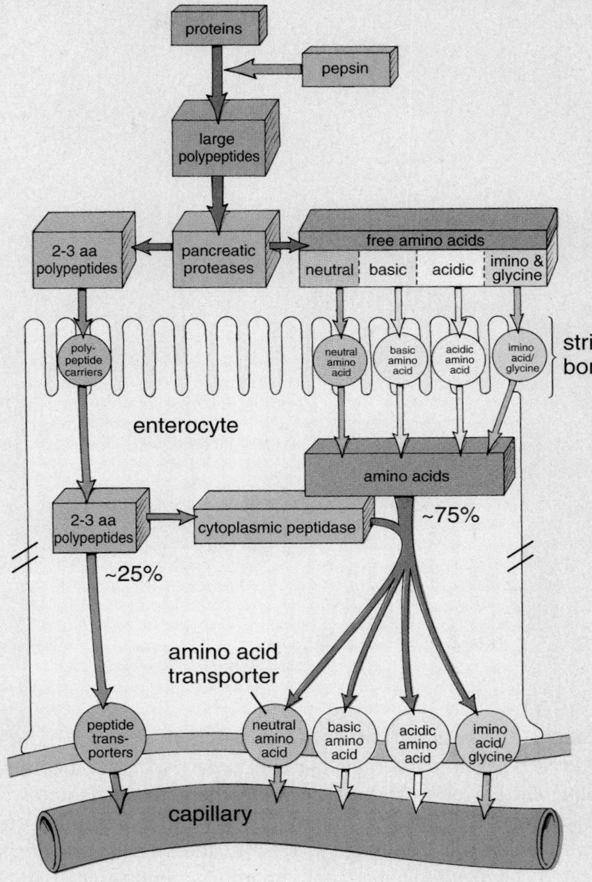

FIGURE 16.31
Diagram showing the digestion and absorption of protein by an enterocyte. Proteins entering the alimentary canal are completely digested into free amino acids and small dipeptide or tripeptide fragments. Protein digestion starts in the stomach with pepsin, which hydrolyzes proteins to large polypeptides. The next step occurs in the small intestine by the action of pancreatic proteolytic enzymes. The activation process is shown in Figure 16.29. Free amino acids are transported by four different amino acid transporters and several dipeptide and tripeptide transporters into the cell and then from the cell into the underlying capillaries of the portal circulation.

externa exhibits three thickened, equally spaced bands known as the ***teniae coli.***

- The external surface of the cecum and colon exhibits sacculations known as ***haustra*** that are visible between the teniae. The mucosa has a "smooth" surface; neither plicae circulares nor villi are present.
- Small fatty projections of the serosa known as ***omental appendices*** are visible on the outer intestinal surface.

Mucosa

The mucosa of the large intestine contains numerous straight tubular intestinal glands (crypts of Lieberkühn) that extend through the full thickness of the mucosa (Fig. 16.33a). The glands consist of simple columnar epithelium, as does the intestinal surface from which they invaginate. Examination of the luminal surface of the large intestine at

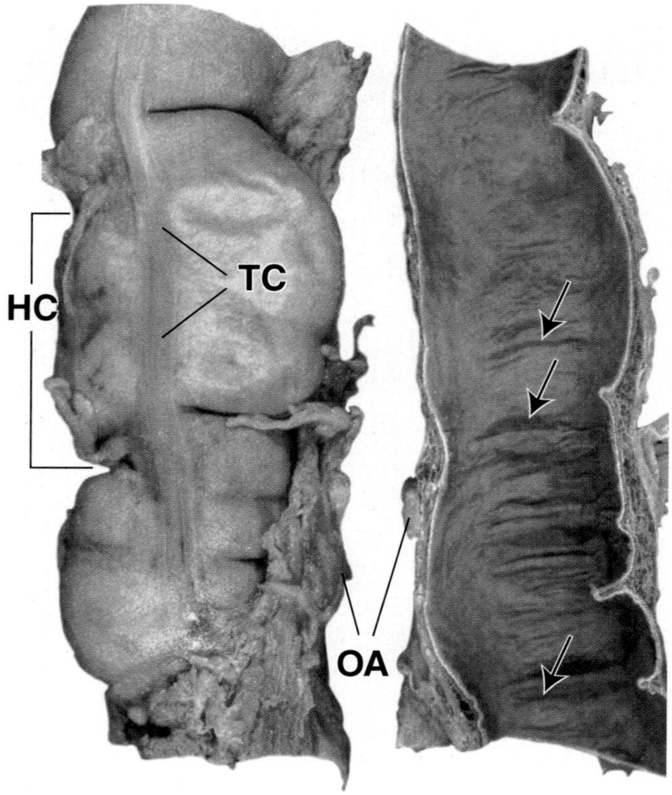

FIGURE 16.32
Photograph of the large intestine. This photograph shows the outer (serosal) surface *(left)* and internal (mucosal) surface *(right)* of the transverse colon. On the outer surface, note the characteristic features of the large intestine: a distinctive smooth muscle band representing one of the three teniae coli *(TC)*; haustra coli *(HC)*, the sacculations of the colon located between the teniae; and omental appendices *(OA)*, small peritoneal projections filled with fat. The smooth mucosal surface shows semilunar folds *(arrows)* formed in response to contractions of the muscularis externa. Compare the mucosal surface as shown here with that of the small intestine (Fig. 16.17).

the microscopic level reveals the openings of the glands, which are arranged in an orderly pattern (Fig. 16.33b).

The principal functions of the large intestine are reabsorption of electrolytes and water and elimination of undigested food and waste

The primary function of the ***columnar absorptive cells*** is reabsorption of water and electrolytes. The morphology of absorptive cells is essentially identical to that of the enterocytes of the small intestine. Reabsorption is accomplished by the same Na^+/K^+-activated ATPase-driven transport system as described for the small intestine.

Elimination of semisolid to solid waste materials is facilitated by the large amounts of mucus secreted by the numerous goblet cells of the intestinal glands. Goblet cells are more numerous in the large intestine than in the small intestine (see Fig. 16.33a). They produce mucin that is secreted continuously to lubricate the bowel, facilitating the passage of the increasingly solid contents.

The mucosal epithelium of the large intestine contains the same cell types as the small intestine except Paneth cells, which are normally absent in humans

Columnar absorptive cells predominate (4:1) over goblet cells in most of the colon, although this is not always apparent in histologic sections (see Fig. 16.33a). The ratio decreases, however, approaching 1:1, near the rectum, where the number of goblet cells increases. Although the absorptive cells secrete glycocalyx at a rapid rate (turnover time is 16 to 24 hours in humans), this layer has not been shown to contain digestive enzymes in the colon. As in the small intestine, however, Na^+/K^+-ATPase is abundant and is localized in the lateral plasma membranes of the absorptive cells. The intercellular space is often dilated, indicating active transport of fluid.

Goblet cells may mature deep in the intestinal gland, even in the replicative zone (Fig. 16.34). They secrete mucus continuously, even to the point where they reach the luminal surface. Here, at the surface, the secretion rate exceeds the synthesis rate, and "exhausted" goblet cells appear in the epithelium. These cells are tall and thin and have a small number of mucinogen granules in the central apical cytoplasm. An infrequently observed cell type, the ***caveolated "tuft" cell***, has also been described in the colonic epithelium; however, this cell may be a form of exhausted goblet cell.

Epithelial Cell Renewal in the Large Intestine

All intestinal epithelial cells in the large intestine derive from a single stem cell population

As in the small intestine, all of the mucosal epithelial cells of the large intestine arise from stem cells located at the bottom of the intestinal gland. The lower third of the gland constitutes the normal replicative zone where newly generated cells undergo 2 to 3 more divisions as they begin their migration up to the luminal surface where they are shed about 5 days later. The intermediate cell types found in the lower third of the intestinal gland are identical to those seen in the small intestine.

The turnover times of the epithelial cells of the large intestine are similar to those of the small intestine, i.e., about 6 days for absorptive cells and goblet cells and up to 4 weeks for enteroendocrine cells. Senile epithelial cells that reach the mucosal surface are shed into the lumen at the midpoint between two adjacent intestinal glands.

Lamina Propria

Although the lamina propria of the large intestine contains the same basic components as the rest of the digestive

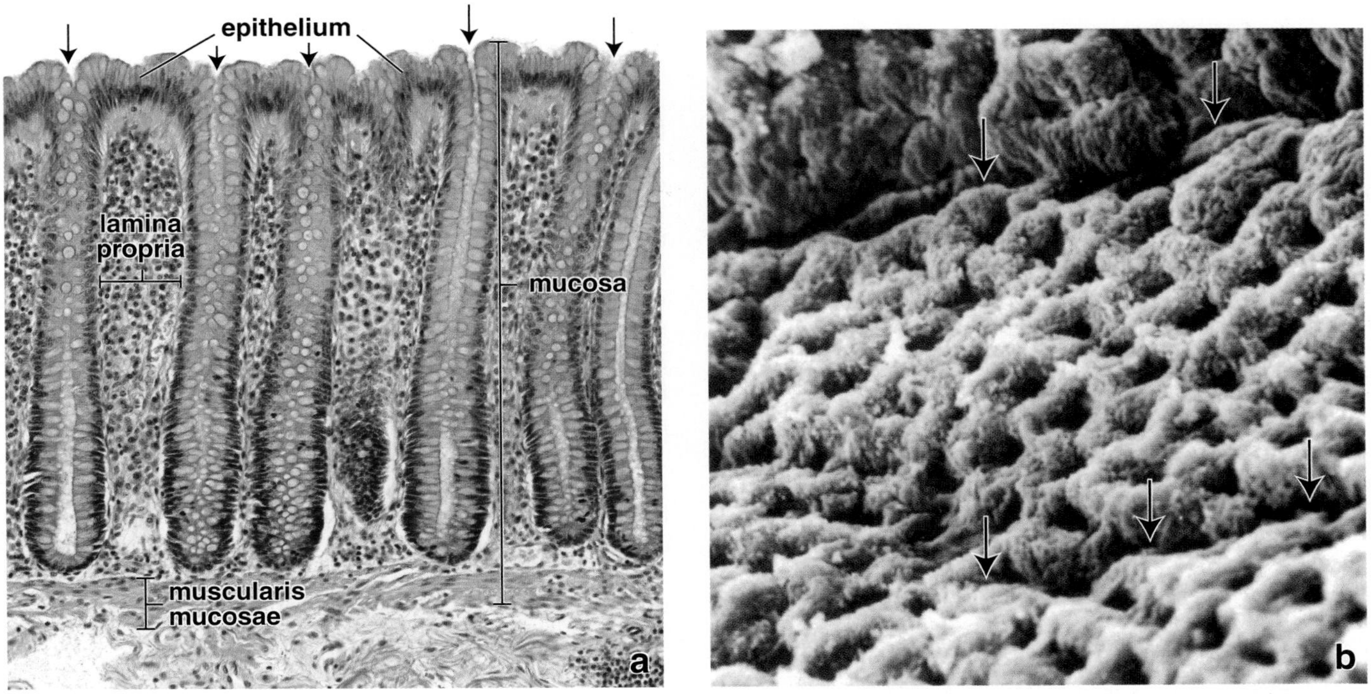

FIGURE 16.33
Mucosa of the large intestine. a. This photomicrograph of a H&E preparation shows the mucosa and part of the submucosa. The surface epithelium is continuous with the straight, unbranched, tubular intestinal glands (crypts of Lieberkühn). The openings of the glands at the intestinal surface are identified *(arrows).* The epithelial cells consist principally of absorptive and goblet cells. As the absorptive cells are followed into the glands, they become fewer in number, whereas the goblet cells increase in number. The highly cellular lamina propria contains numerous lymphocytes and other cells of the immune system. **b.** Scanning electron micrograph of the human mucosal surface of the large intestine. The surface is divided into territories by clefts *(arrows).* Each territory contains 25 to 100 gland openings. ×140. (From Fenoglio CM, Richart RM, Kaye GI. *Gastroenterology* 1975;69: 100–109.)

tract, it demonstrates some additional structural features and greater development of some others. These include

- The ***collagen table***, a thick layer of collagen and proteoglycans that lies between the basal lamina of the epithelium and that of the fenestrated absorptive venous capillaries. This layer is as much as 5 μm thick in the normal human colon and can be up to 3 times that thickness in human hyperplastic colonic polyps. The collagen table participates in regulation of water and electrolyte transport from the intercellular compartment of the epithelium to the vascular compartment.
- Well-developed GALT, which is continuous with that of the terminal ileum. In the large intestine GALT is more extensively developed; large lymphatic nodules distort the regular spacing of the intestinal glands and extend into the submucosa. The extensive development of the immune system in the colon probably reflects the large number and variety of microorganisms and noxious end products of metabolism normally present in the lumen.
- A well-developed ***pericryptal fibroblast sheath***, which constitutes a fibroblast population of regularly replicating cells. They divide immediately beneath the base of the intestinal gland, adjacent to the stem cells found in the epithelium (in both the large and small intestines). The fibroblasts then differentiate and migrate upward in parallel and synchrony with the epithelial cells. Although the ultimate fate of the pericryptal fibroblast is unknown, most of these cells, after they reach the level of the luminal surface, take on the morphologic and histochemical characteristics of macrophages. Some evidence suggests that the macrophages of the core of the lamina propria in the large intestine may arise as a terminal differentiation of the pericryptal fibroblasts
- Absence of lymphatic vessels in the lamina propria. There are no lymphatic vessels in the core of the lamina propria between the intestinal glands. Lymphatic vessels form a network around the muscularis mucosae, as they do in the small intestine, but no vessels or associated smooth muscle cells extend toward the free surface from that layer. The absence of lymphatic vessels from the lamina propria is important to understanding the slow rate of metastasis from certain colon cancers. Cancers that develop in large adenomatous colonic polyps may grow extensively within the epithelium and lamina propria before they even have access to the lymphatic vessels at the level of the muscularis mucosae. Lymphatic vessels are found in the

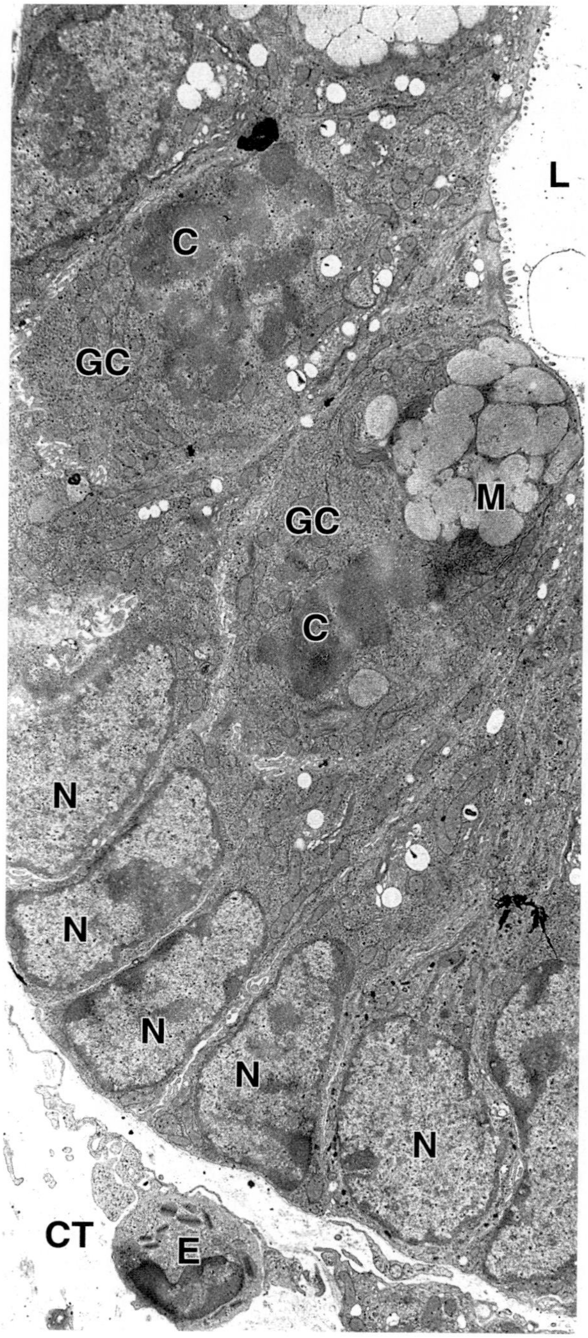

FIGURE 16.34
Electron micrograph of dividing goblet cells. This electron micrograph demonstrates that certain cells of the intestine continue to divide even after they have differentiated. Here, two goblet cells *(GC)* are shown in division. Typically, the dividing cells move away from the basal lamina toward the lumen. One of the goblet cells shows mucinogen granules *(M)* in its apical cytoplasm. The chromosomes *(C)* of the dividing cells are not surrounded by a nuclear membrane. Compare with the nuclei *(N)* of the nondividing intestinal epithelial cells. The lumen of the gland *(L)* is on the right. *CT*, connective tissue; and *E*, eosinophil. ×5,000.

submucosa and as a network around the muscularis externa.

Muscularis Externa

As noted, in the cecum and colon (the ascending, transverse, descending and sigmoid colon), the outer layer of the muscularis externa is, in part, condensed into prominent longitudinal bands of muscle, called ***teniae coli,*** which may be seen at the gross level (see Fig. 16.32). Between these bands, the longitudinal layer forms an extremely thin sheet. In the rectum, anal canal, and vermiform appendix, the outer longitudinal layer of smooth muscle is a uniformly thick layer, as in the small intestine.

Bundles of muscle from the teniae coli penetrate the inner, circular layer of muscle at irregular intervals along the length and circumference of the colon. These apparent discontinuities in the muscularis externa allow segments of the colon to contract independently, leading to the formation of ***saccules (haustra)*** in the colon wall.

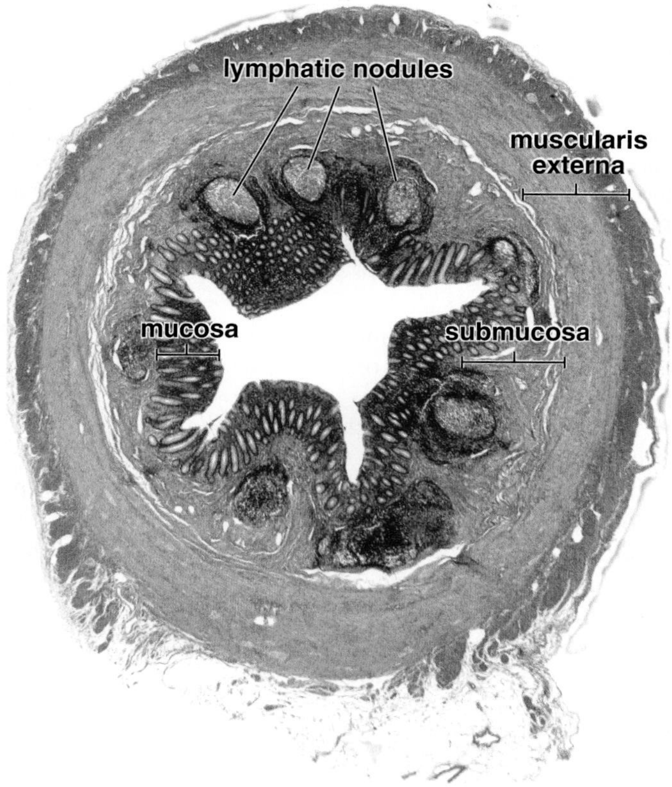

FIGURE 16.35
Photomicrograph of a cross section through the vermiform appendix. The vermiform appendix displays the same four layers as those of the large intestine except that its diameter is smaller. Typically, lymphatic nodules are seen within the entire mucosa and usually extend into the submucosa. Note the distinct germinal centers within the lymphatic nodules. The muscularis externa is composed of a relatively thick circular layer and a much thinner outer longitudinal layer. The appendix is covered by a serosa that is continuous with the mesentery of the appendix (lower right). ×10.

The muscularis externa of the large intestine produces two major types of contraction: segmentation and peristalsis. Segmentation is local and does not result in the propulsion of contents. Peristalsis results in the distal mass movement of the colonic contents. Mass peristaltic movements occur infrequently; in healthy persons, they usually occur once a day to empty the distal colon.

Submucosa and Serosa

The submucosa of the large intestine corresponds to the general description already given. Where the large intestine is directly in contact with other structures (as on much of its posterior surface), its outer layer is an adventitia; elsewhere, the outer layer is a typical serosa.

Cecum and Appendix

The cecum forms a blind pouch just distal to the ileocecal valve; the appendix is a thin, finger-like extension of this pouch. The histology of the cecum closely resembles that of the rest of the colon; the appendix differs from it in having a uniform layer of longitudinal muscle in the muscularis externa (Fig. 16.35). The most conspicuous feature of the appendix is the large number of lymphatic nodules that extend into the submucosa. In many adults, the normal structure of the appendix is lost, and the appendage is filled with fibrous scar tissue.

Rectum and Anal Canal

The ***rectum*** is the dilated distal portion of the alimentary canal. Its upper part is distinguished from the rest of the large intestine by the presence of folds called ***transverse rectal folds.*** The mucosa of the rectum is similar to that of the rest of the distal colon, having straight, tubular intestinal glands with many goblet cells.

The most distal portion of the alimentary canal is the ***anal canal.*** It has an average length of 4 cm and extends from the upper aspect of the pelvic diaphragm to the anus (Fig. 16.36). The upper part of the anal canal has longitudinal folds called ***anal columns.*** Depressions between the

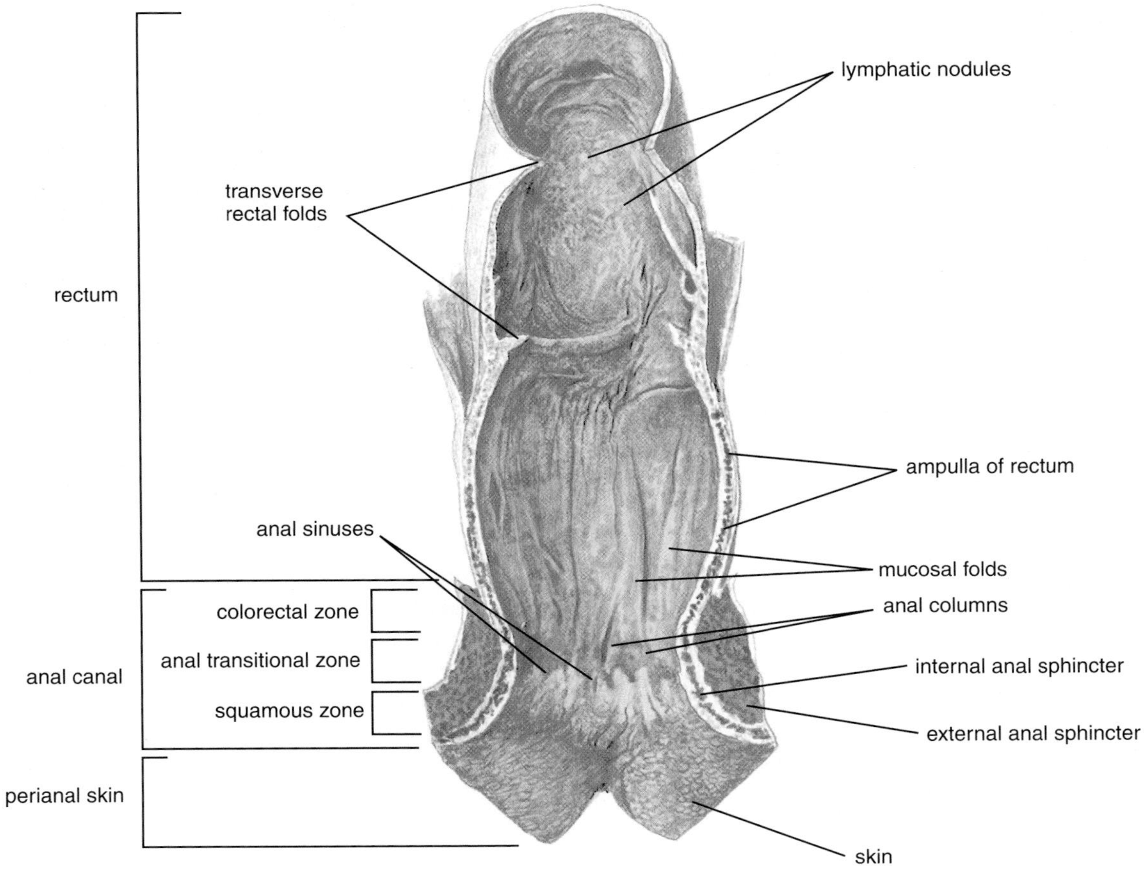

FIGURE 16.36
Drawing of the rectum and anal canal. The rectum and anal canal are the terminal portions of the large intestine. They are lined by the colorectal mucosa that possesses a simple columnar epithelium containing mostly goblet cells and numerous anal glands. In the anal canal the simple columnar epithelium undergoes transition into a stratified columnar (or cuboidal) epithelium and then to a stratified squamous epithelium. This transition occurs in the area referred as the anal transitional zone, which occupies the middle third of the anal canal between the colorectal zone and the squamous zone of the perianal skin.

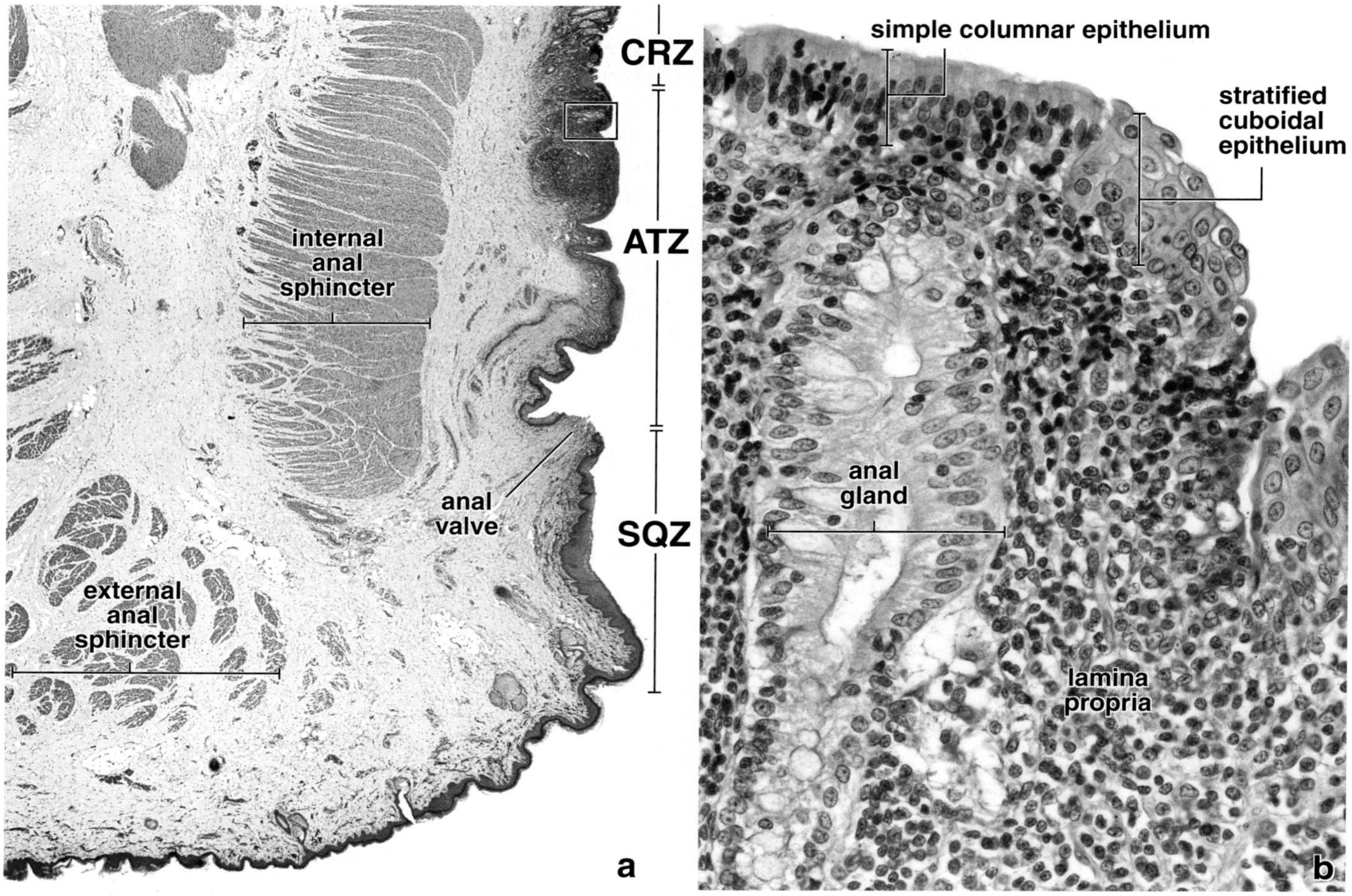

FIGURE 16.37

Photomicrographs of the anal canal. a. This photomicrograph shows a longitudinal section through the wall of the anal canal. Note the three zones in the anal canal: the squamous zone *(SQZ)* containing stratified squamous epithelium; the anal transitional zone *(ATZ)* containing stratified squamous, stratified cuboidal, or columnar epithelium and simple columnar epithelium of the rectal mucosa; and the colorectal zone *(CRZ)* containing only simple columnar epithelium like the rest of the colon. Note the anal valve that demarcates the transition between the ATZ and SQZ. The internal anal sphincter is derived from the thickening of the circular layer of the muscularis externa. A small portion of the external anal sphincter is seen subcutaneously. ×10. **b.** This high magnification of the area indicated by the *rectangle* in *a* shows the area of the anal transitional zone *(ATZ)*. Note the abrupt transition between stratified cuboidal and simple columnar epithelium. The simple columnar epithelium of anal glands extends into the submucosa. These straight, mucus-secreting tubular glands are surrounded by diffuse lymphatic tissue. ×200.

anal columns are called ***anal sinuses.*** The anal canal is divided into three zones according to the character of the epithelial lining:

- *Colorectal zone,* which is found in the upper third of the anal canal and contains simple columnar epithelium with characteristics identical to that in the rectum
- *Anal transitional zone (ATZ),* which occupies the middle third of the anal canal. It represents a transition between the simple columnar epithelium of the rectal mucosa and the stratified squamous epithelium of the perianal skin. The ATZ possesses a stratified columnar epithelium interposed between the simple columnar epithelium and the stratified squamous epithelium, which extends to the cutaneous zone of the anal canal (Fig. 16.37).
- *Squamous zone,* which is found in the lower third of the anal canal. This zone is lined with stratified squamous epithelium that is continuous with that of the perineal skin.

In the anal canal, ***anal glands*** extend into the submucosa and even into the muscularis externa. These branched, straight tubular glands secrete mucus onto the anal surface through ducts lined with stratified columnar epithelium. Sometimes the anal glands are surrounded by diffuse lymphatic tissue. They often lead to the formation of pathologic fistulas (a false opening between the anal canal and the perianal skin).

Large apocrine glands, the ***circumanal glands,*** are found in the skin surrounding the anal orifice. In some animals, the secretion of these glands acts as a sex attractant.

BOX 16.5

Functional Considerations: Immune Functions of the Alimentary Canal

Immunologists have shown that the GALT not only responds to antigenic stimuli but also functions in a monitoring capacity. This function has been partially clarified for the lymphatic nodules of the intestinal tract. The M cells that cover Peyer's patches and lymphatic nodules have a distinctive surface that might be misinterpreted in sections as thick microvilli. The cells are readily identified with the scanning electron microscope because microfolds contrast sharply with the microvilli that constitute the striated border of the adjacent enterocytes.

It has been shown with horseradish peroxidase (an enzyme used as an experimental marker) that the M cells pinocytose protein from the intestinal lumen, transport the pinocytotic vesicles through the cell, and discharge the protein by exocytosis into deep recesses of the adjacent extracellular space (Fig. 16.38). Lymphocytes within the deeply recessed extracellular space sample the luminal protein, including antigens, and thus have the opportunity to stimulate development of specific antibodies against the antigens. The destination of these exposed lymphocytes has not yet been fully determined. Some remain within the local lymphatic tissue, but others may be destined for other sites in the body, such as the salivary and mammary glands. Recall that in the salivary glands, cells of the immune system (plasma cells) secrete IgA, which the glandular epithelium then converts into sIgA. Some experimental observations suggest that antigen contact necessary for the production of IgA by plasma cells occurs in the lymphatic nodules of the intestines.

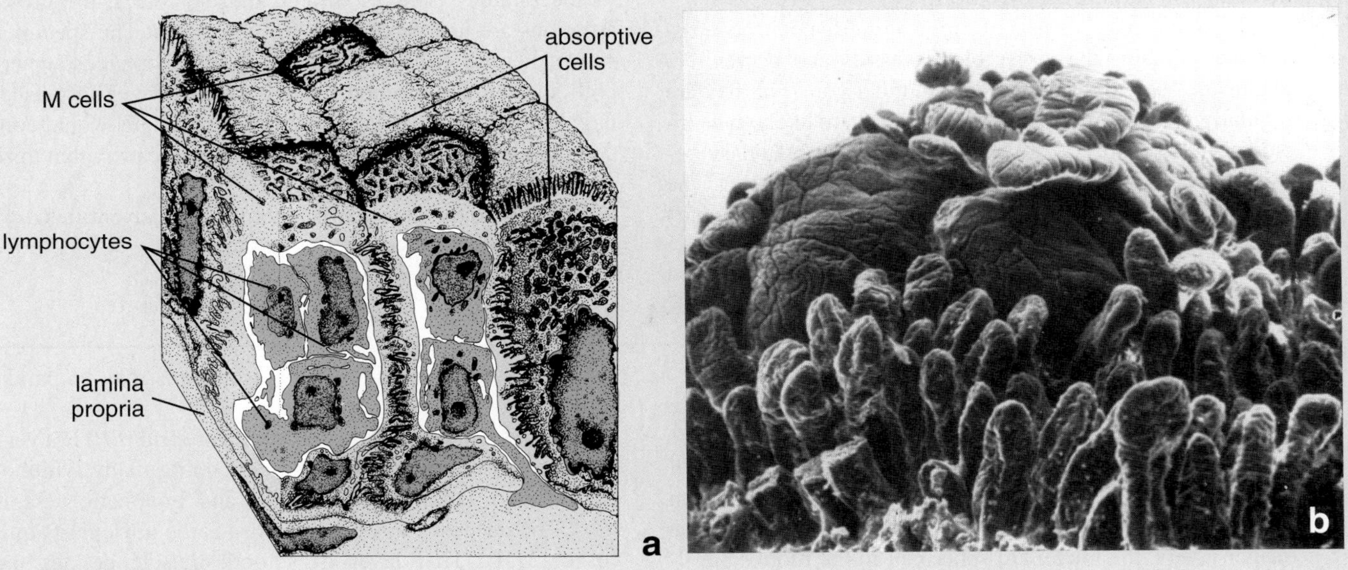

FIGURE 16.38
Diagram of M cells in a lymphatic nodule of the intestine. a. This diagram shows the relationship of the M cells (microfold cells) and absorptive cells to the lymphatic nodule. The M cell is an epithelial cell that displays microfolds rather than microvilli on its apical surface. It has deep recesses within which lymphocytes come close to the lumen of the small intestine. M cells have MHC II molecules on their surface and are therefore considered antigen-presenting cells. Antigen from the intestinal lumen is presented to T lymphocytes residing within the recesses of the M cell. (Based on Owen RL, Nemanic PC, eds. *Scanning Electron Microscopy.* Vol II. O'Hare, IL: AMF, 1978.) **b.** Scanning electron micrograph of a Peyer's patch lymphatic nodule bulging into the lumen of the ileum. Note that the area of the follicle covered by M cells is surrounded by the finger-like projections of the intestinal villi. The surface of the M cells has a smooth appearance. The absence of absorptive cells and mucus-producing goblet cells in the area covered by M cells facilitates immunoreactions to antigens. ×80. (From Owen RL, Johns AL. *Gastroenterology* 1974;66.)

Hair follicles and sebaceous glands are also found at this site.

The submucosa of the anal columns contains the terminal ramifications of the superior rectal artery and the rectal venous plexus. Enlargements of these submucosal veins constitute ***internal hemorrhoids,*** which are related to elevated venous pressure in the portal circulation (portal hypertension). There are no teniae coli at the level of the rectum; the longitudinal layer of the muscularis externa forms a uniform sheet. The muscularis mucosae disappears at about the level of the anal transitional zone (ATZ), where the circular layer of the muscularis externa thickens to form the ***internal anal sphincter.*** The external anal sphincter is formed by striated muscle of the pelvic floor.

PLATE 50. ESOPHAGUS

The esophagus is a muscular tube that conveys food and other substances from the pharynx to the stomach.

Figure 1, esophagus, monkey, H&E ×60; inset ×400.

A cross section of the wall of the esophagus is shown here. The mucosa (*Muc*) consists of stratified squamous epithelium (*Ep*), a lamina propria (*LP*), and muscularis mucosae (*MM*). The boundary between the epithelium and lamina propria is distinct, although uneven, as a result of the presence of numerous deep connective tissue papillae. The basal layer of the epithelium stains intensely, appearing as a dark band that is relatively conspicuous at low magnification. This is, in part, due to the cytoplasmic basophilia of the basal cells. That the basal cells are small results in a high nuclear-cytoplasmic ratio, which further intensifies the hematoxylin staining of this layer.

The submucosa consists of irregular dense connective tissue that contains the larger blood vessels and nerves. No glands are seen in the submucosa in this figure, but they are regularly present throughout this layer and are likely to be included in a section of the wall. Whereas the boundary between the epithelium and lamina propria is striking, the boundary between the mucosa (*Muc*) and submucosa (*SubM*) is less well marked, although it is readily discernable.

The muscularis externa (*ME*) shown here is composed largely of smooth muscle, but it also contains areas of striated muscle. Although the striations are not evident at this low magnification, the more densely stained eosinophilic areas (*asterisks*) prove to be striated muscle when observed at higher magnification. Reference to the **inset,** which is from an area in the lower half of the figure, substantiates this identification.

The **inset** shows circularly oriented striated and smooth muscle. The striated muscle stains more intensely with eosin, but of greater significance are the distribution and number of nuclei. In the midarea of the **inset,** numerous elongated and uniformly oriented nuclei are present; this is smooth muscle (*SM*). Above and below, few elongated nuclei are present; moreover, they are largely at the periphery of the bundles. This is striated muscle (*StM*); the cross-striations are just perceptible in some areas. The specimen shown here is from the middle of the esophagus, where both smooth and striated muscle are present. The muscularis externa of the distal third of the esophagus would contain only smooth muscle, whereas that of the proximal third would consist of striated muscle.

External to the muscularis externa is the adventitia (*Adv*) consisting of dense connective tissue.

Figure 2, esophagus, monkey, H&E ×300.

As in other stratified squamous epithelia, new cells are produced in the basal layer, from which they move to the surface. During this migration, the shape and orientation of the cells change. This change in cell shape and orientation is also reflected in the appearance of the nuclei. In the deeper layers, the nuclei are spherical; in the more superficial layers, the nuclei are elongated and oriented parallel to the surface. That nuclei can be seen throughout the epithelial layer, particularly the surface cells, indicates that the epithelium is not keratinized. In some instances, the epithelium of the upper regions of the esophagus may be parakeratinized or, more rarely, keratinized.

As shown in this figure, the lamina propria (*LP*) is a very cellular, loose connective tissue containing many lymphocytes (*Lym*), small blood vessels, and lymphatic vessels (*LV*). The deepest part of the mucosa is the muscularis mucosae (*MM*). That layer of smooth muscle defines the boundary between mucosa and submucosa. The nuclei of the smooth muscle cells of the muscularis mucosae appear spherical because the cells have been cut in cross section.

KEY

Adv, adventitia
Ep, stratified squamous epithelium
L, longitudinal layer of muscularis externa
LP, lamina propria
LV, lymphatic vessels
Lym, lymphocytes
ME, muscularis externa
MM, muscularis mucosae
Muc, mucosa
SM, smooth muscle
StM, striated muscle
SubM, submucosa
arrows (Fig. 2), lymphocytes in epithelium
asterisks (Fig. 1), areas containing striated muscle in the muscularis externa

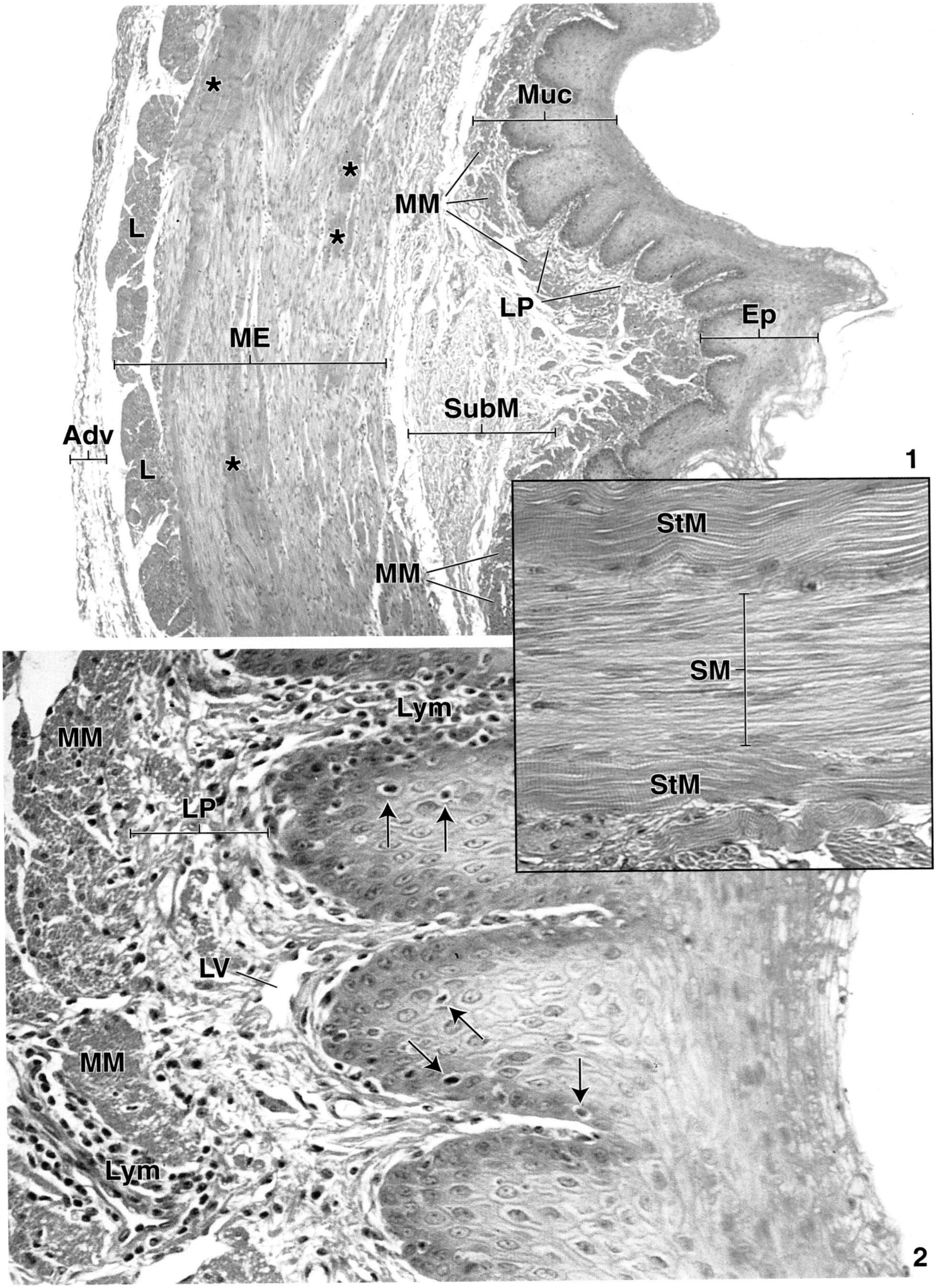
Muc
MM
LP
Ep
ME
SubM
Adv
L
L
MM
1
StM
SM
StM
Lym
MM
LP
LV
MM
Lym
2

PLATE 51. ESOPHAGUS AND STOMACH, CARDIAC REGION

The *esophagogastric junction* marks a change in function from that of a conduit (esophagus) to that of a digestive organ (stomach). The epithelium of the mucosa changes from stratified squamous (protective) to a simple columnar secretory epithelium that forms mucosal glands that secrete mucinogen, digestive enzymes, and hydrochloric acid. The very cellular lamina propria is rich in diffuse lymphatic tissue, emphasizing the role of this layer in the immune system.

Figure 1, esophagogastric junction, H&E ×100. The junction between the esophagus and stomach is shown here. The esophagus is on the right, and the cardiac region of the stomach is on the left. The *large rectangle* marks a representative area of the cardiac mucosa seen at higher magnification in Figure 2; the *smaller rectangle* shows part of the junction examined at higher magnification in Figure 3.

As noted in Plate 50, the esophagus is lined by stratified squamous epithelium *(Ep)* that is indented on its undersurface by deep connective tissue papillae. When these are sectioned obliquely (as five of them have been), they appear as islands of connective tissue within the thick epithelium. Under the epithelium are the lamina propria and the muscularis mucosae *(MM)*. At the junction between the esophagus and the stomach (see also Fig. 3), the stratified squamous epithelium of the esophagus ends abruptly, and the simple columnar epithelium of the stomach surface begins.

The surface of the stomach contains numerous and relatively deep depressions called gastric pits *(P)*, or foveolae, that are formed by epithelium similar to, and continuous with, that of the surface. Glands *(Gl)* open into the bottom of the pits; they are cardiac glands. The entire gastric mucosa contains glands. There are three types of gastric glands: cardiac, fundic, and pyloric. Cardiac glands are in the immediate vicinity of the opening of the esophagus; pyloric glands are in the funnel-shaped portion of the stomach that leads to the duodenum; and fundic glands are throughout the remainder of the stomach.

Figure 2, esophagogastric junction, H&E ×260. The cardiac glands and pits seen in Figure 1 are surrounded by a very cellular lamina propria. At this higher magnification, it can be seen that many cells of the lamina propria are lymphocytes and other cells of the immune system. Large numbers of lymphocytes *(L)* may be localized between the smooth muscle cells of the muscularis mucosae *(MM)*, and thus, the muscularis mucosae in these locations appears to be disrupted.

The cardiac glands *(GL)* are limited to a narrow region around the cardiac orifice. They are not sharply delineated from the fundic region of the stomach that contains parietal and chief cells. Thus, at the boundary, occasional parietal cells are seen in the cardiac glands.

In certain animals (e.g., ruminants and pigs), the anatomy and histology of the stomach are different. In these, at least one part of the stomach is lined with stratified squamous epithelium.

Figure 3, esophagogastric junction, H&E ×440. The columnar cells of the stomach surface and gastric pits *(P)* produce mucus. Each surface and pit cell contains a mucous cup in its apical cytoplasm, thereby forming a glandular sheet of cells named surface mucous cells *(MSC)*. The content of the mucous cup is usually lost during the preparation of the tissue, and thus, the apical cup portion of the cells appears empty in routine H&E paraffin sections such as the ones shown in this plate.

Figure 4, esophagogastric junction, H&E ×440. The epithelium of the cardiac glands *(Gl)* also consists of mucous cells *(MGC)*. As seen in the photomicrograph, the nucleus of the gland cell is typically flattened; one side is adjacent to the base of the cell, while the other side is adjacent to the pale-staining cytoplasm. Again, mucus is lost during processing of the tissue, and this accounts for the pale-staining appearance of the cytoplasm. Although the cardiac glands are mostly unbranched, some branching is occasionally seen. The glands empty their secretions via ducts *(D)* into the bottom of the gastric pits. The cells forming the ducts are columnar, and the cytoplasm stains well with eosin. This makes it easy to distinguish the duct cells from mucous gland cells. Among the cells forming the duct portion of the gland are those that undergo mitotic division to replace both surface mucous and gland cells. Cardiac glands also contain enteroendocrine cells, but they are difficult to identify in routine H&E paraffin sections.

KEY

D, ducts of cardiac glands
Ep, epithelium
Gl (Figs. 1 and 4), cardiac glands
GL (Fig. 2), cardiac glands
L, lymphocytes
LP, lamina propria
MGC, mucous gland cells
MM, muscularis mucosae
MSC, surface mucous cells
P, gastric pits
arrows, intraepithelial lymphocytes

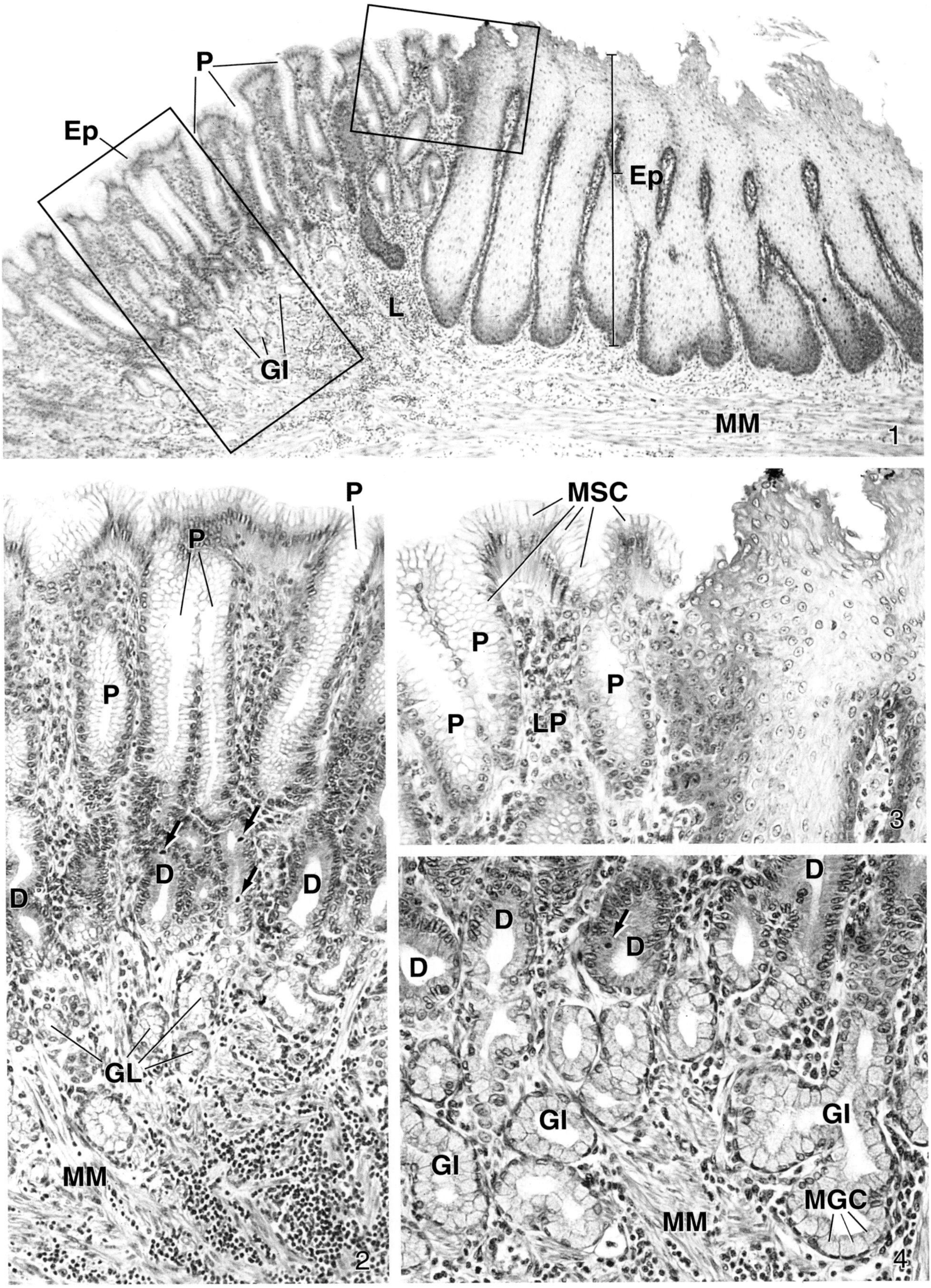
P
Ep
Ep
L
Gl
MM
1
P
P
P
D
D
D
GL
MM
2
MSC
P
P
LP
P
3
D
D
D
D
Gl
Gl
Gl
MM
MGC
4

PLATE 52. STOMACH I

The stomach is divided into three regions: the *cardia,* nearest the esophagus, contains cardiac glands that secrete primarily mucinogen; the *pylorus,* proximal to the *gastrointestinal (pyloric) sphincter* contains *pyloric glands* that secrete a mucinogen that resembles that of the *surface mucous cells;* and the *fundus,* the body or largest part of the stomach that contains the *fundic (gastric) glands.* Fundic glands contain *parietal (oxyntic) cells,* acidophilic cells that secrete 0.16 N HCl; and *chief cells,* basophilic cells that contain acidophilic secretory granules in the apical cytoplasm. The granules contain, principally, pepsinogen. The glands in all parts of the stomach contain *enteroendocrine cells.*

Figure 1, stomach, H&E.

As with other parts of the gastrointestinal tract, the wall of the stomach consists of four layers: a mucosa *(Muc),* a submucosa *(SubM),* a muscularis externa *(ME),* and a serosa. The mucosa is the innermost layer and reveals three distinctive regions *(arrows).* The most superficial region contains the gastric pits; the middle region contains the necks of the glands, which tend to stain with eosin; and the deepest part of the mucosa stains most heavily with hematoxylin. The cell types of the deep (hematoxylin-staining) portion of the fundic mucosa are considered in Figure 3. The cells of all three regions and their staining characteristics are considered in Figure 1 of Plate 53.

The inner surface of the empty stomach is thrown into long folds referred to as rugae. One such cross-sectioned fold is shown here. It consists of mucosa and submucosa *(asterisks).* The rugae are not permanent folds; they disappear when the stomach wall is stretched, as in the distended stomach. Also evident are mamillated areas *(M),* which are slight elevations of the mucosa that resemble cobblestones. The mamillated areas consist only of mucosa without submucosa.

The submucosa and muscularis externa stain predominantly with eosin; the muscularis externa appears darker. The smooth muscle of the muscularis externa gives an appearance of being homogeneous and uniformly solid. In contrast, the submucosa, being connective tissue, may contain areas with adipocytes and contains numerous profiles of blood vessels *(BV).* The serosa is so thin that it is not evident as a discrete layer at this low magnification.

Figure 2, stomach, H&E.

This figure and Figure 3 show the junction between the cardiac and fundic regions of the stomach. This junction can be identified histologically on the basis of the structure of the mucosa. The gastric pits *(P),* some of which are seen opening at the surface *(arrows),* are similar in both regions, but the glands are different. The boundary between cardiac glands *(CG)* and fundic glands *(FG)* is marked by the *dashed line* in each figure.

The full thickness of the gastric mucosa is shown here, as indicated by the presence of the muscularis mucosae *(MM)* deep to the fundic glands. The muscularis mucosae under the cardiac glands is obscured by a large infiltration of lymphocytes forming a lymphatic nodule *(LN).*

Figure 3, stomach, H&E.

This figure provides a comparison between the cardiac and fundic glands at higher magnification. The cardiac glands *(CG)* consist of mucous gland cells arranged as a simple columnar epithelium; the nucleus is in the most basal part of the cell and is somewhat flattened. The cytoplasm appears as a faint network of lightly stained material. The lumina *(L)* of the cardiac glands are relatively wide. On the other hand, the fundic glands *(FG)* (left of the *dashed line*) are small, and a lumen is seen readily only in certain fortuitously sectioned glands. As a consequence, most of the glands appear to be cords of cells. Because this is a deep region of the fundic mucosa, most of the cells are chief cells. The basal portion of the chief cell contains the nucleus and extensive ergastoplasm, thus, its basophilia. The apical cytoplasm, normally occupied by secretory granules that were lost during the preparation of the tissue, stains poorly. Interspersed among the chief cells are parietal cells *(P).* These cells typically have a round nucleus that is surrounded by eosinophilic cytoplasm. Among the cells of the lamina propria are some with pale elongate nuclei. These are smooth muscle cells *(SM)* that extend into the lamina propria from the muscularis mucosae.

KEY

BV, blood vessels
CG, cardiac glands
FG, fundic glands
L, lumen
LN, lymphatic nodule
M, mamillated areas
ME, muscularis externa
MM, muscularis mucosae
Muc, mucosa
P: Fig. 2, gastric pits; Fig. 3, parietal cells
SM, smooth muscle cells
SubM, submucosa
arrows: Fig. 1, three differently stained regions of fundic mucosa; Fig. 2, opening of gastric pits
asterisks, submucosa in ruga
dashed line, boundary between cardiac and fundic glands

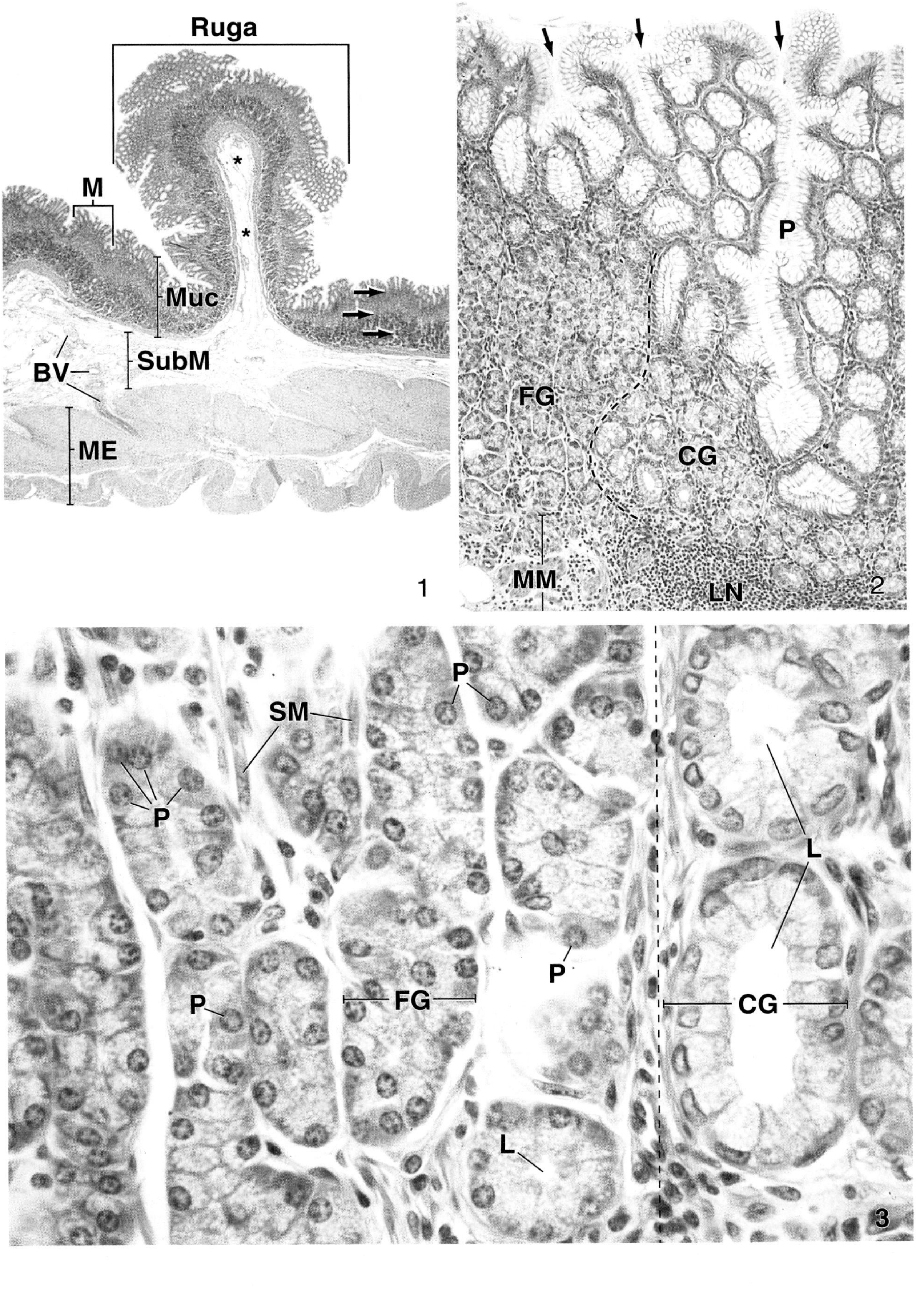
Ruga
M
Muc
SubM
BV
ME
1
FG
CG
P
MM
LN
2
SM
P
FG
CG
L
3

PLATE 53. STOMACH II

The epithelial lining of the alimentary canal is a regularly renewing epithelium; each portion has a characteristic turnover time and stem cell location. In the stomach, stem cells are located in the *mucous neck.* Cells that migrate upward to form the mucous cells of the gastric pit and surface have a turnover time of 3 to 5 days; cells that migrate downward to form the parietal cells, chief cells, and enteroendocrine cells of the glands have a turnover time of about 1 year.

Figure 1, stomach, monkey, H&E ×320.

This figure shows an area of the fundic mucosa that includes the bottom of the gastric pits and the neck and deeper part of the fundic glands. It includes the areas marked by the *arrows* in Figure 1 of Plate 52. The surface mucous cells *(MSC)* of the gastric pits are readily identified because the mucous cup in the apical pole of each cell has an empty, washed-out appearance. Just below the gastric pits are the necks *(N)* of the fundic glands, in which one can identify mucous neck cells *(MNC)* and parietal cells *(PC).* The mucous neck cells produce a mucous secretion that differs from that produced by the surface mucous cells. As seen here, the mucous neck cells display a cytoplasm that is lightly stained; there are no cytoplasmic areas that stain intensely, nor is there a characteristic local absence of staining as in the mucous cup of the surface mucous cells. The mucous neck cells are also the stem cells that divide to give rise to the surface mucous cells and the gland cells.

Parietal cells are distinctive primarily because of the pronounced eosinophilic staining of their cytoplasm. Their nucleus is round, like that of the chief cell, but tends to be located closer to the basal lamina of the epithelium than to the lumen of the gland because of the pear-like shape of the parietal cell.

This figure also reveals the significant characteristics of chief cells *(CC),* namely, the round nucleus in a basal location; the ergastoplasm, deeply stained with hematoxylin (particularly evident in some of the chief cells where the nucleus has not been included in the plane of the section); and the apical, slightly eosinophilic cytoplasm (normally occupied by the secretory granules).

Figure 2, stomach, monkey, H&E ×320.

This figure shows the bottom of the stomach mucosa, the submucosa *(SubM),* and part of the muscularis externa *(ME).* The muscularis mucosae *(MM)* is the deepest part of the mucosa. It consists of smooth muscle cells arranged in at least two layers. As seen in the photomicrograph, the smooth muscle cells immediately adjacent to the submucosa have been sectioned longitudinally and display elongate nuclear profiles. Just above this layer, the smooth muscle cells have been cut in cross section and display rounded nuclear profiles.

The submucosa consists of connective tissue of moderate density. Present in the submucosa are adipocytes *(A),* blood vessels *(BV),* and a group of ganglion cells *(GC).* These particular cells belong to the submucosal plexus (Meissner's plexus *[MP]*). The **inset** shows some of the ganglion cells *(GC)* at higher magnification. These are the large cell bodies of the enteric neurons. Each cell body is surrounded by satellite cells intimately apposed to the neuron cell body. The *arrowheads* point to the nuclei of the satellite cells.

Figure 3, stomach, silver stain ×160.

Enteroendocrine cells constitute a class of cells that can be displayed with special histochemical or silver-staining methods but that are not readily evident in H&E sections. The distribution of cells demonstrable with special silver-staining procedures is shown here *(arrows).* Because of the staining procedure, these cells are properly designated as argentaffin cells. The surface mucous cells *(MSC)* in the section mark the bottom of the gastric pits and establish the fact that the necks of the fundic glands are represented in the section. The argentaffin cells appear black in this specimen. The relatively low magnification permits the viewer to assess the frequency of distribution of these cells.

Figure 4, stomach, silver stain ×640.

At higher magnification, the argentaffin cells *(arrows)* are almost totally blackened by the silver staining, although a faint nucleus can be seen in some cells. The silver stains the secretory product lost during the preparation of routine sections, and accordingly, in H&E–stained paraffin sections the argentaffin cell appears as a clear cell. The special silver staining in this figure and in Figure 3 shows that many of the argentaffin cells tend to be near the basal lamina and away from the lumen of the gland.

KEY

A, adipocytes
BV, blood vessels
CC, chief cells
GC, ganglion cells
ME, muscularis externa
MM, muscularis mucosae
MNC, mucous neck cells
MP, Meissner's plexus
MSC, surface mucous cells
N, neck of fundic glands
PC, parietal cells
SubM, submucosa
arrows, argentaffin cells
arrowheads, nuclei of satellite cells

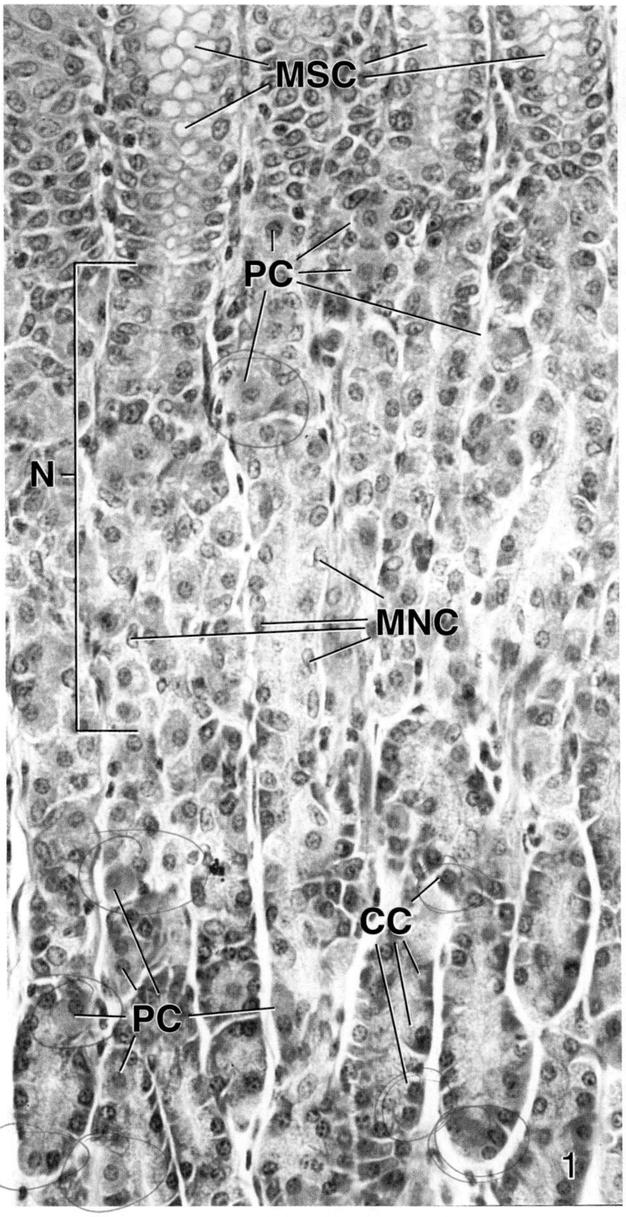
MSC
PC
N
MNC
CC
PC
1

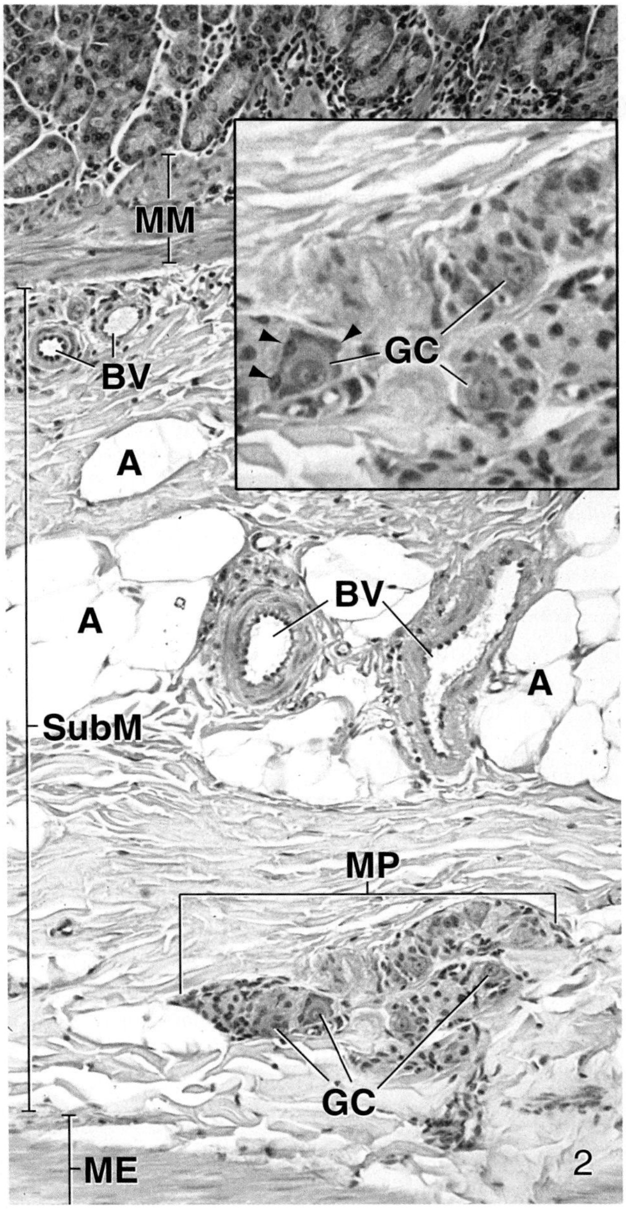
MM
BV
GC
A
BV
A
A
SubM
MP
GC
ME
2

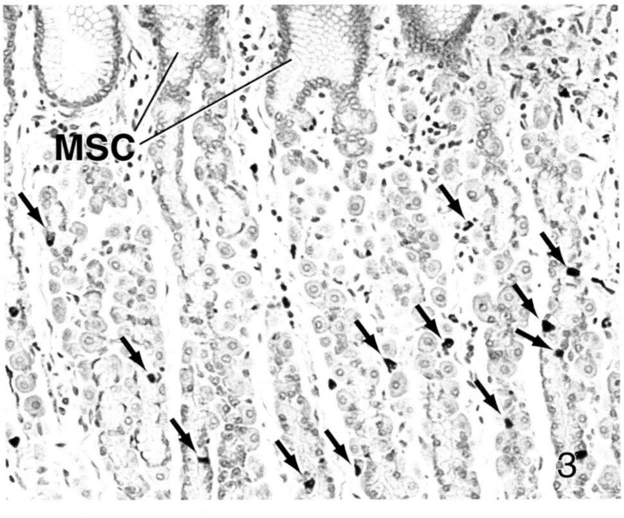
MSC
3

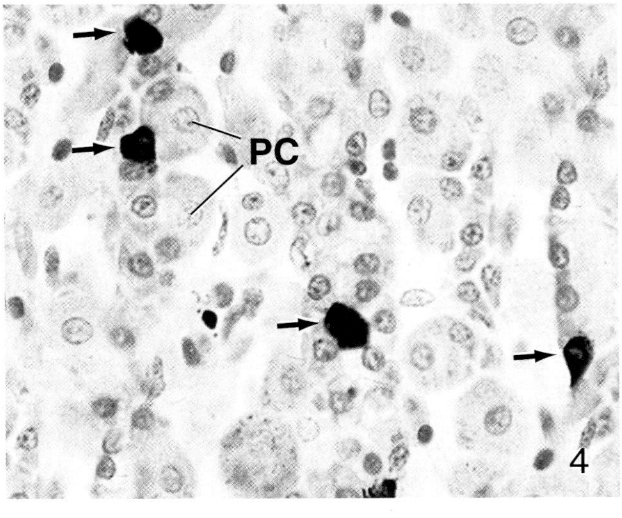
PC
4

PLATE 54. GASTRODUODENAL JUNCTION

The *gastroduodenal (pyloric) junction* marks the entry into the absorptive portion of the alimentary canal. Thickening of the circular layer of muscularis externa at this site forms the *gastroduodenal (pyloric) sphincter* that regulates passage of chyme from stomach to intestine. The mucous secretion of the pyloric glands helps to neutralize the chyme as it enters the intestine.

Figure 1, stomach-duodenum, monkey, H&E ×40.

The junction between the stomach and the duodenum is shown here. Most of the mucosa in the micrograph belongs to the stomach; it is the pyloric mucosa *(PMuc)*. The pyloric sphincter appears as a thickened region of smooth muscle below the pyloric mucosa. On the far right is the duodenal mucosa, the first part of the intestinal mucosa *(IMuc)*. The area marked by the *rectangle* is shown at higher magnification in Figure 2. It provides a comparison of the two mucosal regions and also shows the submucosal glands (Brunner's glands).

The submucosa of the duodenum contains submucosal (Brunner's) glands. These are below the muscularis mucosae; therefore, this structure serves as a useful landmark in identifying the glands. In the stomach, the muscularis mucosae is readily identified as narrow bands of muscular tissue *(MM)*. It can be followed toward the right into the duodenum but is then interrupted in the region between the two *asterisks*.

This figure also shows the thickened region of the gastric muscularis externa, where the stomach ends. This is the pyloric sphincter *(PS)*. Its thickness, mostly due to the amplification of the circular layer of smooth muscle of the muscularis externa, can be appreciated by comparison with the muscularis externa in the duodenum *(ME)*.

Figure 2, stomach-duodenum, monkey ×120.

Examination of this region at higher magnification reveals that in addition to intestinal glands *(IGl)* within the mucosa, there are glands within the duodenal submucosa. These are submucosal (Brunner's) glands *(BGl)*. Some of the glandular elements *(arrows)* can be seen to pass from the submucosa to the mucosa, thereby interrupting the muscularis mucosae *(MM)*. The submucosal glands empty their secretions into the duodenal lumen by means of ducts *(D)*. In contrast, the pyloric glands *(PGl)* are relatively straight for most of their length but are coiled in the deepest part of the mucosa and are sometimes branched. They are restricted to the mucosa and empty into deep gastric pits. The boundary between the pits and glands is, however, hard to ascertain in H&E sections.

With respect to the mucosal aspects of gastroduodenal histology, as mentioned above, the glands of the stomach empty into gastric pits. These are depressions; accordingly, when the pits are sectioned in a plane that is oblique or at right angles to the long axis of the pit, as in this figure, the pits can be recognized as being depressions because they are surrounded by lamina propria. In contrast, the inner surface of the small intestine has villi *(V)*. These are projections into the lumen of slightly varying height. When the villus is cross-sectioned or obliquely sectioned, it is surrounded by space of the lumen, as is one of the villi shown here. In addition, the villi have lamina propria *(LP)* in their core.

Figure 3, stomach-duodenum, monkey ×640.

The *rectangular area* in Figure 2 is considered at higher magnification here. It shows how the epithelium of the stomach differs from that of the intestine. In both cases, the epithelium is simple columnar, and the underlying lamina propria *(LP)* is highly cellular because of the presence of large numbers of lymphocytes. The boundary between gastric and duodenal epithelium is marked by the *arrow*. On the stomach side of the *arrow*, the epithelium consists of surface mucous cells *(MSC)*. The surface cells contain an apical cup of mucous material that typically appears empty in a H&E–stained paraffin section. In contrast, the absorptive cells *(AC)* of the intestine do not possess mucus in their cytoplasm. Although goblet cells are found in the intestinal epithelium and are scattered among the absorptive cells, they do not form a complete mucous sheet. The intestinal absorptive cells also possess a striated border, which is shown in Plate 56.

KEY

AC, absorptive cells
BGl, Brunner's glands
D, ducts
IGl, intestinal glands
IMuc, intestinal mucosa
LP, lamina propria
ME, muscularis externa
MM, muscularis mucosae
MSC, surface mucous cells
PGl, pyloric glands
PMuc, pyloric mucosa
PS, pyloric sphincter
V, villi
arrows: Fig. 2, Brunner's gland element that passes from the submucosa to the mucosa; Fig. 3, boundary between gastric and duodenal epithelium
asterisks, interruption in muscularis mucosae

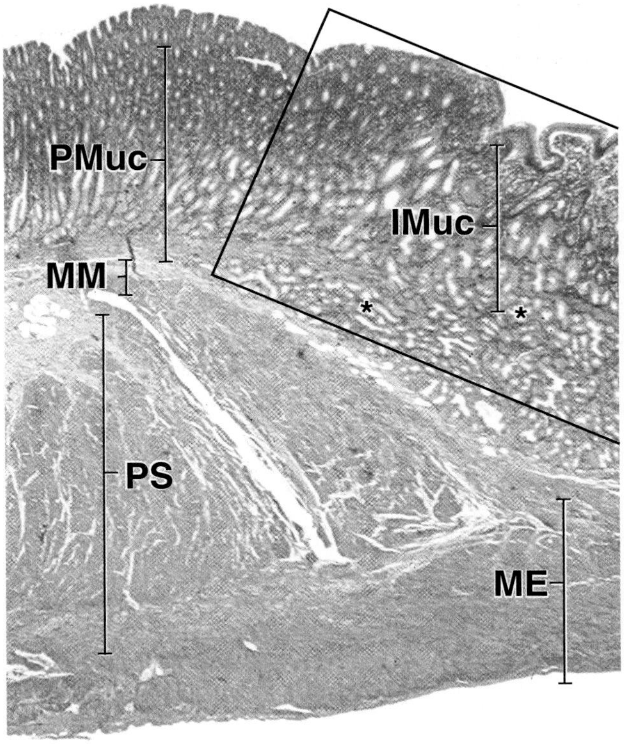

1

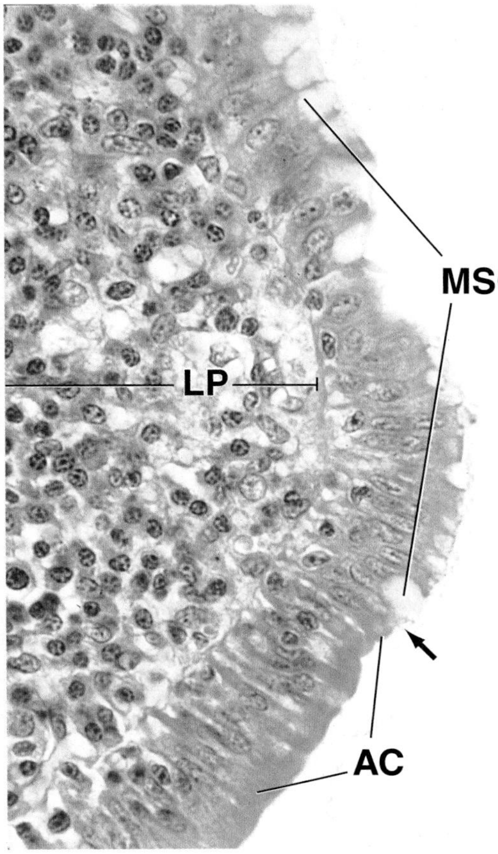

3

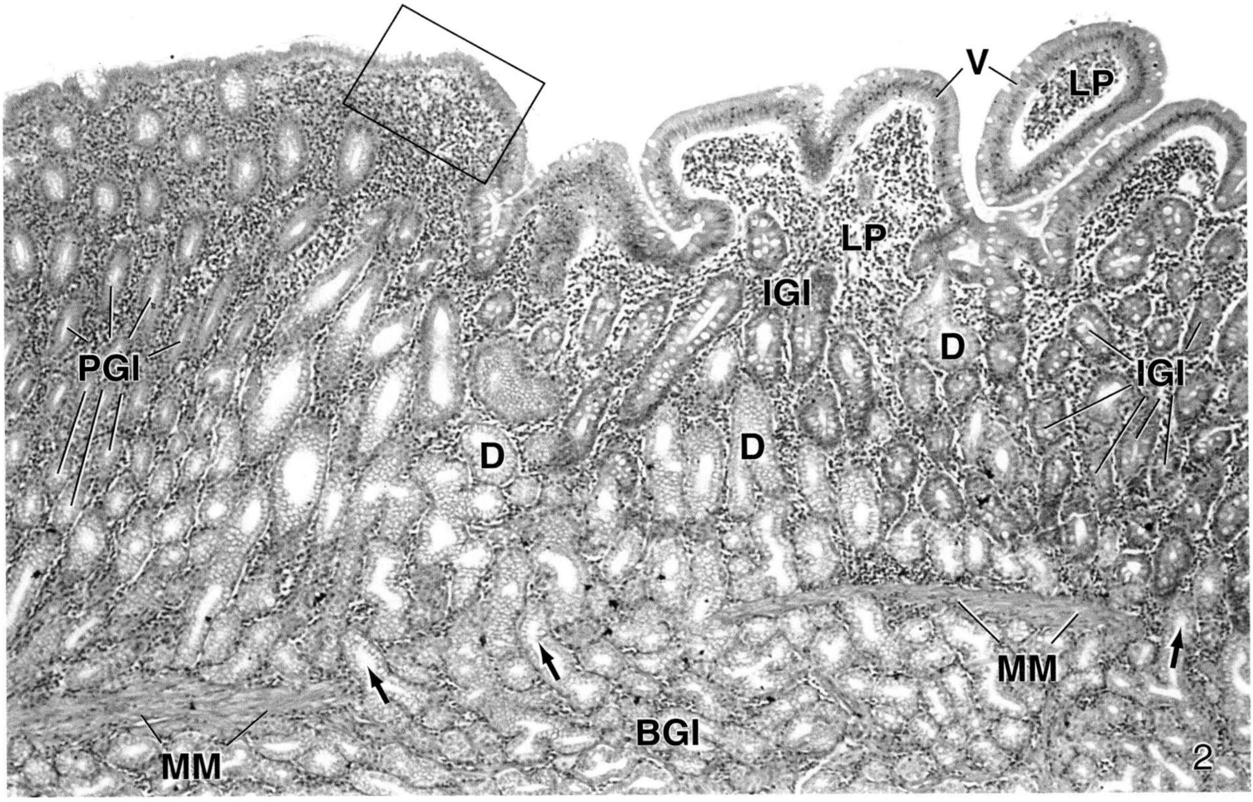

PLATE 55. DUODENUM

The small intestine is the principal site for the digestion of food and absorption of the products of digestion. It is the longest component of the alimentary canal, measuring over 6 m, and is divided into three segments: *duodenum* (~25 cm); *jejunum* (~2.5 m); and *ileum* (~3.5 m). The first portion, the duodenum, receives a partially digested bolus of food (chyme) from the stomach, as well as secretions from the stomach, pancreas, liver, and gallbladder that contain digestive enzymes, enzyme precursors, and other products that aid digestion and absorption.

The small intestine is characterized by *plicae circulares,* permanent transverse folds that contain a core of submucosa, and *villi,* finger-like and leaf-like projections of the mucosa that extend into the lumen. *Microvilli,* multiple finger-like extensions of the apical surface of each intestinal epithelial cell (enterocyte), further increase the surface for absorption of metabolites.

Mucosal glands extend into the lamina propria. They contain the stem cells and developing cells that will ultimately migrate to the surface of the villi. In the duodenum, submucosal glands (Brunner's glands) secrete an alkaline mucus that helps to neutralize the acidic chyme. Enterocytes not only absorb metabolites digested in the intestinal lumen but also synthesize enzymes inserted into the membrane of the microvilli for terminal digestion of disaccharides and dipeptides.

Figure 1, duodenum, monkey, H&E ×120.

This figure shows a segment of the duodenal wall. As in the stomach, the layers of the wall, in order from the lumen, are the mucosa *(Muc),* the submucosa *(SubM),* the muscularis externa *(ME),* and the serosa *(S).* Both longitudinal *(L)* and circular *(C)* layers of the muscularis externa can be distinguished. Although plicae circulares are found in the wall of the small intestine, including the duodenum, none is included in this photomicrograph.

A distinctive feature of the intestinal mucosa is the presence of finger-like and leaf-like projections into the intestinal lumen, called villi. Most of the villi *(V)* shown here display profiles that correspond to their description as finger-like. One villus, however, displays the form of a leaf-like villus *(asterisk).* The *dashed line* marks the boundary between the villi and the intestinal glands (also called crypts of Lieberkühn). The latter extend as far as the muscularis mucosae *(MM).*

Under the mucosa is the submucosa, containing the Brunner's glands *(BGl).* These are branched tubular or branched tubuloalveolar glands whose secretory components, shown at higher magnification in Figure 2, consist of columnar epithelium. A duct *(D)* through which the glands open into the lumen of the duodenum is shown here and, at higher magnification, in Figure 2, where it is marked by an *arrow.*

Figure 2, duodenum, monkey, H&E ×240.

The histologic features of the duodenal mucosa are shown at higher magnification here. Two kinds of cells can be recognized in the epithelial layer that forms the surface of the villus: enterocytes (absorptive cells) and goblet cells *(GC).* Most of the cells are absorptive cells. They have a striated border that will be seen at higher magnification in Plate 56; their elongate nuclei are located in the basal half of the cell. Goblet cells are readily identified by the presence of the apical mucous cup, which appears empty. Most of the dark round nuclei also seen in the epithelial layer covering the villi belong to lymphocytes.

The lamina propria *(LP)* makes up the core of the villus. It contains large numbers of round cells whose individual identity cannot be ascertained at this magnification. Note, however, that these are mostly lymphocytes (and other cells of the immune system), which accounts for the designation of the lamina propria as diffuse lymphatic tissue. The lamina propria surrounding the intestinal glands *(IGl)* similarly consists largely of lymphocytes and related cells. The lamina propria also contains components of loose connective tissue and isolated smooth muscle cells.

The intestinal glands *(IGl)* are relatively straight and tend to be dilated at their base. The bases of the intestinal crypts contain the stem cells from which all of the other cells of the intestinal epithelium arise. They also contain Paneth cells. These cells possess eosinophilic granules in their apical cytoplasm. The granules contain lysozyme, a bacteriolytic enzyme thought to play a role in regulating intestinal microbial flora. The main cell type in the intestinal crypt is a relatively undifferentiated columnar cell. These cells are shorter than the enterocytes of the villus surface; they usually undergo two mitoses before they differentiate into absorptive cells or goblet cells. Also present in the intestinal crypts are some mature goblet cells and enteroendocrine cells.

KEY

BGl, Brunner's glands
C, circular (inner) layer of muscularis externa
D, duct of Brunner's gland
GC, goblet cells
IGl, intestinal glands (crypts)
L, longitudinal (outer) layer of muscularis externa
LP, lamina propria
ME, muscularis externa
MM, muscularis mucosae
Muc, mucosa
S, serosa
SubM, submucosa
V, villi
arrow, duct of Brunner's gland
asterisk, leaf-like villus
dashed line (Fig. 1), boundary between base of villi and intestinal glands

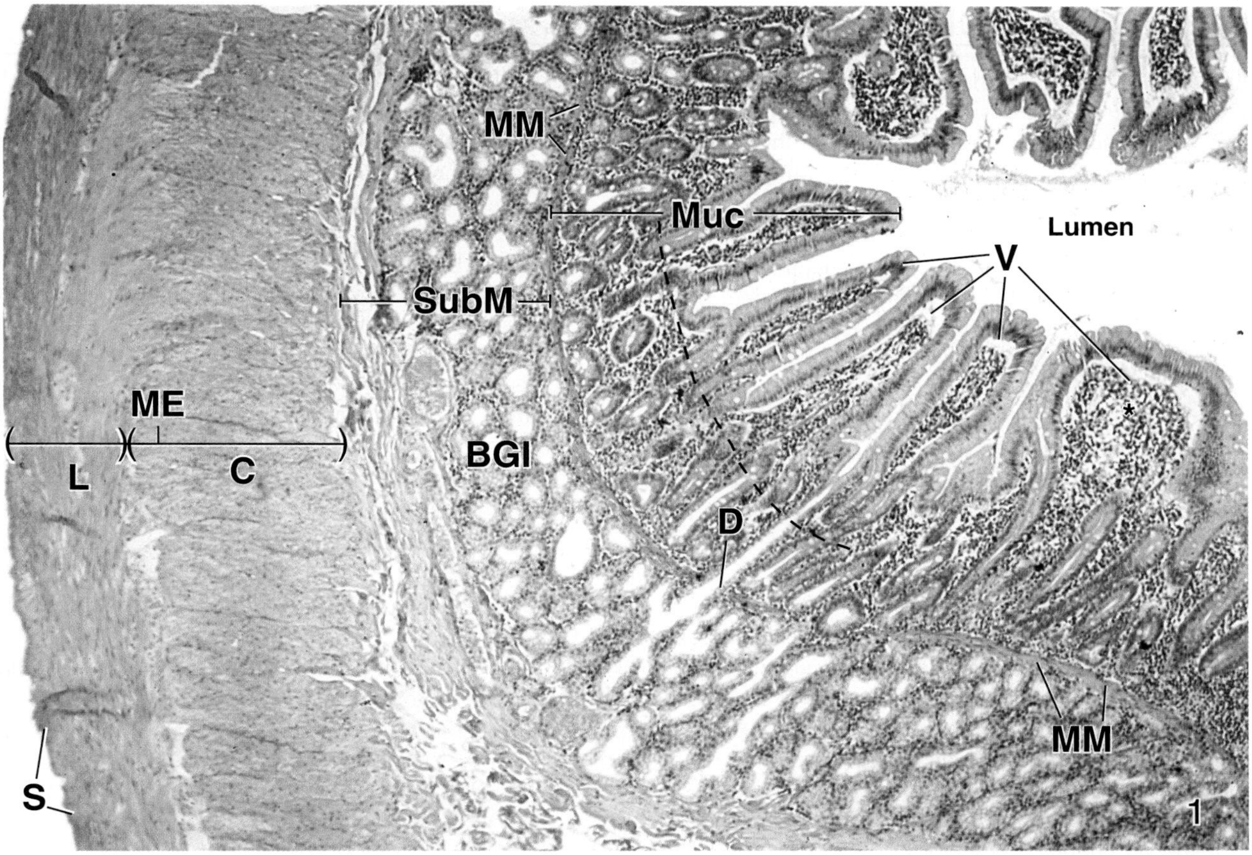
MM
Muc
Lumen
V
SubM
ME
L
C
BGI
D
MM
S
1

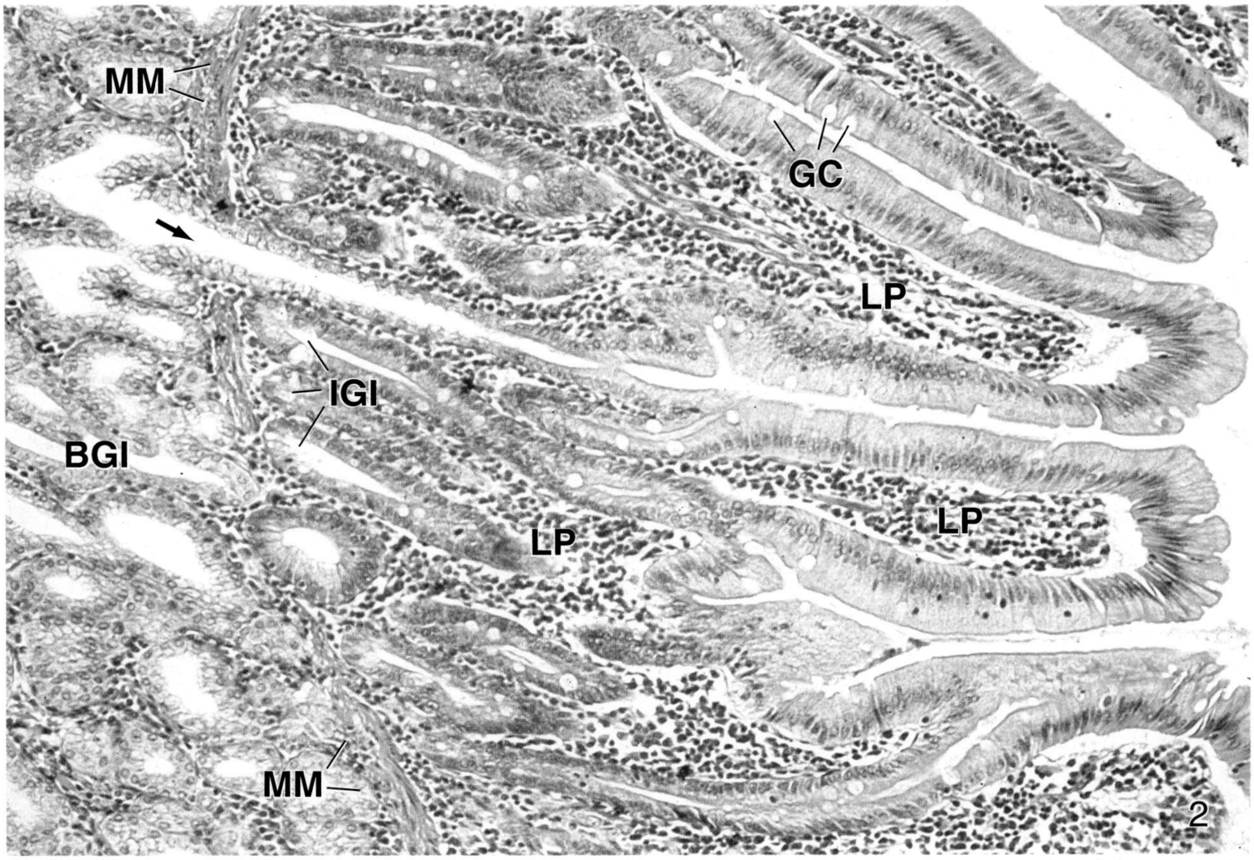
MM
GC
LP
IGI
BGI
LP
LP
MM
2

PLATE 56. JEJUNUM

The jejunum is the principal site of absorption of *nutrients* in the small intestine. The villi are more finger-like than leaf-like and are covered largely with absorptive columnar epithelial cells (enterocytes), although *goblet cells* and *enteroendocrine cells* are also present. The stem cells for all of these cells and the *Paneth cells* that secrete the antibacterial enzyme *lysozyme* are found deep in the intestinal gland. Replicating cells line the lower half of the gland.

Figure 1, jejunum, monkey, H&E ×22.

This is a longitudinal section of the jejunum, showing the permanent circular folds of the small intestine, the plicae circulares *(PC)*. These folds or ridges are mostly arranged with their long axis at roughly right angles to the longitudinal axis of the intestine; therefore, the plicae circulares shown here are cut in cross section. The plicae circulares consist of mucosa *(Muc)* as well as submucosa *(SubM)*. The broad band of tissue external to the submucosa is the muscularis externa *(ME)* and is not included in the plicae. (The serosa cannot be distinguished at this magnification.) Most of the villi *(V)* in this specimen have been cut longitudinally, thereby revealing their full length as well as the fact that some are slightly shorter than others. The shortening is considered to be due to the contraction of smooth muscle cells in the villi. Also seen here are the lacteals *(L)*, which in most of the villi are dilated. Lacteals are lymphatic capillaries that begin in the villi and carry certain absorbed dietary lipids and proteins from the villi to the larger lymphatic vessels of the submucosa.

Figure 2, jejunum, monkey, H&E ×60.

Part of the plica marked by the *bracket* in Figure 1 is shown at higher magnification. Note the muscularis mucosae *(MM)*, the intestinal glands *(Gl)*, and the villi *(V)*. The boundary between the glands and villi is marked by the *dashed line*. Some of the glands are cut longitudinally; some are cut in cross section; most of the villi have been cut longitudinally. In conceptualizing the mucosal structure of the small intestine, it is important to recognize that the glands are epithelial depressions that project into the wall of the intestine, whereas the villi are projections that extend into the lumen. The glands are surrounded by cells of the lamina propria; the villi are surrounded by space of the intestinal lumen. The lamina propria with its lacteal occupies a central position in the villus; the lumen occupies the central position of the gland. Also note that the lumen of the gland tends to be dilated at its base. Studies of enzymatically isolated preparations of mucosa show that the bases of the glands are often divided into two to three finger-like extensions resting on the muscularis mucosae.

Figure 3, jejunum, monkey, H&E ×500.

This figure shows portions of two adjacent villi at higher magnification. The epithelium consists chiefly of enterocytes. These are columnar absorptive cells that typically exhibit a striated border *(SB)*, the light microscopic representation of the microvilli on the apical surface of each enterocyte. The dark band at the base of the striated border is due to the terminal web of the cell, a layer of actin filaments that extends across the apex of the cell to which the actin filaments of the cores of the microvilli attach. The nuclei of the enterocytes have essentially the same shape, orientation, and staining characteristics. Even if the cytoplasmic boundaries were not evident, the nuclei would be an indication of the columnar shape and orientation of the cells. The enterocytes rest on a basal lamina not evident in H&E–stained paraffin sections. The eosinophilic band *(arrow)* at the base of the cell layer, where one would expect a basement membrane, actually consists of flat lateral cytoplasmic processes from the enterocytes. These processes partially delimit the basal-lateral intercellular spaces *(asterisks)* that are dilated, as can be seen here, during active transport of absorbed substrates.

The epithelial cells with an expanded apical cytoplasm in the form of a cup are goblet cells *(GC)*. In this specimen, the nucleus of almost every goblet cell is just at the base of the cup, and a thin cytoplasmic strand (not always evident) extends to the level of the basement membrane. The scattered round nuclei within the epithelium belong to lymphocytes *(Ly)*.

The lamina propria *(LP)* and the lacteal *(L)* are located beneath the intestinal epithelium. The cells forming the lacteal are simple squamous epithelium (endothelium). Two nuclei of these cells *(EC)* appear to be exposed to the lumen of the lacteal; another elongate nucleus slightly removed from the lumen belongs to a smooth muscle cell *(M)* accompanying the lacteals.

KEY

EC, endothelial cell
GC, goblet cell
Gl, intestinal glands (crypts)
L, lacteal
LP, lamina propria
Ly, lymphocytes
M, smooth muscle cell
ME, muscularis externa
MM, muscularis mucosae
Muc, mucosa
PC, plicae circulares
S, serosa
SB, striated border
SubM, submucosa
V, villi
arrow, basal processes of enterocytes
asterisks, basal-lateral intercellular spaces
dashed line, boundary between villi and intestinal glands

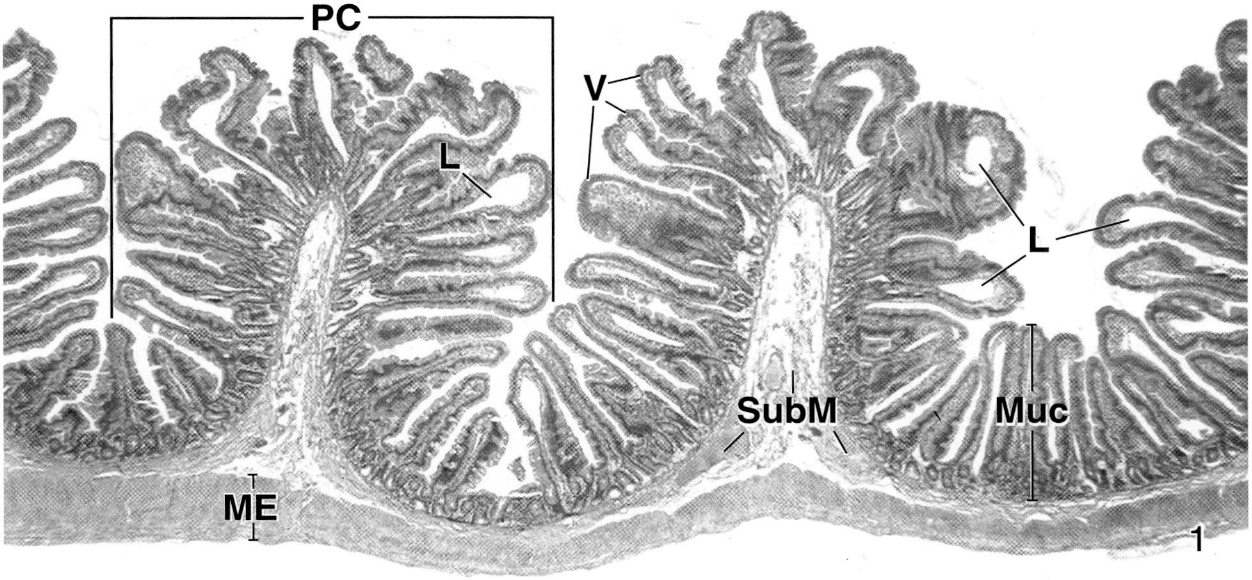
PC
V
L
L
SubM
Muc
ME
1

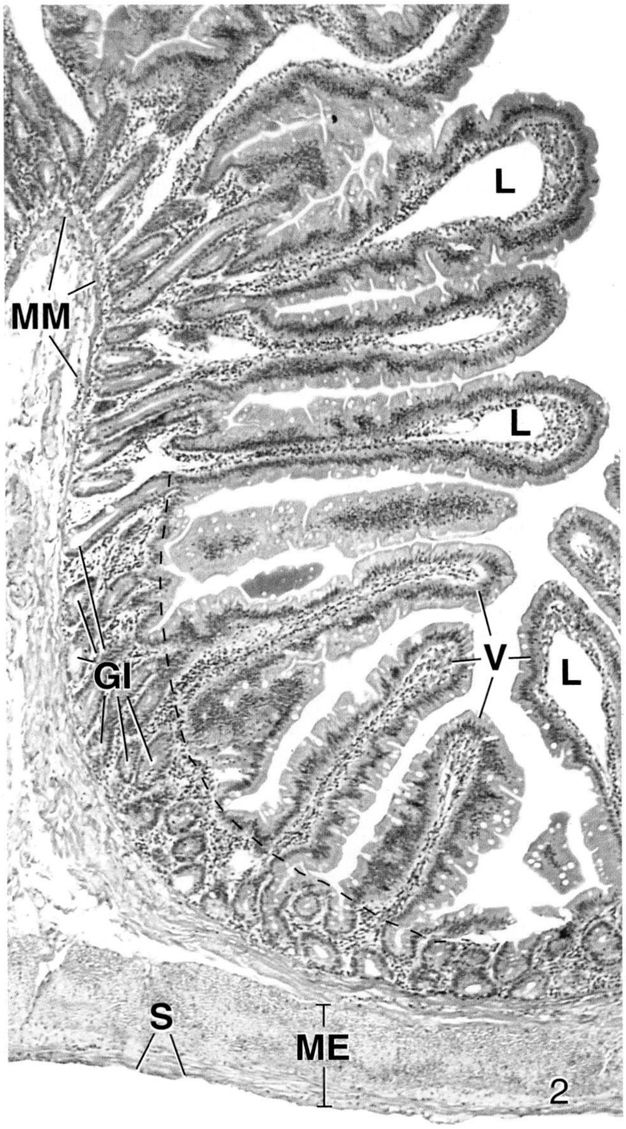
L
MM
L
GI
V
L
S
ME
2

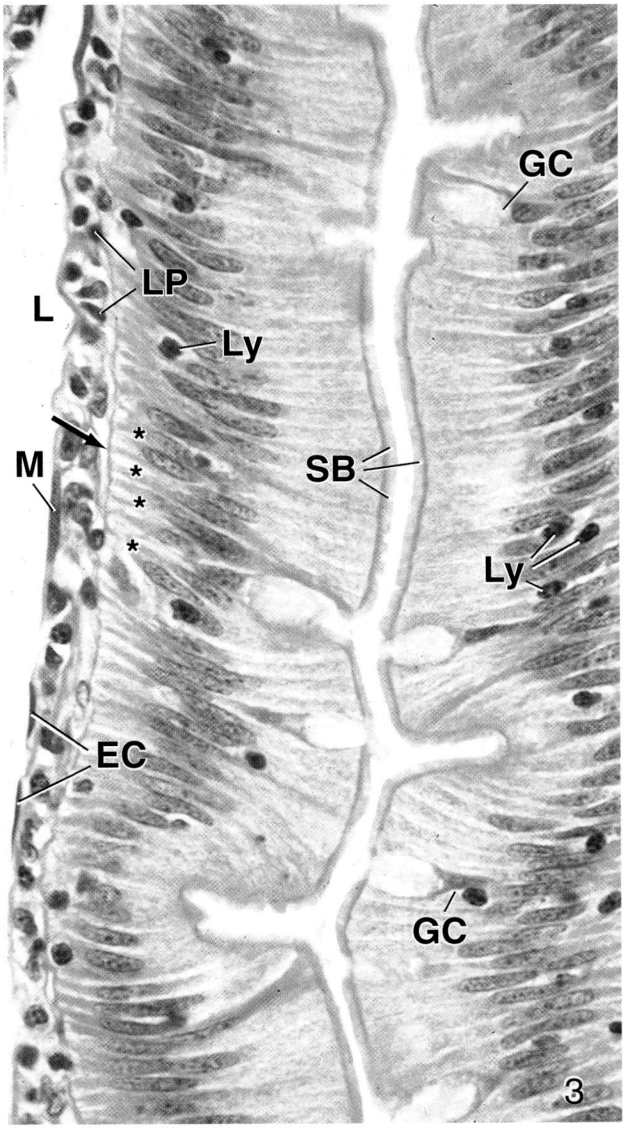
GC
LP
L
Ly
M
SB
Ly
EC
GC
3

PLATE 57. ILEUM

The ileum is the principal site of water and electrolyte reabsorption in the small intestine. It has essentially the same histologic features as the jejunum. Some, however, are emphasized; namely, villi in the ileum are more frequently leaf-like, and lymphatic tissue in the lamina propria is organized into small and large nodes that are found in great number on the antimesenteric side of the ileum. The nodes fuse to form large accumulations of lymphatic tissue called Peyer's patches.

The surface epithelium of the small intestine renews itself every 5 to 6 days. The stem cells are restricted to the bottoms of the mucosal glands, and the zone of cell replication is restricted to the lower half of the gland. The cells migrate onto the villus and are lost from its tip. All of the epithelial cells, absorptive cells, and goblet cells, as well as enteroendocrine cells and Paneth cells, derive from the same stem cell population, but enteroendocrine cells migrate only slowly, and Paneth cells do not migrate.

Figure 1, ileum, monkey, H&E ×20.

For purposes of orientation, the submucosa *(SM)* and muscularis externa *(ME)* have been marked in the cross section through the ileum shown here. Just internal to the submucosa is the mucosa; external to the muscularis externa is the serosa. The mucosa reveals several longitudinally sectioned villi *(V),* which have been labeled, and other unlabeled villi, which can be identified easily on the basis of their appearance as islands of tissue completely surrounded by the space of the lumen. They are, of course, not islands because this appearance is due to the plane of section that slices completely through some of the villi obliquely or in cross section, thereby isolating them from their base. Below the villi are the intestinal glands, many of which are obliquely or transversely sectioned and can be readily identified, as was done in the preceding plates, because they are totally surrounded by lamina propria.

There are about 8 to 10 projections of tissue into the intestinal lumen that are substantially larger than the villi. These are the plicae circulares. As noted above, plicae generally have circular orientation, but they may travel in a longitudinal direction for short distances and may branch. In addition, even if all the plicae are arranged in a circular manner, if the section is somewhat oblique, the plicae will be cut at an angle, as appears to be the case with several plicae in this figure. One of the distinctive features of the small intestine is the presence of single and aggregated lymph nodules in the intestinal wall. Isolated nodules of lymphatic tissue are common in the proximal end of the intestinal canal. As one proceeds distally through the intestines, however, the lymph nodules occur in increasingly larger numbers. In the ileum, large aggregates of lymph nodules are regularly seen; they are referred to as Peyer's patches. Several lymphatic nodules *(LN)* forming a Peyer's patch are shown in this figure. The nodules are partly within the mucosa of the ileum and extend into the submucosa. Although not evident in the figure, the nodules are characteristically located opposite where the mesentery connects to the intestinal tube.

Figure 2, ileum, monkey, H&E ×40.

Sometimes, in a cross section through the intestine, a plica displays a clear cross-sectional profile such as that shown here. Note, again, that the submucosa *(SM)* constitutes the core of the plica. Although many of the villi in this figure present profiles *(V)* that would be expected if the villus were a finger-like projection, others clearly do not. In particular, one villus (marked with three *asterisks*) shows the broad profile of a longitudinally sectioned leaf-like villus. If this same villus were cut at a right angle to the plane shown here, it would appear as a finger-like villus.

Figure 3, ileum, monkey, H&E ×100; inset ×200.

Part of a lymphatic nodule and part of the overlying epithelium are shown here at higher magnification. The lymphocytes and related cells are so numerous that they virtually obscure the cells of the muscularis mucosae. Their location, however, can be estimated as being near the presumptive label *(MM??),* inasmuch as the muscularis mucosae is ordinarily adjacent to the base of the intestinal glands *(Gl).* Moreover, on examination of this area at higher magnification **(inset),** groups of smooth muscle cells *(MM)* can be seen separated by numerous lymphocytes close to the intestinal glands *(Gl).* Clearly, the lymphocytes of the nodule are on both sides of the muscularis mucosae and, thus, within both the mucosa and the submucosa.

In places, the lymph nodule is covered by the intestinal epithelium. Whereas the nature of the epithelium cannot be appreciated fully in the light microscope, electron micrographs (both scanning and transmission) have shown that among the epithelial cells are special cells, designated M cells, that sample the intestinal content (for antigen) and present this antigen to the lymphocytes in the epithelial layer.

KEY

Gl, intestinal glands
LN, lymphatic nodules
ME, muscularis externa
MM, muscularis mucosae
MM??, presumptive location of muscularis mucosae
SM, submucosa
V, villi
asterisks, leaf-like villus

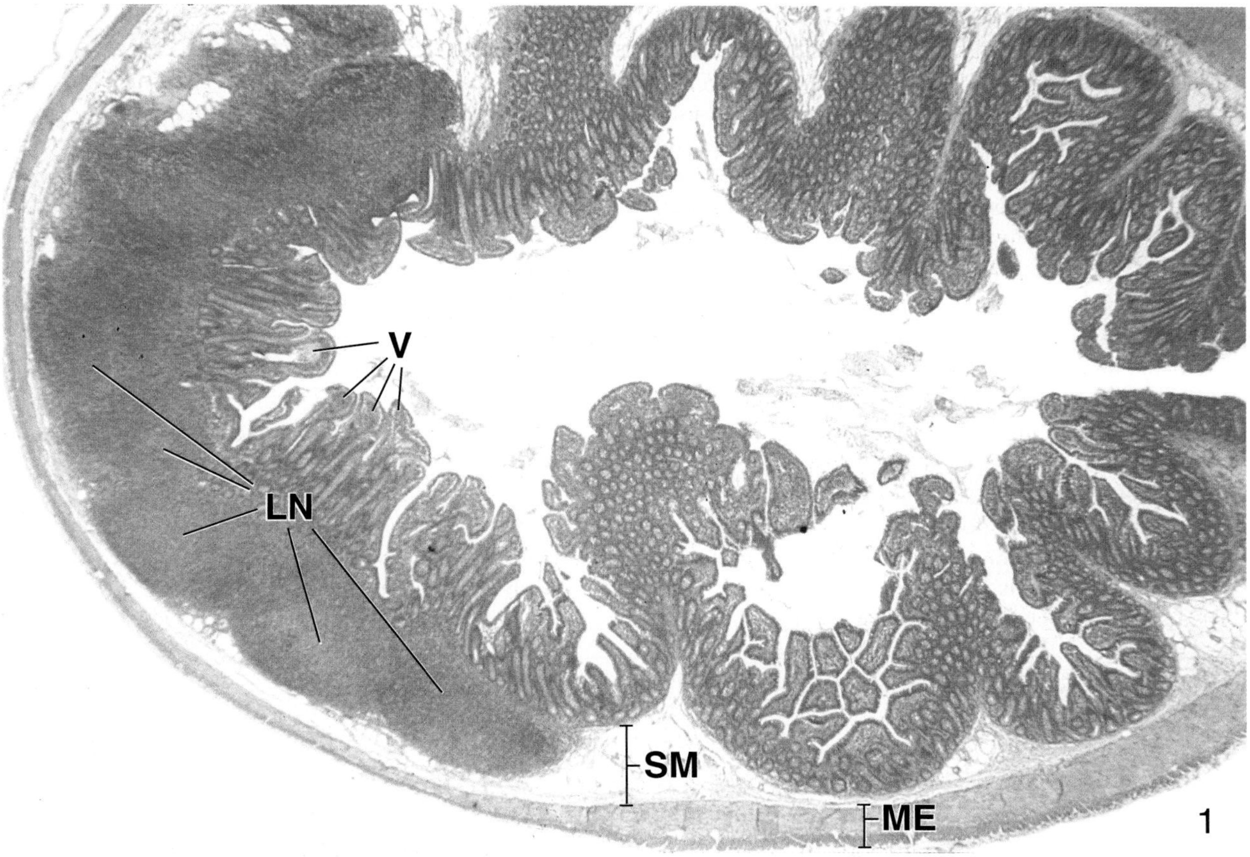
V
LN
SM
ME
1

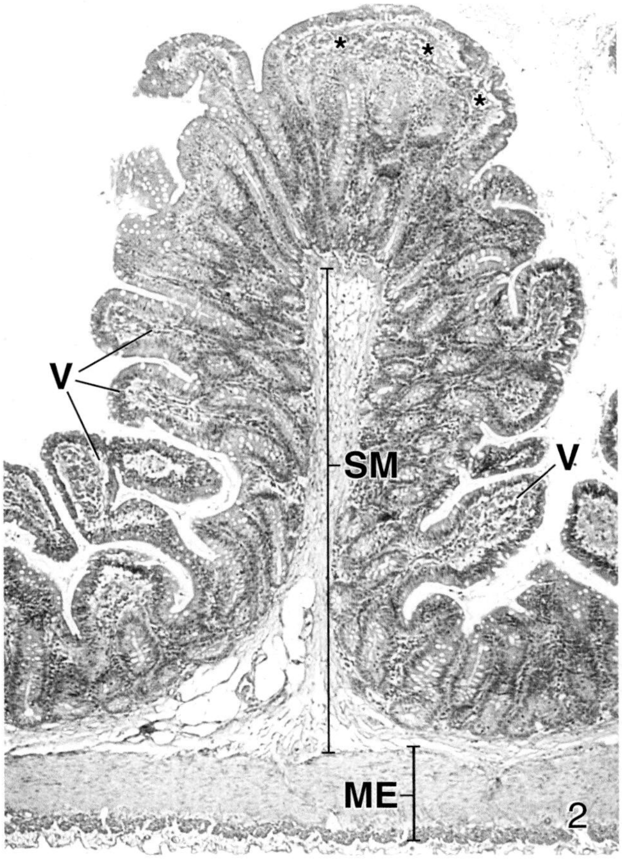
*
*
*
V
SM
V
ME
2

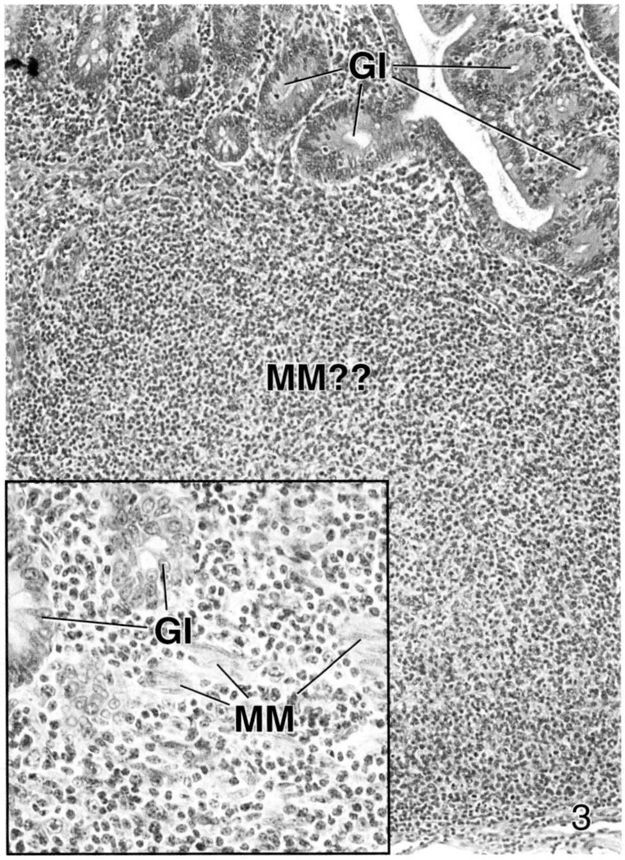
GI
MM??
GI
MM
3

PLATE 58. COLON

The principal functions of the colon are reabsorption of electrolytes and water and elimination of undigested food and other waste. The mucosa has a smooth surface; neither plicae circulares nor villi are present. Numerous simple glands (crypts of Lieberkühn) extend through the full thickness of the mucosa. The glands, as well as the surface, are lined with a simple columnar epithelium that contains goblet cells, absorptive cells, and enteroendocrine cells but does not normally contain Paneth cells. Here, too, stem cells are restricted to the bottoms of the glands (crypts), and the normal zone of replication extends about one third of the height of the crypt.

Figure 1, colon, monkey, H&E ×30.
A cross section through the large intestine is shown at low magnification. It shows the four layers that make up the wall of the colon: the mucosa *(Muc),* the submucosa *(SubM),* the muscularis externa *(ME),* and the serosa *(S).* Although these layers are the same as those in the small intestine, several differences should be noted. The large intestine has no villi, nor does it have plicae circulares. On the other hand, the muscularis externa is arranged in a distinctive manner, and this is evident in the photomicrograph. The longitudinal layer *(ME[l])* is substantially thinner than the circular layer *(ME[c])* except in three locations where the longitudinal layer of smooth muscle is present as a thick band. One of these thick bands, called a tenia coli *(TC),* is shown in this figure. Because the colon is cross-sectioned, the tenia coli is also cross-sectioned. The three teniae coli extend along the length of the large intestine as far as, but not into, the rectum.

The submucosa consists of a rather dense irregular connective tissue. It contains the larger blood vessels *(BV)* and areas of adipose tissue (see *A,* Fig. 2).

Figure 2, colon, monkey, H&E ×140.
The mucosa, shown at higher magnification, contains straight, unbranched, tubular glands (crypts of Lieberkühn) that extend to the muscularis mucosae *(MM).* The *arrows* identify the openings of some of the glands at the intestinal surface. Generally, the lumen of the glands is narrow except in the deepest part of the gland, where it is often slightly dilated (*asterisks,* Fig. 3). Between the glands *(Gl)* is a lamina propria *(LP)* that contains considerable numbers of lymphocytes and other cells of the immune system. Two *rectangles* mark areas of the mucosa that are examined at higher magnification in Figures 3 and 4.

Figure 3, colon, monkey, H&E ×525.
This figure reveals the muscularis mucosae *(MM)* and the cells in the lamina propria *(LP),* many of which can be recognized as lymphocytes and plasma cells. The smooth muscle cells of the muscularis mucosae are arranged in two layers. Note that the smooth muscle cells marked by the *arrowheads* show rounded nuclei; however, other smooth muscle cells appear as more or less rounded eosinophilic areas. These smooth muscle cells have been cut in cross section. Just above these cross-sectioned smooth muscle cells are others that have been cut longitudinally; they display elongate nuclei and elongate strands of eosinophilic cytoplasm.

Figure 4, colon, monkey, H&E ×525.
The cells that line the surface of the colon and the glands are principally absorptive cells *(AC)* and goblet cells *(GC).* The absorptive cells have a thin striated border that is evident where the *arrows* show the opening of the glands. Interspersed among the absorptive cells are the goblet cells *(GC).* As the absorptive cells are followed into the glands, they become fewer, whereas the goblet cells increase in number. Other cells in the gland are enteroendocrine cells, not easily identified in routine H&E–stained paraffin sections, and, in the deep part of the gland, undifferentiated cells of the replicative zone, derived from the stem cells in the base of the crypt. The undifferentiated cells are readily identified if they are undergoing division, by virtue of the mitotic figures *(M)* they display (see Fig. 3).

KEY

A, adipose tissue
AC, absorptive cells
BV, blood vessels
GC, goblet cells
Gl, intestinal glands
LP, lamina propria
M, mitotic figures
ME, muscularis externa
ME(c), circular layer of muscularis externa
ME(l), longitudinal layer of muscularis externa
MM, muscularis mucosae
Muc, mucosa
S, serosa
SubM, submucosa
TC, tenia coli
arrowheads, smooth muscle cells showing rounded nuclei
arrows, opening of intestinal glands
asterisks, lumen of intestinal glands

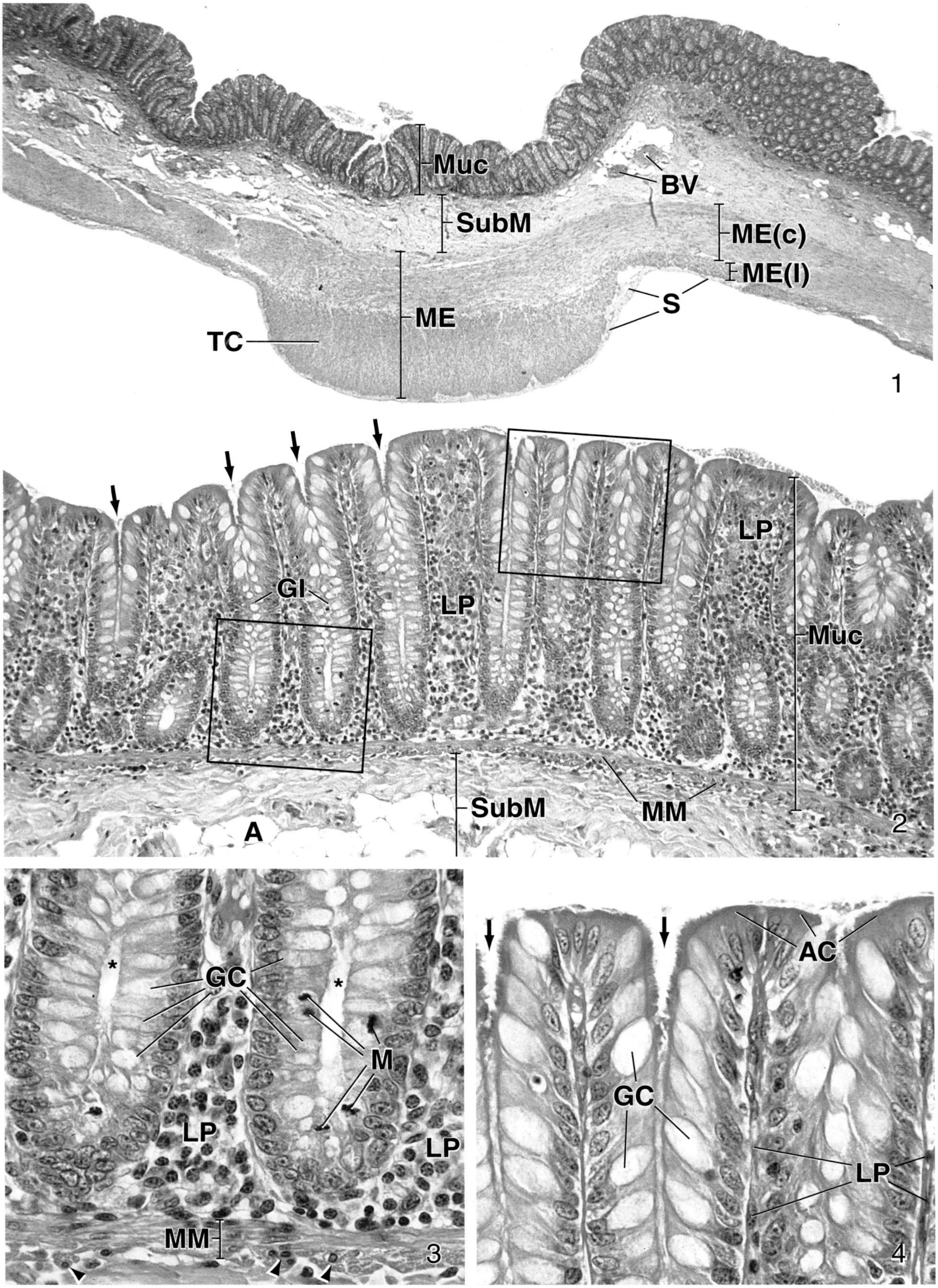
Muc
BV
SubM
ME(c)
ME(l)
S
ME
TC
1
LP
Gl
LP
Muc
SubM
MM
A
2
GC
M
LP
LP
MM
3
AC
GC
LP
4

PLATE 59. APPENDIX

The appendix (vermiform appendix) is typically described as a worm- or finger-like structure *[L. vermis, worm; forma, form]*. It arises from the cecum (the first segment of the large intestine; the others, in order, are the ascending, transverse, and descending colon; the sigmoid colon; the rectum; and the anal canal) and forms a blind-ending tube ranging from 2.5 cm to as much as 13 cm in length (average length of ~8 cm). Because it is a blind-ended pouch, intestinal contents may be trapped or sequestered in the appendix, often leading to inflammation and infection. In infants and children it is both relatively and absolutely longer than in adults and contains numerous lymphatic nodules, suggesting that it has an immunologic role. Recent evidence indicates that it (and the cecum and terminal ileum) may be the "bursa equivalent" in mammals, i.e., the portion of the immature immune system in which potential B lymphocytes achieve immunocompetence (equivalent to the *bursa of Fabricius* in birds).

The wall of the appendix is much like that of the small intestine, having a complete longitudinal layer of muscularis externa, but it lacks both plicae circulares and villi. Thus, the mucosa is similar to that of the colon, having simple glands. Even this resemblance is often obliterated, however, by the large number and size of the lymphatic nodules that usually fuse and extend into the submucosa. In later life, the amount of lymphatic tissue in the appendix regresses, and there is a consequent reduction in size. In many adults, the normal structure is lost, and the appendage is filled with fibrous scar tissue.

Figure 1, appendix, human, H&E ×25.
Cross section of an appendix from a preadolescent, showing the various structures composing its wall. The lumen *(L)*, mucosa *(Muc)*, submucosa *(Subm)*, muscularis externa *(ME)*, and serosa *(S)* are identified.

Figure 2, appendix, human, H&E ×80; inset ×200.
This micrograph is a higher magnification of the *boxed area* in Figure 1. It reveals the straight tubular glands *(Gl)* that extend to the muscularis mucosae. Below is the submucosa *(Subm)* in which the lymphatic nodules *(LN)* and considerable diffuse lymphatic tissue are present. Note the distinct germinal centers *(GC)* of the nodules and the cap region *(Cap)* that faces the lumen. The more superficial part of the submucosa blends and merges with the mucosal lamina propria because of the numerous lymphocytes in these two sites. The deeper part of the submucosa is relatively devoid of lymphocyte infiltration and contains the large blood vessels *(BV)* and nerves. The muscularis externa *(ME)* is composed of a relatively thick circular layer and a much thinner outer longitudinal layer. The serosa *(S)* is only partially included in this micrograph.

The **inset** is a higher magnification of the *rectangular area* in Figure 2. Note that the epithelium of the glands in the appendix is similar to that of the large intestine. Most of the epithelial cells contain mucin; hence, the light appearance of the apical cytoplasm. The lamina propria, as noted, is heavily infiltrated with lymphocytes, and the muscularis mucosae at the base of the glands is difficult to recognize *(arrows)*.

KEY

BV, blood vessel
Cap, cap of lymphatic nodule
GC, germinal center
Gl, gland
L, lumen
LN, lymphatic nodule
ME, muscularis externa
Muc, mucosa
S, serosa
Subm, submucosa
arrows, muscularis mucosae at base of glands

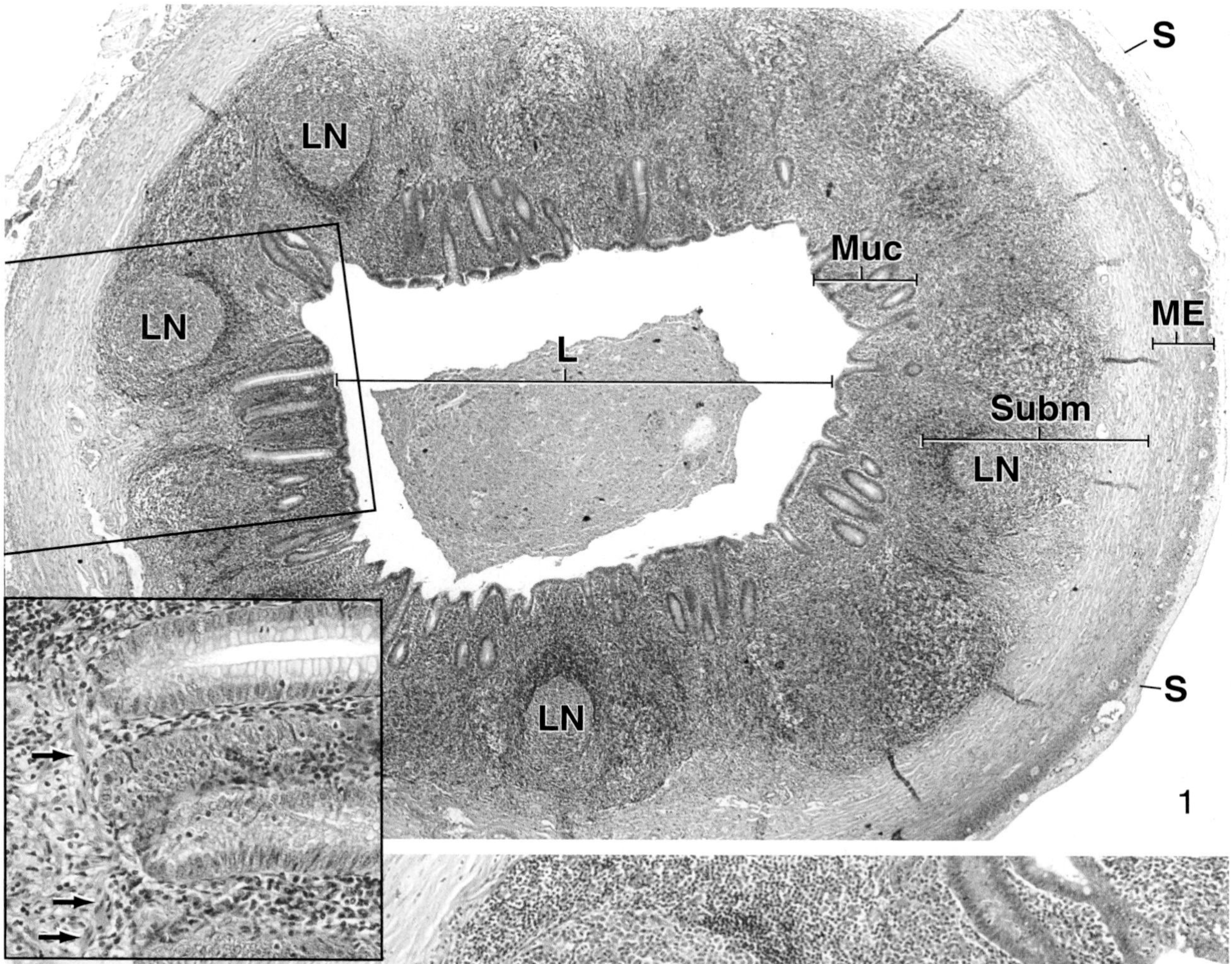
S
LN
LN
Muc
ME
L
Subm
LN
LN
S
1

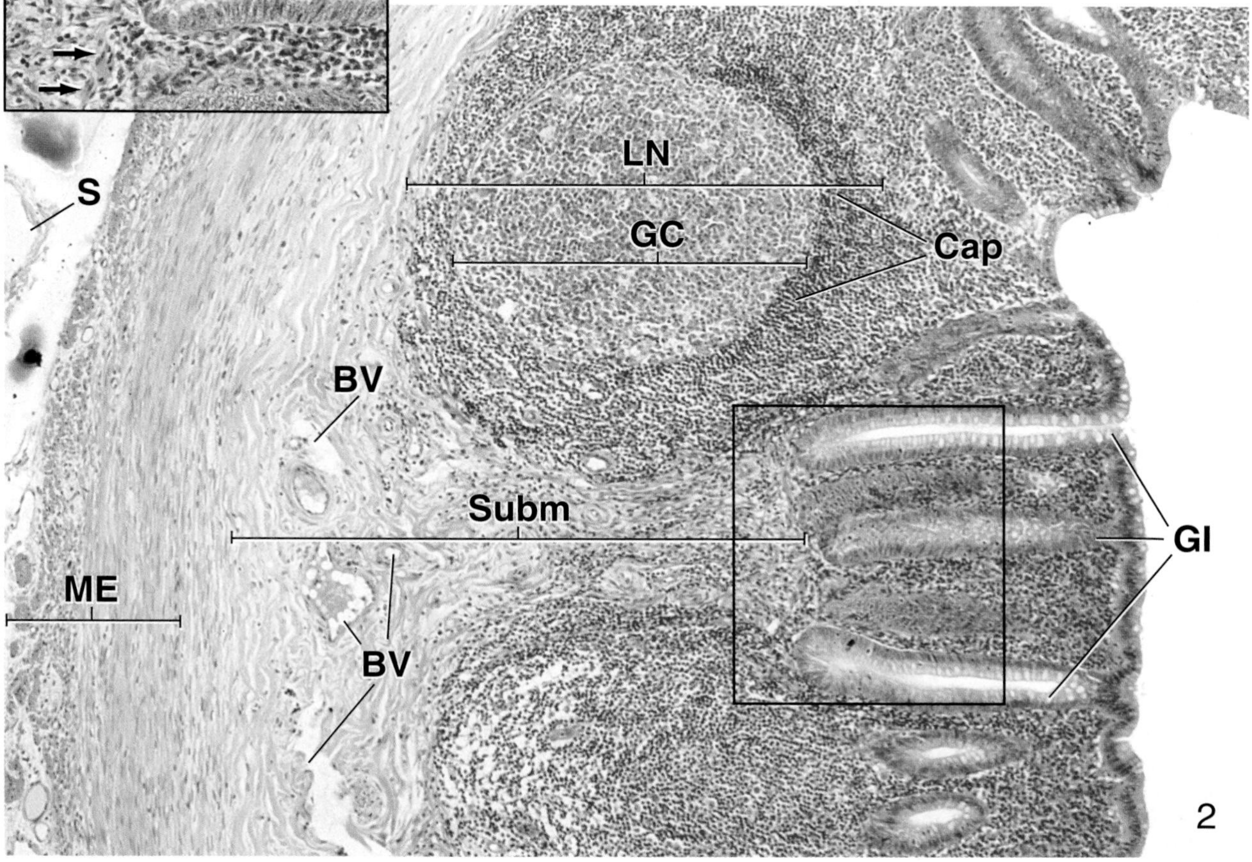
LN
GC
Cap
S
BV
Subm
GI
ME
BV
2

PLATE 60. ANORECTAL JUNCTION

At the anorectal junction, there is a transition from the simple columnar epithelium of the intestinal mucosa to the keratinized stratified squamous epithelium of the skin. Between these two distinctly different epithelia there is a narrow region where the epithelium is first stratified columnar (or stratified cuboidal) and then nonkeratinized stratified squamous.

At the level of the anorectal junction, the muscularis mucosae disappears. At the same level, the circular layer of the muscularis externa thickens to become the internal anal sphincter. The external anal sphincter is formed by the striated muscles of the perineum.

Figure 1, anorectal junction, H&E ×40.

A view of the anorectal junction is shown at low magnification. Mucosa characteristic of the large intestine is seen on the upper left of the micrograph. This region is the upper part of the anal canal, and the intestinal glands are the same as those present in the colon. The muscularis mucosae *(MM)* is readily identified as the narrow band of tissue under the glands. Both the intestinal glands and the muscularis mucosae terminate within the *left rectangular area* of the field, and here, at the *diamond,* there is the first major change in the epithelium. This area is examined at higher magnification in Figure 2. The *right rectangular area* includes the stratified squamous epithelium *(StS)* of the skin and is examined at higher magnification in Figure 3.

Between the two *diamonds* in the *rectangular areas* shown is epithelium of the lower part of the anal canal. Under this epithelium, there is a lymphatic nodule that has a well-formed germinal center. Isolated lymphatic nodules under mucous membranes should not be construed to have fixed locations. Rather, they may or may not be present, according to local demands.

Also, at this low magnification, note the internal anal sphincter muscle *(IAS),* i.e., the thickened, most distal portion of the circular layer of smooth muscle of the muscularis externa. Under the skin on the right is the external anal sphincter muscle *(EAS).* It is composed of striated muscle fibers, which are seen in cross section.

Figure 2, anorectal junction, H&E ×160; inset ×300.

The junction between the simple columnar *(SC)* and the stratified *(ST)* epithelium is marked with the *diamond.* The simple columnar epithelium of the upper part of the anal canal contains numerous goblet cells, and as in the mucosa of the colon, this epithelium is continuous with the epithelium of the intestinal glands *(IG).* These glands continue to about the same point as the muscularis mucosae *(MM).* Characteristically, the lamina propria contains large numbers of lymphocytes *(Lym),* particularly so in the region marked. A higher magnification of the stratified columnar epithelium *(StCol)* and stratified cuboidal epithelium *(StC)* found in the transition zone is shown in the **inset.**

Figure 3, anorectal junction, H&E ×160.

The final change in epithelial type that occurs at the anorectal junction is shown here. On the right is the stratified squamous epithelium of skin *(StS(k)).* The keratinized nature of the surface is apparent. On the other hand, the stratified squamous epithelium *(StS)* below the level of the *diamond* is not keratinized, and nucleated cells can be seen all the way to the surface. Again, numerous lymphocytes *(Lym)* are in the underlying connective tissue, and many have migrated into the epithelium in the nonkeratinized area.

KEY

EAS, external anal sphincter
IAS, internal anal sphincter
IG, intestinal glands
LN, lymphatic nodules
Lym, lymphocytes
MM, muscularis mucosae
SC, simple columnar epithelium
ST, stratified epithelium
StC, stratified cuboidal epithelium
StCol, stratified columnar epithelium
StS, stratified squamous epithelium
StS(k), stratified squamous epithelium (keratinized)
arrow, termination of muscularis mucosae
diamonds, junctions between epithelial types

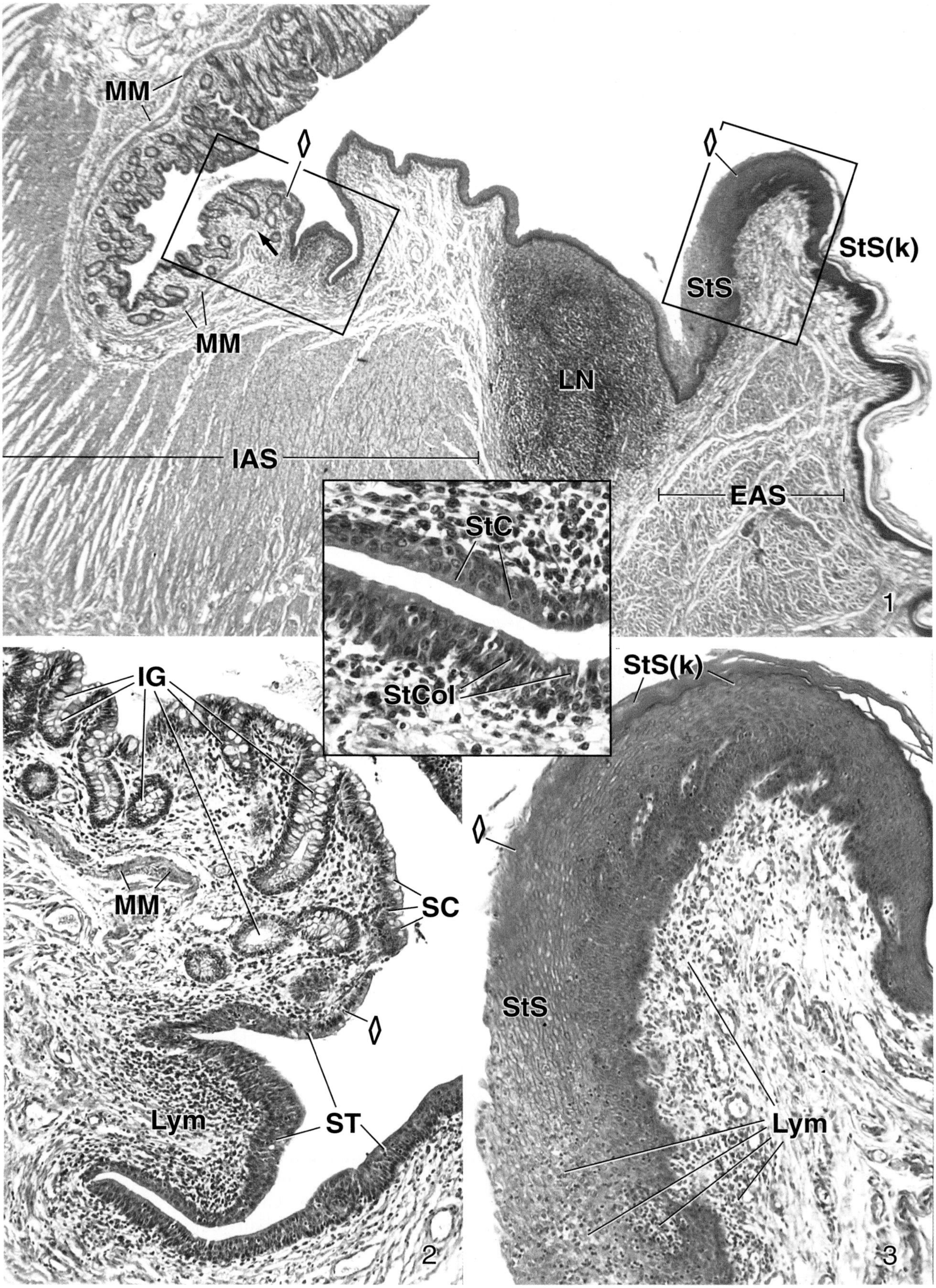
MM
MM
◊
◊
StS(k)
StS
LN
IAS
EAS
StC
StCol
1
IG
MM
SC
◊
Lym
ST
2
StS(k)
◊
StS
Lym
3

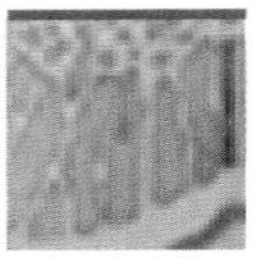
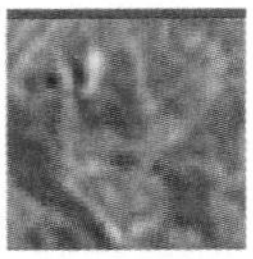
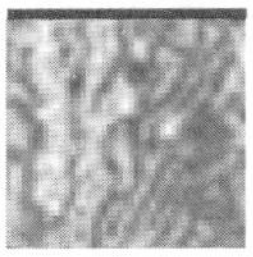

17

Digestive System III: Liver, Gallbladder, and Pancreas

▼ LIVER

Overview

The liver is the largest mass of glandular tissue in the body and the largest internal organ, weighing approximately 1500 g and accounting for nearly 2.5% of adult body weight. It is located in the upper right and partially in the upper left quadrants of the abdominal cavity, protected by the ribcage. The liver is enclosed in a capsule of fibrous connective tissue (Glisson's capsule); a serous covering (visceral peritoneum) surrounds the capsule, except where the liver adheres directly to the diaphragm or the other organs.

The liver is anatomically divided by deep groves into two large lobes (the right and left lobes) and two smaller lobes (the quadrate and caudate lobes) (Fig. 17.1). This anatomic division has only topographic importance because it relates lobes of the liver to other abdominal organs. Division into functional/surgical segments that corresponds to the blood supply and bile drainage is more clinically important.

In the embryo, the liver develops as an ***endodermal evagination*** from the wall of the foregut (specifically the site that will become the duodenum) to form the ***hepatic diverticulum.*** The diverticulum proliferates, giving rise to the ***hepatocytes,*** which become arranged in ***cellular (liver) cords,*** thus forming the parenchyma of the liver. The original stalk of the hepatic diverticulum becomes the ***common bile duct.*** An outgrowth from the common bile duct forms the ***cystic diverticulum*** that gives rise to the ***gallbladder*** and ***cystic duct.***

Liver Physiology

Many circulating plasma proteins are produced and secreted by the liver. The liver plays an important role in the uptake, storage, and distribution of both nutrients and vitamins from the bloodstream. It also maintains the blood glucose level and regulates circulating levels of ***very low density lipoproteins (VLDLs).*** In addition, the liver degrades or conjugates numerous toxic substances and drugs, but it can be overwhelmed by such substances and damaged. The liver is also an exocrine organ; it produces a bile secretion that contains bile salts, phospholipids, and cholesterol. Finally, the liver performs important endocrine-like functions.

The liver produces most of the body's circulating plasma proteins

The circulating plasma proteins produced by the liver include

- ***Albumins,*** which are involved in regulating plasma volume and tissue fluid balance by maintaining the plasma colloid osmotic pressure.
- ***Lipoproteins,*** in particular, VLDLs. The liver synthesizes most VLDLs, which participate in the transport of triglycerides from the liver to other organs. The liver also produces small amounts of other plasma lipoproteins, such as ***low-density lipoproteins (LDLs)*** and ***high-density lipoproteins (HDLs).*** LDLs transport cholesterol esters from the liver to other tissues. HDLs remove cholesterol from the peripheral tissues and transport it to the liver.
- ***Glycoproteins,*** which include proteins involved in iron transport such as ***haptoglobin, transferrin,*** and ***hemopexin.***

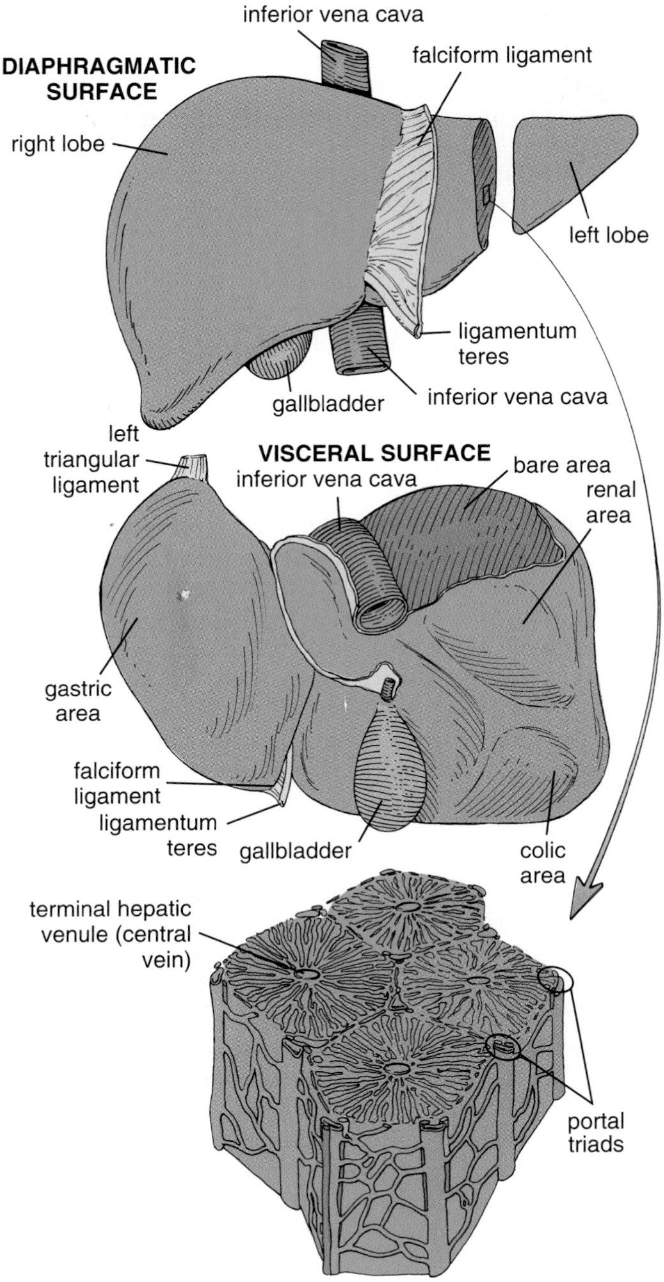

FIGURE 17.1
Anatomic structure of the liver. This diagram shows the gross view of the diaphragmatic and visceral surface of the liver, with labeled anatomic landmarks found on both surfaces. The enlarged cross-sectional area of the liver *(bottom)* shows the general microscopic organization of the liver into lobules. Note the presence of hepatic portal triads at the periphery of each lobule, with the terminal hepatic venule (central vein) in the center of the lobule.

- ***Prothrombin*** and ***fibrinogen,*** important components of the blood-clotting cascade.
- ***Nonimmune α- and β-globulins,*** which also help maintain plasma colloid osmotic pressure and serve as carrier proteins for various substances (see Chapter 9, page 216).

The liver stores and converts several vitamins and iron

Several vitamins are taken up from the bloodstream and are then stored and/or biochemically modified by the liver. They include

- ***Vitamin A (retinol),*** an important vitamin in vision. Vitamin A is the precursor of retinal, which is required for the synthesis of rhodopsin in the eye. The liver plays a major role in the uptake, storage, and maintenance of circulating levels of vitamin A. When the vitamin A levels in the blood decrease, the liver mobilizes its storage sites in the hepatic stellate cells (see page 541). Vitamin A is then released into the circulation in the form of retinol bound to ***retinol-binding protein (RBP).*** The liver also synthesizes RBP; RBP synthesis is regulated by plasma levels of vitamin A. ***Night blindness*** and multiple skin disorders are related to vitamin A deficiency.
- ***Vitamin D (cholecalciferol),*** an important vitamin in calcium and phosphate metabolism. Vitamin D is acquired from dietary vitamin D_3 and is also produced in the skin during exposure to ultraviolet light by conversion of 7-dehydrocholesterol. Unlike vitamin A, vitamin D is not stored in the liver but is distributed to skeletal muscles and adipose tissue. The liver plays an important role in vitamin D metabolism by converting vitamin D_3 to ***25-hydroxycholecalciferol,*** the predominant form of circulating vitamin D. Further conversion takes place in the kidney to 1,25-hydroxycholecalciferol, which is 10 times more active than vitamin D_3. Vitamin D is essential for development and growth of the skeletal system and teeth. Deficiency of vitamin D is associated with ***rickets*** and disorders of bone mineralization.
- ***Vitamin K,*** which is important in hepatic synthesis of prothrombin and several other clotting factors. Like vitamin D, it is derived from two sources: dietary vitamin K and synthesis in the small intestine by intestinal bacterial flora. Vitamin K is transported to the liver with chylomicrons, where it is rapidly absorbed, partially used, and then partially secreted with the VLDL fraction. Vitamin K deficiency is associated with ***hypoprothrombinemia*** and bleeding disorders.

In addition, the liver functions in the storage, metabolism, and homeostasis of iron. It synthesizes almost all of the proteins involved in iron transport and metabolism, including transferrin, haptoglobin, and hemopexin. Transferrin is a plasma iron-transport protein. Haptoglobin binds to free hemoglobin in the plasma, from which the entire complex is removed by the liver to preserve iron. Hemopexin is involved in the transport of free heme in the blood. Iron is stored within the hepatocyte cytoplasm in the form of ***ferritin*** or may be converted to ***hemosiderin granules.*** Recent studies indicate that hepatocytes are the major sites of long-term storage of iron. Iron overload (as in multiple blood transfusions) may lead to ***hemochromatosis,*** a form of liver damage characterized by excessive amounts of hemosiderin in hepatocytes.

The liver degrades drugs and toxins

Hepatocytes are involved in degradation of drugs, toxins, and other proteins foreign to the body (xenobiotics). Many drugs and toxins are not hydrophilic; therefore, they cannot be eliminated effectively from the circulation by the kidneys. The liver converts these substances into more soluble forms. This process is performed by the hepatocytes in two phases:

- ***Phase I,*** called ***oxidation,*** includes hydroxylation (adding an —OH group) and carboxylation (adding a —COOH group) to a foreign compound. This phase is performed in the hepatocyte smooth endoplasmic reticulum (sER) and mitochondria. It involves a series of biochemical reactions with proteins collectively named ***cytochrome P450.***
- ***Phase II,*** or ***conjugation,*** includes conjugation with ***glucuronic acid, glycine,*** or ***taurine.*** This process makes the product of phase I even more water soluble so that it can be easily removed by the kidney.

The liver is involved in many other important metabolic pathways

The liver is important in carbohydrate metabolism as it maintains an adequate supply of nutrients for cell processes. In ***glucose*** metabolism, the liver phosphorylates absorbed glucose from the gastrointestinal tract to ***glucose-6-phosphate.*** Depending on energy requirements, glucose-6-phosphate is either stored in the liver in the form of ***glycogen*** or used in the glycolytic pathways. During fasting, glycogen is broken down by ***glycogenolysis,*** and glucose is released into the bloodstream. In addition, the liver functions in lipid metabolism. ***Fatty acids*** derived from plasma are consumed by hepatocytes using ***β-oxidation*** to provide energy. The liver also produces ***ketone bodies*** that are used as a fuel by other organs (the liver cannot use them as an energy source). The involvement in ***cholesterol*** metabolism (synthesis and uptake from the blood) is also an important function of the liver. Cholesterol is used in formation of bile salts, synthesis of VLDLs, and biosynthesis of organelles. The liver synthesizes most of the ***urea*** in the body from ammonium ions derived from protein and nucleic acid degradation. Finally, the liver is involved in the synthesis and conversion of ***nonessential amino acids*** into essential amino acids.

Bile production is an exocrine function of the liver

The liver is engaged in numerous metabolic conversions involving substrates delivered by blood from the digestive tract, pancreas, and spleen. Some of these products are involved in the production of ***bile***, an exocrine secretion of the liver. Bile contains conjugated and degraded waste products that are returned to the intestine for disposal, as well as substances that bind to metabolites in the intestine to aid in absorption. (Table 17.1) Bile is carried from the parenchyma of the liver by ***bile ducts*** that fuse to form the ***hepatic duct***. The ***cystic duct*** then carries the bile into the ***gallbladder*** where it is concentrated. Bile is returned, via the cystic duct, to the ***common bile duct***, which delivers bile from the liver and gallbladder to the duodenum (see Fig. 17.15).

The endocrine-like functions of the liver are represented by its ability to modify the structure and function of many hormones

The liver modifies the action of hormones released by other organs. The liver's endocrine-like actions involve

- ***Vitamin D***, which is converted by the liver to 25-hydroxycholecalciferol, the predominant form of circulating vitamin D (page 534).
- ***Thyroxine***, a hormone secreted by the thyroid gland as ***tetraiodothyronine*** ***(T_4)***, which is converted in the liver to the biologically active form, ***triiodothyronine*** ***(T_3)***, by deiodination.
- ***Growth hormone (GH)***, a hormone secreted by the pituitary gland. The action of GH is modified by liver-produced ***growth hormone–releasing hormone (GHRH)*** and inhibited by ***somatostatin***, which is secreted by enteroendocrine cells of the gastrointestinal tract.
- ***Insulin and glucagon***, both pancreatic hormones. These hormones are degraded in many organs, but the liver and kidney are the most important sites of their degradation.

Blood Supply to the Liver

To appreciate the myriad functions of the liver introduced above, one must first understand its unique blood supply and how blood is distributed to the hepatocytes. The liver has a dual blood supply consisting of a venous (portal) supply via the ***hepatic portal vein*** and an arterial supply via the ***hepatic artery***. Both vessels enter the liver at a hilum or ***porta hepatis***, the same site at which the common bile duct, carrying the bile secreted by the liver, and the lymphatic vessels leave the liver.

The liver receives the blood that initially supplied the intestines, pancreas, and spleen

The liver is unique among organs because it receives its major blood supply (about 75%) from the ***hepatic portal vein***, which carries venous blood that is largely depleted of oxygen. The blood delivered to the liver by the hepatic portal vein comes from the digestive tract and the major abdominal organs, such as the pancreas and spleen.

The portal blood carried to the liver contains

- Nutrients and toxic materials absorbed in the intestine
- Blood cells and breakdown products of blood cells from the spleen
- Endocrine secretions of the pancreas and enteroendocrine cells of the gastrointestinal tract

Thus, the liver stands directly in the pathway of blood vessels that convey substances absorbed from the digestive tract. While the liver is the first organ to receive metabolic

TABLE 17.1. Composition of Bile

Component	Function
Water	Solute in which other components are carried
Phospholipids (i.e., lecithin) and cholesterol	Metabolic substrates for other cells in the body; precursors of membrane components and steroids; largely reabsorbed in the gut and recycled
Bile salts (also called bile acids): primary (secreted by liver): cholic acid, chenodeoxycholic acid; secondary (converted by bacterial flora in the intestine): deoxycholic acid, lithocholic acid	Emulsifying agents that aid in the digestion and absorption of lipids from the gut and help to keep the cholesterol and phospholipids of the bile in solution, largely recycled, going back and forth between the liver and gut
Bile pigments, principally the glucuronide of the bilirubin produced in the spleen, bone marrow, and liver by the breakdown of hemoglobin	Detoxify bilirubin, the end product of hemoglobin degradation, and carry it to the gut for disposal
Electrolytes: Na^+, K^+, Ca^{2+}, Mg^{2+}, Cl^-, and HCO_3^-	Establish and maintain bile as an isotonic fluid; also largely reabsorbed in the gut

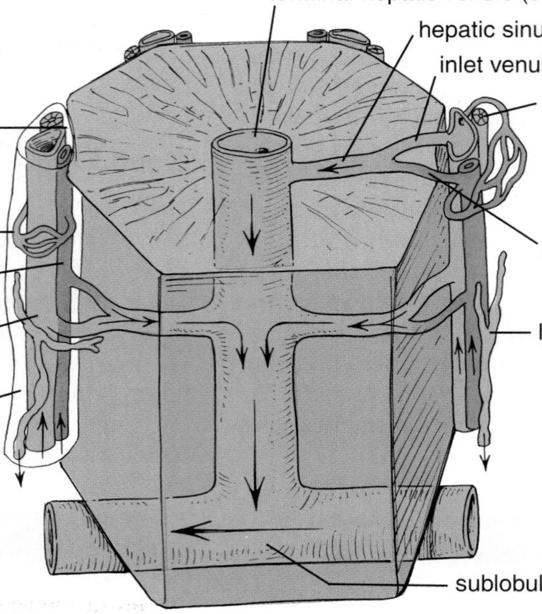

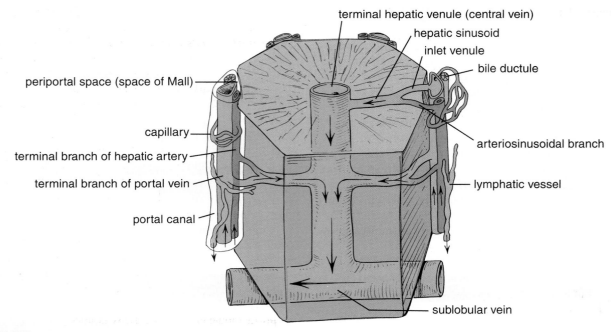

FIGURE 17.2
Blood supply to the liver: the portal triad. The portal triad is composed of the branches of the hepatic artery, portal vein, and bile duct. Blood from the terminal branches of the hepatic artery and portal vein enters the hepatic sinusoids. The mixture of venous and arterial blood is transported by the sinusoids toward the terminal hepatic venule (central vein). From here, blood drains into the sublobular veins, the tributaries of the hepatic vein. Note the small vessels and capillary network in the perivascular connective tissue surrounding each hepatic triad within the portal canal. Also note the periportal space of Mall, located between the portal canal and the outermost hepatocytes. This space is also filled with a small amount of connective tissue in which lymph drainage begins. From here, blind-ended lymphatic capillaries form larger lymphatic vessels that accompany branches of the hepatic artery.

substrates and nutrients, it is also the first exposed to toxic substances that have been absorbed.

The *hepatic artery*, a branch of the celiac trunk, carries oxygenated blood to the liver, providing the remaining 25% of its blood supply. Because blood from the two sources is mixed just before it perfuses the hepatocytes of the liver parenchyma, the liver cells are never exposed to fully oxygenated blood.

Within the liver, the distributing branches of the portal vein and hepatic artery, which supply the ***sinusoidal capillaries (sinusoids)*** that bathe the hepatocytes, and the draining branches of the bile duct system, which lead to the common hepatic duct, course together in a relationship termed the ***portal triad.*** Although a convenient term, it is a misnomer because one or more vessels of the lymphatic drainage system of the liver always travel with the vein, artery, and bile duct. (Fig. 17.2)

The ***sinusoids*** are in intimate contact with the hepatocytes and provide for the exchange of substances between the blood and liver cells. The sinusoids lead to a ***central vein*** that in turn empties into the ***sublobular veins.*** Blood leaves the liver through the ***hepatic veins,*** which empty into the inferior vena cava.

Structural Organization of the Liver

As introduced above, the structural components of the liver include

- ***Parenchyma,*** consisting of organized plates of hepatocytes, which in the adult are normally one cell thick and are separated by sinusoidal capillaries. In young individuals up to 6 years of age, the liver cells are arranged in plates two cells thick.
- ***Connective tissue stroma*** that is continuous with the fibrous capsule of Glisson. Blood vessels, nerves, lymphatic vessels, and bile ducts travel within the connective tissue stroma.
- ***Sinusoidal capillaries (sinusoids),*** the vascular channels between the plates of hepatocytes.
- ***Perisinusoidal spaces (spaces of Disse),*** which lie between the sinusoidal endothelium and the hepatocytes.

With this information as background, one can now consider several ways to describe the organization of these structural elements in order to understand the major functions of the liver.

LIVER LOBULES

There are three ways to describe the structure of the liver in terms of a functional unit: the ***classic lobule***, the ***portal lobule***, and the ***liver acinus***. The classic lobule is the traditional way to describe the organization of the liver parenchyma, and it is relatively easy to visualize. It is based on the distribution of the branches of the portal vein and hepatic artery within the organ and the pathway that blood from them follows as it ultimately perfuses the liver cells.

The classic hepatic lobule is a roughly hexagonal mass of tissue

The ***classic lobule*** (Fig. 17.3) consists of stacks of ***anastomosing plates*** of hepatocytes, one cell thick, separated by the anastomosing system of sinusoids that perfuse the cells with the mixed portal and arterial blood. Each lobule measures about 2.0 × 0.7 mm. At the center of the lobule is a relatively large venule, the ***terminal hepatic venule (central vein)***, into which the sinusoids drain. The plates of cells radiate from the central vein to the periphery of the lobule, as do the sinusoids. At the angles of the hexagon are the ***portal areas (portal canals)***, loose stromal connective tissue characterized by the presence of the portal triads. This connective tissue is ultimately continuous with the fibrous capsule of the liver. The portal canal is bordered by the outermost hepatocytes of the lobule. At the edges of the portal canal, between the connective tissue stroma and the hepatocytes, is a small space called the ***space of Mall***. This space is thought to be one of the sites where lymph originates in the liver.

In some species, e.g., the pig (Fig. 17.4a), the classic lobule is easily recognized because the portal areas are connected by relatively thick layers of connective tissue. In humans, however, there is normally very little interlobular connective tissue, and it is necessary, when examining histologic sections of liver, to draw imaginary lines between portal areas surrounding a central vein to get some sense of the size of the classic lobule (Fig. 17.4b).

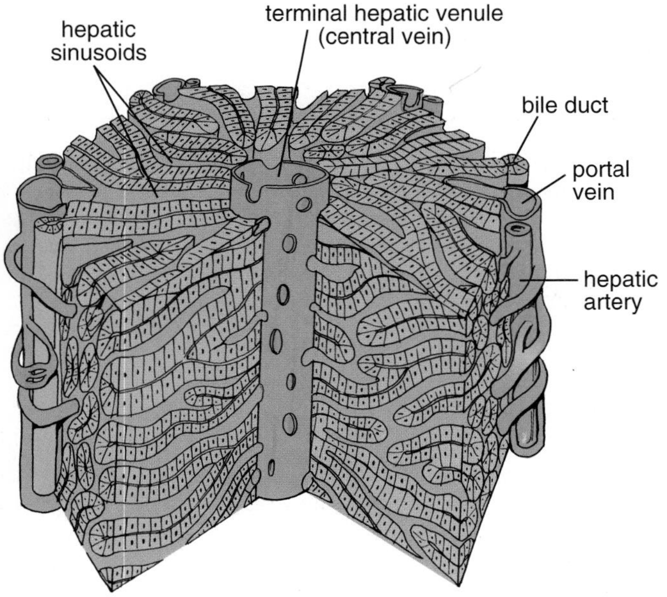

FIGURE 17.3
Diagram of a "classic" liver lobule. A "classic" liver lobule can be schematically diagramed as a six-sided polyhedral prism with portal triads (hepatic artery, portal vein, and bile duct) at each of the corners. The blood vessels of the portal triads send distributing branches along the sides of the lobule, and these branches open into the hepatic sinusoids. The long axis of the lobule is traversed by the terminal hepatic venule (central vein), which receives blood from the hepatic sinusoids. Note that a wedge of the tissue has been removed from the lobule for better visualization of the terminal hepatic venule. Interconnecting sheets or plates of hepatocytes are disposed in a radial pattern from the terminal hepatic venule to the periphery of the lobule.

The portal lobule emphasizes the exocrine functions of the liver

The major exocrine function of the liver is bile secretion. Thus, the morphologic axis of the portal lobule is the interlobular bile duct of the portal triad of the "classic" lobule. Its outer margins are imaginary lines drawn between the three central veins that are closest to that portal triad (Fig. 17.5). These lines define a roughly triangular block of tissue that includes those portions of three classic lobules that secrete the bile that drains into its axial bile duct. This concept allows a description of hepatic parenchymal structure comparable to that of other exocrine glands.

The liver acinus is the structural unit that provides the best correlation between blood perfusion, metabolic activity, and liver pathology

The liver acinus is lozenge shaped and represents the smallest functional unit of the hepatic parenchyma. The ***short axis*** of the acinus is defined by the terminal branches of the portal triad that lie along the border between two classic lobules. The ***long axis*** is a line drawn between the two central veins closest to the short axis. Therefore, in a two-dimensional view (Fig. 17.6) the liver acinus occupies parts of adjacent classic lobules. This concept allows a description of the exocrine secretory function of the liver comparable to that of the portal lobule.

The hepatocytes in each liver acinus are described as being arranged in three concentric elliptical zones surrounding the short axis (see Fig. 17.6).

- ***Zone 1*** is closest to the short axis and the blood supply from penetrating branches of the portal vein and hepatic

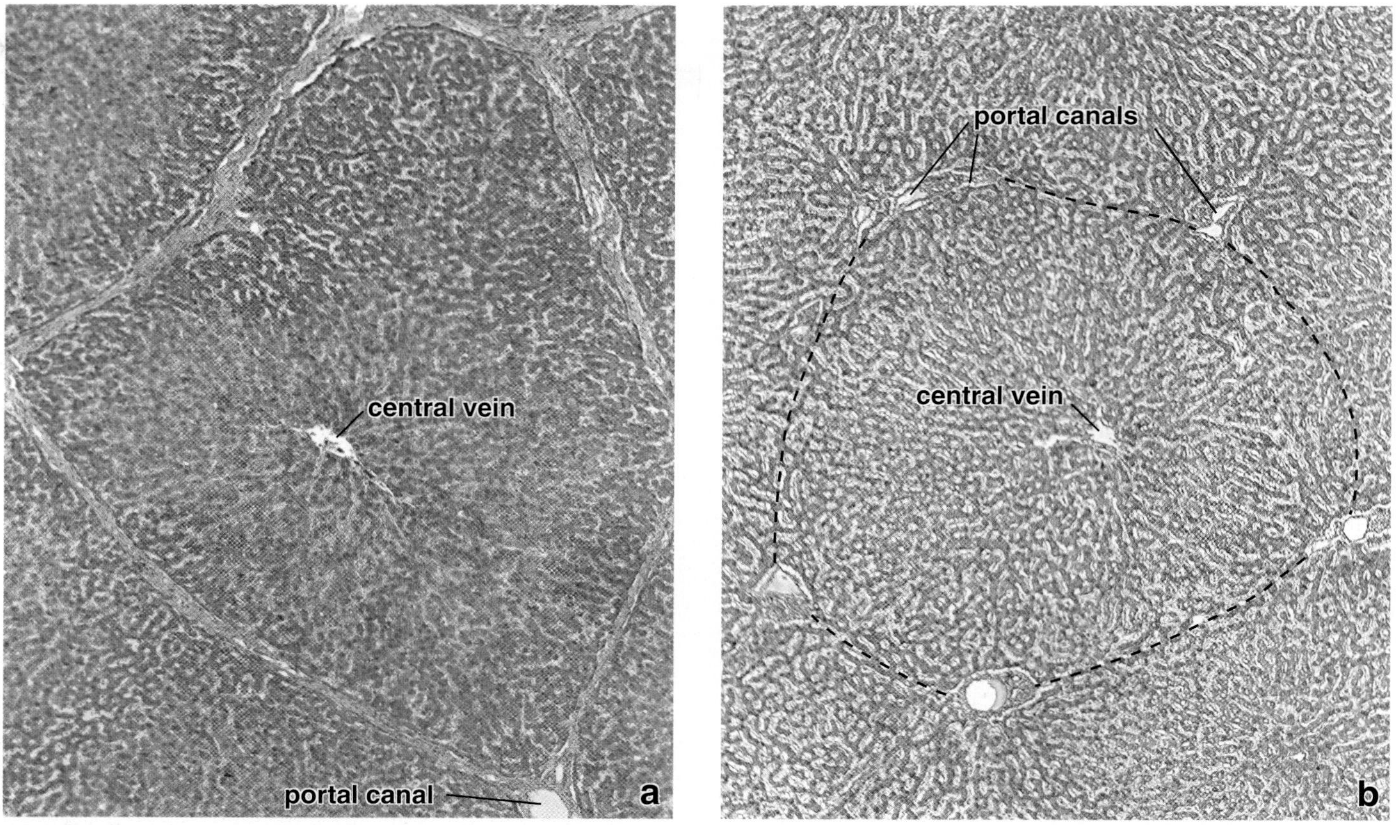

FIGURE 17.4

Photomicrographs of pig and human livers. a. This photomicrograph shows a cross section of a pig liver lobule stained by the Mallory-Azan method to visualize connective tissue components. Note the relatively thick interlobular connective tissue *(stained blue)* surrounding the lobules. The terminal hepatic venule (central vein) is visible in the center of the lobule. ×65. **b.** Photomicrograph of a human liver from a routine H&E preparation. Note that in contrast to the pig liver, the lobules of the human liver lack connective tissue septa. The plates of hepatocytes of one lobule merge with those of adjacent lobules. The boundaries of a lobule can be approximated, however, by drawing a line *(dashed line)* from one portal canal to the next, thus circumscribing the lobule. ×65.

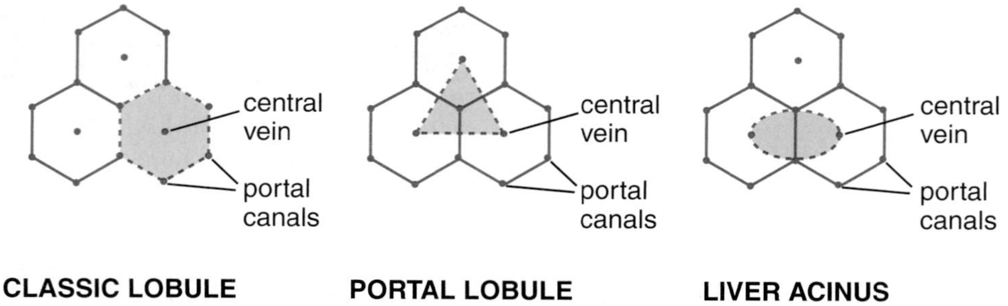

FIGURE 17.5

Comparison of the classic liver lobule, portal lobule, and liver acinus. The *area indicated in blue* shows the territory of each of the three units relating to liver organization and function. The classic lobule has the terminal hepatic venule *(central vein)* at the center of the lobule and the portal canals containing portal triads at the peripheral angles of the lobule. The portal lobule has a portal canal at the center of the lobule and terminal hepatic venules *(central veins)* at the peripheral angles of the lobule. The liver acinus has distributing vessels at the equator and terminal hepatic venules *(central veins)* at each pole.

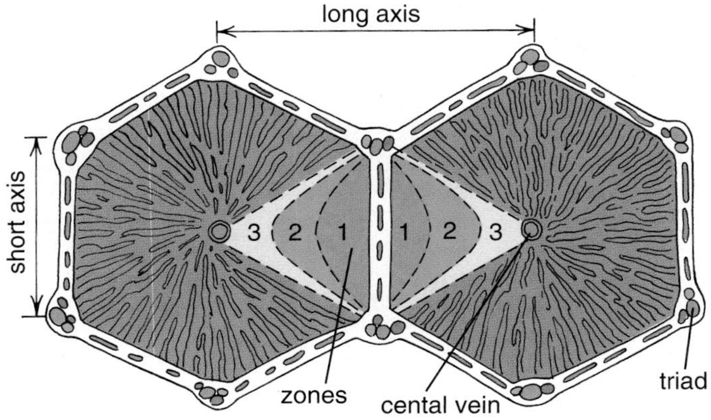

FIGURE 17.6
The liver acinus. The liver acinus is a functional interpretation of liver organization. It consists of adjacent sectors of neighboring hexagonal fields of classic lobules partially separated by distributing blood vessels. The zones, marked 1, 2, and 3, are supplied with blood that is most oxygenated and richest in nutrients in zone 1 and least so in zone 3. The terminal hepatic venules (central veins) in this interpretation are at the edges of the acinus instead of in the center, as in the classic lobule. The vessels of the portal canals, namely, terminal branches of the portal vein and hepatic artery that, along with the smallest bile ducts, make up the portal triad, are shown at the corners of the hexagon that outlines the cross-sectioned profile of the classic lobule.

BOX 17.1

Clinical Correlations: Congestive Heart Failure and Liver Necrosis

Liver injury may be triggered by hemodynamic changes in the circulatory system. In congestive heart failure, the heart is unable to provide sufficient oxygenated blood to meet the metabolic requirements of many tissues and organs, including the liver, which is readily affected by hypoperfusion and hypoxia (low blood oxygen content). Zone 3 of the liver acinus is the first to be affected by this condition. The hepatocytes in this zone are the last to receive blood as it passes along the sinusoids; as a result, these cells receive a blood supply already depleted in oxygen. Examination of a liver biopsy specimen from an individual with congestive heart failure shows a distinct pattern of liver necrosis. Hepatocytes in zone 3, which is located around the central vein, undergo ischemic necrosis. Typically, no noticeable changes are seen in zones 1 and 2, representing the periphery of a classic lobule. Necrosis of this type is referred to as ***centrilobular necrosis***. Figure 17.7 shows the centrilobular portion of a classic lobule. The multiple round vacuoles indicate lipid accumulation, and the atrophic changes are the result of dying hepatocytes undergoing autophagocytosis. Centrilobular necrosis due to hypoxia is referred as ***cardiac cirrhosis***; however, unlike true cirrhosis, nodular regeneration of hepatocytes is minimal.

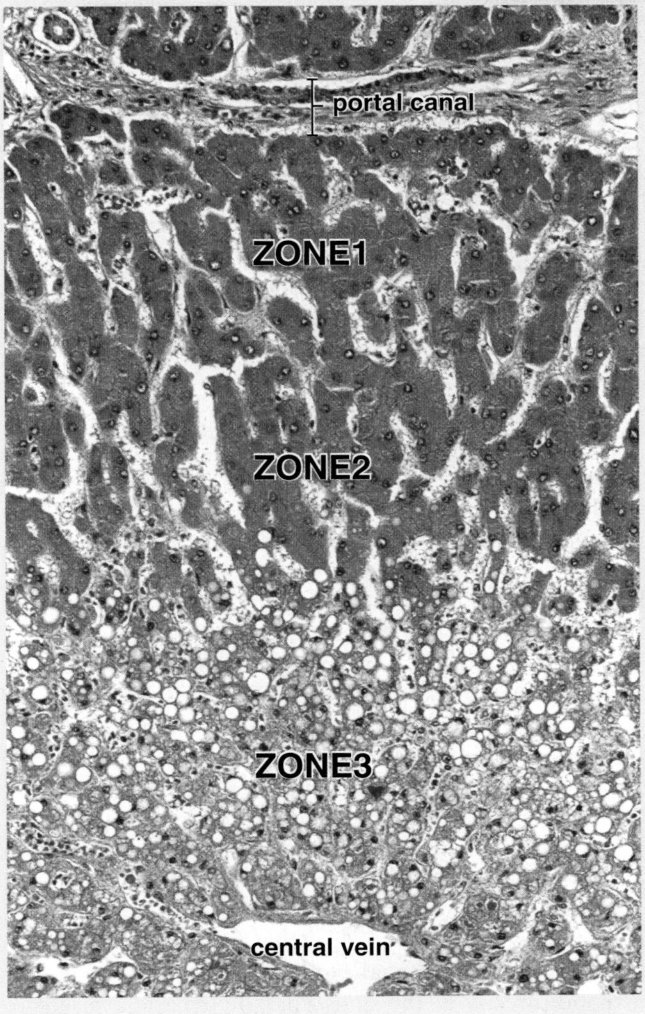

FIGURE 17.7
Photomicrograph of centrilobular necrosis in human liver. This photomicrograph shows a routine H&E liver biopsy specimen from an individual with congestive heart failure. Pathologic changes (referred to as ischemic necrosis) are most severe in hepatocytes in zone 3. This zone surrounds the terminal hepatic venule (central vein). This type of necrosis is referred to as centrilobular necrosis. Note the presence of multiple round vacuoles, which indicates extensive lipid accumulation. No noticeable changes are seen in the periphery of the lobule, i.e., zone 1 and much of zone 2. ×320.

artery. This zone corresponds to the periphery of the classic lobules.

- *Zone 3* is farthest from the short axis and closest to the terminal hepatic vein (central vein). This zone corresponds to the most central part of the classic lobule that surrounds the terminal hepatic vein.
- *Zone 2* lies between zones 1 and 3 but has no sharp boundaries.

The zonation is important in the description and interpretation of patterns of degeneration, regeneration, and specific toxic effects in the liver parenchyma relative to the degree or quality of vascular perfusion of the hepatic cells. As a result of the sinusoidal blood flow, the oxygen gradient, the metabolic activity of the hepatocytes, and the distribution of hepatic enzymes varies across the three zones. The distribution of liver damage due to ischemia and exposure to toxic substances can be explained using this zonal interpretation.

Cells in zone 1 are the first to receive oxygen, nutrients, and toxins from the sinusoidal blood and are the first to show morphologic changes following bile duct occlusion (bile stasis). These cells are also the last to die if circulation is impaired and the first to regenerate. On the other hand, cells in zone 3 are the first to show ischemic necrosis (centrilobular necrosis) in situations of reduced perfusion and the first to show fat accumulation. They are the last to respond to toxic substances and bile stasis. Normal variations in enzyme activity, the number and size of cytoplasmic organelles, and the size of cytoplasmic glycogen deposits are also seen between zones 1 and 3. Cells in zone 2 have functional and morphologic characteristics and responses intermediate to those of zones 1 and 3.

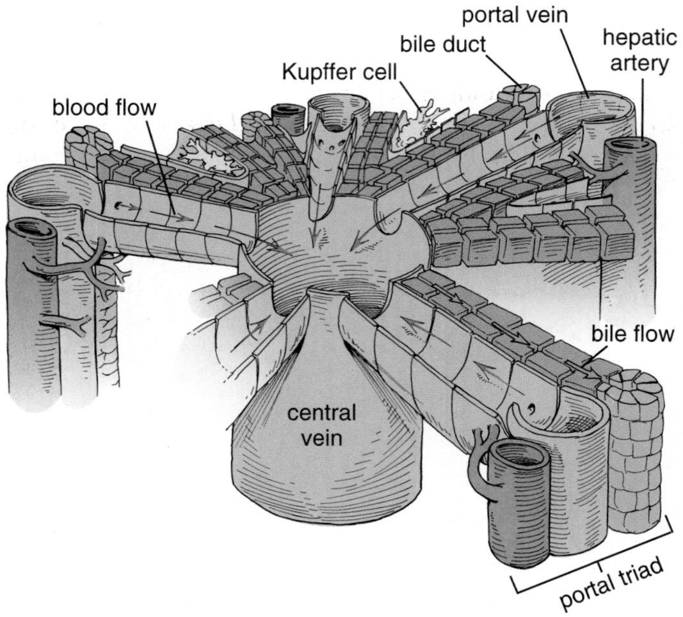

FIGURE 17.8
Diagram of the flow of blood and bile in the liver. This schematic diagram of a part of a classic lobule shows the components of the portal triads, hepatic sinuses, terminal hepatic venule *(central vein)* and associated plates of hepatocytes. *Red arrows* indicate the direction of the blood flow in the sinusoids. Note that the direction of bile flow *(green arrows)* is opposite that of the blood flow.

BLOOD VESSELS OF THE PARENCHYMA

The blood vessels that occupy the portal canals are called interlobular vessels. Only the interlobular vessels that form the smallest portal triads send blood into the sinusoids. The larger interlobular vessels branch into distributing vessels that are located at the periphery of the lobule. These distributing vessels send inlet vessels to the sinusoids (Fig. 17.8). In the sinusoids, the blood flows centripetally toward the central vein. The central vein courses through the central axis of the classic liver lobule, becoming larger as it progresses through the lobule and empties into a sublobular vein. Several sublobular veins converge to form larger hepatic veins that empty into the inferior vena cava.

The structure of the portal vein and its branches within the liver is typical of veins in general. The lumen is much larger than that of the artery associated with it. The structure of the hepatic artery is like that of other arteries, i.e., it has a thick muscular wall. In addition to providing arterial blood directly to the sinusoids, the hepatic artery provides arterial blood to the connective tissue and other structures in the larger portal canals. Capillaries in these larger portal canals return the blood to the interlobular veins before they empty into the sinusoid.

The central vein is a thin-walled vessel receiving blood from the hepatic sinusoids. The endothelial lining of the central vein is surrounded by small amounts of spirally arranged connective tissue fibers. The central vein, so named because of its central position in the classic lobule, is actually the terminal venule of the system of hepatic veins and, thus, is more properly called the **terminal hepatic venule.** The sublobular vein, the vessel that receives blood from the terminal hepatic venules, has a distinct layer of connective tissue fibers, both collagenous and elastic, just external to the endothelium. The sublobular veins as well as the hepatic veins into which they drain, travel alone. Because they are solitary vessels, they can be readily distinguished in a histologic section from the portal veins that are members of a triad. There are no valves in hepatic veins.

Hepatic sinusoids are lined with a thin discontinuous endothelium

The discontinuous sinusoidal endothelium has a discontinuous basal lamina that is absent over large areas. The discontinuity of the endothelium is evident in two ways:

- *Large fenestrae,* without diaphragms, are present within the endothelial cells.

- *Large gaps* are present between neighboring endothelial cells.

Hepatic sinusoids differ from other sinusoids in that a second cell type, the ***stellate sinusoidal macrophage***, or ***Kupffer cell*** (Fig. 17.9), is a regular part of the vessel lining.

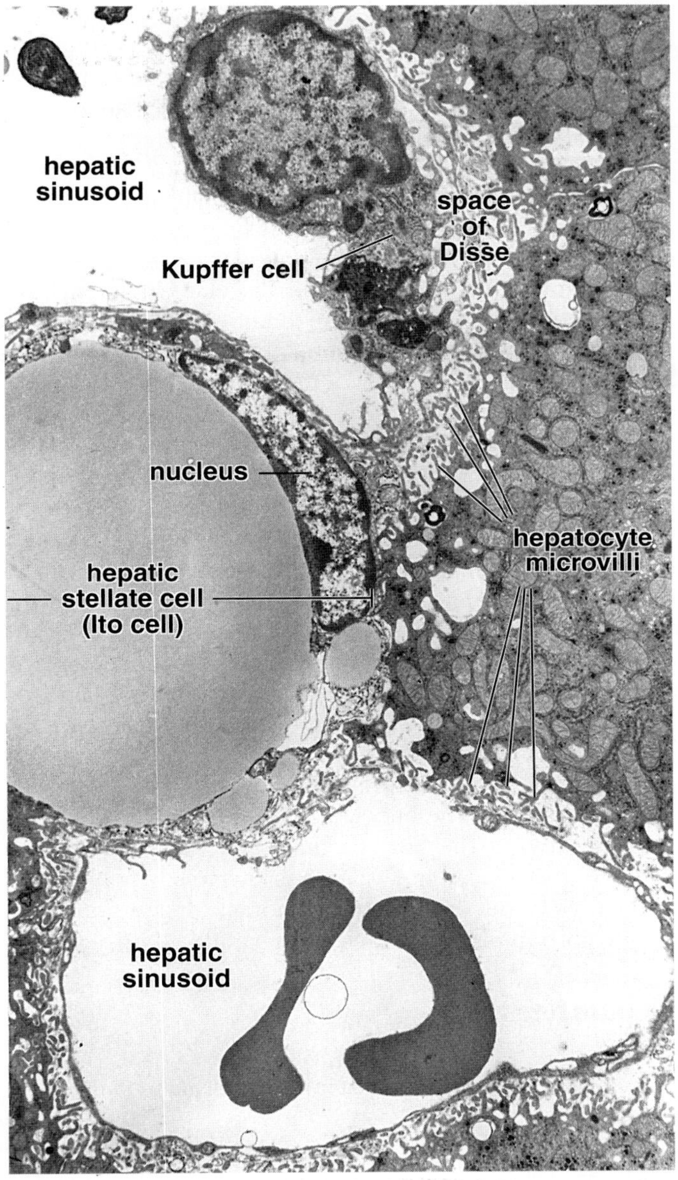

FIGURE 17.9
Electron micrograph of two hepatic sinusoids of the liver. One hepatic sinusoid *(top)* displays a stellate sinusoidal macrophage *(Kupffer cell)*. The remainder of the sinusoid as well as the other sinusoid is lined by thin endothelial cell cytoplasm. Surrounding each sinusoid is the perisinusoidal space *(space of Disse)*, which contains numerous hepatocyte microvilli. Also present in the perisinusoidal space is a hepatic stellate cell *(Ito cell)* with a large lipid droplet and several smaller droplets. Its nucleus conforms to the curve of the lipid droplet. ×6,600.

Kupffer cells belong to the mononuclear phagocytotic system

Like other members of the mononuclear phagocytotic system, Kupffer cells are derived from monocytes. The scanning electron microscope (SEM) and transmission electron microscope (TEM) clearly show that the Kupffer cells form part of the lining of the sinusoid. Previously, they had been described as lying on the luminal surface of the endothelial cells. This older histologic description was probably based on the fact that processes of the Kupffer cells occasionally overlap endothelial processes on the luminal side. Kupffer cells do not form junctions with neighboring endothelial cells.

Processes of Kupffer cells often seem to span the sinusoidal lumen and may even partially occlude it. The presence of red cell fragments and iron in the form of ferritin in the cytoplasm of Kupffer cells suggests that they may be involved in the final breakdown of some damaged or senile red blood cells that reach the liver from the spleen. Some of the ferritin iron may be converted to hemosiderin granules and stored in the cells. This function is greatly increased after splenectomy and is then essential for red blood cell disposal.

PERISINUSOIDAL SPACE (SPACE OF DISSE)

The perisinusoidal space is the site of exchange of materials between blood and liver cells

The *perisinusoidal space (space of Disse)* lies between the basal surfaces of hepatocytes and the basal surfaces of endothelial cells and Kupffer cells that line the sinusoids. Small, irregular microvilli project into this space from the basal surface of the hepatocytes (Fig. 17.10).

The microvilli increase the surface area available for exchange of materials between hepatocytes and plasma by as much as 6 times. Because of the large gaps in the endothelial layer and the absence of a continuous basal lamina, no significant barrier exists between the blood plasma in the sinusoid and the hepatocyte plasma membrane. Proteins and lipoproteins synthesized by the hepatocyte are transferred into the blood in the perisinusoidal space; this pathway is for liver secretions other than bile.

In the fetal liver, the space between blood vessels and hepatocytes contains islands of blood-forming cells. In cases of chronic anemia in the adult, blood-forming cells may again appear in the perisinusoidal space.

The hepatic stellate cells (Ito cells) store vitamin A; however, in pathologic conditions, they differentiate into myofibroblasts and synthesize collagen

The other cell type found in the perisinusoidal space is the ***hepatic stellate cell*** (commonly called an ***Ito cell***). These cells of mesenchymal origin are the primary storage

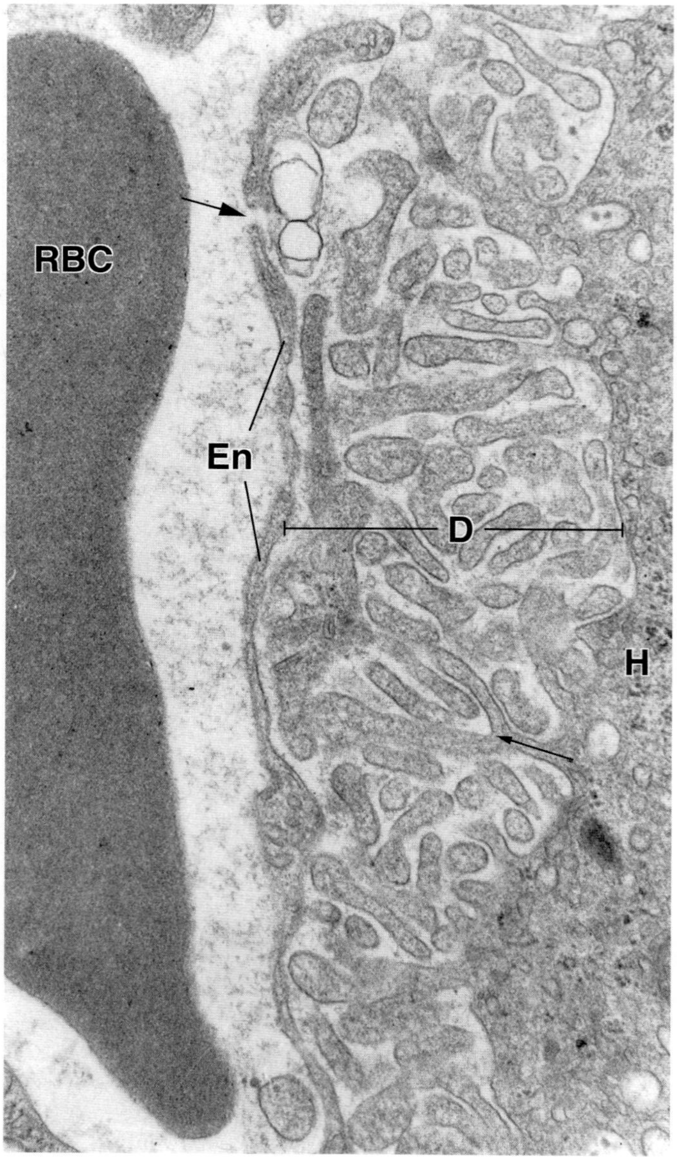

FIGURE 17.10
Electron micrograph showing the perisinusoidal space (of Disse). The perisinusoidal space *(D)* is located between the hepatocytes *(H)* and the sinusoid. A gap *(large arrow)* separates the endothelial cells *(En)* that line the sinusoid. Such gaps allow easy passage of small substances between the sinusoid and the perisinusoidal space. Numerous microvilli extend from the hepatocytes into the perisinusoidal space. These processes are long and frequently branch *(small arrow)*. A red blood cell *(RBC)* is within the sinusoid. ×18,000.

site for hepatic vitamin A in the form of ***retinyl esters*** within cytoplasmic lipid droplets. Vitamin A is released from the hepatic stellate cell as ***retinol*** (alcohol form) bound to ***RBP***. It is then transported from the liver to the retina, where its stereoisomer ***11-***cis ***retinal*** binds to the protein opsin to form ***rhodopsin***, the visual pigment of rods and cones of the retina. For many years, fish liver oils (e.g., cod liver oil) were medically and economically important nutritional sources of vitamin A.

In certain pathologic conditions, such as chronic inflammation or cirrhosis, hepatic stellate cells lose their lipid and vitamin A storage capability and differentiate into cells with characteristics of myofibroblasts. These cells appear to play a significant role in hepatic fibrogenesis; they synthesize and deposit type I and type III collagen within the perisinusoidal space, resulting in liver fibrosis. This collagen is continuous with the connective tissue of the portal space and the connective tissue surrounding the central vein. An increased amount of perisinusoidal fibrous stroma is an early sign of liver response to toxic substances. The cytoplasm of hepatic stellate cells contains contractile elements, such as desmin and smooth muscle α-actin filaments. During cell contraction, they increase the vascular resistance within the sinusoids by constricting the vascular channels, leading to portal hypertension. In addition, hepatic stellate cells play a role in remodeling the extracellular matrix during recovery from liver injury.

Lymphatic Pathway

Hepatic lymph originates in the perisinusoidal space

Plasma that remains in the perisinusoidal space drains to the periportal connective tissue where a small space, the ***space of Mall*** (see Fig. 17.11b), is described between the stroma of the portal canal and the outermost hepatocytes. From this collecting site, the fluid then enters lymphatic capillaries that travel with the other components of the portal triad.

The lymph moves in progressively larger vessels, in the same direction as the bile, i.e., from the level of the hepatocytes, toward the portal canals and eventually to the hilum of the liver. About 80% of the hepatic lymph follows this pathway and drains into the thoracic duct, forming the major portion of the thoracic duct lymph.

Hepatocytes

Hepatocytes make up the anastomosing cell plates of the liver lobule

Hepatocytes are large, polygonal cells measuring between 20 and 30 μm in each dimension. They constitute about 80% of the cell population of the liver.

Hepatocyte nuclei are large and spherical and occupy the center of the cell. Many cells in the adult liver are binucleate; most cells in the adult liver are tetraploid (i.e., they contain the 4*n* amount of DNA). Heterochromatin is present as scattered clumps in the nucleoplasm and as a distinct band under the nuclear envelope. Two or more well-developed nucleoli are present in each nucleus.

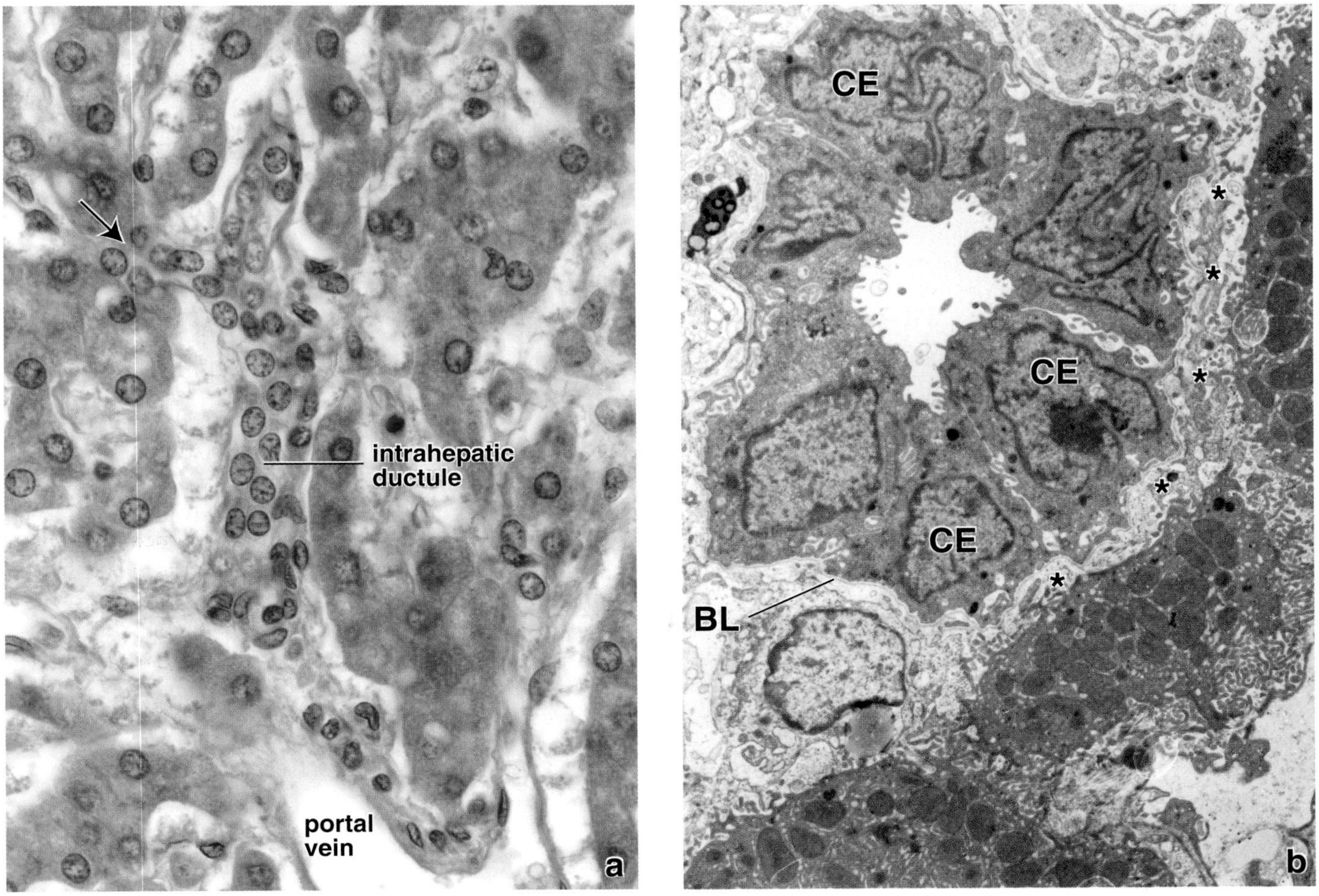

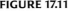

FIGURE 17.11
The intrahepatic ductule (canal of Hering). a. Photomicrograph showing an area near a portal canal. The terminal branch of a portal vein (lower right) accompanied by a small intrahepatic ductule (canal of Hering) are evident. The *arrow* indicates the area where a bile canaliculus is draining into the intrahepatic ductule. Note that the intrahepatic ductule is surrounded by hepatocytes, in contrast to the bile duct, which is embedded in the connective tissue of the portal canal. ×800. **b.** Electron micrograph showing an intrahepatic ductule. The ductule collects bile from the bile canaliculi. It is close to the hepatocytes, but the actual connection between bile canaliculi and the intrahepatic ductule is not evident in this plane of section. The ductule is composed of cuboidal epithelium *(CE)* surrounded by a complete basal lamina *(BL)*. The narrow space *(asterisks)* into which microvilli of hepatocytes project is the periportal space (of Mall), not the perisinusoidal space (of Disse). ×6,000.

Hepatocytes are relatively long-lived for cells associated with the digestive system; their average lifespan is about 5 months. In addition, liver cells are capable of considerable regeneration when liver substance is lost to hepatotoxic processes, disease, or surgery.

The hepatocyte cytoplasm is generally acidophilic. Specific cytoplasmic components may be identified by routine and special staining procedures, including

- Basophilic regions that represent rough endoplasmic reticulum (rER) and free ribosomes.
- Numerous mitochondria; as many as 800 to 1000 mitochondria per cell can be demonstrated by vital staining or enzyme histochemistry
- Multiple small Golgi complexes seen in each cell after specific staining
- Large numbers of peroxisomes demonstrated by immunocytochemistry
- Deposits of glycogen stained by means of the periodic acid–Schiff (PAS) procedure. However, in a well-preserved hematoxylin and eosin (H&E) preparation, glycogen is also visible as irregular spaces, usually giving a fine foamy appearance to the cytoplasm.
- Lipid droplets of various sizes seen after appropriate fixation and Sudan staining. In routinely prepared histologic sections, round spaces are sometimes seen that represent dissolved lipid droplets. The number of lipid

droplets increases after injection or ingestion of certain hepatotoxins, including ethanol.

- Lipofuscin pigment within lysosomes seen with routine H&E staining in various amounts. Well-delineated brown granules can also be visualized by the PAS method.

As noted above, the liver cell is polyhedral; for convenience, it is described as having six surfaces, although there may be more. A schematic section of a cuboidal hepatocyte is shown in Fig. 17.12. Two of its surfaces face the perisinusoidal space. The plasma membrane of two surfaces faces a neighboring hepatocyte and a bile canaliculus. Assuming that the cell is cuboidal, the remaining two surfaces, which cannot be seen in the diagram, would also face neighboring cells and bile canaliculi. The surfaces that face the perisinusoidal space correspond to the basal surface of other epithelial cells; the surfaces that face neighboring cells and bile canaliculi correspond to the lateral and apical surfaces, respectively, of other epithelial cells.

Peroxisomes are numerous in hepatocytes

Hepatocytes have as many as 200 to 300 ***peroxisomes*** per cell. They are relatively large and vary in diameter from 0.2 to 1.0 μm (see Fig. 17.13a). Peroxisomes are a major site of oxygen use and in this way perform a function similar to that of mitochondria. They contain a large amount of oxidase that generates toxic hydrogen peroxide, H_2O_2. The enzyme catalase, also residing within peroxisomes, degrades hydrogen peroxide to oxygen and water. These types of reactions are involved in many detoxification processes occurring in the liver, e.g., detoxification of alcohol. In fact, about one half of the ethanol that is ingested is converted to acetaldehyde by enzymes contained in liver peroxisomes. In humans, ***catalase*** and ***D-amino acid oxidase,*** as well as ***alcohol dehydrogenase,*** are found in peroxisomes. In addition, peroxisomes are also involved in breakdown of fatty acids ***(β-oxidation)*** as well as gluconeogenesis and metabolism of purines.

sER can be extensive in hepatocytes

The sER in hepatocytes may be extensive but varies with metabolic activity (see Fig. 17.13b). The sER contains enzymes involved in degradation and conjugation of toxins and drugs as well as enzymes responsible for synthesizing cholesterol and the lipid portion of lipoproteins. Under conditions of hepatocyte challenge by drugs, toxins, or metabolic stimulants, the sER may become the predominant organelle in the cell. In addition to stimulating sER

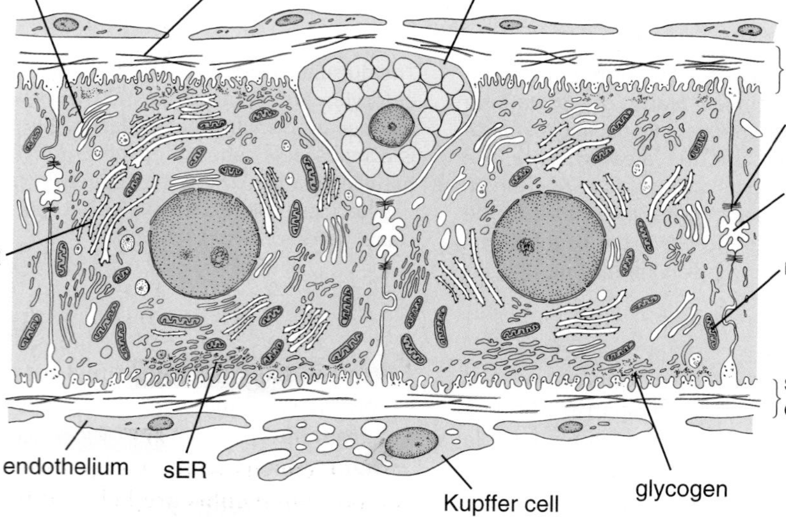

FIGURE 17.12

Schematic diagram of a plate of hepatocytes interposed between hepatic sinusoids. This diagram shows a one-cell-thick plate of hepatocytes interposed between two sinusoids. If it is assumed that the cell is cuboidal, two sides of each cell (shown) would face hepatic sinusoids, two sides of each cell (shown) would face bile canaliculi, and the additional two sides (not shown) would face bile canaliculi. Note the location and features of a hepatic stellate cell *(Ito cell)* filled with cytoplasmic vacuoles containing vitamin A. The sparse collagen fibers found in the perisinusoidal space (of Disse) are produced by the hepatic stellate cells (Ito cells). In certain pathologic conditions, these cells lose their storage vacuoles and differentiate into myofibroblasts that produce collagen fibers, leading to liver fibrosis. Observe that the stellate sinusoidal macrophage *(Kupffer cell)* forms an integral part of the sinusoidal lining.

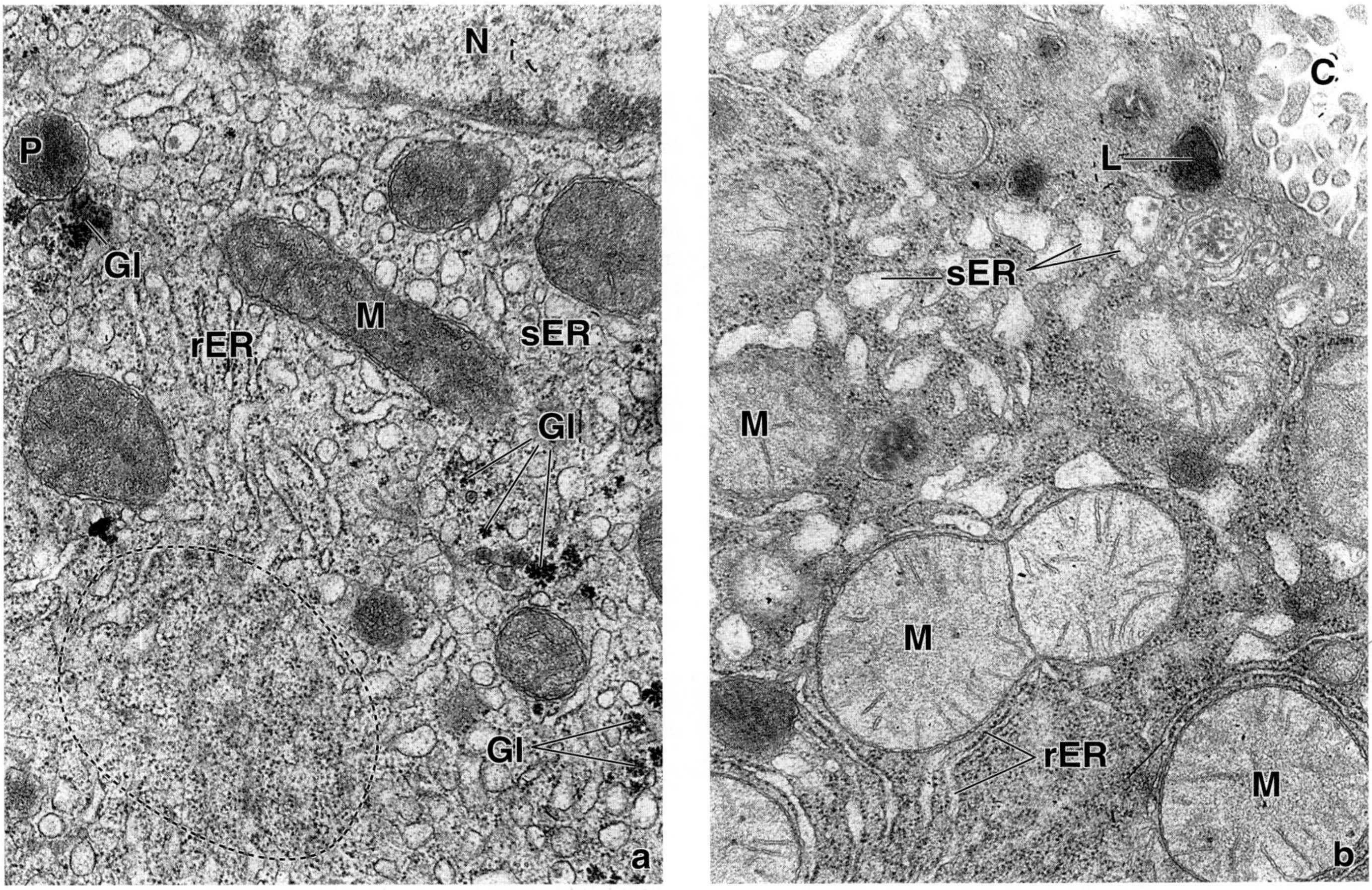

FIGURE 17.13
Electron micrographs of a hepatocyte. a. This electron micrograph shows organelles and other cytoplasmic structures near the nucleus *(N)*. These include a peroxisome *(P)*, mitochondrion *(M)*, glycogen inclusions *(Gl)*, smooth endoplasmic reticulum *(sER)*, and rough endoplasmic reticulum *(rER)*. In the lower left, the membranes of the rER have been cut in a tangential plane showing the ribosomes (encircled by a *dashed line*) on the cytoplasmic face of the membrane. ×12,000. **b.** This micrograph shows a region of cytoplasm near a bile canaliculus *(C)*. It includes a lysosome *(L)*, mitochondria *(M)*, and both sER and rER. Note the microvilli in the bile canaliculus. ×18,000.

activity, certain drugs and hormones induce synthesis of new sER membranes and their associated enzymes. The sER undergoes hypertrophy following administration of alcohol, drugs (i.e, phenobarbital, anabolic steroids, and progesterone), and certain chemotherapeutic agents used to treat cancer.

Stimulation of the sER by ethanol enhances its ability to detoxify other drugs, certain carcinogens, and some pesticides. On the other hand, metabolism by the sER can actually increase the hepatocyte-damaging effects of some toxic compounds, such as carbon tetrachloride (CCl_4) and 3,4-benzpyrene.

The large Golgi apparatus in hepatocytes consists of as many as 50 Golgi units

Examination of hepatocytes with the TEM shows the Golgi to be much more elaborate than those seen in routine histologic specimens. Heavy-metal preparations (Golgi stains) of thick sections of liver give an indication of the extent of the Golgi network. As many as 50 Golgi units, each consisting of three to five closely stacked cisternae, plus many large and small vesicles, are found in hepatocytes. These "units" are actually branches of the tortuous Golgi apparatus seen in heavy-metal preparations. Elements of the Golgi apparatus concentrated near the bile canaliculus are believed to be associated with the exocrine secretion of bile. Golgi cisternae and vesicles near the sinusoidal surfaces of the cell, however, contain electron-dense granules 25 to 80 nm in diameter that are believed to be VLDL and other lipoprotein precursors. These substances are subsequently released into the circulation as part of the endocrine secretory function of the hepatocytes. Similar dense globules are seen in dilated portions of the sER and, occasionally, in the dilated ends of rER cisternae where they are synthesized.

BOX 17.2

Clinical Correlations: Lipoproteins

Lipoproteins are multicomponent complexes of proteins and lipids that are involved in the transport of cholesterol and triglycerides in the blood. Cholesterol and triglycerides do not circulate free in the plasma because lipids, on their own, would be unable to remain in suspension. The association of the protein with the lipid-containing core makes the complex sufficiently hydrophilic to remain suspended in the plasma.

Lipoproteins serve a variety of functions in cellular membranes and in the transport and metabolism of lipids. Lipoprotein precursors are produced in the liver. The lipid component is produced in the sER; the protein component is produced in the rER of the hepatocytes. The lipoprotein complexes pass to the Golgi, where secretory vesicles containing electron-dense lipoprotein particles bud off and are then released at the cell surface bordering the perisinusoidal space to reach the bloodstream. Several hormones, such as estrogen and thyroid hormones, regulate the secretion of lipoproteins.

In general, four classes of lipoproteins have been defined by their characteristic density, molecular weight, size, and chemical composition: ***chylomicrons, VLDLs, LDLs***, and ***HDLs***. These lipoproteins differ in chemical composition and can be isolated from plasma according to their flotation properties, from largest and least dense to smallest and most dense.

Chylomicrons, the lightest of all lipoproteins, are made only in the small intestine. Their main function is to transport the large amount of absorbed fat to the bloodstream.

VLDLs are denser and smaller than chylomicrons; they are synthesized predominately in the liver and to a lesser extent in the small intestine. VLDLs are rich in triglycerides. Their function is to transport most of the triglycerides from the liver to other organs. Liver VLDLs are associated with circulating ***apolipoprotein B-100***, also synthesized in the liver, which aids in secretion of VLDLs. In congenital liver disease, such as ***abetalipoproteinemia***, and to a lesser degree in acute and chronic disorders, the liver is unable to produce apolipoprotein B-100, leading to blockage in the secretion of VLDLs. In liver biopsy specimens from these individuals, large lipid droplets occupy most of the hepatocyte cytoplasm.

LDLs and ***HDLs*** are produced in the plasma; however, small amounts of these fractions are produced by the liver. LDLs are denser than VLDLs, and HDLs are denser than LDLs. The function of LDLs is to transport cholesterol esters from the liver to the peripheral organs. The HDLs are involved in the transport of cholesterol from the peripheral tissues to the liver. High levels of LDL are directly correlated with increased risk of cardiovascular disease; high levels of HDL or low levels of LDL are associated with decreased risk.

Lysosomes concentrated near the bile canaliculus correspond to the peribiliary dense bodies seen in histologic sections

Hepatocyte lysosomes are so heterogeneous that they can only be positively identified, even at the TEM level, by histochemical means. In addition to normal lysosomal enzymes, TEM reveals other components:

- Pigment granules (lipofuscin)
- Partially digested cytoplasmic organelles
- Myelin figures

Hepatocyte lysosomes may also be a normal storage site for iron (as a ferritin complex) and a site of iron accumulation in certain storage diseases.

The number of lysosomes increases in a variety of pathologic conditions, ranging from simple obstructive bile stasis to viral hepatitis and anemia. However, although the range of normal liver function—particularly the rate of bile secretion—is quite wide, no statistically significant morphologic changes take place in the Golgi apparatus or lysosomes of the peribiliary cytoplasm to correlate with the rate of bile secretion.

Biliary Tree

The ***biliary tree*** is the system of conduits of increasing diameter that bile flows through from the hepatocytes to the gallbladder and then to the intestine. The smallest branches of this system are the canaliculi into which the hepatocytes secrete bile.

The bile canaliculus is a small canal formed by apposed grooves in the surface of adjacent hepatocytes

Bile canaliculi form a complete loop around four sides of the idealized six-sided hepatocytes (Fig. 17.14). They are approximately 0.5μm in luminal diameter and are isolated from the rest of the intercellular compartment by tight junctions, which are part of junctional complexes that also include zonulae adherentes and desmosomes. Microvilli of the two adjacent hepatocytes extend into the canalicular lumen. Adenosine triphosphatase (ATPase) and other alkaline phosphatases can be localized on the plasma membranes of the canaliculi, suggesting that bile secretion into this space is an active process. Bile flow is centrifugal, i.e., from the region of the central vein toward the portal canal (a direction opposite to the blood flow). Near the portal canal but still within the lobule, bile canaliculi join to form the short ***intrahepatic ductules***, the ***canals of Hering*** (see Fig. 17.11a), which are lined with cuboidal nonhepatocytic cells. This ductule epithelium is subtended by a complete basal lamina, as is the rest of the distal biliary tree.

Intrahepatic bile ductules carry bile to hepatic ducts

The ductules have a diameter of about 1.0 to 1.5 μm and carry bile through the boundary of the lobule to the ***interlobular bile ducts*** that form part of the portal triad (see Fig. 17.11b). These ducts range from 15 to 40 μm in di-

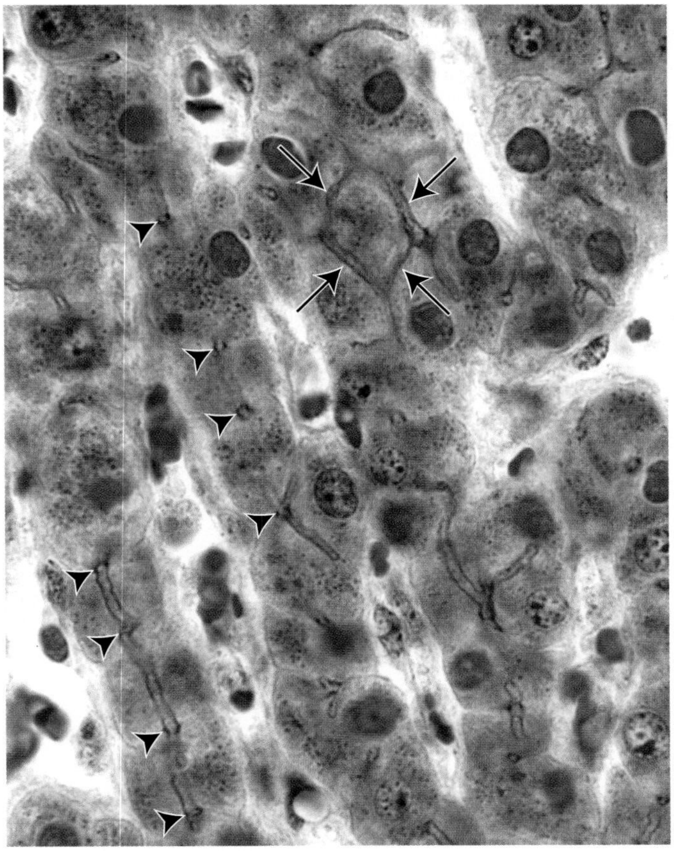

FIGURE 17.14
Photomicrograph of bile canaliculi. This high-magnification photomicrograph shows several one-cell-thick plates of hepatocytes separated by hepatic sinusoids. The plane of section in certain areas is parallel to the bile canaliculi. In this plane, the canaliculi reveal their arrangement on four sides of the hepatocytes (*arrows*). *Arrowheads* indicate those bile canaliculi that appear only in cross-sectional profile. ×1,240.

ameter and are lined by an epithelium that is cuboidal near the lobules and gradually becomes columnar as the ducts near the porta hepatis. The columnar cells have well-developed microvilli, as do those of the extrahepatic bile ducts and gallbladder. As the bile ducts get larger, they gradually acquire a dense connective tissue investment containing numerous elastic fibers. Smooth muscle cells appear in this connective tissue as the ducts approach the hilum. Interlobular ducts join to form the ***right*** and ***left hepatic ducts,*** which in turn join at the hilum to form the ***common hepatic duct*** (Fig. 17.15).

In some individuals, the ***ducts of Luschka*** are located in the connective tissue between the liver and the gallbladder, near the neck of the gallbladder. These ducts connect with the cystic duct, not with the lumen of the gallbladder. They are histologically similar to the intrahepatic bile ducts and may be remnants of aberrant embryonic bile ducts.

Extrahepatic bile ducts carry the bile to the gallbladder and duodenum

The ***common hepatic duct*** is about 3 cm long and is lined with tall columnar epithelial cells that closely resemble those of the gallbladder (described below). All of the layers of the alimentary canal (see page 475) are represented in the duct, except the muscularis mucosae. The ***cystic duct*** connects the common hepatic duct to the gallbladder and carries bile both into and out of the ***gallbladder.*** Distal to the junction with the cystic duct, the fused duct is called the ***common bile duct*** and extends for about 7 cm to the wall of the duodenum at the ***ampulla of Vater.*** A thickening of the muscularis externa of the duodenum at the ampulla constitutes the ***sphincter of Oddi,*** which surrounds the openings of both the common bile duct and the ***pancreatic duct*** (see below) and acts as a valve to regulate the flow of bile and pancreatic juice into the duodenum.

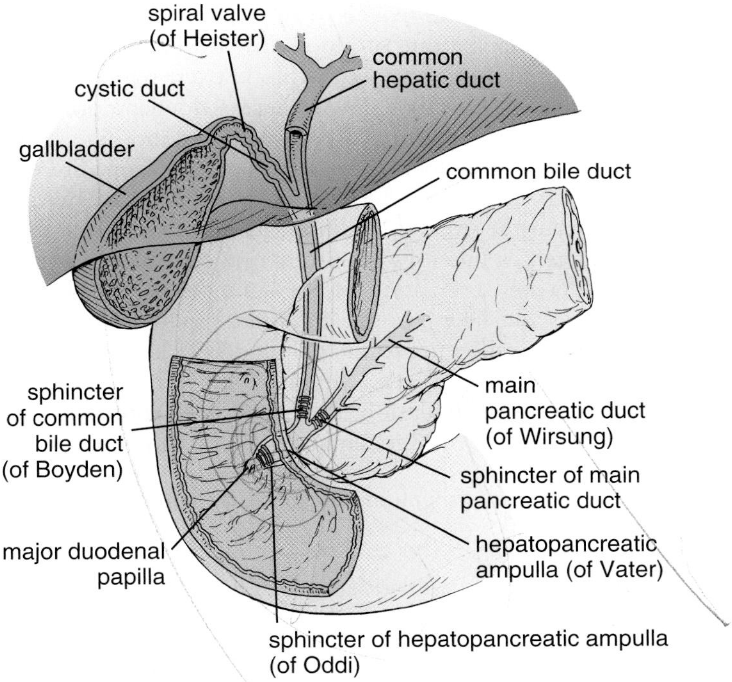

FIGURE 17.15
Diagram showing the relationship of hepatic, pancreatic, and gallbladder ducts. The gallbladder is a blind pouch joined to a single cystic duct in which numerous mucosal folds form the spiral valve (of Heister). The cystic duct joins with the common hepatic duct, and together they form the common bile duct that leads into the duodenum. At the entry to the duodenum, the common bile duct is joined by the main pancreatic duct to form the hepatopancreatic ampulla (of Vater), and together they enter the second part of the duodenum. Sphincters can be found at the distal part of these ducts. The sphincters of the common bile duct (of Boyden), the main pancreatic duct, and the hepatopancreatic ampulla (of Oddi) control the flow of bile and pancreatic secretion into the duodenum. When the common bile duct sphincter contracts, bile cannot enter the duodenum; it backs up and flows into the gallbladder, where it is concentrated and stored.

The adult human liver secretes, on average, about 1 L of bile a day

The composition of bile and the functions of most of its components are listed in Table 17.1. As noted in the table, many components of the bile are recycled via the portal circulation.

- About 90% of the ***bile salts,*** a component of bile, is reabsorbed by the gut and transported back to the liver in the portal blood. The bile salts are then reabsorbed and resecreted by hepatocytes. Hepatocytes also synthesize new bile salts to replace those that are lost.
- ***Cholesterol*** and phospholipid ***lecithin,*** as well as most of the ***electrolytes*** and water delivered to the gut with the bile, are also reabsorbed and recycled.

Bilirubin glucuronide, the detoxified end product of hemoglobin breakdown, is not recycled. It is ultimately excreted with the feces and gives them their color. Failure to absorb bilirubin or failure to conjugate it or secrete glucuronide can produce ***jaundice.***

Bile flow from the liver is regulated by hormonal and neural control. The rate of blood flow to the liver and the concentration of bile salts in the blood exert regulatory effects on the bile flow. Bile flow is increased when hormones such as cholecystokinin (CCK), gastrin, and motilin are released by enteroendocrine cells during digestion. Steroid hormones (i.e., estrogen during pregnancy) decrease bile secretion from the liver. In addition, parasympathetic stimulation increases bile flow by prompting contraction of the gallbladder and relaxation of the sphincter of Oddi. Bile that leaves the liver via the common hepatic duct flows through the cystic duct to the gallbladder. The gallbladder stores and can increase the concentration of bile up to 10-fold. Following stimulation, the gallbladder contracts and delivers the bile to the duodenum via the common bile duct.

The liver has both sympathetic and parasympathetic innervation

The liver (and gallbladder) receives nerves from both sympathetic and parasympathetic divisions of the autonomic nervous system. The nerves enter the liver at the porta hepatis and ramify through the liver in the portal canals along with the members of the portal triad. Sympathetic fibers are believed to innervate blood vessels; parasympathetic fibers are assumed to innervate the large ducts (those that contain smooth muscle in their walls) and possibly blood vessels. The cell bodies of parasympathetic neurons are often present near the porta hepatis.

▼ GALLBLADDER

The gallbladder is a pear-shaped, distensible sac with a volume of about 50 mL in humans (see Fig. 17.15). It is attached to the visceral surface of the liver. The gallbladder is a secondary derivative of the embryonic foregut, arising as an evagination of the primitive bile duct that connects the embryonic liver to the developing intestine.

The gallbladder concentrates and stores bile

The gallbladder is a blind pouch that leads, via a neck, to the cystic duct. Through this duct it receives dilute bile from the hepatic duct. Hormones secreted by the enteroendocrine cells of the small intestine in response to the presence of fat in the proximal duodenum, stimulate contractions of the smooth muscle of the gallbladder. As a result of these contractions, concentrated bile is discharged into the common bile duct, which carries the bile to the duodenum.

Mucosa of the gallbladder has several characteristic features

The empty or partially filled gallbladder has numerous deep mucosal folds (Fig. 17.16). The mucosal surface consists of simple columnar epithelium. The tall epithelial cells exhibit the following features:

- Numerous well-developed ***apical microvilli***
- ***Apical junctional complexes*** that join adjacent cells and form a barrier between the lumen and the intercellular compartment
- Localized ***concentrations of mitochondria*** in the apical and basal cytoplasm
- Complex ***lateral plications*** (Fig. 17.17)

These cells closely resemble the absorptive cells of the intestine.

Both cells share the above characteristics, as well as localization of Na^+/K^+-activated ATPase on their lateral plasma membranes and secretory vesicles filled with glycoproteins in their apical cytoplasm.

The lamina propria of the mucosa is particularly rich in fenestrated capillaries and small venules, but there are no lymphatic vessels in this layer. The lamina propria is also very cellular, containing large numbers of lymphocytes and plasma cells. The characteristics of the lamina propria resemble those of the colon, another organ specialized for the absorption of electrolytes and water.

Mucin-secreting glands are sometimes present in the lamina propria in the normal human gallbladder, especially near the neck of the organ, but they are more commonly found in inflamed gallbladders. Cells that appear identical to enteroendocrine cells of the intestine are also found in these glands.

The wall of the gallbladder lacks a muscularis mucosae and submucosa

External to the lamina propria is a ***muscularis externa*** that has numerous collagen and elastic fibers among the

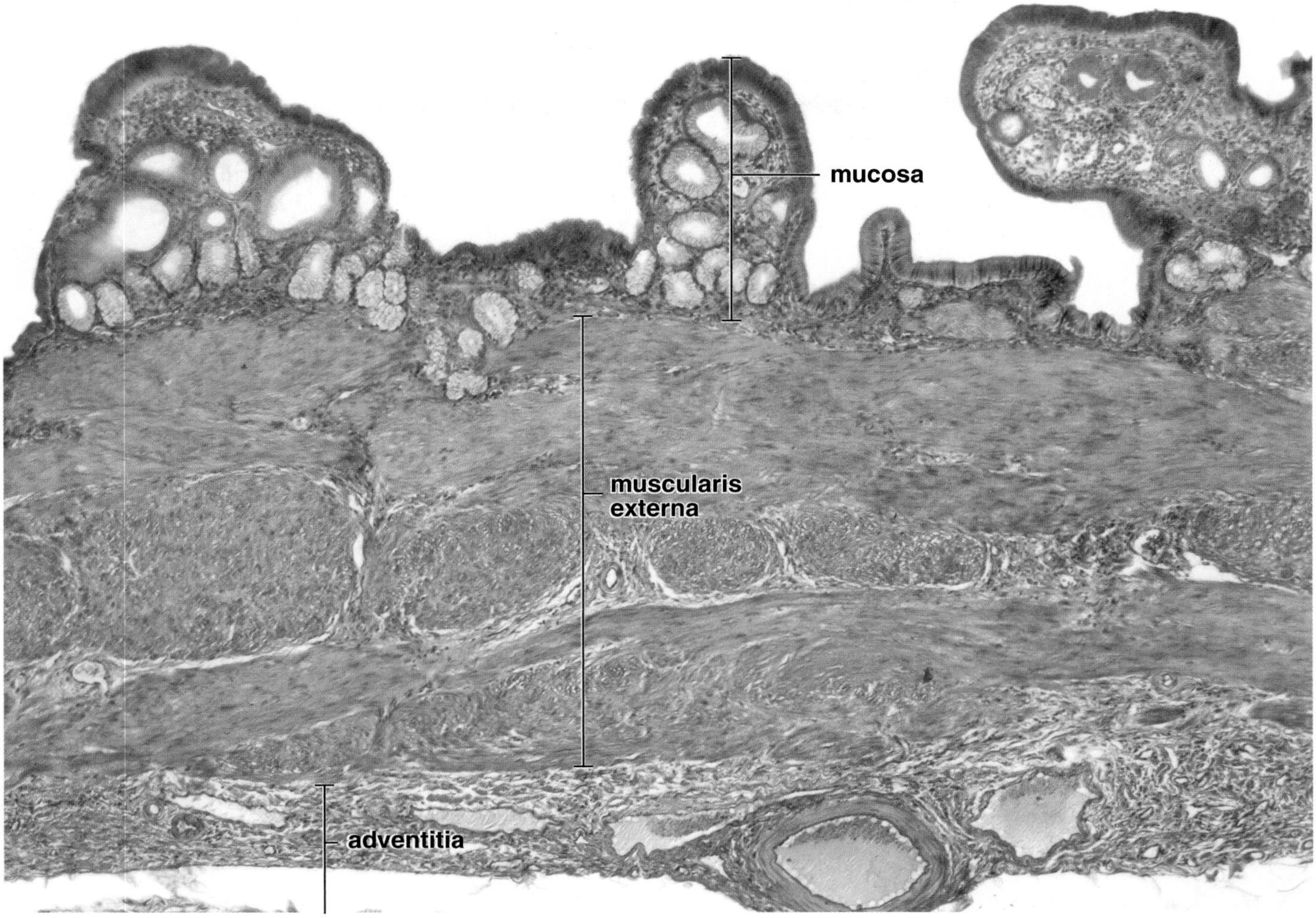

FIGURE 17.16
Photomicrograph of the wall of the gallbladder. The mucosa of the gallbladder consists of a lining of simple columnar epithelial cells and a lamina propria of loose connective tissue, which typically exhibits numerous deep folds in the mucosa. Beneath this layer is a relatively thick layer, the muscularis externa. There is no muscularis mucosae or submucosa. The smooth muscle bundles of the muscularis externa are randomly oriented. External to the muscle is an adventitia containing adipose tissue and blood vessels. The portion of the gallbladder not attached to the liver displays a typical serosa instead of an adventitia. ×175.

bundles of smooth muscle cells. Despite its origin from a foregut-derived tube, the gallbladder does not have a muscularis mucosae or submucosa. The smooth muscle bundles are somewhat randomly oriented, unlike the layered organization of the intestine. Contraction of the smooth muscle reduces the volume of the bladder, forcing its contents out through the cystic duct.

External to the muscularis externa is a thick layer of dense connective tissue (see Fig. 17.16). This layer contains large blood vessels, an extensive lymphatic network, and the autonomic nerves that innervate the muscularis externa and the blood vessels (cell bodies of parasympathetic neurons are found in the wall of the cystic duct). The connective tissue is also rich in elastic fibers and adipose tissue. Where the gallbladder attaches to the liver surface, this layer is referred to as the ***adventitia***. The unattached surface is covered by a ***serosa*** or visceral peritoneum consisting of a layer of mesothelium and a thin layer of loose connective tissue.

In addition, deep diverticula of the mucosa, called ***Rokitansky-Aschoff sinuses***, sometimes extend through the muscularis externa (Fig. 17.18). They are thought to presage pathologic changes. Also, bacteria may accumulate in these sinuses, causing chronic inflammation.

Concentration of the bile requires the coupled transport of salt and water

The epithelial cells of the gallbladder actively transport both Na^+ and Cl^- (and HCO_3^-) from the cytoplasm into

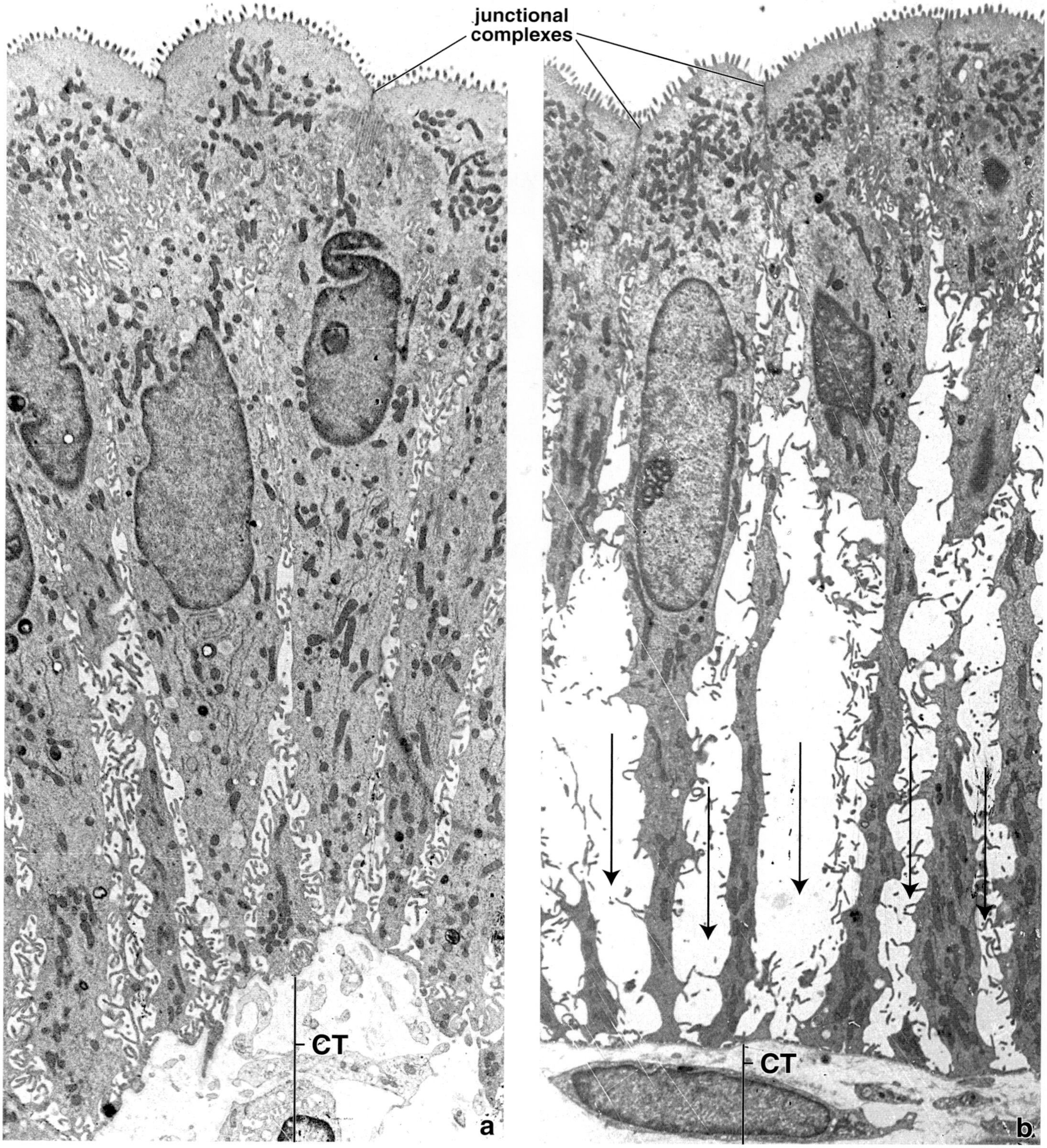

FIGURE 17.17

Electron micrographs of gallbladder epithelium. a. The tall columnar cells display features typical of absorptive cells, with microvilli on their apical surface, an apical junctional complex separating the lumen of the gallbladder from the lateral intercellular space, and numerous mitochondria in the apical portion of the cell. ×3,000. **b.** During active fluid transport, salt is pumped from the cytoplasm into the intercellular space, and water follows the salt. Both salt and water then diffuse into the cell from the lumen. As this process continues, the intercellular space becomes greatly distended *(arrows)*. Fluid moves from the engorged intercellular space *(arrows)* across the basal lamina into the underlying connective tissue *(CT)* and then into blood vessels. The increase in size of the lateral intercellular space during active fluid transport is evident with the light microscope. ×3,000.

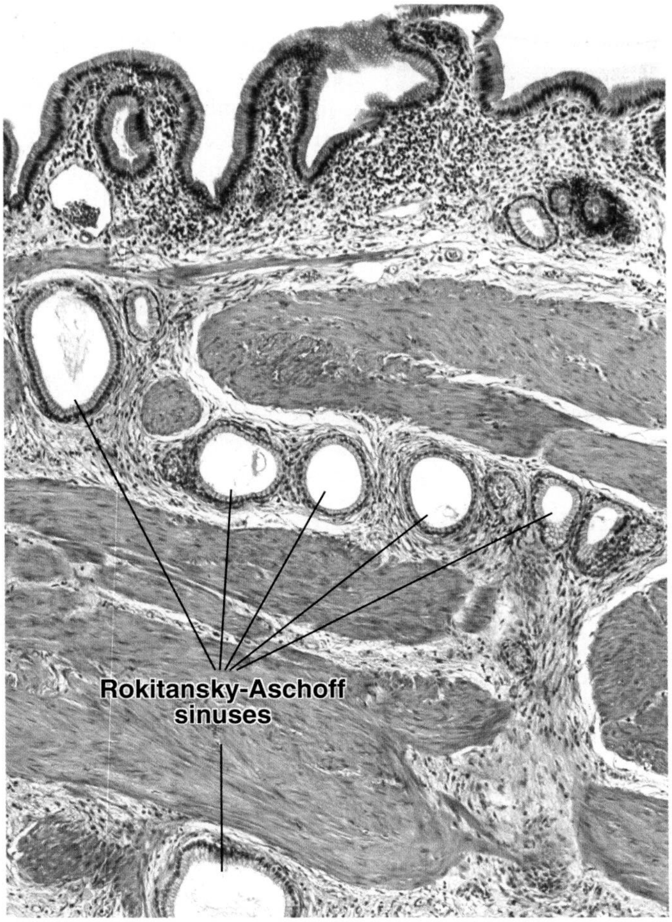

FIGURE 17.18
Photomicrograph of the Rokitansky-Aschoff sinuses in the wall of the gallbladder. This photomicrograph shows deep invaginations of the mucosa extending into the muscularis externa. These invaginations are referred to as Rokitansky-Aschoff sinuses. ×120.

the intercellular compartment of the epithelium. ATPase is located in the lateral plasma membranes of the epithelial cells. This active transport mechanism is essentially identical to that described in Chapter 16 for the enterocytes of the small intestine and the absorptive cells of the colon.

Active transport of Na^+, Cl^-, and HCO_3^- across the lateral plasma membrane into the intercellular (paracellular) compartment causes the concentration of electrolytes in the intercellular space to increase. The increased electrolyte concentration creates an osmotic gradient between the intercellular space and the cytoplasm and between the intercellular space and the lumen. Water moves from the cytoplasm and from the lumen into the intercellular space because of the osmotic gradient, i.e., it moves down its concentration gradient (see Fig. 17.17b). Although the intercellular space can distend to a degree often visible with the light microscope, this ability is limited. The movement of electrolytes and water into the space creates hydrostatic pressure that forces a nearly isotonic fluid out of the intercellular compartment into the subepithelial connective tissue (the lamina propria). The fluid that enters the lamina propria quickly passes into the numerous fenestrated capillaries and the venules that closely underlie the epithelium. Studies of fluid transport in the gallbladder first demonstrated the essential role of the intercellular compartment in transepithelial transport of an isotonic fluid from the lumen to the vasculature.

▼ PANCREAS

Overview

The *pancreas* is an elongate gland described as having a head, body, and tail. The ***head*** is an expanded portion that lies in the C-shaped curve of the duodenum (Fig. 17.19). It is joined to the duodenum by connective tissue. The centrally located ***body*** of the pancreas crosses the midline of the human body, and the ***tail*** extends toward the hilum of the spleen. The ***pancreatic duct (of Wirsung)*** extends through the length of the gland and empties into the duo-

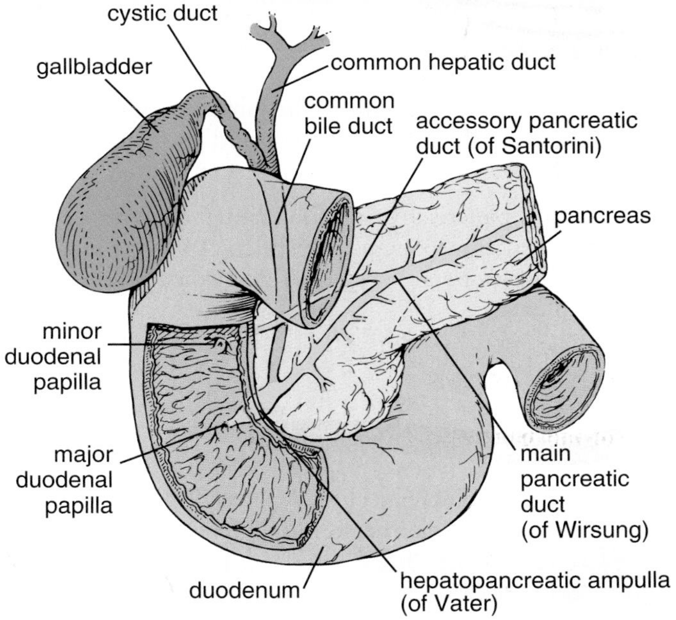

FIGURE 17.19
Diagram of pancreas, duodenum, and associated excretory ducts. The main pancreatic duct (of Wirsung) traverses the length of the pancreas and enters the duodenum after joining with the common bile duct. An accessory pancreatic duct (of Santorini) is commonly present, as shown, and empties into the duodenum at a separate minor duodenal papilla. The site of entry of the common bile duct and main pancreatic duct into the duodenum is typically marked by a major duodenal papilla visible on the inner surface of the duodenum.

denum at the ***hepatopancreatic ampulla (of Vater)*** through which the common bile duct from the liver and gallbladder also enters the duodenum. The ***hepatopancreatic sphincter (of Oddi)*** surrounds the ampulla and not only regulates the flow of bile and pancreatic juice into the duodenum but also prevents reflux of intestinal contents into the pancreatic duct. In some individuals, an ***accessory pancreatic duct (of Santorini)*** is present, a vestige of the pancreas's origin from two embryonic endodermal primordia that evaginate from the foregut.

A thin layer of loose connective tissue forms a capsule around the gland. From this capsule, septa extend into the gland, dividing it into ill-defined lobules. Within the lobules, a stroma of loose connective tissue surrounds the parenchymal units. Between the lobules, larger amounts of connective tissue surround the larger ducts, blood vessels, and nerves. Moreover, in the connective tissue surrounding the pancreatic duct, there are small mucous glands that empty into the duct.

The pancreas is an exocrine and endocrine gland

Unlike the liver, in which the exocrine and secretory (endocrine) functions reside in the same cell, the dual functions of the pancreas are relegated to two structurally distinct components.

- The ***exocrine component*** synthesizes and secretes enzymes into the duodenum that are essential for digestion in the intestine.
- The ***endocrine component*** synthesizes and secretes the hormones ***insulin*** and ***glucagon*** into the blood. These hormones regulate glucose, lipid, and protein metabolism in the body.

The exocrine pancreas is found throughout the organ; within the exocrine pancreas, distinct cell masses called ***islets of Langerhans*** are dispersed and constitute the endocrine pancreas.

Exocrine Pancreas

The exocrine pancreas is a serous gland

The exocrine pancreas closely resembles the parotid gland, with which it can be confused. The secretory units are acinar or tubuloacinar in shape and are formed by a simple epithelium of pyramidal serous cells (Fig. 17.20a). The cells have a narrow free (luminal) surface and a broad basal surface. Periacinar connective tissue is minimal.

The serous secretory cells of the acinus produce the digestive enzyme precursors secreted by the pancreas. Pancreatic acini are unique among glandular acini; the initial duct that leads from the acinus, the ***intercalated duct,*** actually begins within the acinus (Fig. 17.20b). The duct cells located inside the acinus are referred to as ***centroacinar cells.***

The acinar cells are characterized by distinct basophilia in the basal cytoplasm and by acidophilic ***zymogen granules*** in the apical cytoplasm (see Fig. 17.20a). Zymogen granules are most numerous in the pancreas of fasting individuals. The squamous centroacinar cells lack both ergastoplasm and secretory granules; thus, they stain very lightly with eosin. This weak staining helps identify them in routine histologic sections.

Zymogen granules contain a variety of digestive enzymes in an inactive form

Pancreatic enzymes can digest most food substances. The inactive enzymes, or proenzymes, contained in pancreatic zymogen granules are listed below along with the specific substances they digest when activated.

- ***Proteolytic endopeptidases (trypsinogen, chymotrypsinogen)*** and ***proteolytic exopeptidases (procarboxypeptidase, proaminopeptidase)*** digest proteins by cleaving their internal peptide bonds (endopeptidases) or by cleaving amino acids from the carboxyl or amino end of the peptide.
- ***Amylolytic enzymes (α-amylase)*** digest carbohydrates by cleaving the glycosidic linkages of glucose polymers
- ***Lipases*** digest lipids by cleaving ester bonds of triglycerides, producing free fatty acids.
- ***Nucleolytic enzymes (deoxyribonuclease and ribonuclease)*** digest nucleic acids, producing mononucleotides.

The pancreatic digestive enzymes are activated only after they reach the lumen of the small intestine. Initially, the proteolytic activity of enzymes ***(enterokinases)*** in the glycocalyx of the microvilli of the intestinal absorptive cells converts trypsinogen to ***trypsin,*** a potent proteolytic enzyme. Trypsin then catalyzes the conversion of the other inactive enzymes as well as the digestion of proteins in the chyme.

The cytoplasmic basophilia of the pancreatic acinar cells when observed with the TEM appears as an extensive array of rER and free ribosomes. The presence of these numerous organelles correlates with the high level of protein synthetic activity of the acinar cells (Fig. 17.21). A well-developed Golgi apparatus is present in the apical cytoplasm and is involved in concentration and packaging of the secretory products. Mitochondria are small and, although found throughout the cell, are concentrated among the rER cisternae. Acinar cells are joined to one another by junctional complexes at their apical poles, thus forming an isolated lumen into which small microvilli extend from the apical surfaces of the acinar cells and into which the zymogen granules are released by exocytosis.

Duct System of the Exocrine Pancreas

The centroacinar cells (see Fig. 17.20a) are the beginning of the duct system of the exocrine pancreas. They have a

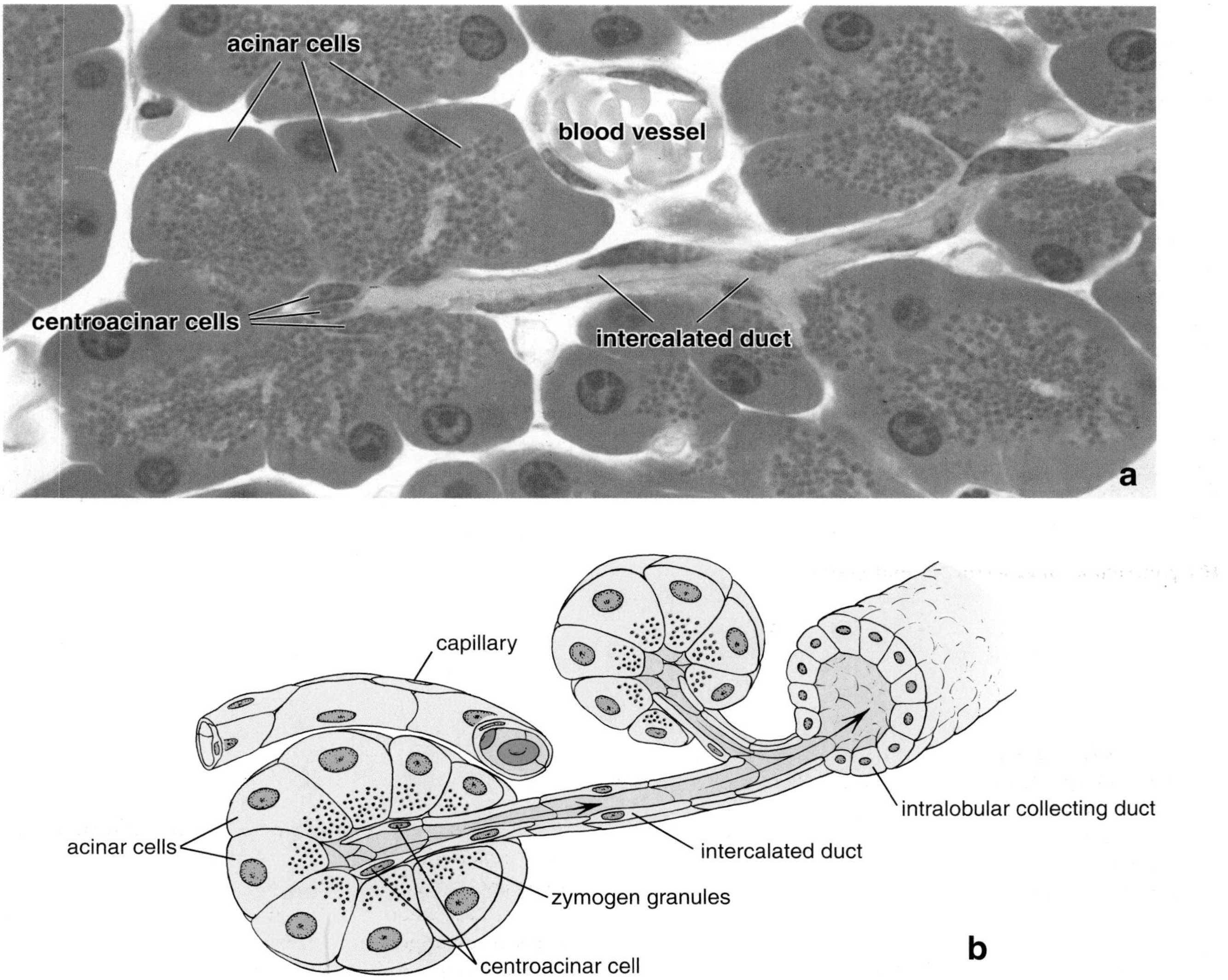

FIGURE 17.20
Pancreatic acinus and its duct system. a. In this photomicrograph of a thin, H&E–stained plastic section, an intercalated duct can be seen beginning within a pancreatic acinus. The cells forming the duct within the acinus are the centroacinar cells. The eosinophilic zymogen granules are clearly seen in the apical cytoplasm of the parenchymal cells. ×860. **b.** In this schematic diagram, observe the beginning of the intercalated duct. Note the location and shapes of the centroacinar cells within the acinus. They represent the initial lining of the intercalated duct, which drains into an intralobular collecting duct.

centrally placed, flattened nucleus and attenuated cytoplasm, which is typical of a squamous cell.

Centroacinar cells are intercalated duct cells located in the acinus

Centroacinar cells are continuous with the cells of the short intercalated duct that lies outside the acinus. The structural unit of the acinus and centroacinar cells resembles a small balloon (the acinus) into which a drinking straw (the intercalated duct) has been pushed. The intercalated ducts are short and drain into intralobular collecting ducts. There are no striated (secretory) ducts in the pancreas.

The complex, branching network of intralobular ducts drains into the larger ***interlobular ducts,*** which are lined with a low columnar epithelium in which enteroendocrine cells and occasional goblet cells may be found. The interlobular ducts, in turn, drain directly into the ***main pancreatic duct,*** which runs the length of the gland parallel to its long axis, giving this portion of the duct system a herringbone-like appearance (see Fig. 17.19). A second large duct, the ***accessory pancreatic duct,*** arises in the head of the pancreas.

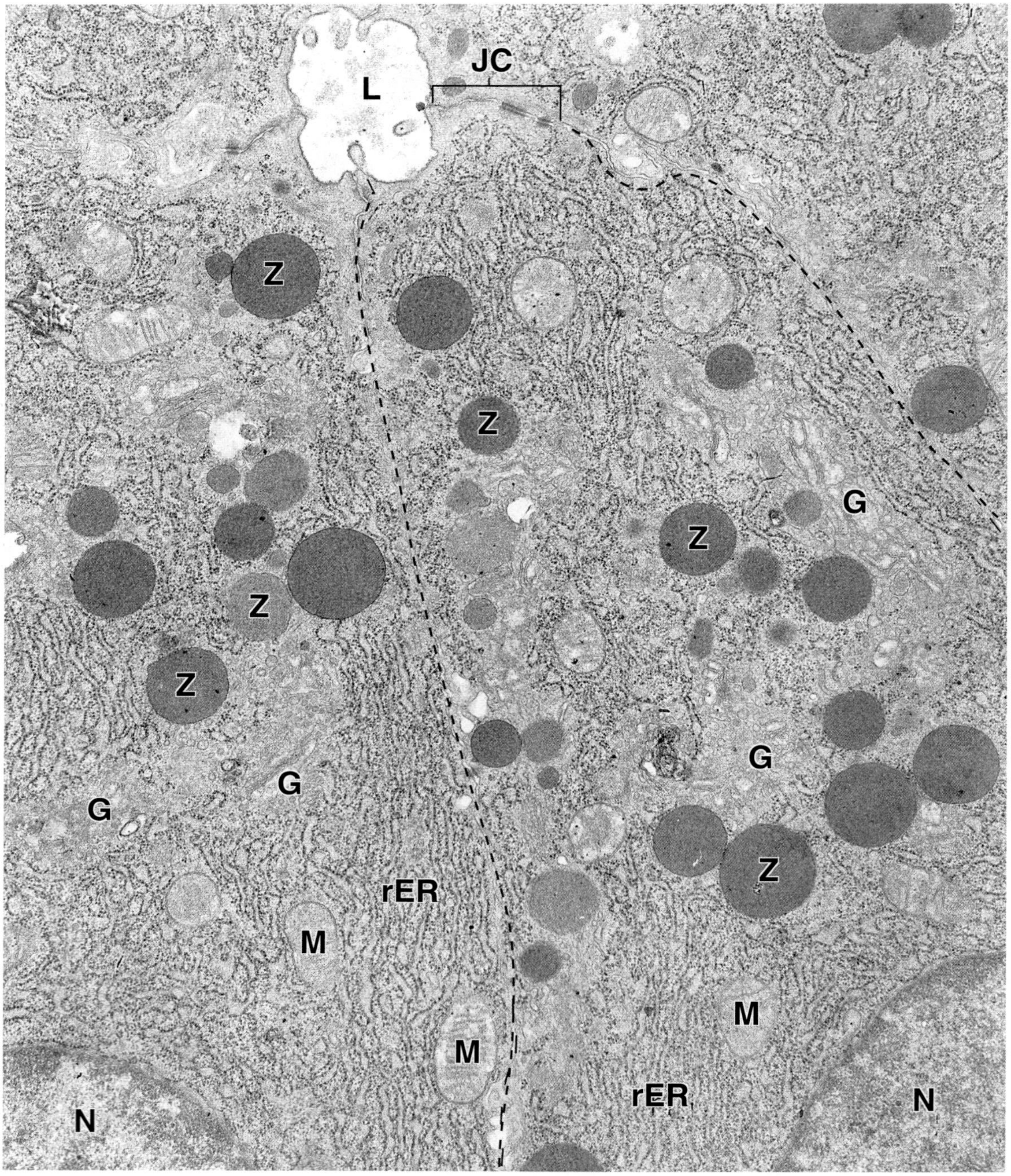

FIGURE 17.21

Electron micrograph of the apical cytoplasm of several pancreatic acinar cells. One pancreatic acinar cell is outlined by the *dashed line.* Nuclei *(N)* of adjoining cells are evident at the bottom left and right of the electron micrograph. The apical cytoplasm contains extensive rough endoplasmic reticulum *(rER),* mitochondria *(M),* zymogen-containing secretory granules *(Z),* and Golgi profiles *(G).* At the apices of these cells, a lumen *(L)* is present, into which the zymogen granules are discharged. A junctional complex *(JC)* is indicated near the lumen. ×20,000.

The intercalated ducts add bicarbonate and water to the exocrine secretion

The pancreas secretes about 1 L of fluid per day, about equal to the initial volume of the hepatic bile secretion. Whereas bile is concentrated in the gallbladder, the entire volume of the pancreatic secretion is delivered to the duodenum. While the acini secrete a small volume of protein-rich fluid, the intercalated duct cells secrete a large volume of fluid rich in sodium and bicarbonate. The bicarbonate

serves to neutralize the acidity of the chyme that enters the duodenum from the stomach and to establish the optimal pH for the activity of the major pancreatic enzymes.

Pancreatic exocrine secretion is under hormonal and neural control

Two hormones secreted by the enteroendocrine cells of the duodenum, ***secretin and CCK***, are the principal regulators of the exocrine pancreas (see Tables 16.1 and 16.2). The entry of the acidic chyme into the duodenum stimulates the release of these hormones into the blood.

- ***Secretin*** is a polypeptide hormone (27 amino acid residues) that stimulates the duct cells to secrete a large volume of fluid with a high HCO_3^- concentration but little or no enzyme content.
- ***CCK*** is a polypeptide hormone (33 amino acid residues) that causes the acinar cells to secrete their proenzymes.

The coordinated action of the two hormones results in the secretion of a large volume of enzyme-rich, alkaline fluid into the duodenum. In addition to hormonal influences, the pancreas also receives autonomic innervation. Sympathetic nerve fibers are involved in regulation of pancreatic blood flow. Parasympathetic fibers stimulate activity of acinar as well as centroacinar cells. Cell bodies of neurons occasionally seen in the pancreas belong to parasympathetic postganglionic neurons.

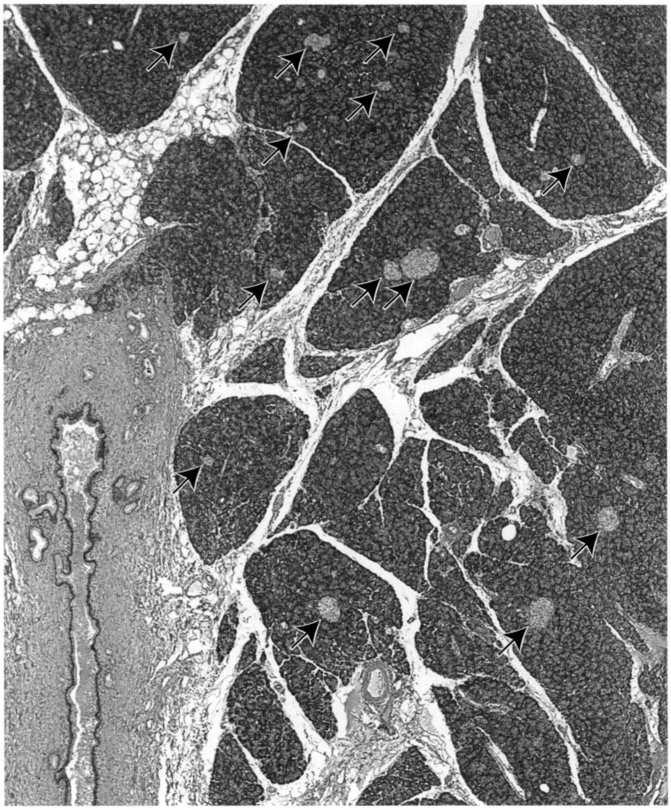

FIGURE 17.22
Photomicrograph of the pancreas. This H&E–stained specimen shows a number of pancreatic lobules separated by connective tissue septa that are continuous with the thin surrounding capsule of the gland. The pancreatic lobules consist largely of the exocrine acini and their intralobular duct system. Most of the lobules exhibit small, round, lighter-staining profiles, which are the islets of Langerhans *(arrows)*. Adjacent to the lobules, at the lower left, is a large interlobular duct that serves the exocrine pancreas. ×25.

Endocrine Pancreas

The endocrine pancreas is a diffuse organ that secretes hormones that regulate blood glucose levels

The islets of Langerhans, the endocrine component of the pancreas, are scattered throughout the organ in cell groupings of varying size (Fig. 17.22). The islets constitute about 1 to 2% of the volume of the pancreas but are most numerous in the tail. Individual islets may contain only a few cells or many hundreds of cells. Their polygonal cells are arranged in short, irregular cords that are profusely invested with a network of fenestrated capillaries. The definitive endocrine cells of the islets develop between 9 and 12 weeks of gestation.

In H&E–stained sections, the islets of Langerhans appear as clusters of pale-staining cells surrounded by more intensely staining pancreatic acini. It is not practical to attempt to identify the several cell types found in the islets in routinely prepared specimens (Fig. 17.23). After Zenker-formol fixation and staining by the Mallory-Azan method, however, it is possible to identify three principal cell types designated A *(alpha)*, B *(beta)*, and D *(delta)* cells (Table 17.2 and Fig. 17.24). With this method, the A cells stain red, the B cells stain brownish orange, and the D cells stain blue. About 5% of the cells appear to be unstained after this procedure. TEM allows identification of the principal cell types by the size and density of their secretory granules.

Islet cells, other than B cells, are counterparts of the enteroendocrine cells of the gastrointestinal mucosa

In addition to the three principal islet cells, three minor islet cell types have also been identified by using a combination of the TEM and immunocytochemistry (Table 17.3). Each cell type can be correlated with a specific hormone, and each has a specific location in the islet.

B cells constitute about 70% of the total islet cells in humans and are generally located in its central portion. They secrete ***insulin*** (see Table 17.2). B cells contain numerous secretory granules about 300 nm in diameter with a dense polyhedral core and a pale matrix. The polyhedral core is believed to be crystallized insulin.

A cells constitute about 15 to 20% of the human islet population and are generally located peripherally in the

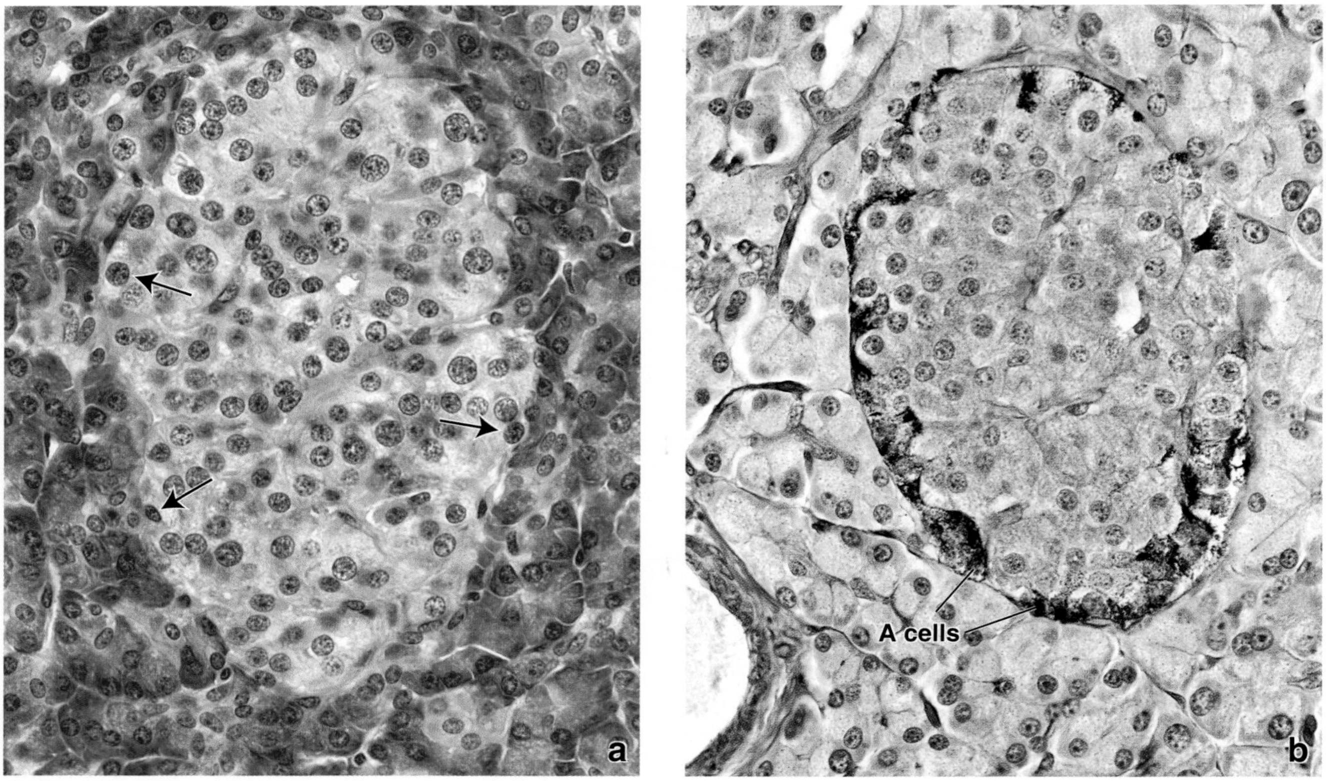

FIGURE 17.23
Photomicrographs of islets of Langerhans. a. In this routine H&E preparation, it is difficult to identify specific islet cell types without special stains. At best, one can identify small cells *(arrows)* at the periphery of the islet that are probably A cells. ×360. **b.** This photomicrograph shows an islet of Langerhans stained with a special Grimelius silver stain that reacts with glucagon-secreting cells. The silver-impregnated A cells are arranged around the periphery of the islet. ×360.

TABLE 17.2. **Principal Cell Types in Pancreatic Islets**

Cell Type	%	Cytoplasmic Staining with Mallory-Azan	Product	Granules (TEM)
A	15–20	Red	Glucagon	About 250 nm; dense, eccentric core surrounded by light substance
B	60–70	Brownish orange	Insulin	About 300 nm; many with dense, crystalline (angular) core surrounded by light substance
D	5–10	Blue	Somatostatin	About 325 nm; homogeneous matrix

TABLE 17.3. **Minor Cell Types in Pancreatic Islets**

Cell Type	Secretion	Location (in Addition to Islet)	Actions
PP cell (F cell)[A]	Pancreatic polypeptide		Stimulates gastric chief cells, inhibits bile secretion and intestinal motility, inhibits pancreatic enzymes and HCO_3^- secretion
D-1 cell	Vasoactive intestinal peptide (VIP)	Also in exocrine acini and duct epithelium[B]	Similar to those of glucagon (hyperglycemic and glycogenolytic); also affects secretory activity and motility in gut; stimulates pancreatic exocrine secretion
EC cell[A]	Secretin, motilin, substance P	Also in exocrine acini and duct epithelium[B]	Secretin: acts locally to stimulate HCO_3^- secretion in pancreatic juice and pancreatic enzyme secretion Motilin: increases gastric and intestinal motility Substance P: has neurotransmitter properties

[A]PP, protein polypeptide; EC, enterochromaffin cell.
[B]This localization further emphasizes the ontogeny of the pancreas from the embryonic gut.

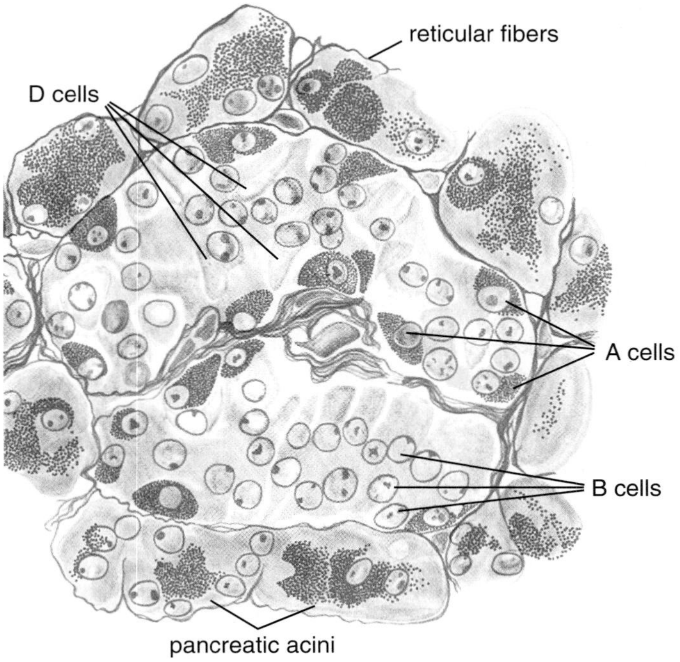

FIGURE 17.24
Diagram of an islet of Langerhans stained by the Mallory-Azan method. A cells display red cytoplasmic staining, B cells (comprising most of the islet cells) display brownish-orange staining, and D cells show a blue cytoplasm.

islets. They secrete ***glucagon*** (see Table 17.2). A cells contain secretory granules about 250 nm in diameter that are more uniform in size and more densely packed in the cytoplasm than the granules of B cells. The granule is the site of stored glucagon (Fig. 17.25).

D cells constitute about 5 to 10% of the total pancreatic endocrine tissue and are also located peripherally in the islets. D cells secrete ***somatostatin***, which is contained in secretory granules that are larger than those of the A and B cells (300 to 350 nm) and contain material of low to medium electron density (see Fig. 17.25).

The minor islet cells constitute about 5% of the islet tissue and may be equivalent to the pale cells seen after Mallory-Azan staining. Their characteristics and functions are summarized in Table 17.3.

Evidence suggests that some cells may secrete more than one hormone. Immunocytochemical staining has localized several hormones in addition to glucagon in the A cell cytoplasm. These include ***gastric inhibitory peptide (GIP), CCK***, and ***adrenocorticotropic hormone (ACTH)-endorphin***. Although there is no clear morphologic evidence for the presence of G cells (gastrin cells) in the islets, ***gastrin*** may also be secreted by one or more of the islet cells. Certain pancreatic islet cell tumors secrete large amounts of gastrin, thereby producing excessive acid secretion in the stomach (Zollinger-Ellison syndrome).

FUNCTIONS OF PANCREATIC HORMONES

All of the hormones secreted by the endocrine pancreas regulate metabolic functions either systemically, regionally (in the gastrointestinal tract), or locally (in the islet itself).

Insulin, the major hormone secreted by the islet tissue, decreases blood glucose levels

Insulin is the most abundant endocrine secretion. Its principal effects are on the liver, skeletal muscle, and adipose tissue. Insulin has multiple individual actions in each of these tissues. In general, insulin stimulates

- ***Uptake of glucose*** from the circulation. Specific cell membrane glucose transporters are involved in this process.
- ***Storage of glucose*** by activation of glycogen synthase and subsequent glycogen synthesis.
- ***Phosphorylation and use of glucose*** by promoting its glycolysis within cells.

Absence or inadequate amounts of insulin lead to elevated blood glucose levels and the presence of glucose in the urine, a condition known as ***diabetes mellitus***.

In addition to its effects on glucose metabolism, insulin stimulates glycerol synthesis and inhibits lipase activity in adipose cells. Circulating insulin also increases the amount of amino acids taken up by cells (which may involve cotransport with glucose) and inhibits protein catabolism. Insulin appears to be essential for normal cell growth and function, as demonstrated in tissue culture systems.

Glucagon, secreted in amounts second only to insulin, increases blood glucose levels

The actions of ***glucagon*** are essentially reciprocal to those of insulin. It stimulates release of glucose into the bloodstream, and stimulates gluconeogenesis (synthesis of glucose from metabolites of amino acids) and glycogenolysis (breakdown of glycogen) in the liver. Glucagon also stimulates proteolysis to promote gluconeogenesis, mobilizes fats from adipose cells, and stimulates hepatic lipase.

Somatostatin inhibits insulin and glucagon secretion

Somatostatin is secreted by the D cells of the islets. It is identical with the hormone secreted by the hypothalamus that regulates somatotropin (growth hormone) release from the anterior pituitary gland. Although the precise role of somatostatin in the islets is unclear, it has been shown to inhibit both insulin and glucagon secretion.

The molecular characteristics of the major and some minor islet hormones are summarized in Table 17.4.

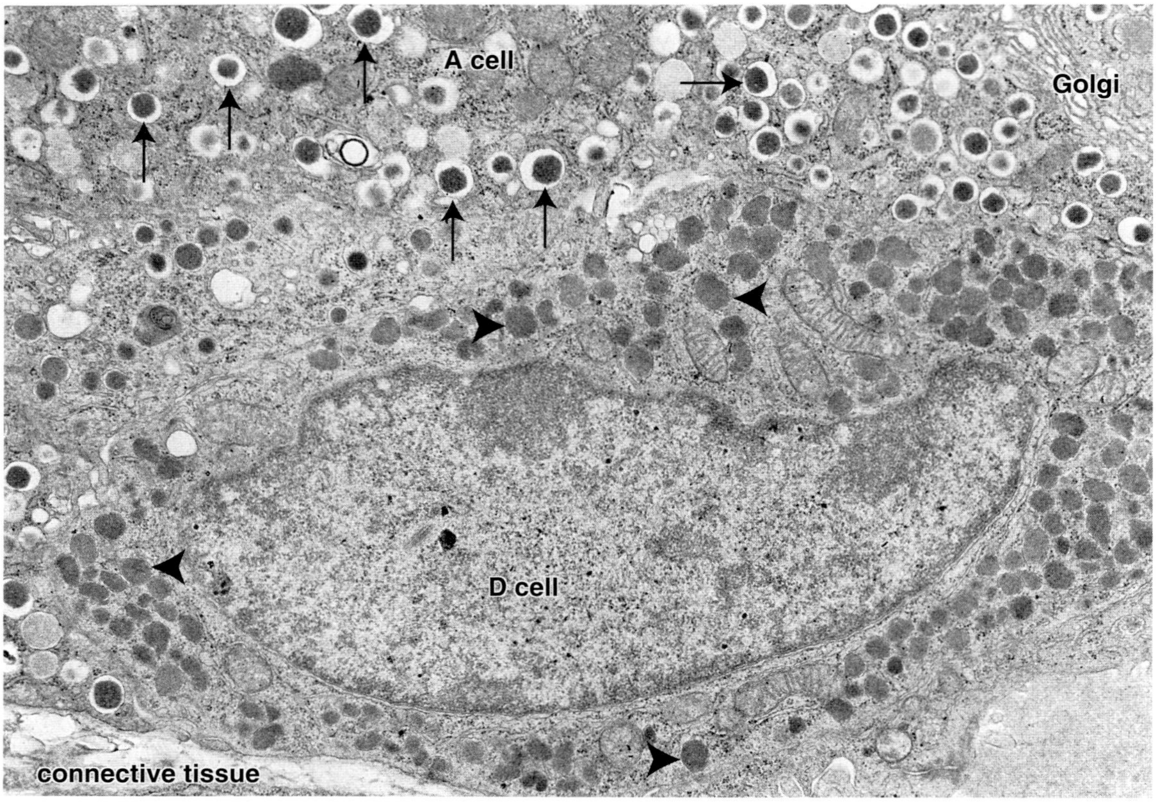

FIGURE 17.25
Electron micrograph of pancreatic islet cells. The portion of the cell in the upper part of the illustration is an A cell. It contains characteristic granules *(arrows)* showing a dense spherical core surrounded by a clear area and then a membrane. This cell also displays a characteristically well-developed Golgi apparatus. The cell in the bottom of the illustration is a D cell. It contains numerous membrane-bounded granules of moderately low density *(arrowheads).* ×15,000.

TABLE 17.4. **Characteristics of Pancreatic Hormones**

Hormone	Molecular Weight (Da)	Structure
Insulin	5700–6000	Two protein chains linked by disulfide bridges: α chain, 21 amino acids; β chain, 30 amino acids
Glucagon	3500	Linear polypeptide: 29 amino acids
Somatostatin	1638	Cyclic polypeptide: 14 amino acids
VIP	3300	Linear polypeptide: 28 amino acids
Pancreatic polypeptide	4200	Linear polypeptide

REGULATION OF ISLET ACTIVITY

A blood glucose level above the normal 70 mg/100 mL (70 mg/dL) stimulates release of insulin from beta cells, leading to uptake and storage of glucose by liver and muscle. The resultant decrease in the blood glucose level stops insulin secretion. Some amino acids also stimulate insulin secretion, either alone or in concert with elevated blood glucose levels. Increased blood fatty acid levels also stimulate insulin release, as do circulating gastrin, CCK, and secretin. CCK and glucagon, released in the islet by the A cells, act as paracrine secretions to stimulate B cell secretion of insulin.

Blood glucose levels below 70 mg/100 mL stimulate release of glucagon; blood glucose levels significantly above 70 mg/100 mL inhibit glucagon secretion. Glucagon is also released in response to low levels of fatty acids in the blood. Insulin inhibits release of glucagon by A cells, but because of the cascading circulation in the islet (see below), this inhibition is effected by a hormonal action of insulin carried in the general circulation.

The islets have both sympathetic and parasympathetic innervation. About 10% of the islet cells have nerve endings directly on their plasma membrane. Well-developed gap junctions are located between islet cells. Ionic events triggered by synaptic transmitters at the nerve endings are carried from cell to cell across these junctions. Autonomic nerves may have direct effects on hormone secretion by A and B cells.

Parasympathetic (cholinergic) stimulation increases secretion of both insulin and glucagon; sympathetic (adrenergic) stimulation increases glucagon release but inhibits insulin release. This neural control of insulin and glucagon may contribute to the availability of circulating glucose in stress reactions.

The blood supply to the pancreas provides a cascading perfusion of the islets and acini

Several arterioles enter the periphery of the islets and branch into fenestrated capillaries. In humans, the capillaries first perfuse the A and D cells, peripherally, before the blood reaches the B cells, centrally. Larger vessels that travel in septa that penetrate the central portion of the islet are also accompanied by A and D cells, so that blood reaching the B cells has always first perfused the A and D cells.

Large **efferent capillaries** leave the islet and branch into the capillary networks that surround the acini of the exocrine pancreas. This cascading flow resembles the portal systems of other endocrine glands (pituitary, adrenal).

Secretions of the islet cells have regulatory effects on the acinar cells:

- Insulin, the vasoactive intestinal peptide (VIP), and CCK stimulate exocrine secretion.
- Glucagon, pancreatic polypeptide (PP), and somatostatin inhibit exocrine secretion.

BOX 17.3

Functional Considerations: Insulin Synthesis, An Example of Posttranslational Processing

Insulin is a small protein consisting of two polypeptide chains joined by disulfide bridges. Its biosynthesis presents a clear example of the importance of posttranslational processing in the achievement of the final, active structure of a protein.

Insulin is originally synthesized as a single 110–amino acid polypeptide chain with a molecular weight of about 12,000 Da. This polypeptide is called ***preproinsulin***. Preproinsulin is reduced to a polypeptide with a molecular weight of about 9000 Da, called ***proinsulin***, as the molecule is inserted into the cisternae of the rER. Proinsulin is a single polypeptide chain of 81 to 86 amino acids that has the approximate shape of the letter G. Two disulfide bonds connect the bar of the G to the top loop.

During packaging and storage of proinsulin in the Golgi apparatus, a cathepsin-like enzyme cleaves most of the side of the loop, leaving the bar of the G as an ***A chain*** of 21 amino acids cross-linked by the disulfide bridges to the top of the loop, which becomes the ***B chain*** of 30 amino acids. The 35–amino acid peptide removed from the loop is called a ***C peptide*** (connecting peptide). It is stored in the secretory vesicles and released with the insulin in equimolar amounts. No function has been identified for the C peptide. However, measurement of circulating levels of C peptide sometimes provides important clinical information on the secretory activity of B cells.

PLATE 61. LIVER I

The liver is the largest mass of glandular tissue in the body and the largest internal organ. It is unique because it receives its major blood supply from the *hepatic portal vein,* which carries venous blood from the small intestine, pancreas, and spleen. Thus the liver is directly in the pathway that conveys materials absorbed in the intestine. This gives the liver the first exposure to metabolic substrates and nutrients; it also makes the liver the first organ exposed to noxious and toxic substances absorbed from the intestine. One of the major roles of the liver is to degrade or *conjugate* toxic substances to render them harmless. It can, however, be seriously damaged by an excess of such substances.

Each liver cell has both exocrine and endocrine functions. The exocrine secretion of the liver, called *bile,* contains conjugated and degraded waste products that are delivered back to the intestine for disposal. It also contains substances that bind to metabolites in the intestine to aid absorption. A series of ducts of increasing diameter and complexity, beginning with *canaliculi* between individual hepatocytes and ending with the *common bile duct,* deliver bile from the liver and gallbladder to the duodenum.

The endocrine secretions of the liver are released directly into the blood that supplies the liver cells; these secretions include albumin, nonimmune α- and β-globulins, prothrombin, and glycoproteins, including fibronectin. Glucose, released from stored glycogen, and *triiodothyronine* (T_3), the more active deiodination product of thyroxine, are also released directly into the blood.

Functional units of the liver, described as lobules or acini, are made up of irregular interconnecting sheets of hepatocytes separated from one another by the blood sinusoids.

Figure 1, liver, human, H&E ×65; inset ×65.

At the low magnification shown here, large numbers of hepatic cells appear to be uniformly disposed throughout the specimen. The hepatic cells are arranged in one-cell-thick plates, but when sectioned, they appear as interconnecting cords one or more cells thick, depending on the plane of section. The sinusoids appear as light areas between the cords of cells; they are more clearly shown in Figure 2 *(asterisks).*

Also present in this figure is a portal canal. It is a connective tissue septum that carries the branches of the hepatic artery *(HA)* and portal vein *(PV),* bile ducts *(BD),* and lymphatic vessels and nerves. The artery and vein, along with the bile duct, are collectively referred to as a *portal triad.*

The hepatic artery and the portal vein are easy to identify because they are found in relation to one another within the surrounding connective tissue of the portal canal. The vein is typically thin walled; the artery is smaller in diameter and has a thicker wall. The bile ducts are composed of a simple cuboidal or columnar epithelium, depending on the size of the duct. Multiple profiles of the blood vessels and bile ducts may be evident in the canal because of either branching or their passage out of the plane of section and then back in again.

The vessel through which blood leaves the liver is the hepatic vein. It is readily identified because it travels alone **(inset)** and is surrounded by an appreciable amount of connective tissue *(CT).* If more than one profile of a vein is present within this connective tissue, but no arteries or bile ducts are present, the second vessel will also be a hepatic vein. Such is the case in the **inset,** where a profile of a small hepatic vein is seen just above the larger hepatic vein *(HV).*

Figure 2, liver, human, H&E ×160.

The terminal hepatic venules or central veins *(CV)* are the most distal radicals of the hepatic vein, and like the hepatic vein, they also travel alone. Their distinguishing features are the sinusoids that penetrate the wall of the vein and the paucity of surrounding connective tissue. These characteristics are shown to advantage in Plate 62.

It is best to examine low-magnification views of the liver to define the boundaries of a lobule. A lobule is best identified when it is cut in cross section. The central vein then appears as a circular profile, and the hepatic cells appear as cords radiating from the central vein. Such a lobule is outlined by the *dashed line* in Figure 1.

The limits of the lobule are defined, in part, by the portal canal. In other directions, the plates of the lobule do not appear to have a limit; i.e., they have become contiguous with plates of an adjacent lobule. One can estimate the dimensions of the lobule, however, by approximating a circle with the central vein as its center and incorporating those plates that exhibit a radial arrangement up to the point where a portal canal is present. If the lobule has been cross-sectioned, the radial limit is set by the location of one or more of the portal canals as indicated by the bile ducts *(BD)* in this figure.

KEY

BD, bile duct
CT, connective tissue
CV, central vein (terminal hepatic venule)
HA, hepatic artery
HV, hepatic vein
L, lymphatic nodule
PV, portal vein
asterisks (Fig. 2), blood sinusoids
dotted line (Fig. 1), approximates the limits of a lobule

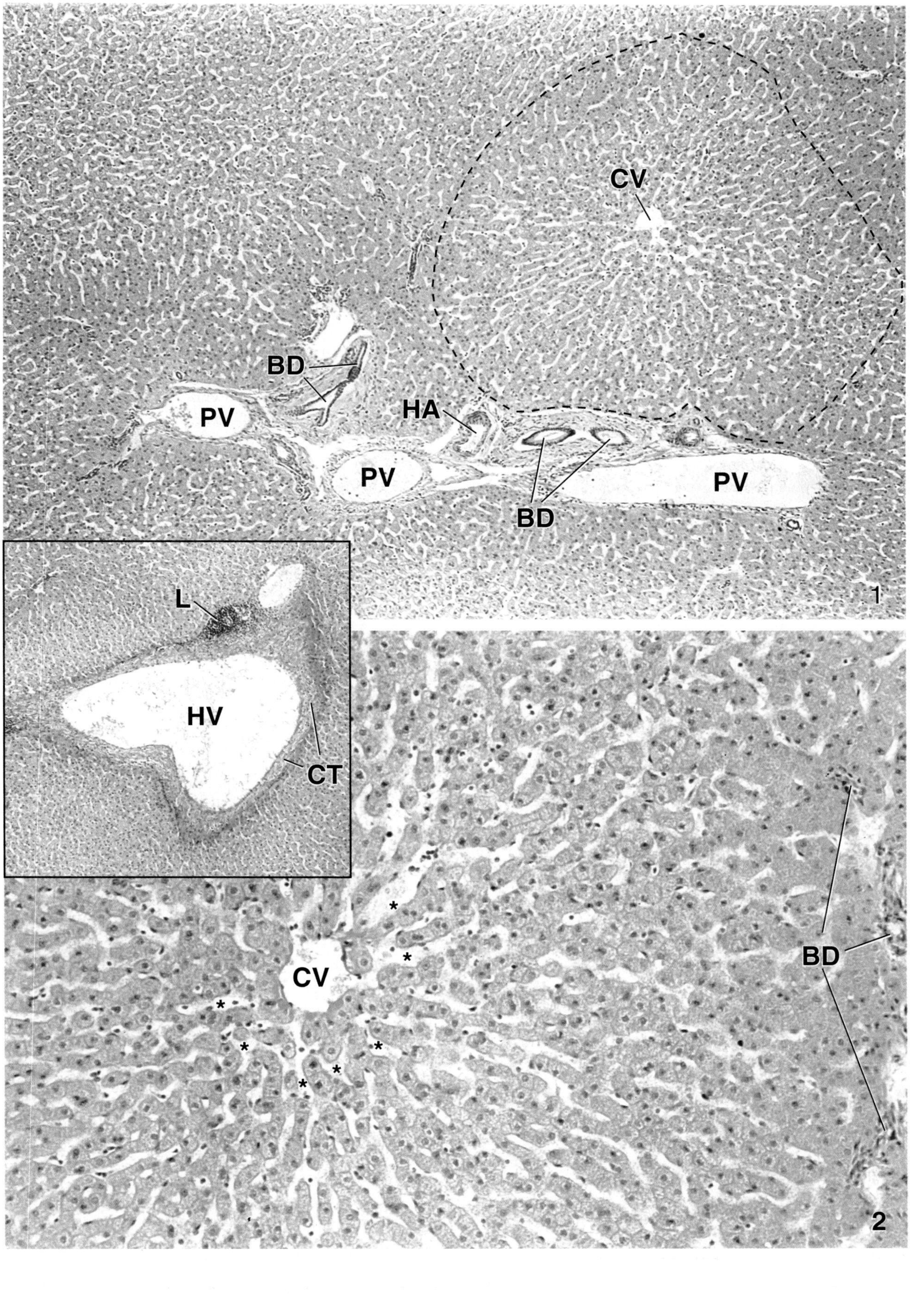
CV
BD
PV
HA
PV
PV
BD
1
L
HV
CT
*
*
CV
*
*
*
*
*
BD
2

PLATE 62. LIVER II

There are three ways of describing the liver parenchyma in terms of a functional unit, *"classic" lobules, portal lobules,* or *acini* (see Fig. 17.5, page 538). The classic lobule is a roughly hexagonal block of tissue that has at its center the terminal hepatic venule (central vein) and at its six corners the *portal canals (portal triads)* containing in each a branch of the portal vein, hepatic artery, and bile duct. The portal lobule is a triangular construct that emphasizes the exocrine secretory function. It has as its axis the bile duct of the portal triad of the classic lobule, and its outer margins are imaginary lines drawn between the central veins closest to that portal triad. The liver acinus provides the best correlation among blood perfusion, metabolic activity, and liver pathology. The acinus is a small diamond- or lozenge-shaped mass of tissue that has as its short axis the fine branches of the portal triad that lie along the border of two classic lobules and as its long axis a line drawn between the two central veins closest to the short axis. The hepatocytes in each acinus are described as arranged in three concentric elliptical zones around the short axis; zone 1 is closest to, and zone 3 is farthest from, the axis.

Figure 1, liver, human, H&E ×500; inset ×800.

The central vein and surrounding hepatocytes from Figure 2 of Plate 61 are shown here at higher magnification. The cytoplasm of the hepatocytes in this specimen has a foamy appearance because of extraction of glycogen and lipid during tissue preparation. The boundaries between individual hepatocytes are discernable in some locations but not between those cells where the knife has cut across the boundary in an oblique plane. Frequently, when cell boundaries are observed at still higher magnification **(inset),** a very small circular or oval profile is observed midway along the boundary. These profiles represent the bile canaliculi *(BC).*

The cells that line the sinusoids *(S)* show little, if any, cytoplasmic detail in routine preparations. Perisinusoidal macrophages (Kupffer cells *[KC]*) are generally recognized by their ovoid nuclei and the projection of the cell into the lumen. The endothelial cell, in contrast, is a squamous cell that has a smaller, attenuated or elongated nucleus. Some nuclei of this description are evident in the micrograph.

The termination of two of the sinusoids and their union with the central vein *(CV)* is indicated by the *curved arrows.* Note that the wall of the vein is strengthened by connective tissue, mostly collagen, which appears as homogeneous eosin-stained material *(asterisks).* Fibroblasts *(F)* within this connective tissue can be identified and distinguished from the endothelial cell *(EN)* lining of the vein.

Figure 2, liver, rat, glutaraldehyde–osmium fixation, toluidine blue ×900.

This figure shows a plastic-embedded liver specimen fixed by the method normally used for electron microscopy. In contrast to the H&E–stained preparation, it demonstrates to advantage the cytologic detail of the hepatocytes and the sinusoids *(S).* The hepatocytes are deeply colored with toluidine blue. Note that the cytoplasm exhibits irregular magenta masses *(arrows).* This is glycogen that has been retained by the glutaraldehyde fixation and stained metachromatically by toluidine blue. Also evident are lipid droplets *(L)* of varying size that have been preserved and stained black by the osmium used as the secondary fixative. The quantities of lipid and glycogen are variable and, under normal conditions, reflect dietary intake. Examination of the hepatocyte cytoplasm also reveals small, punctate, dark-blue bodies contrasted against the lighter-blue background of the cell. These are the mitochondria. Another feature of this specimen is the clear representation of the bile canaliculi *(BC)* between liver cells. They appear as empty circular profiles when cross-sectioned and as elongate channels (lower right) when longitudinally sectioned.

The sinusoidal lining cells are of two distinct types. The Kupffer cells *(KC)* are the more prominent cells. They exhibit a large nucleus and a substantial amount of cytoplasm. They protrude into the lumen and may give the appearance of occluding it. However, they do not block the channel. The surface of the Kupffer cell exhibits a very irregular or jagged contour because of the numerous processes that provide the cell with an extensive surface area. The endothelial cell *(EN)* has a smaller nucleus, attenuated cytoplasm, and a smooth surface contour.

A third cell type, the less frequently observed perisinusoidal lipocyte (Ito cell), is not seen in this micrograph. This cell would appear as a light cell containing numerous lipid droplets. The lipid droplets contain stored vitamin A.

KEY

BC, bile canaliculus
CV, central vein
EN, endothelial cell
F, fibroblast
KC, Kupffer cell
L, lipid droplet
S, sinusoid
arrows (Fig. 2), glycogen
asterisks, connective tissue of central vein
curved arrows, opening of sinusoid into central vein

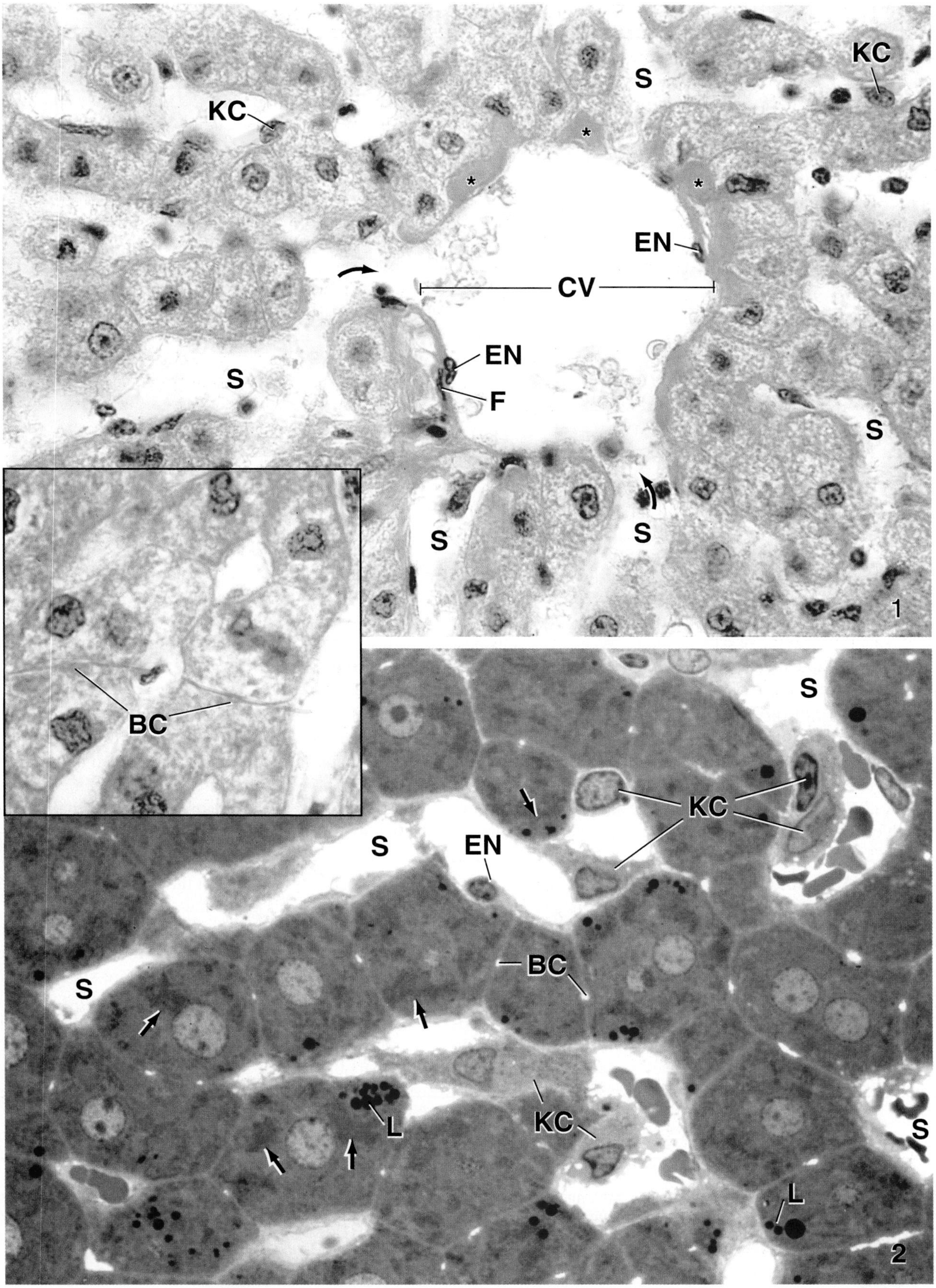
KC
S
KC
*
*
*
EN
CV
EN
S
F
S
S
S
1
BC
S
KC
S
EN
S
BC
L
KC
S
L
2

PLATE 63. GALLBLADDER

The gallbladder concentrates and stores bile for delivery to the duodenum. The bile is concentrated by the active transport of salt from the bile and the passive movement of water in response to the salt transport. The mucosa is characterized by a tall columnar absorptive epithelium that closely resembles that of the intestine and the colon in both its morphology and function. The epithelial cells are characterized by numerous short apical microvilli, apical junctional complexes, concentrations of mitochondria in the apical and basal cytoplasm, and complex lateral plications. In addition, Na^+-K^+–activated ATPase is localized on the lateral plasma membrane of the epithelial cell.

Figure 1, gallbladder, H&E ×45.
The gallbladder is a hollow, pear-shaped organ that concentrates and stores the bile. The full thickness of its wall is shown here. It is composed of a mucosa *(Muc),* muscularis *(Mus),* and adventitia *(Adv)* and, on its free surface (not shown), a serosa. The mucosa is considered at higher magnification in Figure 2. The muscularis consists of interlacing bundles of smooth muscle *(SM).* The adventitia *(Adv)* consists of irregular dense connective tissue through which the larger blood vessels *(BV)* travel and, more peripherally, of varying amounts of adipose tissue *(AT).*

The mucosa is thrown into numerous folds that are particularly pronounced when the muscularis is highly contracted. This is the usual histologic appearance of the gallbladder unless, of course, steps are taken to fix and preserve it in a distended state. Occasionally, the section cuts through a recess in a fold, and the recess may then resemble a gland *(arrows).* The mucosa, however, does not possess glands, except in the neck region, where some mucous glands are present (see Fig. 4).

Figure 2, gallbladder, human, H&E ×325.
The mucosa consists of a tall simple columnar absorptive epithelium *(Ep)* resting on a lamina propria of loose irregular connective tissue *(CT).* The epithelium has characteristics that distinguish it from the absorptive epithelium of other organs, such as the intestines. Only one cell type, tall columnar cells, is present in the epithelial layer (see Fig. 3). The nuclei are in the basal portion of the cell. The cells possess a thin apical striated border. However, this is not always evident in routine H&E–stained sections. The cytoplasm stains rather uniformly with eosin. This is related to its absorptive function and is in contrast to the staining of cells that are engaged in the production of protein. Lastly, with respect to its absorptive function, the epithelial cells frequently exhibit distended intercellular spaces at their basal aspect (see Fig. 3, *arrows*). This is a feature associated with the transport of fluid across the epithelium and, as noted above, commonly seen in intestinal absorptive cells.

Figure 3, gallbladder, human, H&E ×550.
The lamina propria underlying the epithelium is usually very cellular. In this specimen, in addition to lymphocytes *(L),* a relatively common finding, a large number of plasma cells *(PC)* is also present within the lamina propria. (The high concentration of plasma cells suggests chronic inflammation.) Another feature of note in the lamina propria is the presence of several glands and gland-like profiles *(Gl)* other than those seen in the mucosa and noted above. These are readily apparent in Figure 1. Two of these structures, marked by *asterisks* in Figure 1, are shown at higher magnification in Figure 4.

Figure 4, gallbladder, human, H&E ×550.
The smaller of the two gland-like structures is composed of mucous cells *(MC)* and represents a section through a mucous gland. This specimen was taken from a site near the neck of the gallbladder where mucous glands are often present. Note the characteristic flattened nuclei at the base of the cell and the lightly stained appearance of the cytoplasm, features characteristic of mucin-secreting cells. In contrast, the epithelium of the large gland-like profile that is only partially included in the micrograph has rounded or ovoid nuclei. This epithelial-lined structure is not a true gland but represents an invagination of the mucous membrane that extends into and often through the thickness of the muscularis. These invaginations are known as Rokitansky-Aschoff sinuses. Their role or significance, if any, is unknown. (Some authorities contend that they result from disease, but they are also found in small numbers in gallbladders that appear normal in all other respects.)

KEY

Adv, adventitia
AT, adipose tissue
BV, blood vessel
CT, connective tissue, lamina propria
Ep, epithelium
Gl, gland or gland-like structure
L, lymphocytes
MC, mucous cells
Muc, mucosa
Mus, muscularis
PC, plasma cells
SM, smooth muscle
arrows: Fig. 1, recess in luminal surface; Fig. 3, intercellular spaces
asterisks (Fig. 1), gland or gland-like structure

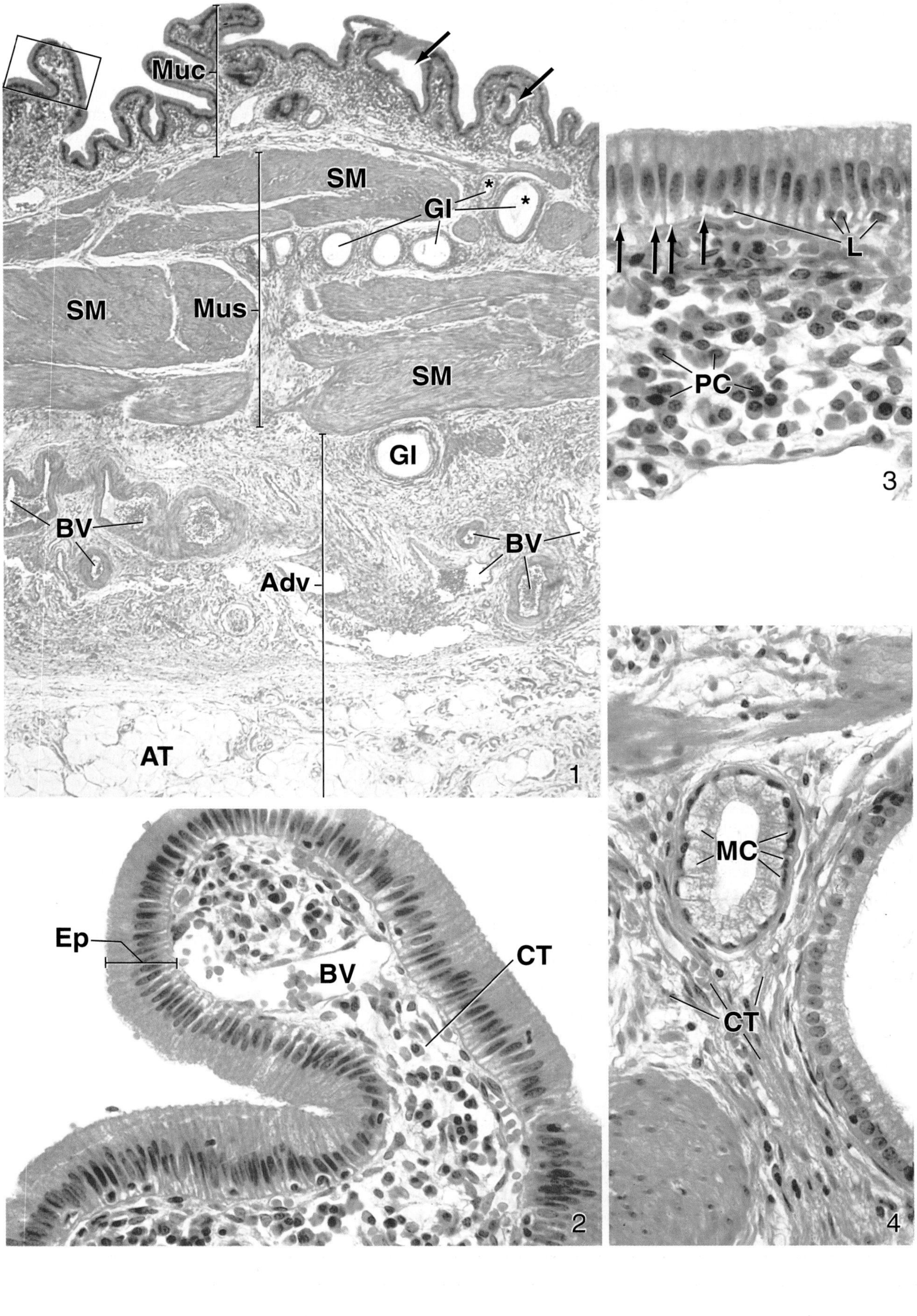
Muc
SM
GI
SM
Mus
SM
GI
BV
BV
Adv
AT
1
Ep
BV
CT
2
L
PC
3
MC
CT
4

PLATE 64. PANCREAS

The pancreas is an elongated extramural digestive gland with a head nestled in the C-shaped bend of the duodenum, a body that crosses the midline of the abdomen, and a tail extending across the back of the abdomen. It is a mixed gland containing both an exocrine component and an endocrine component that have distinctive characteristics. The exocrine component is a compound tubuloacinar gland with a branching network of ducts that convey the exocrine secretions to the duodenum. These secretions consist primarily of inactive forms of potent proteolytic enzymes, as well as amylase, lipase, nucleases, and electrolytes, particularly HCO_3^-.

The endocrine component is isolated as highly vascularized islets of epithelioid tissue (islets of Langerhans). The islet cells secrete a variety of polypeptide and protein hormones, most notably *insulin* and *glucagon,* which regulate glucose metabolism throughout the other tissues of the body. Other hormones secreted by islet cells include *somatostatin, pancreatic polypeptide, vasoactive intestinal peptide, secretin, motilin,* and *substance P.* All of these substances, with the exception of insulin, are also secreted by the population of enteroendocrine cells in the intestine, the organ from which the pancreas is derived during embryonic development. While insulin and glucagon act primarily in endocrine regulation of distant cells, the other hormones (and glucagon) have significant roles in the paracrine regulation of the insulin-secreting B cells of the pancreatic islet.

Figure 1, pancreas, H&E ×160; inset ×360

The pancreas is surrounded by a delicate capsule of moderately dense connective tissue. Septa from the capsule divide the pancreas into lobules, one of which is shown here, bounded by connective tissue *(CT).* Larger blood vessels *(BV)* travel in the connective tissue septa; nerves also travel in the septa, but they are seen infrequently. Within the lobule are the numerous acini of the exocrine component, an intralobular duct *(InD),* intercalated ducts (not readily evident at this low magnification), and islets of Langerhans *(IL).* Also within the lobule are the small blood vessels and the connective tissue serving as a stroma for the parenchymal elements of the gland.

This figure shows an islet of Langerhans *(IL)* among the far more numerous acini. (Islets are most numerous in the tail of the pancreas and least numerous in the head). Cells within the islets are arranged as irregular cords. In routine preparations, it is not possible to identify the various cell types within the islets. Note, however, that B cells are the most numerous; these produce insulin. The next most numerous are A cells; these produce glucagon. The **inset** also shows numerous capillaries *(arrows).* The labels *A* and *B* are not intended to identify specific cells but rather to show those parts of the islets where A and B cells are found in greatest number.

Figure 2, pancreas, H&E ×600.

Acini of the pancreas consist of serous cells. In sections, the acini present circular and irregular profiles. The lumen of the acinus is small, and only in fortuitous sections through an acinus is the lumen included *(asterisks).* The nucleus is characteristically in the base of the acinar cell. There is a region of intense basophilia adjacent to the nucleus. This is the ergastoplasm *(Er),* and it reflects the presence of rER that is active in the synthesis of pancreatic enzymes. Some acini reveal a centrally positioned cell with cytoplasm that shows no special staining characteristics in H&E–stained paraffin sections. These are centroacinar cells *(CC).* They are the beginning of the intercalated ducts.

This figure demonstrates particularly well the morphology and relationships of the intercalated ducts. Note, first, the cross-sectioned intralobular duct *(InD)* consisting of cuboidal epithelium. (There are no striated ducts in the pancreas.) Leading to the intralobular duct is an intercalated duct *(ID),* which is seen in cross section at the furthest distance from the intralobular duct and then, in longitudinal section, in the center of the illustration as it travels toward the intralobular duct. The lumen is evident where the intercalated duct is seen in cross section but is not evident where it is seen in longitudinal section. This is because the plane of section cuts chiefly through the cells rather than the lumen. As a consequence, this figure provides a good view of the nuclei of the duct cells. They are elongate, with their long axis oriented in the direction of the duct. In addition, they display a staining pattern similar to that of centroacinar cells and different from that of nuclei of the parenchymal cells.

Once the cells of the intercalated duct have been identified in one part of the section, their staining characteristics and location can be used to identify the intercalated ducts in other parts of the lobule, several of which are marked *(ID).*

KEY

A, region with most A cells
B, region with most B cells
BV, blood vessels
CC, centroacinar cells
CT, connective tissue
Er, ergastoplasm
ID, intercalated ducts
IL, islets of Langerhans
InD, intralobular duct
arrows, capillaries
asterisks, lumen of acini

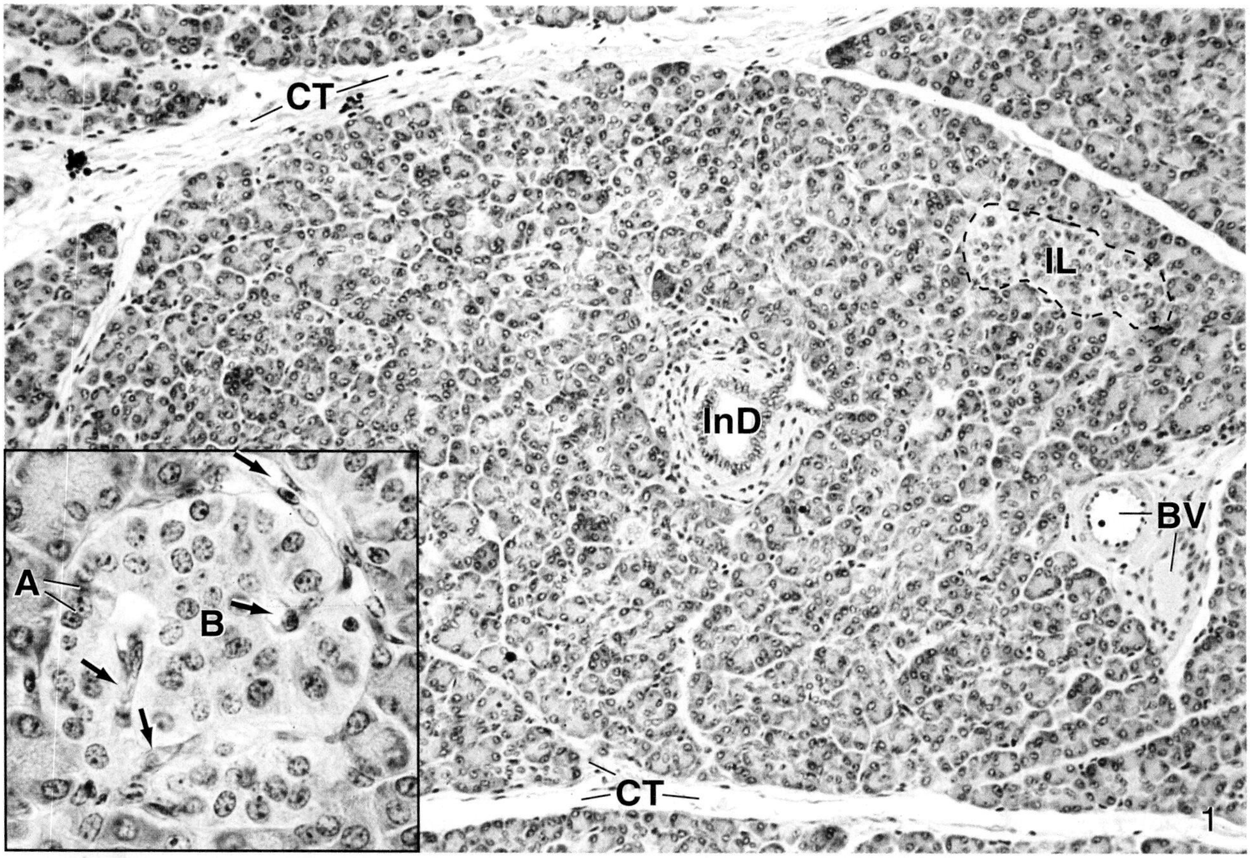
CT
IL
InD
A
B
BV
CT
1

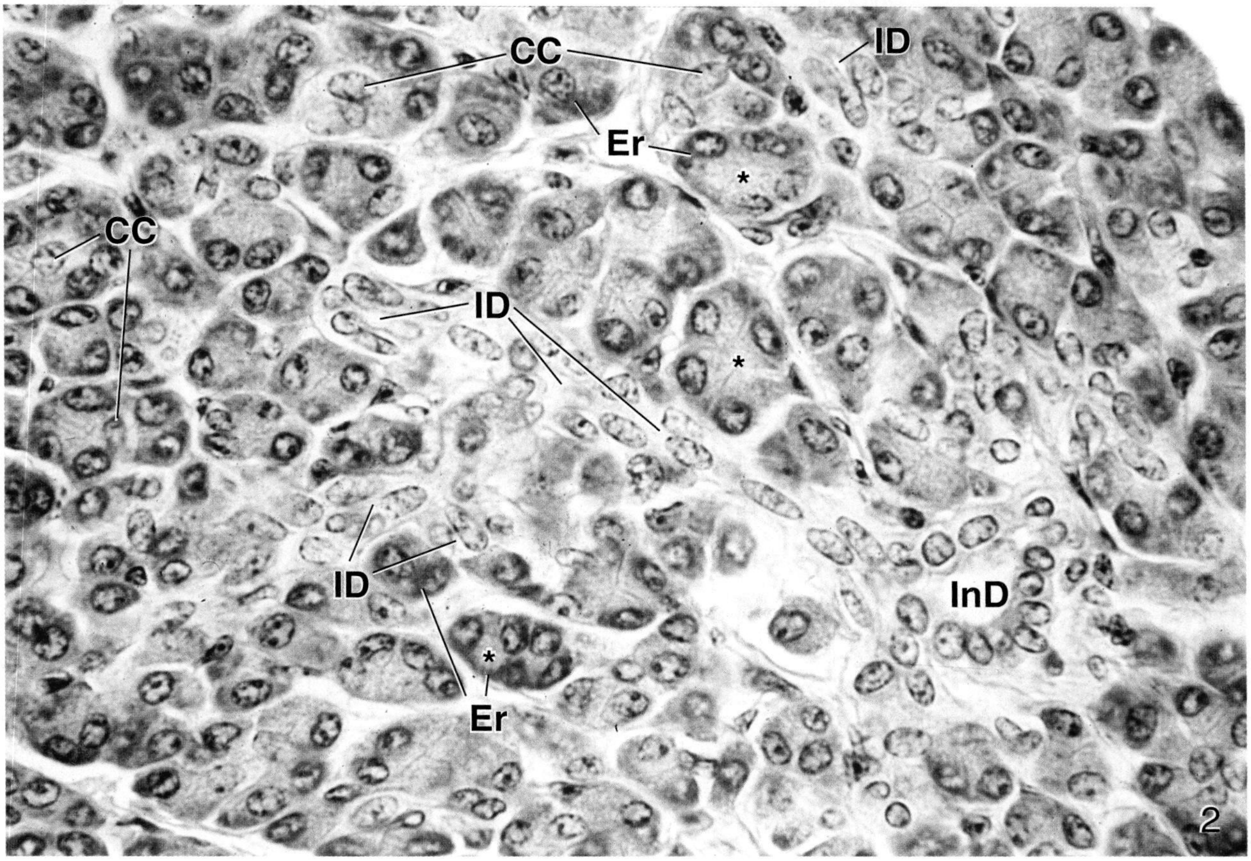
CC
ID
Er
CC
ID
ID
InD
Er
2

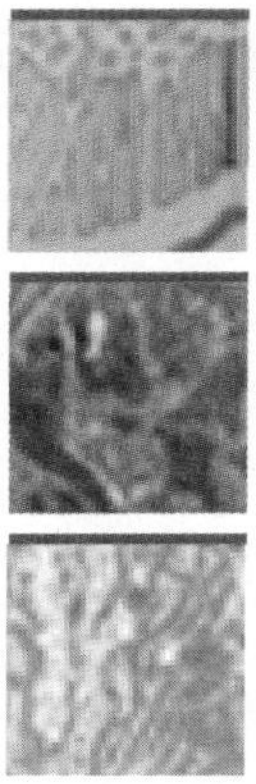

18

Respiratory System

OVERVIEW OF THE RESPIRATORY SYSTEM

The respiratory system consists of the paired lungs and a series of air passages that lead to and from the lungs. Within the lung, the air passages branch into increasingly smaller tubes until the very smallest air spaces, called ***alveoli***, are reached (Fig. 18.1).

Three principal functions are performed by this system: *air conduction, air filtration,* and *gas exchange (respiration)*. The latter occurs in the alveoli. In addition, air passing through the ***larynx*** is used to produce speech, and air passing over the ***olfactory mucosa*** in the ***nasal cavities*** carries stimuli for the sense of smell. The respiratory system also participates to a lesser degree in endocrine functions (hormone production and secretion),

as well as regulation of *immune responses* to inhaled antigens.

The lungs develop in the embryo as a ventral evagination of the foregut; thus, the epithelium of the respiratory system is of endodermal origin. This initial ***respiratory diverticulum*** grows into the thoracic mesenchyme. The bronchial cartilages, smooth muscle, and the other connective tissue elements are derived from the thoracic mesenchyme.

The air passages of the respiratory system consist of a conducting portion and a respiratory portion

The ***conducting portion*** of the respiratory system consists of those air passages that lead to the sites of respiration within the lung where gas exchange takes place. The conducting passages include those located outside as well as within the lungs.

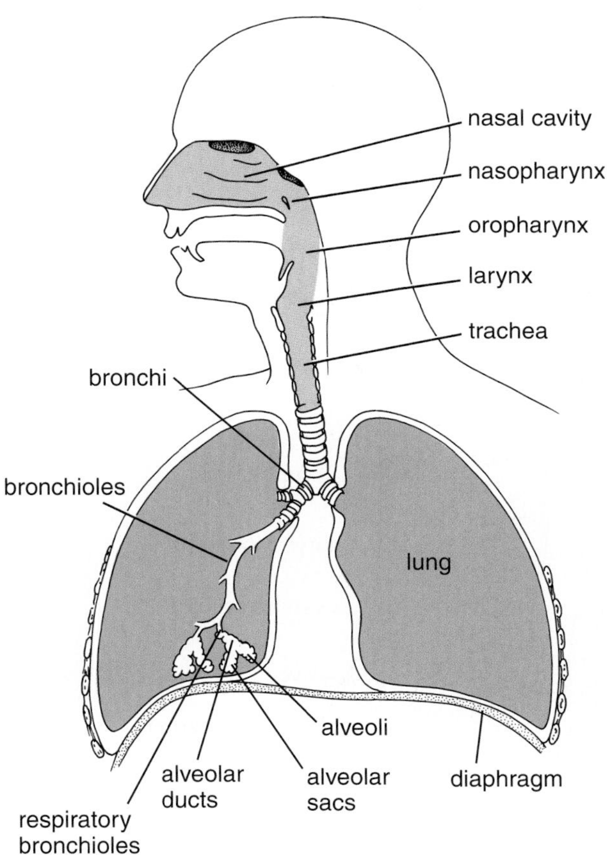

FIGURE 18.1
Diagram of respiratory passages. The nasal cavities, nasopharynx, oropharynx, larynx, trachea, bronchi, and bronchioles constitute the conducting portion of the respiratory system. The respiratory portion of the system, where gas exchange occurs, is composed of respiratory bronchioles, alveolar ducts, alveolar sacs, and alveoli. (Based on Boileau G. *A Method of Anatomy.* Baltimore: Williams & Wilkins, 1980.)

The passages external to the lungs consist of

- ***Nasal cavities*** (and, during forced breathing, the ***oral cavity***)
- ***Nasopharynx*** and ***oropharynx***
- ***Larynx***
- ***Trachea***
- ***Paired main (primary) bronchi***

Within the lungs, the ***main bronchi*** undergo extensive branching to give rise ultimately to the distributing ***bronchioles.*** The bronchioles represent the terminal part of the conducting passages. Collectively, the internal bronchi and the bronchioles constitute the ***bronchial tree.***

The ***respiratory portion*** is that part of the respiratory tract in which ***gas exchange*** occurs. Sequentially, it includes

- ***Respiratory bronchioles***
- ***Alveolar ducts***
- ***Alveolar sacs***
- ***Alveoli***

Blood vessels enter the lung with the bronchi. The arteries branch into smaller vessels as they follow the bronchial tree into the substance of the lung. Capillaries come into intimate contact with the terminal respiratory units, the alveoli. This intimate relationship between the alveolar air spaces and the pulmonary capillaries is the structural basis for gas exchange within the lung parenchyma. The essential features of the lung blood supply are described on page 590.

Air passing through the respiratory passages must be conditioned before reaching the terminal respiratory units. ***Conditioning*** of the air occurs in the conducting portion of the system and includes ***warming, moistening,*** and ***removal of particulate materials.*** Mucous and serous secretions play a major role in the conditioning process. These secretions moisten the air and also trap particles that have managed to slip past the special short thick hairs, called ***vibrissae,*** in the nasal cavities. Mucus, augmented by these serous secretions, also prevents the dehydration of the underlying epithelium by the moving air. Mucus covers almost the entire luminal surface of the conducting passages and is continuously produced by goblet cells and mucus-secreting glands in the walls of the passages. The mucus and other secretions are moved toward the pharynx by means of coordinated sweeping movements of cilia and are then normally swallowed.

▼ NASAL CAVITIES

The ***nasal cavities*** are paired chambers separated by a bony and cartilaginous septum. Each cavity or chamber communicates anteriorly with the external environment

through the ***nares*** (nostrils) and posteriorly with the nasopharynx through the ***choanae*** (Fig. 18.2). The chambers are divided into three regions:

- *Vestibule*
- *Respiratory segment*
- *Olfactory segment*

Vestibule of the Nasal Cavity

The ***vestibule*** communicates anteriorly with the external environment. It is lined with stratified squamous epithelium, a continuation of the skin of the face, and contains a variable number of stiff hairs, vibrissae, that entrap large particulate matter before it is carried in the air stream to the rest of the cavity. Sebaceous glands are also present and their secretions assist in the entrapment of particulate matter. Posteriorly, where the vestibule ends, the stratified squamous epithelium becomes thinner and undergoes a transition to the pseudostratified epithelium that characterizes the respiratory segment. At this site, sebaceous glands are absent.

Respiratory Segment of the Nasal Cavity

The respiratory segment constitutes most of the volume of the nasal cavities. It is lined with a ciliated, pseudostratified columnar epithelium. The underlying lamina propria is attached to the periosteum of the adjacent bone.

The medial wall of the respiratory segment, the ***nasal septum***, is smooth, but the lateral walls are thrown into folds by the presence of three shelf-like, bony projections called ***turbinates*** or ***conchae***. The turbinates play a dual role. They increase surface area as well as cause turbulence in airflow to allow more efficient conditioning of inspired air.

The ciliated, pseudostratified columnar epithelium of the respiratory segment is composed of five cell types:

- ***Ciliated cells***, tall columnar cells with cilia that project into the mucus covering the surface of the epithelium
- ***Goblet cells*** that synthesize and secrete mucus
- ***Brush cells***, a general name for those cells in the respiratory tract that bear short, blunt microvilli

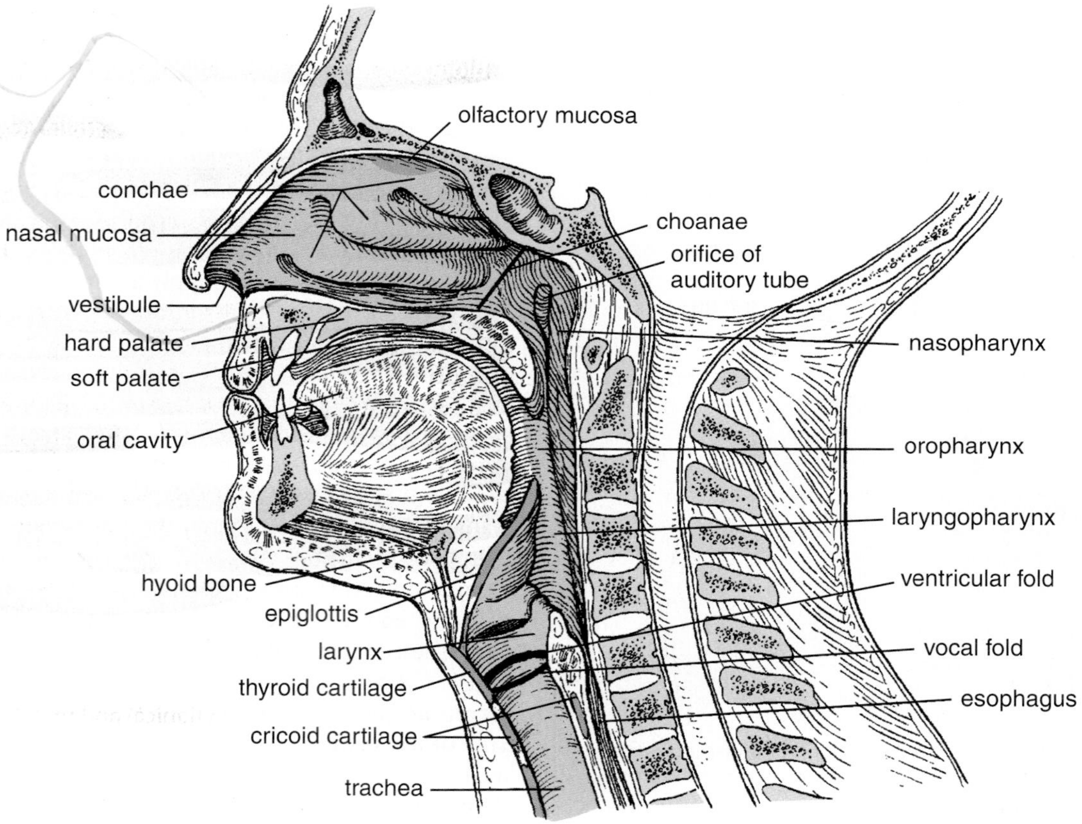

FIGURE 18.2

Diagram of the relationship of the pharynx to the respiratory and digestive systems. The pharynx is divided into three parts: nasopharynx, oropharynx, and laryngopharynx. It is located posterior to the nasal and oral cavities and extends inferiorly past the larynx. The pharynx serves both respiratory and digestive systems. This midsagittal section also transects the cartilages forming the skeleton of the larynx (i.e., epiglottis, thyroid cartilage, and cricoid cartilage). Note the ventricular and vocal folds in the middle of the larynx, approximately at the level of the thyroid cartilage. This part of the larynx represents the narrowest portion of the respiratory system and is responsible for producing sound by audible vibration of the vocal folds.

- *Small granule cells* that resemble basal cells but contain secretory granules
- *Basal cells,* stem cells from which the other cell types arise

The epithelium of the respiratory segment of the nasal cavity is essentially the same as the epithelium lining most of the parts that follow in the conducting system. Because the respiratory epithelium of the trachea is studied and examined in preference to that of the nasal cavity, the above cell types are discussed in the section on the trachea (page 575).

The mucosa of the respiratory segment warms, moistens, and filters inspired air

The lamina propria of the respiratory segment has a rich, vascular network that includes a complex set of capillary loops. The arrangement of the vessels allows the inhaled air to be warmed by blood flowing through the part of the loop closest to the surface. The capillaries that reside near the surface are arranged in rows; the blood flows perpendicular to the airflow, much as one would find in a mechanical heat-exchange system. These same vessels may become engorged and leaky during allergic reactions or viral infections such as the common cold. The lamina propria then becomes distended with fluid, resulting in marked swelling of the mucous membrane with consequent restriction of the air passage, making breathing difficult. The lamina propria also contains mucous glands, many exhibiting serous demilunes. Their secretions supplement that of the goblet cells in the respiratory epithelium.

By increasing surface area, the turbinates increase the efficiency with which the inspired air is warmed. The turbinates also increase the efficiency of filtration of inspired air through the process of **turbulent precipitation.** The air stream is broken into eddies by the turbinates. Particulate matter suspended in the air stream is thrown out of the stream and adheres to the mucus-covered wall of the nasal cavity. Particles trapped in this layer of mucus are transported to the pharynx by means of coordinated sweeping movements of cilia and are then swallowed.

Olfactory Segment of the Nasal Cavity

The *olfactory segment* is located on part of the dome of each nasal cavity and, to a variable extent, the contiguous lateral and medial nasal walls. It is lined with a specialized *olfactory mucosa.* In living tissue, this mucosa is distinguished by its slight yellowish brown color caused by pigment in the *olfactory epithelium* and the associated *olfactory glands.* In humans, the total surface area of the olfactory mucosa is only a few square centimeters; in animals with an acute sense of smell, the total surface area of the olfactory mucosa is considerably more extensive.

The lamina propria of the olfactory mucosa is directly contiguous with the periosteum of the underlying bone. This connective tissue contains numerous blood and lymphatic vessels, unmyelinated olfactory nerves, myelinated nerves, and olfactory glands.

The olfactory epithelium, like the epithelium of the respiratory segment, is also pseudostratified, but it contains very different cell types. Also, it lacks goblet cells (Fig. 18.3). The olfactory epithelium is composed of the following cell types:

- *Olfactory cells, bipolar neurons* that span the thickness of the epithelium
- *Supporting* or *sustentacular cells,* columnar cells that provide mechanical and metabolic support to the olfactory cells
- *Basal cells,* stem cells from which new olfactory cells and supporting cells differentiate
- *Brush cells,* the same cell type that occurs in the respiratory epithelium

Olfactory cells are bipolar neurons that possess an apical projection bearing cilia

The apical (luminal) pole of each *olfactory cell* is a dendritic process that projects above the epithelial surface as a knob-like structure called the *olfactory vesicle.* A number of cilia (10 to 23) with typical basal bodies arise from the olfactory vesicle and extend radially in a plane parallel to the epithelial surface (see Fig. 18.3). The cilia are usually up to 200 μm long and may overlap with cilia of adjacent olfactory cells. The cilia are regarded as nonmotile, although some research suggests that they may have limited motility. The plasma membrane of the cilia contains *odorant-binding proteins* that act as olfactory receptors. Incoming odorant molecules are solubilized in the olfactory mucus and interact with the olfactory receptors to generate an action potential. The basal pole of the cell gives rise to an axonal process that leaves the epithelial compartment to enter the connective tissue, where it joins with axons from other olfactory cells to form the *olfactory nerve (cranial nerve I).* Autoradiographic studies show that olfactory cells have a lifespan of about 1 month. If injured, they are quickly replaced. Olfactory cells (and some neurons of the enteric division of the autonomic nervous system) appear to be the only neurons that are readily replaced during postnatal life.

Supporting cells provide mechanical and metabolic support for the olfactory cells

Supporting cells are the most numerous cells in the olfactory epithelium. The nuclei of these tall columnar or sustentacular cells occupy a more apical position in the epithelium than do those of the other cell types, thus aiding in their identification in the light microscope (see Fig. 18.3). They have numerous microvilli on their apical surface, and abundant mitochondria. Numerous profiles of smooth endoplasmic reticulum (sER) and, to a more lim-

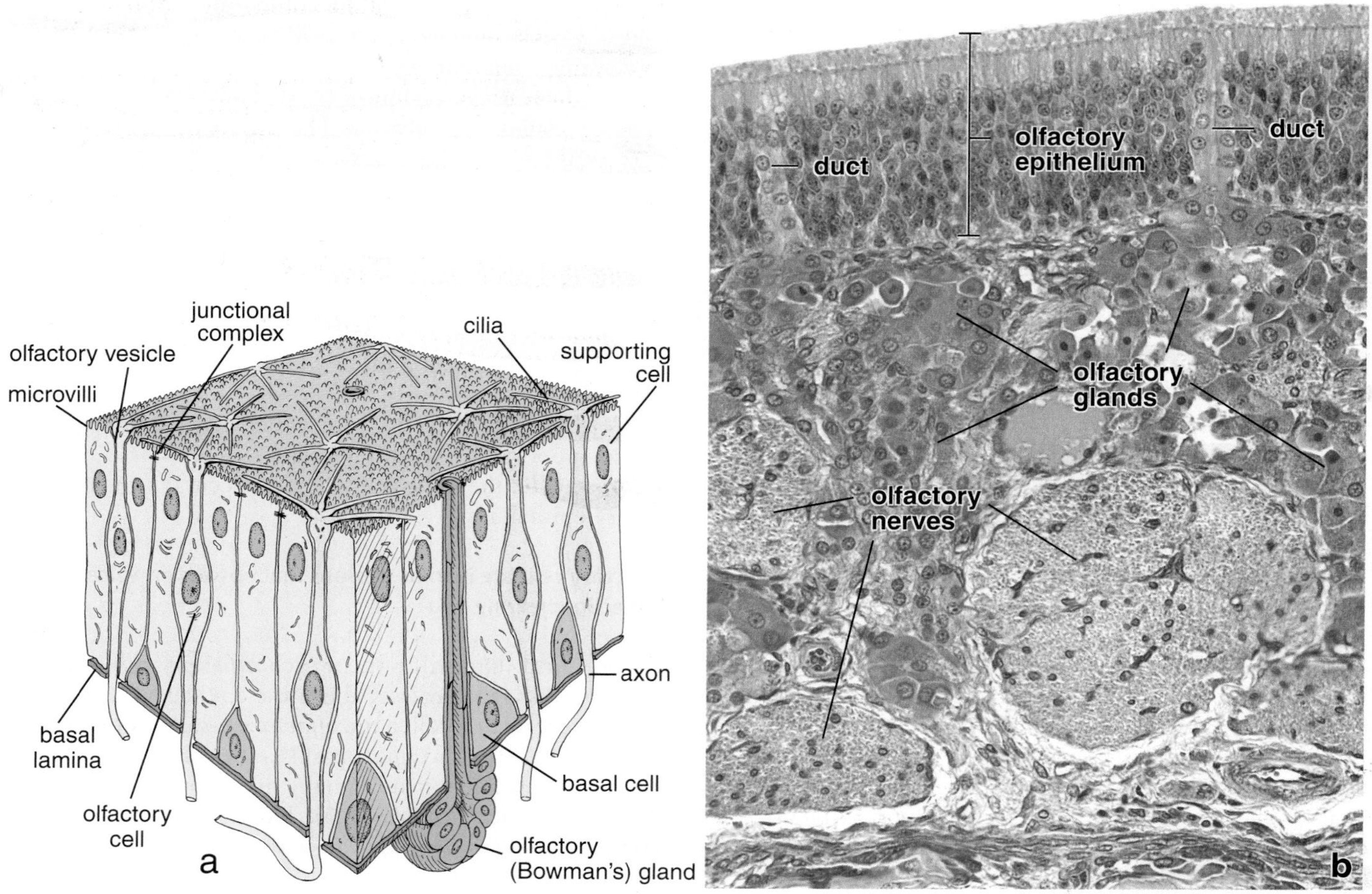

FIGURE 18.3
Olfactory mucosa of the nasal cavity. a. This diagram shows the three major cell types located within the olfactory epithelium: the olfactory cell, supporting (sustentacular) cell, and basal cell. The olfactory cell is the receptor cell; it has an apical expansion, the olfactory vesicle, from which long, nonmotile cilia extend. At its basal surface it extends an axon into the connective tissue that joins with axons of other olfactory cells to form an olfactory nerve. The basal cells are small and cuboidal. They are restricted to the basal part of the epithelium. The supporting cells, in contrast, are columnar and extend the full thickness of the epithelium; their nuclei are located in the upper portion of the cell. Note the olfactory (Bowman's) gland and its duct that empties on the surface of the mucosa. **b.** Photomicrograph of the olfactory mucosa. The olfactory epithelium exhibits nuclei through much of its thickness, but the individual cell types to which they belong are not discernable. The underlying connective tissue is largely occupied by numerous olfactory (Bowman's) glands, olfactory nerves, and blood vessels. Note that the ducts of the olfactory glands extend from the secretory portion of the gland to the epithelial surface. ×240.

ited extent, rough endoplasmic reticulum (rER) are observed in the cytoplasm. They also possess lipofuscin granules. Adhering junctions are present between these cells and the olfactory cells, but gap and tight junctions are absent. The supporting cells function in a manner comparable to that of glial cells, providing both metabolic and physical support to the olfactory cells.

Brush cells are columnar cells specialized for transduction of general sensation

The olfactory epithelium also contains cells present in much smaller numbers, called ***brush cells***. As noted, these cells are present in the epithelium of other parts of the conducting air passages. With the electron microscope, brush cells exhibit large, blunt microvilli at their apical surface, a feature that gives them their name. The basal surface of a brush cell is in synaptic contact with nerve fibers that penetrate the basal lamina. The nerve fibers are terminal branches of the ***trigeminal nerve (cranial nerve V)*** that function in general sensation rather than olfaction. Brush cells appear to be involved in transduction of general sensory stimulation of the mucosa.

Basal cells are progenitors of the other mature cell types

Basal cells are small, rounded cells located close to the basal lamina. Their nuclei are frequently invagi-

nated and lie at a level below those of the olfactory cell nuclei. The cytoplasm contains few organelles, a feature consistent with their role as a reserve or stem cell. A feature consistent with their differentiation into supporting cells is the observation of processes in some basal cells that partially ensheathe the first portion of the olfactory cell axon. They thus maintain a relationship to the olfactory cell even in their undifferentiated state.

Olfactory glands are a characteristic feature of the olfactory mucosa

The *olfactory glands (Bowman's glands)*, a characteristic feature of the mucosa, are branched tubuloalveolar serous glands that deliver their proteinaceous secretions via ducts onto the olfactory surface (see Fig. 18.3). Lipofuscin granules are prevalent in the gland cells, and in combination with the lipofuscin granules in the supporting cells of the olfactory epithelium, they give the mucosa its natural yellow-brown coloration. Short ducts composed of cuboidal cells lead from the glands and pass through the basal lamina into the olfactory epithelium, where they continue to the epithelial surface to discharge their contents.

The serous secretion of the olfactory glands serves as a trap and solvent for odoriferous substances. Constant flow from the glands rids the mucosa of remnants of detected odoriferous substances so that new scents can be continuously detected as they arise.

The identifying feature of the olfactory region of the nasal mucosa in a histologic preparation is the olfactory nerves in combination with olfactory glands in the lamina propria. The nerves are particularly conspicuous because of the relatively large diameter of the individual unmyelinated fibers that they contain (see Fig. 18.3).

Paranasal Sinuses

Paranasal sinuses are air-filled spaces in the bones of the walls of the nasal cavity

The ***paranasal sinuses*** are extensions of the respiratory segment of the nasal cavity and are lined by respiratory epithelium. The sinuses are named for the bone in which they are found, i.e., the ethmoid, frontal, sphenoid, and maxillary bones. The sinuses communicate with the nasal cavities via narrow openings onto the respiratory mucosa. The mucosal surface of the sinuses is a thin, ciliated, pseudostratified columnar epithelium with numerous goblet cells. Mucus produced in the sinuses is swept into the nasal cavities by coordinated ciliary movements. The sinuses are often subject to acute infection following viral infection of the upper respiratory tract. Severe infections may require physical drainage.

▼ PHARYNX

The pharynx connects the nasal and oral cavities to the larynx and esophagus. It serves as a passageway for air and food and acts as a resonating chamber for speech. The pharynx is located posterior to the nasal and oral cavities and is divided regionally into the ***nasopharynx*** and ***oropharynx***, respectively (see Fig. 18.2). The ***auditory (Eustachian) tubes*** connect the nasopharynx to each middle ear. Diffuse lymphatic tissue and lymphatic nodules are present in the wall of the nasopharynx. The concentration of lymphatic nodules at the junction between the superior and posterior walls of the pharynx is called the ***pharyngeal tonsil***.

▼ LARYNX

The passageway for air between the oropharynx and trachea is the *larynx* (see Fig. 18.2). This complex tubular segment of the respiratory system is formed by irregularly shaped plates of hyaline and elastic cartilage (the epiglottis and the vocal processes of the arytenoid cartilages). In addition to serving as a conduit for air, the larynx serves as the organ for speech *(phonation)*.

Vocal folds control the flow of air through the larynx and vibrate to produce sound

The ***vocal folds***, also referred to as ***vocal cords***, are two folds of mucosa that project into the lumen of the larynx (Fig. 18.4). They are oriented in an anteroposterior direction and define the lateral boundaries of the opening of the larynx, the ***rima glottis***. A supporting ligament and skeletal muscle, the ***vocalis muscle***, is contained within each vocal fold. Ligaments and the ***intrinsic laryngeal muscles*** join the adjacent cartilaginous plates and are responsible for generating tension in the vocal folds and for opening and closing the glottis. The ***extrinsic laryngeal muscles*** insert on cartilages of the larynx but originate in extralaryngeal structures. These muscles move the larynx during swallowing *(deglutition)*.

Expelled air passing through the glottis can be induced to cause the vocal folds to vibrate. The vibrations are altered by modulating the tension on the vocal folds and by changing the degree of glottal opening. This alteration of the vibrations produces sounds of different *pitch*.

The ventricular folds located above the vocal folds are the "false vocal cords"

Above the vocal folds is an elongated recess in the larynx called the ***ventricle***. Immediately above the ventricle is another pair of mucosal folds, the ***ventricular folds***, or

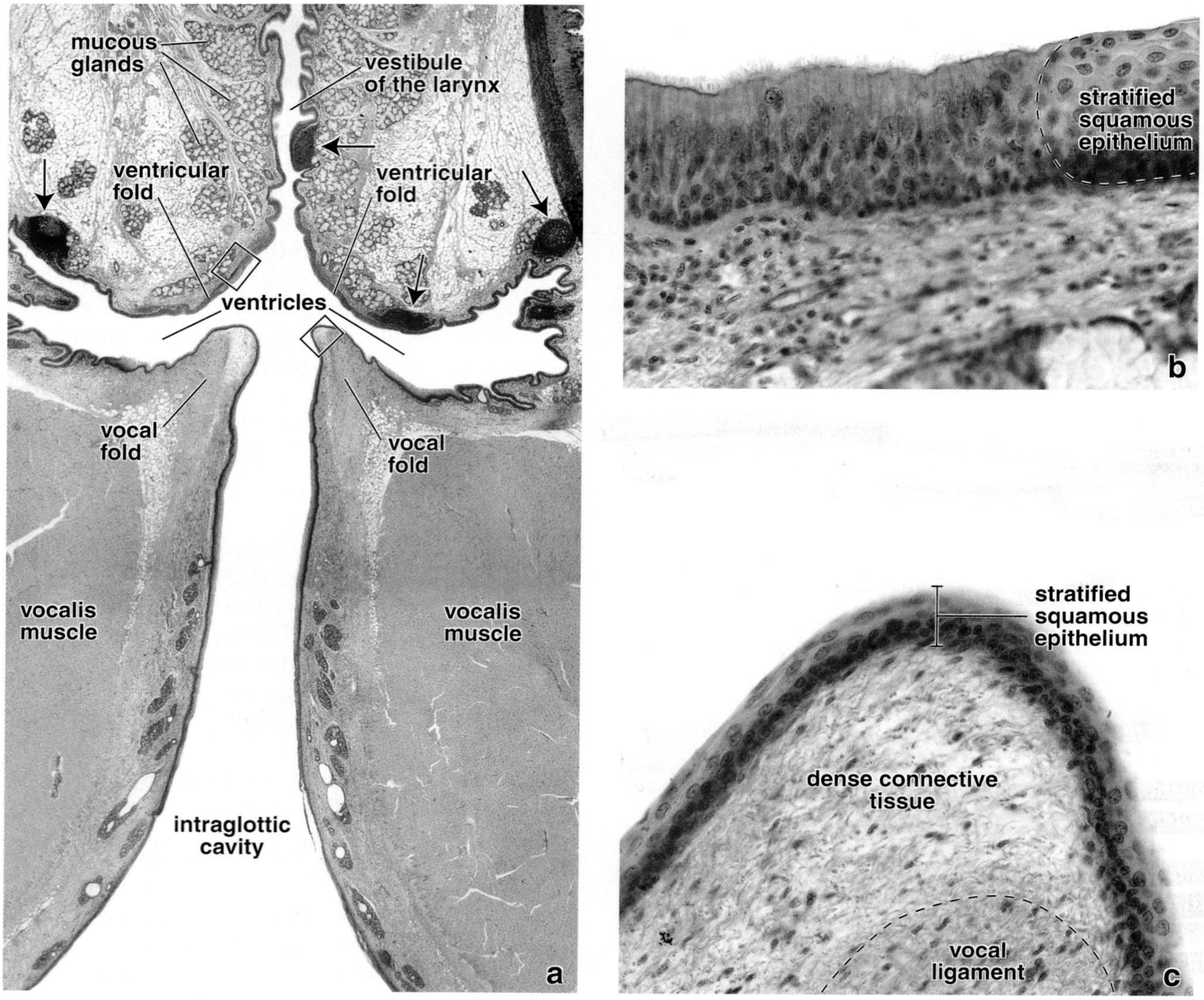

FIGURE 18.4

Photomicrograph of a frontal section of the larynx. a. This photomicrograph shows three parts of the larynx: the vestibule above the ventricular folds, the ventricles between the vestibular folds and superior to the vocal folds, and the infraglottic cavity that extends from the vocal folds to the cricoid cartilage. Note that mucous glands are prominent in the ventricular folds and are covered by the typical pseudostratified ciliated epithelium. The vocal fold is composed of the epithelium, vocal ligament, and underlying vocalis muscle. Numerous lymph nodules are also present within the mucosa of the larynx *(arrows)*. ×10. **b.** High magnification of the area of the ventricular fold indicated by the *upper rectangle* in *a* shows on the left the pseudostratified ciliated epithelium that lines most of the larynx. Many nonsmoking adults and virtually all smokers exhibit patches of stratified squamous epithelium, as seen on the right of the micrograph. ×240. **c.** High magnification of the area of the vocal fold indicated by the *lower rectangle* in *a* reveals normal stratified squamous epithelium at this site. Just beneath the epithelium is the connective tissue known as Reinke's space. This clinically important site lacks lymphatic vessels and is poorly vascularized. The vocal ligament, inscribed by the *dashed line,* is seen at the bottom of the micrograph. ×240.

false vocal cords (see Fig. 18.5). These folds do not have the intrinsic muscular investment of the true vocal cords and, therefore, do not modulate in phonation. They and the ventricle, however, are important in creating sound *resonance*.

Stratified squamous and ciliated pseudostratified columnar epithelium line the larynx

The luminal surface of the vocal cords is covered with stratified squamous epithelium, as is most of the epiglottis.

BOX 18.1

Clinical Correlations: Metaplasia

In human respiratory mucosa, ciliated pseudostratified epithelium may change to stratified squamous epithelium. This transformation is a normal occurrence on the rounded, more exposed portions of the turbinates, on the vocal folds, and in certain other regions. Changes in the character of the respiratory epithelium may, however, occur in other ciliated epithelial sites when the pattern of airflow is altered or when forceful airflow occurs, as in chronic coughing. Typically, in ***chronic bronchitis*** and ***bronchiectasis***, the respiratory epithelium changes in certain regions to a stratified squamous form. The altered epithelium is more resistant to physical stress and insult, but it is less effective functionally. In smokers, a similar epithelial change occurs. Initially, the cilia on ciliated cells lose their synchronous beating pattern due to noxious elements in smoke. As a result, removal of mucus is impaired. To compensate, the individual begins to cough, thereby facilitating the expulsion of accumulated mucus in the airway, particularly in the trachea. With time, the number of ciliated cells decreases because of chronic coughing. This reduction in ciliated cells further impairs the normal epithelium and results in its replacement with stratified squamous epithelium at affected sites in the airway.

Epithelial alterations of this kind are referred to as ***metaplasia***, i.e., a reversible change from one type of fully differentiated adult cell to a different type of adult cell. A given mature cell does not change to another type of mature cell; rather, basal cell proliferation gives rise to the new differentiated cell type. These cellular changes are considered to be controlled and adaptive.

The epithelium serves to protect the mucosa from abrasion caused by the rapidly moving air stream. The rest of the larynx is lined with the ciliated, pseudostratified columnar epithelium that characterizes the respiratory tract (see Fig. 18.4). The connective tissue of the larynx contains mixed mucoserous glands that secrete through ducts onto the laryngeal surface.

▼ TRACHEA

The *trachea* is a short, flexible, air tube about 2.5 cm in diameter and about 10 cm long. It serves as a conduit for air; additionally, its wall assists in conditioning inspired air. The trachea extends from the larynx to about the middle of the thorax, where it divides into the two *main (primary) bronchi*. The lumen of the trachea stays open because of the arrangement of the series of cartilaginous rings.

The wall of the trachea consists of four definable layers:

- *Mucosa*, composed of a ciliated, pseudostratified epithelium and an elastic, fiber-rich lamina propria
- *Submucosa*, composed of a slightly denser connective tissue than the lamina propria
- *Cartilaginous layer*, composed of C-shaped hyaline cartilages
- *Adventitia*, composed of connective tissue that binds the trachea to adjacent structures

A unique feature of the trachea is the presence of a series of C-shaped hyaline cartilages that are stacked one on top of each other to form a supporting structure (Fig. 18.5). These cartilages, which might be described as a skeletal framework, prevent collapse of the tracheal lumen, particularly during expiration. Fibroelastic tissue and smooth muscle, the *trachealis muscle*, bridge the gap between the free ends of the C-shaped cartilages at the posterior border of the trachea, adjacent to the esophagus.

Tracheal Epithelium

Tracheal epithelium is similar to respiratory epithelium in other parts of the conducting airway

Ciliated columnar cells, mucous (goblet) cells, and basal cells are the principal cell types in the tracheal epithelium (Figs. 18.6 and 18.7). Brush cells are also present but in small numbers, as are small granule cells.

- *Ciliated cells*, the most numerous of the tracheal cell types, extend through the full thickness of the epithelium. Cilia appear in histologic sections as short, hairlike profiles projecting from the apical surface. Each cell has approximately 250 cilia. Immediately below the cilia is a dark line formed by the aggregated ciliary basal bodies (Fig. 18.8). The cilia provide a coordinated sweeping motion of the mucous coat from the farthest reaches of the air passages toward the pharynx. In effect, the ciliated cells function as a "*mucociliary escalator*" that serves as an important protective mechanism for removing small inhaled particles from the lungs.
- *Mucous cells* are similar in appearance to intestinal goblet cells and are, thus, often referred to by the same name. They are interspersed among the ciliated cells and also extend through the full thickness of the epithelium (see Fig. 18.8). They are readily seen in the light microscope after they have accumulated mucinogen granules in their cytoplasm. Although the mucinogen is typically washed out in hematoxylin and eosin (H&E) preparations, the identity of the cell is made apparent by the remaining clear area in the cytoplasm and the lack of cilia at the apical surface. In contrast to ciliated cells, the

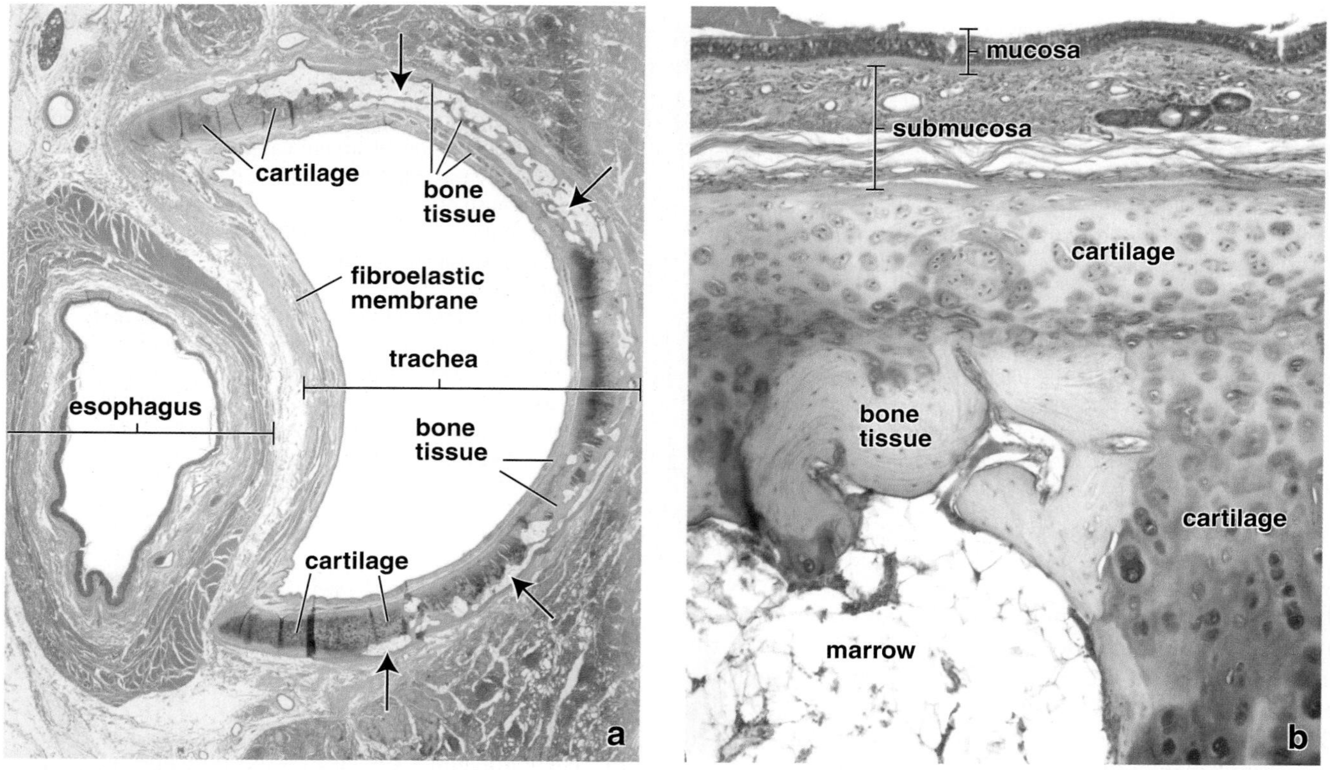

FIGURE 18.5
Photomicrograph of a section of the trachea and esophagus. a. This specimen, obtained from an elderly individual, shows the relationship between the trachea and the esophagus at the base of the neck. The cartilaginous tracheal rings, which keep the trachea patent, have a C-shaped appearance. The cartilage gap, where the trachea is adjacent to the esophageal wall, is spanned by a fibroelastic membrane. It contains the trachealis muscle and numerous seromucous glands. In this specimen, the tracheal ring has been transformed, in part, to bone, a process that occurs in aging. The darker-staining material represents cartilage, whereas the lighter-staining material has been replaced by bone tissue. The very light areas *(arrows)* are marrow spaces. ×3.25. **b.** This high-magnification photomicrograph shows an area of the tracheal ring that has partially transformed into bone. The top of the micrograph shows the tracheal mucosa and submucosa. Below is part of the tracheal ring. In this particular region, however, a substantial portion of the cartilage has been replaced by bone tissue and marrow. The bone tissue exhibits typical lamellae and osteocytes. The cartilage tissue, in contrast, exhibits nests of chondrocytes. ×100.

number of mucous cells increases during chronic irritation of the air passages.

- ***Brush cells*** have the same general features as those described for the respiratory epithelium of the nasal cavity (Fig. 18.9a). They are columnar cells that bear blunt microvilli. The basal surface of the cells is in synaptic contact with an afferent nerve ending (epitheliodendritic synapse). Thus, the brush cell is regarded as a receptor cell.
- ***Small granule cells*** are respiratory representatives of the general class of enteroendocrine cells of the gut and gut derivatives (Fig. 18.9b). Their presence is explained by the development of the respiratory tract and lungs from an evagination of the primitive foregut. Small granule cells usually occur singly in the trachea and are sparsely dispersed among the other cell types. They are difficult to distinguish from basal cells in the light microscope without special techniques such as silver staining, which reacts with the granules. The nucleus is located near the basement membrane; the cytoplasm is somewhat more extensive than that of the smaller basal cells. With the transmission electron microscope (TEM), a thin, tapering cytoplasmic process is sometimes observed extending to the lumen. Also, with the TEM, the cytoplasm exhibits numerous, membrane-bounded, dense-core granules. In one type of small granule cell the secretion is a catecholamine. A second cell type produces polypeptide hormones such as serotonin, calcitonin, and gastrin-releasing peptide (bombesin). Some small granule cells appear to be innervated. The function of these cells is not well understood. Some are present in groups in association with nerve fibers, forming neuroepithelial bodies, which are thought to function in reflexes regulating the airway or vascular caliber.
- ***Basal cells*** serve as a reserve cell population that maintains individual cell replacement in the epithelium. Basal cells tend to be prominent because their nuclei form a row in close proximity to the basal lamina. Although nuclei of other cells reside at this same general level within the epithelium, they are relatively sparse. Thus, most of the nuclei near the basement membrane belong to basal cells.

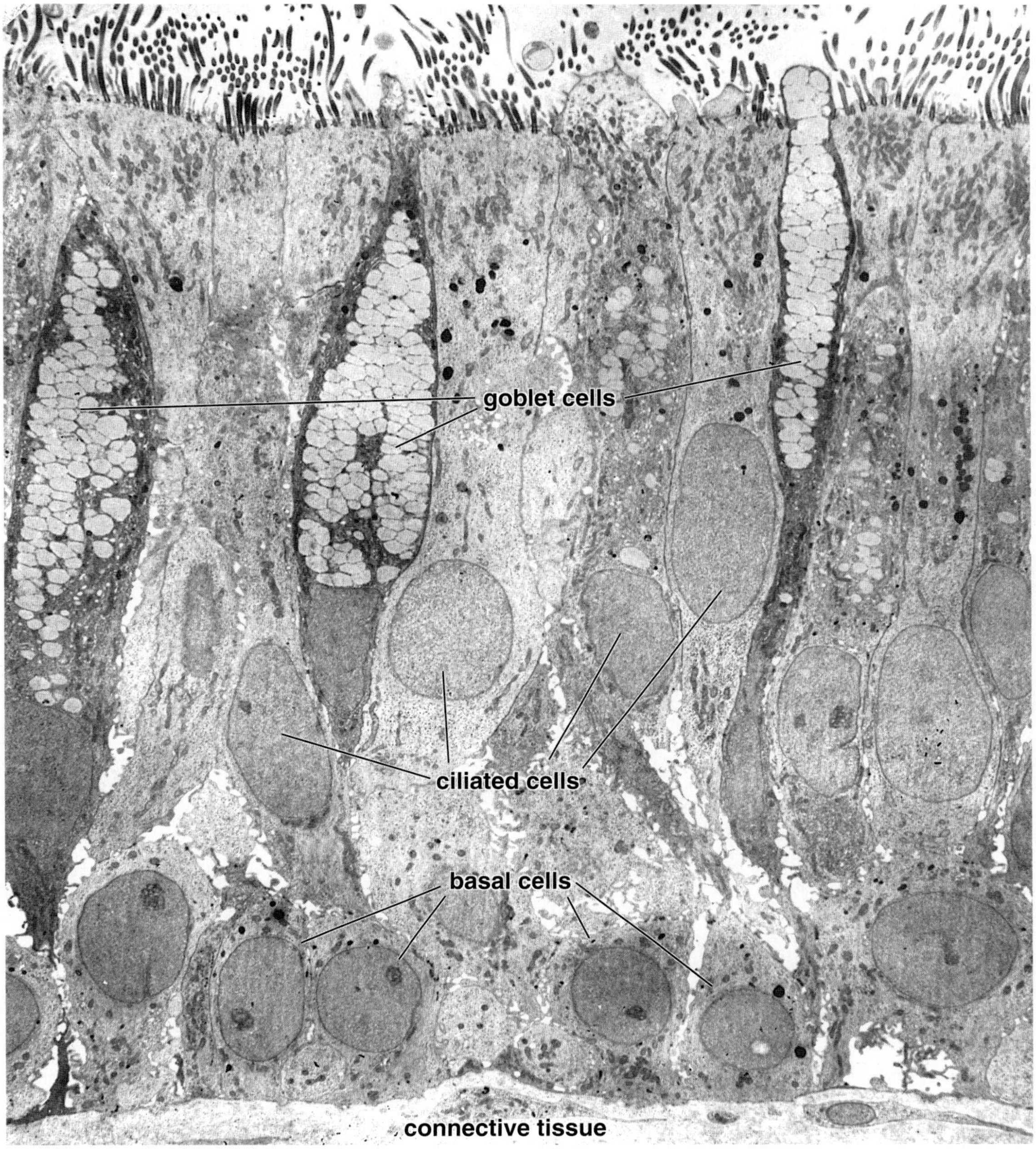

FIGURE 18.6
Electron micrograph of human trachea. This electron micrograph shows the three main cell types of this respiratory epithelium. They are represented by ciliated epithelial cells extending to the surface, where they possess cilia; goblet cells with mucinogen granules; and basal cells, which are confined to the basal portion of the epithelial layer near the connective tissue. ×1,800. (Courtesy of Dr. Johannes A. G. Rhodin.)

Basement Membrane and Lamina Propria

A thick "basement membrane" is characteristic of tracheal epithelium

Located beneath the tracheal epithelium is a distinctive layer typically referred to as a "basement membrane." It usually appears as a glassy or homogeneous light-staining layer approximately 25 to 40 μm thick (see Fig. 18.8). Electron microscopy reveals that it consists of densely packed collagenous fibers that lie immediately under the epithelial basal lamina. Structurally, it can be regarded as an unusually thick and dense reticular lamina and, as such, is part of the lamina propria. In smokers, particularly

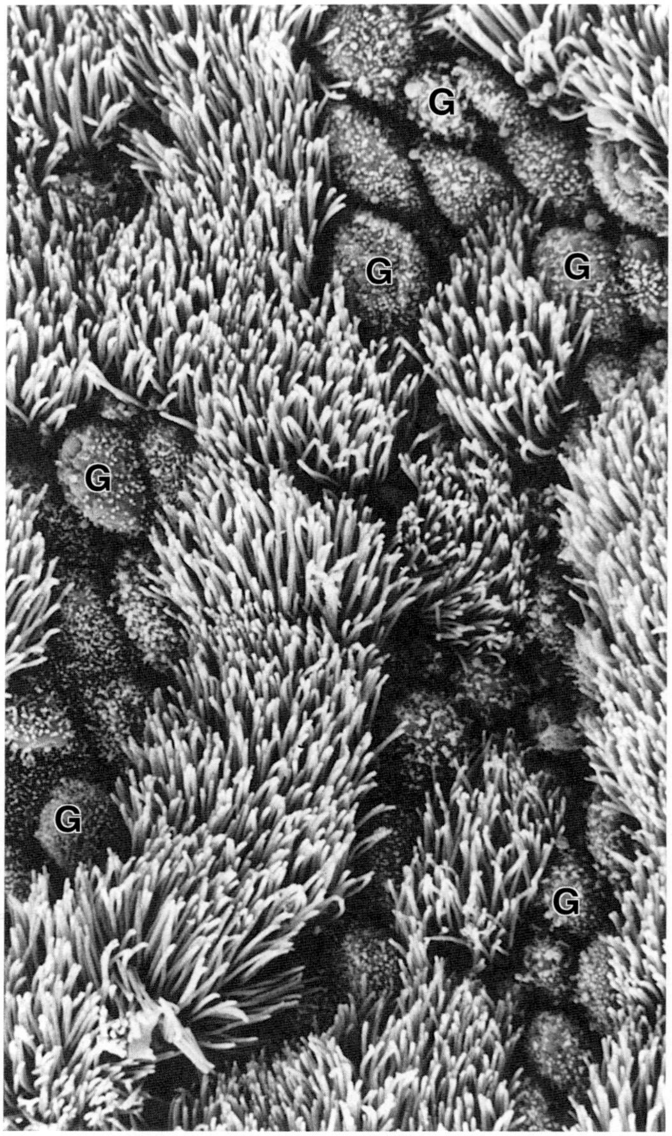

FIGURE 18.7
Scanning electron micrograph of the luminal surface of a bronchus. The nonciliated cells are the goblet cells *(G).* Their surface is characterized by small blunt microvilli that give a stippled appearance to the cell at this low magnification. The cilia of the many ciliated cells occupy the remainder of the micrograph. Note how all are "synchronously" arrayed (i.e., uniformly leaning in the same direction) appearing just as they were when fixed at a specific moment during their wave-like movement. ×1,200.

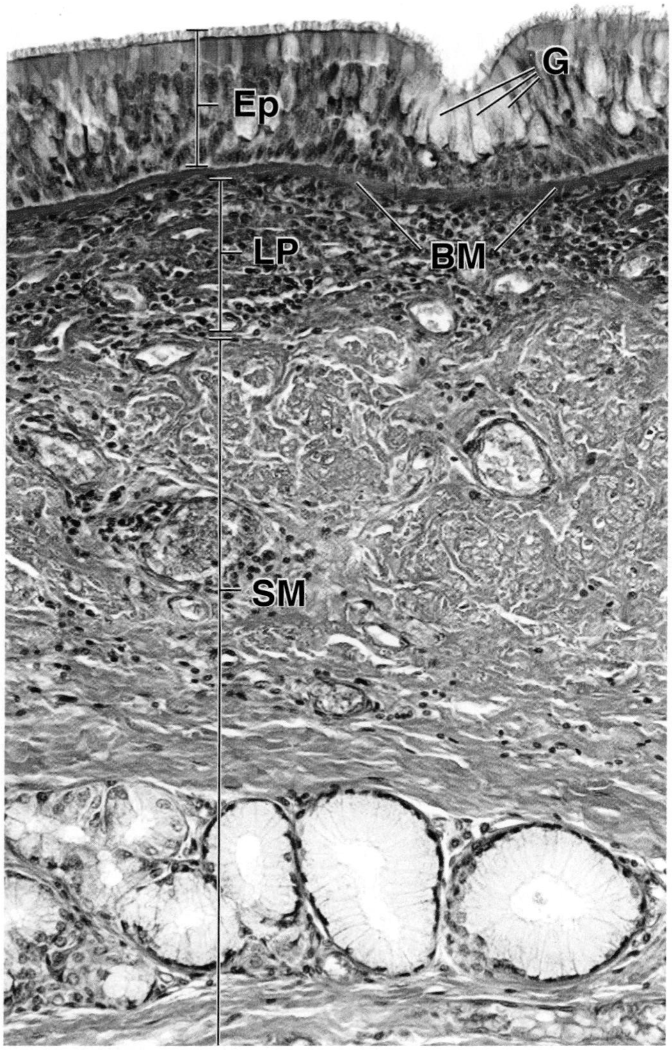

FIGURE 18.8
Photomicrograph of tracheal epithelium. Three major cell types are evident in the tracheal epithelium *(Ep):* ciliated columnar cells; mucus-secreting goblet cells *(G)* interspersed between the ciliated cells; and basal cells, which are close to the basement membrane *(BM).* The ciliated columnar cells extend from the basement membrane to the surface. At their free surface they contain numerous cilia that, together, give the surface a brush-like appearance. At the base of the cilia is a dense eosinophilic line. This is due to the linear aggregation of structures referred to as basal bodies, located at the proximal end of each cilium. Although basement membranes are not ordinarily seen in H&E preparations, a structure identified as such is seen regularly under the epithelium in the human trachea. The underlying lamina propria *(LP)* consists of loose connective tissue. The more deeply located submucosa *(SM)* contains dense irregular connective tissue with blood and lymphatic vessels, nerves, and numerous mucus-secreting tracheal glands. × 400.

those who experience chronic coughing, this layer may be considerably thicker, a response to mucosal irritation.

The lamina propria, excluding that part just designated as basement membrane, appears as a typical loose connective tissue. It is very cellular, containing numerous lymphocytes, many of which infiltrate the epithelium. Plasma cells, mast cells, eosinophils, and fibroblasts are the other cell types readily observed in this layer. Lymphatic tissue, in both diffuse and nodular forms, is consistently present in the lamina propria and submucosa of the tracheal wall. It is also present in other parts of the respiratory system involved primarily with air conduction. This lymphatic tissue is the developmental and functional equivalent of the ***bronchus-associated lymphatic tissue (BALT).***

The boundary between mucosa and submucosa is defined by an elastic membrane

Interspersed among the collagenous fibers are numerous elastic fibers. Where the lamina propria ends, the elastic material is more extensive, and in specimens stained for these fibers, a distinct band of elastic material is seen. This band or ***elastic membrane*** marks the boundary between the lamina propria and submucosa. In H&E preparations, however, the boundary is not obvious.

The submucosa is unlike that of most other organs, where this connective tissue typically has a dense character. In the trachea, the submucosa is a relatively loose connective tissue similar in appearance to the lamina propria, which makes it difficult to determine where it begins. Diffuse lymphatic tissue and lymphatic nodules characteristically extend into this layer from the lamina propria. The submucosa contains the larger distributing vessels and lymphatics of the tracheal wall.

Submucosal glands composed of mucus-secreting acini with serous demilunes are also present in the submucosa. Their ducts consist of a simple cuboidal epithelium and extend through the lamina propria to deliver their product, largely glycoproteins, on the epithelial surface. The glands are especially numerous in the cartilage-free gap on the posterior portion of the trachea. Some penetrate the muscle layer at this site and, therefore, also lie in the adventitia. The submucosal layer ends where its connective tissue fibers blend with the perichondrium of the cartilage layer.

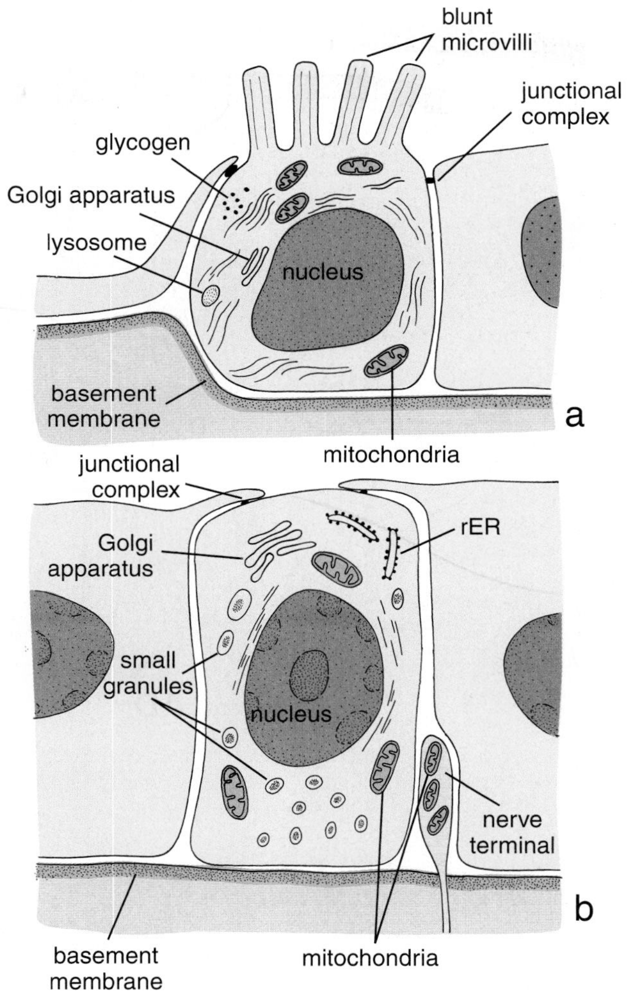

FIGURE 18.9
Diagram of a brush cell and small granule cell. a. The brush cell, as illustrated here, is interposed between type I and type II alveolar cells of an alveolus. Blunt microvilli are distinctive features of the brush cell. The cytoplasm typically shows a Golgi apparatus, lysosomes, mitochondria, and glycogen inclusions. **b.** This small granule cell is shown located between two Clara cells, as in a terminal or respiratory bronchiole. The cell contains small secretory vesicles, most of which are in the basal portion of the cell. In addition to the vesicles, the most conspicuous organelles of the cell are rough-surfaced endoplasmic reticulum *(rER)*, a Golgi apparatus, and mitochondria. A nerve terminal is shown within the epithelium adjacent to the cell.

The tracheal cartilages and trachealis muscle separate submucosa from adventitia

The tracheal cartilages, which number about 16 to 20 in humans, represent the next layer of the tracheal wall. As noted, the cartilages are C shaped. They sometimes anastomose with adjacent cartilages, but their arrangement provides flexibility to the tracheal pipe and also maintains patency of the lumen. With age, the hyaline cartilage may be partially replaced by bone tissue (see Fig. 18.5), causing it to lose much of its flexibility.

The ***adventitia***, the outer layer, lies peripheral to the cartilage rings and trachealis muscle. It binds the trachea to adjacent structures in the neck and mediastinum and contains the largest blood vessels and nerves that supply the tracheal wall, as well as the larger lymphatics that drain the wall.

▼ BRONCHI

The trachea divides into two branches forming the ***main (primary) bronchi.*** Anatomically, these divisions are more frequently described as simply the ***right and left main bronchi***, terms that are more useful because of the physical difference between the two. The right bronchus is wider and significantly shorter than the left. On entering the hilum of the lung, each main bronchus divides into the ***lobar bronchi (secondary bronchi)***. The left lung is divided into two lobes; the right lung is divided into three lobes. Thus, the right bronchus divides into three lobar bronchial branches, and the left into two lobar bronchial branches, with each branch supplying one lobe. The left lung is further divided into 8 ***bronchopulmonary segments*** and the right lung into 10 such segments. Thus, in the right lung the lobar bronchi give rise to 10 ***segmental bronchi (tertiary bronchi)***; the lobar bronchi of the left lung give rise to 8 segmental bronchi.

A segmental bronchus and the lung parenchyma that it supplies constitute a ***bronchopulmonary segment***. The sig-

nificance of the bronchopulmonary segment in the human lung becomes apparent when considering the need for surgical resection, which may be required in certain disease states. The segments, each with its own blood supply and connective tissue septa, are convenient subunits that facilitate surgical resection.

Initially, the bronchi have the same general histologic structure as the trachea. At the point where the bronchi enter the lungs to become intrapulmonary bronchi, the structure of the bronchial wall changes. The cartilage rings are replaced by cartilage plates of irregular shape. The plates are distributed in a linear array around the entire circumference of the wall, giving the bronchi a circular or cylindrical shape in contrast to the ovoid shape with a flattened posterior wall of the trachea. As the bronchi decrease in size because of branching, the cartilage plates become smaller and less numerous. The plates ultimately disappear at the point where the airway reaches a diameter of about 1 mm, whereupon the branch is designated a *bronchiole.*

Bronchi can be identified by their cartilage plates and a circular layer of smooth muscle

The second change observed in the wall of the intrapulmonary bronchus is the addition of smooth muscle to form a complete circumferential layer. The smooth muscle becomes an increasingly conspicuous layer as the amount of cartilage diminishes. Initially, the smooth muscle is arranged in interlacing bundles forming a continuous layer. In the smaller bronchi, the smooth muscle may appear discontinuous.

Because the smooth muscle forms a separate layer, namely, a muscularis, the wall of the bronchus can be regarded as having five layers:

- *Mucosa,* composed of a pseudostratified epithelium with the same cellular composition as the trachea. The height of the cells decreases as the bronchi decrease in diameter. In H&E specimens the "basement membrane" is conspicuous in the primary bronchi but quickly diminishes in thickness and disappears as a discrete structure. The lamina propria is similar to that of the trachea but is reduced in amount in proportion to the diameter of the bronchi.
- *Muscularis,* a continuous layer of smooth muscle in the larger bronchi. It is more attenuated and loosely organized in smaller bronchi, where it may appear discontinuous because of its spiral course. Contraction of the muscle maintains the appropriate diameter of the airway.
- *Submucosa* remains as a relatively loose connective tissue. Glands are present as well as adipose tissue in the larger bronchi.
- *Cartilage layer* consists of discontinuous cartilage plates that become smaller as the bronchial diameter diminishes.
- *Adventitia* is moderately dense connective tissue that is continuous with that of adjacent structures, such as pulmonary artery and lung parenchyma.

BRONCHIOLES

The bronchopulmonary segments are further subdivided into ***pulmonary lobules;*** each lobule is supplied by a ***bronchiole.*** Delicate connective tissue septa that partially separate adjacent lobules may be represented on the surface of the lung as faintly outlined polygonal areas. ***Pulmonary acini*** are smaller units of structure that make up the lobules. Each acinus consists of a ***terminal bronchiole*** and the ***respiratory bronchioles*** and ***alveoli*** that it aerates (see Fig. 18.10). The smallest functional unit of pulmonary structure is thus the ***respiratory bronchiolar unit.*** It con-

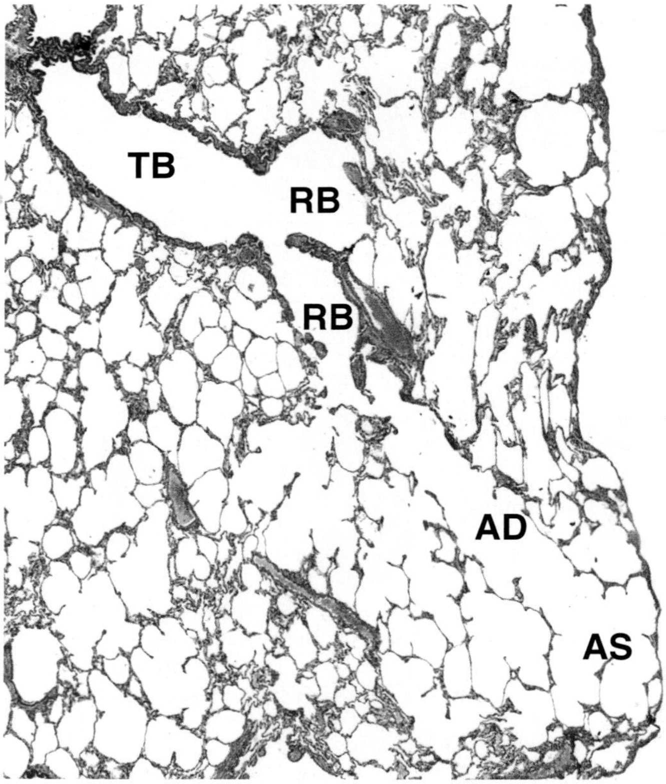

FIGURE 18.10
Photomicrograph showing the respiratory portion of the bronchial tree. In this photomicrograph a terminal bronchiole *(TB)* is shown longitudinally sectioned as it branches into two respiratory bronchioles *(RB).* The terminal bronchiole is the most distal part of the conducting portion of the respiratory system and is not engaged in gas exchange. The respiratory bronchiole engages in gas exchange and is the beginning of the respiratory portion of the bronchial tree. Respiratory bronchioles give rise to alveolar ducts *(AD),* which are elongate airways that have almost no walls, only alveoli surrounding the duct space. Alveolar sacs *(AS)* are spaces at the termination of the alveolar ducts that, likewise, are surrounded by alveoli. $\times 120$.

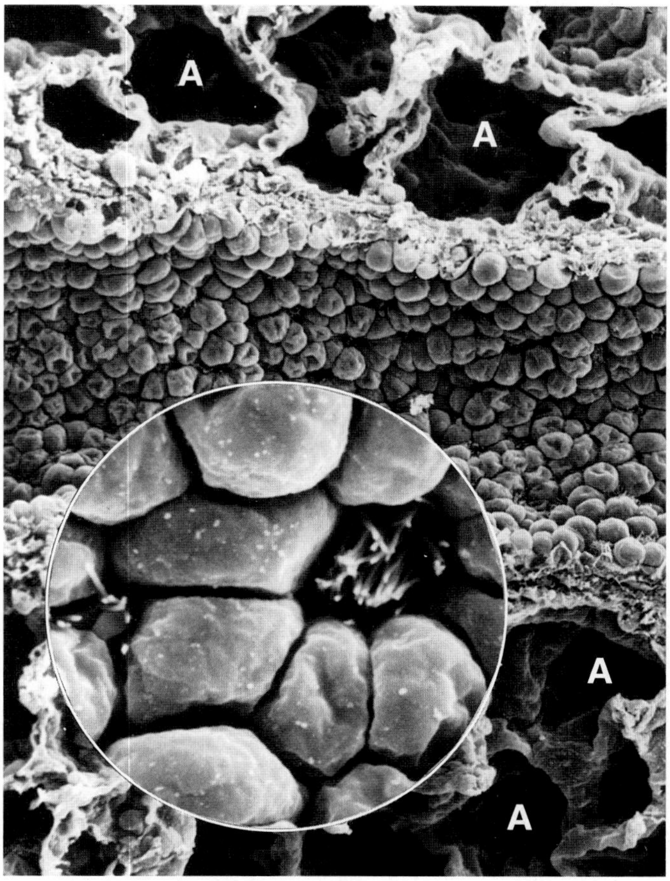

FIGURE 18.11
Scanning electron micrograph of a terminal bronchiole. This scanning photomicrograph shows a longitudinal section throughout the terminal bronchiole and surrounding alveoli *(A)*. Note that the apical surfaces of the Clara cells possess no cilia and have a characteristic dome-shaped appearance. ×150. The **inset** shows some of the Clara cells at a higher magnification and the cilia of a neighboring ciliated cell, which are present in very small numbers at this level. Note the relatively few cilia present on these small cells. ×1,200.

sists of a single respiratory bronchiole and the alveoli that it supplies.

Bronchiolar Structure

Bronchioles are air-conducting ducts that measure 1 mm or less in diameter. The larger bronchioles represent branches of the segmental bronchi. These ducts branch repeatedly, giving rise to the smaller ***terminal bronchioles*** that also branch. The terminal bronchioles finally give rise to the ***respiratory bronchioles.***

Cartilage plates and glands are not present in bronchioles

The larger-diameter bronchioles initially have a ciliated, pseudostratified columnar epithelium that gradually transforms into a simple ciliated columnar epithelium as the duct narrows. Goblet cells are still present in the largest bronchioles but are not present in the terminal bronchioles that follow. An exception is in smokers and others exposed to irritants in the air. There are no subepithelial glands in bronchioles. Cartilage plates, characteristic of bronchi, are absent in bronchioles. Instead, small elements of cartilage may be present, particularly at branching points. A relatively thick layer of smooth muscle is present in the wall of all bronchioles.

Small bronchioles have a simple cuboidal epithelium. The smallest conducting bronchioles, the ***terminal bronchioles,*** are lined with a simple cuboidal epithelium in which ***Clara cells*** are interspersed among the ciliated cells (see Fig. 18.11). Clara cells increase in number as the ciliated cells decrease along the length of the bronchiole. Occasional brush cells and small granule cells are also present. A small amount of connective tissue underlies the epithelium, and a circumferential layer of smooth muscle underlies the connective tissue in the conducting portions.

Clara cells are nonciliated cells that have a characteristic rounded or dome-shaped apical surface projection. They display TEM characteristics of protein-secreting cells (Fig. 18.12). They have a well-developed basal rER, a lateral or supranuclear Golgi apparatus, secretory granules that stain for protein, and numerous cisternae of sER in the apical

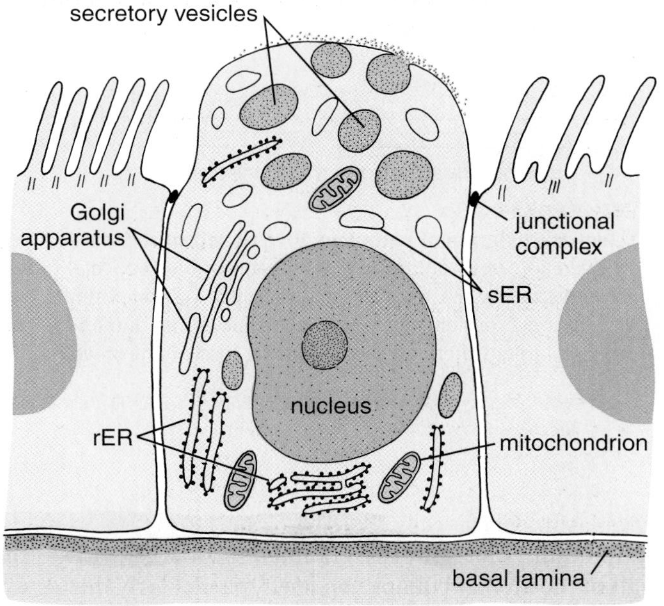

FIGURE 18.12
Diagram of a Clara cell between bronchiolar ciliated epithelial cells. The nucleus is in a basal location. Rough-surfaced endoplasmic reticulum *(rER)*, a Golgi apparatus, and mitochondria are chiefly in basal and paranuclear locations of the cell. Smooth-surfaced endoplasmic reticulum *(sER)* and secretory vesicles are chiefly in the apical cytoplasm. One of the secretory vesicles is shown discharging its contents onto the surface of the cell.

BOX 18.2

Clinical Correlations: Cystic Fibrosis

Cystic fibrosis (mucoviscidosis) is a chronic obstructive pulmonary disease of children and young adults. It is an autosomal recessive disorder that affects the viscosity of the secretion of the exocrine glands. Almost all exocrine glands secrete abnormally viscid mucus that obstructs the glands and their excretory ducts. The primary cause of cystic fibrosis is a genetic defect in the ***Cl^- channel protein,*** which results in abnormal epithelial transport of Cl^-.

The course of the disease is largely determined by the degree of pulmonary involvement. At birth, the lungs are normal. However, the defective Cl^- channel protein in the bronchial epithelium causes decreased Cl^- secretion and increased Na^+ and water reabsorption from the lumen (Fig. 18.13). As a result, the "mucociliary escalator" malfunctions, with consequent accumulation of an unusually thick, viscous mucous secretion. The pulmonary lesion is probably initiated by obstruction of the bronchioles. Bronchiolar obstruction blocks the airways and leads to thickening of the bronchiole walls and to other degenerative changes in the alveoli. Because fluids remain trapped in the lungs, individuals with cystic fibrosis have frequent respiratory tract infections. The recent cloning of the cystic fibrosis gene could lead to the use of gene therapy in the future.

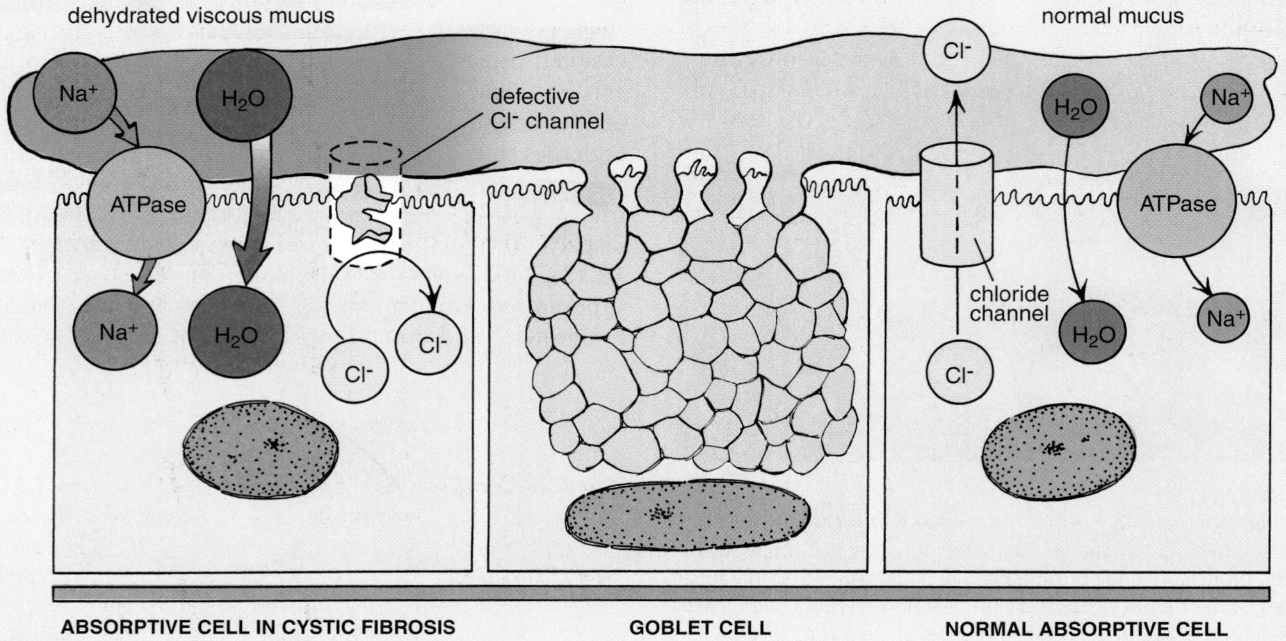

FIGURE 18.13
Schematic diagram of pathology in cystic fibrosis. In cystic fibrosis, secretion of Cl^- anions into the lumen of the bronchial tree is markedly decreased because of a defective or nonexistent chloride channel protein. Na^+ resorption from the lumen of the bronchial tree is then increased, causing movement of water into the cell. As a result, the mucous layer within the bronchial tree becomes dehydrated and viscous. This thick mucus is difficult to move by the mucociliary escalator mechanism, and it clogs the lumen of the bronchial tree, obstructing airflow.

cytoplasm. Clara cells secrete a surface-active agent, a lipoprotein, that prevents luminal adhesion should the wall of the airway collapse on itself, particularly during expiration. In addition, Clara cells produce a 16-kDa protein known as *Clara cell protein (CC16)*, which is an abundant component of the airway secretion. CC16 is used as a measurable pulmonary marker in bronchoalveolar lavage fluid and serum. Secretion of CC16 into the bronchial tree decreases in lung injury (because of damage of Clara cells), while serum levels of CC16 may increase because of leakage across the air–blood barrier.

Bronchiolar Function

3

Respiratory bronchioles are the first part of the bronchial tree that allows gas exchange

Respiratory bronchioles constitute a transitional zone in the respiratory system; they are involved in both air conduction and gas exchange. They have a narrow diameter and are lined by cuboidal epithelium. The epithelium of the initial segments of the respiratory bronchioles contains both ciliated cells and Clara cells (see Fig. 18.11). Distally,

Clara cells predominate. Occasional brush cells and dense-core granule cells are also present along the length of the respiratory bronchiole. Scattered, thin-walled outpocketings, ***alveoli***, extend from the lumen of the respiratory bronchioles (see Fig. 18.10). Alveoli are the sites at which air leaves and enters the bronchiole to allow gas exchange.

▼ ALVEOLI

Alveoli are the site of gas exchange

The surface area available for gas exchange is increased by the lung ***alveoli***. Alveoli are the terminal air spaces of the respiratory system and are the actual sites of gas exchange between the air and the blood. Each alveolus is surrounded by a network of capillaries that brings blood into close proximity to inhaled air inside the alveolus. About 150 to 250 million alveoli are found in each adult lung; their combined internal surface area is approximately 75 m^2, roughly the size of a tennis court. Each alveolus is a thin-walled polyhedral chamber approximately 0.2 mm in diameter that is confluent with an alveolar sac (Fig. 18.14).

- ***Alveolar ducts*** are elongate airways that have almost no walls, only alveoli, as their peripheral boundary. Rings of smooth muscle are present in the knob-like interalveolar septa (see below).
- ***Alveolar sacs*** are spaces surrounded by clusters of alveoli. The surrounding alveoli open into these spaces.

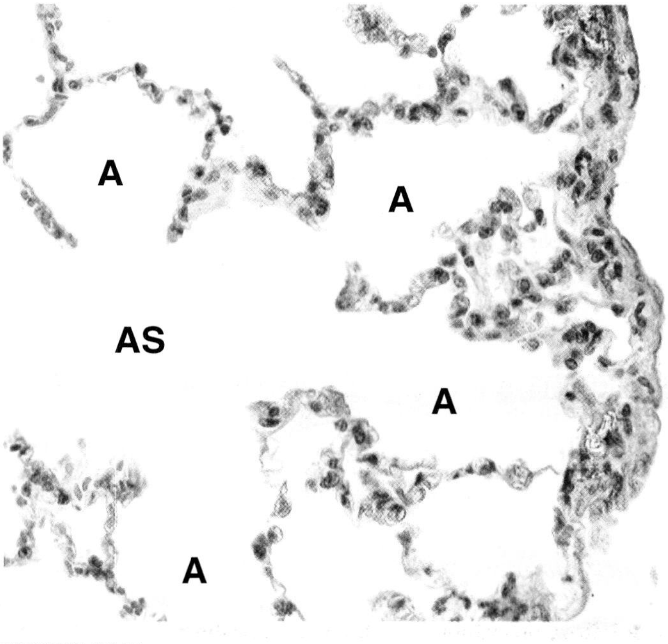

FIGURE 18.14
Photomicrograph showing an alveolar sac with adjacent alveoli. This photomicrograph shows the terminal components of the respiratory system, namely, the alveolar sac *(AS)* and the surrounding alveoli *(A)*. The alveoli are surrounded and separated from one another by a thin connective tissue layer, the interalveolar septa, containing blood capillaries. On the right is the lung surface, which is covered by visceral pleura containing simple squamous epithelium and an underlying layer of connective tissue. ×360.

Alveolar sacs usually occur at the termination of an alveolar duct but may occur anywhere along its length. Alveoli are surrounded and separated from one another by an exceedingly thin connective tissue layer that contains blood capillaries. The tissue between adjacent alveolar air spaces is called the ***alveolar septum*** or ***septal wall*** (Fig. 18.15).

Alveolar epithelium is composed of type I and II alveolar cells and occasional brush cells

The alveolar surface forms a vulnerable biologic interface that is subject to many destabilizing surface forces and to continuous exposure to inhaled particles, pathogens, and toxins. The alveolar epithelium is composed of several specialized cells and their products, some of which play defensive and protective roles:

- ***Type I alveolar cells***, also known as ***type I pneumocytes***, are extremely thin squamous cells that line most (95%) of the surface of the alveoli (see Fig. 18.15). These cells are joined to one another and to the other cells of the alveolar epithelium by occluding junctions (Fig. 18.16). The junctions form an effective barrier between the air space and the components of the septal wall. Type I alveolar cells are not capable of cell division.
- ***Type II alveolar cells***, also called ***type II pneumocytes*** or ***septal cells***, are secretory cells. These cuboidal cells are interspersed among the type I cells but tend to congregate at septal junctions. Type II cells are as numerous as type I cells, but because of their different shape they cover only about 5% of the alveolar air surface. Like Clara cells, type II cells tend to bulge into the air space (see Fig. 18.16). Their apical cytoplasm is filled with granules that are resolved with the TEM (Fig. 18.17) as stacks of parallel membrane lamellae, the ***lamellar bodies***. They are rich in a mixture of phospholipids, neutral lipids, and proteins that is secreted by exocytosis to form an alveolar lining, surface-active agent called ***surfactant***. In addition to secretion of surfactant, type II alveolar cells are progenitor cells for type I alveolar cells. Following lung injury, they proliferate and restore both types of alveolar cells within the alveolus. Hyperplasia of type II alveolar cells is an important marker of alveolar injury and repair of alveoli.
- ***Brush cells*** are also present in the alveolar wall, but they are few in number. They may serve as receptors that monitor air quality in the lung.

Surfactant decreases the alveolar surface tension and actively participates in the clearance of foreign materials

The surfactant layer produced by type II alveolar cells reduces the surface tension at the air–epithelium interface.

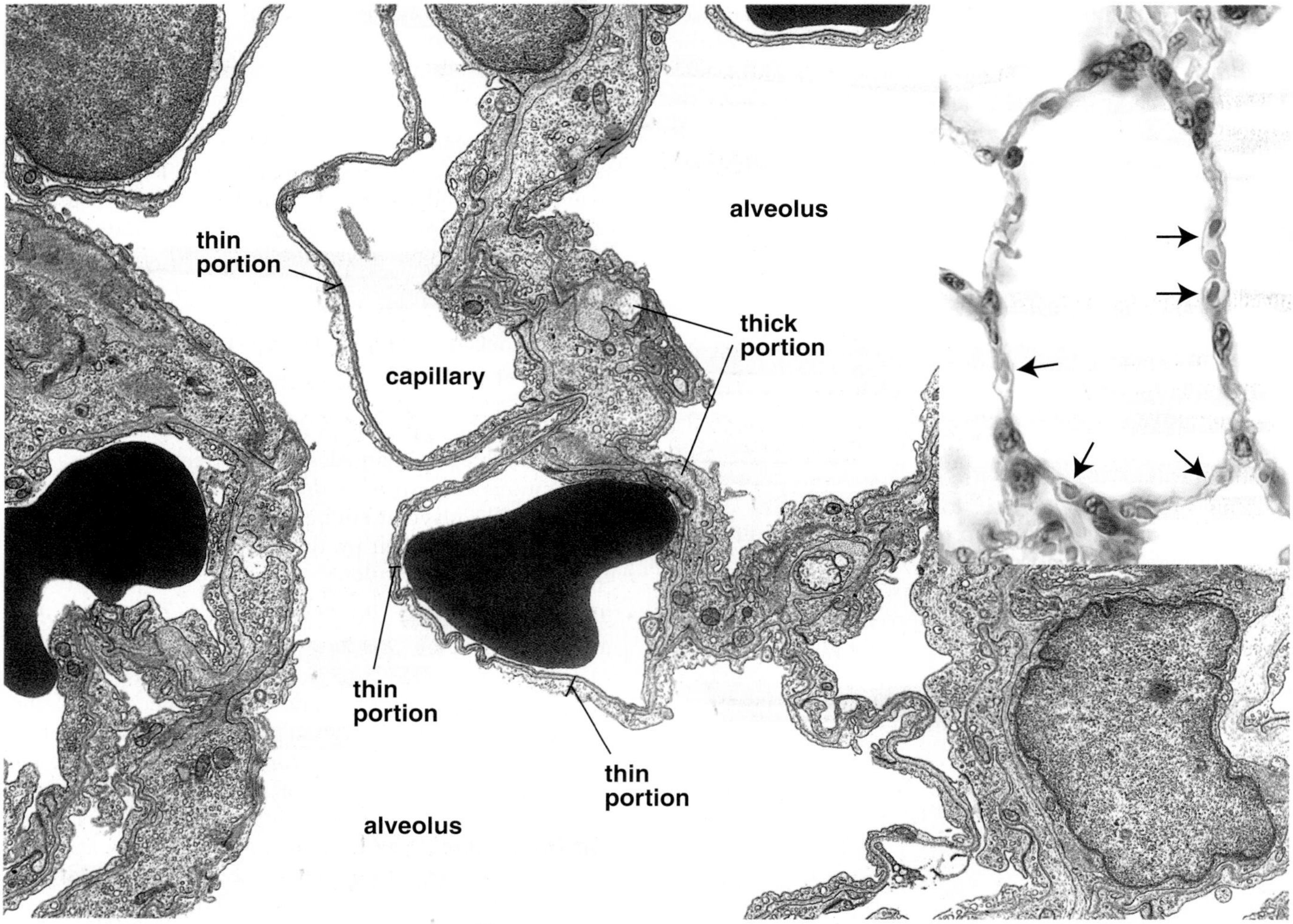

FIGURE 18.15
Electron micrograph of lung alveoli. This electron micrograph shows two alveolar spaces separated by an alveolar septum containing capillaries, some of which contain red blood cells. Note the areas of thin and thick portions of the alveolar septum. These are shown at a higher magnification in Figure 18.19. ×5,800. **inset.** Photomicrograph of an alveolus for comparison with the alveolar wall as seen in an electron micrograph. *Arrows* indicate alveolar capillaries containing red blood cells. ×480.

The most critical agent for air space stability is a specific phospholipid called ***dipalmitoylphosphatidylcholine (DPPC)***, which accounts for almost all surface tension–reducing properties of surfactant. Surfactant synthesis in the fetus occurs after the 35th week of gestation and is modulated by a variety of hormones, including cortisol, insulin, prolactin, and thyroxine. Without adequate secretion of surfactant, the alveoli would collapse on each successive exhalation. Such collapse occurs in premature infants whose lungs have not developed sufficiently to produce surfactant, causing neonatal respiratory distress syndrome (RDS). Prophylactic administration of exogenous surfactant at birth to extremely premature infants and administration to symptomatic newborns reduces the risk of RDS. In addition, administration of cortisol to mothers with threatened premature delivery decreases neonatal mortality.

Surfactant proteins help organize the surfactant layer and modulate alveolar immune responses

In addition to phospholipids, hydrophobic proteins are necessary for the structure and function of surfactant. These proteins are

- ***Surfactant protein A (SP-A)***, the most abundant surfactant protein. SP-A is responsible for surfactant homeostasis (regulating synthesis and secretion of surfactant by type II alveolar cells). It also modulates immune responses to viruses, bacteria, and fungi.
- ***Surfactant protein B (SP-B)***, an important protein for the transformation of the lamellar body into the thin surface film of surfactant. SP-B is a critical surfactant-organizing protein responsible for adsorption and spreading of surfactant onto the surface of the alveolar epithelium.

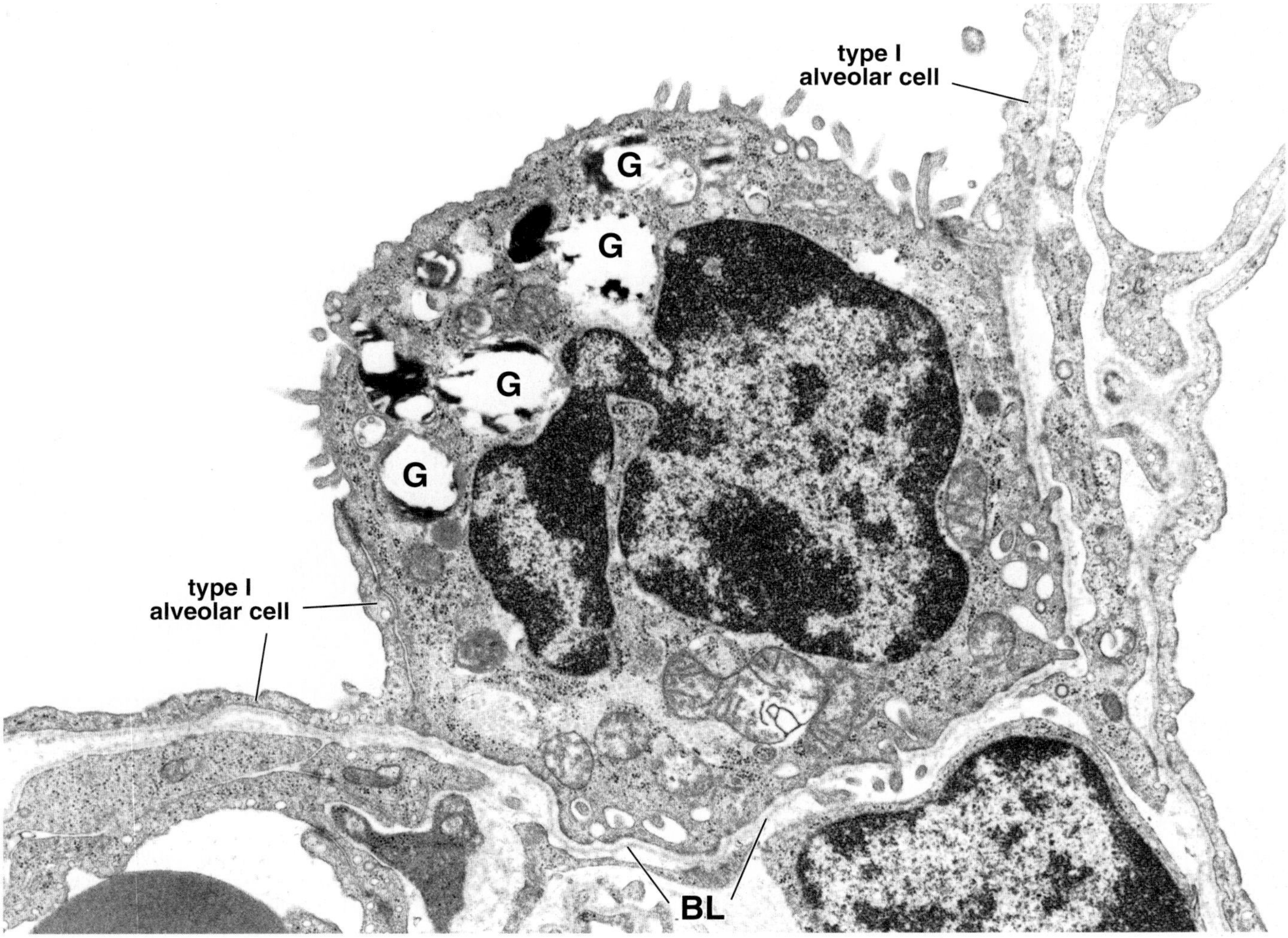

FIGURE 18.16
Electron micrograph of a type II alveolar cell. The type II alveolar cell has a dome-shaped apical surface with a number of short microvilli at its periphery and a relatively smooth-contoured apical center. The lateral cell margins are overlain to a variable degree by the type I alveolar cells that are joined to the type II cell by occluding junctions. Both cell types rest on the basal lamina *(BL)*. The secretory vesicles *(G)* in this specimen are largely dissolved, but their lamellar character is shown to advantage in Figure 18.17b. ×24,000.

- ***Surfactant protein C (SP-C),*** which represents only 1% of the total mass of surfactant protein. Along with SP-B, SP-C aids in orientation of DPPC within the surfactant and maintenance of the thin film layer within the alveoli.
- ***Surfactant protein D (SP-D),*** a primary protein involved in host defense. It binds to various microorganisms (e.g., Gram-negative bacteria) and to lymphocytes. SP-D participates in a local inflammatory response as the result of acute lung injury and with SP-A modulates an allergic response to various inhaled antigens.

The alveolar septum is the site of the air–blood barrier

The ***air–blood barrier*** refers to the cells and cell products across which gases must diffuse between the alveolar and capillary compartments. The thinnest air–blood barrier consists of a thin layer of surfactant, a type I epithelial cell and its basal lamina, and a capillary endothelial cell and its basal lamina. Often, these two basal laminae are fused (Fig. 18.18). Connective tissue cells and fibers that may be present between the two basal laminae widen the air–blood barrier. These two arrangements produce a ***thin portion*** and a ***thick portion*** of the barrier (Fig. 18.19). It is thought that most gas exchange occurs across the thin portion of the barrier. The thick portion is thought to be a site in which tissue fluid can accumulate and even cross into the alveolus. Lymphatic vessels in the connective tissue of the terminal bronchioles drain fluid that accumulates in the thick portion of the septum.

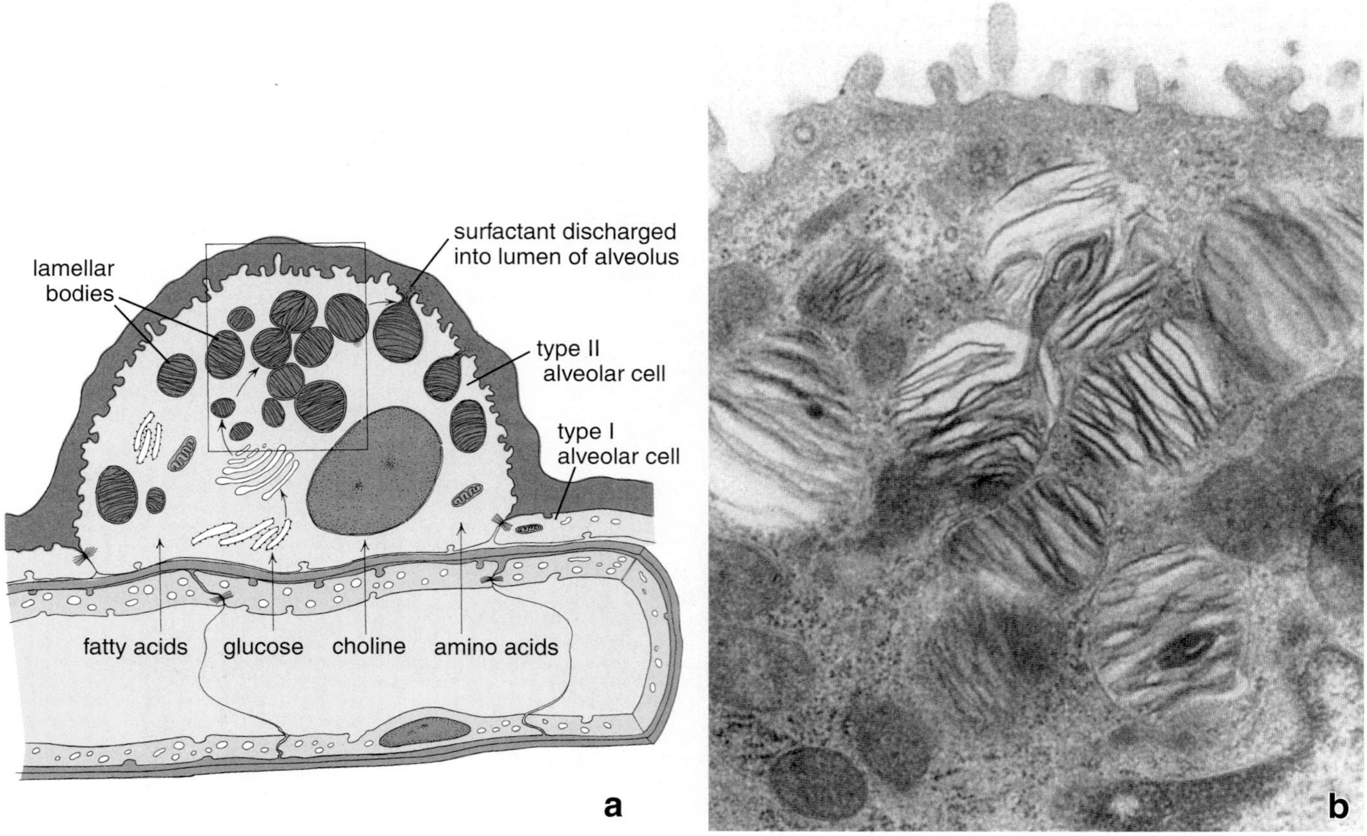

FIGURE 18.17
Diagram of a type II alveolar cell and electron micrograph of lamellar bodies. a. Surfactant is an oily mixture of proteins, phospholipids, and neutral lipids that are synthesized in the rER from precursors in the blood. These precursors are glucose, fatty acids, choline, and amino acids. The protein constituents of surfactant are produced in the rER and stored in the cytoplasm within lamellar bodies, which are discharged into the lumen of the alveolus. With the aid of surfactant protein, surfactant is distributed, on the surface of epithelial cells lining the alveolus, as a thin film that reduces the surface tension. **b.** Higher-magnification electron micrograph showing the typical lamellar pattern of the secretory vesicles of type II alveolar cells. These vesicles contain the pulmonary surfactant precursor proteins. ×38,000. (Courtesy of Dr. A. Mercuri.)

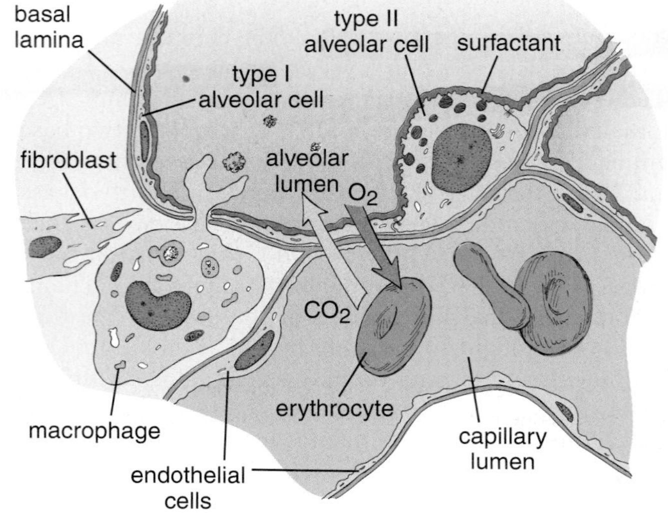

FIGURE 18.18
Diagram of the interalveolar septum. This diagram shows the thick and thin portions of the interalveolar septum. The thin portion forms the air–blood barrier and is responsible for most of the gas exchange that occurs in the lung. *Arrows* indicate the direction of CO_2 and O_2 exchange between the alveolar air space and the blood. The thick portion of the interalveolar septum plays an important role in fluid distribution and its dynamics. It contains connective tissue cells. Note the macrophage in the thick portion that extends its processes into the lumen of the alveolus.

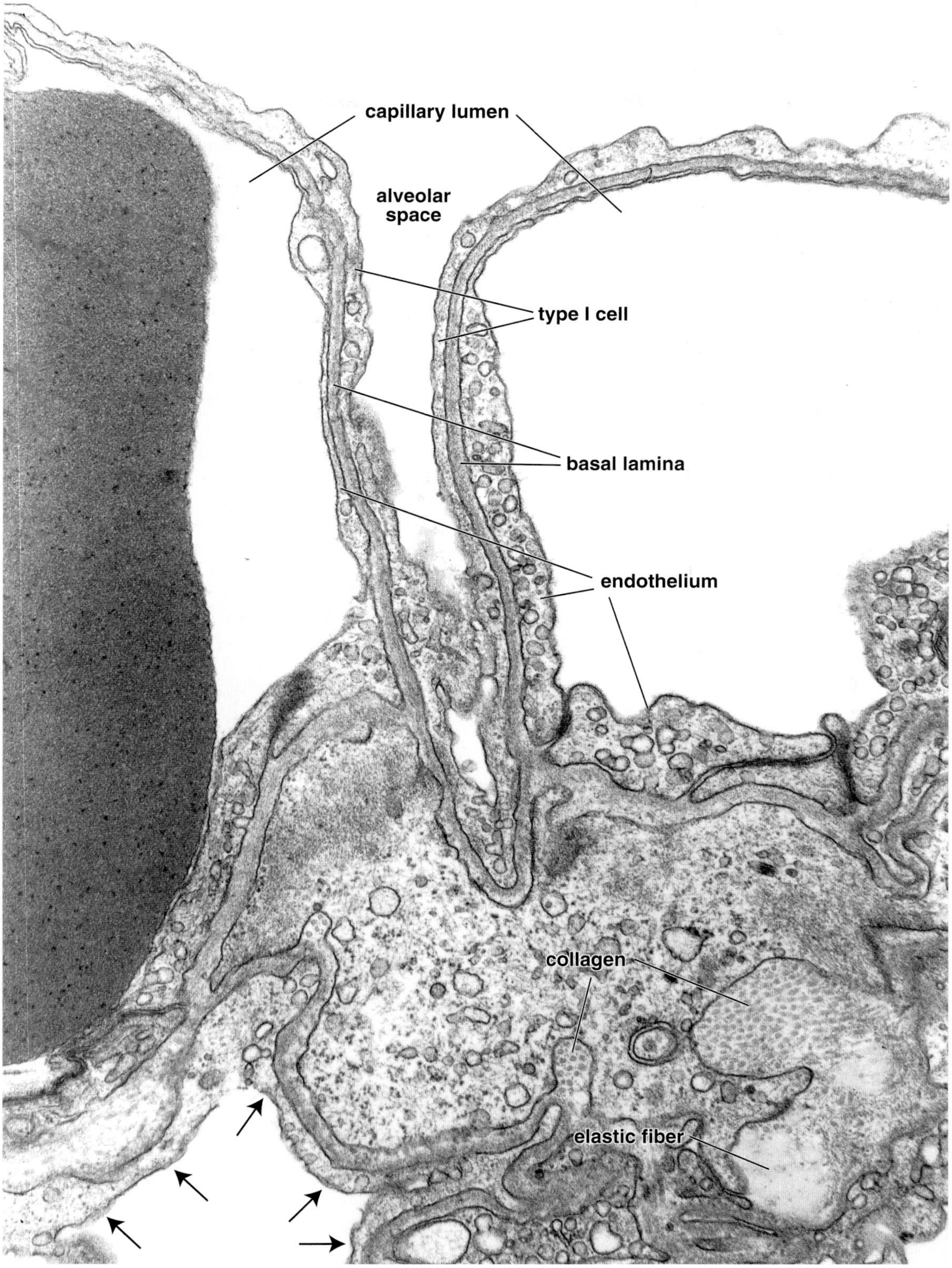

FIGURE 18.19

Electron micrograph of the alveolar septum. This high-magnification micrograph shows the thin portion of the air–blood barrier where it consists of type I alveolar cells, capillary endothelium, and the fused basal lamina shared by both cells. In the thick portion, the type I alveolar cell *(arrows)* rests on a basal lamina, and on the opposite side is connective tissue in which collagen fibrils and elastic fibers are evident. ×33,000.

BOX 18.3

Clinical Correlations: Emphysema and Pneumonia

Emphysema is a condition of the lung characterized by permanent enlargement of the air spaces distal to the terminal bronchiole. This enlargement is caused by chronic obstruction of airflow, most often because of narrowing of the bronchioles, and is accompanied by destruction of the alveolar wall (Fig. 18.20). Thus, significant area for gas exchange is lost in this disease. Emphysema is relatively common; it is seen in about half of all autopsies and is easily recognized. Pathologists identify several types of emphysema. The severity of the disease is clinically more important, however, than recognition of the specific type. Emphysema is often caused by chronic inhalations of foreign particulate material such as coal dust, textile fibers, and construction dust. The most common cause, however, is cigarette smoking.

The destruction of the alveolar wall may be associated with excess lysis of elastin and other structural proteins in the alveolar septa. Elastase and other proteases are derived from lung neutrophils, macrophages, and monocytes. A specific genetic disease, α_1-antitrypsin deficiency, causes a particularly severe form of emphysema in both heterozygous and homozygous individuals. It is usually fatal in homozygotes if untreated, but its severity can be reduced by supplying the enzyme inhibitor exogenously.

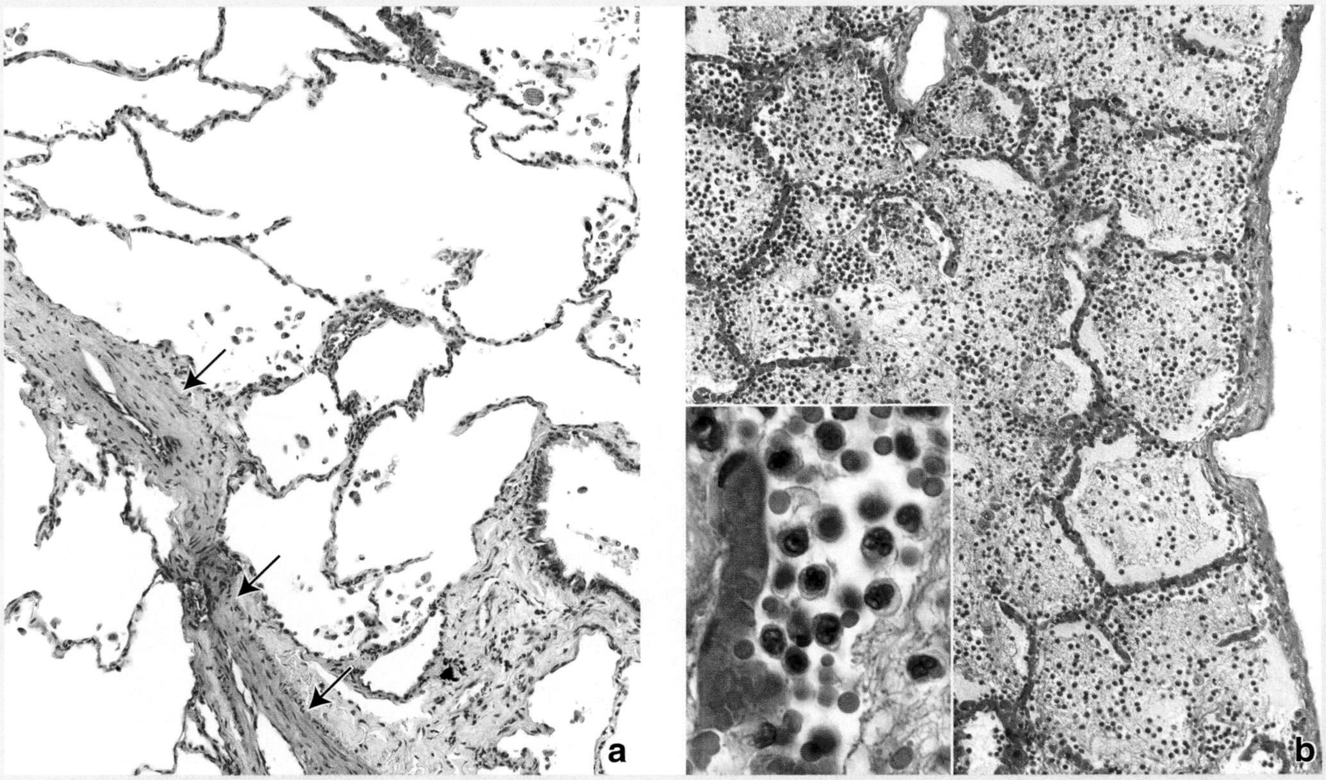

FIGURE 18.20

Photomicrographs of emphysema and pneumonia. a. This photomicrograph from the lung of an individual with emphysema shows the partial destruction of interalveolar septa, resulting in permanent enlargement of the air spaces. Note that the changes in the lung parenchyma are accompanied by thickening of the wall of the pulmonary vessels *(arrows)* and the presence of numerous cells within the air spaces. These cells are the alveolar macrophages and are shown at higher magnification in Figure 18.21. ×240. **b.** This photomicrograph from the lung of an individual in the early stages of acute pneumonia (inflammation of the lung). Note that the air spaces are filled with exudate containing white blood cells (mainly neutrophils), red blood cells, and fibrin. The capillaries in the alveolar septum are enlarged and congested with red blood cells. Pathologists recognize this stage as the red hepatization stage of the pneumonia. At this stage, the affected portion of the lung on gross examination appears red (because of enlarged capillaries), firm (because of the lack of air spaces), and heavy (because of the presence of exudate within the alveoli); the term *hepatization* stems from the tissue's resemblance to the liver. ×240. **inset.** Part of an alveolus at a higher magnification. Note the enlarged, congested capillary within the alveolar septum. The air space is filled with neutrophils and red blood cells. The lower right corner shows early organization of the intra-alveolar exudate; observe that the developing fibrin network contains entrapped neutrophils and several red blood cells. ×420.

Alveolar macrophages remove inhaled particulate matter from the air spaces and red blood cells from the septum

Alveolar macrophages are unusual in that they function both in the connective tissue of the septum and in the air space of the alveolus (Fig. 18.21). In air spaces, they scavenge the surface to remove inhaled particulate matter, e.g., dust and pollen, thus giving them one of their alternate names, dust cells. Alveolar macrophages are derived from blood monocytes and belong to the mononuclear phagocytotic system (page 144). They phagocytize red blood cells that may enter the alveoli in heart failure (see Fig. 18.21). Some engorged macrophages pass up the bronchial tree in the mucus and are disposed of by swallowing or expectoration when they reach the pharynx. Other macrophages return to or remain in the septal connective tissue, where, filled with accumulated phagocytized material, they may remain for much of an individual's life. Thus, at autopsy, the lungs of urban dwellers as well as smokers will usually show many alveolar and septal macrophages filled with carbon particles, anthracotic pigment, and birefringent needle-like particles of silica. Alveolar macrophages also phagocytose infectious organisms such as *Mycobacterium tuberculosis,* which can be recognized in the cells in appropriately stained specimens. These bacilli are not digested by macrophages, however, and other infections or conditions that damage alveolar macrophages can lead to release of the bacteria and recurrent tuberculosis.

Collateral air circulation through alveolar pores allows air to pass between alveoli

Scanning electron microscopic studies of alveolar structure show openings in the interalveolar septa that allow circulation of air from one alveolus to another. These ***alveolar pores (of Kohn)*** can be of great significance in some pathologic conditions in which obstructive lung disease blocks the normal pathway of air to the alveoli. The alveoli distal to the blockage may continue to be aerated, via the pores, from an adjacent lobule or acinus.

A basic summary of information related to the respiratory system is included in Table 18.1.

TABLE 18.1. **Divisions of the Bronchial Tree and Summary of Its Histologic Features**

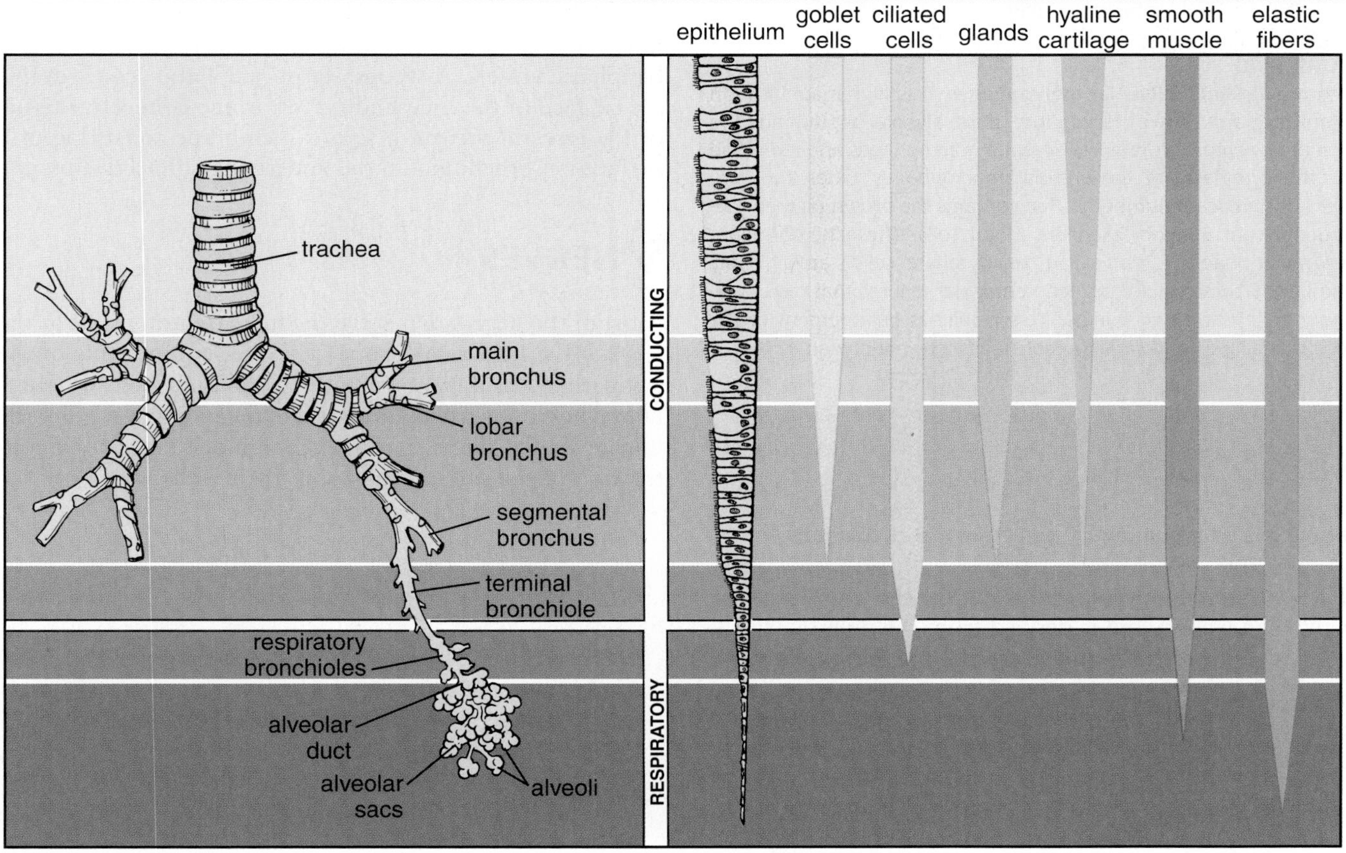

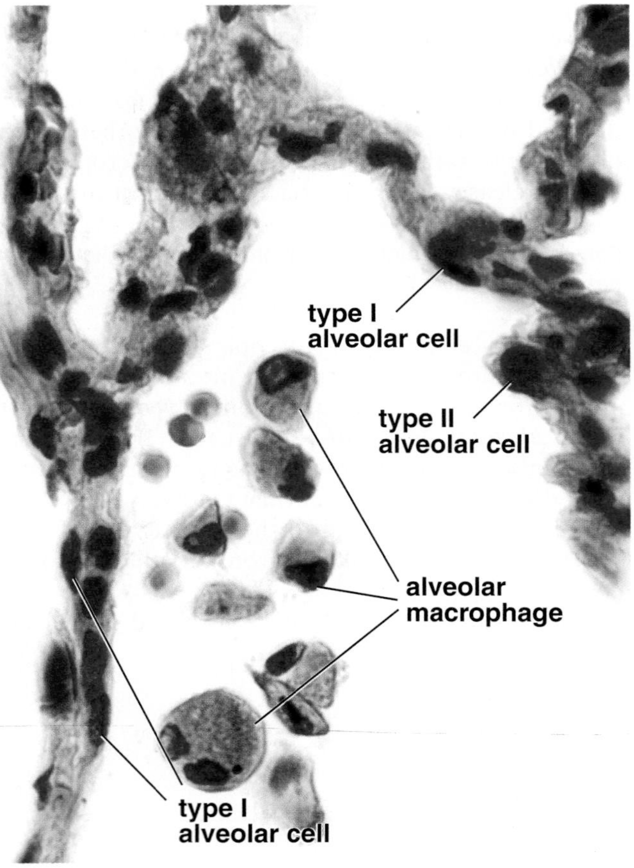

FIGURE 18.21
Photomicrograph of alveolar macrophages. This high-magnification photomicrograph shows the structure of the alveolar septum and the lumen of an alveolus containing alveolar macrophages and red blood cells. The cytoplasm of the alveolar macrophages, when they are present in significant numbers, often contains the brown pigment hemosiderin from phagocytosed red blood cells. These hemosiderin-laden macrophages (often called "heart failure cells") are typically found in heart disease, mostly left ventricular failures that cause pulmonary congestion and edema. This results in enlargement of the alveolar capillaries and small hemorrhages into the alveoli. ×560.

▼ BLOOD SUPPLY

The lung has both pulmonary and bronchial circulations

The ***pulmonary circulation*** supplies the capillaries of the alveolar septum and is derived from the pulmonary artery that leaves the right ventricle of the heart. The branches of the pulmonary artery travel with those of the bronchi and bronchioles and carry blood down to the capillary level at the alveoli. This blood is oxygenated and collected by pulmonary venous capillaries that join to form venules. They ultimately form the four pulmonary veins that return blood to the left atrium of the heart. The pulmonary venous system is located at a distance from the respiratory passages at the periphery of the bronchopulmonary segments.

The ***bronchial circulation,*** via bronchial arteries that branch from the aorta, supplies all of the lung tissue other than the alveoli, i.e., the walls of the bronchi and bronchioles and the connective tissue of the lung other than that of the alveolar septum. The finest branches of the bronchial arterial tree also open into the pulmonary capillaries. Therefore, the bronchial and pulmonary circulations anastomose at about the level of the junction between the conducting and respiratory passages. Bronchial veins drain only the connective tissue of the hilar region of the lungs. Most of the blood reaching the lungs via the bronchial arteries leaves the lungs via the pulmonary veins.

▼ LYMPHATIC VESSELS

A dual lymphatic drainage of the lungs parallels the dual blood supply. One set of lymphatic vessels drains the parenchyma of the lung and follows the air passages to the hilum. Lymph nodes are found along the route of the larger lymphatic vessels. A second set of lymphatic vessels drains the surface of the lung and travels in the connective tissue of the ***visceral pleura,*** a serous membrane consisting of a surface mesothelium and the underlying connective tissue.

▼ NERVES

Most of the nerves that serve the lung are not visible at the level of the light microscope. They are components of the sympathetic and parasympathetic divisions of the autonomic nervous system and mediate reflexes that modify the dimensions of the air passages (and blood vessels) by contraction of the smooth muscle in their walls.

PLATE 65. OLFACTORY MUCOSA

Olfactory mucosa is located in the roof and part of the walls of the nasal cavity. Its pseudostratified epithelium is thicker than that of nonsensory epithelium, and it serves as the receptor for smell. Olfactory epithelium consists of *olfactory cells, supporting (sustentacular) cells, basal cells,* and *brush cells* (see Fig. 18.3, page 582).

Olfactory cells are bipolar neurons. The apex of the cell is expanded into the olfactory vesicle from which nonmotile cilia, the actual receptors, extend into surface secretions. The base of the cell tapers into an axonal process that enters the lamina propria and joins axons from other receptor cells to form the olfactory nerve. Large, cuboidal Schwann cells are a prominent feature of these axons, giving the nerve an unusual appearance.

Supporting cells are columnar cells with apical microvilli. They attach to the receptor cells through adhering junctions and provide mechanical and metabolic support to the olfactory cells. Basal cells are stem cells from which new olfactory and supporting cells differentiate. Brush cells are the same cell type that occurs in nonsensory respiratory epithelium.

The lamina propria is directly contiguous with periosteum. It contains numerous blood and lymphatic vessels, unmyelinated and myelinated nerves, and olfactory (Bowman's) glands. These are tubuloalveolar serous glands whose watery secretion serves as a trap and solvent for odorant substances and continuously washes the olfactory surface.

Figure 1, olfactory mucosa, human, Azan ×75.

This low-magnification orientation micrograph shows part of the wall of the nasal cavity. The olfactory mucosa *(OM)* and adjacent ethmoid bone *(EB)* are indicated. The olfactory mucosa is directly attached to the bone tissue; no submucosa is present. In this specimen, however, the mucosa is separated from the bone tissue because of shrinkage, a frequently encountered artifact. The olfactory epithelium *(OEp)* is pseudostratified, like respiratory epithelium; however, it is typically thicker. Note the respiratory epithelium *(REp)* included in the lower right of the micrograph. The feature that is most useful in identifying olfactory mucosa is the presence of numerous large, unmyelinated nerves *(N)* and extensive olfactory (Bowman's) glands *(BG)* in the connective tissue of the mucosa. Note that the adjacent respiratory mucosa lacks the nerves and exhibits a relative paucity of glands.

Figure 2, olfactory mucosa, human, Azan ×375.

At this higher magnification, it is possible to distinguish in a general way the three principal cell types of the olfactory epithelium on the basis of nuclear location and appearance, as well as by certain cytoplasmic characteristics. For example, the nuclei of the supporting cells *(SC)* are relatively dense and are located closest to the epithelial surface. They are arranged in an almost discrete single layer. The supporting cell has a cylindrical shape and extends from the basement membrane through the full thickness of the epithelium. Immediately beneath this layer are the cell bodies of the olfactory receptor cells *(OC)*. They lie at different levels within the thickness of the epithelium. Careful examination of the nuclei of these bipolar neuronal cells reveals that they contain more euchromatin than the nuclei of the supporting cells and often exhibit several nucleoli. In this preparation, the nucleoli appear as small round red bodies. In some cases, particularly when there is shrinkage, the thin tapering dendritic process that extends to the olfactory surface may be observed. Similarly, an axonal process may sometimes be observed extending basally. The basal cells *(BC)*, the least numerous of the principal cell types, are characterized by their small round nuclei and scant cytoplasm. They are irregularly spaced and lie in proximity to the basement membrane.

The lamina propria contains numerous blood vessels (capillaries *[C]*, veins *[V]*), lymphatics, olfactory nerves *(N)*, and olfactory (Bowman's) glands *(BG)*. The Bowman's glands are branched tubuloalveolar structures. They exhibit a very small lumen *(arrows)*. The duct elements extend from the secretory portion of the gland beginning in close proximity to the overlying epithelium *(arrowhead)* and pass directly through the epithelium to deliver their secretions at the surface. The ducts are very short, making it difficult to identify them. The very thin axonal processes *(AP)* of the olfactory cells are sometimes evident within the lamina propria prior to being ensheathed by Schwann cells to form the prominent olfactory nerves. The nuclei present within the olfactory nerves represent Schwann cell nuclei *(ScC)*.

KEY

A (Fig. 1), artery
AP, axonal process
BC, basal cells
BG, Bowman's glands
C, capillary
EB, ethmoid bone
ES, ethmoid sinus
N, olfactory nerves
OC, olfactory cells
OEp, olfactory epithelium
OM, olfactory mucosa
REp, respiratory epithelium
SC, supporting cell nuclei
ScC, Schwann cell nuclei
V (Fig. 2), vein
arrows, lumina of Bowman's glands
arrowhead, duct of a Bowman's gland entering epithelium

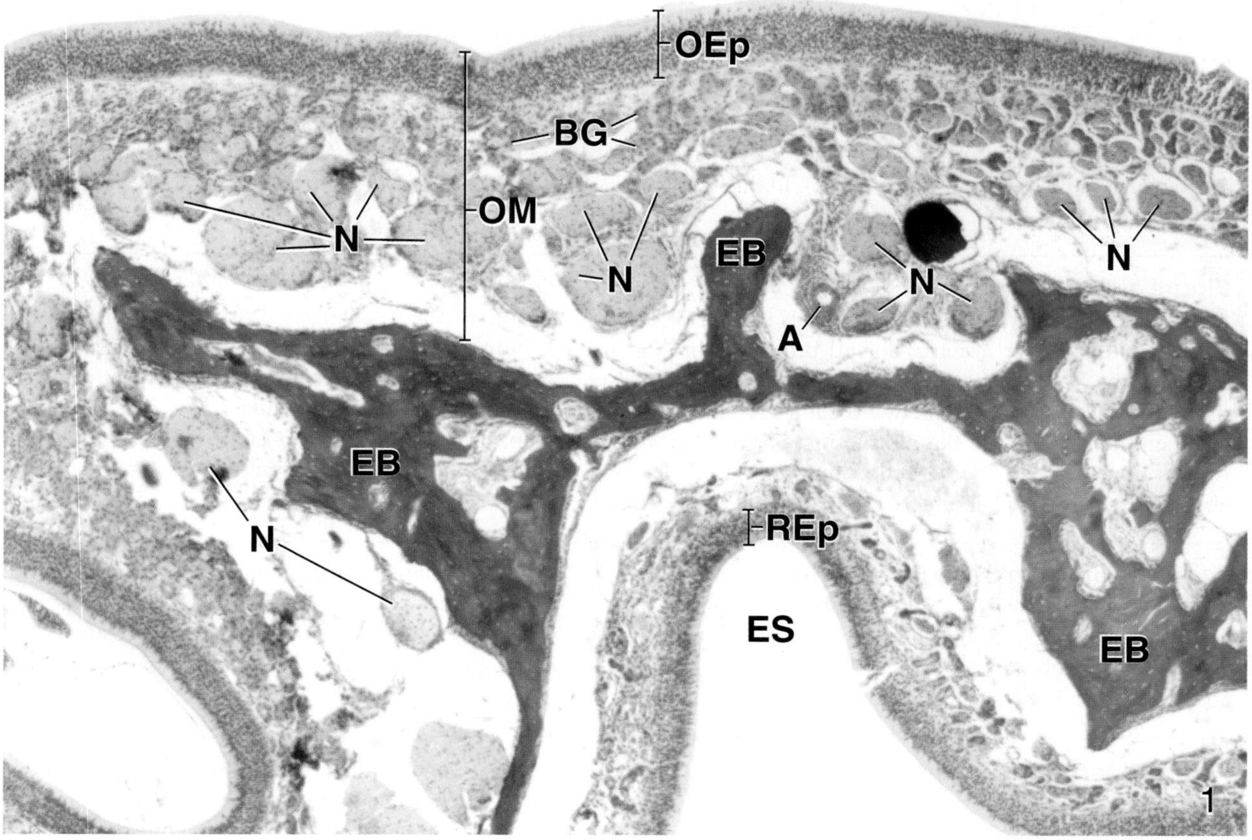
OEp
BG
OM
N
N
EB
N
N
A
EB
REp
N
ES
EB
1

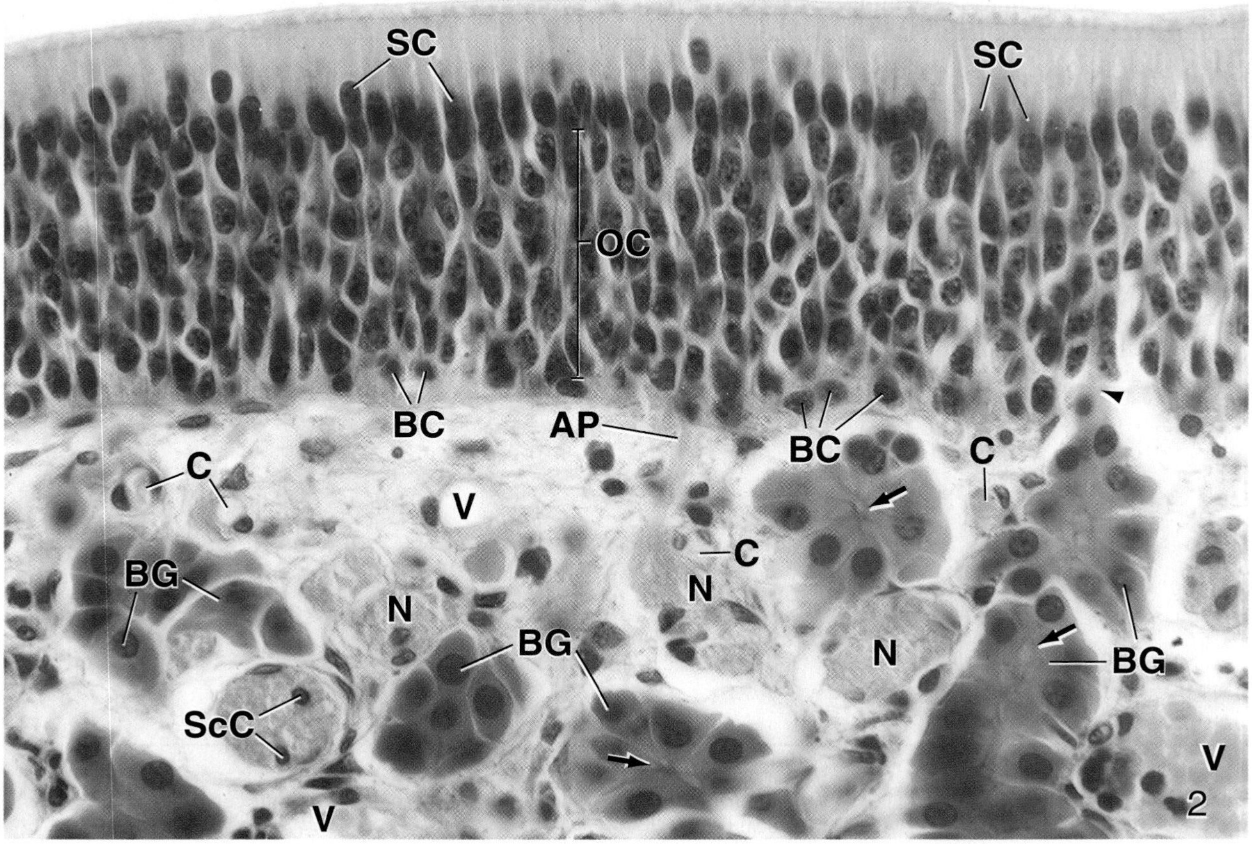
SC
SC
OC
BC
AP
BC
C
C
V
C
C
BG
N
N
BG
N
BG
ScC
V
V
2

PLATE 66. LARYNX

The larynx is the passageway for air between the oropharynx and the trachea that functions in the production of sound. It consists of a cartilaginous framework to which both extrinsic and intrinsic muscles are attached and a mucosal surface that varies in character from pseudostratified to stratified squamous in regions subject to abrasion by the air stream. The muscles move certain cartilages with respect to others, thus increasing or decreasing the opening of the glottis and increasing or decreasing the tension on the vocal folds (cords). In this way, vibrations of different wavelengths are generated in the passing air, and sound is produced.

Figure 1, larynx, monkey, H&E ×15.

The vocal folds are ridge-like structures that are oriented in an anteroposterior (ventral-dorsal) direction. In frontal sections, the vocal folds *(VF)* are cross-sectioned, giving the appearance seen here. The two vocal folds and the space between them constitute the glottis. Just above each vocal fold is an elongated recess called the ventricle *(V),* and above the ventricle is another ridge called the *ventricular fold (VnF)* or, sometimes, the *false vocal fold.* Below and lateral to the vocal folds are the vocalis muscles *(VM).* Within the vocal fold is a considerable amount of elastic material, although it is usually not evident in routine H&E preparations. This elastic material is part of the vocal ligament. It lies in an anteroposterior direction within the substance of the vocal fold and plays an important role in phonation.

Figure 2, larynx, monkey, H&E ×160.

The surfaces of a vocal fold and the facing ventricular fold within *rectangle 1* in Figure 1 are turned 90° clockwise and shown at higher magnification in this figure. Medially, both are lined by stratified squamous epithelium *(SSE).* Here, the contact between surfaces is considerable. Laterally, the surfaces consist of stratified columnar epithelium *(SCE).* The contact between these surfaces is less wearing. Small glands *(Gl)* are in the lamina propria of the laryngeal mucosa.

Figure 3, larynx, monkey, H&E ×160.

Rectangle 2 in Figure 1 is shown at higher magnification in this figure. It shows the junction between the stratified squamous epithelium *(SSE),* with its flat surface cells, and the stratified columnar epithelium *(SCE),* with its columnar surface cells. The lamina propria consists of loose connective tissue in which glands *(Gl)* are present.

Figure 4, larynx, monkey, H&E ×160.

Just below the portion of the larynx shown in Figure 1, the epithelium changes again, giving way, below, to the ciliated pseudostratified columnar epithelium *(PSE)* shown here. Note the cylinders of cytoplasm that clearly indicate the columnar nature of the surface cells. In the upper part of the figure, the epithelium is stratified columnar; in the lower part of the figure, it is pseudostratified columnar. This distinction is difficult to make from the examination of a single sample such as that shown here, and other information is needed to make the assessment. The additional information is the presence of cilia on the pseudostratified columnar epithelium; this epithelium is typically ciliated. Although not evident in the photomicrographs, note that stratified columnar epithelium has a very limited distribution, usually occurring between stratified squamous epithelium and some other epithelial types (e.g., pseudostratified columnar here or simple columnar at the anorectal junction, Plate 60).The lamina propria is a loose cellular connective tissue, and it also shows some glands *(Gl).*

KEY

Gl, glands
PSE, pseudostratified columnar epithelium
SCE, stratified columnar epithelium
SSE, stratified squamous epithelium
V, ventricles
VF, vocal folds
VM, vocalis muscles
VnF, ventricular folds

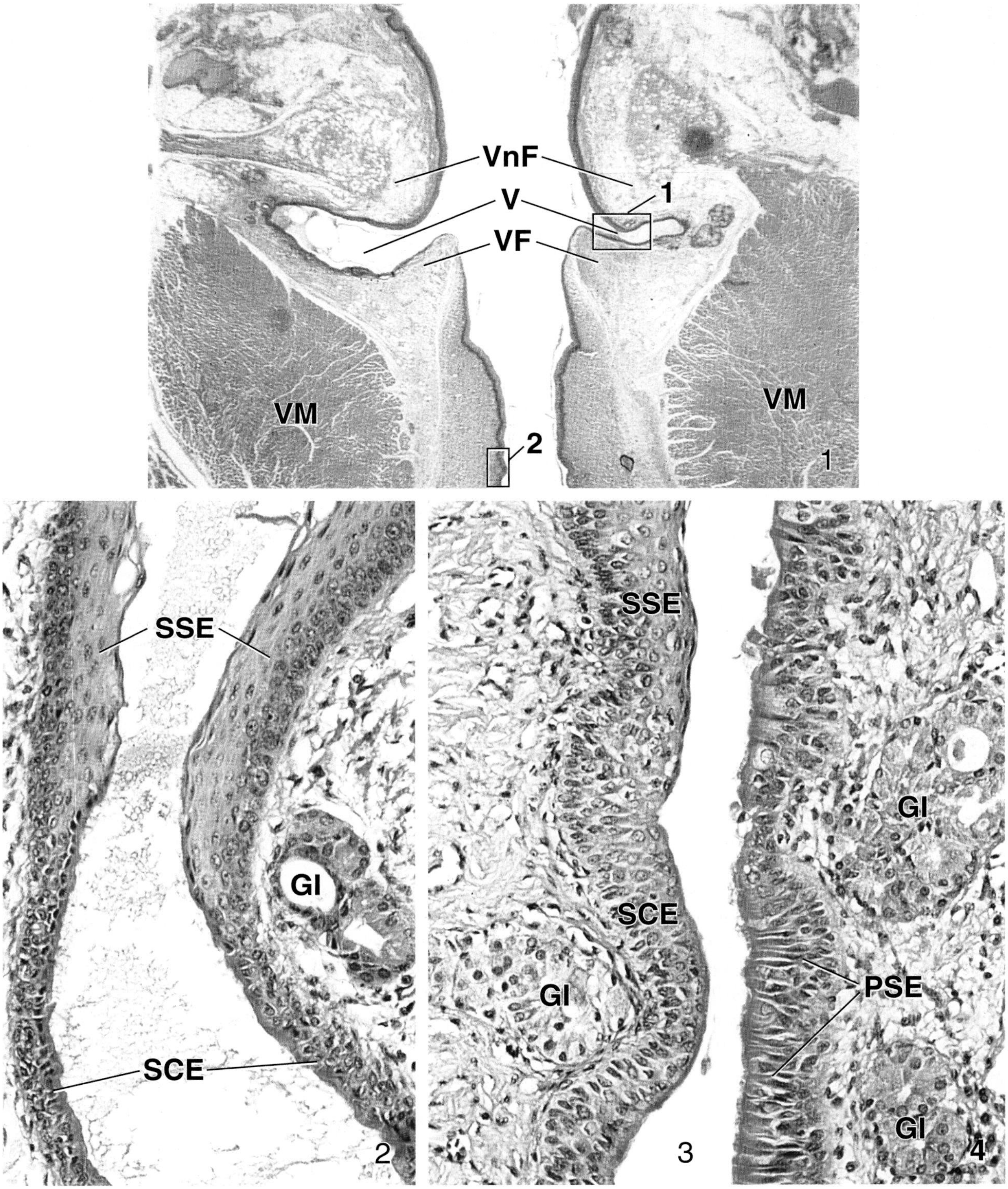
VnF
V
VF
1
VM
VM
2
1
SSE
GI
SCE
2
SSE
SCE
GI
3
GI
PSE
GI
4

PLATE 67. TRACHEA

The *trachea* is a short tube about 2.5 cm in diameter and about 10 cm long. It extends from the larynx to about the middle of the thorax, where it divides into the two *primary bronchi (extrapulmonary bronchi).* Its major function is to serve as a conduit for air. The lumen of the trachea is held open by a series of C-shaped hyaline cartilages that are stacked on one another to form a supporting structure. Fibroelastic tissue and smooth muscle (the *trachealis muscle*) bridge the gap between the free ends of the cartilages at the posterior border of the trachea, adjacent to the esophagus. Typical respiratory (ciliated pseudostratified columnar) epithelium lines the trachea and primary bronchi.

On entering the lungs, the primary bronchi become the *intrapulmonary bronchi,* which branch immediately to give rise to the *lobar bronchi (secondary bronchi)* that supply the two lobes of the left lung and the three lobes of the right lung. Within the lung, the C-shaped cartilages are replaced by an investment of (sometimes overlapping) cartilaginous plates that completely surround the bronchi.

Figure 1, trachea, human, H&E ×90.
This low-magnification micrograph of the posterior wall of the human trachea shows the pseudostratified ciliated columnar epithelium *(EP)* subtended by a well-developed basement membrane *(Bm).* The basement membrane, which consists of tightly packed, fine collagen fibers, is actually an unusually thick and dense reticular layer and is, thus, part of the lamina propria. It is particularly distinct in the human trachea and may thicken with chronic irritation, as in smokers. Numerous goblet cells *(GC)* are evident as clear ovoid spaces in the respiratory epithelium. A thin lamina propria *(LP)* and a dense thick submucosa *(SM)* underlie the respiratory epithelium. Seromucous glands *(Gl)* are seen on both sides of the trachealis muscle *(TM),* a band of smooth muscle that fills the gap between the posterior ends of the C-shaped tracheal cartilages (not shown) and serves to separate the trachea from the esophagus. Adipose tissue *(Ad)* is also present in the submucosa between the esophagus and trachea.

Figure 2, trachea, human H&E ×65.
This micrograph shows the wall of the trachea at the level of one end of the C-shaped tracheal cartilage *(TC).* The portion of the pseudostratified ciliated columnar epithelium *(EP)* does not exhibit as many goblet cells as are seen in the figure above. However, the basement membrane *(Bm)* is clear, as are the cellular lamina propria *(LP)* and the submucosa *(SM)* of the trachea. Again, seromucous glands *(Gl)* are evident beneath the submucosa. The ends of the bundles of the trachealis muscle *(TM)* are located toward the posterior midline from the glands. A small lymphatic nodule *(LN)* is located adjacent to the end of one of the bundles. A significant amount of adipose tissue *(Ad)* is found in the connective tissue between the trachealis muscle and the wall of the esophagus (not shown in this figure).

Figure 3, trachea, human, H&E ×250; inset ×500.
In this higher-magnification micrograph of the tracheal wall and in the **inset,** the cilia of the pseudostratified ciliated columnar epithelium *(EP)* are particularly well demonstrated, as is the dense line *(BB)* formed by the basal bodies of the cilia in the apical cytoplasm of the epithelial cells. Goblet cells *(GC)* are easily recognized, and the displacement of the flattened nucleus *(N)* toward the base of the cell is well demonstrated. The thickness and the density of the basement membrane *(Bm)* are more easily seen here than in the lower-magnification views in the other figures. A venule *(V)* containing red cell ghosts is seen in the middle of the submucosa, and some inflammatory cells *(IC),* probably lymphocytes, are seen adjacent to the vein as well as distributed lightly through the submucosa and more densely in the lamina propria. Portions of the seromucous glands *(Gl)* are just visible at the bottom edge of the figure.

KEY

Ad, adipose tissue
BB, brush border
Bm, basement membrane
C, cilia
EP, epithelium
GC, goblet cells
Gl, glands
IC, inflammatory cells
LN, lymphatic nodule
LP, lamina propria
N, nuclei of goblet cells
SM, submucosa
TC, tracheal cartilage
TM, trachealis muscle
V, vein

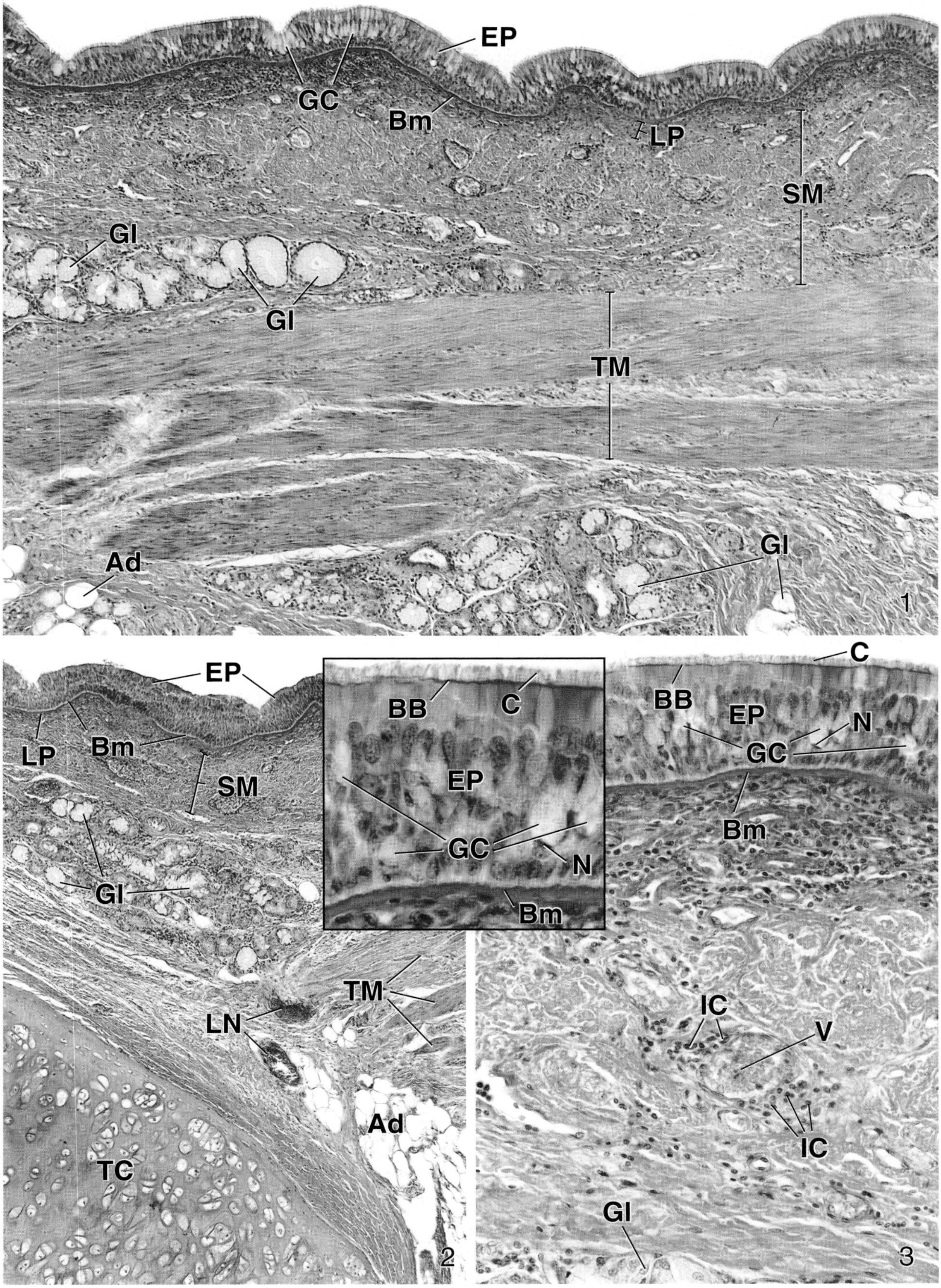
EP
GC
Bm
LP
SM
Gl
Gl
TM
Ad
Gl
1
EP
LP
Bm
SM
Gl
TM
LN
Ad
TC
2
BB
C
EP
GC
N
Bm
C
BB
EP
N
GC
Bm
IC
V
IC
Gl
3

PLATE 68. BRONCHIOLE AND END RESPIRATORY PASSAGES

The primary bronchus that enters each lung divides into smaller secondary and tertiary bronchi. As the bronchi become smaller, some components of the wall are lost or reduced in amount. Ultimately, the respiratory passage has distinctly different features than those of a bronchus, and it is called a *bronchiole.* The features that characterize the bronchiole are the absence of cartilage, loss of submucosal glands, and gradual disappearance of goblet cells. The epithelium changes from pseudostratified columnar to simple ciliated columnar, and some columnar cells even lack cilia. Smooth muscle occupies a relatively larger portion of the bronchiolar wall than of the bronchial wall.

The smallest diameter conducting bronchioles, the *terminal bronchioles,* are lined with simple ciliated cuboidal epithelium in which Clara cells, cells that secrete a surface-active agent that prevents luminal adhesion of bronchiolar walls during expiration, are found among the ciliated cells. *Respiratory bronchioles* are the first part of the bronchial tree that allows gas exchange to occur. Respiratory bronchioles constitute a transition zone in which both air conduction and gas exchange occur. Scattered, thin-walled evaginations of the lumen of the respiratory bronchiole are called *alveoli;* these are the structures in which gas exchange between the air passages and the blood capillaries occurs.

Figure 1, bronchiole, H&E ×75.

A typical bronchiole is shown here. Characteristically, blood vessels *(BV)* are adjacent to the bronchiole. The main features of the bronchiolar wall that are evident in the figure are bundles of smooth muscle *(SM)* and the lining epithelium (shown at higher magnification in Plate 69). Higher magnification would reveal that the epithelium is ciliated. The connective tissue is minimal and, at this low magnification, not conspicuous. Nevertheless, it is present and separates the muscle into bundles (i.e., the muscle layer is not a single continuous layer). The connective tissue contains collagenous and some elastic fibers. Glands are not present in the wall of the bronchiole. Surrounding the bronchiole, comprising most of the lung substance, are the air spaces or alveoli of the lung.

Figure 2, bronchiole and respiratory bronchioles, H&E ×75.

In this figure, a short length of a bronchiole *(B)* is shown longitudinally sectioned as it branches into two respiratory bronchioles *(RB).* The last portion of a bronchiole that leads into respiratory bronchioles is called a terminal bronchiole. It is not engaged in exchange of air with the blood; the respiratory bronchiole does engage in air exchange. *Arrows* mark the place where the terminal bronchiole ends. Not uncommonly, as shown here, cartilage *(C)* is found in the bronchiolar wall where branching occurs. Blood vessels *(BV)* and a nodule of lymphocytes *(L)* are adjacent to the bronchiole.

The respiratory bronchiole has a wall composed of two components: One consists of recesses that have a wall similar to that of the alveoli and are thus capable of gas exchange; the other has a wall formed by small cuboidal cells that appear to rest on a small bundle of eosinophilic material. This is smooth muscle surrounded by a thin investment of connective tissue. Both of these components are shown at higher magnification in Plate 69.

Figure 3, alveoli, H&E ×75.

The most distal component of the respiratory passage is the alveolus. Groups of alveoli clustered together and sharing a common opening are referred to as an *alveolar sac (AS).* Alveoli that form a tube are referred to as *alveolar ducts (AD).*

The outer surface of lung tissue is the serosa *(S);* it consists of a lining of mesothelial cells resting on a small amount of connective tissue. This is the layer that gross anatomists refer to as the *visceral pleura.*

KEY

AD, alveolar ducts
AS, alveolar sacs
B, bronchiole
BV, blood vessels
C, cartilage
L, nodule of lymphocytes
RB, respiratory bronchiole
S, serosa
SM, smooth muscle
arrows, end of terminal bronchiole

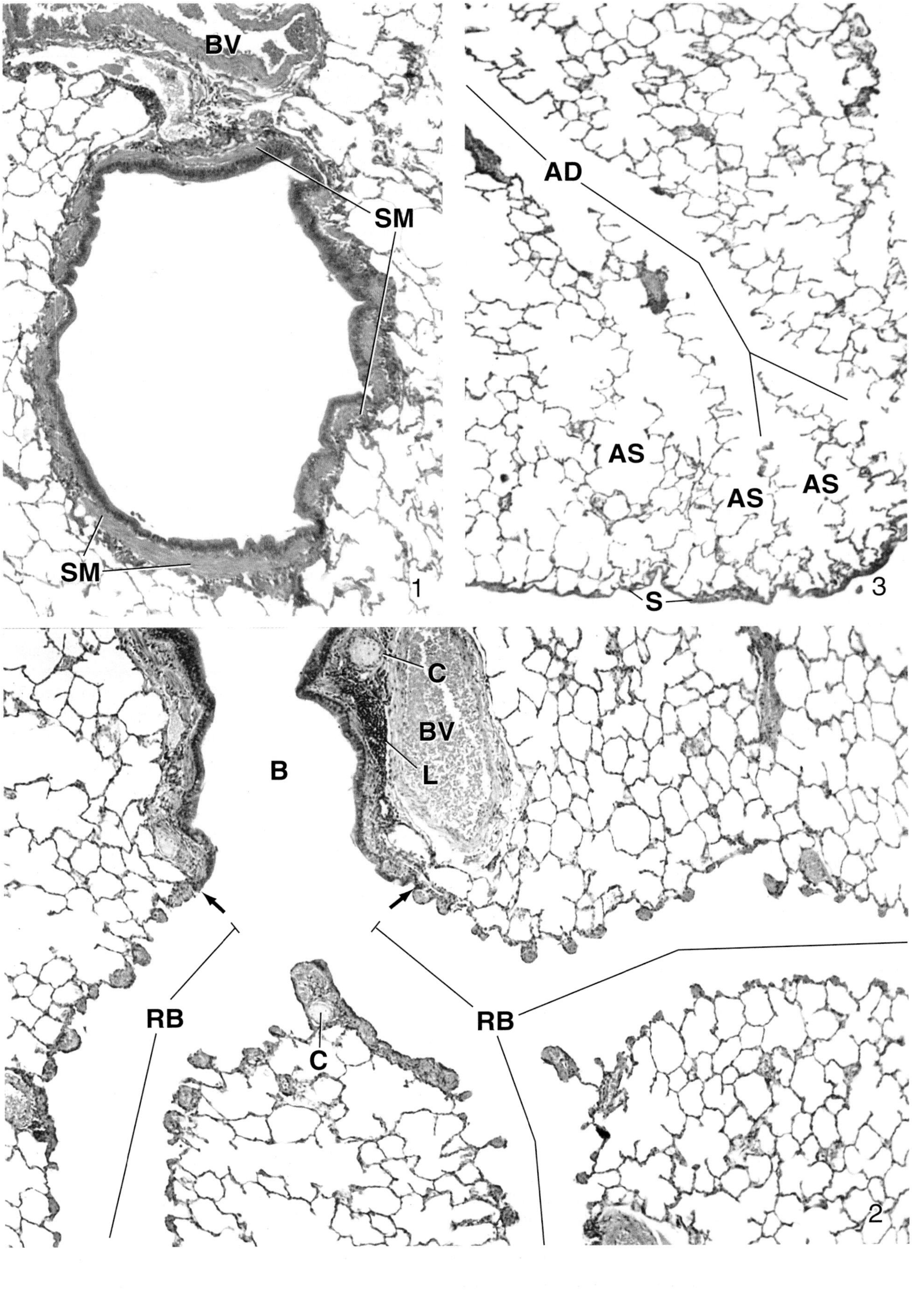
BV
SM
SM
SM
1
AD
AS
AS
AS
S
3
C
BV
B
L
RB
RB
C
2

PLATE 69. WALL OF TERMINAL BRONCHIOLE, RESPIRATORY BRONCHIOLE, AND ALVEOLUS

Respiratory bronchioles continue to divide to form *alveolar ducts,* passages lined solely with rows of alveoli that have rings of smooth muscle in knob-like interalveolar septa. The alveolar ducts terminate in *alveolar sacs,* enlarged spaces surrounded by clusters of alveoli that open into the spaces. The alveoli are lined with *type I alveolar cells,* extremely thin squamous cells that cover about 95% of the alveolar surface, and with *type II alveolar cells,* cuboidal cells that secrete *surfactant,* a surface-active agent that reduces surface tension at the air–epithelium surface. The tissue between adjacent alveoli is called the *alveolar septum.* This consists of the alveolar epithelial cells and their basal lamina, the basal lamina of the underlying capillary endothelium and the endothelial cells, themselves, and any other connective tissue elements that may lie between the two basal laminae. The alveolar septum is the site of the *air–blood barrier.*

Figure 1, terminal bronchiole, H&E ×550.

The histologic features of the terminal bronchiolar wall are shown here. Ciliated epithelium extends from the top of the figure to the *diamond.* This is ciliated pseudostratified columnar epithelium (PsEp). Some basal cells are still present and, therefore, the designation pseudostratified columnar. Elsewhere, the epithelium might be ciliated simple columnar, and just before it becomes a respiratory bronchiole, the epithelium may include cuboidal or low columnar nonciliated cells. These nonciliated cells are Clara cells (*CC,* beyond the *diamond*). Clara cells produce a surface-active agent that is instrumental in expansion of the lungs. The smooth muscle *(SM)* in the bronchiolar wall is organized in bundles; other cells under the epithelium and around the smooth muscle belong to the connective tissue.

Figure 2, respiratory bronchiole, H&E ×550.

The wall of a respiratory bronchiole is shown here and in Figure 3. The alveoli *(A)* are terminal air spaces on the left in each of the two figures. The lumen of the respiratory bronchiole is on the right. Characteristically, the wall of the respiratory bronchiole consists of alternating thick and thin regions. The thick regions are similar to the wall of the bronchiole except that cuboidal Clara cells instead of columnar epithelium form the surface. Thus, as seen here, Clara cells *(CC)* are the surface-lining cells of the thick regions, and smooth muscle bundles *(SM)* are under the Clara cells, with a small amount of intervening connective tissue. The thin regions have a wall similar to the alveolar wall; this is considered below.

Figure 3, respiratory bronchiole, H&E ×550.

The respiratory bronchiole shown in Figure 3 is slightly more distal than the area seen in Figure 2. Structurally, it shows essentially the same features as those seen in Figure 2 except that there are fewer Clara cells and the smooth muscle is somewhat thinner.

Figure 4, alveolus, H&E ×800.

The alveolar wall is shown in Figure 4. The central component of the wall is the capillary *(C)* and, in certain locations, associated connective tissue. On each side, where it faces the alveolus *(A),* a flat squamous cell is interposed between the capillary and the air spaces. This is a pneumocyte type I cell. In some places, the type I cell is separated from the capillary endothelial cell by a single basal lamina shared by the two cells. This is the thin portion of the alveolar–capillary complex, readily seen in the upper part of the figure *(arrows).* Gas exchange occurs through the thin portion of the alveolar–capillary complex. Elsewhere, connective tissue is interposed between the pneumocyte type I cell and the endothelial cell of the capillary; each of these epithelial cells retains its own basal lamina.

A second cell type, the pneumocyte type II cell or septal cell *(SC),* also lines the alveolar air space. This cell typically displays a rounded (rather than flattened) shape, and the nucleus is surrounded by a noticeable amount of cytoplasm, some of which may appear clear. The septal cell produces a surface-active agent different from that of the Clara cell, which also acts in permitting the lung to expand.

KEY

A, alveolus
C, capillary
CC, Clara cells
PsEp, pseudostratified squamous epithelium
SC, septal cell
SM, smooth muscle
arrows (Fig. 4), thin portion of alveolar–capillary complex
diamond, junction between pseudostratified columnar epithelium and Clara cells

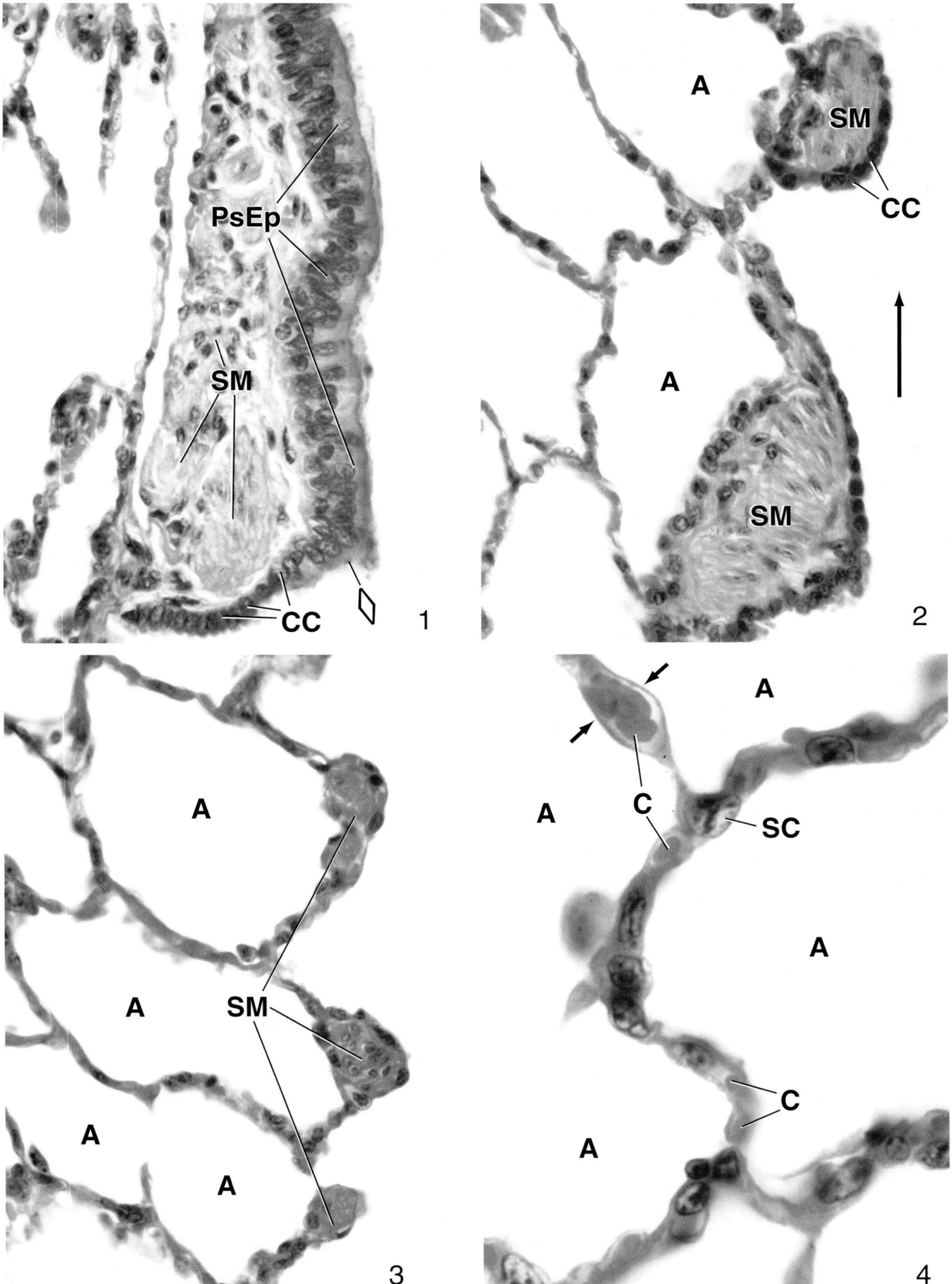
PsEp
SM
CC
1
A
SM
CC
A
SM
2
A
SM
A
A
A
3
A
A
C
SC
A
C
A
4

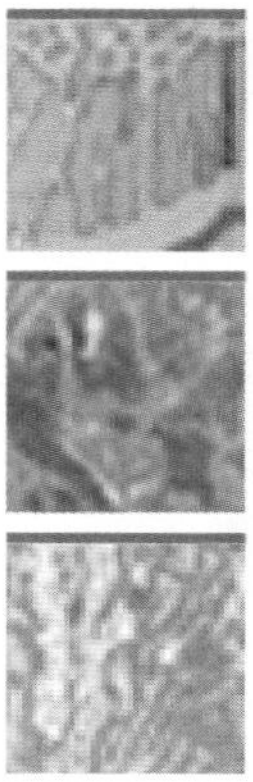

19

Urinary System

OVERVIEW OF THE URINARY SYSTEM

The urinary system consists of the paired ***kidneys;*** paired ***ureters,*** which lead from the kidneys to the ***bladder;*** and the ***urethra,*** which leads from the bladder to the exterior of the body.

The kidneys conserve body fluid and electrolytes and remove metabolic waste

Like the lungs and liver, the kidneys retrieve essential materials and dispose of wastes. They conserve water, essential electrolytes, and metabolites, and they remove certain waste products of metabolism from the body. The kidneys play an important role in regulating and maintaining the composition and volume of extracellular fluid. They also are essential in maintaining acid–base balance by excreting H^+ when bodily fluids become too acidic or excreting bicarbonate when bodily fluids become too basic.

The kidneys are highly vascular organs; they receive approximately 25% of the cardiac output. The kidneys produce ***urine,*** initially an ***ultrafiltrate*** of the blood, which is then modified by selective resorption and specific secretion by the cells of the kidney. The final urine is conveyed by the ureters to the urinary bladder, where it is stored until discharged via the urethra.

The final urine contains water and electrolytes as well as waste products, such as urea, uric acid, and creatinine, and breakdown products of various substances.

The kidney also functions as an endocrine organ

Endocrine activities of the kidneys include

- Synthesis and secretion of the glycoprotein hormone ***erythropoietin,*** which regulates red blood cell formation in response to decreased blood oxygen concentration. Erythropoietin acts on specific receptors expressed on the surface of CFU-E (colony-forming units for erythrocytes) cells in the bone marrow.
- Synthesis and secretion of the acid protease ***renin,*** an enzyme involved in control of blood pressure and blood volume. Renin cleaves circulating angiotensinogen to release ***angiotensin I.***
- Hydroxylation of ***25-OH vitamin D_3,*** a steroid precursor produced in the liver, to hormonally active ***1,25-$(OH)_2$ vitamin D_3.*** This step is regulated primarily by parathyroid hormone (PTH), which stimulates activity of the enzyme 1α-hydroxylase and increases the production of the active hormone.

BOX 19.1

Functional Considerations: Vitamin D

Despite its name, vitamin D is actually an inactive precursor that undergoes a series of transformations to become the fully active hormone that regulates plasma calcium levels. In the human body vitamin D is derived from two sources:

- ***Skin,*** in which ***vitamin D_3 (cholecalciferol)*** is rapidly produced by the action of ultraviolet light on the precursor 7-dehydrocholesterol. The skin is the major source of vitamin D_3, especially in regions where food is not supplemented with vitamin D. Typically, a half to 2 hours exposure to sunlight per day can provide enough vitamin D to fulfill daily body requirements for this vitamin.
- ***Diet,*** from which vitamin D_3 is absorbed by the small intestine in association with chylomicrons.

In the blood vitamin D_3 is bound to ***vitamin D–binding protein*** and transported to the liver. The first transformation occurs in the liver and involves hydroxylation of vitamin D_3 to form ***25-OH vitamin D_3.*** This compound is released into the bloodstream and undergoes a second hydroxylation in the kidney to produce the highly active ***1,25-$(OH)_2$ vitamin D_3.*** The process is regulated indirectly by an increase in plasma Ca^{2+} concentration, which triggers secretion of PTH, or directly by a decrease in circulating phosphates, which in turn stimulates activity of 1α-hydroxylase responsible for conversion of 25-OH vitamin D_3 into active 1,25-$(OH)_2$ vitamin D_3. Active 1,25-$(OH)_2$ vitamin D_3 stimulates intestinal absorption of Ca^{2+} and phosphate and mobilization of Ca^{2+} from bones. It is therefore necessary for normal development and growth of bones and teeth. The related compound ***vitamin D_2 (ergocalciferol)*** undergoes the same conversion steps as vitamin D_3 and produces the same biologic effects.

Vitamin D_3 deficiency results in ***rickets,*** a disease that causes abnormal bone ossification. In addition, patients on prolonged renal hemodialysis are often supplemented with vitamin D_3 and calcium to avoid severe disturbance of calcium homeostasis as a result of secondary hyperparathyroidism, a condition prevalent in these patients.

GENERAL STRUCTURE OF THE KIDNEY

The kidneys are large, reddish, bean-shaped organs located on either side of the spinal column in the retroperitoneal space of the posterior abdominal cavity. They extend from the 12th thoracic to the 3rd lumbar vertebrae, with the right kidney positioned slightly higher. Each kidney measures approximately 10 cm long × 6.5 cm wide (from concave to convex border) × 3 cm thick. On the upper pole of each kidney, embedded within the renal fascia and a thick protective layer of perirenal adipose tissue, lies an ***adrenal gland.*** The medial border of the kidney is concave and contains a deep vertical fissure, called the ***hilum,*** through which the renal vessels and nerves pass and through which the expanded, funnel-shaped origin of the ureter, called the ***renal pelvis,*** exits. A section through the kidney shows the relationship of these structures as they lie just within the hilum of the kidney in a space called the ***renal sinus*** (Fig. 19.1). Although not shown in the illustration, the space between and around these structures is filled largely with loose connective tissue and adipose tissue.

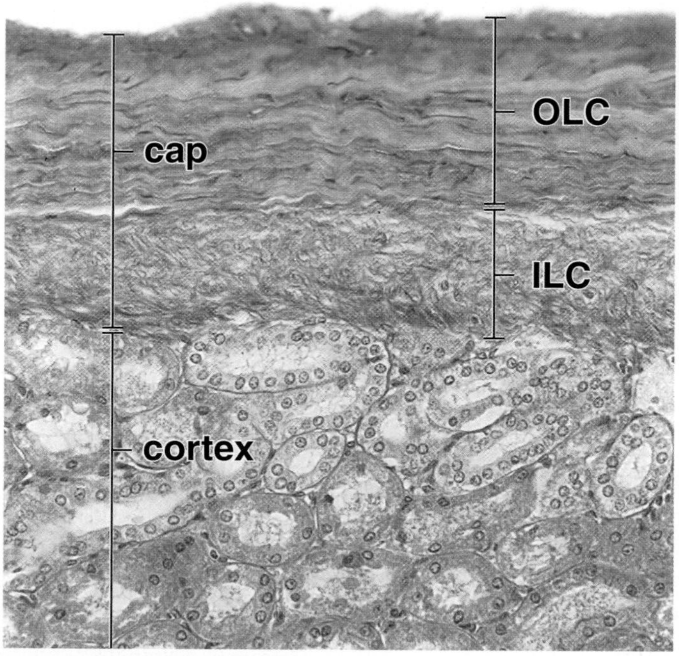

FIGURE 19.2
Photomicrograph of human kidney capsule. This photomicrograph of a Mallory-Azan–stained section shows the capsule *(cap)* and part of the underlying cortex. The outer layer of the capsule *(OLC)* is composed of dense connective tissue. The fibroblasts in this part of the capsule are relatively few in number; their nuclei appear as narrow, elongate, red-staining profiles against a blue background representing the stained collagen fibers. The inner layer of the capsule *(ILC)* consists of large numbers of myofibroblasts whose nuclei appear as round or elongate, red-staining profiles, depending on their orientation within the section. Note that the collagen fibers in this layer are relatively sparse and that the myofibroblast nuclei are more abundant than those of the fibroblasts in the outer layer of the capsule. ×180.

Capsule

The kidney surface is covered by a connective tissue ***capsule.*** The capsule consists of two distinct layers: an outer layer of fibroblasts and collagen fibers, and an inner layer with a cellular component of myofibroblasts (Fig. 19.2). The contractility of the myofibroblasts may aid in resisting volume and pressure variations that can accompany variations in kidney function. Its specific role, however, is not known. The capsule passes inward at the hilum, where it forms the connective tissue covering of the sinus and becomes continuous with the connective tissue forming the walls of the calyces and renal pelvis (see Fig. 19.1).

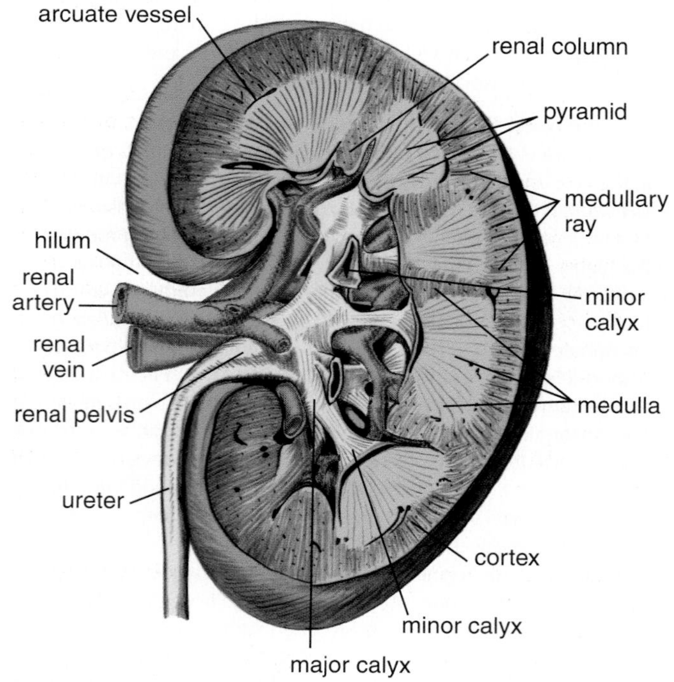

FIGURE 19.1
Diagram of kidney structure. The diagram represents a hemisection of a kidney, revealing its structural organization.

Cortex and Medulla

Examination with the naked eye of the cut face of a fresh, hemisected kidney reveals that its substance can be divided into two distinct regions:

- *Cortex,* the outer reddish brown part
- *Medulla,* the much lighter-colored inner part

The color seen in the cut surface of the unfixed kidney reflects the distribution of blood in the organ. Approxi-

mately 90 to 95% of the blood passing through the kidney is in the cortex; 5 to 10% is in the medulla.

The cortex is characterized by renal corpuscles and their associated tubules

The cortex consists of *renal corpuscles* along with the *convoluted* and *straight tubules* of the *nephron,* the *collecting tubules, collecting ducts,* and an extensive vascular supply. The nephron is the basic functional unit of the kidney and is described below. The renal corpuscles are spherical structures, barely visible with the naked eye. They constitute the beginning segment of the nephron and contain a unique capillary network called a *glomerulus.*

Examination of a section cut through the cortex at an angle perpendicular to the surface of the kidney reveals a series of vertical striations that appear to emanate from the medulla (see Fig 19.1). These striations are the *medullary rays* (of Ferrein). Their name reflects their appearance, as the striations seem to radiate from the medulla. Approximately 400 to 500 medullary rays project into the cortex from the medulla.

Each medullary ray is an aggregation of straight tubules and collecting ducts

Each medullary ray contains *straight tubules* of the nephrons and *collecting ducts.* The regions between medullary rays contain the renal corpuscles, the convoluted tubules of the nephrons, and the collecting tubules. These areas are referred to as *cortical labyrinths.* Each nephron and its *collecting tubule* (which connects to a *collecting duct* in the medullary ray) form the *uriniferous tubule.*

The medulla is characterized by straight tubules, collecting ducts, and a special capillary network, the vasa recta

The straight tubules of the nephrons and the collecting ducts continue from the cortex into the medulla. They are accompanied by a capillary network, the *vasa recta,* that runs in parallel with the various tubules. These vessels represent the vascular part of the *countercurrent exchange system* that regulates the concentration of the urine.

The tubules in the medulla, because of their arrangement and differences in length, collectively form a number of conical structures called *pyramids.* Usually 8 to 12 but as many as 18 pyramids may be present in the human kidney. The bases of the pyramids face the cortex, and the apices face the renal sinus. Each pyramid is divided into an *outer medulla* (adjacent to the cortex) and an *inner medulla.* The outer medulla is further subdivided into an *inner stripe* and an *outer stripe.* The zonation and stripes are readily recognized in a sagittal section through the pyramid of a fresh specimen. They reflect the location of distinct parts of the nephron at specific levels within the pyramid (Fig. 19.3).

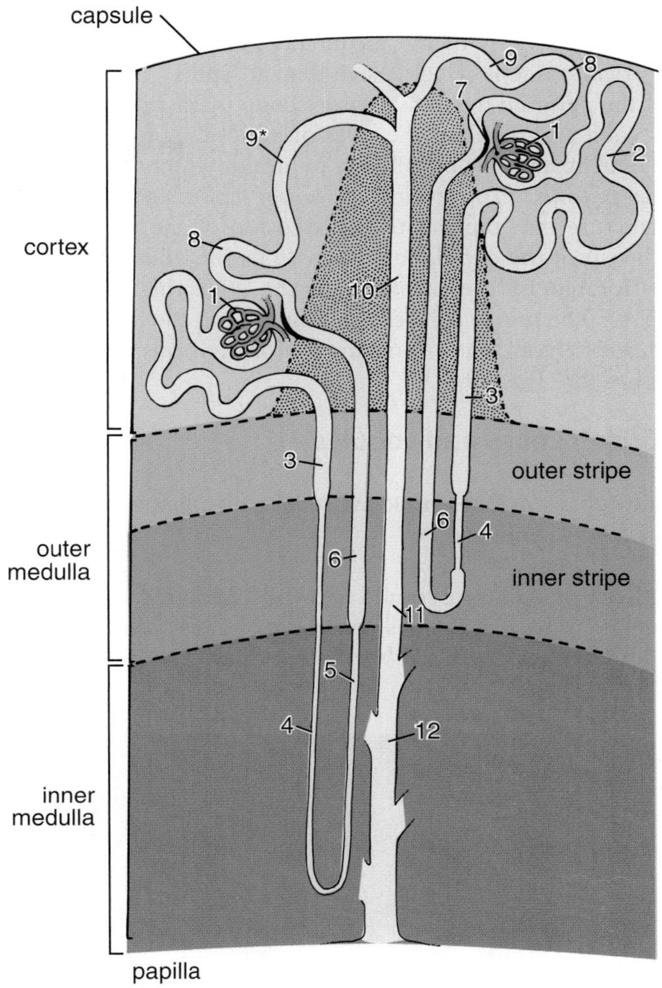

FIGURE 19.3
Diagram of two types of nephrons in the kidney and their associated collecting duct systems. A long-looped nephron is shown on the left, and a short-looped nephron is shown on the right. The relative position of the cortex, medulla, papilla, and capsule are indicated. The inverted cone-shaped area in the cortex represents a medullary ray. The parts of the nephron are indicated by number: *1,* renal corpuscle including the glomerulus and Bowman's capsule; *2,* proximal convoluted tubule; *3,* proximal straight tubule; *4,* descending thin limb; *5,* ascending thin limb; *6,* thick ascending limb (distal straight tubule); *7,* macula densa located in the final portion of the thick ascending limb; *8,* distal convoluted tubule; *9,* connecting tubule; *9*,* collecting tubule that forms an arch (arched collecting tubule); *10,* cortical collecting duct; *11,* outer medullary collecting duct; and *12,* inner medullary collecting duct. (Modified from Kriz W, Bankir L. *Kidney Int* 1988;33:1–7.)

The renal columns represent cortical tissue contained within the medulla

The caps of cortical tissue that lie over the pyramids are sufficiently extensive that they extend peripherally around the lateral portion of the pyramid, forming the *renal columns* (of Bertin). Although renal columns contain the

same components as the rest of the cortical tissue, they are regarded as part of the medulla. In effect, the amount of cortical tissue is so extensive that it "spills" over the side of the pyramid much as a large scoop of ice cream extends beyond and overlaps the sides of an ice cream cone.

The apical portion of each pyramid, which is known as the ***papilla***, projects into a ***minor calyx***, a cup-shaped structure that represents an extension of the renal pelvis. The tip of the papilla, also known as the ***area cribrosa***, is perforated by the openings of the collecting ducts (Fig. 19.4). The minor calyces are branches of the two or three ***major calyces*** that in turn are major divisions of the renal pelvis (see Fig. 19.1).

Kidney Lobes and Lobules

The number of lobes in a kidney equals the number of medullary pyramids

Each medullary pyramid and the associated cortical tissue at its base and sides (one half of each adjacent renal column) constitutes a ***lobe*** of the kidney. The lobar organization of the kidney is conspicuous in the developing fetal kidney (Fig. 19.5). Each lobe is reflected as a convexity on the outer surface of the organ, but they usually disappear after birth. The surface convexities typical of the fetal kidney may persist, however, until the teenage years and, in some cases, into adulthood. Each human kidney contains 8 to 18 lobes. Kidneys of some animals possess only one pyramid; these kidneys are classified as unilobar, in contrast to the multilobar kidney of the human.

A lobule consists of a collecting duct and all the nephrons that it drains

The lobes of the kidney are further subdivided into ***lobules*** consisting of a central medullary ray and surrounding cortical material (Fig. 19.6). Although the center or axis of a lobule is readily identified, the boundaries between adjacent lobules are not obviously demarcated from one another by connective tissue septa. The concept of the lobule has an important physiologic basis; the medullary ray containing the collecting duct for a group of nephrons that drain into that duct constitutes the renal secretory

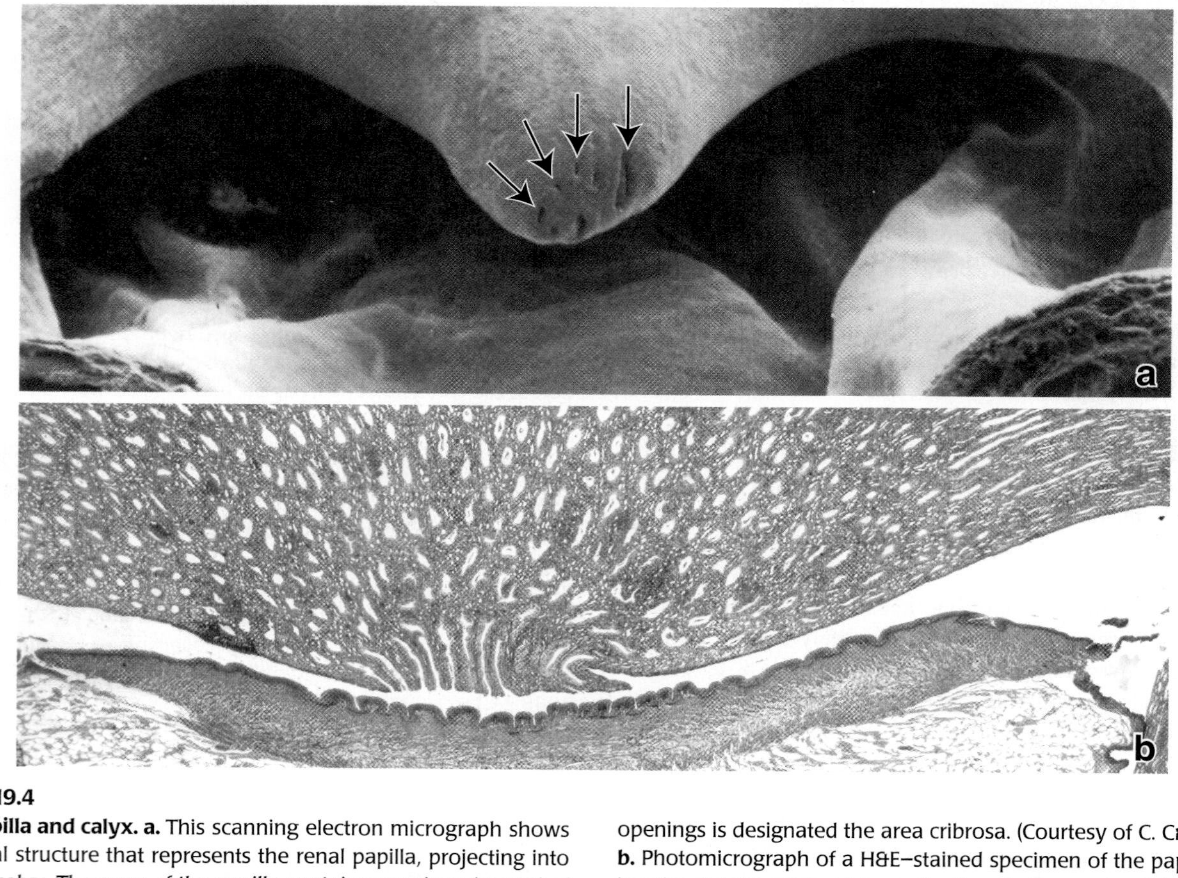

FIGURE 19.4
Renal papilla and calyx. a. This scanning electron micrograph shows the conical structure that represents the renal papilla, projecting into the renal calyx. The apex of the papilla contains openings *(arrows)* of the collecting ducts (of Bellini). These ducts deliver urine from the pyramids to the minor calyx. The surface of the papilla containing the openings is designated the area cribrosa. (Courtesy of C. Craig Tisher.) **b.** Photomicrograph of a H&E–stained specimen of the papilla, showing the distal portion of the collecting ducts opening into the minor calyx. ×120.

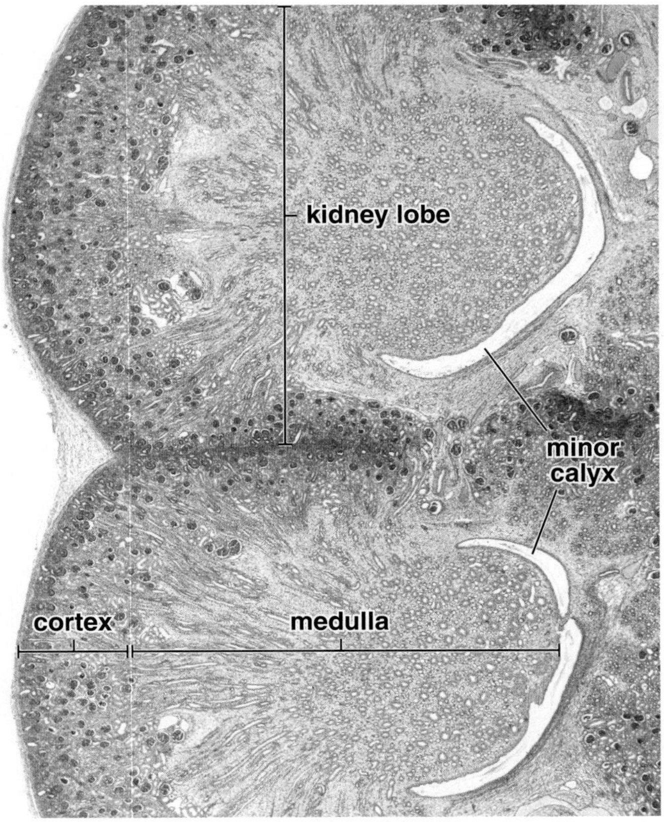

FIGURE 19.5
Photomicrograph of fetal kidney. This photomicrograph of a H&E–stained human fetal kidney shows the cortex, the medulla, and two associated pyramids. Note each surface convexity corresponds to a kidney lobe. During postnatal life the lobar convexities disappear and the kidney then exhibits a smooth surface. ×30.

unit. It is the equivalent of a glandular secretory unit or lobule.

The Nephron

The nephron is the structural and functional unit of the kidney

The nephron is the fundamental structural and functional unit of the kidney (see Fig. 19.3). Each human kidney contains approximately 2 million nephrons. Nephrons are responsible for the production of urine and correspond to the secretory part of other glands. The collecting ducts are responsible for the final concentration of the urine and are analogous to the ducts of exocrine glands that modify the concentration of the secretory product. Unlike the typical exocrine gland in which the secretory and duct portions arise from a single epithelial outgrowth, nephrons and their collecting tubules arise from separate primordia and only later become connected.

General Organization of the Nephron

The nephron consists of the renal corpuscle and a tubule system

As stated above, the ***renal corpuscle*** represents the beginning of the nephron. It consists of the ***glomerulus***, a tuft of capillaries composed of 10 to 20 capillary loops, surrounded by a double-layered epithelial cup, the ***renal*** or ***Bowman's capsule***. Bowman's capsule is the initial portion of the nephron where blood flowing through the glomerular capillaries undergoes filtration to produce the ***glomerular ultrafiltrate***. The glomerular capillaries are supplied by an ***afferent arteriole*** and are drained by an ***efferent arteriole*** that then branches, forming a new capillary network to supply the kidney tubules. The site where the afferent and efferent arterioles penetrate and exit from the parietal layer of Bowman's capsule is called the ***vascular pole***. Opposite this site is the ***urinary pole*** of the renal corpuscle, where the proximal convoluted tubule begins (see Fig. 19.6).

Continuing from Bowman's capsule, the remaining parts of the nephron (the tubular parts) are

- ***Proximal thick segment***, consisting of the ***proximal convoluted tubule (pars convoluta)*** and the ***proximal straight tubule (pars recta)***
- ***Thin segment***, which constitutes the thin part of the loop of Henle
- ***Distal thick segment***, consisting of the ***distal straight tubule (pars recta)*** and the ***distal convoluted tubule (pars convoluta)***

The distal convoluted tubule connects to the collecting tubule, often through a ***connecting tubule***, thus forming the ***uriniferous tubule***, i.e., the nephron plus collecting tubule (see Fig. 19.3).

Tubes of the Nephron

The tubular segments of the nephron are named according to the course that they take (convoluted or straight), location (proximal or distal), and wall thickness (thick or thin)

Beginning from Bowman's capsule, the sequential parts of the nephron consist of the following tubules:

- ***Proximal convoluted tubule*** originates from the urinary pole of Bowman's capsule. It follows a very tortuous or convoluted course and then enters the medullary ray to continue as the proximal straight tubule.
- ***Proximal straight tubule***, commonly referred to as the ***thick descending limb*** of the loop of Henle, descends into the medulla.
- ***Thin descending limb*** is the continuation of the proximal straight tubule within the medulla. It makes a hairpin turn and returns toward the cortex.

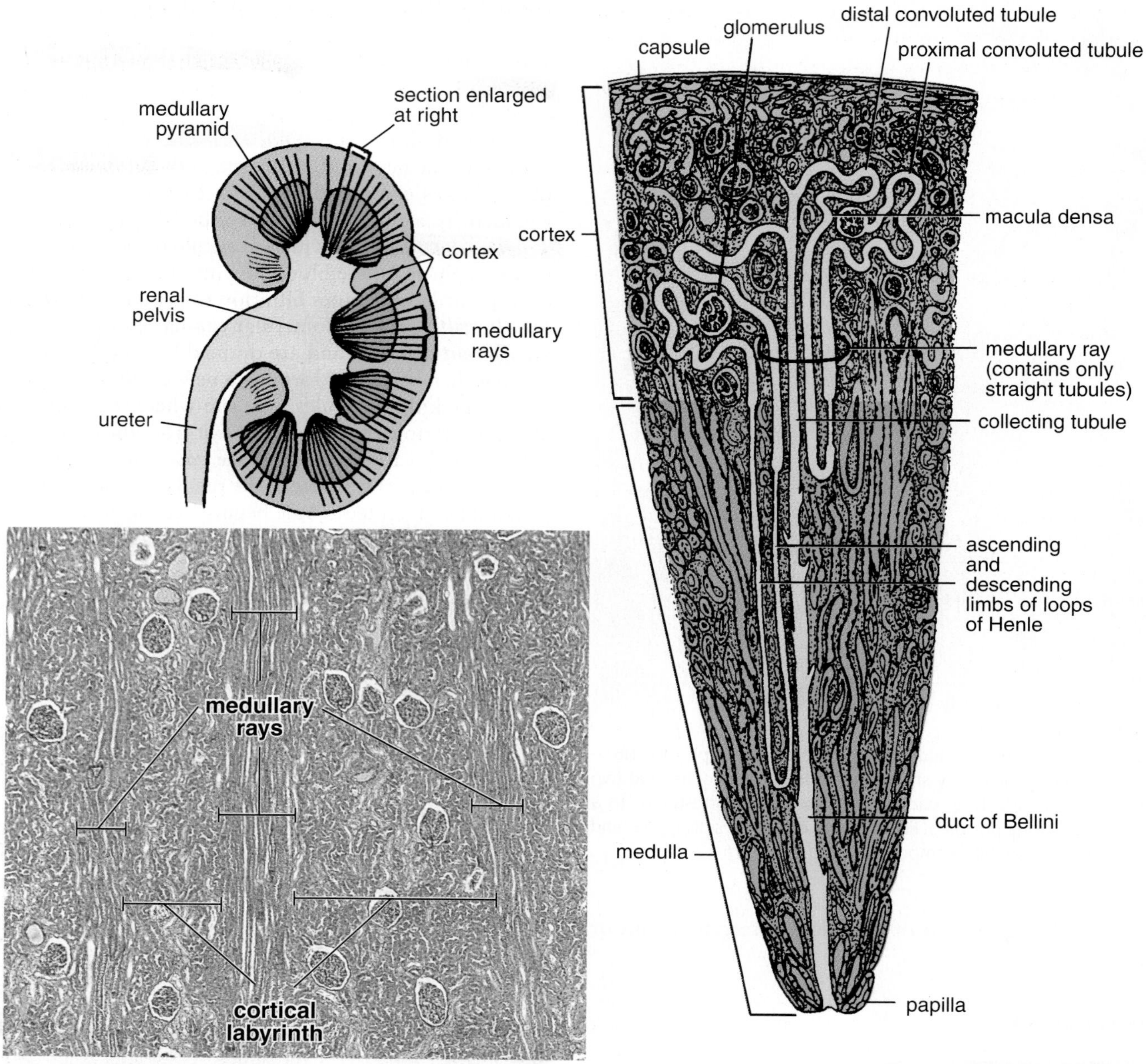

FIGURE 19.6

Diagrams and photomicrograph of an adult human kidney. The *diagram* in the *upper left* is a hemisection of the adult human kidney included for orientation. The *diagram* on the *right* represents an enlarged portion emphasizing the relationship of two nephrons and their collecting tubules and ducts *(yellow)* to the cortex and medulla. The upper nephron, a midcortical nephron, extends only a short distance into the medulla and possesses a short thin segment in the loop of Henle. The lower nephron, a juxtamedullary nephron, has a long loop of Henle that extends deep into the medulla. Both nephrons drain into the collecting tubules in the medullary ray. The photomicrograph shows a section of the cortex. It is organized into a series of medullary rays containing straight tubules and collecting tubules and between them the cortical labyrinths containing the renal corpuscles and their associated proximal and distal convoluted tubules. A kidney lobule consists of a medullary ray at its center and half of the adjacent cortical labyrinth on either side. ×60.

- ***Thin ascending limb*** is the continuation of the thin descending limb after its hairpin turn.
- ***Distal straight tubule,*** which is also referred to as the ***thick ascending limb*** of the loop of Henle, is the continuation of the thin ascending limb. The distal straight tubule ascends through the medulla and enters the cortex in the medullary ray to reach the vicinity of its renal corpuscle of origin. The distal straight tubule then leaves the medullary ray and makes contact with the vascular pole of its parent renal corpuscle. At this point,

the epithelial cells of the tubule adjacent to the afferent arteriole of the glomerulus are modified to form the ***macula densa.*** The distal tubule then leaves the region of the corpuscle and becomes the distal convoluted tubule.

- ***Distal convoluted tubule*** is less tortuous than the proximal convoluted tubule; thus, in a section showing the cortical labyrinth, there are fewer distal tubule profiles than proximal tubule profiles. At its termination, the distal convoluted tubule empties into a collecting duct that lies in the medullary ray via either an ***arched collecting tubule*** or a shorter tubule simply called the ***connecting tubule.***

The loop of Henle forms the entire U-shaped portion of a nephron

The proximal straight tubule, the thin descending limb with its hairpin turn, the thin ascending limb, and the distal straight tubule are collectively called the *loop of Henle.* In some nephrons, the thin descending and ascending segments are extremely short; therefore the hairpin turn may be made by the distal straight tubule.

Types of Nephrons

Several types of nephrons are identified, based on the location of their renal corpuscles in the cortex (see Fig. 19.3):

- ***Subcapsular*** or ***cortical nephrons*** have their renal corpuscles located in the outer part of the cortex. They have short loops of Henle, extending only into the outer medulla. They are typical of the nephrons described above, wherein the hairpin turn occurs in the distal straight tubule.
- ***Juxtamedullary nephrons*** make up about one-eighth of the total nephron count. Their renal corpuscles occur in proximity to the base of a medullary pyramid. They have long loops of Henle and long ascending thin segments that extend well into the inner region of the pyramid. These structural features are essential to the urine-concentrating mechanism, which is described below.
- ***Intermediate*** or ***midcortical nephrons*** have their renal corpuscles in the midregion of the cortex. Their loops of Henle are of intermediate length.

Collecting Tubules and Ducts

The collecting tubules begin in the cortical labyrinth, as either ***connecting tubules*** or ***arched collecting tubules,*** and proceed to the medullary ray where they join the ***collecting ducts.*** The collecting ducts within the cortex are referred to as ***cortical collecting ducts.*** When cortical collecting ducts reach the medulla they are referred to as ***medullary collecting ducts.*** These ducts travel to the apex of the pyramid, where they merge into larger collecting ducts (up to 200 μm), the ***papillary ducts (ducts of Bellini)*** that open into the minor calyx (see Fig. 19.4). The area on the papilla that contains the openings of these collecting ducts is called the ***area cribrosa.***

In summary, the gross appearance of the kidney parenchyma reflects the structure of the nephron. The renal corpuscle and the proximal and the distal convoluted tubules are all located in and make up the substance of the cortical labyrinths. The portions of the straight proximal and straight distal tubules and the descending thin and ascending thin limbs of the loop of Henle in the cortex are located in and make up the major portion of the medullary rays. The thin descending and thin ascending limbs of the loop of Henle are always located in the medulla. Thus, the arrangement of the nephrons (and the collecting tubules and ducts) accounts for the characteristic appearance of the cut surface of the kidney, as can be seen in Figure 19.2.

Filtration Apparatus of the Kidney

The renal corpuscle contains the filtration apparatus of the kidney

The renal corpuscle is spherical and has an average diameter of 200 μm. It consists of the glomerular capillary tuft and the surrounding visceral and parietal epithelial layers of Bowman's capsule (Figs. 19.7 and 19.8). The filtration apparatus, enclosed by the parietal layer of Bowman's capsule, consists of three components:

- ***Endothelium of the glomerular capillaries,*** which possesses numerous fenestrations (Fig. 19.9). These fenestrations are larger (70 to 90 nm in diameter), more numerous, and more irregular in outline than fenestrations in other capillaries. Moreover, the diaphragm that spans the fenestrations in other capillaries is absent in the glomerular capillaries. Endothelial cells of glomerular capillaries possess a large number of aquaporin-1 (AQP-1) water channels that allow the fast movement of water through the epithelium.
- ***Glomerular basement membrane (GBM),*** a thick (300 to 350 nm) basal lamina that is the joint product of the endothelium and the podocytes, the cells of the visceral layer of Bowman's capsule. Because of its thickness, it is prominent in histologic sections stained with the periodic acid–Schiff (PAS) procedure (see Fig. 1.2, page 7). The GBM is the principal component of the filtration barrier.
- ***Visceral layer of Bowman's capsule,*** which contains specialized cells called ***podocytes*** or ***visceral epithelial cells.*** These cells extend processes around the glomerular cap-

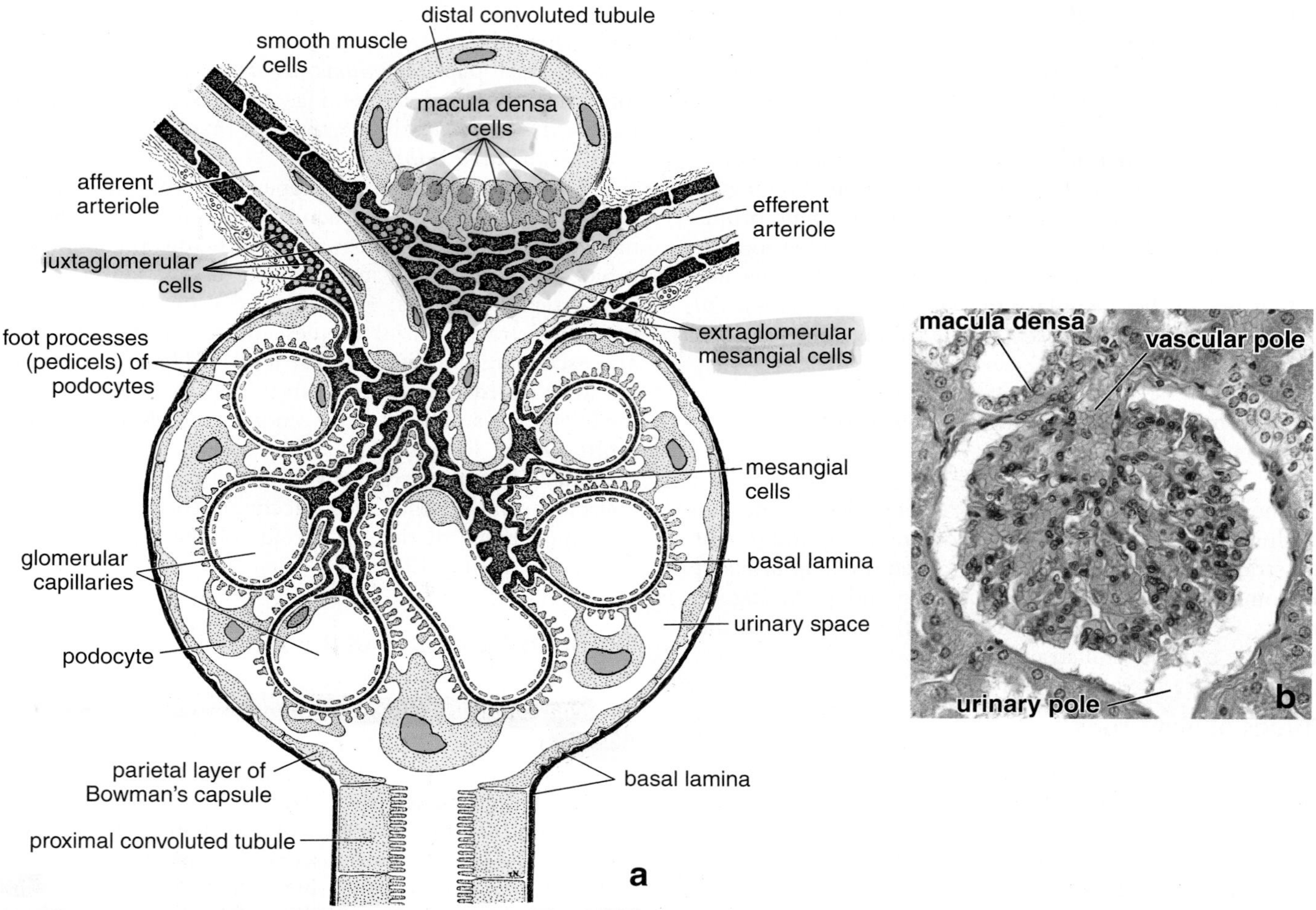

FIGURE 19.7

Structure of the renal corpuscle. a. This schematic diagram shows the organization of the renal corpuscle and the structures associated with it at the vascular and urinary poles. Mesangial cells are associated with the capillary endothelium of the glomerulus and the glomerular basement membrane. The macula densa cells of the distal tubule are shown intimately associated with the juxtaglomerular cells of the afferent arteriole and the extraglomerular mesangial cells. (Modified from Kriz W, Sakai T. Morphological aspects of glomerular function. In: *Nephrology: Proceedings of the Tenth International Congress of Nephrology.* London: Bailliere-Tindall, 1987.) **b.** Photomicrograph of a H&E–stained specimen showing a renal corpuscle. The macula densa is seen in close proximity to the vascular pole. ×160.

illaries (Fig. 19.10). The podocytes arise during embryonic development from one of the blind ends of the developing nephron through invagination of the end of the tubule to form a double-layered epithelial cup. The inner cell layer, i.e., the visceral cell layer, lies in apposition to a capillary network, the glomerulus, which forms at this site. The outer layer of these cells, the parietal layer, forms the squamous cells of Bowman's capsule. The cup eventually closes to form the spherical structure containing the glomerulus. As they differentiate, the podocytes extend processes around the capillaries and develop numerous secondary processes called ***pedicels*** or ***foot processes.*** The foot processes interdigitate with foot processes of neighboring podocytes, a feature that can be clearly demonstrated with the scanning electron microscope (SEM) (Figs. 19.11, a and b). The elongated spaces between the interdigitating foot processes, called ***filtration slits,*** are about 25 nm wide and allow the ultrafiltrate from the blood to enter Bowman's space. The foot processes contain numerous actin ***filaments*** that are thought to help regulate the size and patency of the filtration slits. An additional factor that may influence the passage of substances through the filtration slits is the presence of a thin membrane similar to the diaphragm of capillary fenestrations. This membrane, the ***filtration slit membrane,*** spans the slits (Fig. 19.12, *inset*). The filtration apparatus may thus be described as a ***semipermeable barrier*** having two discontinuous cellular layers applied to either side of a continuous extracellular layer, the basal lamina.

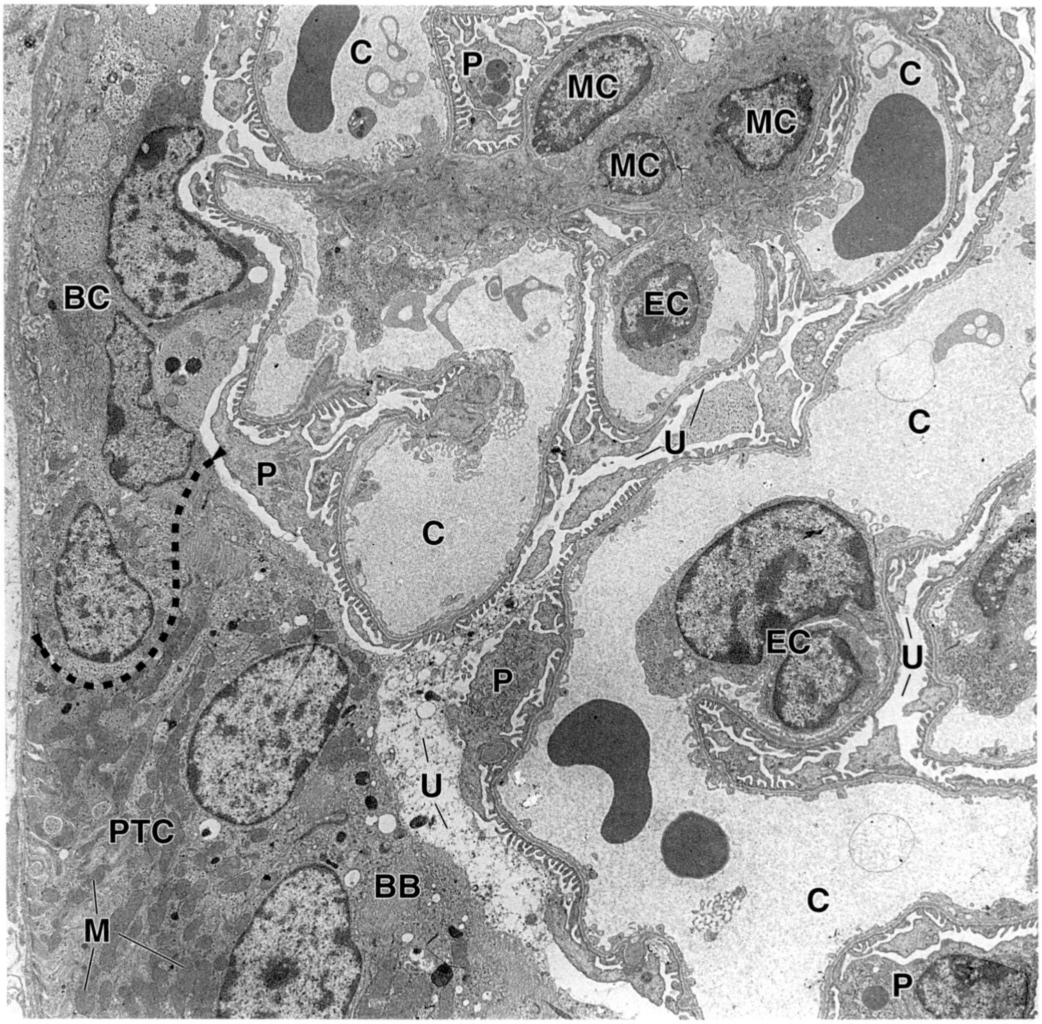

FIGURE 19.8

Transmission electron micrograph of a glomerulus in the region of the urinary pole. The nuclear and perinuclear regions of the endothelial cells *(EC)* that line the glomerular capillaries *(C)* bulge into the vascular lumen. On the outer surface of the capillaries are the processes of the podocytes *(P)*. External to the podocytes is the urinary space *(U)*. Bowman's capsule *(BC)* is shown on the left; it is continuous at the *dashed line* (marked by *arrowheads*) with the tubule cells of the proximal tubule *(PTC)*. Note the numerous mitochondria *(M)* in the base of these cells and the brush border *(BB)* at the apex, projecting into the urinary space. The nuclei of three adjacent mesangial cells *(MC)* can be seen in the upper right of the micrograph. ×4,700.

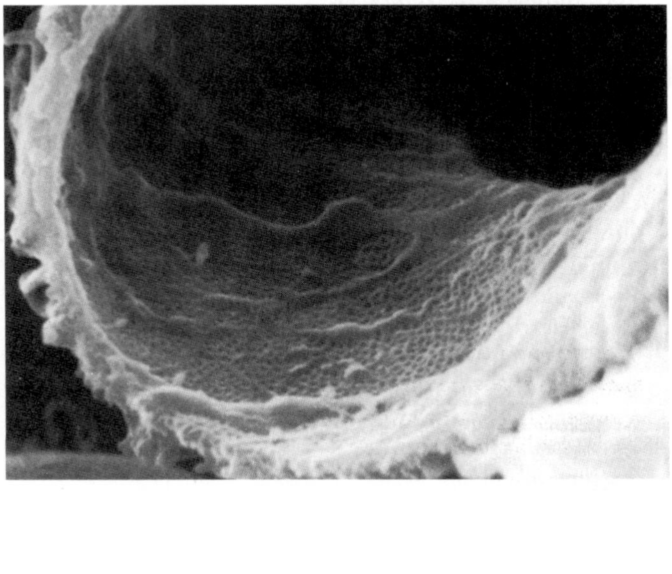

FIGURE 19.9

Scanning electron micrograph of the interior surface of a glomerular capillary. The wall of the capillary shows horizontal ridges formed by the cytoplasm of the endothelial cell. Elsewhere, fenestrations are seen as numerous dark oval and circular profiles. ×5,600. (Courtesy of C. Craig Tisher.)

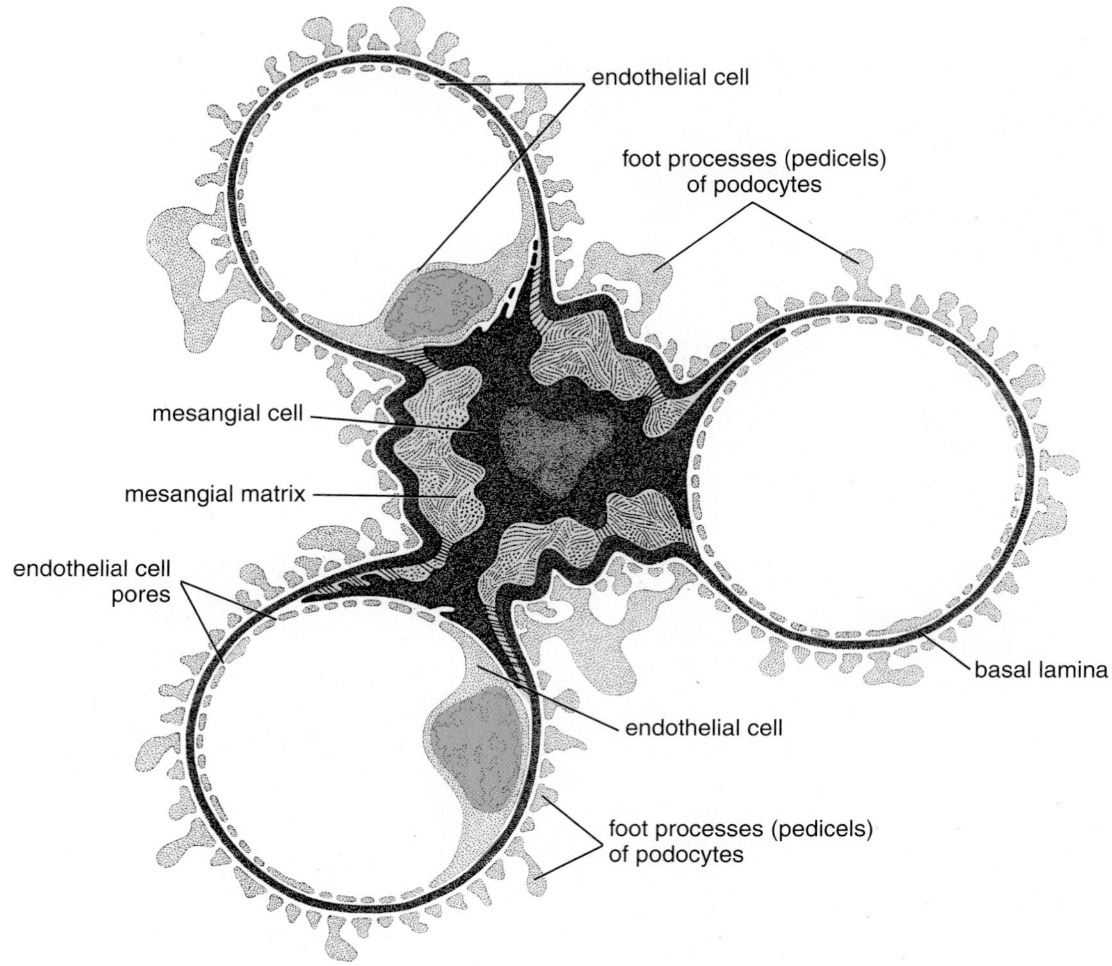

FIGURE 19.10
Schematic diagram showing the relationship between the intraglomerular mesangial cells and the glomerular capillaries. The mesangial cell and its surrounding matrix are enclosed by the basal lamina of the glomerular capillaries. Note that the mesangial cells are in the same compartment as the endothelium and that they can be intimately associated with the basal lamina as well as with the endothelial cells. (Modified from Sakai T, Kriz W. *Anat Embryol* 1987; 176:373–386.)

The glomerular basement membrane acts as a physical barrier and an ion-selective filter

The GBM contains type IV collagen, sialoglycoproteins, and other noncollagenous glycoproteins (e.g., laminin, fibronectin, entactin), as well as proteoglycans and glycosaminoglycans, particularly heparan sulfate (Fig. 19.13). These components are localized in particular portions of the GBM:

- The ***lamina rara externa,*** adjacent to the podocyte processes. It is particularly rich in polyanions, such as heparan sulfate, that specifically impede the passage of negatively charged molecules.
- The ***lamina rara interna,*** adjacent to the capillary endothelium. Its molecular features are similar to those of the lamina rara externa.
- The ***lamina densa,*** the overlapping portion of the two basal laminae, sandwiched between the laminae rarae. It contains type IV collagen, which is organized into a network that acts as a physical filter. The laminin and other proteins present in the lamina rara interna and externa are involved in the attachment of the endothelial cells and podocytes to the GBM.

The GBM restricts the movement of particles, usually proteins, larger than approximately 70,000 daltons or 3.6 nm radius, e.g., albumin or hemoglobin. Although albumin is not a usual constituent, it may sometimes be found in urine, indicating that the size of albumin is close to the effective pore size of the filtration barrier. The polyanionic glycosaminoglycans of the laminae rarae restrict the movement of anionic particles and molecules across the GBM, even those smaller than 70,000 daltons. Despite the ability of the filtration barrier to restrict protein, several grams of protein do pass through the barrier each day. This protein is reabsorbed by endocytosis in the proximal convoluted tubule. The presence of significant amounts of albumin or hemoglobin in the urine (***albuminuria*** or ***hematuria***) indicates physical or functional damage to the GBM. In such cases (e.g., ***di-***

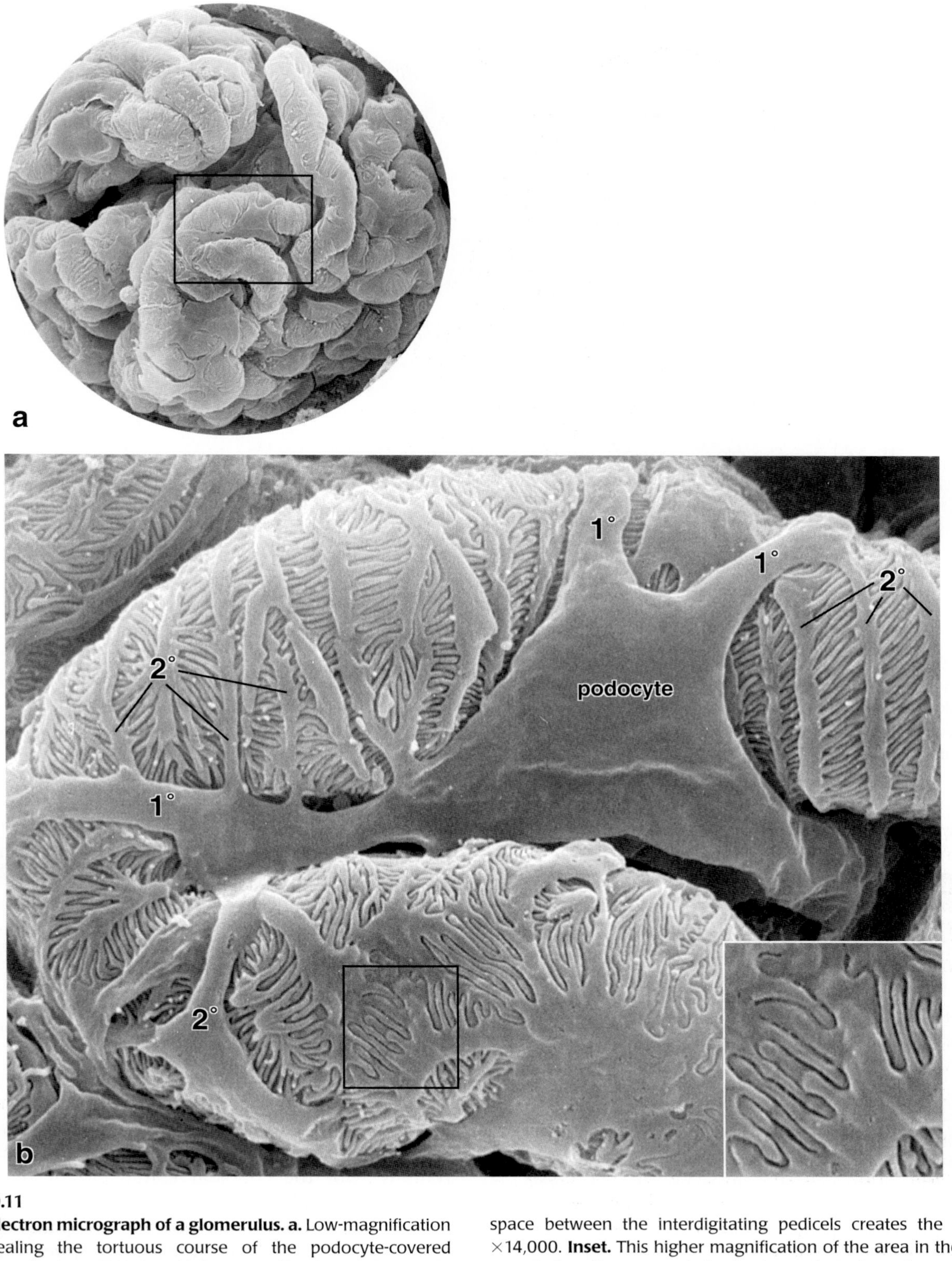

FIGURE 19.11

Scanning electron micrograph of a glomerulus. a. Low-magnification image revealing the tortuous course of the podocyte-covered glomerular capillaries. ×700. **b.** A higher magnification of the area in the *rectangle* in *a.* Note the podocyte and its processes embracing the capillary wall. The primary processes *(1°)* of the podocyte give rise to secondary processes *(2°),* which in turn give rise to the pedicels. The space between the interdigitating pedicels creates the slit pores. ×14,000. **Inset.** This higher magnification of the area in the *rectangle* reveals the slit pores and clearly shows that alternating pedicels belong to the secondary process of one cell; the intervening pedicels belong to the adjacent cell. ×6,000.

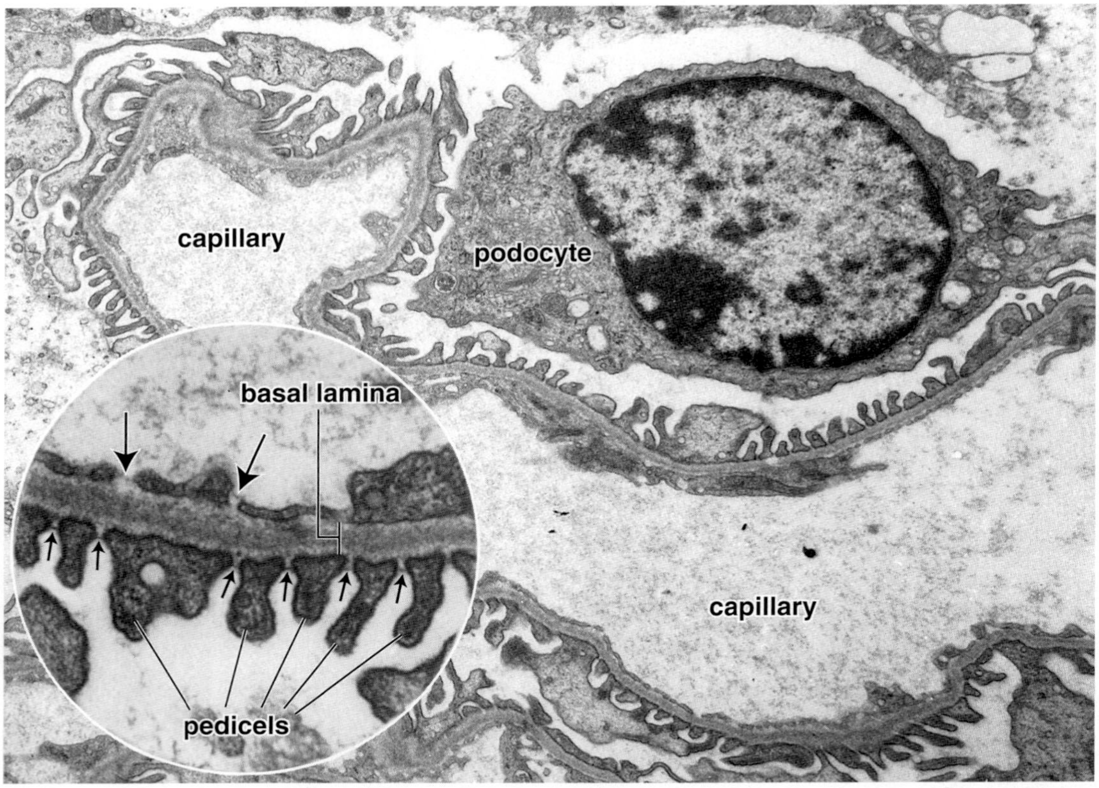

FIGURE 19.12
Transmission electron micrograph of a glomerular capillary and adjacent podocyte. The pedicels of the podocytes rest on the basal lamina adjacent to the capillary endothelium, and together, the three components—capillary endothelium, basal lamina, and podocyte—form a filtration apparatus. ×5,600. **Inset.** The *large arrows* point to the fenestrations in the endothelium. On the other side of the basal lamina are the pedicels of the podocytes. Note the slit membrane *(small arrows)* spanning the gap between adjacent pedicels. ×12,000.

abetic nephropathy) the number of anionic sites, especially in the lamina rara externa, is significantly reduced.

The narrow slit pores formed by the pedicels and the filtration slit membranes also act as physical barriers to bulk flow and free diffusion. The glycoproteins of the filtration slit membrane and of the glycocalyx of the pedicels probably act in a manner similar to that of the glycosaminoglycans of the laminae rarae of the GBM. Lastly, the fenestrae of the capillary endothelium restrict the movement of blood cells and other formed elements of the blood from the capillaries. In addition to the structural barriers, the flow rate and the pressure of the blood in the glomerular capillaries also have an effect on the filtration function of the renal corpuscle.

BOX 19.2

Clinical Correlations: Urinalysis

Urinalysis is an important part of the examination of patients with suspected renal disease. Part of this analysis includes the determination of the amount of protein excreted in the urine. The excretion of excessive amounts of protein, i.e., ***proteinuria*** (albuminuria), is an important diagnostic sign of renal disease. Normally, less than 150 mg of protein is excreted in the urine each day. Although excessive excretion of protein almost always indicates renal disease, extreme exercise, such as jogging, or severe dehydration may produce increased proteinuria in individuals without renal disease.

Simple squamous epithelium constitutes the parietal layer of Bowman's capsule

The ***parietal layer of Bowman's capsule*** contains ***parietal epithelial cells*** and forms a simple squamous epithelium. At the urinary pole of the renal corpuscle, it is continuous with the cuboidal epithelium of the proximal convoluted tubule (see Figs. 19.7 and 19.8).

The space between the visceral and parietal layers of Bowman's capsule is called the ***urinary space*** or ***Bowman's space*** (see Fig. 19.8). It is the receptacle for the ultrafiltrate produced by the filtration apparatus of the renal corpuscle. At the urinary pole of the renal corpuscle, the urinary space is continuous with the lumen of the proximal convoluted tubule.

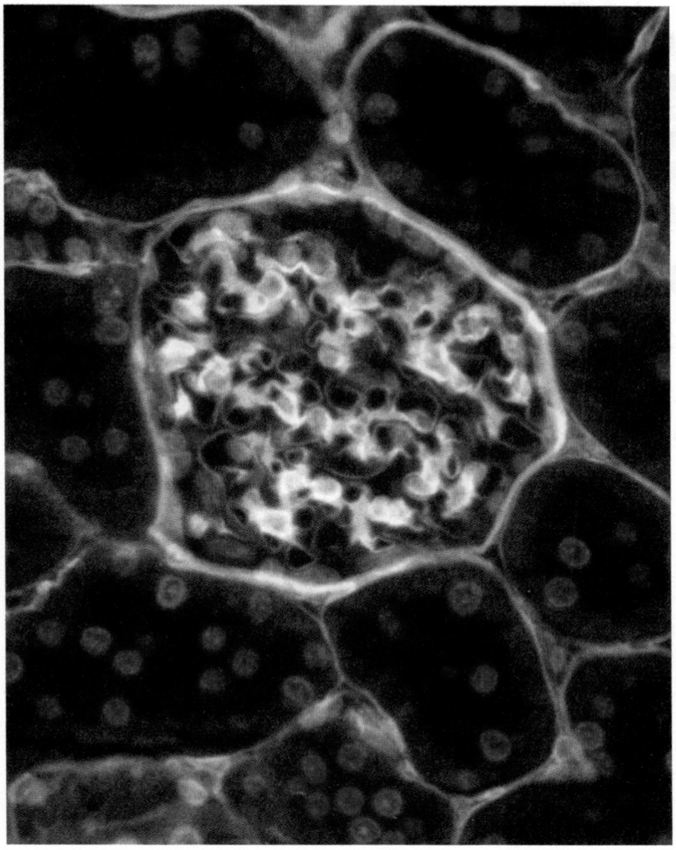

FIGURE 19.13
Immunofluorescent-stained glomerulus. This triple-exposure micrograph of a normal adult rat glomerulus is immunostained with two different antibodies. One antibody recognizes specific extracellular components, namely, basement membrane heparan sulfate proteoglycan (BM-HSPG, rhodamine label). The other antibody recognizes basement membrane chondroitin sulfate proteoglycan (BM-CSPG, fluorescein label). Because it is a triple-exposure micrograph, a yellow color occurs where the two fluorescent labels exactly codistribute. The blue fluorescence is nuclear counterstaining with Hoechst nuclear stain. The micrograph shows that compartmentalization occurs with respect to glomerular proteoglycan populations. The glomerular capillary basement membrane is composed exclusively of BM-HSPG, whereas the mesangial matrix *(yellow)* contains both BM-HSPG and BM-CSPG. Bowman's capsule appears to be strongly stained by only BM-CSPG antibodies. ×360. (Courtesy of Dr. Kevin J. McCarthy.)

Mesangium

The renal corpuscle contains an additional group of cells called ***mesangial cells.*** These cells and their extracellular matrix constitute the ***mesangium.*** It is most obvious at the vascular stalk of the glomerulus and at the interstices of adjoining glomerular capillaries. Mesangial cells are positioned much the same as pericytes, in that they are enclosed by the basal lamina of the glomerular capillaries (see Fig. 19.10). The mesangial cells are not entirely confined to the renal corpuscle; some are located outside the corpuscle along the vascular pole, where they are also designated as ***lacis cells*** and form part of what is called the ***juxtaglomerular apparatus*** (see Fig. 19.7).

Although all of the functions of mesangial cells are not yet fully understood, the following functions have been demonstrated:

- ***Phagocytosis.*** Mesangial cells remove trapped residues and aggregated proteins from the GBM, thus keeping the glomerular filter free of debris.
- ***Structural support.*** Mesangial cells provide support for the podocytes in the areas where the epithelial basement membrane is absent or incomplete.
- ***Secretion.*** Mesangial cells synthesize and secrete a variety of molecules such as interleukin-1 (IL-1) and platelet-derived growth factor (PDGF), which play a central role in response to glomerular injury.

The primary function of the mesangial cells is believed to be to clean the GBM. Clinically, it has been observed that mesangial cells proliferate in certain kidney diseases in which abnormal amounts of protein and protein complexes are trapped in the basement membrane. Mesangial cells are contractile. Thus, they may also play a role in regulating glomerular blood flow.

Embryologically, mesangial and juxtaglomerular cells (discussed below) are derived from smooth muscle cell precursors. Although mesangial cells are clearly phagocytotic, they are unusual in the sense that they are not derived from the usual precursor cells of the mononuclear phagocytotic system, the blood-borne monocytes.

Juxtaglomerular Apparatus

The juxtaglomerular apparatus includes the macula densa, the juxtaglomerular cells, and the extraglomerular mesangial cells

Lying directly adjacent to the afferent and efferent arterioles and adjacent to some extraglomerular mesangial cells at the vascular pole of the renal corpuscle is the terminal portion of the distal straight tubule of the nephron. At this site the wall of the tubule contains cells that are referred to collectively as the ***macula densa.*** When viewed in the light microscope, the cells of the macula densa are distinctive, in that they are narrower and usually taller than other distal tubule cells. The nuclei of these cells appear crowded, even to the extent that they appear partially superimposed over one another, thus the name "macula densa."

In this same region, the smooth muscle cells of the adjacent afferent arteriole (and, sometimes, the efferent arteriole) are modified. They contain secretory granules, and their nuclei are spherical, as opposed to the typical elongate smooth muscle cell nucleus. These ***juxtaglomerular cells*** (see Fig. 19.7) require special stains to reveal the secretory vesicles in the light microscope.

> BOX 19.3
>
> **Clinical Correlations: Renin–Angiotensin–Aldosterone System and Hypertension**
>
> For years, cardiologists and nephrologists believed that ***chronic essential hypertension***, the most common form of hypertension, was somehow related to an abnormality in the renin–angiotensin–aldosterone system. However, 24-hour urine renin levels in such patients were usually normal. Not until a factor in the venom of a South American snake was shown to be a potent inhibitor of ACE in the lung did investigators have both a clue to the cause of chronic essential hypertension and a new series of drugs with which to treat this common disease.
>
> The "lesion" in chronic essential hypertension is now believed to be excessive production of angiotensin II in the lung. Development of the so-called ***ACE inhibitors***—captopril, enalapril, and related derivatives of the original snake venom factor—has revolutionized the treatment of chronic essential hypertension. These antihypertensive drugs do not cause the often-dangerous side effects of the diuretics and β-blockers that were previously the most commonly used drugs for control of this condition.

The juxtaglomerular apparatus regulates blood pressure by activating the renin–angiotensin–aldosterone system

In certain physiologic (low sodium intake) or pathologic conditions (decrease in volume of circulating blood due to hemorrhage or reduction in renal perfusion due to compression of the renal arteries) juxtaglomerular cells are responsible for activating the ***renin–angiotensin–aldosterone system***. This system plays an important role in maintaining sodium homeostasis and renal hemodynamics. The granules of the juxtaglomerular cells contain an aspartyl protease, called ***renin***, which is synthesized, stored, and released into the bloodstream from the modified smooth muscle cells. In the blood, renin catalyzes the hydrolysis of circulating α_2-globulin, ***angiotensinogen***, to produce the decapeptide ***angiotensin I***. Then

- Angiotensin I is converted to the active octapeptide ***angiotensin II*** by ***angiotensin-converting enzyme (ACE)*** present on the endothelial cells of lung capillaries.
- Angiotensin II stimulates the synthesis and release of the hormone ***aldosterone*** from the ***zona glomerulosa of the adrenal gland*** (see page 665).
- Aldosterone, in turn, acts on collecting ducts to increase reabsorption of sodium and concomitant reabsorption of water, thereby raising blood volume and pressure.
- Angiotensin II is also a potent vasoconstrictor that has a regulatory role in the control of renal and systemic vascular resistance.

The juxtaglomerular apparatus functions both as an endocrine organ that helps to regulate blood composition and volume and as a sensor of blood composition and volume. Decreased blood volume or decreased sodium concentration in the blood are believed to be stimuli for the release of renin by the juxtaglomerular cells. The cells of the macula densa monitor NaCl concentration in the afferent arteriole and regulate the release of renin by the juxtaglomerular cells in a paracrine manner. An increase in blood volume sufficient to cause stretching of the juxtaglomerular cells in the afferent arteriole may be the stimulus that closes the feedback loop and stops secretion of renin.

▽ KIDNEY TUBULE FUNCTION

As the glomerular ultrafiltrate passes through the uriniferous and collecting tubules of the kidney, it undergoes changes that involve both active and passive absorption, as well as secretion.

- Certain substances within the ultrafiltrate are reabsorbed, some partially (e.g., water, sodium, and bicarbonate) and some completely (e.g., glucose).
- Other substances (e.g., creatinine and organic acids and bases) are added to the ultrafiltrate (i.e., the primary urine) by secretory activity of the tubule cells.

Thus, the volume of the ultrafiltrate is reduced substantially, and the urine is made hyperosmotic. The long ***loops of Henle*** and the ***collecting tubules*** that pass parallel to similarly arranged blood vessels, the ***vasa recta***, serve as the basis for the ***countercurrent multiplier mechanism*** that is instrumental in concentrating the urine, thereby making it hyperosmotic.

Proximal Convoluted Tubule

The proximal convoluted tubule is the initial and major site of reabsorption

The ***proximal convoluted tubule*** receives the ultrafiltrate from the urinary space of Bowman's capsule. The cuboidal cells of the proximal convoluted tubule have the elaborate surface specializations associated with cells engaged in absorption and fluid transport. They exhibit the following features:

- A ***brush border***, composed of relatively long, closely packed, and straight microvilli (Fig. 19.14)
- A ***junctional complex***, consisting of a narrow, tight junction that seals off the intercellular space from the lumen of the tubule and a zonula adherens that maintains the adhesion between neighboring cells
- ***Plicae*** or ***folds*** located on the lateral surfaces of the cells, which are large flattened processes, alternating with similar processes of adjacent cells (see Fig. 19.14)
- Extensive ***interdigitation of basal processes*** of adjacent cells (Figs. 19.15 and 19.16)

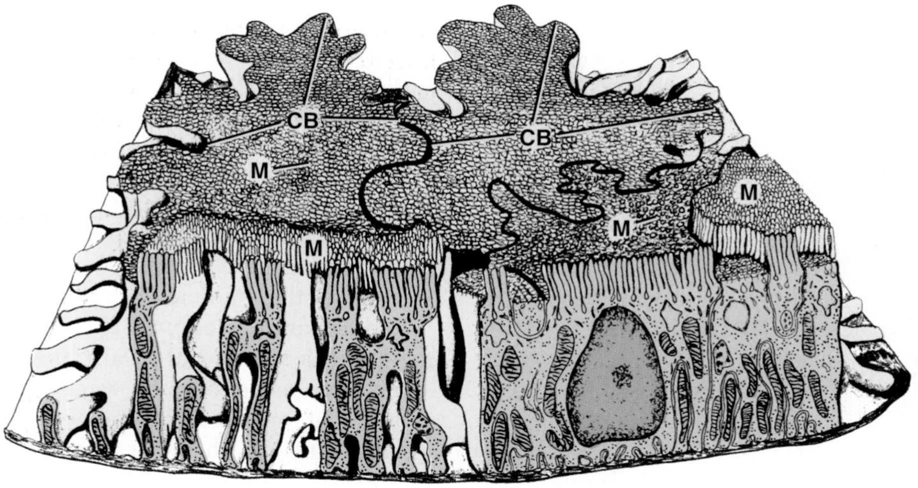

FIGURE 19.14

Drawing of proximal convoluted tubule cells. The drawing, at the electron microscopic level, shows the sectioned face on the right and a three-dimensional view of the basolateral surface of a cell with a partial cut face on the left. Here the interdigitating parts of the adjoining cell have been removed to show the basolateral interdigitations. Some of the interdigitating processes extend the full height of the cell. The processes are long in the basal region and create an elaborate extracellular compartment adjacent to the basal lamina. Apically, the microvilli *(M)* constitute the brush border. In some locations, the microvilli have been omitted, thereby revealing the convoluted character of the apical cell boundary *(CB)*. (Based on Bulger RE. *Am J Anat* 1965;116:253.)

- *Basal striations*, consisting of elongate mitochondria concentrated in the basal processes and oriented vertically to the basal surface (see Fig. 19.15)

In well-fixed histologic preparations, the basal striations and the apical brush border help to distinguish the cells of the proximal convoluted tubule from those of the other tubules.

At the very base of the proximal convoluted tubule cell, in the interdigitating processes, bundles of 6-nm microfilaments are present (see *arrows*, Figs. 19.15 and 19.16). These actin filaments may play a role in regulating the movement of fluid from the basolateral extracellular space across the tubule basal lamina toward the adjacent peritubular capillary.

The proximal convoluted tubule reabsorbs about 150 L of fluid per day or about 80% of the ultrafiltrate. Two ma-

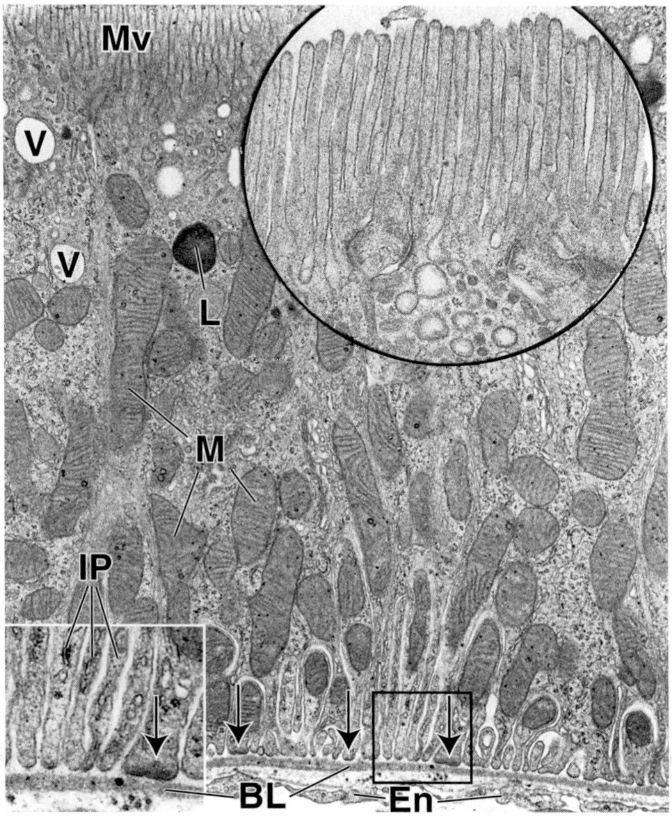

FIGURE 19.15

Electron micrograph of a proximal tubule cell. The apical surface of the cell shows the closely packed microvilli *(Mv)* that collectively are recognized as the brush border in the light microscope. Many vesicles *(V)* are evident in the apical cytoplasm. Also present in the apical region of the cell are lysosomes *(L)*. The nucleus has not been included in the plane of section. Extensive numbers of longitudinally oriented mitochondria *(M)* are present in the cell within the interdigitating processes. The mitochondria are responsible for the appearance of the basal striations seen in the light microscope, particularly if the extracellular space is enlarged. The electron micrograph also reveals a basal lamina and a small amount of connective tissue and the fenestrated endothelium *(En)* of an adjacent peritubular capillary. ×15,000. **Upper inset.** This higher magnification of the microvilli shows the small endocytotic vesicles that have pinched off from the plasma membrane at the base of the microvilli. ×32,000. **Lower inset.** A higher magnification of the basal portion of the interdigitating processes *(IP)* below the reach of the mitochondria. The extreme basal aspect of these processes reveals a dense material *(arrows)* that represents bundles of actin filaments (see Fig. 19.16). ×15,000.

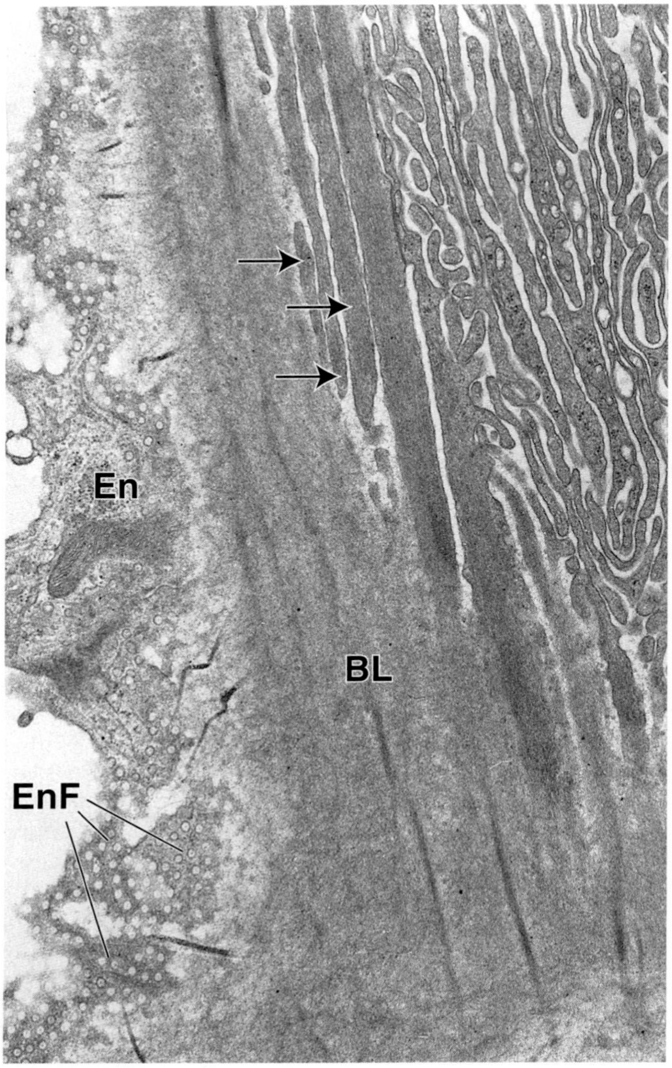

FIGURE 19.16
Electron micrograph of a proximal convoluted tubule cell. This section is almost tangential and slightly oblique to the base of a proximal convoluted tubule cell and the subjacent basal lamina and capillary. In the left part of the micrograph is the capillary endothelium *(En)*. Characteristically, the endothelium possesses numerous fenestrations *(EnF)*, and in this plane of section, the fenestrations are seen en face, displaying circular profiles. The plane of section also makes the basal lamina *(BL)* appear as a broad band of homogenous material. To the right of the basal lamina are the interdigitating basal processes of the proximal tubule cells. The long, straight processes contain longitudinally oriented actin filaments *(arrows)*. In this plane of section, the basal extracellular space appears as a maze between the cellular processes. ×32,000.

jor proteins are responsible for fluid reabsorption in the proximal convoluted tubules:

- ***Na^+/K^+-ATPase pumps,*** transmembrane proteins that are localized in the lateral folds of the plasma membrane. They are responsible for the *reabsorption of Na^+*, which is the major driving force for reabsorption of water in the proximal convoluted tubule. As in the intestinal and gallbladder epithelia, this process is driven by active transport of Na^+ into the lateral intercellular space. Active transport of Na^+ is followed by passive diffusion of Cl^- to maintain electrochemical neutrality. The accumulation of NaCl in the lateral intercellular spaces creates an osmotic gradient that draws water from the lumen into the intercellular compartment. This compartment distends as the amount of fluid in it increases; the lateral folds separate to allow this distension.
- ***AQP-1,*** a small (~30 kDa) transmembrane protein that functions as a molecular water channel in the cell membrane of proximal convoluted tubules. Movement of water through these membrane channels does not require the high energy of Na^+/K^+-ATPase pumps. Immunocytochemical methods can be used to demonstrate the presence of these proteins.

The hydrostatic pressure that builds up in the distended intercellular compartment, presumably aided by contractile activity of the actin filaments in the base of the tubule cells, drives an essentially isosmotic fluid across the tubule basement membrane into the renal connective tissue. Here, the fluid is reabsorbed into the vessels of the ***peritubular capillary network.***

The proximal convoluted tubule also reabsorbs amino acids, sugars, and polypeptides

As in the intestine, the microvilli of proximal convoluted tubule cells are covered with a well-developed glycocalyx that contains several ATPases, peptidases, and high concentrations of disaccharidases. In addition to amino acids and monosaccharides, the ultrafiltrate also contains small peptides and disaccharides. The latter adsorb on the glycocalyx for further digestion before internalization of the resulting amino acids and monosaccharides (including glucose). Also, as in the gut, amino acid and glucose resorption depend on active Na^+ transport.

Proteins and large peptides are endocytosed in the proximal convoluted tubule

Deep tubular invaginations are present between the microvilli of the proximal convoluted tubule cells. Proteins in the ultrafiltrate, on reaching the tubule lumen, bind to the glycocalyx that covers the plasma membrane of the invaginations. Then endocytotic vesicles containing the bound protein bud from the invaginations and fuse in the apical cytoplasm to form large protein-containing early endosomes (see Fig. 19.15). These early endosomes are destined to become lysosomes, and the endocytosed proteins are degraded by acid hydrolases. The amino acids produced in the lysosomal degradation are recycled into the circulation

BOX 19.4

Functional Considerations: Structure and Function of Aquaporin Water Channels

AQPs are a recently recognized family of small, hydrophobic, transmembrane proteins that mediate water transport in the kidney and other organs. To date, 10 proteins have been characterized and cloned. The molecular size of AQPs ranges from 26 to 34 kDa. Each protein consists of six transmembrane domains arranged to form a distinct pore. The sites where AQPs are expressed implicate their role in water transport, such as renal tubules (water reabsorption), brain and spinal cord (cerebrospinal fluid reabsorption), lacrimal apparatus (secretion and resorption of tears), and eye (aqueous humor secretion and reabsorption). Most AQPs are selective for the passage of water (AQP-1, AQP-2, AQP-4, AQP-5, AQP-6, and AQP-8), whereas others, such as AQP-3, AQP-7, and AQP-9, called aquaglyceroporins, also transport glycerol and other larger molecules in addition to water. Prominent members of the AQP family include

- ***AQP-1***, expressed in kidney (proximal convoluted tubules) and other cell types such as hepatocytes and red blood cells.
- ***AQP-2***, present in the terminal portion of the distal convoluted tubules and in the epithelium of collecting tubules and ducts. AQP-2 is under the regulation of antidiuretic hormone (ADH) and is thus known as an ADH-regulated water channel. Mutation of the AQP-2 gene has been linked to ***congenital nephrogenic diabetes insipidus***.
- ***AQP-3*** and ***AQP-4*** have also been detected in the basolateral cell surface of the light cells of kidney collecting ducts as well in the gastrointestinal epithelium (AQP-3) and the brain and spinal cord (AQP-4).

Current research into the function and structure of the AQP proteins may lead to the development of water channel blockers that could be used to treat hypertension, congestive heart failure, and brain swelling and to regulate intracranial or intraocular pressure.

via the intercellular compartment and the interstitial connective tissue.

Also, the pH of the ultrafiltrate is modified in the proximal convoluted tubule by the reabsorption of bicarbonate and by the specific secretion into the lumen of exogenous organic acids and organic bases derived from the peritubular capillary circulation.

Proximal Straight Tubule

The cells of the proximal straight tubule (i.e., the thick descending limb of the loop of Henle) are not as specialized for absorption as are those of the proximal convoluted tubule. They are shorter, with a less well developed brush border and with fewer and less complex lateral and basal-lateral processes. The mitochondria are smaller than those of the cells of the convoluted segment and are randomly distributed in the cytoplasm. There are fewer apical invaginations and endocytotic vesicles, as well as fewer lysosomes.

Thin Segment of Loop of Henle

As noted above, the length of the thin segment varies with the location of the nephron in the cortex. Juxtamedullary nephrons have the longest limbs; cortical nephrons have the shortest. Furthermore, various cell types are present in the thin segment. In the light microscope it is possible to detect at least two kinds of thin segment tubules, one with a more squamous epithelium than the other. Electron microscopic examination of the thin segments of various nephrons reveals further differences, namely, the existence of four types of epithelial cells (Fig. 19.17):

- *Type I* epithelium is found in the thin descending and ascending limbs of the loop of Henle of short-looped nephrons. It consists of a thin, simple epithelium. The cells have almost no interdigitations with neighboring cells and few organelles.
- *Type II* epithelium, found in the thin descending limb of long-looped nephrons in the cortical labyrinth, consists of taller epithelium. These cells possess abundant organelles and have many small, blunt microvilli. The extent of lateral interdigitation with neighboring cells varies by species.
- *Type III* epithelium, found in the thin descending limb in the inner medulla, consists of a thinner epithelium. The cells have a simpler structure and fewer microvilli than type II epithelial cells. Lateral interdigitations are absent.
- *Type IV* epithelium, found at the bend of long-looped nephrons and through the entire thin ascending limb, consists of a low, flattened epithelium without microvilli. The cells possess few organelles.

The specific functional roles of the four cell types in the thin segment are not yet clear, although this segment is part of the countercurrent exchange system that functions in concentrating urine. Morphologic differences, such as microvilli, mitochondria, and degree of cellular interdigitation, probably reflect specific active or passive roles in this process.

The thin descending and ascending limbs of the loop of Henle differ in structural and functional properties

Studies of ultrafiltrate entering the thin descending limb and leaving the thin ascending limb of the loop of Henle reveal dramatic changes in its osmolality. The ultrafiltrate that enters the thin descending limb is isosmotic whereas the ultrafiltrate leaving the thin ascending limp is hypoosmotic to plasma. This change is achieved

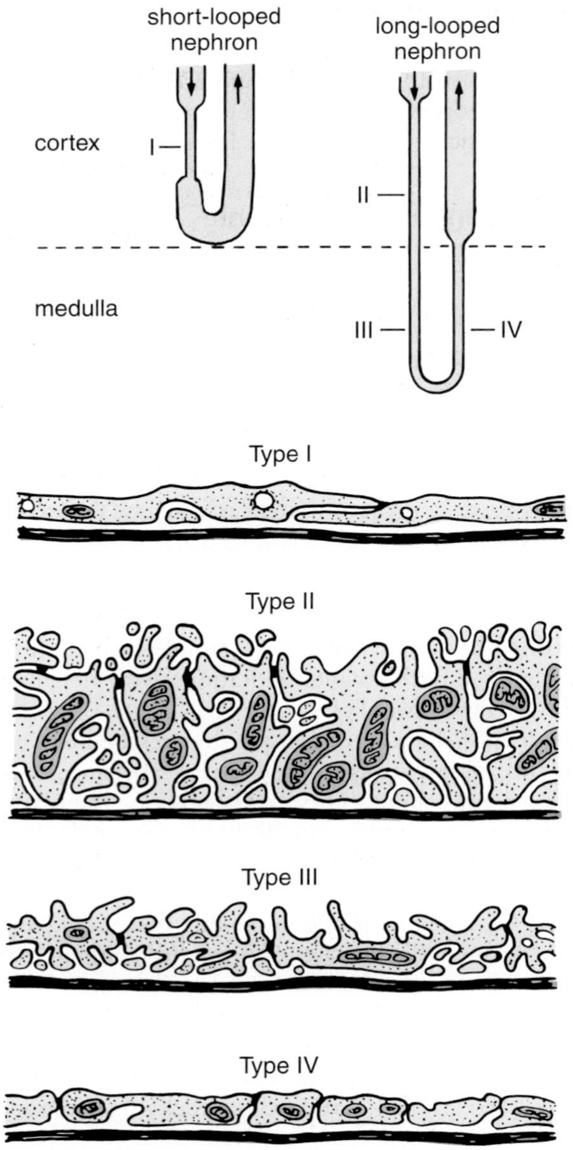

FIGURE 19.17
Schematic diagram of loop-of-Henle thin-limb epithelial cells. *Roman numerals (I-IV)* identify the various segments of the epithelium and the region where they are found in the thin limb of the short and long loops of Henle. The diagrams of the epithelium do not include nuclear regions of the epithelial cells. (Modified from Madsen KM, Tisher CC. *Kidney Hormones* 1986;3:45–100.)

by reabsorbing more salts than water. The two limbs of the loop of Henle have different permeabilities and thus different functions:

- The ***thin descending limb*** of the loop of Henle is permeable, permitting free passage or equilibration of salt and water between the lumen of the nephron and the peritubular connective tissue. Because the interstitial fluid in the medulla is hyperosmotic, water diffuses out of, and salt diffuses into, the nephron at this site. The cells of this limb do not actively transport significant amount of ions; thus changes in osmolarity are the result of passive movement of water into the peritubular connective tissue and of salt and urea into the thin descending limb.
- The ***thin ascending limb*** of the loop of Henle also has active function but allows passive diffusion of NaCl into the interstitium. Cl^- ion diffuses into the interstitium following its concentration gradient through the Cl^--conducting channels. Although the energy from ATP is required to open these channels, the movement of Cl^- is not an example of active transport and does not require Cl^--stimulated ATPase activity. Counter ions, in this case Na^+ (the majority) and K^+, follow passively in order to maintain electrochemical neutrality. The hyperosmolarity of the interstitium is directly related to the transport activity of the cells in this limb of the loop of Henle. As in most pump systems, a counter ion, in this case Na^+, follows passively to maintain electrochemical neutrality. Further, the thin ascending limb is largely ***impermeable*** to water, so that at this site, as the salt concentration increases in the interstitium, the interstitium becomes hyperosmotic and the fluid in the lumen of the nephron becomes hypoosmotic.

Distal Straight Tubule

The distal straight tubule is a part of the ascending limb of the loop of Henle

The ***distal straight tubule (thick ascending limb)***, as previously noted, is a part of the ascending limb of the loop of Henle and includes both medullary and cortical portions, with the latter located in the medullary rays. The distal straight tubule, like the ascending thin limb, transports ions from the tubular lumen to the interstitium. The apical cell membrane in this segment has electroneutral transporters (synporters) that allow Cl^-, Na^+, and K^+ to enter the cell from the lumen. Na^+ is actively transported across the extensive basal-lateral plications by the Na^+/K^+-ATPase pumps; Cl^- and K^+ diffuse out from the intracellular space by the Cl^- and K^+ channels. Some K^+ ions leak back into the tubular fluid throughout K^+ channels, causing the tubular lumen to be positively charged in respect to the interstitium. This positive gradient provides the driving force for the reabsorption of many other ions such as Ca^{2+} and Mg^{2+}. Note that this significant movement of ions occurs without the movement of water through the wall of the distal straight tubule, resulting in separation of water from its solutes.

In routine histologic preparations, the large cuboidal cells of the distal straight tubule stain lightly with eosin,

and the lateral margins of the cells are indistinct. The nucleus is located in the apical portion of the cell and sometimes, especially in the straight segment, causes the cell to bulge into the lumen. As noted above, these cells have extensive basal-lateral plications, and there are numerous mitochondria associated with these basal folds (Fig. 19.18). They also have considerably fewer and less well developed microvilli than proximal straight tubule cells (compare Figs. 19.15 and 19.18).

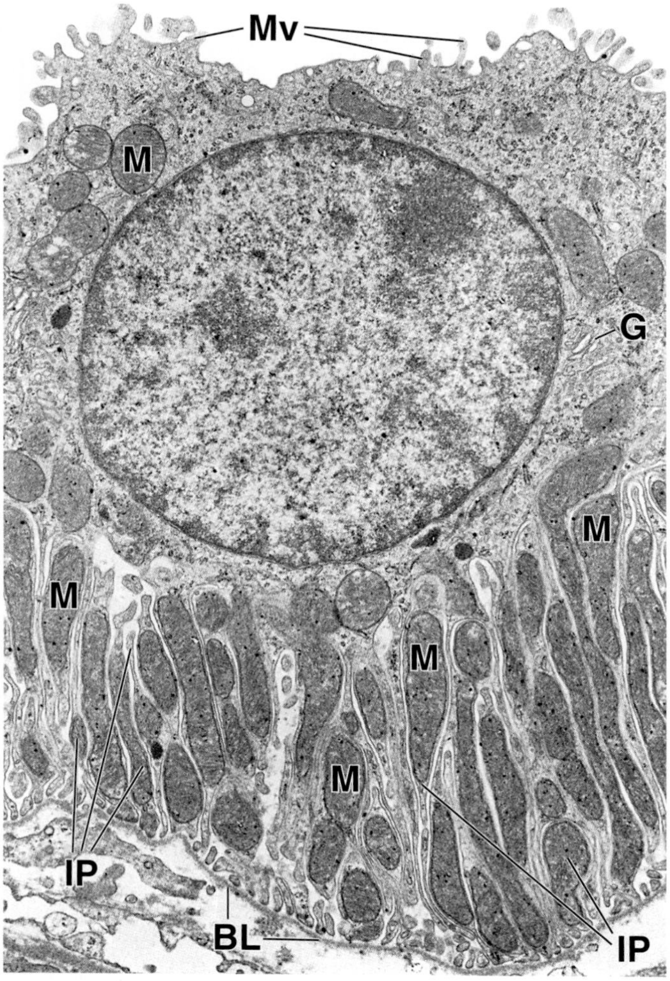

FIGURE 19.18
Electron micrograph of a distal convoluted tubule cell. The apical surface of the cell displays some microvilli *(Mv)*, but they are not sufficiently long or numerous to give the appearance of a brush border (compare with Fig. 19.15). The nucleus and Golgi apparatus *(G)* are in the upper portion of the cell. Mitochondria *(M)* are chiefly in the basal region of the cell within the interdigitating processes *(IP)*. As in the proximal tubule cell, the mitochondria account for the appearance of basal striations in the light microscope. A basal lamina *(BL)* is seen adjacent to the basal surface of the cell. ×12,000.

Distal Convoluted Tubule

The distal convoluted tubule exchanges Na^+ for K^+ under aldosterone regulation

The ***distal convoluted tubule,*** located in the cortical labyrinth, is only about one third as long (~5 mm) as the proximal convoluted tubule. This short tubule is responsible for

- ***Reabsorption of Na^+ and secretion of K^+*** into the ultrafiltrate to conserve Na^+
- ***Reabsorption of bicarbonate ion,*** with concomitant secretion of hydrogen ion, leading to further acidification of the urine
- ***Conversion of ammonia to ammonium ion,*** which then enters the urea cycle that counteracts the toxic effects of ammonia

Aldosterone, secreted by the adrenal gland and released under stimulation by angiotensin II, increases the reabsorption of Na^+ and secretion of K^+. These effects increase blood volume and blood pressure in response to increased blood Na^+ concentration.

Collecting Tubules and Collecting Ducts

The ***collecting tubules*** as well as the ***cortical*** and ***medullary collecting ducts*** are composed of simple epithelium. The collecting tubules and cortical collecting ducts have flattened cells, somewhat squamous to cuboidal in shape. The medullary collecting ducts have cuboidal cells, with a transition to columnar cells as the ducts increase in size. The collecting tubules and ducts are readily distinguished from proximal and distal tubules by virtue of the cell boundaries that can be seen in the light microscope.

Two distinct types of cells are present in the collecting tubules and collecting ducts:

- ***Light cells,*** also called ***collecting duct or CD cells,*** are the principal cells of the system. They are pale-staining cells with true basal infoldings rather than processes that interdigitate with those of adjacent cells. They possess a single cilium and relatively few short microvilli (Fig. 19.19). They contain small, spherical mitochondria. These cells possess an abundance of ADH-regulated water channels, AQP-2, which are responsible for water permeability of the collecting ducts. In addition, aquaporins AQP-3 and AQP-4 are present within the basolateral membrane of these cells.
- ***Dark cells,*** also called ***intercalated (IC) cells,*** occur in considerably smaller numbers. They have many mitochondria, and their cytoplasm appears denser. Microplicae, cytoplasmic folds, are present on their apical surface, as well as microvilli. The microplicae are readily observed with the SEM but may be mistaken for mi-

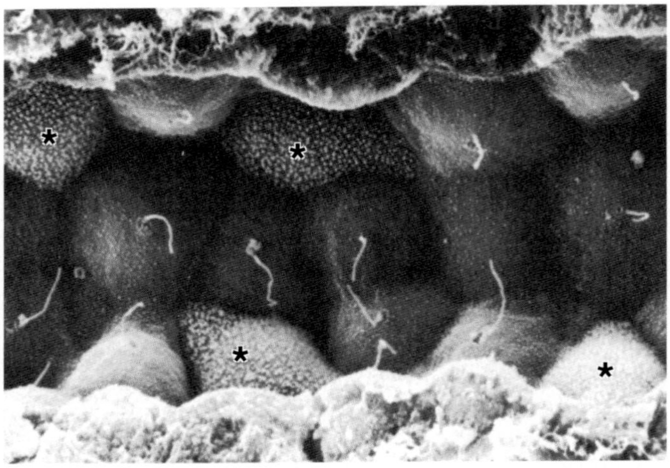

FIGURE 19.19
Scanning electron micrograph of a collecting tubule. This micrograph shows dark cells *(asterisks),* with numerous short lamellipodia or microridges on their surface, and light cells, each with a single cilium on its free surface along with small microvilli. The terms "light" and "dark" refer to the staining character of sectioned cells and not to the density differences reflecting charge characteristics of the coated surface of the specimen. (Courtesy of C. Craig Tisher.)

crovilli with the transmission electron microscope (TEM) (see Fig. 19.19). They do not show basal infoldings but have basally located interdigitations with neighboring cells. Numerous vesicles are present in the apical cytoplasm.

The cells of the collecting ducts gradually become taller as the ducts pass from the outer to the inner medulla and become columnar in the region of the renal papilla. The number of dark cells gradually decreases until none are present in the ducts as they approach the papilla.

▼ INTERSTITIAL CELLS

The connective tissue of the kidney parenchyma, called ***interstitial tissue***, surrounds the nephrons, ducts, and blood and lymphatic vessels. This tissue increases considerably in amount from the cortex (where it constitutes approximately 7% of the volume) to the inner region of the medulla and papilla (where it may constitute more than 20% of the volume).

In the cortex, two types of interstitial cells are recognized: cells that resemble fibroblasts, found between the basement membrane of the tubules and the adjacent peritubular capillaries, and occasional macrophages. In their intimate relationship with the base of the tubular epithelial cells, the fibroblasts resemble the subepithelial fibroblasts of the intestine. These cells synthesize and secrete the collagen and glycosaminoglycans of the extracellular matrix of the interstitium.

In the medulla, the principal interstitial cells resemble myofibroblasts. They are oriented to the long axes of the tubular structures and may have a role in compressing these structures. The cells contain prominent bundles of actin filaments, abundant rough endoplasmic reticulum (rER), a well-developed Golgi complex, and lysosomes. Prominent lipid droplets in the cytoplasm appear to increase and decrease in relation to the diuretic state. Some evidence suggests that these cells may secrete a hormone-like material that reduces blood pressure, but this sub-

BOX 19.5

Functional Considerations: Hormonal Regulation of Collecting Duct Function

Water permeability of the epithelium of the collecting ducts is regulated by ***antidiuretic hormone (ADH*** or ***vasopressin)***, a hormone produced in the ***hypothalamus*** and released from the ***posterior lobe of the pituitary gland***. ADH increases the permeability of the collecting duct to water, thereby producing more concentrated urine. At the molecular level, ADH acts on ADH-regulated water channels, AQP-2, located in the epithelium of the terminal portion of the distal convoluted tubule and in the epithelium of the collecting tubules and ducts. However, the action of ADH is more significant in the collecting tubules and collecting ducts. ADH binds to receptors on the cells of these tubules and triggers the following actions:

- ***Translocation of the AQP-2–containing intracytoplasmic vesicles*** into the apical cell surface—a short-term effect. This results in an increased number of available AQP-2 channels at the cell surface, thus increasing water permeability of the epithelium.
- ***Synthesis of AQP-2s*** and their insertion into the apical cell membrane—a long-term effect.

An increase in plasma osmolality or a decrease in blood volume stimulates release of ADH, as does nicotine.

In the absence of ADH, copious, dilute urine is produced. This condition is called ***central diabetes insipidus (CDI)***. Recent studies indicate that mutation of two genes encoding AQP-2 and ADH receptors is responsible for a form of CDI called ***nephrogenic diabetes insipidus***. In this disease, the kidney does not respond to ADH because of defective AQP-2 and ADH receptor proteins synthesized by the collecting tubule and duct epithelial cells. Excess water consumption can also inhibit ADH release, thereby promoting the production of a large volume of hypoosmotic urine.

Increased secretion of ADH can produce an extremely hyperosmotic urine, thereby conserving water in the body. Inadequate consumption of water or loss of water due to sweating, vomiting, or diarrhea stimulates release of ADH. This leads to an increase in the permeability of the epithelium of the distal and collecting tubules and promotes the production of a small volume of hyperosmotic urine.

stance has been neither isolated nor characterized. In addition, prostaglandins and prostacyclin may also be synthesized in the interstitium.

HISTOPHYSIOLOGY OF THE KIDNEY

The countercurrent multiplier system creates hyperosmotic urine

The term *countercurrent* indicates a flow of fluid in adjacent structures in opposite directions. The ability to excrete hyperosmotic urine depends on the ***countercurrent multiplier system*** that involves three structures:

- *Loop of Henle,* which acts as a ***countercurrent multiplier.*** The ultrafiltrate moves within the descending limb of the thin segment of the loop toward the renal papilla and moves back toward the corticomedullary junction within the ascending limb of the thin segment. The osmotic gradients of the medulla are established along the axis of the loop of Henle.
- *Vasa recta,* form loops parallel to the loop of Henle. They act as ***countercurrent exchangers*** of water and solutes between the descending part (arteriolae rectae) and ascending part (venulae rectae) of the vasa recta. The vasa recta help to maintain the osmotic gradient of the medulla.
- *Collecting duct* in the medulla acts as an ***osmotic equilibrating device.*** Modified ultrafiltrate in the collecting ducts can be further equilibrated with the hyperosmotic medullary interstitium. The level of equilibration depends on activation of ADH-dependent water channels (AQP-2).

A standing gradient of ion concentration produces hyperosmotic urine by a countercurrent multiplier effect

The loop of Henle creates and maintains a gradient of ion concentration in the medullary interstitium that increases from the corticomedullary junction to the renal papilla. As noted above, the thin descending limb of the loop of Henle is freely permeable to Na^+, Cl^-, and water, whereas the ascending limb of the loop of Henle is impermeable to water. Further, the thin ascending limb cells add Na^+ and Cl^- to the interstitium.

Because water cannot leave the thin ascending limb, the interstitium becomes hyperosmotic relative to the luminal contents. Although some of the Cl^- and Na^+ of the interstitium diffuses back into the nephron at the thin descending limb, the ions are transported out again in the thin ascending limb and distal straight tubule (thick ascending limb). This produces the ***countercurrent multiplier effect.*** Thus, the concentration of NaCl in the interstitium gradually increases down the length of the loop of Henle and, consequently, through the thickness of the medulla from the corticomedullary junction to the papilla.

Vasa recta containing descending arterioles and ascending venules act as countercurrent exchangers

For an understanding of the countercurrent exchange mechanism, it is necessary to resume the description of the renal circulation at the point at which the efferent arteriole leaves the renal corpuscle.

The efferent arterioles of the renal corpuscles of most of the cortex branch to form the capillary network that surrounds the tubular portions of the nephron in the cortex, the ***peritubular capillary network.*** The efferent arterioles of the juxtamedullary renal corpuscles form several unbranched arterioles that descend into the medullary pyramid. These ***arteriolae rectae*** make a hairpin turn deep in the medullary pyramid and ascend as the ***venulae rectae.*** Together, the descending arterioles and the ascending venules are called the ***vasa recta.*** The arteriolae rectae form capillary plexuses lined by fenestrated endothelium that supply the tubular structures at the various levels of the medullary pyramid.

Interaction between collecting ducts, loops of Henle, and vasa rectae is required for concentrating urine by the countercurrent exchange mechanism

Because the thin ascending limb of the loop of Henle has a high level of transport activity and because it is impermeable to water, the modified ultrafiltrate that ultimately reaches the distal convoluted tubule is *hypoosmotic.* When ADH is present, the distal convoluted tubules, the collecting tubules, and the collecting ducts are highly permeable to water. Therefore, within the cortex, in which the interstitium is isosmotic with blood, the modified ultrafiltrate within the distal convoluted tubule equilibrates and also becomes isosmotic, partly by loss of water to the interstitium and partly by addition of ions other than Na^+ and Cl^- to the ultrafiltrate. In the medulla, increasing amounts of water leave the ultrafiltrate as the collecting ducts pass through the increasingly hyperosmotic interstitium on their course to the papillae.

As noted above, the vasa recta also form loops in the medulla that parallel the loop of Henle. This arrangement ensures that the vessels provide circulation to the medulla without disturbing the osmotic gradient established by transport of Cl^- in the epithelium of the ascending limb of the loop of Henle.

The vasa recta form a ***countercurrent exchange system*** in the following manner: Both the arterial and venous sides of the loop are thin-walled vessels that form plexuses of fenestrated capillaries at all levels in the medulla. As the arterial vessels descend through the medulla, the blood loses water to the interstitium and gains salt from the interstitium so that at the tip of the loop, deep in the medulla, the blood is essentially in equilibrium with the hyperosmotic interstitial fluid.

As the venous vessels ascend toward the corticomedullary junction, the process is reversed, i.e., the hyperosmotic blood loses salt to the interstitium and gains water from the interstitium. This passive countercurrent exchange of water and salt between the blood and the interstitium occurs *without expenditure of energy* by the endothelial cells. The energy that drives this system is the same energy that drives the multiplier system, namely, the movement of Na^+ and Cl^- out of the cells of the water-impermeable ascending limb of the loop of Henle. The countercurrent exchange system and other movement of molecules in different parts of the nephron are shown in Figure 19.20.

BLOOD SUPPLY

Some aspects of the blood supply of the kidney have been described in relation to specific functions, i.e., glomerular filtration, control of blood pressure, and countercurrent exchange. It remains, however, to provide an overall description of the blood supply of the kidney.

Each kidney receives a large branch from the abdominal aorta, called the ***renal artery***. The renal artery branches within the renal sinus and sends ***interlobar*** branches into the substance of the kidney (Fig. 19.21). The interlobar arteries travel between the pyramids as far as the cortex and

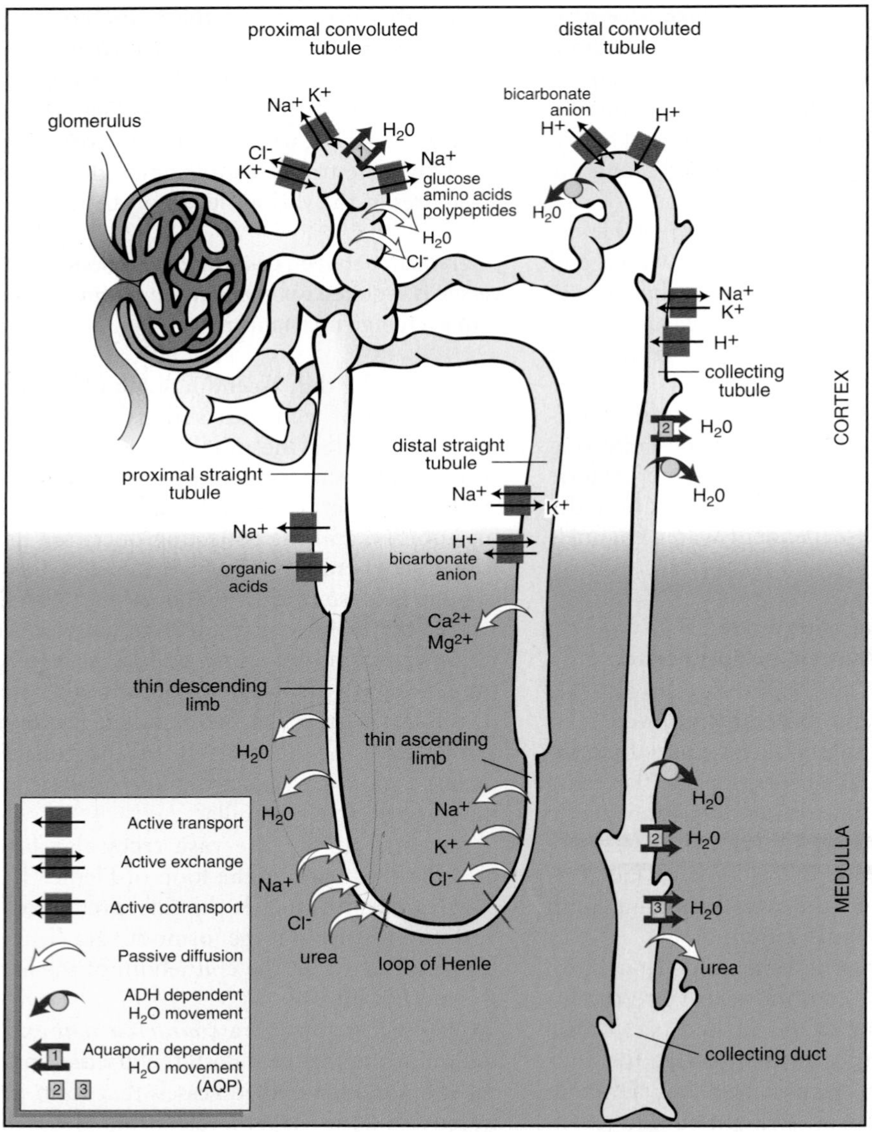

FIGURE 19.20

Diagram showing movement of substances into and out of the nephron and collecting system. The *symbols* indicate the mode of transport as noted in the key.

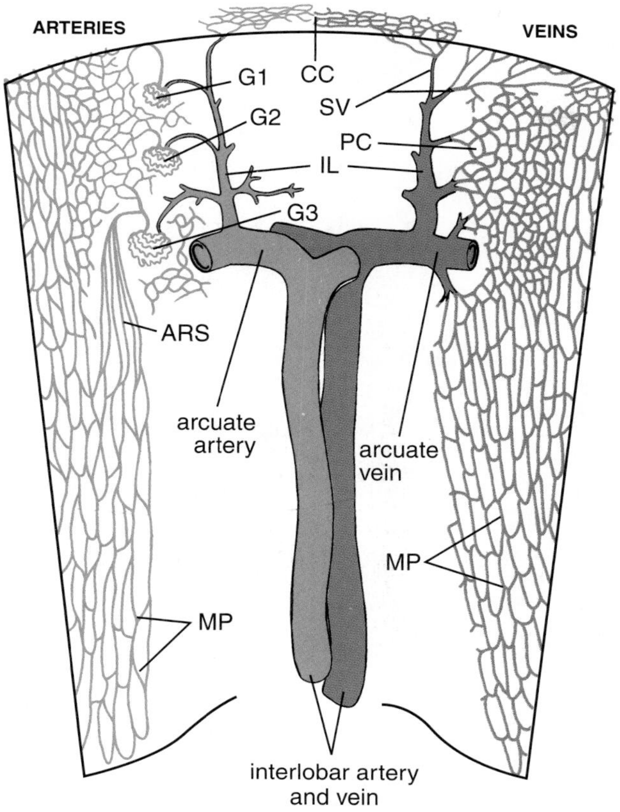

FIGURE 19.21
Schematic diagram of the renal blood supply. The renal artery gives rise to interlobar arteries that branch into arcuate arteries at the border between the medulla and cortex. Interlobular arteries *(IL)* branch from the arcuate arteries and travel toward the renal capsule, giving off afferent arterioles to the glomeruli *(G)*. Glomeruli in the outer part of the cortex *(G1, G2)* send efferent arterioles to the peritubular capillaries *(PC)* that surround the tubules in the cortex; glomeruli near the medulla *(G3)*, the juxtamedullary glomeruli, send efferent arterioles almost entirely into the medullary plexus *(MP)* of capillaries via the arteriolae rectae spuriae *(ARS)*. Blood returns from the capillaries via veins that enter the arcuate veins. Stellate veins *(SV)* near the capsule drain both the capsular *(CC)* and the peritubular capillaries.

then turn to follow an arched course along the base of the pyramid between the medulla and the cortex. Thus, these interlobar arteries are designated ***arcuate arteries.***

Interlobular arteries branch from the arcuate arteries and ascend through the cortex toward the capsule. Although the boundaries between lobules are not distinct, the interlobular arteries, when included in a section cut perpendicular to the vessel, are located midway between adjacent medullary rays, traveling in the cortical labyrinth. As they traverse the cortex toward the capsule, the interlobular arteries give off branches, the ***afferent arterioles,*** one to each glomerulus. A single afferent arteriole may spring directly from the interlobular artery, or a common stem from the interlobular artery may branch to form several afferent arterioles. Some interlobular arteries terminate near the periphery of the cortex, whereas others enter the kidney capsule to provide its arterial supply.

Afferent arterioles give rise to the capillaries that form the glomerulus. The glomerular capillaries reunite to form an ***efferent arteriole*** that, in turn, gives rise to a second network of capillaries, the ***peritubular capillaries.*** The arrangement of these capillaries differs according to whether they originate from cortical or juxtamedullary glomeruli.

- ***Efferent arterioles from cortical glomeruli*** lead into a peritubular capillary network that surrounds the local uriniferous tubules (see *G1* and *G2*, Fig. 19.21).
- ***Efferent arterioles from juxtamedullary glomeruli*** descend into the medulla alongside the loop of Henle; they break up into smaller vessels that continue toward the apex of the pyramid but make hairpin turns at various levels to return again as straight vessels toward the base of the pyramid (see *G3* Fig. 19.21). Thus, the efferent arterioles from the juxtamedullary glomeruli give rise to ***vasa recta*** involved in the countercurrent exchange system and their peritubular capillary network. These vessels are described in the explanation of the countercurrent exchange system (page 623).

Generally, venous flow in the kidney follows a reverse course to arterial flow, with the veins running in parallel with the corresponding arteries (see Fig. 19.21). Thus,

- ***Peritubular cortical capillaries*** drain into ***interlobular veins,*** which in turn drain into ***arcuate veins, interlobar veins,*** and the ***renal vein.***
- The ***medullary vascular*** network drains into ***arcuate veins*** and so forth.
- ***Peritubular capillaries*** near the kidney surface and ***capillaries of the capsule*** drain ***into stellate veins*** (so called for their pattern of distribution when viewed from the kidney surface), which drain into ***interlobular veins,*** and so forth.

▼ LYMPHATIC VESSELS

The kidneys contain two major networks of lymphatic vessels. These networks are not usually visible in routine histologic sections but can be demonstrated by experimental methods. One network is located in the outer regions of the cortex and drains into larger lymphatic vessels in the capsule. The other network is located more deeply in the substance of the kidney and drains into large lymphatic vessels in the renal sinus. There are numerous anastomoses between the two lymphatic networks.

NERVE SUPPLY

The fibers that form the renal plexus are derived mostly from the sympathetic division of the autonomic nervous system. They cause contraction of vascular smooth muscle and consequent vasoconstriction.

- *Constriction of the afferent arterioles* to the glomeruli reduces the filtration rate and decreases the production of urine.
- *Constriction of the efferent arterioles* from the glomeruli increases the filtration rate and increases the production of urine.
- Loss of sympathetic innervation leads to increased urinary output.

It is evident, however, that the extrinsic nerve supply is not necessary for normal renal function. Although the nerve fibers to the kidney are cut during renal transplantation, transplanted kidneys subsequently function normally.

URETER, URINARY BLADDER, AND URETHRA

All excretory passages, except the urethra, have the same general organization

On leaving the collecting ducts at the ***area cribrosa***, the urine enters a series of structures that do not modify it but are specialized for its storage and passage to the exterior of the body. The urine flows sequentially to a ***minor calyx***, a ***major calyx***, and the ***renal pelvis***, and leaves each kidney through the ***ureter*** to the ***urinary bladder***, where it is stored. The urine is finally voided through the ***urethra***.

All of these excretory passages, except the urethra, have the same general structures, namely, a mucosa (lined by transitional epithelium), muscularis, and adventitia (or, in some regions, a serosa).

Transitional epithelium lines the calyces, ureters, bladder, and the initial segment of the urethra

Transitional epithelium (urothelium) lines the excretory passages leading from the kidney. This stratified epithelium is essentially impermeable to salts and water. The epithelium begins in the minor calyces as two cell layers and increases to an apparent four to five layers in the ureter (Fig. 19.22) and as many as six or more layers in the empty bladder. However, when the bladder is distended, as few as three layers are seen. This change reflects the ability of the cells to accommodate to distension. The cells in the distended bladder, particularly the large surface cells and those in the layers below, flatten and unfold to accommodate the increasing surface area. As the individual cells unfold and flatten, the resulting appearance is the "true" three layers.

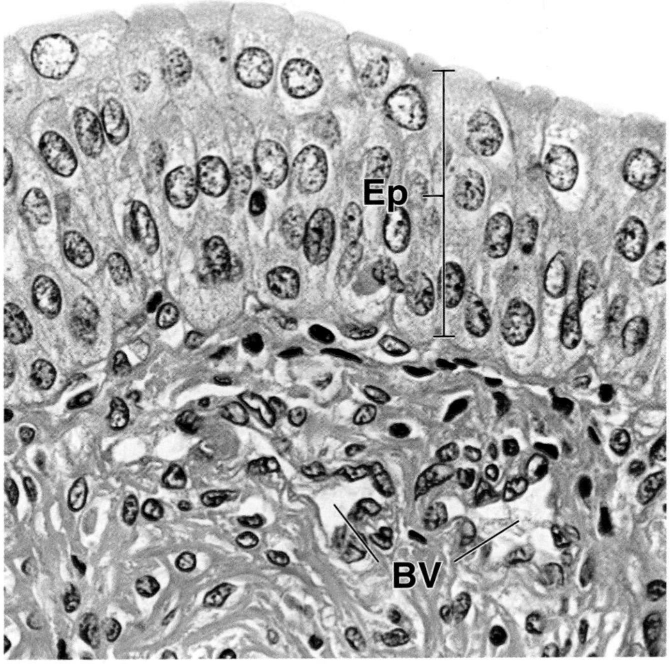

FIGURE 19.22
Photomicrograph of transitional epithelium (urothelium). This H&E–stained specimen shows the 4- to 5-cell-layer thickness of the epithelium in the relaxed ureter. The surface cells exhibit a rounded or dome-shaped profile. The connective tissue below the epithelium *(Ep)* is relatively cellular and contains a number of lymphocytes. Blood vessels *(BV)* are also abundant in this area. ×450.

In routine histologic sections obtained from the empty bladder, the surface epithelial cells are usually cuboidal and bulge into the lumen. They are frequently described as "dome-shaped" cells because of the curvature of the apical surface (see Fig. 19.22). When examined with the TEM, the plasma membrane exhibits an unusual feature, e.g., modified areas of the plasma membrane called ***plaques*** are seen (Fig. 19.23). These plaques appear to be more rigid and thicker (up to 12 nm) than the rest of the apical plasma membrane. Actin filaments are observed stretching from the inner surface of the plaques into the cytoplasm. In the undistended urinary bladder the plaques give the luminal surface of cells an irregular scalloped contour (Fig. 19.24). Each cell appears to fold inward upon itself. As a result of this folding, the plaques appear as a series of ***fusiform vesicles.*** Their lumina, however, are in continuity with the cell's exterior. As the bladder distends, the fusiform vesicles unfold and become part of the surface as the cell stretches and flattens (Fig. 19.25).

Smooth muscle of the urinary passages is arranged in bundles

A dense collagenous lamina propria underlies the urothelium throughout the excretory passages. Neither a muscularis mucosae nor a submucosal layer is present in

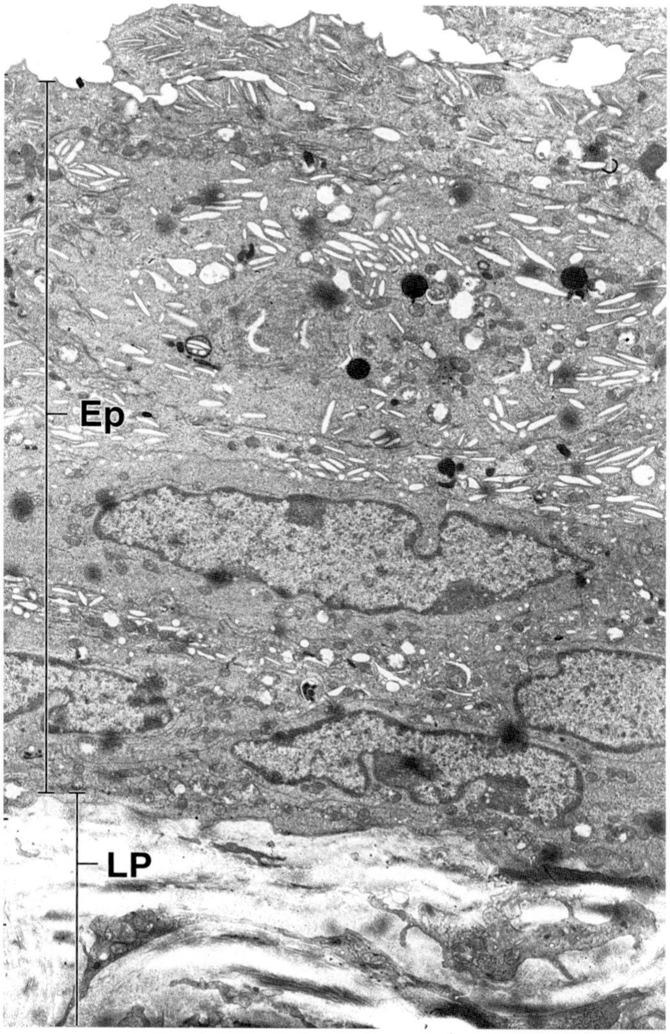

FIGURE 19.23
Transmission electron micrograph of urinary bladder epithelium. The mucous membrane of the urinary bladder consists of transitional epithelium *(Ep)* with an underlying lamina propria *(LP)*. The epithelial cells contain unique fusiform vesicles, which are evident here at this relatively low magnification. These are seen at higher magnification in Figure 19.24. ×5,000.

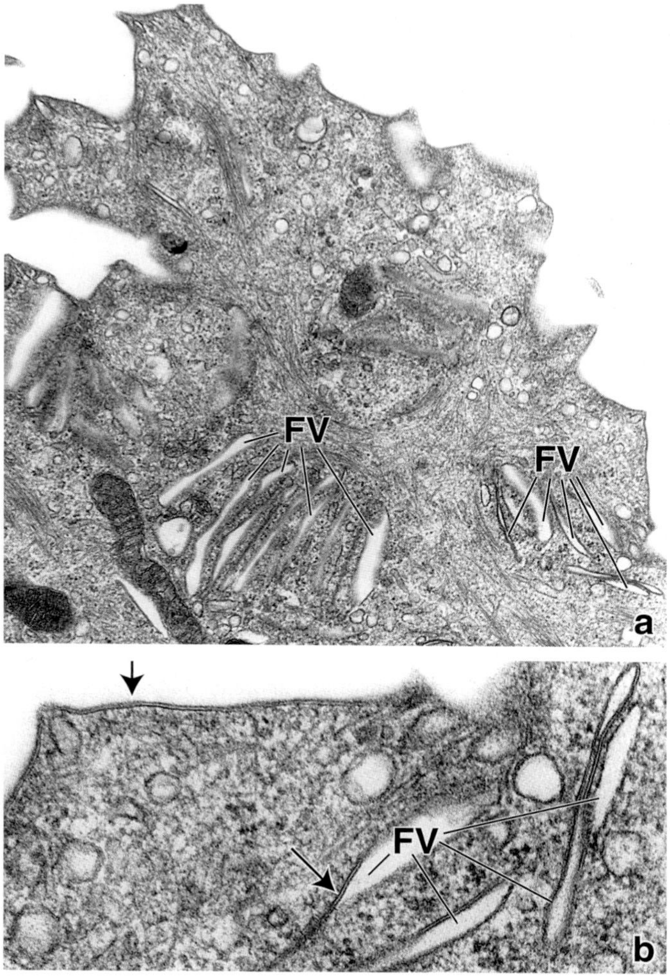

FIGURE 19.24
Transmission electron micrograph of the apical portion of a transitional epithelial cell. a. The cytoplasm displays small vesicles, filaments, and mitochondria, but the most distinctive feature of the cell is its fusiform vesicles *(FV)*. ×27,000. **b.** The higher magnification shows that the membrane forming the vesicles appears to be similar to the plasma membrane of the cell surface *(arrows)*. Both membranes are thickened and give the impression of possessing a degree of rigidity greater than that of plasma membrane in other locations. The thickened plasma membrane represents a sectioned view of a surface plaque. The fusiform vesicles are formed by the infolding of the plaques in the cells of the relaxed urinary bladder. ×60,000.

their walls. In the tubular portions (ureters and urethra), usually two layers of smooth muscle lie beneath the lamina propria:

- The inner layer is arranged in a loose spiral described as a ***longitudinal layer***.
- The outer layer is arranged in a tight spiral described as a ***circular layer***.

Note that this arrangement of the smooth muscle is opposite that of the muscularis externa of the intestinal tract. The smooth muscle of the urinary passages is mixed with connective tissue, so that it forms parallel bundles rather than pure muscular sheets. Peristaltic contractions of the smooth muscle move the urine from the minor calyces through the ureter to the bladder.

Ureters

Each ureter conducts urine from the renal pelvis to the urinary bladder and is approximately 24 to 34 cm long. The distal part of the ureter enters the urinary bladder and follows an oblique path through the wall of the bladder. Transitional epithelium (urothelium) lines the luminal surface of

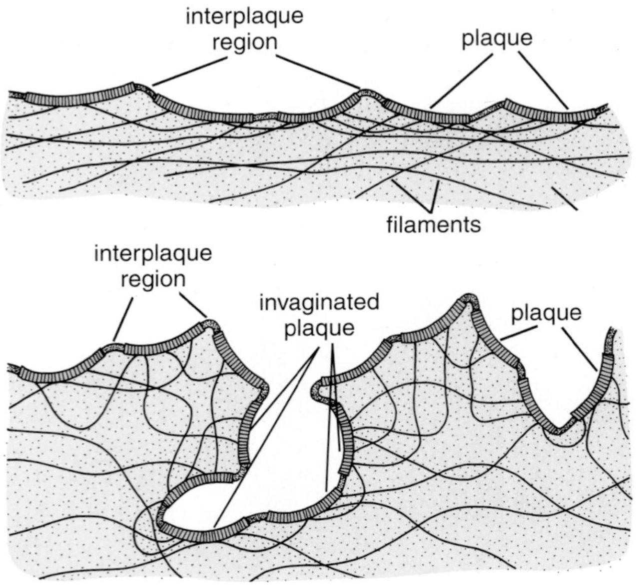

FIGURE 19.25
Diagrams of the luminal surface of transitional epithelial cells. The *upper drawing* depicts part of a surface cell in a distended bladder; the *lower drawing* depicts the same cell as it would appear in a relaxed bladder. The plasma membrane is thickened in regions to form plaques. The interplaque regions consist of membrane that is not thickened. In the relaxed bladder, the plaques are invaginated into the cell, and although they retain their continuity with the surface, the invaginated plaques typically appear as isolated fusiform vesicles in electron micrographs. Filaments attached to the undersurface of the plaques may prevent undue stretching in the distended bladder. (Modified from Staehelin LA, Chlapowski FJ, Bonneville MA. *J Cell Biol* 1972;53:73–91.)

the wall of the ureter. The remainder of the wall is composed of smooth muscle and connective tissue. The smooth muscle is arranged in three layers: an inner longitudinal layer, a middle circular layer, and an outer longitudinal layer. However, the outer longitudinal layer is present only at the distal end of the ureter. Usually, the ureter is embedded in the retroperitoneal adipose tissue. The adipose tissue, vessels, and nerves form the adventitia of the ureter.

As the bladder distends with urine, the openings of the ureters are compressed, reducing the possibility of reflux of urine into the ureters. Contraction of the smooth muscle of the bladder wall also compresses the openings of the ureters into the bladder. This action helps prevent the spread of infection from the bladder and urethra, frequent sites of chronic infection (particularly in females), to the kidney.

In the terminal portion of the ureters, a thick outer layer of longitudinal muscle is present in addition to the two listed above, particularly in the portion of the ureter that passes through the bladder wall. Most descriptions of the bladder musculature indicate that this longitudinal layer continues into the wall of the bladder to form a principal component of its wall. The smooth muscle of the bladder however, is not as clearly separated into distinctive layers.

Urinary Bladder

The bladder is a distensible reservoir for urine, located in the pelvis, posterior to the pubic symphysis; its size and shape change as it fills. It contains three openings, two for the ureters (ureteric orifices) and one for the urethra (internal urethral orifice). The triangular region defined by these three openings, the ***trigone,*** is relatively smooth and constant in thickness, whereas the rest of the bladder wall is thick and folded when the bladder is empty and thin and smooth when the bladder is distended. These differences reflect the embryologic origins of the trigone and the rest of the bladder wall: the trigone is derived from the embryonic mesonephric ducts, and the major portion of the wall originates from the cloaca.

The smooth muscle of the bladder wall forms the ***detrusor muscle.*** Toward the opening of the urethra, the muscle fibers form the involuntary ***internal urethral sphincter,*** a ring-like arrangement of muscle around the opening of the urethra. The smooth muscle bundles of the detrusor muscle are less regularly arranged than that of the tubular portions of the excretory passages, and thus, the muscle and collagen bundles are randomly mixed. Contraction of the detrusor muscle of the bladder compresses the entire organ and forces the urine into the urethra.

The bladder is innervated by both sympathetic and parasympathetic divisions of the autonomic nervous system:

- *Sympathetic fibers* form a plexus in the adventitia of the bladder wall. These fibers probably innervate blood vessels in the wall.
- *Parasympathetic fibers* originate from S_2 to S_4 segments of the spinal cord and travel with pelvic splanchnic nerves into the bladder. They end in terminal ganglia in the muscle bundles and the adventitia and are the efferent fibers of the ***micturition reflex.***
- *Sensory fibers* from the bladder to the sacral portion of the spinal cord are the afferent fibers of the micturition reflex.

Urethra

The ***urethra*** is the fibromuscular tube that conveys urine from the urinary bladder to the exterior through the ***external urethral orifice.*** The size, structure, and functions of the urethra differ in males and females.

In the male, the urethra serves as the terminal duct for both the urinary and genital systems. It is about 20 cm long and has three distinct segments:

- ***Prostatic urethra*** extends for 3 to 4 cm from the neck of the bladder through the prostate gland (see page 707). It is lined with transitional epithelium (urothelium). The ejaculatory ducts of the genital system enter the poste-

rior wall of this segment, and many small prostatic ducts also empty into this segment.

- ***Membranous urethra*** extends for about 1 cm from the apex of the prostate gland to the bulb of the penis. It passes through the ***urogenital diaphragm*** of the pelvic floor as it enters the perineum. Skeletal muscle of the urogenital diaphragm surrounding the membranous urethra forms the ***external (voluntary) sphincter of the urethra.*** Transitional epithelium ends in the membranous urethra. This segment is lined with a stratified or pseudostratified columnar epithelium that resembles the epithelium of the genital duct system more than it resembles the epithelium of the more proximal portions of the urinary duct system.
- ***Penile (spongy) urethra*** extends for about 15 cm through the length of the penis and opens on the body surface at the ***glans penis.*** The penile urethra is surrounded by the ***corpus spongiosum*** as it passes through the length of the penis. It is lined with pseudostratified columnar epithelium except at its distal end, where it is lined with stratified squamous epithelium continuous with that of the skin of the penis. ***Ducts of the bulbourethral glands*** (Cowper's glands) and of the mucus-secreting ***urethral glands*** (glands of Littré) empty into the penile urethra.

In the female, the urethra is short, measuring 3 to 5 cm in length from the bladder to the vestibule of the vagina, where it normally terminates just posterior to the clitoris. The mucosa is traditionally described as having longitudinal folds. As in the male urethra, the lining is initially transitional epithelium, a continuation of the bladder epithelium, but changes to stratified squamous epithelium before its termination. Some investigators have reported the presence of stratified columnar and pseudostratified columnar epithelium in the midportion of the female urethra.

Numerous small ***urethral glands,*** particularly in the proximal part of the urethra, open into the urethral lumen. Other glands, the ***paraurethral glands,*** which are homologous to the prostate gland in the male, secrete into the common ***paraurethral ducts.*** These ducts open on each side of the external urethral orifice. They produce an alkaline secretion. The lamina propria is a highly vascularized layer of connective tissue that resembles the corpus spongiosum in the male. Where the urethra penetrates the urogenital diaphragm (membranous part of the urethra), the striated muscle of this structure forms the external (voluntary) urethral sphincter.

PLATE 70. KIDNEY I

The urinary system consists of the paired *kidneys,* the paired *ureters,* which lead from the kidneys to the *urinary bladder,* and the *urethra,* which leads from the bladder to the exterior of the body. The kidneys conserve body fluid and electrolytes and remove metabolic wastes such as urea, uric acid, creatinine, and breakdown products of various substances. They produce *urine,* initially an ultrafiltrate of blood that is modified by selective resorption and specific secretion by kidney tubule cells. The kidneys also function as endocrine organs, producing *erythropoietin,* a growth factor that regulates red blood cell formation, and *renin,* a hormone involved in blood pressure and blood volume control. They also hydroxylate *vitamin D,* a steroid prohormone, to produce its active form.

Each kidney is a flattened, bean-shaped structure approximately 10 cm long, 6.5 cm wide (from convex to concave border), and 3 cm thick. The concave medial border of each kidney contains a hilum, an indented region through which blood vessels, nerves, and lymphatic vessels enter and leave the kidney. The funnel-shaped origin of the ureter, the *renal pelvis,* also leaves the kidney at the hilum. A cut, hemisected fresh kidney reveals two distinct regions: a cortex, the reddish-brown outer region, and a medulla, a much lighter inner part continuous with the renal pelvis. The cortex is characterized by *renal corpuscles* and their tubules, including the convoluted and straight tubules of the *nephron,* the *collecting tubules,* and an extensive vascular supply.

Figure 1, kidney, human, fresh specimen ×3.

A section through the hilum is shown here. The hilar region of the kidney is below, and the convex lateral border is above. The outer part of the kidney (except at the hilum) has a reddish-brown appearance; this is the cortex. It is easily distinguished from the inner portion, the medulla, which is further divided into an outer portion *(OM),* identified here by the presence of straight blood vessels, the vasa recta *(VR),* and an inner portion *(IM),* which has a light appearance. The medulla consists of pyramidal structures, the pyramids, which have their base facing the cortex and their apex in the form of a papilla *(P)* facing the hilar region of the kidney. The pyramids are separated, sometimes only partially in this figure, by cortical material that is designated the renal columns *(RC).* Note, also, that the two pyramids depicted in the illustration share the same papilla. Most of the pyramid belonging to the other papilla, on the left, has not been included in the plane of the section. The papillae are free tips of the pyramids that project into the first of a series of large collecting vessels, the minor calyces *(MC);* the inner surface of the calyx is white. Minor calyces drain into major calyces, and in turn, these open into the renal pelvis, which funnels into the ureter.

An interesting feature in this specimen is that the blood has been retained in many of the vessels, thereby allowing for visualization of several renal vessels in their geographic location. Among the vessels that can be identified in the cut face of the kidney shown here are the interlobular vessels *(IV)* within the cortex; the arcuate veins *(AV)* at the base of the pyramids; and, in the medulla, the vessels going to and from the capillary network of the pyramid. The latter vessels, both arterioles and venules, are relatively straight and are designated collectively as the vasa recta *(VR).*

Figure 2, kidney, human, H&E ×20.

A histologic section including the cortex and part of the medulla is shown here. Located at the boundary between the two (partly marked by the *dashed line*) are numerous profiles of arcuate arteries *(AA)* and arcuate veins *(AV).* The most distinctive feature of the renal cortex, regardless of the plane of section, is the presence of the renal corpuscles *(RC).* These are spherical structures composed of a glomerulus (glomerular vascular tuft) surrounded by the visceral and parietal epithelium of Bowman's capsule. Also seen in the cortex are groups of tubules that are more or less straight and disposed in a radial direction from the base of the medulla *(arrows);* these are the medullary rays. In contrast, the medulla presents profiles of tubular structures that are arranged as gentle curves in the outer part of the medulla, turning slightly to become straight in the inner part of the medulla. The disposition of the tubules (and blood vessels) gives the cut face of the pyramid a slightly striated appearance that is also evident in the gross specimen (Fig. 1).

KEY

AA, arcuate arteries
AV, arcuate veins
IM, inner medulla
IV, interlobular vessels
MC, minor calyx
OM, outer medulla
P, papilla
RC: Fig. 1, renal column; Fig. 2, renal corpuscles
VR, vasa recta
arrows, medullary rays
dashed line (Fig. 2), boundary between cortex and medulla

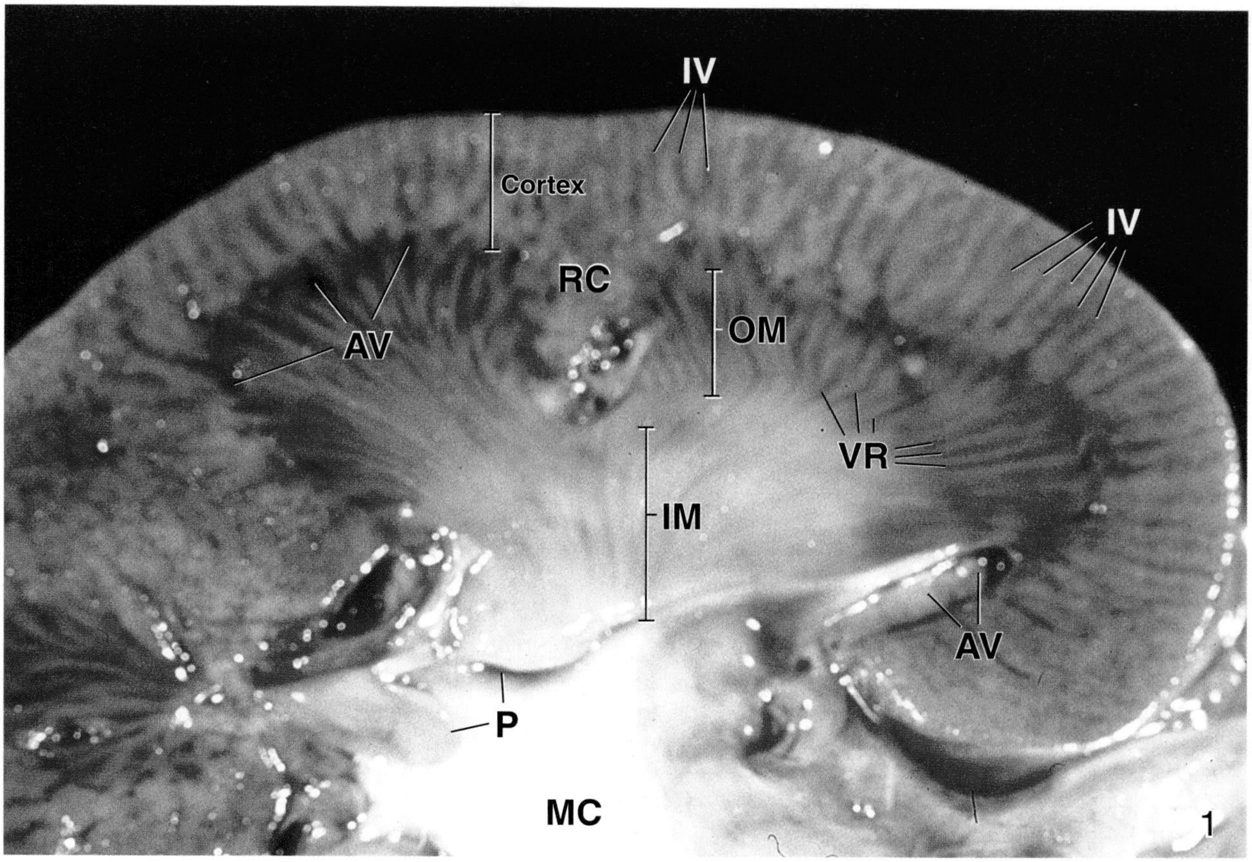
IV
Cortex
IV
RC
AV
OM
VR
IM
AV
P
MC
1

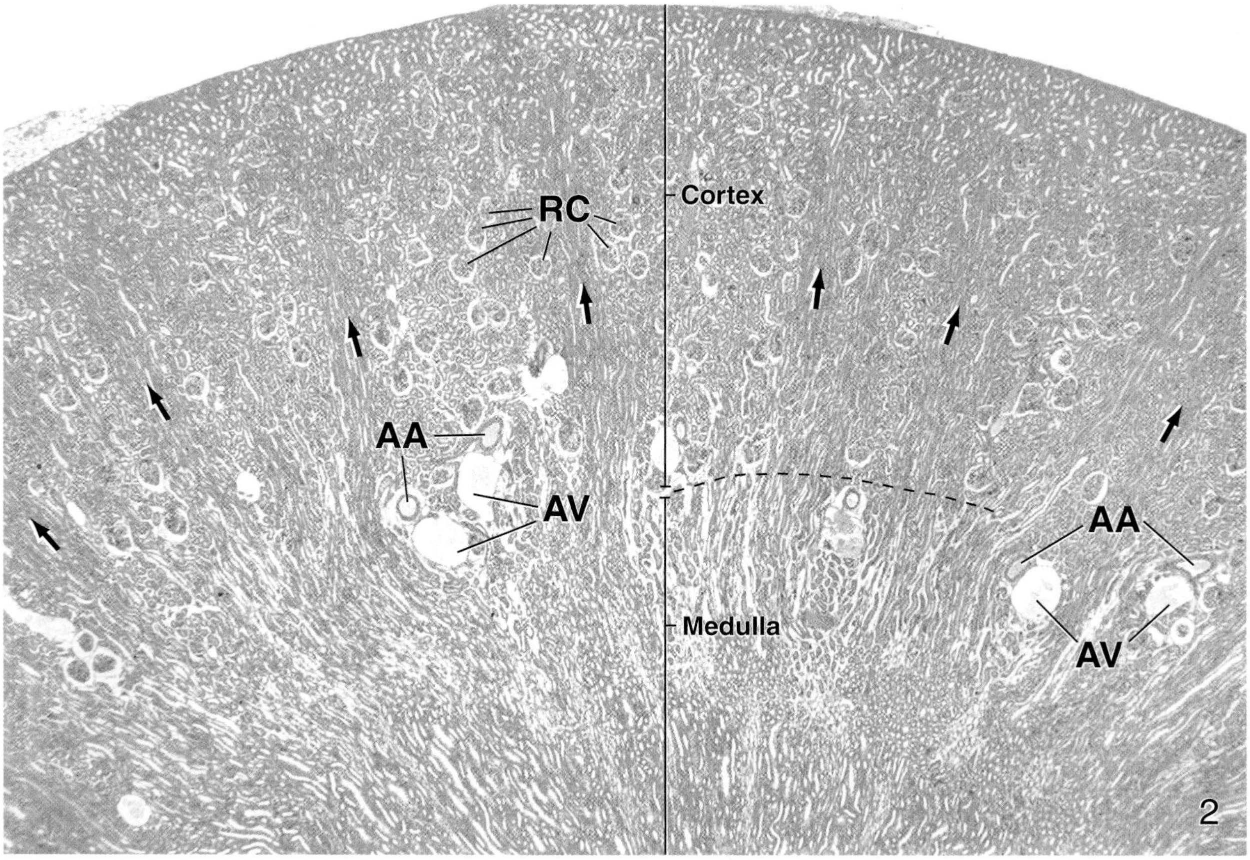
Cortex
RC
AA
AV
AA
AV
Medulla
2

PLATE 71. KIDNEY II

The *nephron* is the functional unit of the kidney. There are about 2 million nephrons in each human kidney. They are responsible for the production of urine and correspond to the secretory part of other glands. The *collecting tubules,* responsible for the final concentration of the urine, are analogous to the ducts of exocrine glands. The nephron is made up of the *renal corpuscle* and the *renal tubule.* The renal corpuscle consists of the *glomerulus,* a tuft of 10 to 20 capillary loops, surrounded by a double-layered epithelial cup, the *renal* or *Bowman's capsule.* The glomerular capillaries are supplied at the *vascular pole* of Bowman's capsule by an *afferent arteriole* and drained by an *efferent arteriole* that leaves Bowman's capsule at the vascular pole and then branches to form a new capillary network to supply the kidney tubules. The opposite pole of Bowman's capsule, the urinary pole, is where the filtrate leaves the renal capsule. The tubular parts of the nephron are the *proximal thick segment* (consisting of the *proximal convoluted tubule* and the *proximal straight tubule*), the *thin segment,* which constitutes the *thin limb of the loop of Henle,* and the *distal thick segment,* consisting of the *distal straight tubule* and the *distal convoluted tubule.* The loop of Henle is the U-shaped portion of the nephron consisting of the thick straight portions of the proximal and distal tubules and the thin segment between them. The distal convoluted tubule joins the *collecting tubule.* The nephron and the collecting tubule constitute the *uriniferous tubule.*

Figure 1, kidney, human, H&E ×60.

The renal cortex can be divided into regions referred to as the cortical labyrinth *(CL)* and the medullary rays *(MR).* The cortical labyrinth contains the renal corpuscles *(RC),* which appear as relatively large spherical structures. Surrounding each renal corpuscle are the proximal and distal convoluted tubules. They are also part of the cortical labyrinth. The convoluted tubules, particularly the proximal, because of their tortuosity, present a variety of profiles, most of which are oval or circular; others, more elongate, are in the shape of a J, a C, or even an S. The medullary rays are composed of groups of straight tubules oriented in the same direction and appear to radiate from the base of the pyramid. When the medullary rays are cut longitudinally, as they are in this figure, the tubules present elongated profiles. The medullary rays contain proximal thick segments (descending limb of Henle's loop), distal thick segments (ascending limbs of Henle's loop), and collecting tubules.

Figure 2, kidney, human, H&E ×120.

This figure presents another profile of the renal cortex, at a somewhat higher magnification, cut in a plane at a right angle to the section in Figure 1. The peripheral part of the micrograph shows the cortical labyrinth in which the tubules display chiefly round and oval profiles but also some that are more elongate and curved. The appearance is the same as the cortical labyrinth areas of Figure 1. A renal corpuscle *(RC)* is also present in the cortical labyrinth. In contrast, the profiles presented by the tubules of the medullary ray in this figure are quite different from those seen in Figure 1. All of the tubules bounded by the *dashed line* belong to the medullary ray *(MR),* and all are cut in cross section.

A general survey of the tubules within the medullary ray reveals that several distinct types can be recognized on the basis of the size of the tubule, shape of the lumen, and size of the tubule cells. These features as well as those of the cortical labyrinth are considered in Plate 72.

KEY

CL, cortical labyrinth
MR, medullary ray
RC, renal corpuscle
dashed line, approximate boundary of the medullary ray

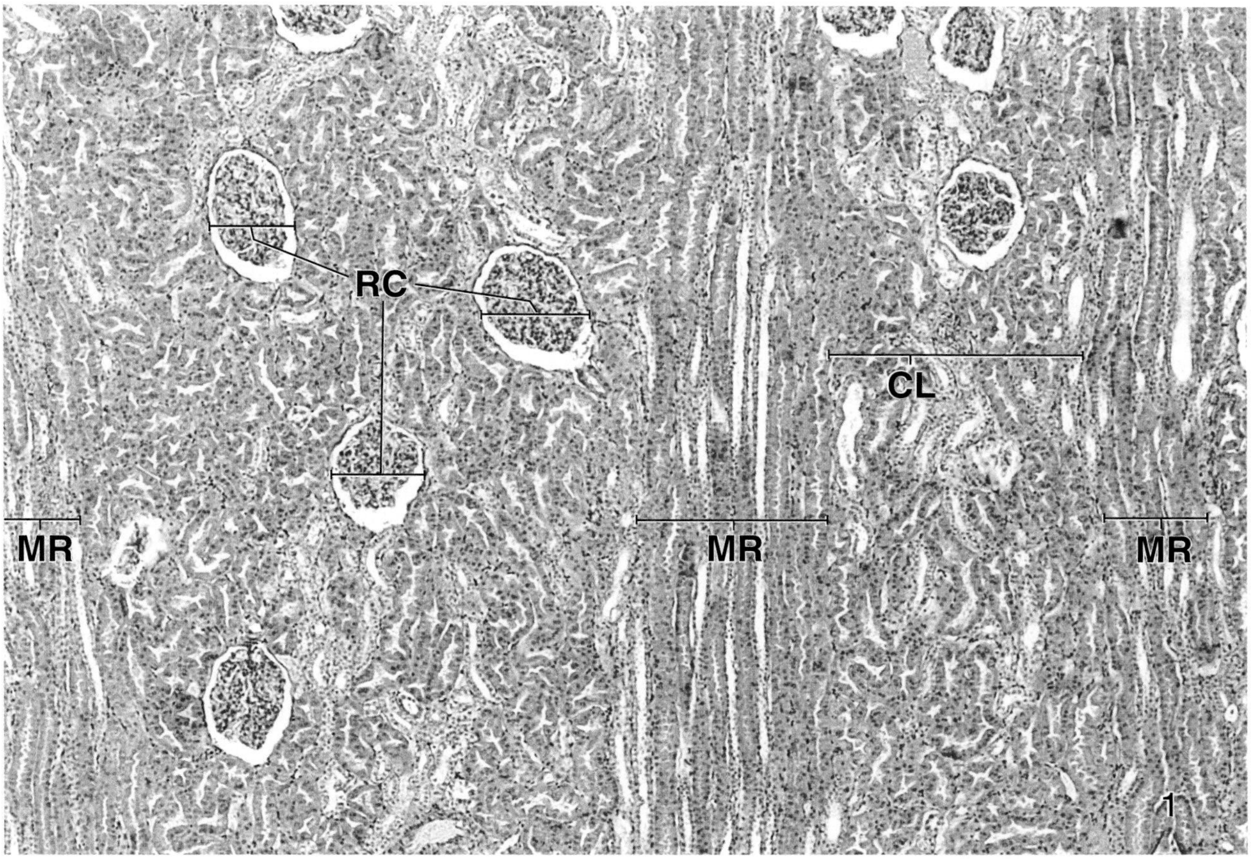
RC
CL
MR
MR
MR
1

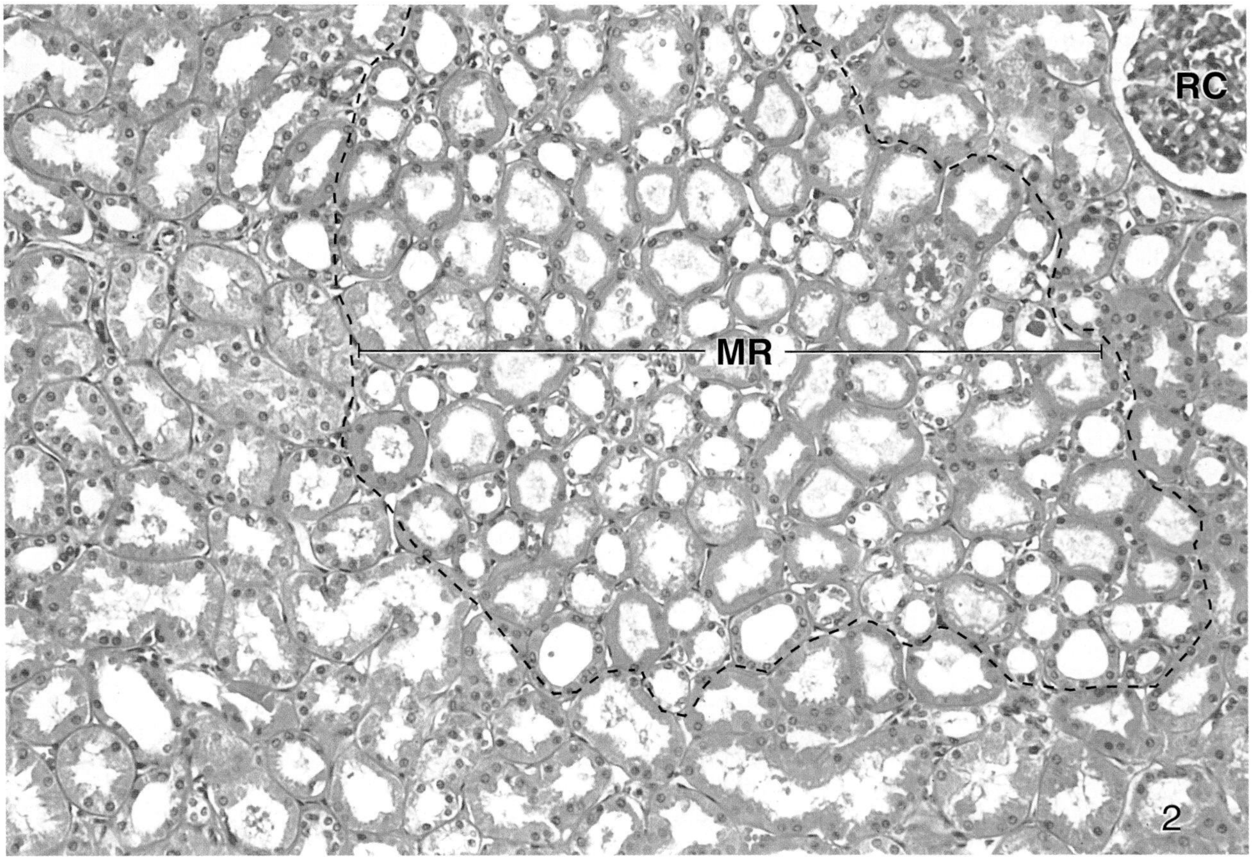
RC
MR
2

PLATE 72. KIDNEY III

Proximal and distal convoluted tubules display features that aid in their identification in H&E–stained paraffin sections. Proximal tubules generally have a larger diameter than distal tubules have; cross sections of the lumen often appear stellate. A brush border (apical microvilli) is often visible on the proximal tubule cells. Also, the proximal convoluted tubule is more than twice as long as the distal convoluted tubule; thus, the majority of tubular profiles in the cortical labyrinth will be of proximal tubules.

Mesangial cells and their extracellular matrix constitute the *mesangium* of the renal corpuscle. They underlie the endothelium of the capillaries of the *glomerular tuft* and extend to the vascular pole, where they become part of the *juxtaglomerular apparatus.* The terminal portion of the distal thick segment of the nephron lies close to the afferent arteriole. Tubule epithelial cells closest to the arteriole are thinner, taller, and more closely packed than other tubule cells and constitute the *macula densa.* Arterial smooth muscle cells opposite the macula densa are modified into *juxtaglomerular cells* that secrete *renin* in response to decreased blood NaCl concentration.

Figure 1, kidney, human, H&E ×240.

In this figure, an area of cortical labyrinth, there are six distal convoluted *(DC)* tubule profiles. The proximal tubules (unlabeled) have a slightly larger outside diameter than the distal tubules have. The proximal tubules have a brush border, whereas the distal tubules have a cleaner, sharper luminal surface. The lumen of the proximal tubules is often star shaped; this is not the case with distal tubules. Typically, fewer nuclei appear in a cross section of a proximal tubule than in an equivalent segment of a distal tubule.

Most of the above points can also be utilized in distinguishing the straight portions of the proximal and distal thick segments in the medullary rays, as shown in Figure 2.

Figure 2, kidney, human, H&E ×240.

In this figure, all of the tubular profiles are rounded except for a proximal convoluted tubule *(PC)* included in the lower right corner of the figure (it belongs to the adjacent cortical labyrinth). Second, the number of proximal *(P)* and distal *(D)* tubular profiles are about equal in the medullary ray, as is shown by the labeling of each tubule in this figure. Note that, in contrast to the distal tubules, the proximal tubules display a brush border and have a larger outside diameter, with many displaying a star-shaped lumen. The medullary ray also contains collecting tubules *(CT).* They are considered in Plate 73.

Figures 3 and 4, kidney, human, H&E ×360.

The renal corpuscle appears as a spherical structure whose periphery is composed of a thin capsule that encloses a narrow clear-appearing space, the urinary space *(asterisks),* and a capillary tuft or glomerulus that appears as a large cellular mass. The capsule of the renal corpuscle, known as the renal or Bowman's capsule, actually has two parts: a parietal layer, which is marked *(BC),* and a visceral layer. The parietal layer consists of simple squamous epithelial cells. The visceral layer consists of cells, called podocytes *(Pod),* that lie on the outer surface of the glomerular capillary. Except where they clearly line the urinary space, as the labeled cells do in Figure 3, podocytes may be difficult to distinguish from the capillary endothelial cells. To complicate matters, the mesangial cells are also a component of the glomerulus. In general, nuclei of podocytes are larger and stain less intensely than do the endothelial and mesangial cell nuclei.

A distal *(DC)* and two proximal *(PC)* convoluted tubules are marked in Figure 3. The cells of the distal tubule are more crowded on one side. These crowded cells constitute the macula densa *(MD)* that lies adjacent to the afferent arteriole.

In Figure 4, both the vascular pole and the urinary pole of the renal corpuscle are evident. The vascular pole is characterized by the presence of arterioles *(A),* one of which is entering or leaving *(double-headed arrow)* the corpuscle. The afferent arteriole possesses modified smooth muscle cells with granules, the juxtaglomerular cells (not evident in Fig. 4). At the urinary pole, the parietal layer of Bowman's capsule is continuous with the beginning of the proximal convoluted tubule *(PC).* Here, the urinary space of the renal corpuscle continues into the lumen of the proximal tubule, and the lining cells change from simple squamous to simple cuboidal or low columnar with a brush border.

KEY

A, arteriole
BC, Bowman's capsule (parietal layer)
CT, collecting tubule
D, distal thick segment (straight portion)
DC, distal convoluted tubule
MD, macula densa
P, proximal thick segment (straight portion)
PC, proximal convoluted tubule
Pod, podocyte (visceral layer of Bowman's capsule)
asterisks, urinary space
double-headed arrow (Fig. 4), blood vessel at vascular pole of renal corpuscle

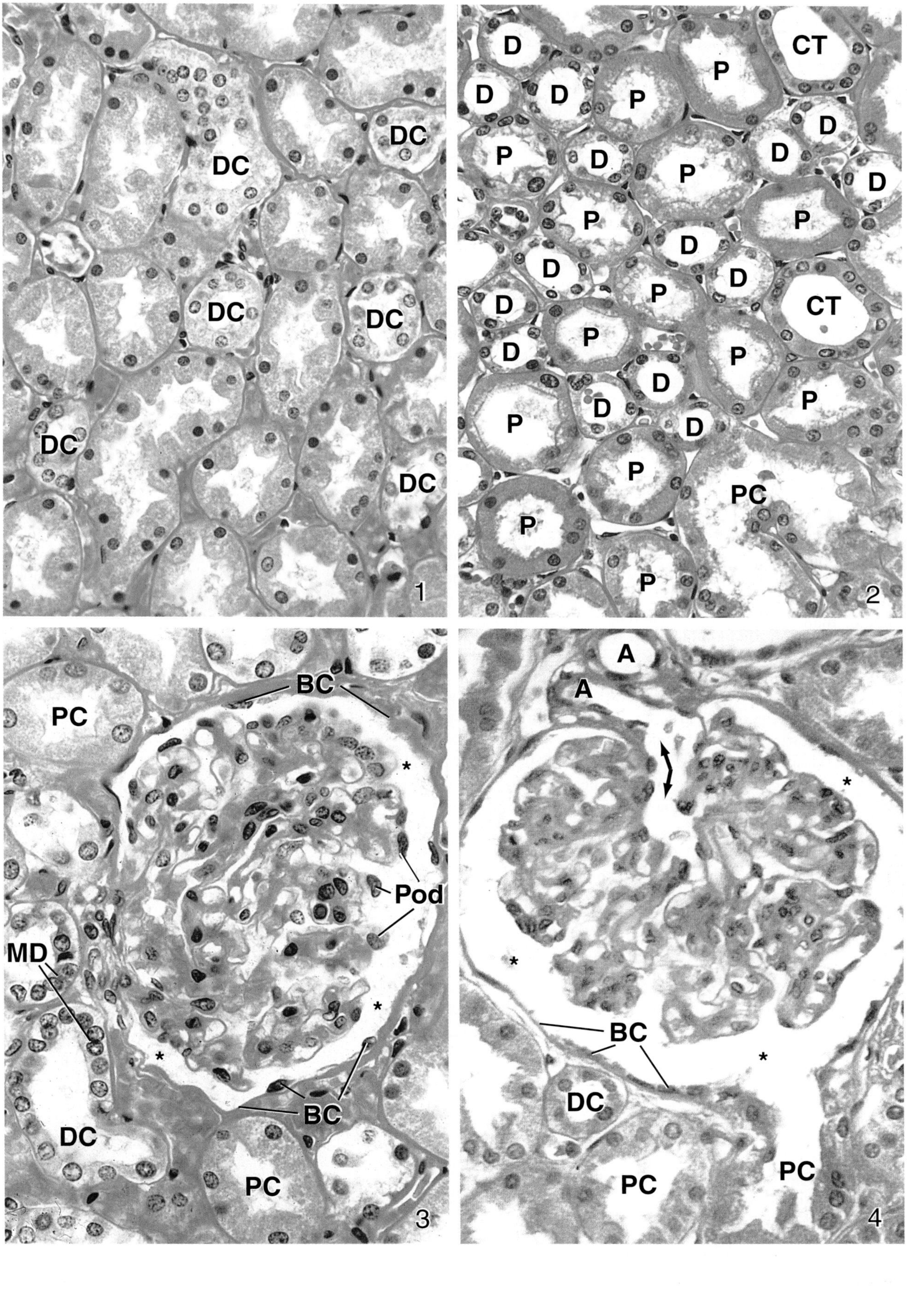
DC
DC
DC
DC
DC
DC
1
D
P
CT
D
D
P
D
P
D
D
P
D
P
D
P
D
D
P
D
CT
D
D
P
D
P
D
P
D
D
P
P
PC
P
P
2
BC
PC
Pod
MD
BC
DC
PC
3
A
A
BC
DC
PC
PC
4

PLATE 73. KIDNEY IV

Renal corpuscles are restricted to the cortical labyrinth. The medulla contains the thick straight segments of proximal and distal tubules, along with their thin segments, the collecting tubules and ducts, and the blood vessels that run in parallel with them. These structures function as the *countercurrent multiplier* and *countercurrent exchange* systems that, ultimately, produce hypertonic urine. The final urine drains from the papillary ducts (of Bellini) into calyces that then empty into the renal pelvis.

Figure 1, kidney, human, H&E ×240.

A section through the outer portion of the medulla is shown in this figure. This region contains proximal and distal thick segments, thin segments, and collecting tubules. All of the tubules are parallel, and all are cut in cross section; thus, they present circular profiles. The proximal *(P)* thick segments display typical star-shaped lumina and a brush border (or the fragmented apical cell surface from which the brush border has been partially broken). These tubules have outside diameters that are generally larger than those of the distal tubules *(D)*. As mentioned previously and as shown here, the distal tubules display a larger number of nuclei than do comparable segments of proximal tubule cells. Note, also, that the lumen of the distal tubule is more rounded and the apical surface of the cells is sharper. The collecting tubules *(CT)* have outer diameters that are about the same as those of the proximal tubules and larger than those of distal tubules. The cells forming the collecting tubules are cuboidal and smaller than those of proximal tubules; thus, they also display a relatively larger number of nuclei than do comparable segments of proximal tubule cells. Count them! Finally, boundaries between the cells that constitute the collecting tubules are usually evident *(asterisks)*; this serves as one of the most dependable features for the identification of collecting tubules.

The thin segments *(T)* have the thinnest walls of all renal tubules seen in the medulla. They are formed by a low cuboidal or simple squamous epithelium, as seen here, and the lumina are relatively large. Occasionally, a section includes the region of transition from a thick to a thin segment and can be recognized even in a cross section through the tubule. One such junction is evident in this figure (the tubule with *two arrows* in the lumen). On one side, the tubule cell *(left-pointing arrow)* is characteristic of the proximal segment; it possesses a distinctive brush border. The other side of the tubule *(right-pointing arrow)* is composed of low cuboidal cells that resemble the cells forming the thin segments. In addition to the renal and collecting tubules, there are many other small tubular structures in this figure. Thin-walled and lined by endothelium, they are small blood vessels.

Figure 2, kidney, human, H&E ×20.

This figure shows a renal pyramid at low magnification. The pyramid is a conical structure composed principally of medullary straight tubules, ducts, and the straight blood vessels (vasa recta). The *dashed line* at the left of the micrograph is placed at the junction between cortex and medulla; thus, it marks the base of the pyramid. Note the arcuate vessels *(AV)* that lie at the boundary of cortex and medulla. They define the boundary line. The few renal corpuscles *(RC)*, upper left, belong to the medulla. They are referred to as juxtamedullary corpuscles.

The pyramid is somewhat distorted in this specimen, as evidenced by regions of longitudinally sectioned tubules, lower left, and cross-sectioned and obliquely sectioned tubules in other regions. In effect, part of the pyramid was bent, thus the change in the plane of section of the tubules.

The apical portion of the pyramid *(arrowhead)*, known as the renal papilla, is lodged in a cup- or funnel-like structure referred to as the calyx. It collects the urine that leaves the tip of the papilla from the papillary ducts (of Bellini). (The actual tip of the papilla is not seen within the plane of section, nor are the openings of the ducts at this low magnification.) The surface of the papilla that faces the lumen of the calyx is simple columnar or cuboidal epithelium *(SCEp)*. (In places, this epithelium has separated from the surface of the papilla and appears as a thin strand of tissue.) The calyx is lined by transitional epithelium *(TEp)*. Although not evident at the low magnification shown here, the boundary between the columnar epithelium covering the papilla and the transitional epithelium covering the inner surface of the calyx is marked by the *diamonds*.

KEY

AV, arc ate vessels
CT ting tubules
ck segment
hick segment
uscle
olumnar epithelium

T, thin segment
TEp, transitional epithelium
arrowhead, location of apex of pyramid
asterisks, boundaries between cells of a collecting tubule

diamonds, boundary between a transitional and a columnar epithelium
left-pointing arrow (Fig. 1), proximal tubule cell
right-pointing arrow (Fig. 1), thin segment cell

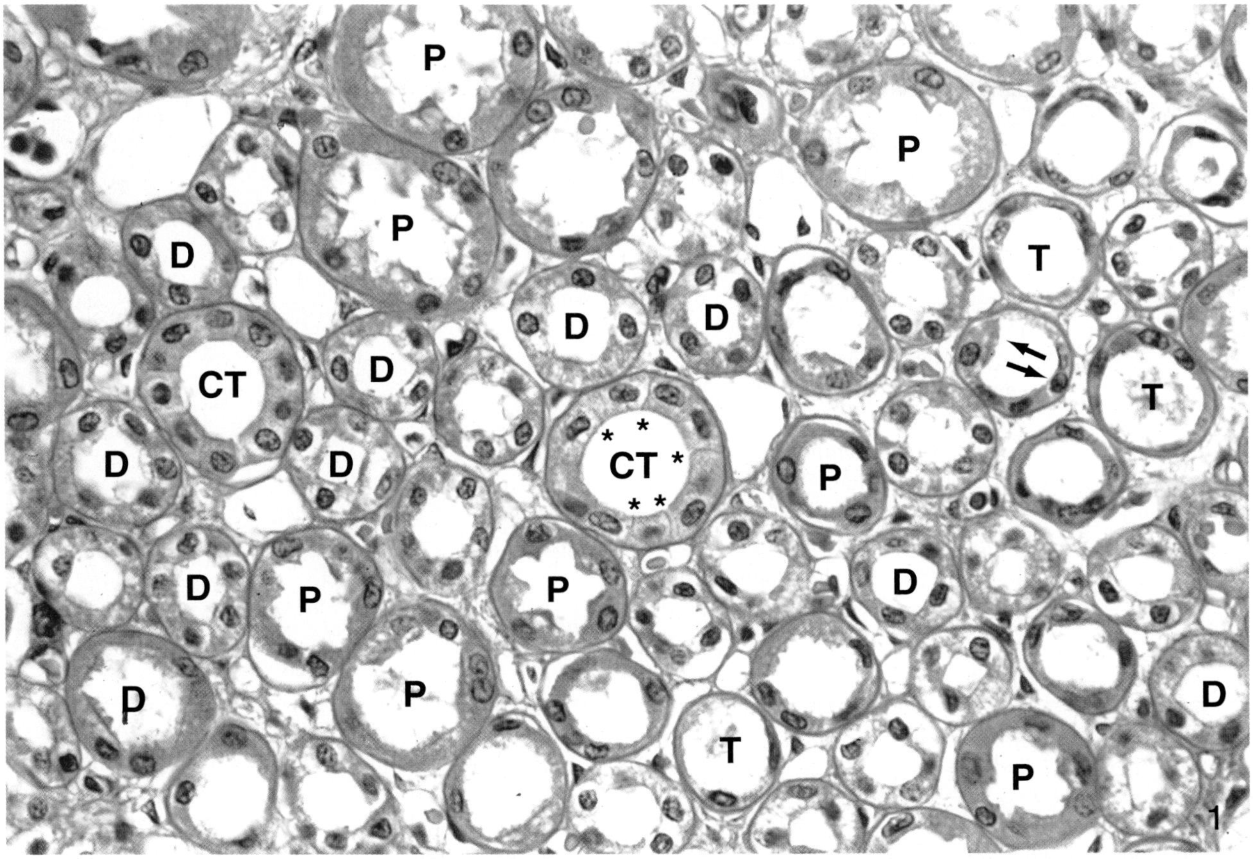
P
P
P
D
T
D
D
CT
D
T
D
CT
D
P
D
P
P
D
P
D
T
P
1

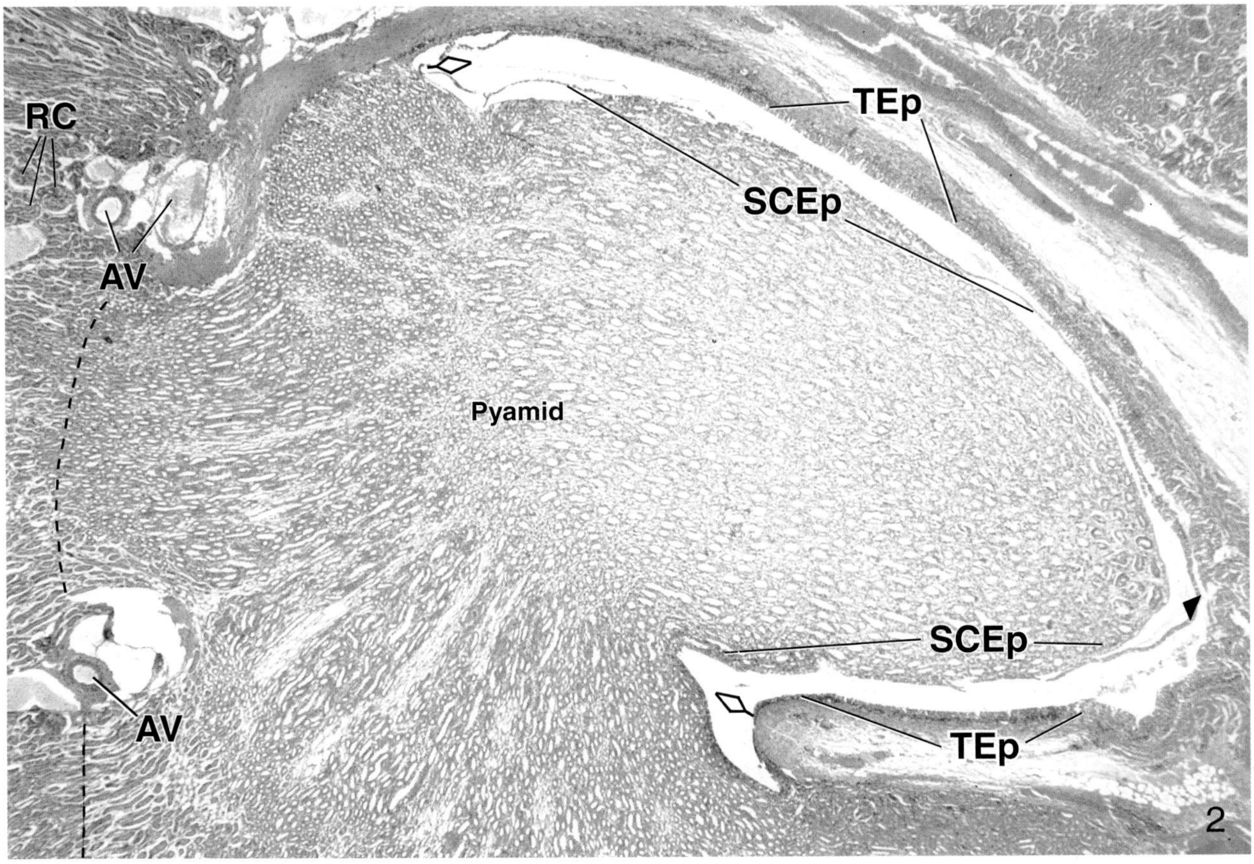
RC
TEp
SCEp
AV
Pyamid
SCEp
AV
TEp
2

PLATE 74. URETER

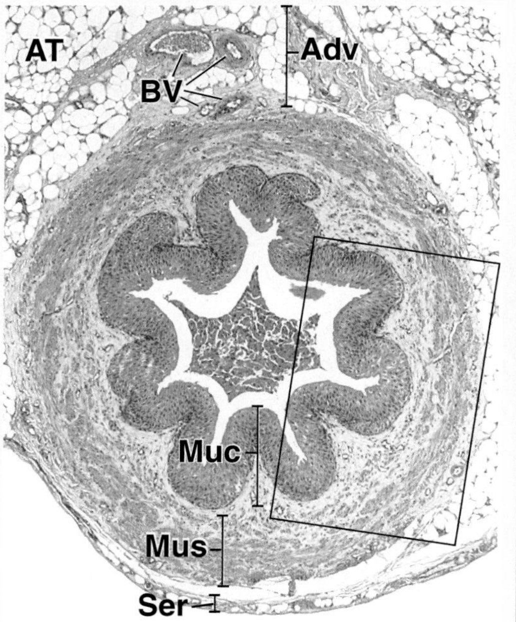

The ureters are paired tubular structures that convey urine from the kidneys to the urinary bladder. They are lined with *transitional epithelium,* an impervious layer that lines the urinary excretory passages from the renal calyces through the urethra. The ability of this epithelium to become thinner and flatter allows all of these passages to accommodate to distension by the urine.

The epithelium rests on a dense collagenous lamina propria, which in turn, rests on an inner longitudinal and an outer circular layer of smooth muscle. Regular peristaltic contractions of this muscle contribute to the flow of urine from the kidney to the urinary bladder.

As shown in this low-power orientation micrograph, the wall of the ureter consists of a mucosa *(Muc),* a muscularis *(Mus),* and an adventitia *(Adv).* Note that the ureters are located behind the peritoneum of the abdominal cavity in their course to the bladder. Thus, a serosa *(Ser)* may be found covering a portion of the circumference of the tube. Also, because of contraction of the smooth muscle of the muscularis, the luminal surface is characteristically folded, thus creating a star-shaped lumen.

Figure 1, ureter, monkey, H&E ×160.

The wall of the ureter from the *rectangular area* in the orientation micrograph is examined at higher magnification in this figure. One can immediately recognize the thick epithelial lining, which appears distinct and sharply delineated from the remainder of the wall. This is the transitional epithelium *(Ep).* The remainder of the wall is made up of connective tissue *(CT)* and smooth muscle. The latter can be recognized as the darker-staining layer. The section also shows some adipose tissue *(AT),* a component of the adventitia.

The transitional epithelium and its supporting connective tissue constitute the mucosa *(Muc).* A distinct submucosa is not present, although the term is sometimes applied to the connective tissue that is closest to the muscle.

The muscularis *(Mus)* is arranged as an inner longitudinal layer *(SM(l)),* a middle circular layer *(SM(c)),* and an outer longitudinal layer *(SM(l)).* However, the outer longitudinal layer is present only at the lower end of the ureter. In a cross section through the ureter, the inner and outer smooth muscle layers are cut in cross section, whereas the middle circular layer of the muscle cells is cut longitudinally. This is as they appear in this figure.

Figure 2, ureter, monkey, H&E ×400.

This figure shows the inner longitudinal smooth muscle layer *(SM(l))* at higher magnification. Note that the nuclei appear as round profiles, indicating that the muscle cells have been cross-sectioned. This figure also shows the transitional epithelium to advantage. The surface cells are characteristically the largest, and some are binucleate *(arrow).* The basal cells are the smallest, and typically, the nuclei appear crowded because of the minimal cytoplasm of each cell. The intermediate cells appear to consist of several layers and are composed of cells larger in size than the basal cells but smaller than the surface cells.

KEY

Adv, adventitia
AT, adipose tissue
BV, blood vessels
CT, connective tissue
Ep, transitional epithelium
Muc, mucosa
Mus, muscularis
Ser, serosa
SM(c), circular layer of smooth muscle
SM(l), longitudinal layer of smooth muscle
arrow (Fig. 2), binucleate surface cell

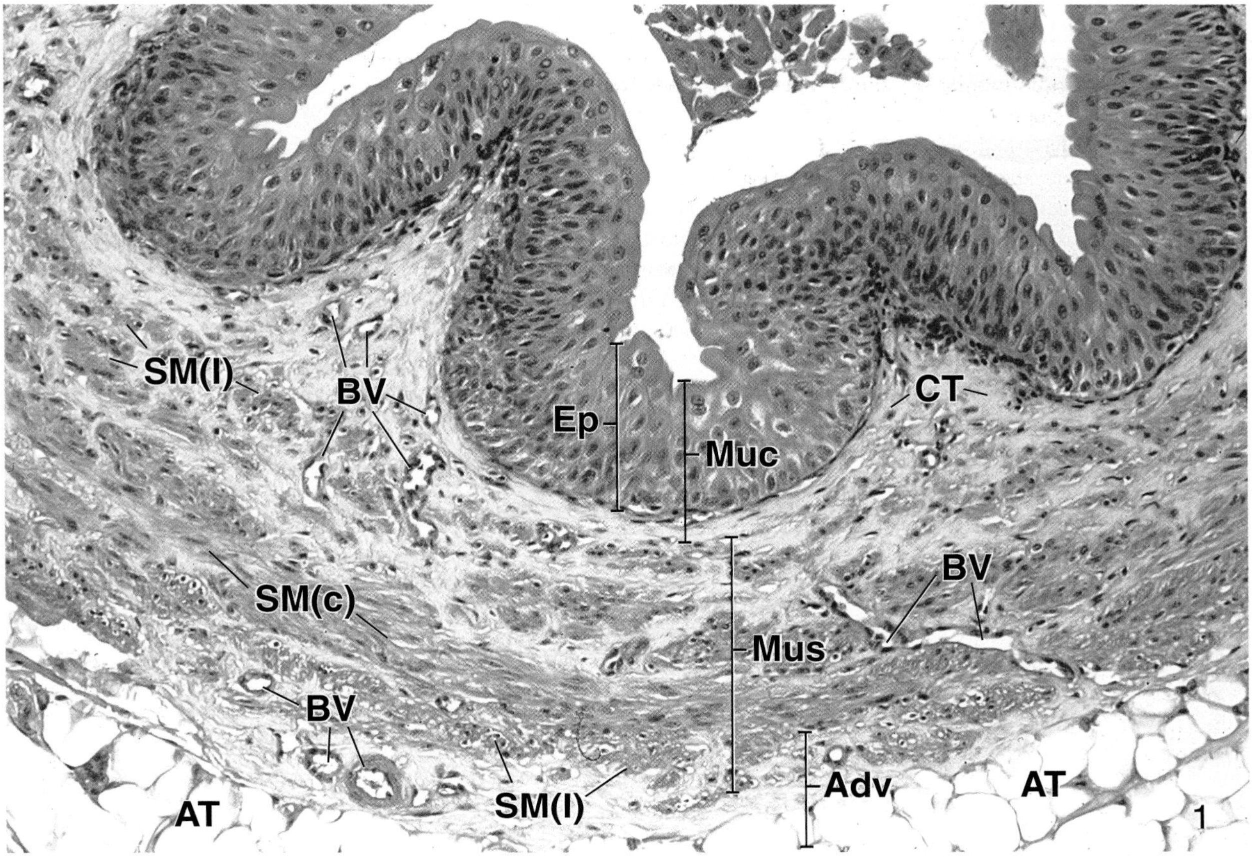
SM(l)
BV
Ep
Muc
CT
SM(c)
BV
Mus
BV
AT
SM(l)
Adv
AT
1

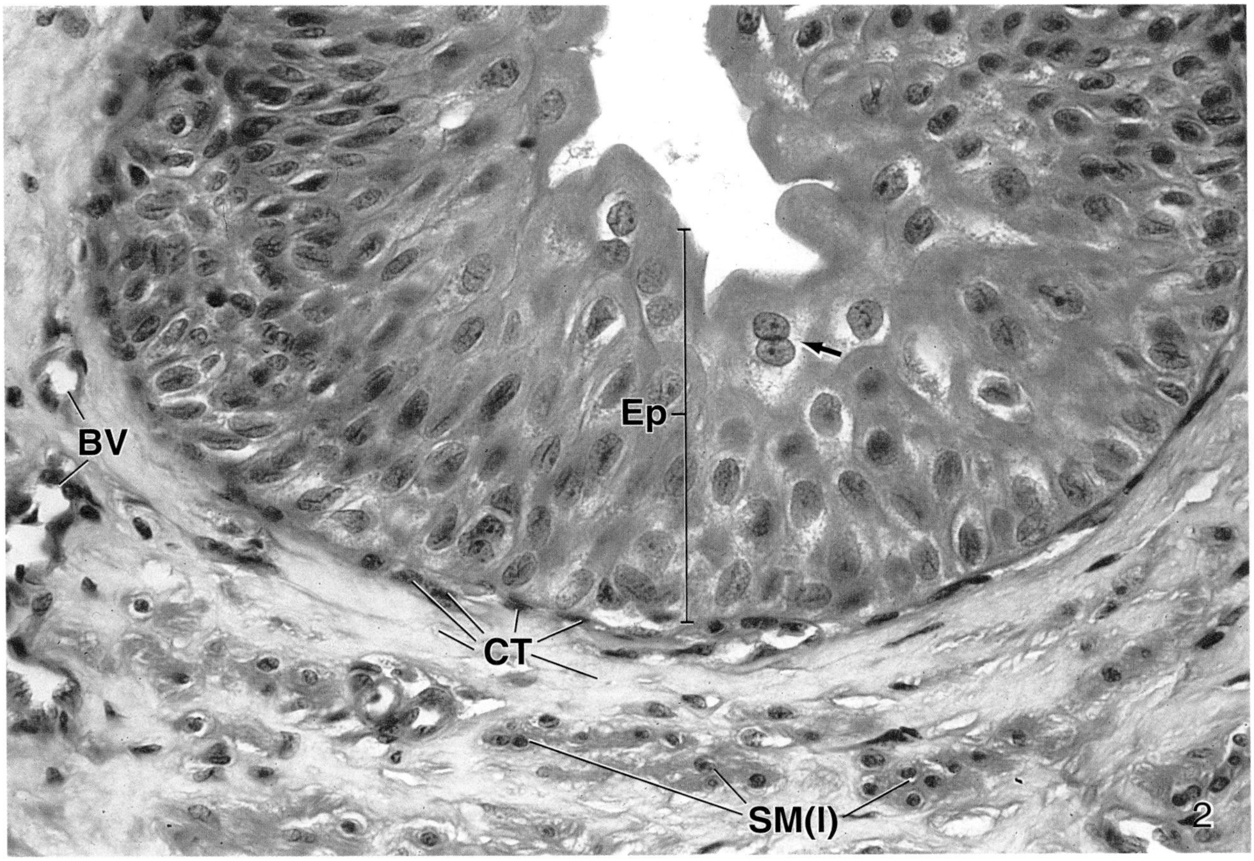
Ep
BV
CT
SM(l)
2

PLATE 75. URINARY BLADDER

The urinary bladder receives the urine from the two ureters and stores it until neural stimulation causes it to contract and expel the urine via the urethra. It, too, is lined with transitional epithelium. Beneath the epithelium and its underlying connective tissue, the wall of the urinary bladder contains smooth muscle that is usually described as being arranged as an inner longitudinal layer, a middle circular layer, and an outer longitudinal layer. As in most distensible hollow viscera that empty their contents through a narrow aperture, the smooth muscle in the wall of the urinary bladder is less regularly arranged than the description indicates, allowing contraction to reduce the volume relatively evenly throughout the bladder.

This orientation micrograph of the urinary bladder reveals the full thickness of the bladder wall. The luminal surface epithelium is at the top of the micrograph. One of the ureters can be seen as it passes through the bladder wall to empty its contents into the bladder lumen. Most of the tissue to the sides and below the ureteral profile is smooth muscle.

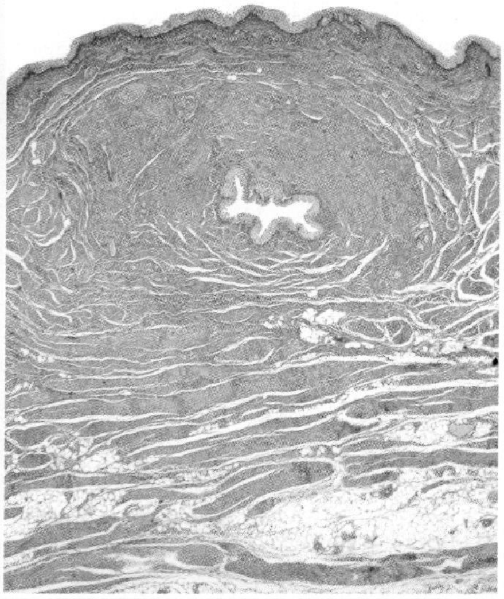

Figure 1, urinary bladder, human, H&E ×60.
This micrograph shows most of the entire thickness of the urinary bladder. An unusual feature is the presence of one of the ureters (*U*) as it is passing through the bladder wall to empty its contents into the bladder lumen. The transitional epithelium (*Ep*) lining the bladder is seen on the right. Beneath the epithelium is a relatively thick layer of connective tissue (*CT*) containing blood vessels (*BV*) of various sizes. Note that the connective tissue stains somewhat denser than the smooth muscle of the underlying muscularis (*M*). The epithelium and connective tissue constitute the mucosa of the bladder. The muscularis consists of smooth muscle arranged in three indistinct layers. It should be noted that as the ureter passes through the bladder wall, it carries with it a layer of longitudinally oriented smooth muscle (*SM(L)*). Medium-size arteries (*A*) and veins (*V*) are occasionally seen in the muscularis.

Figure 2, urinary bladder, human, H&E ×250.
This higher magnification of the *left rectangle* of Figure 1 shows the transitional epithelium (*Ep*) and the underlying connective tissue (*CT*) that represent the mucosa of the ureter. Adjacent to the mucosa are bundles of longitudinally sectioned smooth muscle (*SM(L)*) that belong to the ureter. A small lymphatic vessel (*Lym*) is present in the connective tissue adjacent to the smooth muscle. Note the lymphocytes, identified by their small round densely stained nuclei, within the lumen of the vessel.

Figure 3, urinary bladder, human, H&E ×250.
This higher magnification of the *right rectangle* of Figure 1 shows the bladder epithelium (*Ep*) and the underlying connective tissue (*CT*) of the bladder wall. The transitional epithelium is often characterized by the presence of surface cells that exhibit a "dome" shape. In addition, many of these cells are binucleate (*arrows*). The thickness of transitional epithelium is variable. When the bladder is fully distended, as few as three cell layers are seen. Here, in the contracted bladder, it appears that there are as many as ten cell layers, a result of the cells folding over one another as the smooth muscle contracts and the lining surface is reduced. The connective tissue consists of bundles of collagen fibers interspersed with varying numbers of lymphocytes identified by their densely stained round nuclei. A vein (*V*) filled with red blood cells is also evident in the mucosal connective tissue.

KEY

A, artery
BV, blood vessel
CT, connective tissue
Ep, transitional epithelium
Lym, lymphatic vessel
M, muscularis
SM(L), longitudinally cut smooth muscle
U, ureter
V, vein
arrows, binucleate cells

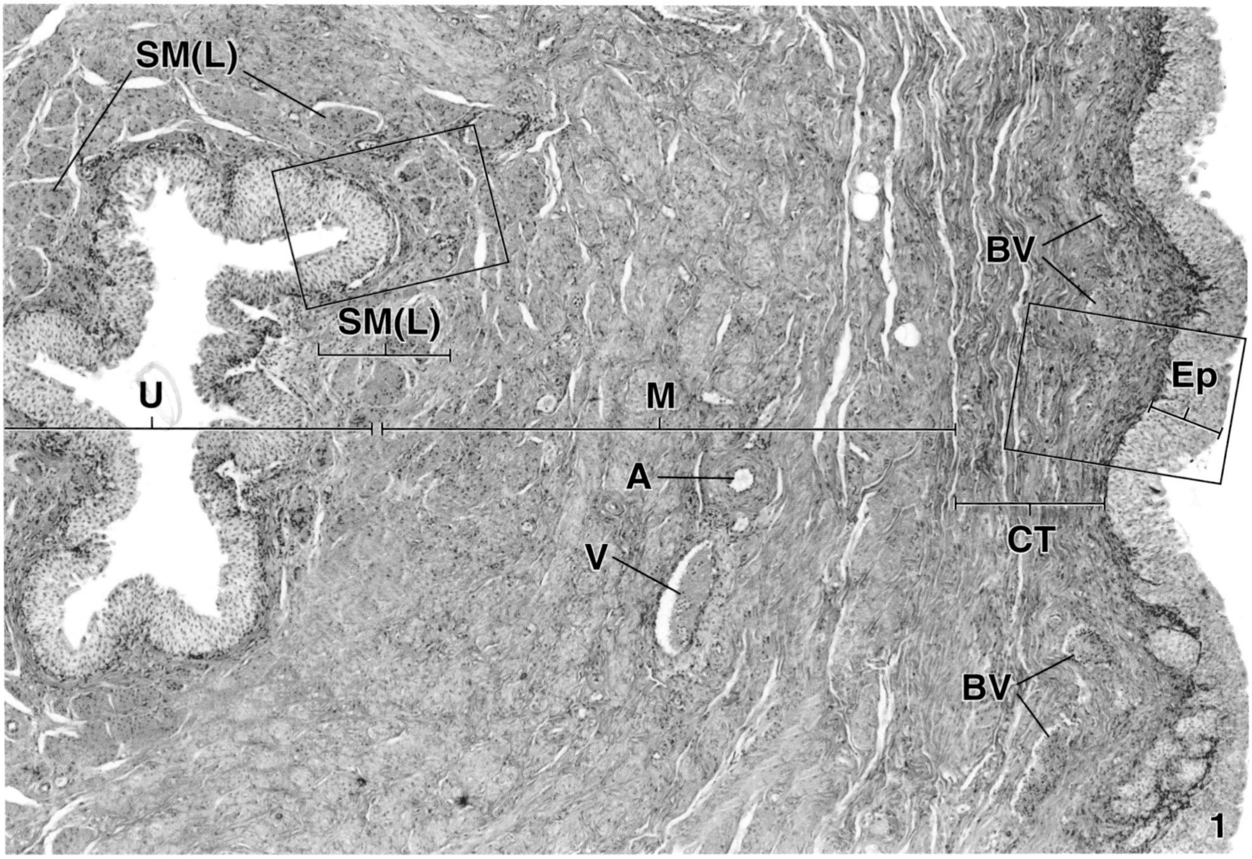
SM(L)
SM(L)
U
M
A
V
BV
Ep
CT
BV
1

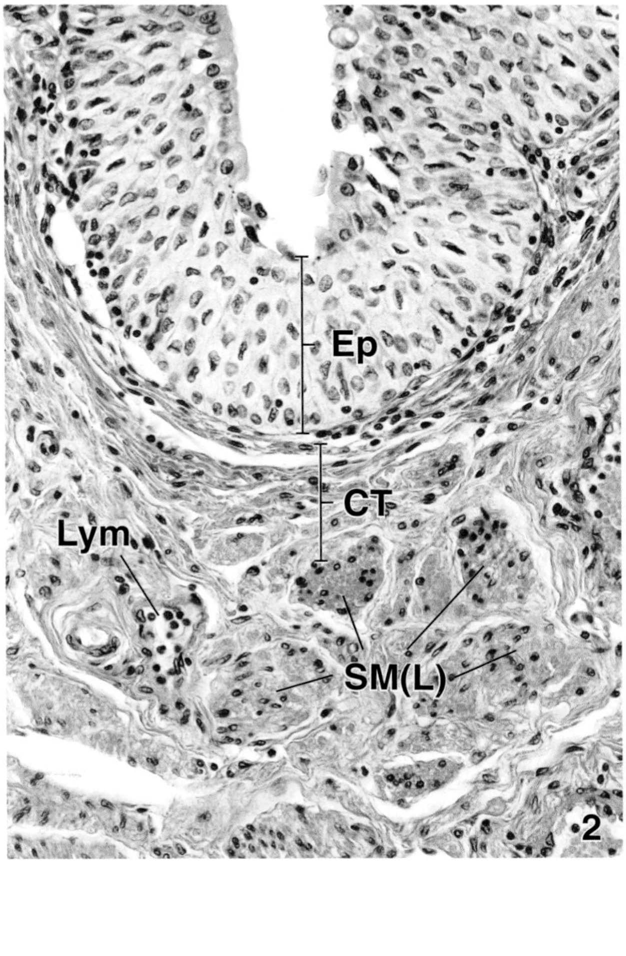
Ep
CT
Lym
SM(L)
2

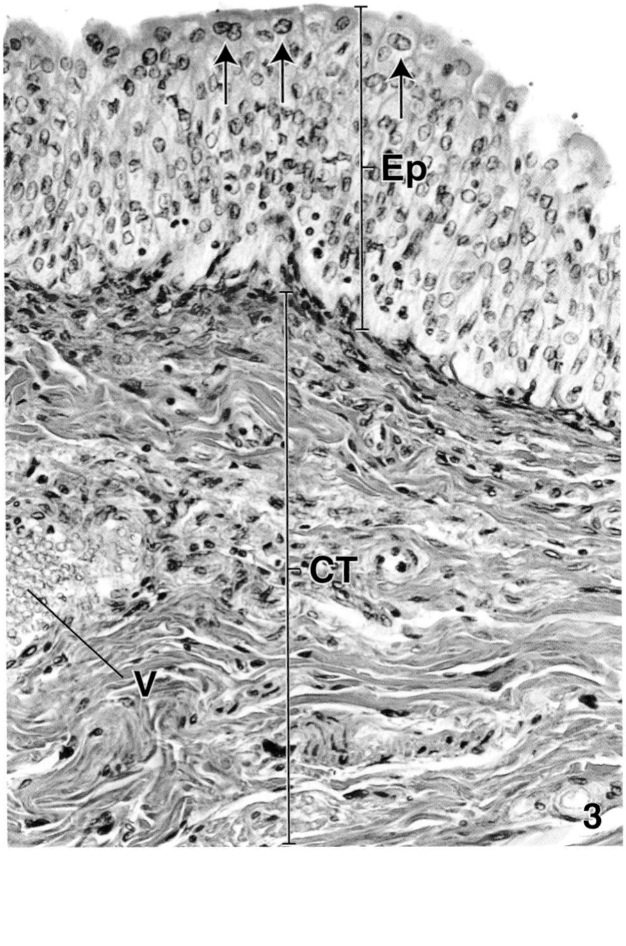
Ep
CT
V
3

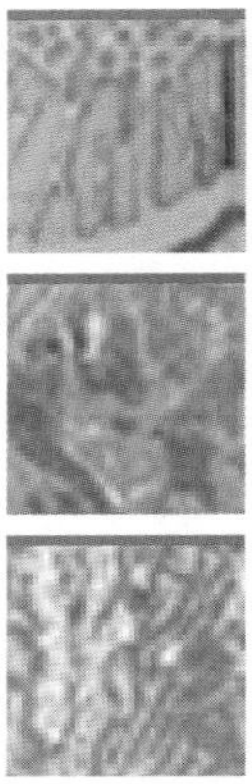

20

Endocrine Organs

▼ OVERVIEW OF THE ENDOCRINE SYSTEM

The ***endocrine system*** produces various secretions called ***hormones*** *[Gr. hormaein, to excite]* that serve as effectors to regulate the activities of various cells, tissues, and organs in the body. Its functions are essential in maintaining homeostasis and coordinating body growth and development. The function of the endocrine system is similar to that of the nervous system; both communicate information to peripheral cells and organs. Communication in the nervous system is through transmission of neural impulses along nerve cell processes and the discharge of neurotransmitter. Communication in the endocrine system is through

hormones, which are carried to their destination via connective tissue spaces and the vascular system. These two systems are functionally interrelated. The endocrine system produces a slower and more prolonged response than the nervous system. Both systems may act simultaneously on the same target cells and tissues, and some nerve cells secrete hormones. The ***hypothalamus,*** a part of the brain, coordinates most endocrine functions of the body and serves as one of the major controlling centers of the autonomic nervous system.

In general, a hormone is described as a biologic substance acting on specific target cells

In the classic definition, a hormone is a secretory product of endocrine cells and organs that passes into the circulatory system (bloodstream) for transport to target cells. Recent research shows that a variety of hormones and hormonally active substances are not always discharged into the bloodstream but are released into connective tissue spaces where they may act on adjacent cells or diffuse to nearby target cells that express receptors specific for that particular hormone.

Hormones include three classes of compounds

Cells of the endocrine system release over 100 hormones and hormonally active substances that are chemically divided into three classes of compounds:

- ***Steroids,*** cholesterol-derived compounds, are synthesized and secreted by cells of the ovaries, testes, and adrenal cortex. These hormones are released into the bloodstream and transported to target cells with the help of plasma proteins or specialized carrier proteins such as ***androgen-binding protein.***
- ***Small peptides, proteins, and glycoproteins*** are synthesized and secreted by cells of the hypothalamus, pituitary gland, thyroid gland, parathyroid gland, pancreas, and scattered enteroendocrine cells of the gastrointestinal tract and respiratory system. Hormones in this group, when released into the circulation, dissolve readily in the blood and do not require special transport proteins.
- ***Amino acid analogues and derivatives,*** including the ***catecholamines*** (norepinephrine and epinephrine), are synthesized and secreted by many neurons as well as cells of the adrenal medulla. Also included in this group of compounds are ***thyroid hormones,*** the ***iodinated amino acids*** that are synthesized and secreted by the thyroid gland. When released into the circulation, catecholamines dissolve readily in the blood, in contrast to thyroid hormones, which bind to serum proteins and a specialized carrier protein, ***thyroxin-binding protein.***

Hormones interact with specific hormone receptors to alter biologic activity of the target cells

The first step in hormone action on a target cell is its binding to a specific hormone receptor. Two groups of hormone receptors have been identified:

- ***Cell surface receptors,*** which interact with peptide hormones or catecholamines that are unable to penetrate the cell membrane. Activation of these receptors as a result of hormone binding rapidly generates large quantities of small intracellular molecules called ***second messengers,*** such as ***cyclic adenosine monophosphate (cAMP), 1,2-diacylglycerol (DAG), inositol triphosphate*** (IP_3), and Ca^{2+}. Second messengers amplify the signal initiated by hormone–receptor interaction and are produced by activation of one of several second-messenger systems. Examples of such systems include the adenylate cyclase/cAMP system (for most protein hormones and catecholamines), the tyrosine kinase system (for insulin and epidermal growth factor [EGF]), the phosphatidylinositol system (for certain hormones and neurotransmitters), and activation of ion channels (as with most neurotransmitters). The second-messenger molecules produced in the cascade reactions of these systems alter the cell's metabolism and produce hormone-specific responses (Fig. 20.1).
- ***Intracellular receptors,*** which are localized within the cell (mainly within the nucleus), are used by steroids and thyroid hormones that can easily penetrate both plasma and nuclear membranes. Their receptors consist of large multiprotein complexes of chaperons containing three binding domains: a hormone-binding region, a DNA-binding region, and an amino-terminal region. Binding of the hormone to these receptors causes allosteric transformation of the receptor into a form that binds to chromosomal DNA and activates or inhibits RNA polymerase activity. Transcription of mRNA is either increased or decreased, leading to the production of new proteins that regulate cell metabolism. Therefore, hormones acting on intracellular receptors influence gene expression directly, without the help of a second messenger (see Fig. 20.1).

Hormone-secreting cells are present in many organs to regulate their activity

This chapter primarily describes the discrete endocrine glands that release their hormones for delivery to the bloodstream for transport to target cells and organs. In other chapters, the endocrine function of cells within the gonads, liver, kidney, and gastrointestinal system are discussed. The cells of the gastroenteropancreatic (GEP) system (see page 491) constitute the largest collection of endocrine cells in the body. In addition to their endocrine

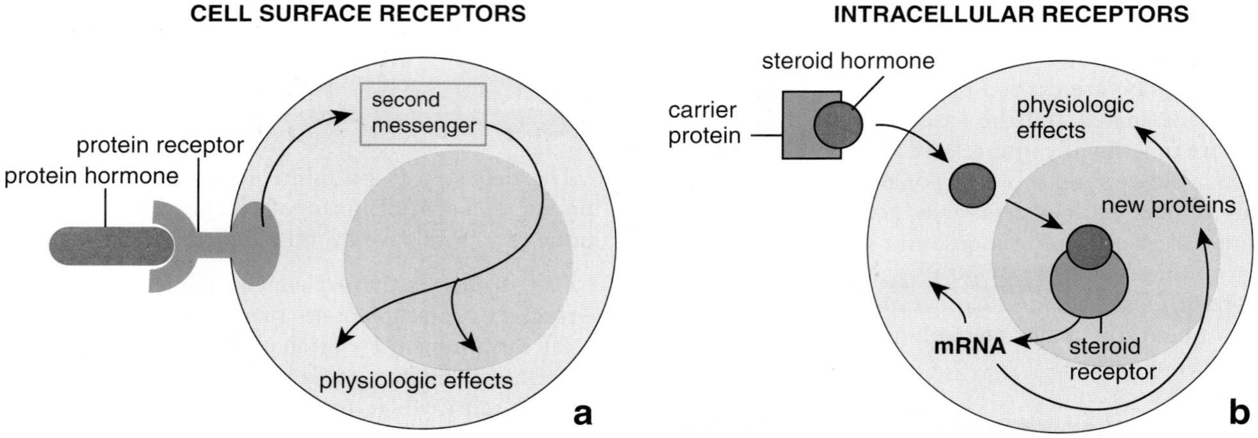

FIGURE 20.1
General mechanisms of hormone action. a. This schematic diagram shows the basis for protein hormone action involving cell surface receptors. Hormone molecules bind to the receptor and initiate synthesis of second-messenger molecules. These molecules, in turn, activate a cascade of reactions that produce hormone-specific responses in the stimulated cell. **b.** This diagram shows the mechanism of action of steroid hormones, which use intracellular receptors. Binding of the hormone to this receptor causes allosteric transformation of the receptor into a form that binds to DNA. This binding leads to mRNA transcription and production of new proteins that produce hormone-specific responses in the stimulated cell.

function, cells of the GEP system exercise ***paracrine*** control of the activity of adjacent epithelial cells by diffusion of peptide secretions through the extracellular spaces.

▽ PITUITARY GLAND (HYPOPHYSIS)

The ***pituitary gland*** and the hypothalamus, the portion of the brain to which the ***pituitary gland*** is attached, are morphologically and functionally linked in the endocrine and neuroendocrine control of other endocrine glands. Because they play central roles in a number of regulatory feedback systems, they are often called the "master organs" of the endocrine system.

Gross Structure and Development

The pituitary gland is composed of glandular epithelial tissue and neural (secretory) tissue

The ***pituitary gland*** is a pea-sized, compound endocrine gland that weighs 0.5 g in males and 1.5 g in multiparous females. It is centrally located at the base of the brain, where it lies in a saddle-shaped depression of the sphenoid bone called the ***sella turcica***. A short stalk, the ***infundibulum***, and a vascular network connect the pituitary gland to the hypothalamus.

The pituitary gland has two functional components (Fig. 20.2):

- ***Anterior lobe (adenohypophysis)***, the glandular epithelial tissue
- ***Posterior lobe (neurohypophysis)***, the neural secretory tissue

These two portions are of different embryologic origin. The anterior lobe of the pituitary gland is derived from an evagination of the ***ectoderm of the oropharynx*** toward the brain ***(Rathke's pouch)***. The posterior lobe of the pituitary gland is derived from a downgrowth (the future infundibulum) of ***neuroectoderm of the floor of the third ventricle*** (the diencephalon) of the developing brain (Fig. 20.3).

The anterior lobe of the pituitary gland consists of three derivatives of Rathke's pouch:

- ***Pars distalis***, which comprises the bulk of the anterior lobe of the pituitary gland and arises from the thickened anterior wall of the pouch
- ***Pars intermedia***, a thin remnant of the posterior wall of the pouch that abuts the pars distalis
- ***Pars tuberalis***, which develops from the thickened lateral walls of the pouch and forms a collar or sheath around the infundibulum

The embryonic infundibulum gives rise to the posterior lobe of the pituitary gland. The posterior lobe of the pituitary gland consists of

- ***Pars nervosa***, which contains neurosecretory axons and their endings
- ***Infundibulum***, which is continuous with the ***median eminence*** and contains the neurosecretory axons forming the ***hypothalamohypophyseal tracts***.

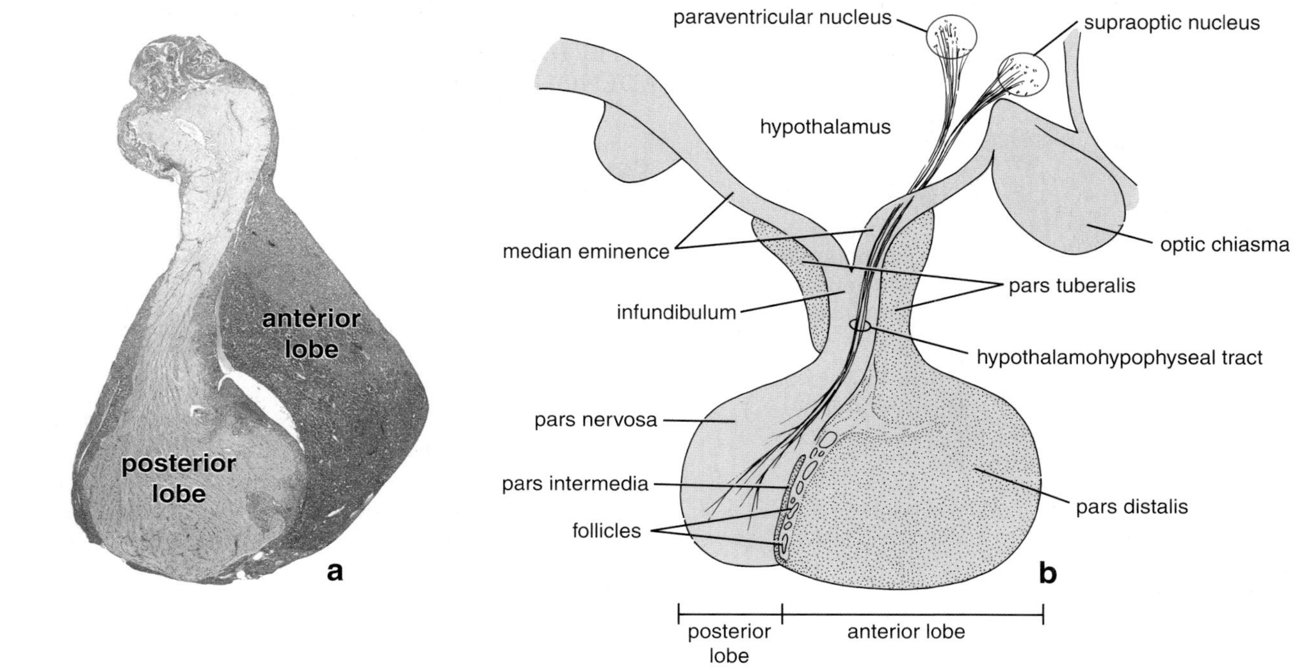

FIGURE 20.2
Pituitary gland. a. Photomicrograph of a human pituitary gland. The pituitary gland lobes can be identified on the basis of their appearance, location, and relation to each other. ×7. **b.** Drawing of a human pituitary and related regions of the hypothalamus. The anterior lobe of the pituitary gland consists of the pars distalis, pars tuberalis, and pars intermedia; the posterior lobe of the pituitary gland consists of the infundibulum and pars nervosa.

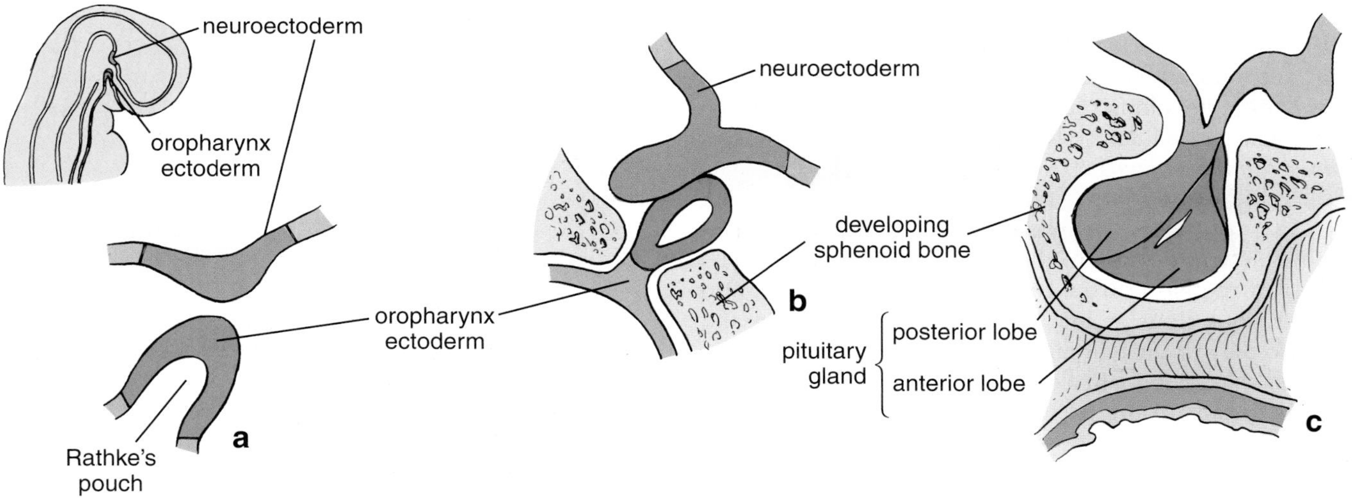

FIGURE 20.3
Development of the pituitary gland. This diagram shows sequential stages (**a** to **c**) in the development of the pituitary gland.

Blood Supply

Knowledge of the unusual blood supply of the pituitary gland is important to understanding its functions. The pituitary blood supply is derived from two sets of vessels (Fig. 20.4):

- ***Superior hypophyseal arteries*** supply the pars tuberalis, median eminence, and infundibular stem. These vessels arise from the internal carotid arteries and posterior communicating artery of the circle of Willis.
- ***Inferior hypophyseal arteries*** primarily supply the pars nervosa. These vessels arise solely from the internal carotid arteries. An important functional observation is that *most of the anterior lobe of the pituitary gland has no direct arterial supply.*

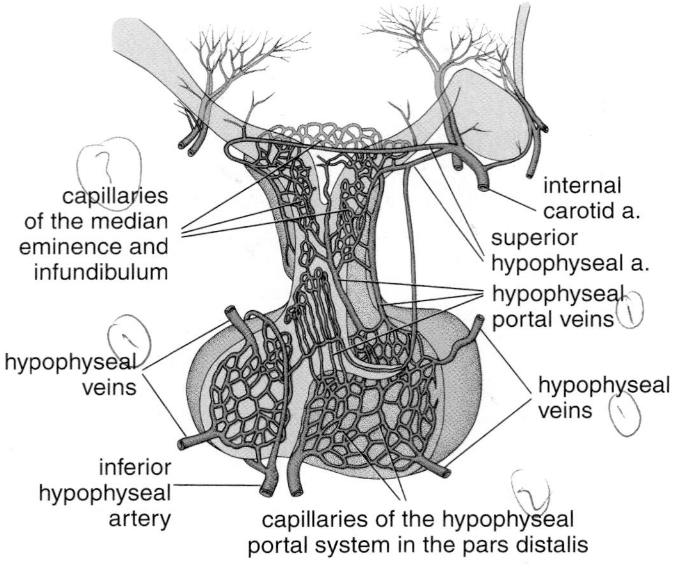

FIGURE 20.4
Diagram of the blood supply to the pituitary gland. The hypophyseal portal veins begin in the capillary beds of the median eminence and infundibulum and end in the capillaries of the pars distalis.

The *hypothalamohypophyseal portal system* provides the crucial link between the hypothalamus and the pituitary gland

The arteries that supply the pars tuberalis, median eminence, and infundibular stem give rise to fenestrated capillaries (the *primary capillary plexus*). These capillaries drain into portal veins, called the ***hypophyseal portal veins***, which run along the pars tuberalis and give rise to a second fenestrated sinusoidal capillary network (the *secondary capillary plexus*). This system of vessels carries the neuroendocrine secretions of hypothalamic nerves from their sites of release in the median eminence and infundibular stem directly to the cells of the pars distalis.

Most of the blood from the *pituitary gland* drains into the cavernous sinus at the base of the diencephalon and then into the systemic circulation. Some evidence suggests, however, that blood can flow via short portal veins from the pars distalis to the pars nervosa and that blood from the pars nervosa may flow toward the hypothalamus. These short pathways provide a route by which the hormones of the anterior lobe of the pituitary gland could provide feedback directly to the brain without making the full circuit of the systemic circulation.

Nerve Supply

The nerves that enter the infundibular stem and pars nervosa from the hypothalamic nuclei are components of the posterior lobe of the pituitary gland (see below). The nerves that enter the anterior lobe of the pituitary gland are postganglionic fibers of the autonomic nervous system and have vasomotor function.

Structure and Function of the Pituitary Lobes

ANTERIOR LOBE OF THE PITUITARY GLAND (ADENOHYPOPHYSIS)

The anterior lobe of the pituitary gland regulates other endocrine glands and some nonendocrine tissues

Most of the anterior lobe of the pituitary gland has the typical organization of endocrine tissue. The cells are organized in clumps and cords separated by fenestrated sinusoidal capillaries of relatively large diameter. These cells respond to signals from the hypothalamus and synthesize and secrete a number of pituitary hormones. Four hormones of the anterior lobe—adrenocorticotropic hormone (ACTH), thyroid-stimulating (thyrotropic) hormone (TSH, thyrotropin), follicle-stimulating hormone (FSH), and luteinizing hormone (LH)—are called ***tropic hormones*** because they regulate the activity of cells in other endocrine glands throughout the body (Fig. 20.5).

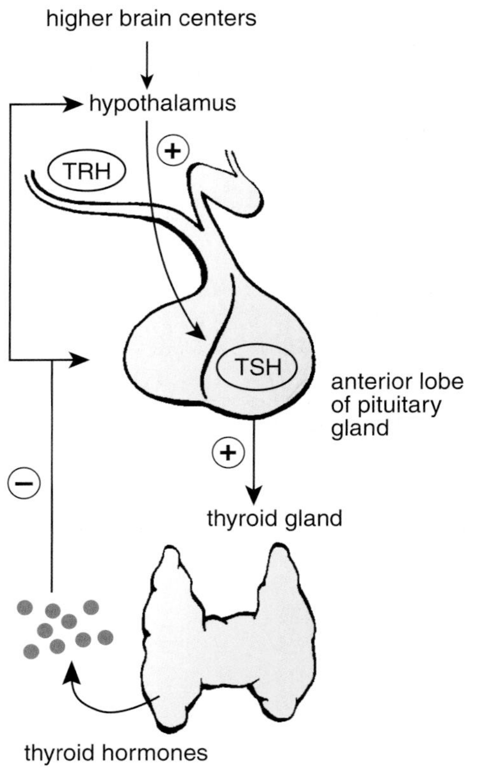

FIGURE 20.5
Interaction of the hypothalamus, anterior lobe of the pituitary gland, and thyroid gland. Production of thyroid hormones is regulated through a negative feedback system. The thyroid hormone can feed back on the system and inhibit further release of thyroid hormones. Such inhibition occurs at the level of the anterior lobe and the hypothalmus. The system is activated in response to low thyroid hormone levels or in response to metabolic needs. *TRH,* thyrotropin-releasing hormone; and *TSH,* thyroid-stimulating hormone.

The two remaining hormones of the anterior lobe, growth hormone (GH) and prolactin (PRL), are not considered tropic because they act directly on target organs that are not endocrine in nature. The general character and effects of the pituitary hormones of the anterior lobe are summarized in Table 20.1.

Pars Distalis

The cells within the ***pars distalis*** vary in size, shape, and staining properties. The cells are arranged in cords and nests with interweaving capillaries. Early descriptions of the cells within the pars distalis were based solely on the staining properties of secretory vesicles within the cells. Using mixtures of acidic and basic dyes (Fig. 20.6), histologists identified three types of cells according to their staining reaction, namely, ***basophils*** (10%), ***acidophils*** (40%), and ***chromophobes*** (50%). However, this classification contains no information regarding the hormonal secretory activity or functional role of these cells.

Histochemical, physiologic, and immunocytochemical methods better define the functions of the cell types in the pars distalis

The three methods used to define the functions of the different cell types of the pars distalis are

- ***Histochemistry.*** The use of histochemical stains for specific chemical groups, such as the periodic acid–Schiff (PAS) reaction for carbohydrates of glycoproteins, trichrome stains (Mallory's, Cleveland-Wolfe, etc.), and other empirically derived combinations of stains (e.g., aldehyde-fuchsin), enables investigators to characterize the cells further. Acidophils and basophils have been subdivided into smaller groups that more closely correlate staining properties with function, as summarized in Table 20.2.
- ***Histophysiologic studies.*** The cells in Table 20.2 are characterized as acidophils and basophils on the basis of their staining characteristics. The role of the cells, however, was identified by combining information on staining properties with changes in the number, size, and staining intensity of the cells as the target organs of the pituitary hormones were physiologically manipulated. Pathologic conditions were also correlated with the absence or overgrowth of specific hypophyseal cells. These physiologic and pathologic observations have led to the recognition that many of the cells originally identified as chromophobes are actually transiently degranulated forms of secretory cells.
- ***Electron microscopy and immunocytochemistry.*** Ultrastructurally, the cells of the anterior lobe of the pituitary gland show relatively distinctive characteristics based on comparison of cell size and shape, degree of development of cytoplasmic organelles, and secretory vesicle size, density, and distribution (Table 20.3).

Five functional cell types are identified in the pars distalis on the basis of immunocytochemical reactions

All known hormones of the anterior lobe of the pituitary gland are small proteins or glycoproteins. This important

TABLE 20.1. **Hormones of the Anterior Lobe of the Pituitary Gland**

Hormone	Composition	MW (kDa)	Major Functions
Growth hormone (somatotropin, GH)	Straight-chain protein (191 aa)	21,700	Stimulates liver and other organs to synthesize and secrete insulin-like growth factor I (IGF-I), which in turn stimulates division of progenitor cells located in growth plates and in skeletal muscles, resulting in body growth
Prolactin (PRL)	Straight-chain protein (198 aa)	22,500	Promotes mammary gland development; initiates milk formation; stimulates and maintains secretion of casein, lactalbumin, lipids, and carbohydrates into the milk
Adrenocorticotropic hormone (ACTH)	Small polypeptide (39 aa)	4,000	Maintains structure and stimulates secretion of glucocorticoids and gonadocorticoids by the zona fasciculata and zona reticularis of the adrenal cortex
Follicle-stimulating hormone (FSH)	2-chain glycoprotein[A] (α, 92 aa; β, 111 aa)	28,000	Stimulates follicular development in the ovary and spermatogenesis in the testis
Luteinizing hormone (LH)	2-chain glycoprotein[A] (α, 92 aa; β, 116 aa)	28,300	Regulates final maturation of ovarian follicle, ovulation, and corpus luteum formation; stimulates steroid secretion by follicle and corpus luteum; in males, essential for maintenance of and androgen secretion by the Leydig (interstitial) cells of the testis
Thyrotropic hormone (TSH)	2-chain glycoprotein[A] (α, 92 aa; β, 112 aa)	28,000	Stimulates growth of thyroid epithelial cells; stimulates production and release of thyroglobulin and thyroid hormones

[A]The α chains of FSH, LH, and TSH are identical and encoded by a single gene; the β chains are specific for each hormone.

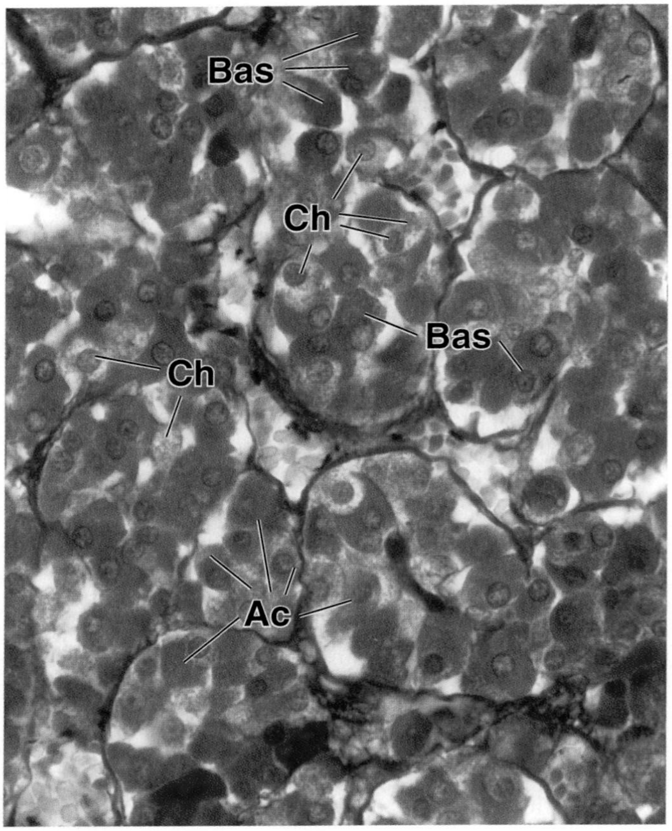

FIGURE 20.6
This specimen of the pars distalis is stained with brilliant crystal scarlet, aniline blue, and Martius yellow to distinguish the various cell types and connective tissue stroma. The cords of cells are surrounded by a delicate connective tissue stroma stained *blue.* The sinusoidal capillaries are seen in close association with the parenchyma and contain erythrocytes stained *yellow.* In the region shown here, the acidophils *(Ac)* are the most numerous cell type present. Their cytoplasm stains *cherry red.* The basophils *(Bas)* stain *blue.* The chromophobes *(Ch),* though few in number in this particular region, are virtually unstained. ×640.

fact has led to definitive identification of specific cell types by immunocytochemistry. These studies have classified cells of anterior lobe of the pituitary gland into five cell types:

- ***Somatotropes*** *(GH cells)* are most commonly found within the pars distalis and constitute approximately 50% of the parenchymal cells in the anterior lobe of the pituitary gland. These medium-sized, oval cells exhibit round, centrally located nuclei and produce ***GH (somatotropin).*** The presence of eosinophilic vesicles in their cytoplasm classifies them into the acidophil cell type. Two hypothalamic hormones regulate the release of GH from somatotropes: ***growth hormone–releasing hormone (GHRH)*** and ***somatostatin,*** which inhibits GH release from the somatotropes. Hormonally active tumors that originate from somatotropes are associated with hypersecretion of GH and cause gigantism in children and acromegaly in adults.
- ***Lactotropes (PRL cells, mammotropes)*** constitute 15 to 20% of the parenchymal cells in the anterior lobe of the pituitary gland. These are large, polygonal cells with oval nuclei. They produce ***PRL.*** In their storage phase, lactotropes exhibit numerous acidophilic vesicles (the histologic feature of an acidophil). When the content of these vesicles is released, the cytoplasm of the lactotrope does not stain (the histologic feature of a chromophobe). Secretion of PRL is under inhibitory control by ***dopamine,*** the catecholamine produced by the hypothalamus. However, thyrotropin-releasing hormone (TRH) and ***vasoactive inhibitory peptide (VIP)*** are known to stimulate synthesis and secretion of PRL. During pregnancy and lactation these cells undergo hypertrophy and hyperplasia, causing the pituitary gland to increase in size. These processes account for the larger size of the pituitary gland in the multiparous female.

TABLE 20.2. **Staining Characteristics of Cells Found in the Anterior Lobe of the Pituitary Gland**

Cell Type	Percentage of Total Cells	General Staining	Specific Staining	Product
Somatotrope (GH cell)	50	Acidophil	Orange G (PAS −)	Growth hormone (GH)
Lactotrope (PRL cell)	15–20	Acidophil	Orange G (PAS −) Herlant's erythrosin Brooke's carmosine	Prolactin (PRL)
Corticotrope (ACTH cell)	15–20	Basophil	Lead hematoxylin (PAS +)	Proopiomelanocortin (POMC), which is cleaved in human into adrenocorticotropic hormone (ACTH) and β-lipotrophic hormone (β-LPH)
Gonadotrope (FSH and LH cells)	10	Basophil	Aldehyde-fuchsin Aldehyde-thionine (PAS +)	Follicle-stimulating hormone (FSH) and luteinizing hormone (LH)
Thyrotrope (TSH cell)	~5	Basophil	Aldehyde-fuchsin Aldehyde-thionine (PAS +)	Thyrotropic hormone (TSH)

TABLE 20.3. Electron Microscopic Characteristics of Cells Found in the Anterior Lobe of the Pituitary Gland

Cell Type	Size/Shape	Nucleus/Location	Secretory Vesicle Size/ Characteristics	Other Cytoplasmic Characteristics
Somatotrope	Medium/oval	Round/central, with prominent nucleoli	Dense: 350 nm, closely packed	None
Lactotrope	Large/polygonal	Oval/central	Inactive: 200 nm, sparse Active: dense, pleomorphic, 600 nm, sparse	Lysosomes increase after lactation
Corticotrope	Medium/polygonal	Round/eccentric	100–300 nm	Lipid droplets, large lysosomes, perinuclear bundles of intermediate filaments
Gonadotrope	Small/oval	Round/eccentric	Dense: 200–250 nm	Prominent Golgi apparatus, distended rER cysternae
Thyrotrope	Large/polygonal	Round/eccentric	Dense: <150 nm	Prominent Golgi apparatus with numerous vesicles

- *Corticotropes (ACTH cells)* also constitute 15 to 20% of the parenchymal cells in the anterior lobe of the pituitary gland. These polygonal, medium-sized cells with round and eccentric nuclei produce a precursor molecule of ***ACTH***, known as ***proopiomelanocortin (POMC)***. These cells stain as basophils and also exhibit a strong positive reaction with PAS reagent, because of the carbohydrate moieties associated with POMC. POMC is further cleaved by proteolytic enzymes within the corticotrope into several fragments, namely **ACTH, *β-lipotrophic hormone (β-LPH), melanocyte-stimulating hormone (MSH), β-endorphin,*** and ***enkephalin.*** ACTH release is regulated by ***corticotropin-releasing hormone (CRH)*** produced by the hypothalamus.
- *Gonadotropes (FSH and LH cells)* constitute about 10% of the parenchymal cells in the anterior lobe of the pituitary gland. These small, oval cells with round and eccentric nuclei produce both ***LH*** and ***FSH.*** They are scattered throughout the pars distalis and stain intensely with both basic stains (thus classifying them as the basophil cell type) and PAS reagent. Many gonadotropes are capable of producing both FSH and LH. However, immunocytochemical studies indicate that some gonadotropes may produce only one hormone or the other. The release of FSH and LH is regulated by ***gonadotropin-releasing hormone (GnRH)*** produced by the hypothalamus. Both FSH and LH play an important role in male and female reproduction, which is discussed in Chapters 21 and 22.
- *Thyrotropes (TSH cells)* constitute about 5% of the parenchymal cells in the anterior lobe of the pituitary gland. These large, polygonal cells with round and eccentric nuclei produce ***TSH (thyrotropic hormone,*** thyrotropin). They exhibit cytoplasmic basophilia (basophils) and stain positively with PAS reagent. Release of TSH is also under the hypothalamic control of ***TRH,*** which also stimulates secretion of PRL. TSH acts on the follicular cells of the thyroid gland and stimulates production of thyroglobulin and thyroid hormones.

Pars Intermedia

The ***pars intermedia*** surrounds a series of small cystic cavities that represent the residual lumen of Rathke's pouch. The parenchymal cells of the pars intermedia surround colloid-filled follicles. The cells lining these follicles appear to be derived from various secretory cells. Transmission electron microscopy reveals that these cells form apical junctional complexes and have vesicles larger than those found in the pars distalis. The nature of this follicular colloid is yet to be determined; however, often, cell debris is found within it. The pars intermedia contains basophils and chromophobes (Fig. 20.7). Frequently, the basophils and cysts extend into the pars nervosa.

The function of the pars intermedia cells in humans remains unclear. From studies of other species, however, it is known that basophils have scattered vesicles in their cytoplasm that contain either α- or β-endorphin (a morphine-related compound). In frogs, the basophils produce MSH, which stimulates pigment production in melanocytes and pigment dispersion in melanophores. In humans, MSH is not a distinct, functional hormone but is a byproduct of β-LPH posttranslational processing. Because MSH is found in the human pars intermedia in small amounts, the basophils of the pars intermedia are assumed to be corticotropes.

Pars Tuberalis

The ***pars tuberalis*** is an extension of the anterior lobe along the pituitary stalk. It is a highly vascular region containing veins of the hypothalamohypophyseal system. The parenchymal cells are arranged in small clusters or cords in association with the blood vessels. Nests of squamous cells and small follicles lined with cuboidal cells are scattered in this region. These cells often show immunoreactivity for ACTH, FSH, and LH.

BOX 20.1

Functional Considerations: Pituitary Secretion and Hypothalamic Regulating Hormones

The release of hormones from the anterior lobe of the pituitary gland is under significant control by the hypothalamus, which regulates release of ***hypothalamic regulating hormones*** into the hypophyseal portal veins. These hypothalamic regulating hormones can stimulate or inhibit secretion of pituitary hormones. The hypothalamic regulating hormones are produced in the cells of the hypothalamus in response to circulating levels of hormones. Thus, the cells of the anterior lobe of the pituitary gland can be selectively inhibited or stimulated. A simple ***negative feedback system*** controls the synthesis and discharge of the releasing hormones. Consider the production of thyroid hormone (see Fig. 20.5). If blood levels of thyroid hormone are high, TRH is not produced or released. If blood levels of thyroid hormone are low, the hypothalamus discharges TRH into the hypothalamohypophyseal portal system. Release of TRH stimulates specific cells within the anterior lobe of the pituitary gland to produce TSH, which, in turn, stimulates the thyroid to produce and release more thyroid hormone. As the thyroid hormone level rises, the negative feedback system stops the hypothalamus from discharging TRH. Most of the tropic hormones produced by the anterior lobe of the pituitary gland are regulated by releasing hormones. PRL production is primarily regulated by the inhibitory effect of dopamine; i.e., PRL secretion is tonically inhibited by the release of dopamine by the hypothalamus.

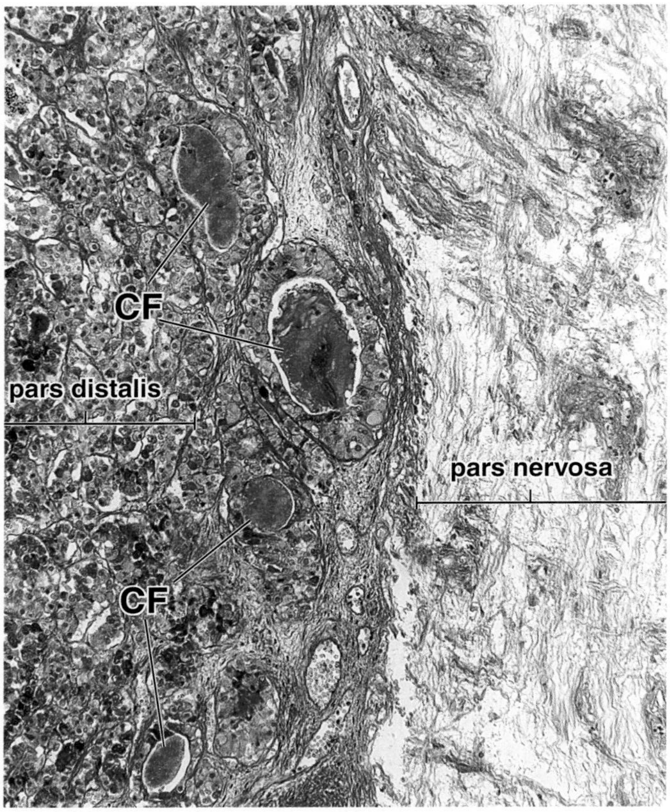

FIGURE 20.7
Photomicrograph of the pars intermedia of an adult human pituitary gland. This photomicrograph of a toluidine blue–stained specimen shows the pars intermedia located between the pars distalis (on the left) and pars nervosa (on the right). In humans, this portion of the gland is somewhat rudimentary. However, a characteristic feature of the pars intermedia is the presence of different-sized follicles filled with colloid *(CF)* and small groups of cells consisting of chromophobes and basophils. ×120.

POSTERIOR LOBE OF THE PITUITARY GLAND (NEUROHYPOPHYSIS)

The posterior lobe of the pituitary gland is an extension of the central nervous system (CNS) that stores and releases secretory products from the hypothalamus

The posterior lobe of the pituitary gland, also known as the neurohypophysis, consists of the ***pars nervosa*** and the ***infundibulum*** that connects it to the hypothalamus. The pars nervosa, the neural lobe of the pituitary, contains nonmyelinated axons and their nerve endings of approximately 100,000 ***neurosecretory neurons*** whose cell bodies lie in the ***supraoptic*** and ***paraventricular nuclei*** of the hypothalamus. The axons form the ***hypothalamohypophyseal*** tract and are unique in two respects. First, they do not terminate on other neurons or target cells but end in close proximity to the fenestrated capillary network of the pars nervosa. Second, they contain ***secretory vesicles*** in all parts of the cells, i.e., the cell body, axon, and axon terminal. These vesicles may be specifically stained with the aldehyde-fuchsin, aldehydethionine, and chrome-hematoxylin methods; by specific procedures for the disulfide groups of cystine; and more specifically by immunochemical reactions. Because of their intense secretory activity, the neurons have well-developed Nissl bodies and, in this respect, resemble ventral horn and ganglion cells.

The posterior lobe of the pituitary gland is *not an endocrine gland.* Rather, it is a *storage site for neurosecretions* of the neurons of the *supraoptic* and *paraventricular nuclei* of the hypothalamus. The nonmyelinated axons convey neurosecretory products to the pars nervosa. Other neurons from the hypothalamic nuclei (described below) also release their secretory products into the fenestrated capillary network of the infundibulum, the first capillary bed of the hypothalamohypophyseal portal system.

Electron microscopy reveals three morphologically distinct neurosecretory vesicles in the nerve endings of the pars nervosa

Three sizes of membrane-bounded vesicles are present in the pars nervosa:

- Neurosecretory vesicles with diameters ranging between 10 and 30 nm accumulate in the axon terminals. They

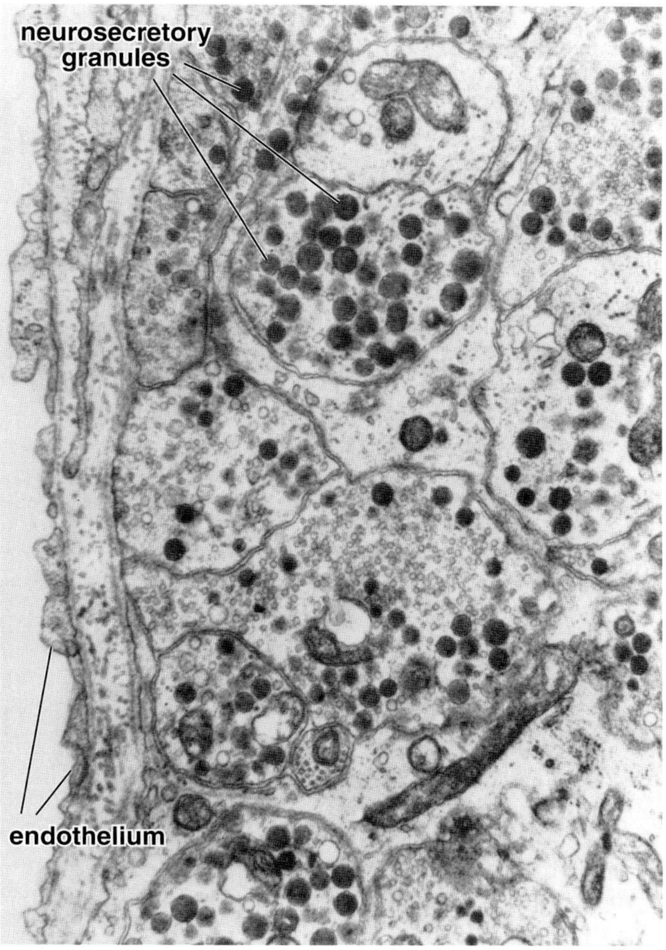

FIGURE 20.8
Electron micrograph of rat posterior lobe. Neurosecretory granules and small vesicles are present in the terminal portions of the axonal processes of the hypothalamohypophyseal tract fibers. Capillaries with fenestrated endothelium are present in close proximity to the nerve endings. ×20,000. (Courtesy of Drs. Sanford L. Palay and P. Orkland.)

also form accumulations that dilate portions of the axon near the terminals (Fig. 20.8). These dilations, called ***Herring bodies***, are visible in the light microscope (Fig. 20.9).

- Nerve terminals also contain 30-nm vesicles that contain acetylcholine. These vesicles may play a specific role in the release of neurosecretory vesicles.
- Larger, 50- to 80-nm vesicles that resemble the dense core vesicles of the adrenal medulla and adrenergic nerve endings are present in the same terminal as the other membrane-bounded vesicles.

The membrane-bounded neurosecretory vesicles that aggregate to form Herring bodies contain either ***oxytocin*** or ***antidiuretic hormone (ADH, vasopressin)*** (Table 20.4). Each hormone is a small peptide of nine amino acid residues. The two hormones differ in only two of these residues. Each vesicle also contains ATP and a ***neurophysin***, a protein that binds to the hormone by noncovalent bonds. Oxytocin and ADH are synthesized as part of a large molecule that includes the hormone and its specific neurophysin. The large molecule is proteolytically cleaved into the hormone and neurophysin as it travels from the perikaryon to the axon terminal. Immunocytochemical staining demonstrates that oxytocin and ADH are secreted by different cells in the hypothalamic nuclei.

ADH controls blood pressure by altering the permeability of the collecting tubules in the kidney

ADH's original name, vasopressin, was derived from the observation that large nonphysiologic doses increase blood pressure by promoting the contraction of smooth muscle in small arteries and arterioles. The primary physiologic effect of ADH is to increase the permeability of the distal portions of the nephron, i.e., the distal convoluted tubule

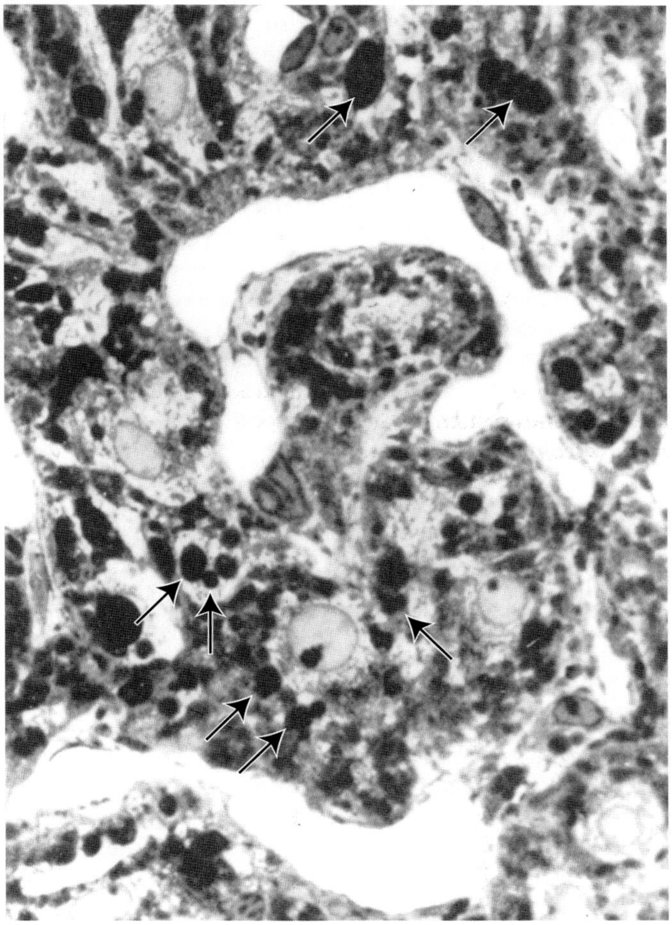

FIGURE 20.9
Photomicrograph of rat posterior lobe. *Arrows* indicate dark rounded masses called Herring bodies that are present in nerve endings adjacent to the capillaries. ×1,100. (Courtesy of Drs. Sanford L. Palay and P. Orkland.)

TABLE 20.4. **Hormones of the Posterior Lobe of the Pituitary Gland**

Hormone	Composition	Source	Major Functions
Oxytocin	Polypeptide containing 9 amino acids	Cell bodies of neurons located in the supraoptic and paraventricular nuclei of the hypothalamus[A]	Stimulates activity of the contractile cells around the ducts of the mammary glands to eject milk from the glands; stimulates contraction of smooth muscle cells in the pregnant uterus
Antidiuretic hormone (ADH; vasopressin)	Polypeptide containing 9 amino acids; two forms: arginine-ADH (most common in humans) and lysine-ADH	Cell bodies of neurons located in the supraoptic and paraventricular nuclei of the hypothalamus[A]	Decreases urine volume by increasing reabsorption of water by collecting ducts of the kidney; decreases the rate of perspiration in response to dehydration; increases blood pressure by stimulating contractions of smooth muscle cells in the wall of arterioles

[A]Immunocytochemical studies indicate that oxytocin and ADH are produced by separate sets of neurons within the supraoptic and paraventricular nuclei of the hypothalamus. Biochemical studies have demonstrated that the supraoptic nucleus contains equal amounts of both hormones, whereas the paraventricular nucleus contains more oxytocin than ADH, but less than the amount found in the supraoptic nucleus.

and collecting ducts by acting on ADH-regulated water channels (AQP-2) (see page 619), causing rapid resorption of water across the tubule epithelium. In the absence or reduced production of ADH, most commonly due to lesions of the hypothalamus or posterior lobe of the pituitary gland, large volumes of dilute urine are produced. Individuals with this condition, called ***diabetes insipidus***, produce up to 20 L of urine per day and have extreme thirst.

Plasma osmolality and blood volume are monitored by specialized receptors of the cardiovascular system (e.g., carotid bodies and juxtaglomerular apparatus). An increase in osmolality or a decrease in blood volume stimulates ADH release. Additionally, the cell bodies of the hypothalamic secretory neurons may also serve as osmoreceptors, initiating ADH release. Pain, trauma, emotional stress, and drugs, such as nicotine, also stimulate release of ADH.

Oxytocin promotes contraction of smooth muscle of the uterus and myoepithelial cells of the breast

Oxytocin is a more potent promoter of smooth muscle contraction than is ADH. Its primary effect includes promotion of contraction of

- Uterine smooth muscle during orgasm, menstruation, and parturition
- Myoepithelial cells of the secretory alveoli and alveolar ducts of the mammary gland

Oxytocin secretion is triggered by neural stimuli that reach the hypothalamus. These stimuli initiate a neurohumoral reflex that resembles a simple sensorimotor reflex. In the uterus, the neurohumoral reflex is initiated by distension of the vagina and cervix. In the breast, the reflex is initiated by nursing (suckling). Contraction of the myoepithelial cells that surround the base of the alveolar secretory cells and cells of the larger ducts causes milk to be released and pass through the ducts that open onto the nipple, i.e., milk ejection (see page 762).

The pituicyte is the only cell specific to the posterior lobe of the pituitary gland

In addition to the numerous axons and terminals of the hypothalamic neurosecretory neurons, the posterior lobe of the pituitary gland contains fibroblasts, mast cells, and specialized glial cells called ***pituicytes***, associated with the fenestrated capillaries. These cells are irregular in shape, with many branches, and resemble astroglial cells. Their nuclei are round or oval, and pigment vesicles are present in the cytoplasm. Like astroglia, they possess specific intermediate filaments called glial fibrillary acidic protein (GFAP). Pituicytes often have processes that terminate in the perivascular space. Because of their many processes and relationships to the blood, the pituicyte serves a supporting role similar to that of astrocytes in the rest of the CNS (see page 299).

The hypothalamus regulates hypophyseal function

The hypothalamus produces numerous neurosecretory products. In addition to oxytocin and ADH, hypothalamic neurons secrete polypeptides that promote and inhibit the secretion and release of hormones from the anterior lobe of the pituitary gland (Table 20.5). These hypothalamic polypeptides also accumulate in nerve endings near the median eminence and infundibular stalk and are released into the capillary bed of the hypothalamohypophyseal portal system for transport to the pars distalis.

A feedback system regulates endocrine function at two levels: hormone production in the pituitary gland and hypothalamic releasing hormone production in the hypothalamus

The circulating level of a specific secretory product of a target organ, a hormone or its metabolite, may act directly on the cells of the anterior lobe of the pituitary gland or

TABLE 20.5. **Hypothalamic Regulating Hormones**

Hormone	Composition	Source	Major Functions
Growth hormone–releasing hormone (GHRH)	Two forms in human: polypeptides containing 40 and 44 amino acids	Cell bodies of neurons located in the arcuate nucleus of hypothalamus[A]	Stimulates secretion and gene expression of GH by somatotropes
Somatostatin	Polypeptide containing 14 amino acids	Cell bodies of neurons located in the periventricular, paraventricular, and arcuate nuclei of hypothalamus[A]	Inhibits secretion of GH by somatotropes
Dopamine	Catecholamine (amino acid derivative)	Cell bodies of neurons located in the arcuate nucleus of hypothalamus[A]	Inhibits secretion of PRL by lactotropes
Corticotropin-releasing hormone (CRH)	Polypeptide containing 41 amino acids	Cell bodies of neurons located in the arcuate, periventricular, and medial paraventricular nuclei of hypothalamus[A]	Stimulates secretion of ACTH by corticotropes; stimulates gene expression for POMC in corticotropes
Gonadotropin-releasing hormone (GnRH)	Polypeptide containing 10 amino acids	Cell bodies of neurons located in the arcuate, ventromedial, dorsal, and paraventricular nuclei of hypothalamus[A]	Stimulates secretion of LH and FSH by gonadotropes
Thyrotropin-releasing hormone (TRH)	Polypeptide containing 3 amino acids	Cell bodies of neurons located by the ventromedial, dorsal, and paraventricular nuclei of hypothalamus[A]	Stimulates secretion and gene expression of TSH by thyrotropes; stimulates synthesis and secretion of PRL

[A] Immunocytochemical studies indicate that oxytocin and ADH are produced by separate sets of neurons within the supraoptic and paraventricular nuclei of the hypothalamus. Biochemical studies have demonstrated that the supraoptic nucleus contains equal amounts of both hormones, whereas the paraventricular nucleus contains more oxytocin than ADH, but less than the amount found in the supraoptic nucleus.

the hypothalamus to regulate the secretion of hypothalamic releasing hormones (see Fig. 20.5). The two levels of feedback allow exquisite sensitivity in the control of secretory function. The hormone itself normally regulates the secretory activity of the cells in the hypothalamus and pituitary gland that regulate its secretion.

In addition, information from most physiologic and psychologic stimuli that reach the brain also reaches the hypothalamus. The hypothalamic-hypophyseal feedback loop provides a regulatory path whereby general information from the CNS contributes to the regulation of the anterior lobe of the pituitary gland and, consequently, to the regulation of the entire endocrine system. The secretion of hypothalamic regulatory peptides is the primary mechanism by which changes in emotional state are translated into changes in the physiologic homeostatic state.

PINEAL GLAND

The ***pineal gland*** (pineal body, epiphysis cerebri) is an endocrine or neuroendocrine gland that regulates daily body rhythm. It develops from neuroectoderm of the posterior portion of the roof of the diencephalon and remains attached to the brain by a short stalk. In humans, it is located at the posterior wall of the third ventricle near the center of the brain. The pineal gland is a flattened, pine cone–shaped structure, hence its name (Fig. 20.10). It measures 5 to 8 mm high and 3 to 5 mm in diameter and weighs between 100 and 200 mg.

The pineal gland contains two types of parenchymal cells: pinealocytes and interstitial (glial) cells

Pinealocytes are the chief cells of the pineal gland. They are arranged in clumps or cords within lobules formed by connective tissue septa that extend into the gland from the pia mater that covers its surface. These cells have a large, deeply infolded nucleus with one or more prominent nucleoli and contain lipid droplets within their cytoplasm. When examined with the transmission electron microscope (TEM), pinealocytes show typical cytoplasmic organelles along with numerous, dense-cored, membrane-bounded vesicles in their elaborate, elongated cytoplasmic processes. The processes also contain numerous parallel bundles of microtubules. The expanded, club-like endings of the processes are associated with the blood capillaries. This feature strongly suggests neuroendocrine activity.

The ***interstitial (glial) cells*** constitute about 5% of the cells in the gland. They have staining and ultrastructural features that closely resemble those of astrocytes and are reminiscent of the pituicytes of the posterior lobe of the pituitary gland.

In addition to the two cell types, the human pineal gland is characterized by the presence of calcified concretions, called ***corpora arenacea*** or ***brain sand*** (Fig. 20.11). These concretions appear to be derived from precipitation of calcium phosphates and carbonates on carrier proteins that are released into the cytoplasm when the pineal secretions are exocytosed. The concretions are recognizable in childhood and increase in number with age. Because they are opaque to x-rays and located in the midline of the brain,

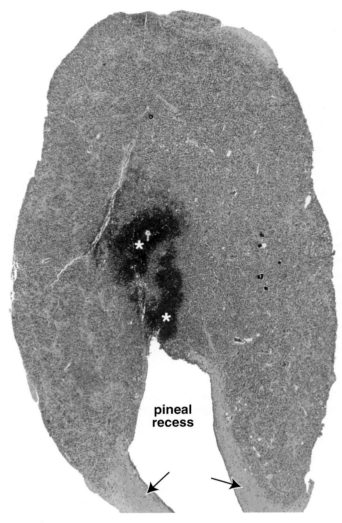

FIGURE 20.10
Photomicrograph of infant pineal gland. This H&E–stained section is from a median cut through the pine cone–shaped gland. The conical anterior end of the gland is at the top of the micrograph. The *arrows* indicate the part of the gland that connects with the posterior commissure. The gland is formed by an evagination of the posterior portion of the roof of the third ventricle (diencephalon). The dark areas indicated by *asterisks* are due to bleeding within the gland. ×25.

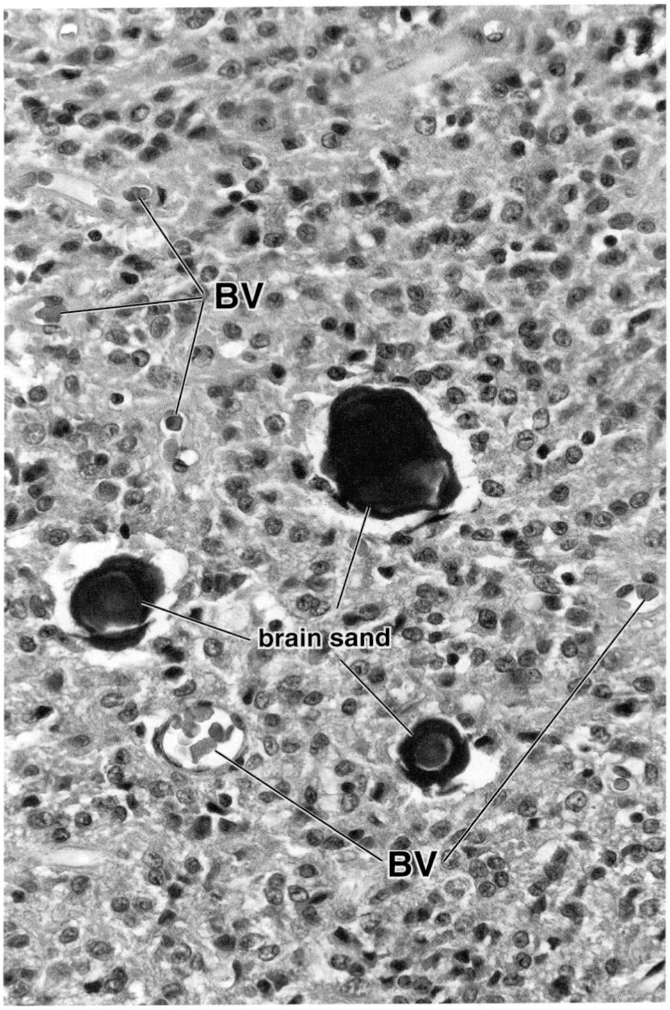

FIGURE 20.11
Photomicrograph of human pineal gland. This higher-magnification photomicrograph shows the characteristic concretions called brain sand or corpora arenacea. Pinealocytes (chief cells of the pineal gland) account for the majority of the cells seen in the specimen. They are arranged in clumps or cords. Those blood vessels *(BV)* that contain red blood cells are readily apparent; numerous other blood vessels are also present but are not recognized at this magnification without evidence of the blood cells. ×250.

they serve as convenient markers in radiographic and ***computed tomography studies.***

The human pineal gland relates light intensity and duration to endocrine activity

The pineal gland is a photosensitive organ and an important timekeeper and regulator of the day/night cycle (circadian rhythm). It obtains information about light and dark cycles from the retina via the ***retinohypothalamic tract,*** which connects in the suprachiasmatic nucleus with sympathetic neural tracts traveling into the pineal gland. During the day, light impulses inhibit the production of the major pineal gland hormone, ***melatonin.*** Therefore, pineal activity, as measured by changes in the plasma level of melatonin, increases during darkness and decreases during light. In humans, these circadian changes of melatonin secretion play an important role in regulating daily body rhythms.

Because melatonin is released in the dark it regulates reproductive function in mammals by inhibiting the steroidogenic activity of the gonads (Table 20.6). Production of gonadal steroids is regulated by the inhibitory action of melatonin on neurosecretory neurons located in the hypothalamus (arcuate nucleus) that produce GnRH. Inhibition of GnRH causes a decrease in the release of FSH

TABLE 20.6. **Hormones of the Pineal Gland**

Hormone	Composition	Source	Major Functions
Melatonin	Indolamine (*N*-acetyl-5-methoxytryptamine)	Pinealocytes	Regulates daily body rhythms and day/night cycle (circadian rhythms); inhibits secretion of GnRH and regulates steroidogenic activity of the gonads particularly as related to the menstrual cycle; in animals, influences seasonal sexual activity

and LH from the anterior lobe of the pituitary gland. In addition to melatonin, extracts of pineal glands from many animals contain numerous neurotransmitters such as ***serotonin, norepinephrine, dopamine, histamine,*** and hypothalamic regulating hormones such as ***somatostatin,*** and ***TRH.*** Clinically, tumors that destroy the pineal gland are associated with precocious (early-onset) puberty.

Animal studies demonstrate that information relating to the length of daylight reaches the pineal gland from photoreceptors in the retina. The pineal gland thus influences seasonal sexual activity. Recent studies in humans suggest that the pineal gland has a role in adjusting to sudden changes in day length, such as those experienced by travelers who suffer from *jet lag*. In addition, the pineal gland may play a role in altering emotional responses to reduced day length during winter in temperate and subarctic zones (seasonal affective disorder, or SAD).

▽ THYROID GLAND

The thyroid gland is located in the anterior neck region adjacent to the larynx and trachea

The ***thyroid gland*** is a bilobate endocrine gland located in the anterior neck region and consists of two large ***lateral lobes*** connected by an ***isthmus,*** a thin band of thyroid tissue. The two lobes, each ~5 cm in length, 2.5 cm in width, and 20 to 30 g in weight, lie on either side of the larynx and upper trachea. The isthmus crosses anterior to the upper part of the trachea. A ***pyramidal lobe*** often extends upward from the isthmus. A thin connective tissue capsule surrounds the gland. It sends trabeculae into the parenchyma that partially outline irregular lobes and lobules. Secretory ***follicles*** constitute the functional units of the gland.

The thyroid gland develops from the endodermal lining of the floor of the primitive pharynx

The thyroid gland begins to develop during the fourth week of gestation from a primordium originating as an endodermal thickening of the floor of the primitive pharynx. The primordium grows caudally and forms a duct-like invagination known as the ***thyroglossal duct.*** The thyroglossal duct descends through the tissue of the neck to its final destination in front of the trachea, where it divides into two lobes. During this downward migration, the thyroglossal duct undergoes atrophy, leaving an embryologic remnant, the pyramidal lobe of the thyroid, which is present in about 40% of the population. About the ninth week of gestation, endodermal cells differentiate into plates of ***follicular cells*** that become arranged into follicles. By week 14, well-developed follicles lined by the follicular cells contain colloid in their lumen. During week 7, epithelial cells lining the invagination of the fourth branchial pouches (sometimes called the fifth branchial pouches) known as the ***ultimobranchial bodies*** start their migration toward the developing thyroid gland and become incorporated into the lateral lobes. After fusing with the thyroid, ultimobranchial body cells disperse among the follicles, giving rise to ***parafollicular cells*** that become incorporated into the follicular epithelium.

The thyroid follicle is the structural unit of the thyroid gland

A ***thyroid follicle*** is a roughly spherical cyst-like compartment with a wall formed by a simple cuboidal or low columnar epithelium, the ***follicular epithelium.*** Hundreds of thousands of follicles that vary in diameter from about 0.2 to 1.0 mm constitute nearly the entire mass of the human thyroid gland. The follicles contain a gel-like mass called ***colloid*** (Fig. 20.12). The apical surfaces of the follicular cells are in contact with the colloid, and the basal surfaces rest on a typical basal lamina.

Follicular epithelium contains two types of cells: follicular and parafollicular cells

The parenchyma of the thyroid gland is composed of epithelium containing two types of cells:

- ***Follicular cells (principal cells)*** are responsible for production of the thyroid hormones T_4 and T_3. These cells vary in shape and size according to the functional state of the gland. In routine hematoxylin and eosin (H&E) preparations follicular cells exhibit a slightly basophilic basal cytoplasm with spherical nuclei containing one or more prominent nucleoli. The Golgi apparatus has a supranuclear position. Lipid droplets and PAS-positive droplets can be identified with appropriate staining. At the ultrastructural level the follicle cells reveal organelles commonly associated with both secretory and absorptive

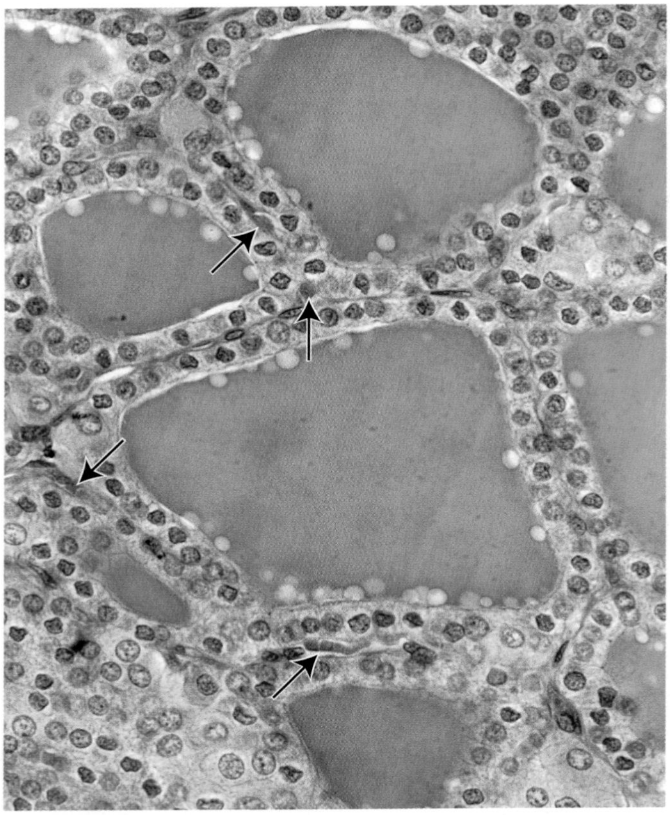

FIGURE 20.12
Thyroid gland. This photomicrograph of a human thyroid is from a section stained with H&E. It shows the colloid-containing follicles of the gland. Each follicle consists of a single layer of epithelial cells surrounding a central mass of colloid. The *arrows* indicate some of the blood capillaries between the follicles. ×500.

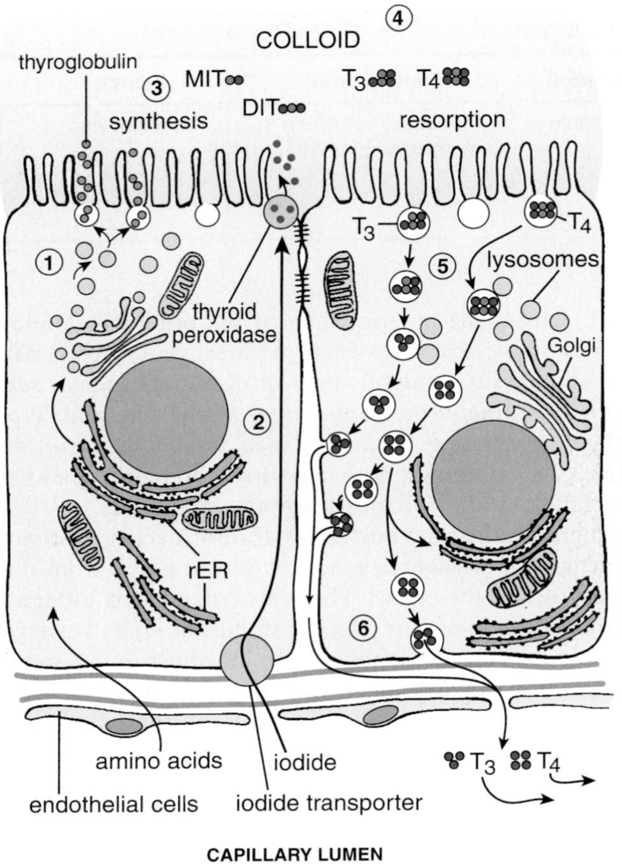

FIGURE 20.13
Diagram of steps in thyroid hormone synthesis. This diagram depicts two follicle cells: one in the process of thyroglobulin synthesis (on the left) and the other in the process of thyroglobulin resorption (on the right). The *numbers,* which are described more fully in the text, indicate the sequential steps that occur: *1,* synthesis and secretion of thyroglobulin; *2,* uptake and concentration of iodide from the blood, oxidation to iodine, and release into the colloid; *3,* iodination of thyroglobulin in the colloid; *4,* formation of T_3 and T_4 hormones in the colloid by oxidative coupling reactions; *5,* resorption of colloid by receptor-mediated endocytosis; and *6,* release of T_4 and T_3 from the cell into the circulation.

cells (shown schematically in Fig. 20.13), including typical junctional complexes at the apical end of the cell and short microvilli on the apical cell surface. Numerous profiles of rough-surfaced endoplasmic reticulum (rER) are present in the basal region. Small vesicles are present in the apical cytoplasm that are morphologically similar to vesicles associated with the Golgi apparatus. Abundant lysosomes and endocytotic vesicles, identified as ***colloidal resorption droplets***, are also present in the apical cytoplasm.

- ***Parafollicular cells (C cells)*** are located in the periphery of the follicular epithelium and lie within the follicle basal lamina. These cells have no exposure to the follicle lumen. They secrete ***calcitonin***, a hormone that regulates calcium metabolism. In routine H&E preparations, C cells are pale staining and occur as solitary cells or small clusters of cells. Human parafollicular cells are difficult to identify with light microscopy. At the electron microscope level, the parafollicular cells reveal numerous small secretory vesicles, which range in diameter from 60 to 550 nm, and a prominent Golgi apparatus (Fig. 20.14).

An extensive network of fenestrated capillaries derived from the superior and inferior thyroid arteries surrounds the follicles. Blind-ended lymphatic capillaries are present in the interfollicular connective tissue and may also provide a second route for conveying the hormones from the gland.

Thyroid gland function is essential to normal growth and development

The thyroid gland produces three hormones, each of which is essential to normal metabolism and homeostasis (Table 20.7):

- ***Thyroxine (tetraiodothyronine, T_4)*** and ***triiodothyronine (T_3)*** are synthesized and secreted by the follicular

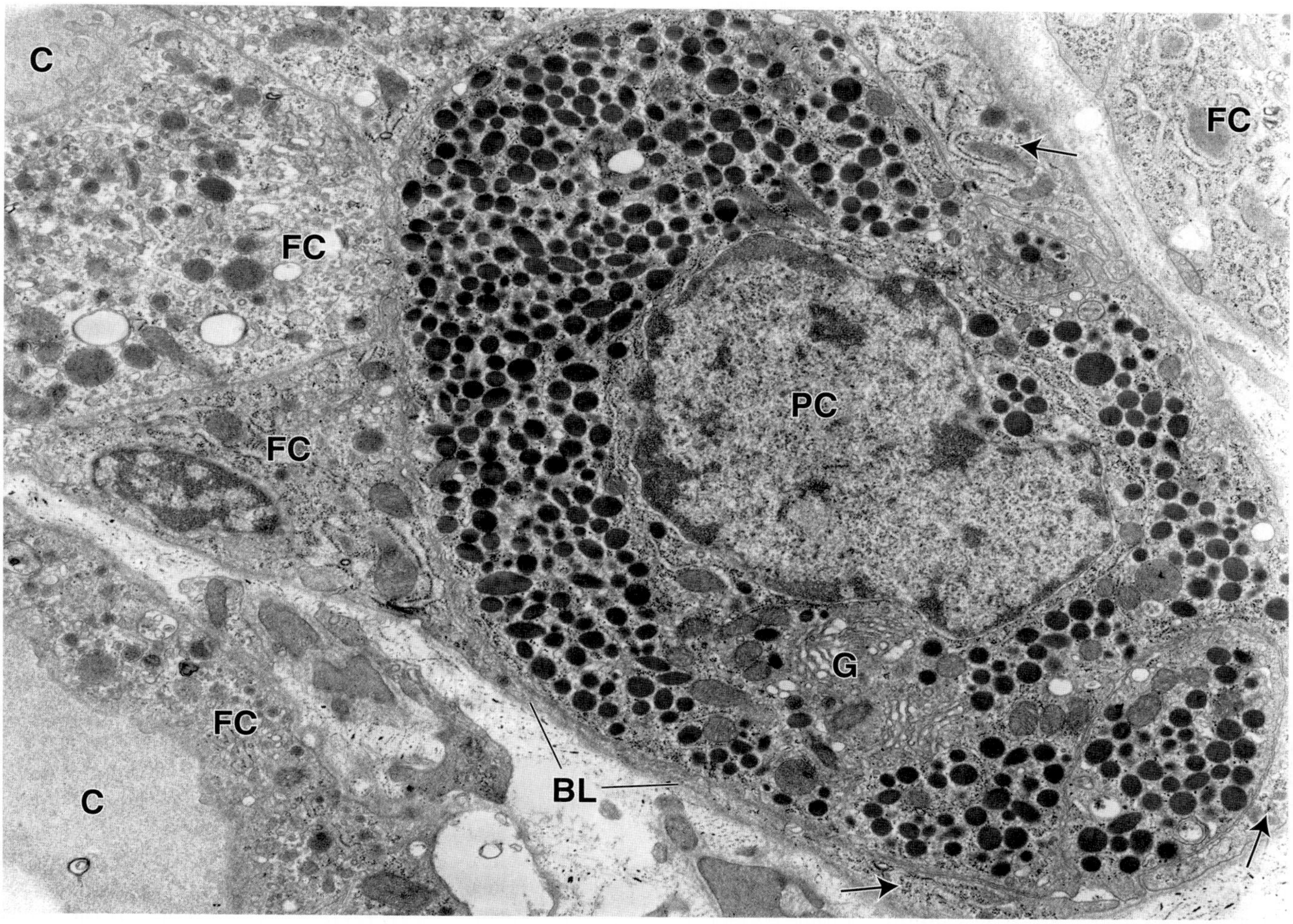

FIGURE 20.14
Electron micrograph of a parafollicular cell. Cytoplasmic processes of follicular cells *(arrows)* partially surround the parafollicular cell *(PC)*, which contains numerous electron-dense granules and a prominent Golgi apparatus *(G)*. A basal lamina *(BL)* is associated with the follicular cells *(FC)*. A portion of the central mass of colloidal material *(C)* in two adjacent follicles can be seen in the left corners of the micrograph. ×12,000. (Courtesy of Dr. Emmanuel-Adrien Nunez.)

TABLE 20.7. **Hormones of the Thyroid Gland**

Hormone	Composition	Source	Major Functions
Thyroxine (tetraiodothyronine, T_4) and triiodothyronine (T_3)[A]	Iodinated tyrosine derivatives	Follicular cells (principal cells)	Regulates tissue basal metabolism (increases rate of carbohydrate use, protein synthesis and degradation, and fat synthesis and degradation); regulates heat production; influences body and tissue growth and development of the nervous system in the fetus and young child[B]; increases absorption of carbohydrates from the intestine
Calcitonin (thyrocalcitonin)	Polypeptide containing 32 amino acids	Parafollicular cells (C cells)	Decreases blood calcium levels by inhibiting bone resorption and stimulating absorption of calcium by the bones

[A]Thyroid gland secretes substantially more T_4 than T_3; however about 40% of T_4 is peripherally converted to T_3, which acts more rapidly and is a more potent hormone.
[B]Deficiency of T_3 and T_4 during development results in fewer and smaller neurons, defective myelination, and mental retardation.

cells. Both hormones regulate cell and tissue basal metabolism and heat production and influence body growth and development. Secretion of these hormones is regulated by TSH released from the anterior lobe of the pituitary gland.

- ***Calcitonin (thyrocalcitonin)*** is synthesized by the parafollicular cells (C cells) and is a physiologic antagonist to parathyroid hormone (PTH). Calcitonin lowers blood calcium levels by suppressing the resorptive action of osteoclasts and promotes calcium deposition in bones by increasing the rate of osteoid calcification. Secretion of calcitonin is regulated directly by blood calcium levels. High levels of calcium stimulate secretion; low levels inhibit it. Secretion of calcitonin is unaffected by the hypothalamus and pituitary gland. Although calcitonin is used to treat patients with hypercalcemia, no clinical disease has been associated with its deficiency or even its absence after total thyroidectomy.

The principal component of colloid is thyroglobulin, an inactive storage form of thyroid hormones

The principal component of colloid is a large (660 kDa) iodinated glycoprotein called ***thyroglobulin*** containing about 120 tyrosine residues. Colloid also contains several enzymes and other glycoproteins. It stains with both basic and acidic dyes and is strongly PAS positive. Thyroglobulin is not a hormone. It is an inactive storage form of the thyroid hormones. Active thyroid hormones are liberated from thyroglobulin and released into the fenestrated blood capillaries that surround the follicles only after further cellular processing. The thyroid is unique among endocrine glands because it stores large amounts of its secretory product extracellularly.

Synthesis of thyroid hormone involves several steps

The synthesis of the two major thyroid hormones, thyroxine (T_4) and T_3 takes place in the thyroid follicle in a series of discrete steps (see Fig. 20.13):

1. ***Synthesis of thyroglobulin.*** The precursor of thyroglobulin is synthesized in the rER of the follicular epithelial cells; it is glycosylated there and in the Golgi apparatus before it is packaged into vesicles and secreted by exocytosis into the lumen of the follicle.
2. ***Resorption, diffusion, and oxidation of iodide.*** Follicular epithelial cells actively transport ***iodide*** from the blood into their cytoplasm using ATP-dependent ***iodide transporters.*** These cells can establish an intracellular concentration of iodide that is 30 to 40 times greater than that of the serum. Iodide ions then diffuse rapidly toward the apical cell membrane where they are oxidized to ***iodine,*** the active form of iodide. This process occurs in the apical cytoplasm and is catalyzed by membrane-bound ***thyroid peroxidase.*** After oxidation the iodine is then released into the colloid.
3. ***Iodination of thyroglobulin.*** One or two iodine atoms are then added to the specific tyrosine residues of thyroglobulin. This process occurs in the colloid at the microvillar surface of the follicular cells and is also catalyzed by thyroid peroxidase. Addition of one iodine atom to a single tyrosine residue forms ***monoiodotyrosine (MIT).*** Addition of a second iodine atom to the MIT residue forms a ***diiodotyrosine (DIT) residue.***
4. ***Formation of T_3 and T_4 by oxidative coupling reactions.*** The thyroid hormones are formed by oxidative coupling reactions of two iodinated tyrosine residues in close proximity. For example, when neighboring DIT and MIT residues undergo a coupling reaction, T_3 is formed; when two DIT residues react with each other, T_4 is formed. After iodination, T_4 and T_3 as well as the DIT and MIT residues that are still linked to a thyroglobulin molecule are stored as the colloid within the lumen of the follicle.
5. ***Resorption of colloid.*** In response to TSH, follicular cells take up thyroglobulin from the colloid by a process of receptor-mediated endocytosis. Large endocytotic vesicles called ***colloidal resorption droplets*** are present at this stage in the apical region of the follicular cells. They gradually migrate to the basal surface of the cells, where they fuse with lysosomes. Thyroglobulin is then degraded by lysosomal proteases into constituent amino acids and carbohydrates, leaving free T_4, T_3, DIT, and MIT molecules. If the levels of TSH remain high, the amount of colloid in the follicle is reduced because it is synthesized, secreted, iodinated, and resorbed too rapidly to accumulate.
6. ***Release of T_4 and T_3 into the circulation and recycling processes.*** T_4 and T_3 are liberated from thyroglobulin by lysosomal action in a T_4-to-T_3 ratio of 20:1. They cross the basal membrane and enter the blood and lymphatic capillaries. Most of the released hormones are immediately bound to either a specific plasma protein (54 kDa), ***thyroxin-binding protein*** (70%), or a nonspecific prealbumin fraction of serum protein (25%), leaving only small amounts (~5%) of free circulating hormones that are metabolically active. Only the follicular cells are capable of producing T_4, whereas most T_3, which is five times more active than T_4, is produced through conversion from T_4 by organs such as the kidney, liver, and heart. The free circulating hormones also function in the feedback system that regulates the secretory activity of the thyroid. Once uncoupled from thyroglobulin, DIT and MIT molecules are further deiodinated within the cytoplasm of the follicular cells to release the amino acid tyrosine and iodide, which are then available for recycling.

BOX 20.2

Functional Considerations: Feedback Control of Thyroid Hormone Synthesis

Synthesis of T_3 and T_4 is regulated by a simple feedback system. The secretion of thyroid hormones is controlled by the release of TSH from the anterior lobe of the pituitary gland into the bloodstream. Under the influence of TSH, thyroid follicular epithelial cells increase in size and activity. The cells become more columnar, and the iodide transporters and extracellular iodination of thyroglobulin are stimulated. In addition, thyroglobulin synthesis, endocytosis, and lysosomal breakdown increase, resulting in the release of large amounts of thyroid hormones. Low levels of free T_3 and T_4 initiate the release of TRH from the hypothalamus. In turn, TRH stimulates thyrotropes in the anterior lobe of the pituitary gland to secrete TSH. High serum levels of free T_3 and T_4 inhibit the synthesis and release of TSH.

Thyroid hormones play an essential role in normal fetal development

In humans, thyroid hormones are essential to normal growth and development. In normal pregnancy both T_3 and T_4 cross the placental barrier and are critical in the early stages of brain development. In addition, the fetal thyroid gland begins to function during the fourteenth week of gestation and also contributes additional thyroid hormones. Thyroid hormone deficiency during fetal development results in irreversible damage to the CNS, including reduced numbers of neurons, defective myelination, and mental retardation. If maternal thyroid deficiency is present prior to the development of the fetal thyroid gland, the mental retardation is severe. Recent studies reveal that thyroid hormones also stimulate gene expression for GH in the somatotropes. Therefore, in addition to neural abnormalities, a generalized stunted body growth is typical. The combination of these two abnormalities is called ***congenital hypothyroidism*** (cretinism).

BOX 20.3

Clinical Correlations: Abnormal Thyroid Function

The most common symptom of thyroid disease is a ***goiter***, the enlargement of the thyroid gland. It may indicate either hypothyroidism or hyperthyroidism.

Hypothyroidism can be caused by insufficient dietary iodine ***(iodine-deficiency goiter, endemic goiter)*** or by one of several inherited autoimmune diseases, such as ***Hashimoto's thyroiditis***. The low levels of circulating thyroid hormone stimulate release of excessive amounts of TSH, which cause hypertrophy of the thyroid through synthesis of more thyroglobulin. Adult hypothyroidism is called ***myxedema*** and is characterized by mental and physical sluggishness and edema of the connective tissue.

In ***hyperthyroidism (toxic goiter, Graves' disease)***, thyroid cells are stimulated and increase in number and size. However, there is little colloid. Thyroid hormones secreted at abnormally high rates cause an increase in metabolism. Often, toxic amounts of hormones are produced (thyrotoxicosis). Levels of TSH are usually normal in hyperthyroidism. In some cases, an abnormal immunoglobulin called long-acting thyroid stimulator (LATS) appears to bind to the TSH receptors on the follicular cells, which leads to continuous stimulation of the cells.

PARATHYROID GLANDS

The parathyroid glands are small endocrine glands closely associated with the thyroid. They are ovoid, a few millimeters in diameter, and arranged in two pairs, constituting the ***superior*** and ***inferior parathyroid glands***. They are usually located in the connective tissue on the posterior surface of the lateral lobes of the thyroid gland. However, the number and location may vary. In 2 to 10% of individuals, additional glands are associated with the thymus.

Structurally, each parathyroid gland is surrounded by a thin connective tissue capsule that separates it from the thyroid. Septa extend from the capsule into the gland to divide it into poorly defined lobules and to separate the densely packed cords of cells. The connective tissue is more evident in the adult, with the development of fat cells that increase with age and ultimately constitute as much as 60 to 70% of the glandular mass.

The glands receive their blood supply from the inferior thyroid arteries or from anastomoses between the superior and inferior thyroid arteries. Typical of endocrine glands, rich networks of fenestrated blood capillaries and lymphatic capillaries surround the parenchyma of the parathyroids.

Parathyroid glands develop from the endodermal cells derived from the third and fourth branchial pouches

Embryologically, the inferior parathyroid glands (and the thymus) are derived from the third branchial pouch; the superior glands, from the fourth branchial pouch. Normally, the inferior parathyroids separate from the thymus and come to lie below the superior parathyroids. Failure of these structures to separate results in the atypical association of the parathyroids with the thymus in the adult. The principal (chief) cells differentiate during embryonic development and are functionally active in regulating fetal calcium metabolism. The oxyphil cells differentiate later at puberty.

Principal cells and oxyphil cells constitute the epithelial cells of the parathyroid gland

- ***Principal (chief) cells***, the more numerous of the parenchymal cells of the parathyroid (Fig. 20.15), are re-

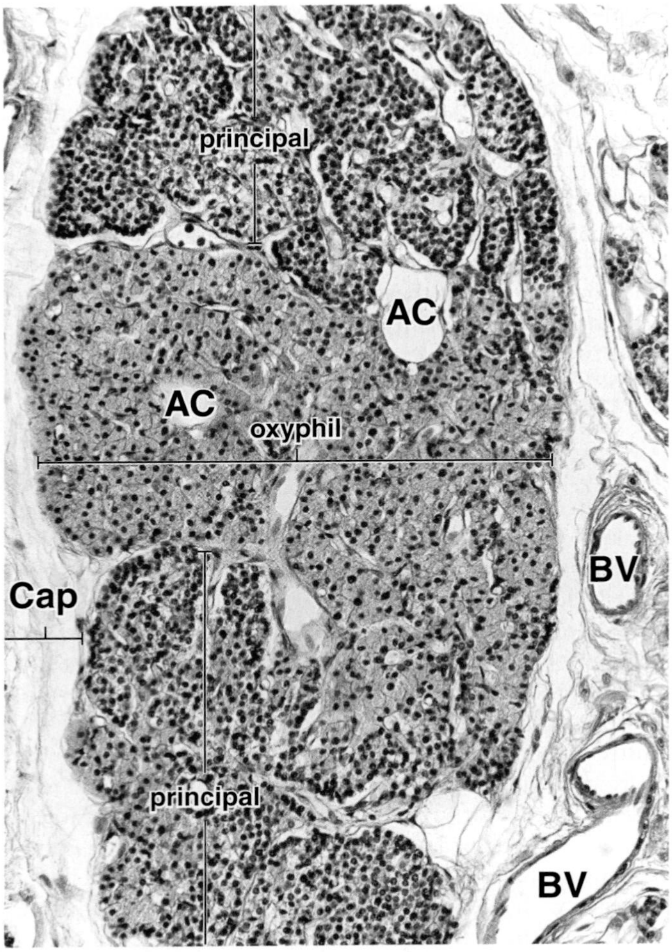

FIGURE 20.15
Photomicrograph of human parathyroid gland. This H&E–stained specimen shows the gland with part of its connective tissue capsule *(Cap)*. The blood vessels *(BV)* are located in the connective tissue septum between lobes of the gland. The principal cells are arranged in two masses *(top and bottom)* and are separated by a large cluster of oxyphil cells *(center)*. The oxyphil cells are the larger cell type with prominent eosinophilic cytoplasm. They may occur in small groups or in larger masses, as seen here. The principal cells are more numerous. They are smaller, having less cytoplasm, and consequently exhibit closer proximity of their nuclei. Adipose cells *(AC)* are present in variable, though limited, numbers. ×175.

sponsible for the secretion of PTH. They are small, polygonal cells, with a diameter of 7 to 10 μm and a centrally located nucleus. The pale-staining, slightly acidophilic cytoplasm contains lipofuscin-containing vesicles, large accumulations of glycogen, and lipid droplets. Small, dense, membrane-limited vesicles seen with the TEM or after using special stains with the light microscope are thought to be the storage form of PTH.

- ***Oxyphil cells*** constitute a minor portion of the parenchymal cells and are not known to have a secretory role. They are found singly or in clusters; the cells are more rounded, considerably larger than the principal cells, and have a distinctly acidophilic cytoplasm (see Fig. 20.15). Mitochondria, often with bizarre shapes and sizes, almost fill the cytoplasm and are responsible for the strong acidophilia of these cells. No secretory vesicles and little if any rER are present. Cytoplasmic inclusion bodies consist of occasional lysosomes, lipid droplets, and glycogen distributed among the mitochondria.

PTH regulates calcium and phosphate levels in the blood

The parathyroids function in the regulation of calcium and phosphate levels. ***PTH***, or ***parathormone***, is essential for life. Therefore, care must be taken during thyroidectomy to leave some functioning parathyroid tissue. If the glands are totally removed, death will ensue because muscles, including the laryngeal and other respiratory muscles, go into tetanic contraction as the blood calcium level falls.

PTH is an 84–amino acid linear peptide (Table 20.8). It binds to a specific PTH receptor on target cells that interacts with G protein to activate a second-messenger system. PTH release causes the level of calcium in the blood to increase. Simultaneously, it reduces the concentration of serum phosphate. Secretion of PTH is regulated by the serum calcium level through a simple feedback system. Low levels of serum calcium stimulate secretion of PTH; high levels of serum calcium inhibit its secretion.

PTH functions at several sites:

- ***Bone resorption*** is stimulated by PTH. The hormone activates osteolysis by osteoclasts during which calcium

TABLE 20.8. **Parathyroid Hormone**

Hormone	Composition	Source	Major Functions
Parathyroid hormone (parathormone, PTH)	Polypeptide containing 84 amino acids	Principal (chief cells)[A]	Increases blood calcium level in three ways: (1) promotes calcium release from bone (increases relative number of osteoclasts), (2) acts on kidney to stimulate calcium reabsorption by distal tubule while inhibiting phosphate reabsorption in the proximal tubule, (3) increases formation of hormonally active 1,25-dihydroxycholecalciferol (1,25-$(OH)_2$ vitamin D_3) in the kidney, which promotes tubular reabsorption of calcium

[A]Some evidence suggests that oxyphil cells, which first appear in the parathyroid gland at about 4 to 7 years of age and increase in number after puberty, may also produce PTH.

and phosphate are both released from calcified bone matrix into the extracellular fluid.

- ***Kidney excretion of calcium*** is decreased by PTH stimulation of tubular reabsorption, thus conserving calcium.
- ***Urinary phosphate excretion*** is increased by PTH secretion, thus lowering phosphate concentration in the blood and extracellular fluids.
- ***Kidney conversion of 25-OH vitamin*** D_3 to hormonally active ***1,25-(OH)***$_2$ ***vitamin*** D_3 is regulated primarily by PTH, which stimulates activity of 1-α-hydroxylase and increases the production of active hormone.
- ***Intestinal absorption of calcium*** is increased under the influence of PTH. Vitamin D_3, however, has a greater effect than PTH on intestinal absorption of calcium.

PTH and calcitonin have reciprocal effects in the regulation of blood calcium levels

Although PTH increases blood calcium levels, the peak increase following its release is not reached for several hours. PTH appears to have a rather slow, long-term homeostatic action. Calcitonin, however, rapidly lowers blood calcium levels and has its peak effect in about 1 hour; therefore, it has a rapid, acute homeostatic action.

▼ ADRENAL GLANDS

The *adrenal (suprarenal) glands* secrete both steroid hormones and catecholamines. They have a flattened triangular shape and are embedded in the perirenal fat at the superior poles of the kidneys.

The adrenal glands are covered with a thick connective tissue capsule from which trabeculae extend into the parenchyma, carrying blood vessels and nerves. The secretory parenchymal tissue is organized into *cortical* and *medullary* regions (Fig 20.16):

- The *cortex* is the steroid-secreting portion. It lies beneath the capsule and constitutes nearly 90% of the gland by weight.
- The *medulla* is the catecholamine-secreting portion. It lies deep to the cortex and forms the center of the gland.

Parenchymal cells of the cortex and medulla are of different embryologic origin

Embryologically, the cortical cells originate from mesodermal mesenchyme, whereas the medulla originates from neural crest cells that migrate into the developing gland (Fig. 20.17). Although embryologically distinct, the two portions of the adrenal gland are functionally related (see below). The parenchymal cells of the adrenal cortex are controlled, in part, by the anterior lobe of the pituitary gland and function in regulating metabolism and maintaining normal electrolyte balance (Table 20.9).

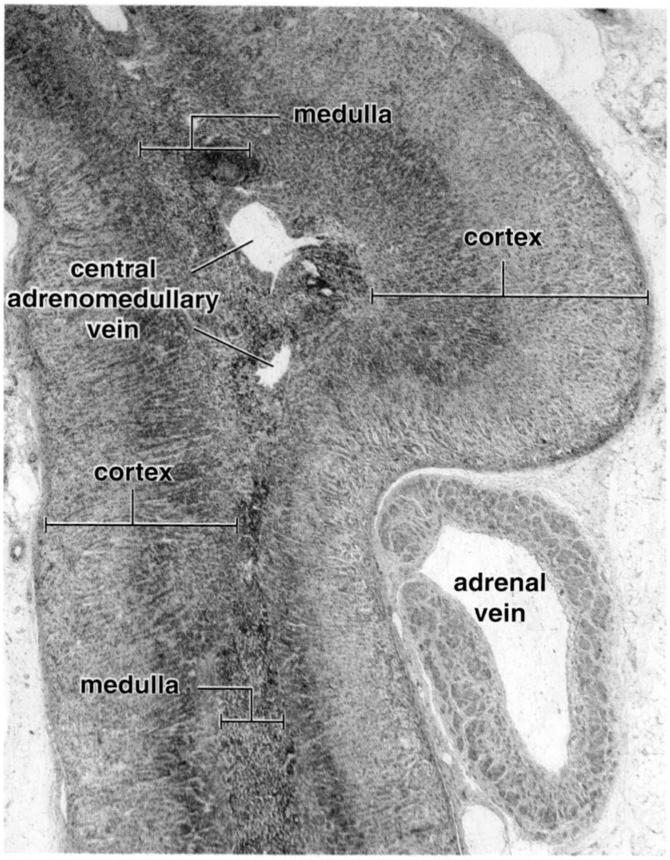

FIGURE 20.16
Photomicrograph of the adrenal gland. This low-power micrograph of a H&E–stained specimen shows the full thickness of the adrenal gland with the cortex seen on both surfaces and a central region containing the medulla. Within the medulla are profiles of the central vein. Note that the deeper portion of the cortex stains darker than the outer portion, a reflection of the washed-out lipid in the zona glomerulosa and outer region of the zona fasciculata. This section also includes a cross section of the adrenal vein, which is characterized by the longitudinally arranged bundles of smooth muscle in its wall. ×20.

Blood Supply

The adrenal glands are supplied with blood by the superior, middle, and inferior suprarenal arteries. These vessels branch before entering the capsule, to produce many small arteries that penetrate the capsule. In the capsule, the arteries branch to give rise to three principal patterns of blood distribution (Figs. 20.18 and 20.19). The vessels form a system that consists of

- *Capsular capillaries* that supply the capsule
- *Fenestrated cortical sinusoidal capillaries* that supply the cortex and then drain into the fenestrated medullary capillary sinusoids
- *Medullary arterioles* that traverse the cortex, traveling within the trabeculae, and bring arterial blood to the *medullary capillary sinusoids*

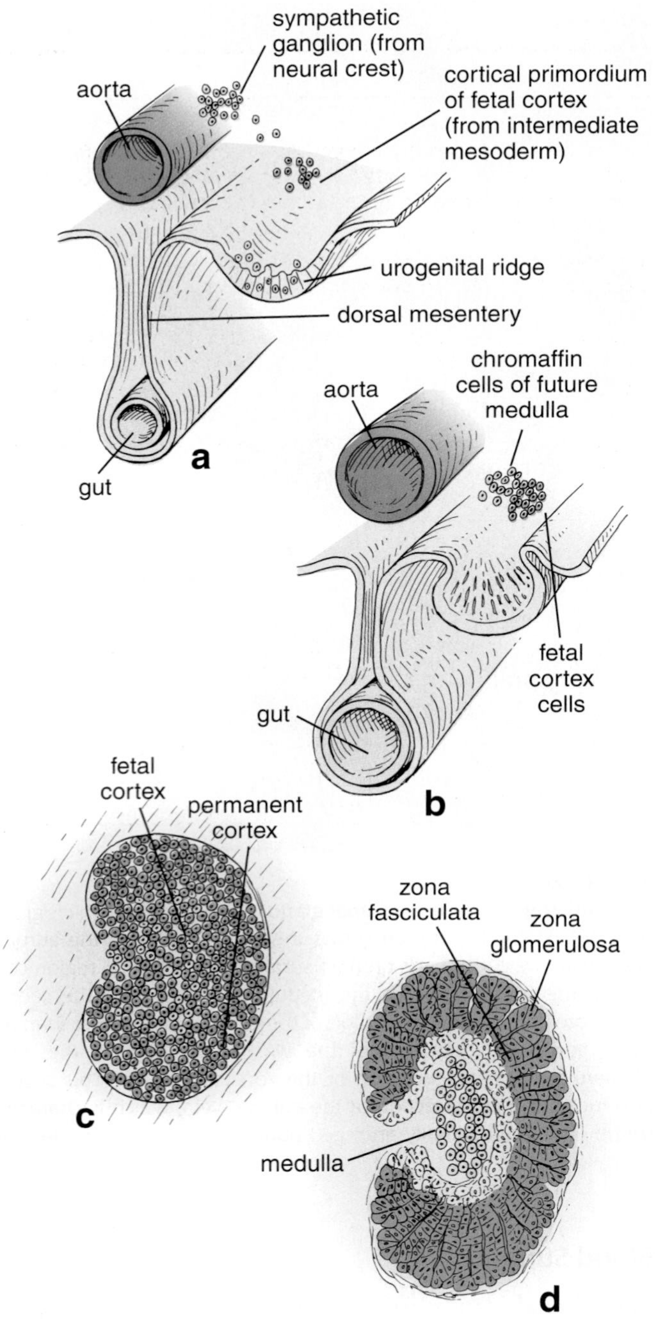

FIGURE 20.17
Development of the adrenal gland. a. In this early stage, the cortex is shown developing from cells of the intermediate mesoderm, and the medulla is shown differentiating from cells in the neural crest and migrating from the neighboring sympathetic ganglion. Note that the gland develops between the root of the dorsal mesentery of the primitive gut and the developing urogenital ridges. **b.** Mesodermal cells from the fetal cortex surround the cells of the developing medulla. **c.** At this stage (about 7 months of development), the fetal cortex occupies about 70% of the cortex. The permanent cortex develops outside the fetal cortex. **d.** The fully developed adrenal cortex is visible at the age of 4 months. The permanent cortex replaces the fetal cortex, which at this age has completely disappeared. Note the fully developed zonation of the permanent cortex.

The medulla thus has a dual blood supply: arterial blood from the medullary arterioles and "venous" blood from the cortical sinusoidal capillaries that have already supplied the cortex. The venules that arise from the cortical and medullary sinusoids drain into the small ***adrenomedullary collecting veins*** that join to form the large ***central adrenomedullary vein***, which then drains directly into the inferior vena cava on the right side and into the left renal vein on the left side. In humans, the central adrenomedullary vein and its tributaries are unusual in that they have a tunica media containing conspicuous, longitudinally oriented bundles of smooth muscle cells. Synchronous contraction of longitudinal smooth muscle bundles along the central adrenomedullary vein and its tributaries cause the volume of the adrenal gland to decrease . This volume decrease enhances the efflux of hormones from the adrenal medulla into the circulation, an action comparable to squeezing a wet sponge.

Lymphatic vessels are present in the capsule and the connective tissue around the larger blood vessels in the gland. Lymphatic vessels have also been demonstrated in the parenchyma of the adrenal medulla. Recent physiologic studies indicate an important role of the lymph vessels in distributing high-molecular-weight secretory products of chromaffin cells, such as chromogranin A, into the circulation.

Cells of the Adrenal Medulla

Chromaffin cells located in the adrenal medulla are innervated by preganglionic sympathetic neurons

The central portion of the adrenal gland, the ***medulla***, is composed of a parenchyma of large, pale-staining epithelioid cells called ***chromaffin cells (medullary cells)***; connective tissue; numerous sinusoidal blood capillaries; and nerves. The chromaffin cells are, in effect, modified neurons (see Box 20.4). Numerous myelinated, preganglionic sympathetic nerve fibers pass directly to the chromaffin cells of the medulla. When nerve impulses carried by the sympathetic fibers reach the catecholamine-secreting chromaffin cells, they release their secretory products. Therefore, chromaffin cells are considered the equivalent of postganglionic neurons. However, they lack axonal processes. Experimental studies reveal that when chromaffin cells are grown in culture, they extend axon-like processes. However, axonal growth can be inhibited by glucocorticoids—hormones secreted by the adrenal cortex. Thus, the hormones of the adrenal cortex exert control over the morphology of the chromaffin cells and prevent them from forming neural processes. Chromaffin cells therefore more closely resemble typical endocrine cells, in that their secretory product enters the bloodstream via the fenestrated capillaries.

Ganglion cells are also present in the medulla. Their axons extend peripherally to the parenchyma of the adrenal cortex to modulate its secretory activity and innervate

TABLE 20.9. **Hormones of the Adrenal Glands**

Hormone	Composition	Source	Major Functions
Adrenal cortex			
Mineralocorticoids (95% of mineralocorticoid activity in aldosterone)	Steroid hormones (cholesterol derivatives)	Parenchymal cells of the zona glomerulosa	Aid in controlling electrolyte homeostasis (act on distal tubule of kidney to increase sodium reabsorption and decrease potassium reabsorption); function in maintaining the osmotic balance in the urine and in preventing serum acidosis
Glucocorticoids (corticosterone, and cortisol; 95% of glucocorticoid activity in cortisol)	Steroid hormones (cholesterol derivatives)	Parenchymal cells of the zona fasciculata (and to a lesser extent of the zona reticularis)	Promote normal metabolism, particularly carbohydrate metabolism (increase rate of amino acid transport to liver, promote removal of protein from skeletal muscle and its transport to the liver, reduce rate of glucose metabolism by cells and stimulate glycogen synthesis by liver, stimulate mobilization of fats from storage deposits for energy use); provide resistance to stress; suppress inflammatory response and some allergic reactions
Gonadocorticoids (dehydroepiandrosterone [DHEA] is a major sex steroid produced in both men and women)	Steroid hormones (cholesterol derivatives)	Parenchymal cells of the zona reticularis (and to a lesser extent of the zona fasciculata)	Induce weak masculinizing effect; at normal serum levels usually their function is insignificant
Adrenal medulla			
Norepinephrine and epinephrine (in human, 80% epinephrine)	Catecholamines (amino acid derivatives)	Chromaffin cells	Sympathomimetic (produce effects similar to those induced by the sympathetic division of the autonomic nervous system)[A]: increase heart rate, increase blood pressure, reduce blood flow to viscera and skin; stimulate conversion of glycogen to glucose; increase sweating; induce dilation of bronchioles; increase rate of respiration; decrease digestion; decrease enzyme production by digestive system glands; decrease urine production

[A]The catecholamines influence the activity of glandular epithelium, cardiac muscle, and smooth muscle located in the walls of blood vessels and viscera.

blood vessels, and extend outside the gland to the splanchnic nerves innervating abdominal organs.

Chromaffin cells of the adrenal medulla have a secretory function

Chromaffin cells are organized in ovoid clusters and short interconnecting cords. The blood capillaries are arranged in intimate relation to the parenchyma. They originate either from the cortical capillaries or, as branches, from the cortical arterioles.

Ultrastructurally, the chromaffin cells are characterized by numerous secretory vesicles with diameters of 100 to 300 nm, profiles of rER, and a well-developed Golgi apparatus. The secretory material in the vesicles can be stained specifically to demonstrate histochemically that the catecholamines epinephrine and norepinephrine secreted by the chromaffin cells are produced by different cell types (Fig. 20.20). The TEM also reveals two populations of

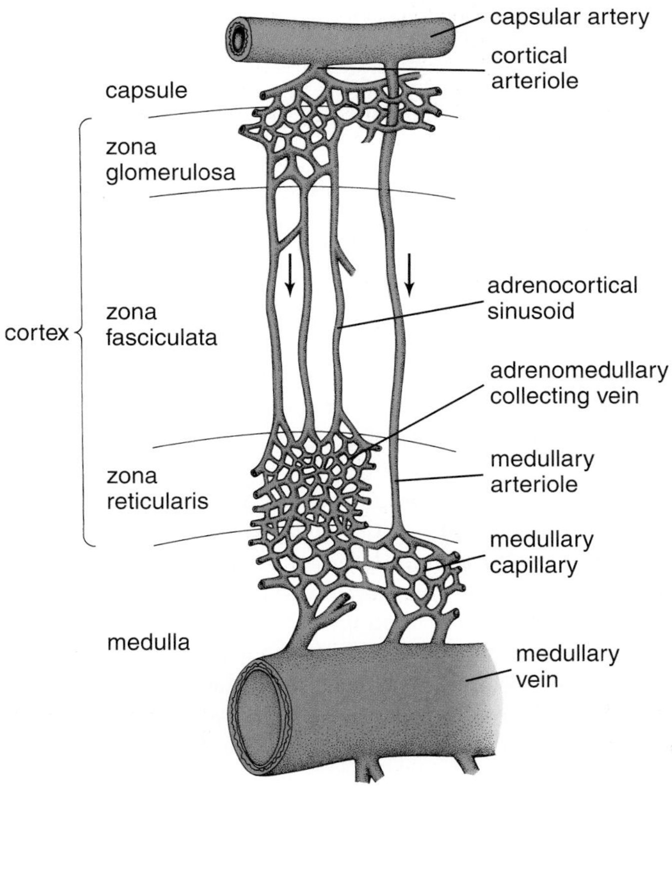

FIGURE 20.18
Diagram illustrating the blood supply to the human adrenal gland. The region of the capsule, the zones within the cortex, and the medulla are indicated. (Modified from Warwick R, Williams PL, eds. *Gray's Anatomy*. 35th ed. Edinburgh: Churchill Livingstone, 1973.)

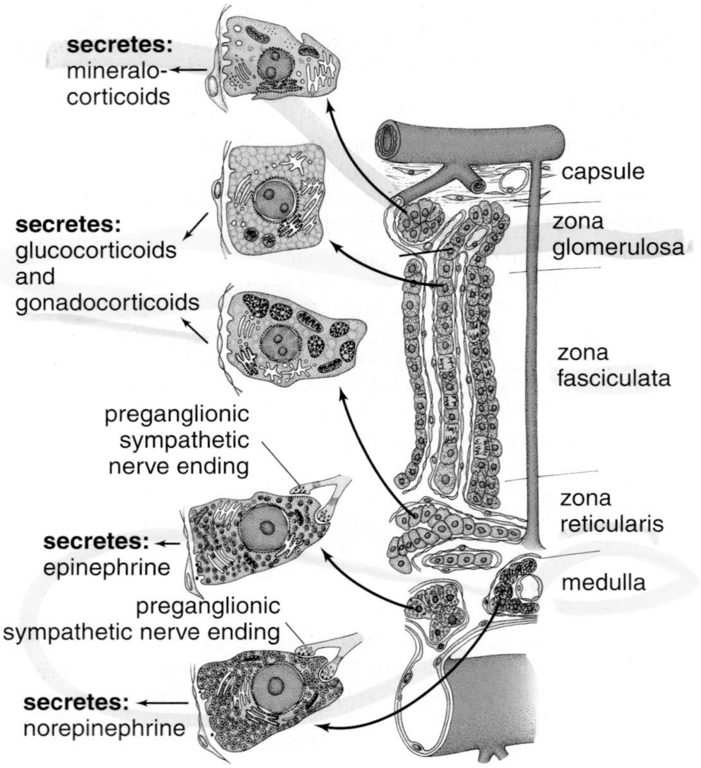

FIGURE 20.19
Diagram illustrating the organization of the cells within the adrenal gland and their relationship to the blood vessels. Refer to Figure 20.18 for identification of the blood vessels. The ultrastructural features of the basic cell types and their secretions are noted. (Modified from Warwick R, Williams PL, eds. *Gray's Anatomy.* 35th ed. Edinburgh: Churchill Livingstone, 1973.)

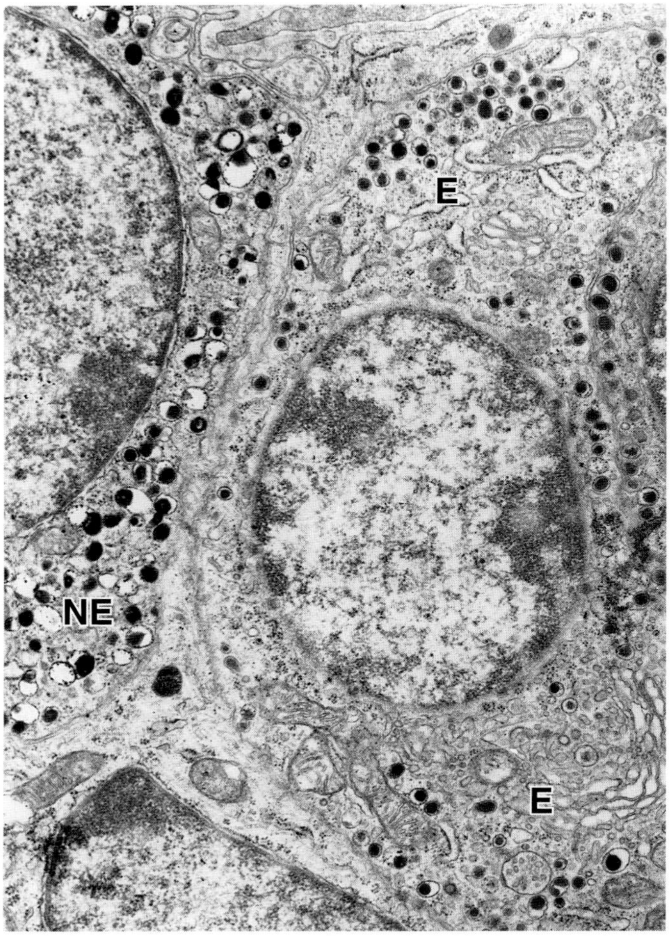

FIGURE 20.20
Electron micrograph of medullary cells. Two types of medullary cells are present. The norepinephrine-secreting cells *(NE)* are identified by their vesicles, which contain a very dense core. The epinephrine-secreting cells *(E)* possess vesicles with less intensely staining granules. ×15,000.

chromaffin cells distinguished by the nature of their membrane-bounded vesicles:

- One population of cells contains only large ***dense core vesicles.*** These cells secrete norepinephrine.
- The other population of cells contains vesicles that are smaller, more homogeneous, and less dense. These cells secrete epinephrine.

Exocytosis of the secretory vesicles is triggered by release of acetylcholine from preganglionic sympathetic axons that synapse with each chromaffin cell

Epinephrine and norepinephrine account for less than 20% of the contents of the medullary secretory vesicles. The vesicles also contain large amounts of soluble 48-kDa proteins, called ***chromogranins,*** that appear to impart the density to the vesicle contents. These proteins, along with ATP and Ca^{2+}, may help to bind the low-molecular-weight catecholamines and are released with the hormones during exocytosis. The catecholamines, synthesized in the cytosol, are transported into the vesicles through the action of a magnesium-activated ATPase in the membrane of the vesicle. Drugs such as ***reserpine,*** which cause depletion of catecholamines from the vesicles, may act by inhibiting this transport mechanism.

Glucocorticoids secreted in the cortex induce the conversion of norepinephrine to epinephrine in chromaffin cells

Glucocorticoids produced in the adrenal cortex reach the medulla directly through the continuity of the cortical and medullary sinusoidal capillaries. They induce the enzyme that catalyzes the methylation of norepinephrine to produce epinephrine. The nature of the blood flow correlates with regional differences in distribution of norepinephrine- and epinephrine-containing chromaffin cells. The epinephrine-containing cells are more numerous in ar-

eas of the medulla supplied with blood that has passed through the cortical sinusoids and thus contains secreted glucocorticoids. In some species, the norepinephrine-containing cells are more numerous in those regions of the medulla supplied by capillaries derived from the cortical arterioles.

The catecholamines, in concert with the glucocorticoids, prepare the body for the "fight-or-flight" response

The sudden release of catecholamines establishes conditions for maximum use of energy and thus maximum physical effort. Both epinephrine and norepinephrine stimulate glycogenolysis (release glucose into the bloodstream) and mobilization of free fatty acids from adipose tissue. The release of catecholamines also causes an increase in blood pressure, dilation of the coronary blood vessels, vasodilation of vessels supplying skeletal muscle, vasoconstriction of vessels conveying blood to the skin and gut, an increase in heart rate and output, and an increase in the rate and depth of breathing.

Zonation of the Adrenal Cortex

The adrenal cortex is divided into three zones on the basis of the arrangement of its cells (Fig. 20.21):

- ***Zona glomerulosa,*** the narrow outer zone that constitutes up to 15% of the cortical volume
- ***Zona fasciculata,*** the thick middle zone that constitutes nearly 80% of the cortical volume
- ***Zona reticularis,*** the inner zone that constitutes only 5 to 7% of the cortical volume but is thicker than the glomerulosa because of its more central location

ZONA GLOMERULOSA

The cells of the ***zona glomerulosa*** are arranged in closely packed ovoid clusters and curved columns that are continuous with the cellular cords in the zona fasciculata. Cells of the zona glomerulosa are relatively small and columnar or pyramidal. Their spherical nuclei appear closely packed and stain densely. In humans, some areas of the cortex may lack a recognizable zona glomerulosa. A rich network of fenestrated sinusoidal capillaries surrounds each cell cluster. The cells have abundant smooth-surfaced endoplasmic reticulum (sER), multiple Golgi complexes, large mitochondria with shelf-like cristae, free ribosomes, and some rER. Lipid droplets are sparse.

The zona glomerulosa secretes aldosterone that functions in the control of blood pressure

The cells of the zona glomerulosa secrete ***mineralocorticoids,*** compounds that function in the regulation of sodium and potassium homeostasis and water balance. The principal secretion, ***aldosterone,*** acts on the distal tubules of the nephron in the kidney, the gastric mucosa, and the salivary and sweat glands to stimulate resorption of sodium at these sites, as well as to stimulate excretion of potassium by the kidney.

> **BOX 20.4**
>
> **Functional Considerations: Chromaffin Cells**
>
> Chromaffin cells (so named because they react with chromate salts) of the adrenal medulla are part of the amine precursor uptake and decarboxylation (APUD) system of cells. The chromaffin reaction is thought to involve oxidation and polymerization of the catecholamines contained within the secretory vesicles of these cells. Classically, chromaffin cells have been defined as being derived from neuroectoderm, innervated by preganglionic sympathetic nerve fibers, and capable of synthesizing and secreting catecholamines. Chromaffin cells are found in the adrenal medulla, paravertebral and prevertebral sympathetic ganglia, and various other locations. The scattered groups of chromaffin cells located among or near the components of the autonomic nervous system are called ***paraganglia.***

The renin–angiotensin–aldosterone system provides feedback control of the zona glomerulosa

The zona glomerulosa is under feedback control of the ***renin–angiotensin–aldosterone system.*** The juxtaglomerular cells in the kidney release renin in response to a decrease in blood pressure or a low blood sodium level. Circulating renin catalyzes the conversion of circulating ***angiotensinogen*** to ***angiotensin I,*** which in turn is converted by angiotensin-converting enzyme (ACE) in the lung to ***angiotensin II.*** Angiotensin II then stimulates the cells of the zona glomerulosa to secrete aldosterone. As the blood pressure, sodium concentration, and blood volume then increase in response to aldosterone, release of renin from the juxtaglomerular cells is inhibited. Drugs that inhibit ACE in the lung are effective in the treatment of chronic essential hypertension.

ZONA FASCICULATA

The cells of the ***zona fasciculata*** are large and polyhedral. They are arranged in long straight cords, one or two cells thick, that are separated by sinusoidal capillaries. The cells of the zona fasciculata have a lightly staining spherical nucleus. Binucleate cells are common in this zone. TEM studies reveal characteristics typical of steroid-secreting cells, i.e., a highly developed sER (more so than cells of the zona glomerulosa) and mitochondria with tubular cristae. They

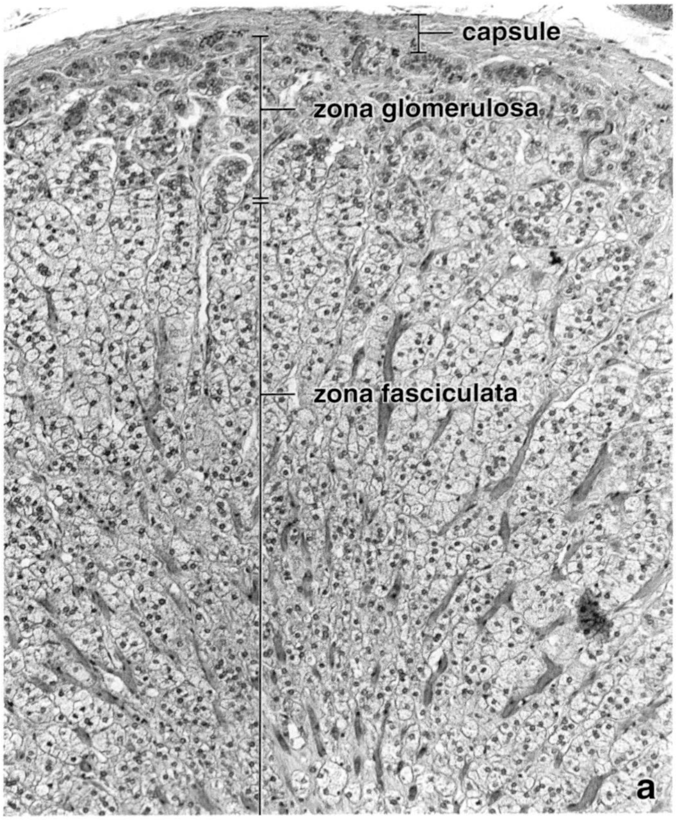

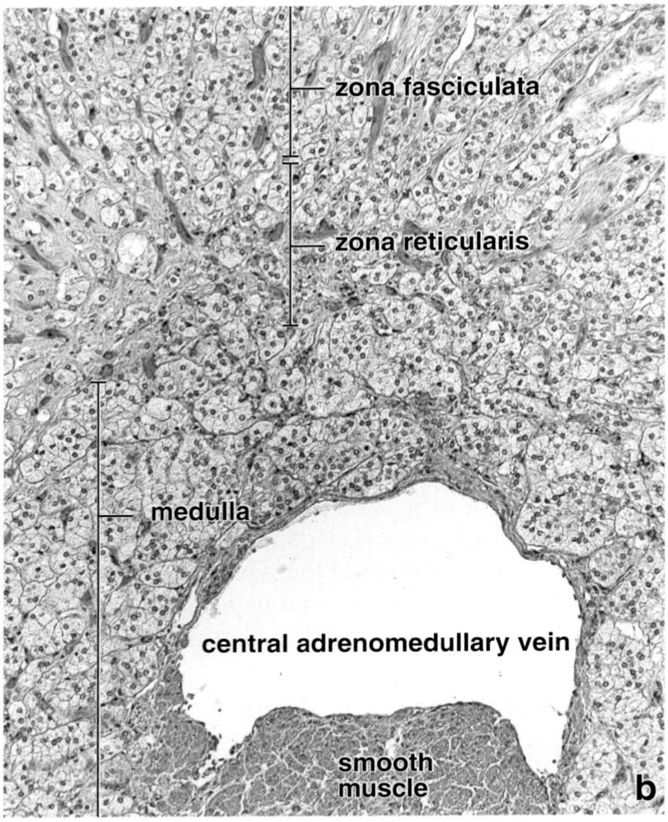

FIGURE 20.21
Photomicrographs of the cortex and medulla of the human adrenal gland. a. This photomicrograph shows a H&E–stained specimen of the outer cortex. It includes the connective tissue capsule, the zona glomerulosa, and the zona fasciculata. Continuous with the zona glomerulosa are the straight cords of cells that characterize the zona fasciculata. Between the cords are the capillaries and the less numerous arterioles. The red linear stripes represent capillaries that are engorged with red blood cells. ×120. **b.** The deep parts of the zona fasciculata, zona reticularis, and medulla are shown here. Note that the linear arrays of the cords in the zona fasciculata give way to irregular groups of cells of the zona reticularis. The medulla, in contrast, consists of ovoid groups of cells and short interconnecting cords of cells. A central adrenomedullary vein is also seen here. Note the thick longitudinally sectioned smooth muscle in part of its wall. ×120.

also have a well-developed Golgi apparatus and numerous profiles of rER that may give a slight basophilia to some parts of the cytoplasm (Fig. 20.22). In general, however, the cytoplasm is acidophilic and contains numerous lipid droplets, although it usually appears vacuolated in routine histologic sections because of the extraction of lipid during dehydration. The lipid droplets contain neutral fats, fatty acids, cholesterol, and phospholipids that are precursors for the steroid hormones secreted by these cells.

The principal secretion of the zona fasciculata is glucocorticoids that regulate glucose and fatty acid metabolism

The zona fasciculata secretes ***glucocorticoids***, so called because of their role in regulating ***gluconeogenesis (glucose synthesis)*** and ***glycogenesis (glycogen polymerization)***. One of the glucocorticoids secreted by the zona fasciculata, ***cortisol (hydrocortisone)***, acts on many different cells and tissues to increase the metabolic availability of glucose and fatty acids, both of which are immediate sources of energy. Within this broad function, glucocorticoids may have different, even opposite effects in different tissues:

- ***In the liver***, glucocorticoids stimulate conversion of amino acids to glucose, stimulate the polymerization of glucose to glycogen, and promote the uptake of amino acids and fatty acids.
- ***In adipose tissue***, glucocorticoids stimulate the breakdown of lipids to glycerol and free fatty acids.
- ***In other tissues***, they reduce the rate of glucose use and promote the oxidation of fatty acids.
- ***In cells*** such as fibroblasts, they inhibit protein synthesis and even promote protein catabolism to provide amino acids for conversion to glucose in the liver.

Glucocorticoids depress the immune and inflammatory responses and, as a result of the latter, inhibit wound healing. They depress the inflammatory response by suppress-

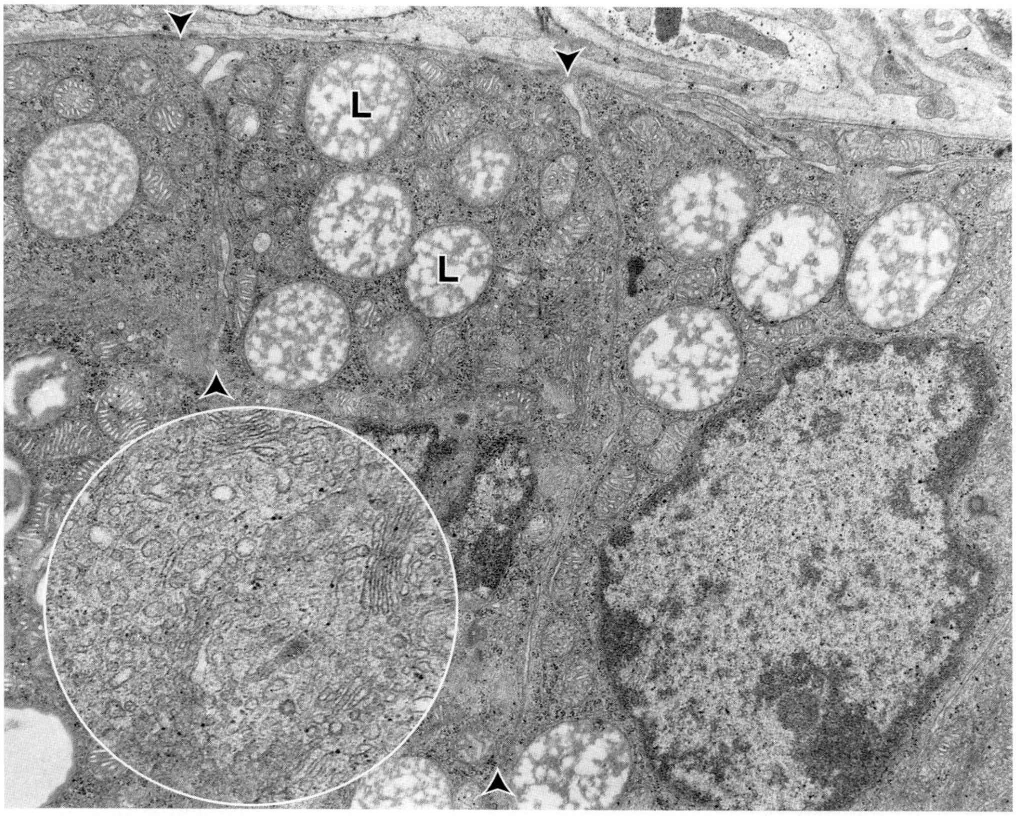

FIGURE 20.22
Electron micrograph of cells in the zona fasciculata. The boundary between adjacent cells of the cord is indicated by the *arrowheads.* Lipid droplets *(L)* are numerous (the lipid has been partially extracted). ×15,000. **Inset.** A higher magnification of an area in the cell at the top of the micrograph reveals the extensive sER that is characteristic of steroid-secreting cells. Portions of the Golgi apparatus are also evident. ×40,000.

ing interleukin-1 (IL-1) and IL-2 production by lymphocytes and macrophages. Glucocorticoids also stimulate destruction of lymphocytes in lymph nodes and inhibit mitosis by transformed lymphoblasts. Cells of the zona fasciculata also secrete small amounts of gonadocorticoids, principally androgens.

ACTH regulates secretion of the zona fasciculata

The secretion and production of glucocorticoids and sex steroids by the zona fasciculata is under feedback control of the CRH–ACTH system. ACTH is necessary for cell growth and maintenance and also stimulates steroid synthesis and increases blood flow through the adrenal gland. Exogenous ACTH maintains the structure and function of the zona fasciculata after hypophysectomy. In animals, administration of ACTH causes hypertrophy of the zona fasciculata.

Circulating glucocorticoids may act directly on the pituitary gland, but they most commonly exert their feedback control on neurons in the arcuate nucleus of the hypothalamus, causing the release of CRH into the hypothalamohypophyseal portal circulation. Evidence also suggests that circulating glucocorticoids and the physiologic effects that they produce stimulate higher brain centers that, in turn, cause the hypothalamic neurons to release CRH.

ZONA RETICULARIS

The zona reticularis produces glucocorticoids and androgens

The cells of the ***zona reticularis*** are noticeably smaller than those of the zona fasciculata, and their nuclei are more deeply stained. They are arranged in anastomosing cords separated by fenestrated capillaries. The cells have relatively few lipid droplets. Both light and dark cells are seen. Dark cells have abundant large lipofuscin pigment granules, and deeply staining nuclei are evident. The cells in this zone are small because they have less cytoplasm than the cells in the zona fasciculata; thus the nuclei appear more closely packed. They exhibit features of steroid-secreting cells, namely, a well-developed sER and numerous elongated mitochondria with tubular cristae, but they have little rER.

The principal secretions of the zona reticularis are weak androgens

The principal secretion of the cells in the zona reticularis consists of weak androgens, mostly ***dehydroepiandrosterone (DHEA)***. The cells also secrete some glucocorticoids, in much smaller amounts than those of the zona fasciculata. Here, too, the principal glucocorticoid secreted is cortisol.

BOX 20.5

Functional Considerations: Cholesterol

Cholesterol is the basic precursor of corticosteroid hormones. It is synthesized from cholesterol esters stored in lipid droplets within the cytoplasm of adrenal cortical cells. Steroid hormones are synthesized from cholesterol esters by removal of part of the side chain and modifications at specific sites on the remainder of the molecule. The enzymes catalyzing these modifications are located in different zones of the cortex as well as in different cytoplasmic sites within the cells. A precursor molecule may move from the sER to a mitochondrion and back again several times before the definitive molecular structure of a given corticosteroid is obtained.

Cholesterol esters removed from cytoplasmic lipid droplets and used in steroid hormone synthesis are quickly replenished from the cholesterol esters contained within ***low-density lipoproteins (LDLs)*** carried in the bloodstream. These esters are the primary source of the cholesterol used in corticosteroid synthesis. In addition, a small portion of cholesterol used for hormone synthesis comes from de novo synthesis of cholesterol by the adrenal cortical cells. Under conditions of short-term or prolonged ACTH stimulation, the lipid stores in adrenal cortical cells are recruited for corticosteroid synthesis.

The zona reticularis is also under feedback control of the CRH–ACTH system and atrophies after hypophysectomy. Exogenous ACTH maintains the structure and function of the zona reticularis after hypophysectomy.

Fetal Adrenal Gland

The fetal adrenal gland consists of an outer narrow permanent cortex and an inner thick fetal cortex or fetal zone

Once fully established, the fetal adrenal gland is unusual in terms of its organization and its large size relative to other developing organs. The gland arises from mesodermal cells located between the root of the mesentery and the developing gonad zone (see Fig. 20.17a). The mesodermal cells penetrate the underlying mesenchyme and give rise to a large eosinophilic cell mass that will become the functional fetal cortex or zone (see Fig. 20.17b). Later, a second wave of cells proliferates from the mesenchyme and surrounds the primary cell mass (see Fig. 20.17c). By the fourth fetal month, the adrenal gland reaches its maximum mass in terms of body weight and is only slightly smaller than the adjacent kidney. At term, the adrenal glands are equivalent in size and weight to those of the adult and produce 100 to 200 mg of steroid compounds per day, about twice that of the adult adrenals.

The histologic appearance of the fetal adrenal gland is superficially similar to that of the adult adrenal gland. During late fetal life, most of the gland consists of cords of large eosinophilic cells that constitute approximately 80% of its mass. This portion of the gland, referred to as the ***fetal cortex (zone),*** arises from the initial mesodermal cell migration. The remainder of the gland is composed of the peripheral layer of small cells with scanty cytoplasm. This portion, referred to as the ***permanent cortex,*** arises from the secondary mesodermal cell migration. The narrow permanent cortex, when fully established in the embryo, appears similar to the adult zona glomerulosa. The cells are arranged in arched groups that extend into short cords. They, in turn, become continuous with the cords of the underlying fetal zone (Fig. 20.23). In H&E preparations, the cytoplasm of the cells in the permanent cortex exhibits some basophilia; in combination with the closely packed nuclei, this gives this part of the gland a blue appearance, in contrast to the eosinophilic staining of the fetal zone.

With the TEM, the cells of the permanent cortex exhibit small mitochondria with shelf-like cristae, abundant ribosomes, and small Golgi profiles. The cells of the fetal zone, in contrast, are considerably larger and are arranged in irregular cords of varying width. With the TEM, these cells exhibit spherical mitochondria with tubular cristae, small lipid droplets, an extensive sER that accounts for the eosinophilia of the cytoplasm, and multiple Golgi profiles. Collectively, these features are characteristic of steroid-secreting cells.

The fetal adrenal lacks a definitive medulla. Chromaffin cells are present but are scattered among the cells of the fetal zone and are difficult to recognize in H&E preparations. The chromaffin cells originate from the neural crest (see Fig. 20.17a) and invade the fetal zone at the time of its formation (see Fig. 20.17b). They remain in this location in small, scattered cell clusters during fetal life (see Fig. 20.17c).

The blood supply to both the permanent cortex and the fetal zone is through sinusoidal capillaries that course between the cords and join to form larger venous channels in the center of the gland. Unlike the postnatal adrenal, arterioles are absent in the parenchyma of the fetal adrenal gland.

Functionally, the fetal adrenal gland is under the control of the CRH–ACTH feedback system through the fetal pituitary. It interacts with the placenta to function as a steroid-secreting organ because it lacks certain enzymes necessary for steroid synthesis that are present in the placenta. Similarly, the placenta lacks certain en-

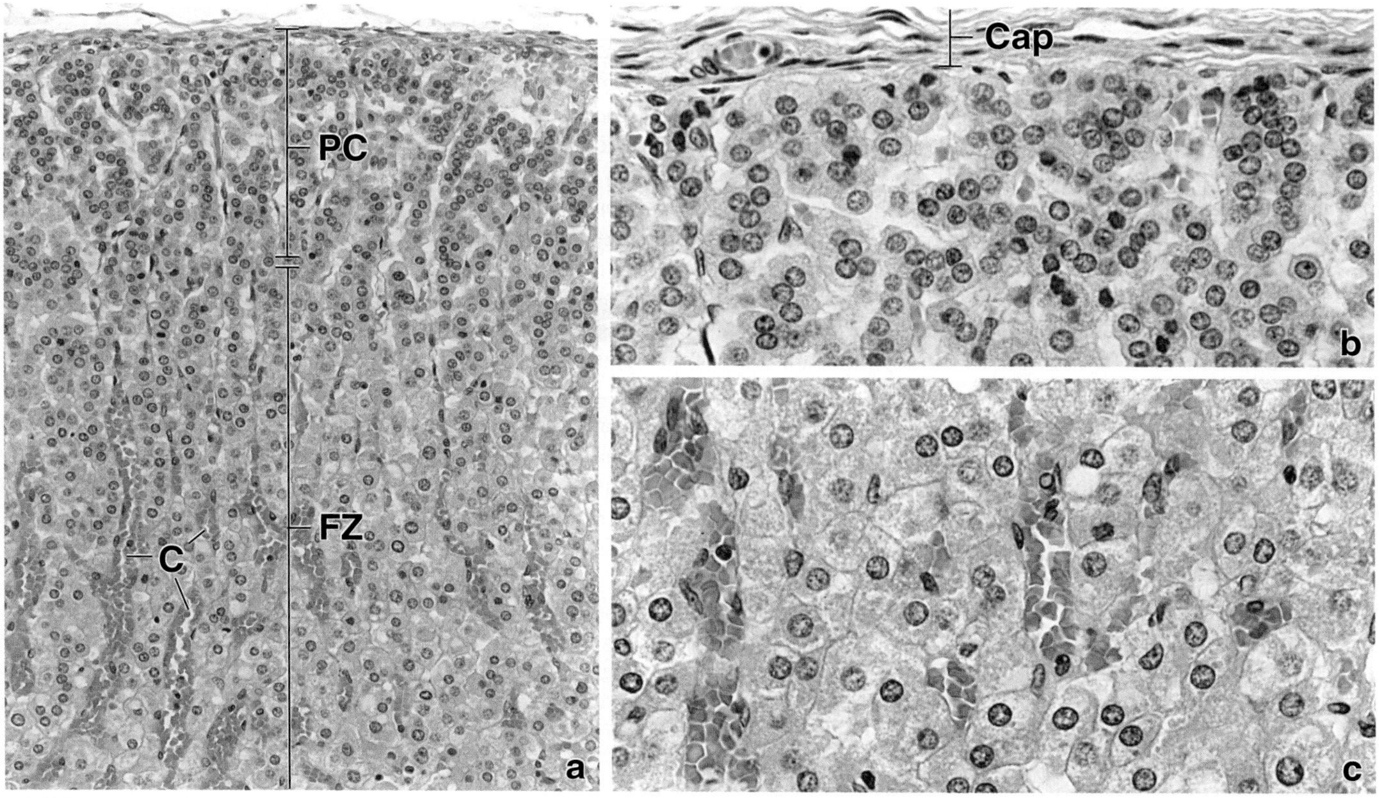

FIGURE 20.23
Photomicrographs of a human fetal adrenal gland. a. Low-power micrograph of a H&E–strained section of a fetal adrenal gland. The permanent cortex *(PC)* is indicated in the upper portion of the micrograph. Below is the fetal zone *(FZ)* in which the cells are arranged in anastomosing linear cords. Some of the capillaries *(C)* are engorged with red blood cells, thereby making them more apparent. ×100. **b.** Higher-power micrograph of the same specimen showing the capsule *(Cap)* and the underlying permanent cortex. The cells are arranged in arched groups that extend into short cords. Note the close proximity of the nuclei and the small amount of cytoplasm in these cells. ×200. **c.** This micrograph shows the cells of the fetal zone at the same magnification as in *b*. Note the slightly larger size of the nuclei and the considerable amount of cytoplasm in each of the fetal zone cells. Also note the eosinophilia of the cytoplasm, compared with the more basophilic cytoplasm of the cells of the permanent cortex. ×200. (Original specimen courtesy of Dr. William H. Donnelly.)

zymes necessary for steroid synthesis that are present in the fetal adrenal gland. Thus, the fetal adrenal gland is part of a ***fetal-placental unit***. Precursor molecules are transported back and forth between the two organs to enable synthesis of glucocorticoids, aldosterone, androgens, and estrogens.

At birth, the fetal cortex undergoes a rapid involution that reduces the gland within the first postnatal month to about a quarter of its previous size. The permanent cortex grows and matures to form the characteristic zonation of the adult cortex. With the involution and disappearance of the fetal zone cells, the chromaffin cells aggregate to form the medulla.

PLATE 76. PITUITARY I

The pituitary gland is located in a bony fossa in the floor of the cranial cavity. It is connected by a stalk to the base of the brain. Although joined to the brain, only part of the gland, the *neurohypophysis,* develops from the neural ectoderm. The larger part of the pituitary, the *adenohypophysis,* develops from oral ectoderm as a diverticulum of the buccal epithelium, called *Rathke's pouch.*

The adenohypophysis regulates other endocrine glands. It is composed of clumps and cords of epithelioid cells, separated by large-diameter fenestrated capillaries. The neurohypophysis is a nerve tract whose terminals store and release secretory products synthesized by their cell bodies in the *supraoptic* and *paraventricular nuclei.* The secretions contain either *oxytocin* or *vasopressin* (*antidiuretic hormone* [ADH]). Other neurons from the hypothalamus release secretions into the fenestrated capillaries of the infundibulum, the first capillary bed of the *hypophyseal portal system* that carries blood to the fenestrated capillaries of the adenohypophysis. These hypothalamic secretions regulate the activity of the adenohypophysis.

Figure 1, pituitary, human, H&E ×50.

This specimen is a sagittal section of the pituitary gland. The neurohypophysis, the posterior lobe of the gland, is delineated by the *dashed line* (indicated by *arrows)* that separates it from the adenohypophysis. The pars nervosa (*PN*) is the expanded portion of the neurohypophysis that is continuous with the infundibulum. The pars tuberalis (*PT*) is located around the infundibular stem but may cover the pars nervosa to a variable extent. The pars intermedia (*PI*) is a narrow band of tissue that lies between the pars distalis (*PD*) and the pars nervosa. It borders a small cleft (*Cl*) that constitutes the remains of the lumen of Rathke's pouch. The pars distalis, the anterior lobe of the gland, is its largest part. It contains a variety of cell types that are not uniformly distributed. This accounts for differences in staining (light and dark staining areas) that are seen throughout the pars distalis.

Each of the components of the adenohypophysis; i.e., the pars distalis, pars tuberalis, and pars intermedia, when examined at higher magnification, exhibit features at the cellular level that aid in their identification. These features are described in the following figures as well as those on Plate 77.

Figure 2, pituitary, human, H&E ×375.

This photomicrograph shows a region of the pars distalis that is rich in acidophils *(A).* Basophils *(B)* are present in this area in lesser numbers. The acidophils are readily identified by the acidophilic staining of their cytoplasm, in contrast to the basophils whose cytoplasm is clearly basophilic. Chromophobes *(C)* are also very numerous in this field. The cytoplasm stains poorly in contrast to that of the acidophils and basophils. The cells are arranged in cords and clumps, between which are capillaries *(Cap),* some of which can be recognized, but most are in a collapsed state and difficult to visualize at this magnification.

Figure 3, pituitary, human, H&E ×375.

This photomicrograph shows a region of the pars distalis that is rich in basophils *(B).* At this particular site, there are no recognizable acidophils (at other sites, it is possible to find a more equal distribution of acidophils and basophils, though, typically, one cell type outnumbers the other in a given region). Chromophobes *(C)* are also relatively numerous at this site. In this particular region, the chromophobe nuclei are readily apparent, but the cytoplasm of the cells is difficult to discern.

Figure 4, pituitary, human, PAS/aniline blue-black ×80.

This photomicrograph shows a small portion of the pars distalis *(PD);* the remainder reveals the pars intermedia *(PI).* The pars distalis shown here contains numerous capillaries filled with red blood cells, thus producing the bright red appearance. The pars intermedia contains a number of small cysts *(Cy).* The cells that make up the pars intermedia, which is relatively small in humans, consist of small basophils and chromophobes. The basophils have taken up the blue stain, thus making them prominent. To the extreme right is a less cellular area, the pars nervosa *(PN).*

KEY

A, acidophils
B, basophils
C, chromophobes
Cap, capillaries
Caps, capsule
Cl, cleft
Cy, cysts
PD, pars distalis
PI, pars intermedia
PN, pars nervosa
PT, pars tuberalis

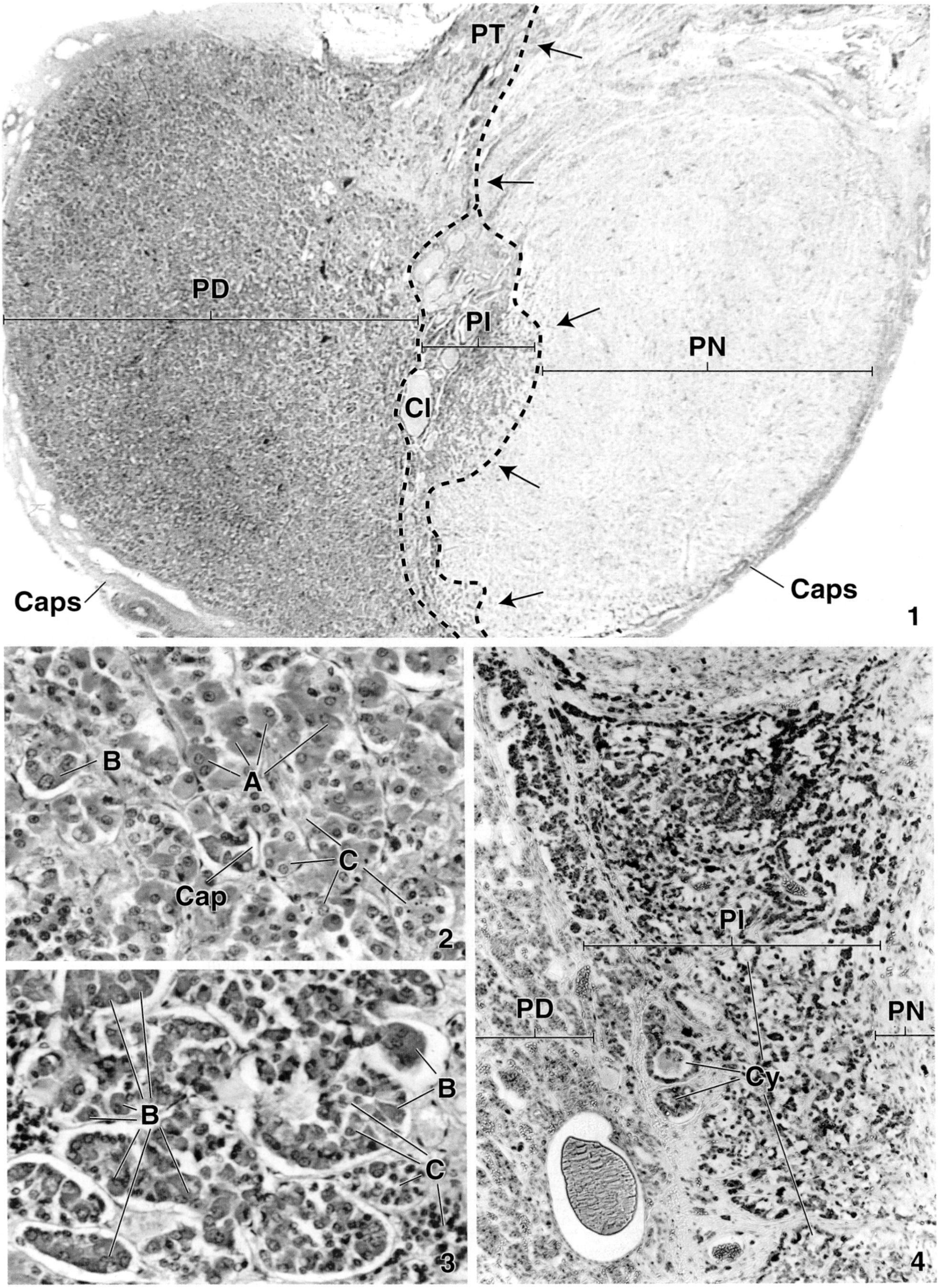
PT
PD
PI
PN
Cl
Caps
Caps
1
B
A
C
Cap
2
B
B
C
3
PI
PD
PN
Cy
4

PLATE 77. PITUITARY II

The parenchyma of the *pars distalis* consists of two general cell types: *chromophobes* and *chromophils.* Chromophobes stain poorly; chromophils stain well. Chromophils are further subdivided into *acidophils* and *basophils.* Basophils stain with basic dyes or hematoxylin, whereas the cytoplasm of the acidophil stains with acid dyes such as eosin. The cytoplasm of basophils also stains with the periodic acid–Schiff (PAS) reaction because of the glycoprotein in its secretory granules.

Acidophils can be further subdivided into two groups on the basis of special cytochemical and ultrastructural features. One group, called *somatotropes,* produces the growth hormone, *somatotropic hormone* (STH); the other group of acidophils, called *mammotropes* or *luteotropes,* produces the lactogenic hormone, *luteotropic hormone* (LTH). The groups of basophils can also be distinguished with the electron microscope and with special cytochemical procedures. One group produces the *thyroid-stimulating hormone* (TSH); another produces the gonadotropic hormones, *follicle-stimulating hormone* (FSH) and *luteinizing hormone* (LH); and a third group produces *adrenocorticotropic hormone* (ACTH) and *lipotropic hormone* (LPH). Chromophobes are also a heterogeneous group of cells. Many are considered to be depleted acidophils or basophils; one group of chromophobes, however, may produce ACTH.

Figure 1, pituitary, human, Mallory ×360; inset ×1200.

This photomicrograph of the pars distalis is from an area where there is an almost equal distribution of acidophils *(A)* and basophils *(B).* The clumps and cords of cells are delineated by strands of connective tissue (stained blue) that surround them. A number of engorged capillaries *(Cap)* containing red blood cells (stained yellow) are also seen. The acidophil cytoplasm in this preparation stains a reddish or rust color. The basophils stain a reddish blue to deep blue, and the chromophobes *(C)* exhibit a pale-blue color. The **inset** shows the three general cell types at higher magnification. The secretory granules of the acidophils *(A)* and basophils *(B)* are just discernable. It is the granules that stain and provide the overall coloration to the two cell types. In contrast, the chromophobe *(C)* lacks granules and simply reveals a pale-blue background color.

Figure 2, pituitary, human, H&E ×325.

The neurohypophysis seen here contains cells called pituicytes, and unmyelinated nerve fibers form the supraoptic and paraventricular nuclei of the hypothalamus. The pituicytes are comparable with neuroglial cells of the central nervous system. The nuclei are round to oval; the cytoplasm extends from the nuclear region of the cell as long processes. In H&E preparations such as this, the cytoplasm of the pituicyte cannot be distinguished from the unmyelinated nerve fibers. The hormones of the neurohypophysis, oxytocin and antidiuretic hormone (ADH) (also called vasopressin), are formed in the hypothalamic nuclei and pass via the fibers of the hypothalamohypophyseal tract to the neurohypophysis, where they are stored in the expanded nerve terminal portion of the nerve fibers. The stored neurosecretory material appears as Herring bodies *(HB).* In H&E preparations, the Herring bodies simply appear as small islands of eosin-stained substance. Interspersed among the nerve fibers are capillaries *(Cap).*

Figure 3, pituitary, human, PAS/aniline blue-black ×250; inset ×700.

In this specimen, the aniline blue has stained the nuclei of the pituicytes; the nerve fibers have taken up some of the stain to give a light-blue background. With this staining technique, the Herring bodies *(HB)* appear as the dark black islands. The **inset** shows the Herring body near the bottom of the micrograph at high magnification. The granular texture of the Herring body as seen here is a reflection of the accumulated secretory granules in the nerve terminals. Also of note in this specimen are the capillaries *(Cap),* which are prominent as a result of the contrasting red staining of the red blood cells within them.

KEY

A, acidophils
B, basophils
C, chromophobes
Cap, capillaries
HB, Herring bodies

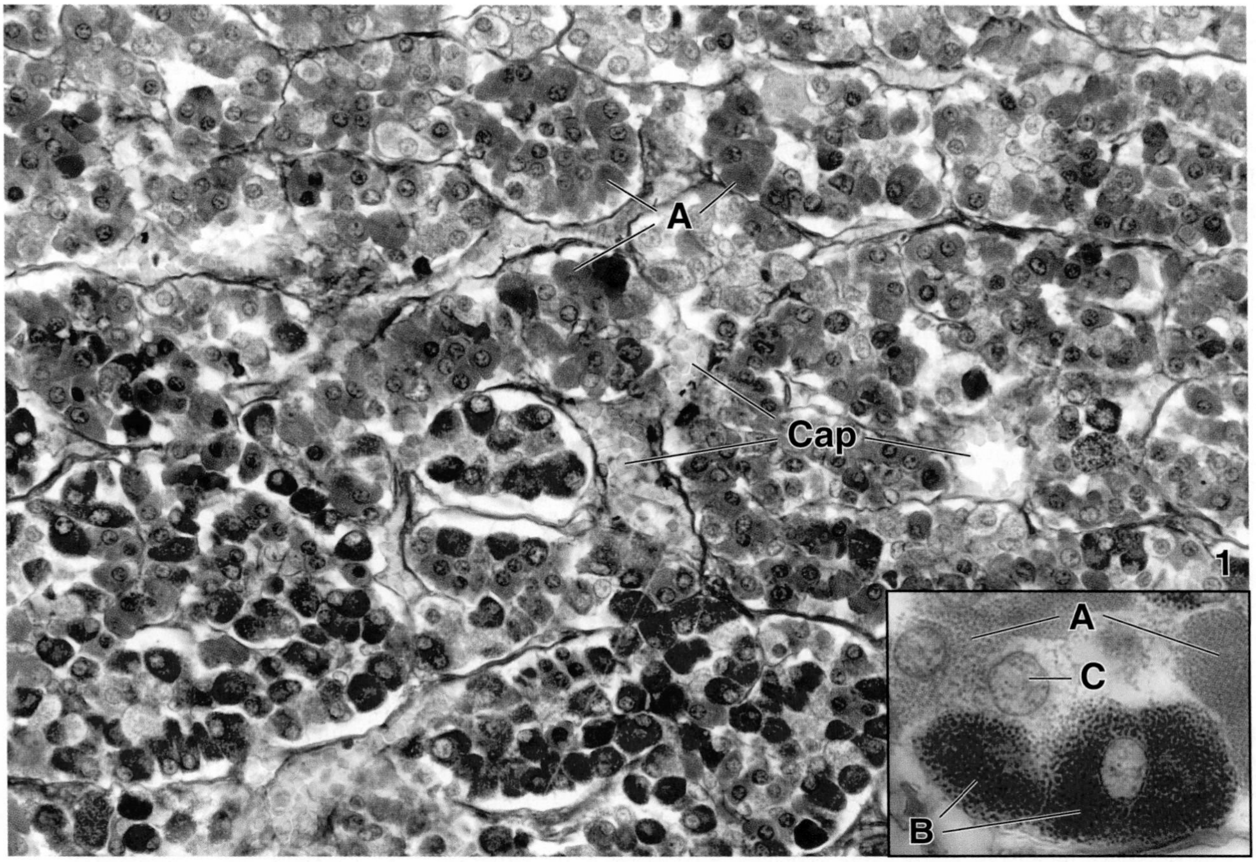
A
Cap
A
C
B
1

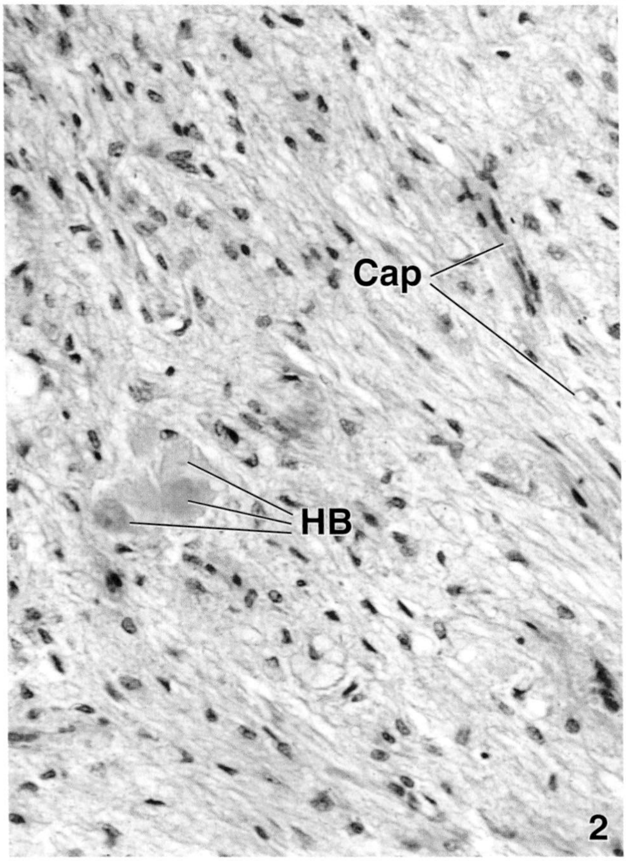
Cap
HB
2

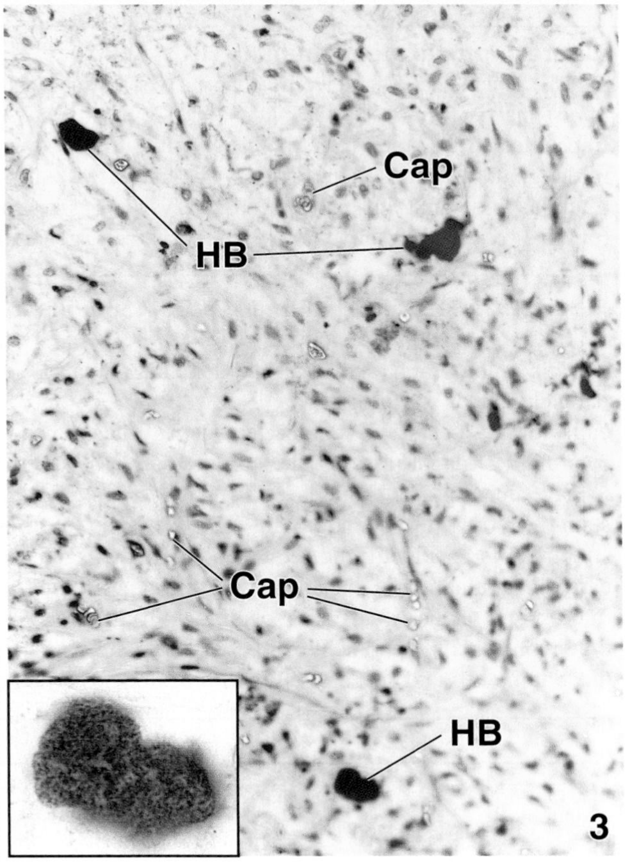
Cap
HB
Cap
HB
3

PLATE 78. PINEAL GLAND

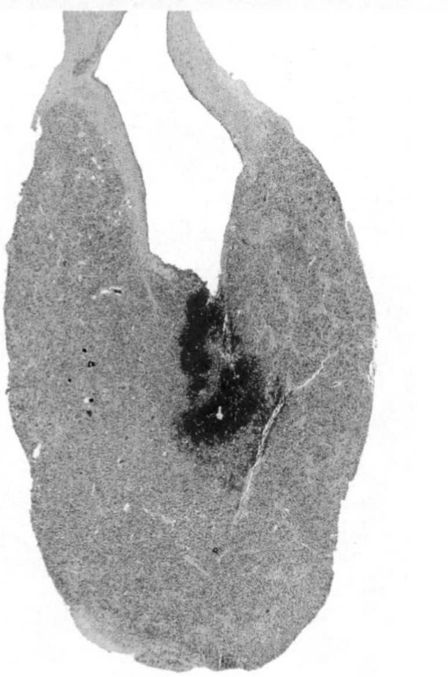

The *pineal gland (pineal body, epiphysis cerebri)* is located in the brain above the superior colliculi. It develops from neuroectoderm but, in the adult, bears little resemblance to nerve tissue.

Two cell types have been described within the pineal gland: parenchymal cells and glial cells. The full extent of these cells cannot be appreciated without the application of special methods. Those would show that the glial cells and the parenchymal cells have processes and that the processes of the parenchymal cells are expanded at their periphery. The parenchymal cells are more numerous. In an H&E preparation, the nuclei of the parenchymal cells are pale staining. The nuclei of the glial cells, on the other hand, are smaller and stain more intensely.

Although the physiology of the pineal gland is not well understood, the secretions of the gland evidently have an antigonadal effect. For example, hypogenitalism has been reported in pineal tumors that consist chiefly of parenchymal cells, whereas sexual precocity is associated with glial cell tumors (presumably, the parenchymal cells have been destroyed). In addition, experiments with animals indicate that the pineal gland has a neuroendocrine function whereby the pineal gland serves as an intermediary that relates endocrine function (particularly gonadal function) to cycles of light and dark. The external photic stimuli reach the pineal gland via optical pathways that connect with the superior cervical ganglion. In turn, the superior cervical ganglion sends postganglionic nerve fibers to the pineal gland. The extent to which these findings with laboratory animals apply to humans is not yet clear.

Recent studies in humans suggest that the pineal gland has a role in adjusting to sudden changes in day length, such as those experienced by travelers who suffer from jet lag, and a role in regulating emotional responses to reduced day length during winter in temperate and subarctic zones (seasonal affective disorder [SAD]).

Figure 1, pineal gland, human, H&E ×180.

The pineal gland is surrounded by a very thin capsule (*Cap*) that is formed by the pia mater. Connective tissue trabeculae (*CT*) extend from the capsule into the substance of the gland dividing it into lobules. The lobules (*L*) appear often as indistinct groups of cells of varying size surrounded by the connective tissue. Blood vessels, generally small arteries (*A*) and veins (*V*), course through the connective tissue. The arteries give rise to capillaries that surround and penetrate the lobules to supply the parenchyma of the gland. In this specimen and even at this low magnification, the capillaries (*C*) are prominent as a consequence of the red blood cells present in their lumina.

Figure 2, pineal gland, human, H&E ×360; inset ×700.

This micrograph shows at higher magnification the parenchyma of the pineal gland as well as a component called brain sand (*BS*) or corpora arenacea. When viewed at even higher magnifications, the corpora arenacea are seen to have an indistinct lamellated structure. Typically, they stain heavily with hematoxylin. The presence of these structures is an identifying feature of the pineal gland. A careful examination of the cells within the gland at the light microscopic level reveals two specific cell types. One cell type represents the parenchymal cells. These are by far the most numerous and are referred to as pinealocytes (or chief cells of the pineal gland). Pinealocytes are modified neurons. Their nuclei are spherical and are relatively lightly stained because of the amount of euchromatin that they contain. The second cell type is the interstitial cell or glial cell that constitutes a relatively small percentage of the cells in the gland. Their nuclei are smaller and more elongate than those of the pinealocytes. The **inset** reveals several glial cells (*G*) that can be identified by their more densely staining nuclei. The majority of the nuclei of the other cells seen here belong to pinealocytes. Also seen in the **inset** are several fibroblasts (*F*) that are present within a trabecula.

KEY

A, artery
BS, brain sand
C, capillary
Cap, capsule
CT, connective tissue
F, fibroblast
G, glial cell
L, lobule
V, vein

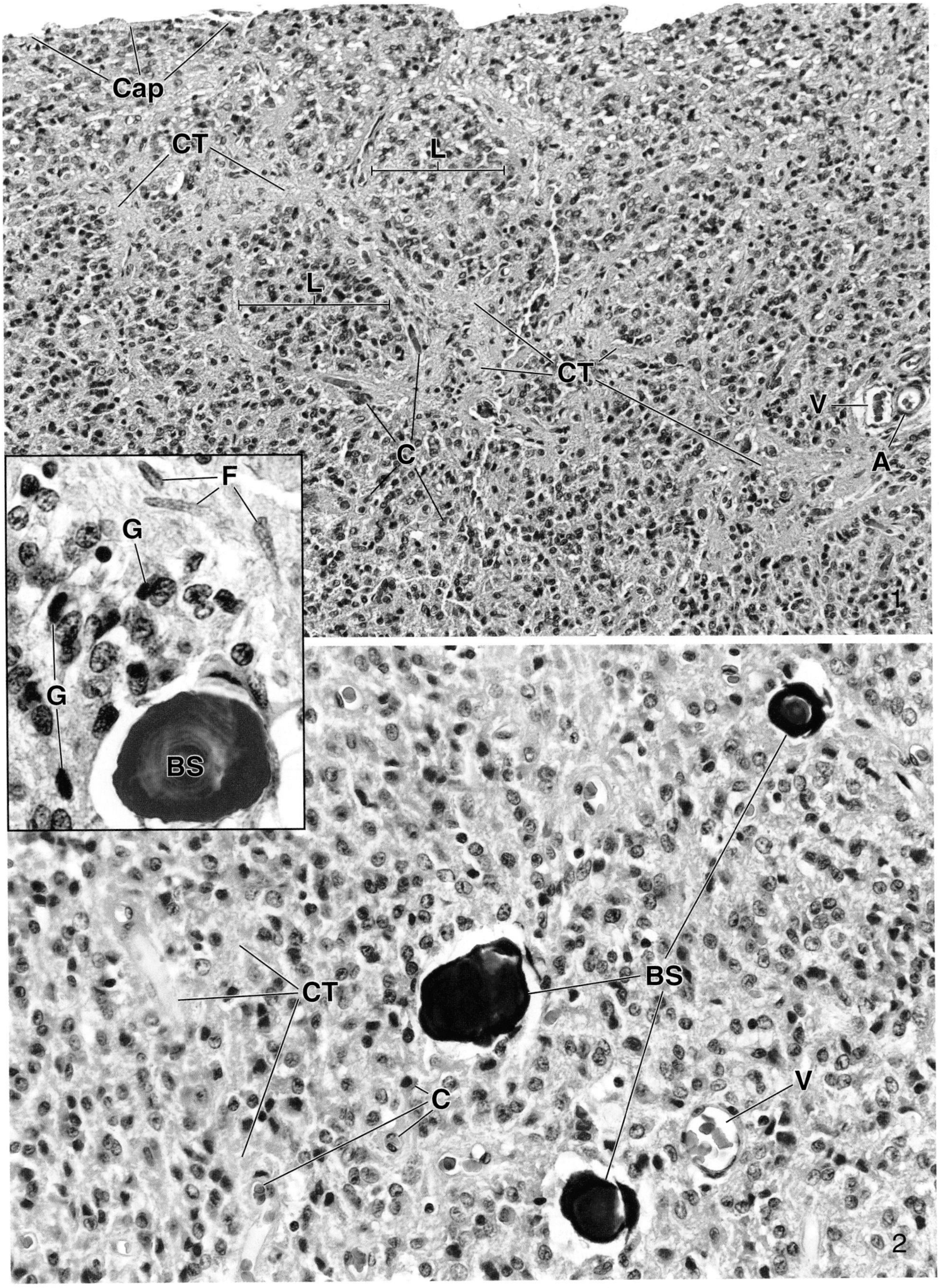
Cap
CT
L
L
CT
V
A
C
1
F
G
G
BS
CT
BS
C
V
2

PLATE 79. PARATHYROID AND THYROID GLANDS

The parathyroid glands are usually four in number. Each is surrounded by a capsule and lies on or is partially embedded in the thyroid gland. Connective tissue trabeculae extend from the capsule into the substance of the gland.

The parathyroid glands elaborate a hormone that influences calcium and bone metabolism. Injection of parathyroid hormone into laboratory animals results in the release of calcium from bone by the action of osteocytes (osteocytic osteolysis) and osteoclasts (osteoclasia). Removal of parathyroid glands results in a rapid drop in blood calcium levels.

The thyroid gland is located in the neck in close relation to the upper part of the trachea and the lower part of the larynx. It consists of two lateral lobes that are joined by a narrow isthmus. The follicle, which consists of a single layer of cuboidal or low columnar epithelium surrounding a colloid-filled space, is the functional unit of the thyroid gland. A rich capillary network is present in the connective tissue that separates the follicles. The connective tissue also contains lymphatic capillaries.

Figure 1, parathyroid gland, human, H&E ×320.
As seen here, the larger blood vessels are associated with the trabeculae (*BV*) and, occasionally, adipose cells (*A*). The parenchyma of the parathyroid glands appears as cords or sheets of cells separated by capillaries and delicate connective tissue septa.

Two parenchymal cell types can be distinguished in routine H&E sections: chief cells (principal cells) and oxyphil cells. The chief cells (*CC*) are more numerous. They contain a spherical nucleus surrounded by a small amount of cytoplasm. Oxyphil cells (*OC*) are less numerous. They are conspicuously larger than chief cells but have a slightly smaller and more intensely staining nucleus. Their cytoplasm stains with eosin, and the boundaries between the cells are usually well marked. Moreover, the oxyphils are arranged in groups of variable size that appear scattered about in a much larger field of chief cells. Even with low magnification it is often possible to identify clusters of oxyphil cells because a unit area contains fewer nuclei than a comparable unit area of chief cells, as is clearly evident in this figure. Oxyphil cells appear during the end of the first decade of life and become more numerous around puberty. A further increase may be seen in older individuals.

Figure 2, thyroid gland, human, H&E ×200.
A histologic section of the thyroid gland is shown here. The follicles (*F*) vary somewhat in size and shape and appear closely packed. The homogeneous mass in the center of each follicle is the colloid. The thyroid cells appear to form a ring around the colloid. Although the individual cells are difficult to distinguish at this magnification, the nuclei of the cells serve as an indication of their location and arrangement.

Large groups of cells are seen in association with some follicles. Where the nuclei are of the same size and staining characteristics, one can conclude that in these sties, the section includes the wall of the follicle (*arrows*) in a tangential manner without including the lumen.

KEY

A, adipose cells
BV, blood vessels
CC, chief cells
CT, connective tissue
F, follicles
OC, oxyphil cells
arrows, tangential section of follicle wall
asterisks, shrinkage artifact

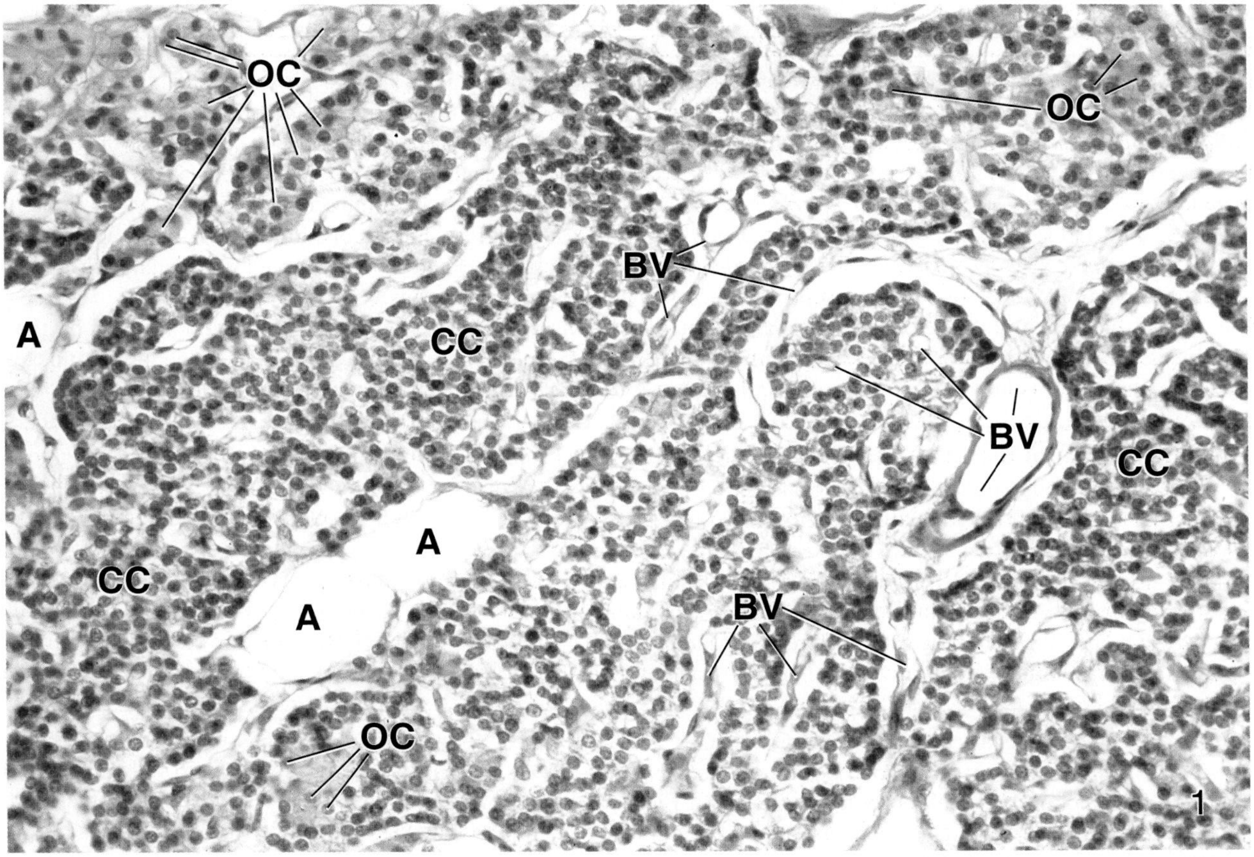
OC
OC
BV
A
CC
BV
CC
A
CC
A
BV
OC
1

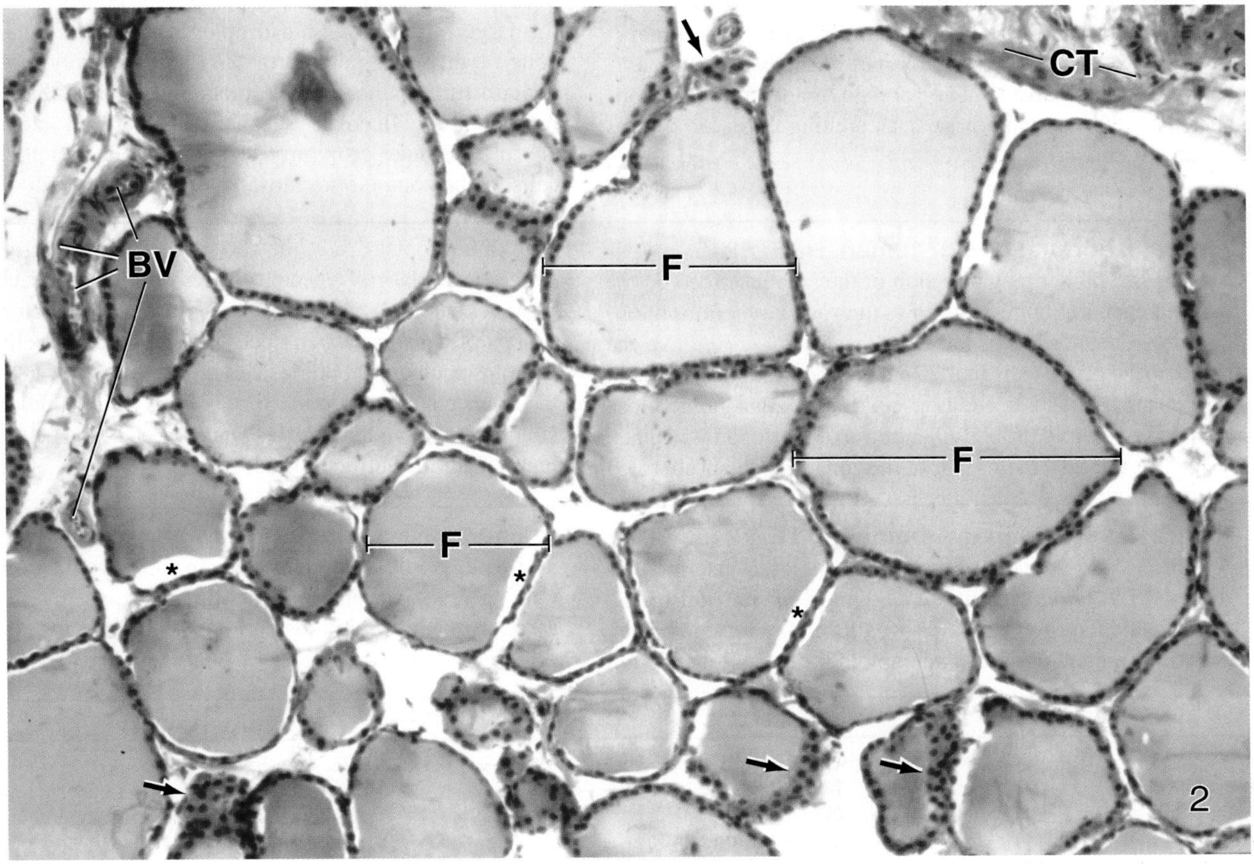
CT
BV
F
F
F
*
*
*
2

PLATE 80. ADRENAL GLAND I

There are two adrenal glands, one at the upper pole of each kidney. The gland is a composite of two distinct structural and functional components: a *cortex* and a *medulla.* The cortex develops from mesoderm and secretes *steroid hormones;* the medulla develops from neuroectoderm of the neural crest and secretes *catecholamines.*

The cortex is divided into three zones according to the type and arrangement of its parenchymal cells. These are designated *zona glomerulosa, zona fasciculata,* and *zona reticularis.* The zona glomerulosa constitutes 15% of the cortical volume. It secretes *mineralocorticoids* (*aldosterone* and *deoxycorticosterone*). The zona fasciculata constitutes nearly 80% of the cortical volume. It secretes the *glucocorticoids* (*cortisol, cortisone,* and *corticosterone*) and a small amount of adrenal androgens. The zona reticularis (5 to 7% of cortical volume) produces most of the adrenal androgens.

The zona fasciculata and the zona reticularis are regulated by *adrenocorticotropic hormone* (ACTH) secreted by the adenohypophysis in response to *corticotropin-releasing factor (CRF)* produced by the hypothalamus. The zona glomerulosa is not regulated by ACTH but is under feedback control of the *renin–angiotensin system* that also regulates blood pressure.

Figure 1, adrenal gland, human, H&E ×45.
This low-magnification micrograph of a section through the partial thickness of an adrenal gland shows the outer capsule *(Cap),* the cortex *(Cort)* from one surface of the gland, the underlying medulla *(Med),* and a very small portion of the cortex from the other surface of the gland *(Cort, bottom center).* The cortex has a distinctly different appearance in both structural organization and staining characteristics. From the inner portion, the medulla, note the lighter appearance of the medullary tissue. A small amount of adipose tissue *(AT)* in which the gland is partially embedded is seen at the upper center of the micrograph. The corticomedullary boundary *(dashed lines)* has a wave-like contour, a reflection of the irregular shape of the gland. Within the medulla are a number of relatively large blood vessels *(BV).* These are the medullary veins that drain both the cortex and the medulla.

Figure 2, adrenal gland, human, H&E ×180.
This is a higher magnification of a portion of the capsule and the full thickness of the cortex from an area in Figure 1. The capsule consists of dense connective tissue in which the larger arteries *(A)* travel to give rise to smaller vessels that will supply the cortex and medulla. The zona glomerulosa *(ZG)* is located at the outer part of the cortex, immediately under the capsule. The parenchyma of this zone consists of small cells that appear as arching cords or as oval groups of cells.

The zona fasciculata *(ZF)* consists of radially oriented cords and sheets of cells, usually two cells in width, that extend toward the medulla. The cells of the outer part of the zona fasciculata are generally larger than those of the inner portion of this zone and typically stain poorly because of the large number of lipid droplets that they contain. The cells of the zona reticularis *(ZR)* are relatively small and contain little or no lipid droplets and, consequently, stain prominently with eosin. Because of their small size, the nuclei are in close proximity to one another, much like the cells of the zona glomerulosa.

Figure 3, adrenal gland, human, H&E ×245.
This is a higher magnification of the area inscribed by the *left rectangle* in Figure 2. It shows the zona glomerulosa *(ZG)* and the outer portion of the zona fasciculata *(ZF).* Note the smaller size of the cells in the zona glomerulosa than those in the zona fasciculata. In addition, cells of the zona glomerulosa contain fewer lipid droplets than those of the zona fasciculata. Typically, the cells in this part of the zona fasciculata are filled with lipid droplets, thus, the very poor staining characteristic of their cytoplasm. Delicate connective tissue trabeculae *(arrows)* extend from the capsule to surround the glomerular groups of cells and extend between the cords of cells in the zona fasciculata. Capillaries and arterioles are located within the connective tissue trabeculae. Usually, the capillaries are collapsed and, without the presence of red blood cells in their lumina, are thus difficult to identify.

Figure 4, adrenal gland, human, H&E ×245.
This is a higher magnification of the area inscribed by the *right rectangle* in Figure 2. This deep portion of the zona fasciculata *(ZF)* reveals smaller cells, although they are still arranged in cords and contain lipid droplets, though in lesser amounts. The cells of the zona reticularis *(ZR)* are arranged in irregular anastomosing cords and contain at best only a small amount of lipid and, consequently, their cytoplasm stains with eosin.

KEY

A, arteries
AT, adipose tissue
BV, blood vessels
Cap, capsule
Cort, cortex
Med, medulla
ZF, zona fasciculata
ZG, zona glomerulosa
ZR, zona reticularis
arrows, connective tissue trabeculae
dashed line, corticomedullary boundary

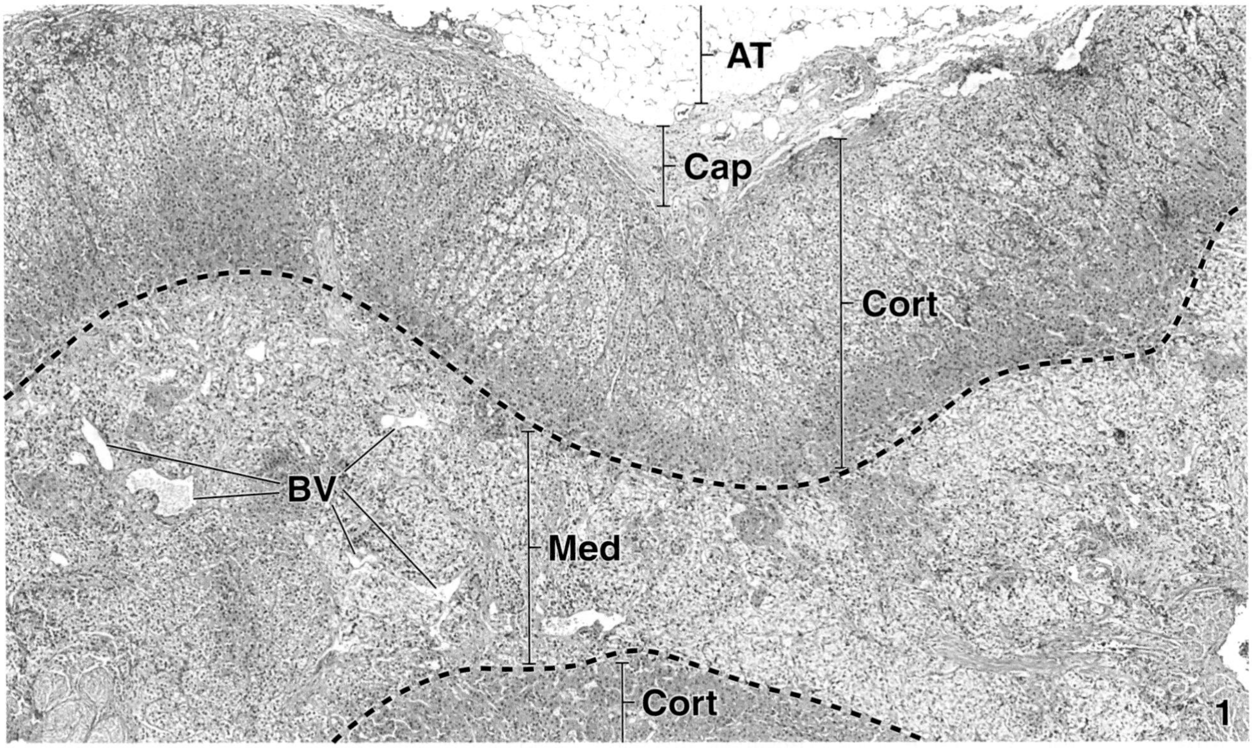
AT
Cap
Cort
BV
Med
Cort
1

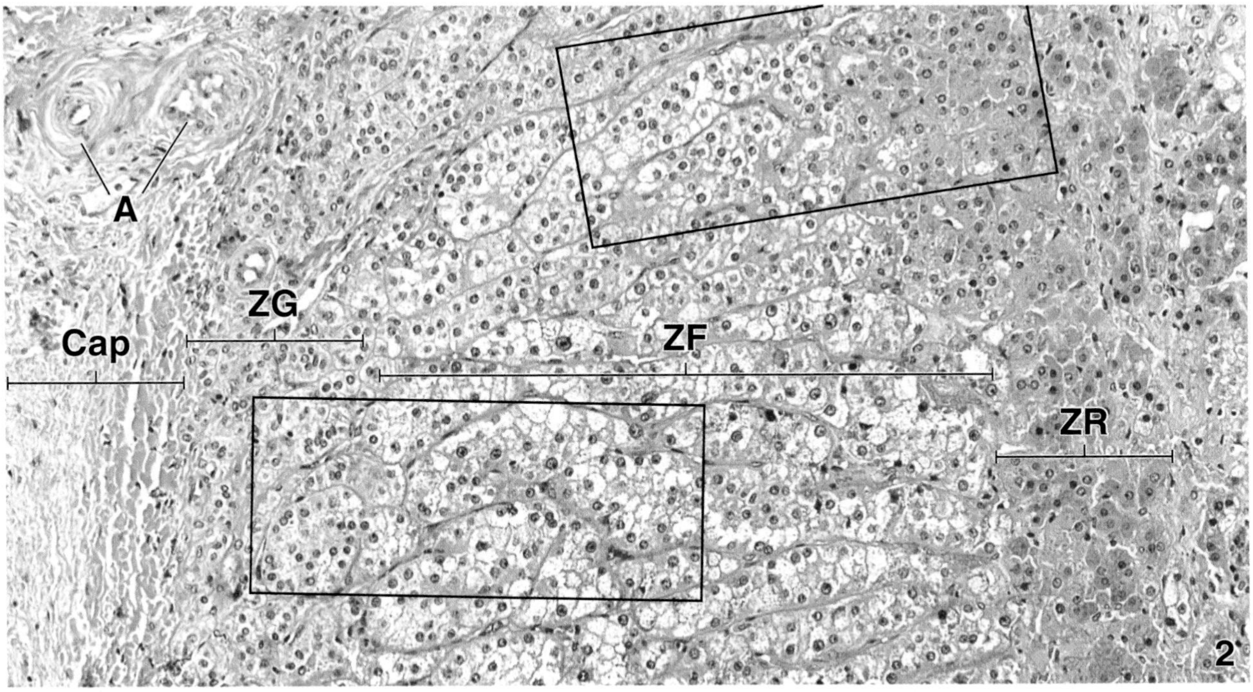
A
ZG
Cap
ZF
ZR
2

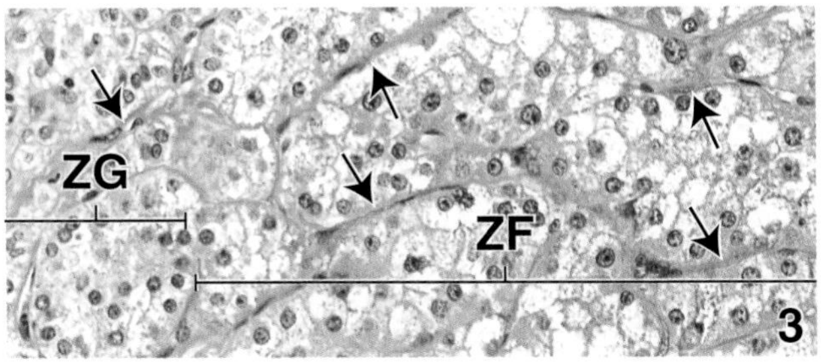
ZG
ZF
3

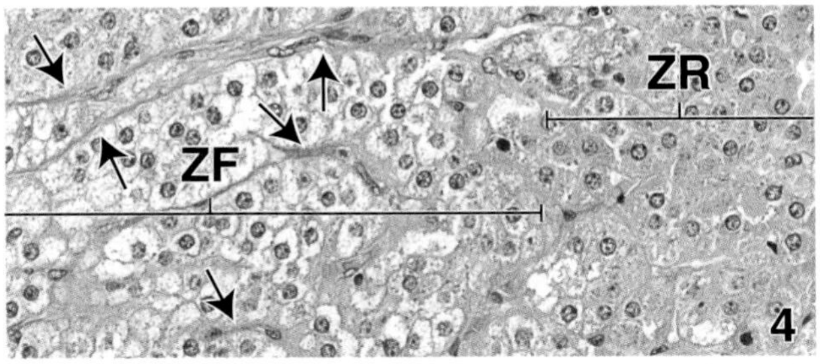
ZR
ZF
4

PLATE 81. ADRENAL GLAND II

The cells of the *adrenal medulla* develop from the same source as the postganglionic cells of the sympathetic nervous system. They are directly innervated by preganglionic cells of the sympathetic system and may be regarded as modified postganglionic cells that are specialized to secrete. These cells produce the catecholamines *epinephrine* and *norepinephrine.*

The adrenal medulla receives its blood supply via two routes: by arterioles that pass through the cortex and by capillaries that continue from the cortex, a type of portal circulation. Thus, some of the blood supplying the medulla contains cortical secretions that regulate medullary function. Blood leaves the medulla via the medullary vein. Its structure is unusual in that the tunica media of the vessel contains prominent bundles of longitudinally oriented smooth muscle, the contraction of which facilitates rapid outflow of blood when medullary catecholamines are released.

Figure 1, adrenal gland, human, H&E ×175; inset ×250.

This moderately low power photomicrograph shows the cells of the adrenal medulla. The medullary cells are organized in ovoid groups and short interconnecting cords. The cytoplasm of the medullary cells may stain with different intensity. The cytoplasm of some cells is very poorly stained, appearing almost clear, whereas others show greater intensity of eosin staining. In this photomicrograph, a portion of the wall, namely, the tunica media *(TM)* of a medullary vein, can be seen. The nature of the medullary veins is described in Figure 2. The **inset** shows the ovoid groups of medullary cells at a higher magnification. Between these groups of cells are capillaries *(Cap)* that, as in the cortex, can be identified when they contain red blood cells as shown here.

Figure 2, adrenal gland, human, H&E ×125.

This micrograph shows a medullary vein *(MV)* that drains the adrenal medulla. The tunica media *(TM)* is unusually thick. The smooth muscle that constitutes this part of the vessel wall is in the form of bundles that are arranged longitudinally, i.e., in the same direction as the vessel. Thus, the muscle seen here is cut in cross section, as is the vein. While the medullary vein occupies most of the micrograph, medullary cells *(MC)* can be seen in several locations surrounding the vein. The portion of the figure outlined by the *rectangle* is seen at higher magnification in Figure 3.

Figure 3, adrenal gland, human, H&E ×350.

This higher-magnification view of the *rectangle* in Figure 2 shows part of the lumen *(L)* of the medullary vein at the bottom of the field. The tunica intima *(TI)* of the vessel is relatively thin but may contain a variable amount of connective tissue. The smooth muscle *(SM)* of the tunica media *(TM)* is readily seen here as being arranged in bundles and appears in cross section. There is no discrete tunica adventitia in the smaller medullary veins. Instead, its connective tissue blends in with surrounding structures. Ganglion cells *(GC)* are frequently found in proximity to the wall of the medullary vein. They are large cells with a moderately basophilic cytoplasm. Because of the large size of the cell, the nucleus is often missed in the section, and only the cell cytoplasm is seen.

KEY

Cap, capillary
GC, ganglion cells
L, lumen of medullary vein
MC, medullary cells
MV, medullary vein
SM, smooth muscle
TI, tunica intima
TM, tunica media

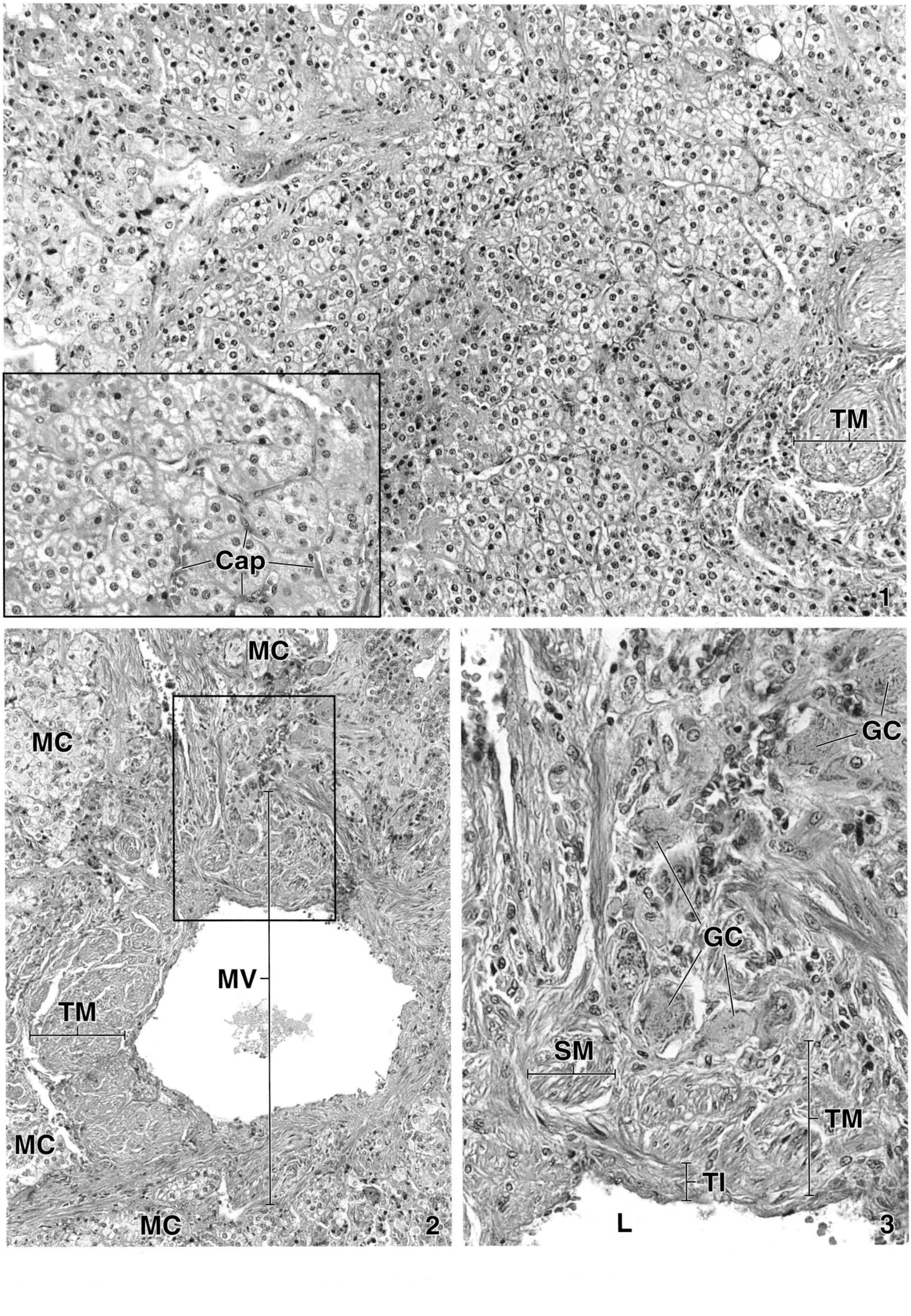
TM
Cap
1
MC
MC
MV
TM
MC
MC
2
GC
GC
SM
TM
TI
L
3

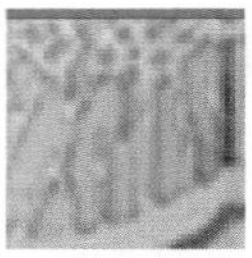
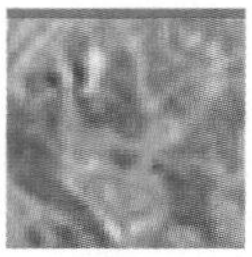

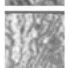

21

Male Reproductive System

OVERVIEW OF THE MALE REPRODUCTIVE SYSTEM

The male reproductive system consists of the testes, genital excurrent ducts, accessory sex glands, and penis (Fig. 21.1). The accessory sex glands include the seminal vesicles, prostate, and bulbourethral glands. The two primary functions of the testis are the production of sperm, male gametes *(**spermatogenesis**)* and synthesis of androgens, or sex hormones *(**steroidogenesis**)*. Androgens, mainly testosterone, are essential for spermatogenesis, play an important role in embryonic development of the male embryo into the phenotypic male fetus, and are responsible for sexual dimorphism (male physical and behavioral characteristics). The events of cell division that occur during production of male gametes, as well as those of the female, the ova, involve both normal division, *mitosis,* and reduction division, *meiosis.*

A brief description of mitosis and meiosis is included in Chapter 2, page 68. A basic understanding of these processes is essential to understand the production of gametes in both the male and the female.

TESTIS

The adult ***testes*** are paired ovoid organs that lie within the ***scrotum,*** located outside the body cavity. Testes are suspended by the spermatic cords and tethered to the scrotum by scrotal ligaments, the remnants of the gubernaculum (see below).

Development of the Testis

The testes develop on the posterior wall of the abdomen and later descend into the scrotum

Genetic sex is determined at fertilization by the presence or absence of the Y chromosome. The testes, however, do not form until the seventh week of development. ***Gonadal sex*** is determined by the presence of the ***SRY gene*** located in the ***sex-determining region*** of the short arm of the Y chromosome. A specific DNA-binding protein, called the ***testis-determining factor (TDF),*** encoded by the SRY gene, has been found to be directly responsible for testicular development and differentiation.

The testes develop in close association with the urinary system retroperitoneally, on the posterior wall of the abdominal cavity. Testes (like ovaries) are derived from three sources:

- ***Intermediate mesoderm*** that forms the urogenital ridges on the posterior abdominal wall
- ***Mesodermal epithelium (coelomic mesothelium)*** that lines the urogenital ridges

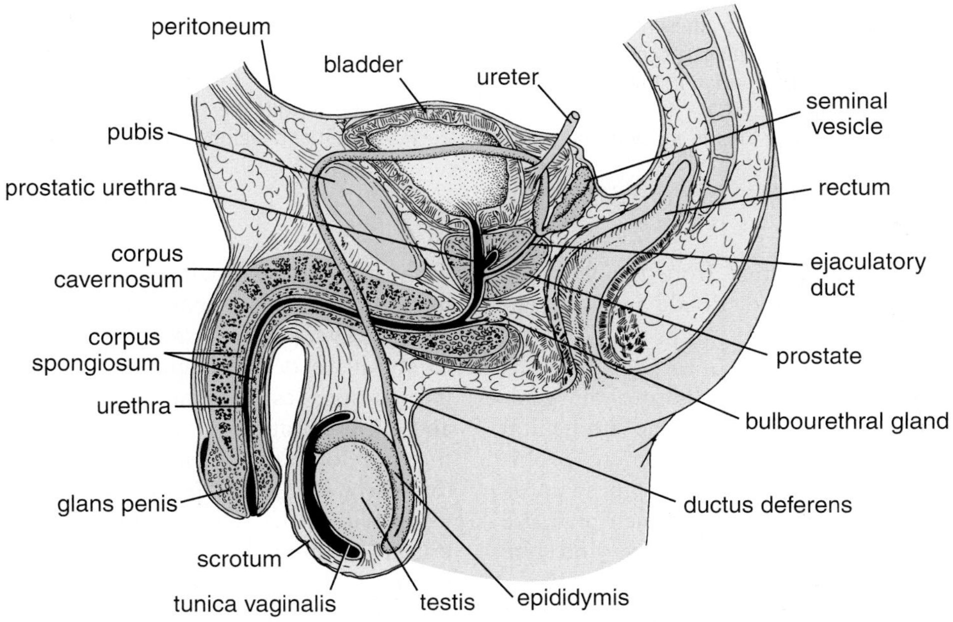

FIGURE 21.1
Schematic diagram demonstrating the components of the male reproductive system. Midline structures are depicted in sagittal section; bilateral structures including the testis, epididymis, ductus deferens, and seminal vesicle are shown intact.

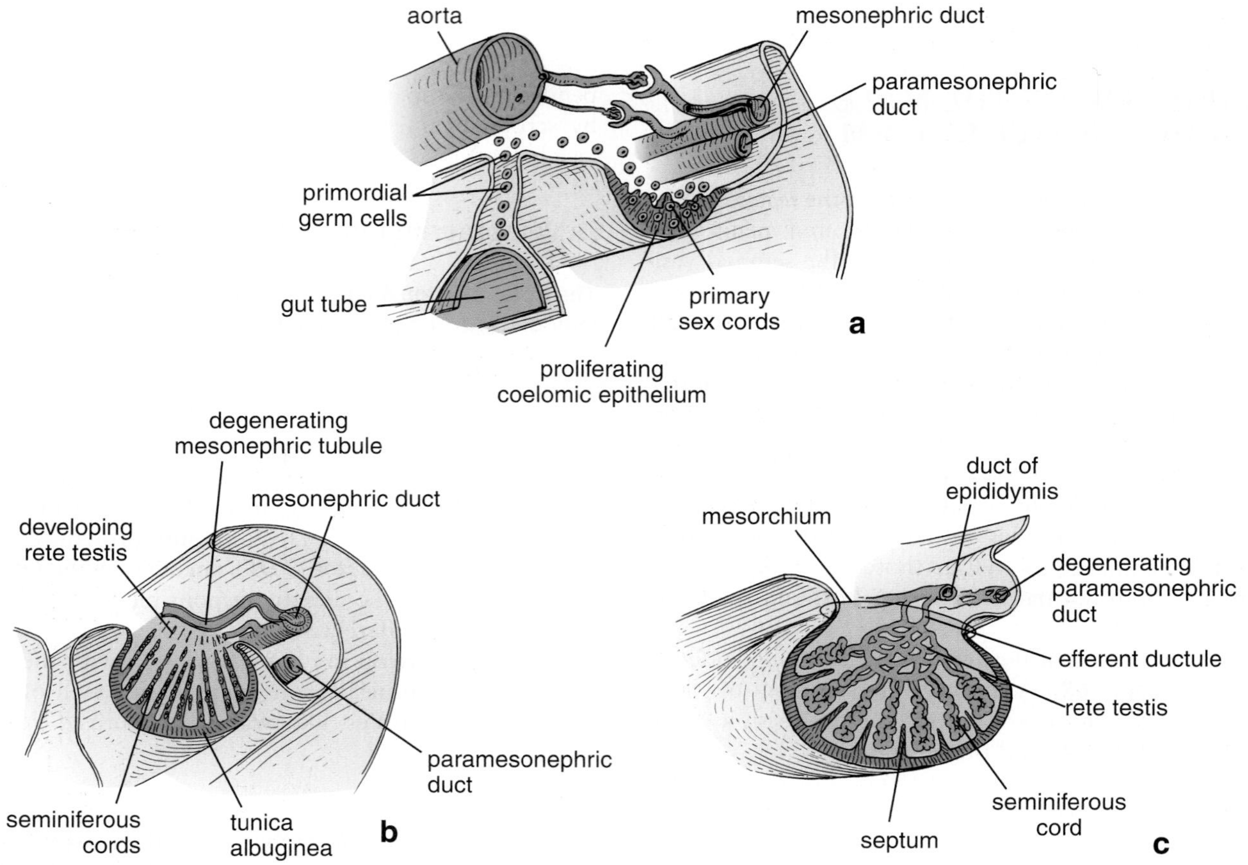

FIGURE 21.2
Schematic diagram of the stages of testicular development. a. This diagram shows the 5-week embryo in the stage of indifferent gonads. The gonadal ridges visible on the posterior abdominal wall are being infiltrated by primordial germ cells *(green)* that migrate from the yolk sac. Most of the developing gonad is formed by mesenchyme derived from the coelomic epithelium. The primordial germ cells become incorporated in the primary sex cords. **b.** At a later stage, under hormonal influence of testis-determining factor (TDF), the developing gonad initiates production of testosterone. This is followed by differentiation of the primary sex cords into seminiferous cords. At the same time, the developing gonad produces Müllerian-inhibiting factor (MIF), which causes regression of the paramesonephric duct and those structures derived from it. Note that the mesonephric tubules come in close contact with the developing rete testis. **c.** Final stages of testicular development. The tunica albuginea surrounding the testis contributes to development of the testicular septa. The rete testis connects with the seminiferous cords and with the excurrent duct system that develops from the mesonephric duct and tubules.

- ***Primordial germ cells*** that migrate from the yolk sac into developing gonads, where they divide and differentiate into spermatogonia

Migration of the primordial germ cells into the genital ridges induces mesodermal cells of the urogenital ridges and cells of the coelomic mesothelium to proliferate and form the ***primary sex cords.*** Later, these cords differentiate into the ***seminiferous cords,*** which give rise to the ***seminiferous tubules, straight tubules,*** and ***rete testis*** (Fig. 21.2).

In the first stage of development, the testes develop on the posterior abdominal wall from indifferent primordia of ***urogenital ridges*** that are identical in both sexes. During this ***indifferent stage*** an embryo has the potential to develop into either a male or female. Early in male development, mesenchyme separating the seminiferous cords gives rise to ***Leydig (interstitial) cells*** that produce ***testosterone*** to stimulate development of the indifferent primordium into a testis. Testosterone is also responsible for the growth and differentiation of the mesonephric (Wolffian) ducts that develop into the male genital excurrent ducts. Also in this early stage, the ***Sertoli (sustentacular) cells*** that develop within the seminiferous cords produce another important hormonal substance, called ***Müllerian-inhibiting factor (MIF).*** MIF's molecular structure is similar to that of transforming growth factor β (TGF-β). It is a large glycoprotein that inhibits cell division of the paramesonephric (Müllerian) ducts, which in turn inhibits development of female reproductive organs (Fig. 21.3).

Development and differentiation of the external genitalia (also from the sexually indifferent stage) occur at the same time and result from the action of ***dihydrotestosterone (DHT)***, a product of the conversion of testosterone by 5α-reductase. Without DHT, regardless of the genetic or gonadal sex, the external genitalia will develop along the female template. The appearance of testosterone, MIF, and DHT in the developing male embryo determines its ***hormonal sex.***

At approximately the 26th week of gestation, the testes descend from the abdomen into the scrotum. This migration of testes is due to differential growth of the abdominal cavity combined with the action of testosterone that causes shortening of the ***gubernaculum***, the testosterone-sensitive ligament connecting the inferior pole of each testis with the developing scrotum. The testes descend into the scrotum by passing through the ***inguinal canal***, the narrow passage between the abdominal cavity and the scrotum. Descent of the testis is sometimes obstructed, resulting in ***cryptorchidism***, or ***undescended testes.*** This condition is common (30%) in premature newborns and about 1% of full-term newborns. Cryptorchidism can lead to irreversible histologic changes in the testis and increases the risk of testicular cancer. Therefore, an undescended testis requires surgical correction. Orchiopexy (placement in the scrotal sac) should be performed, preferably before histologic changes become irreversible at approximately 2 years of age.

Spermatogenesis requires that the testes be maintained below normal body temperature

As the testes descend from the abdominal cavity into the scrotum, they carry with them blood vessels, lymphatic vessels, autonomic nerves, and an extension of the abdominal peritoneum called the ***tunica vaginalis,*** which covers their anterolateral surface. Within the scrotum the temperature of the testes is 2 to 3°C below body temperature. This lower temperature is essential for spermatogenesis, but is not required for hormone production (steroidogenesis), which can occur at normal body temperature. If the testes are maintained at higher temperatures (e.g., because

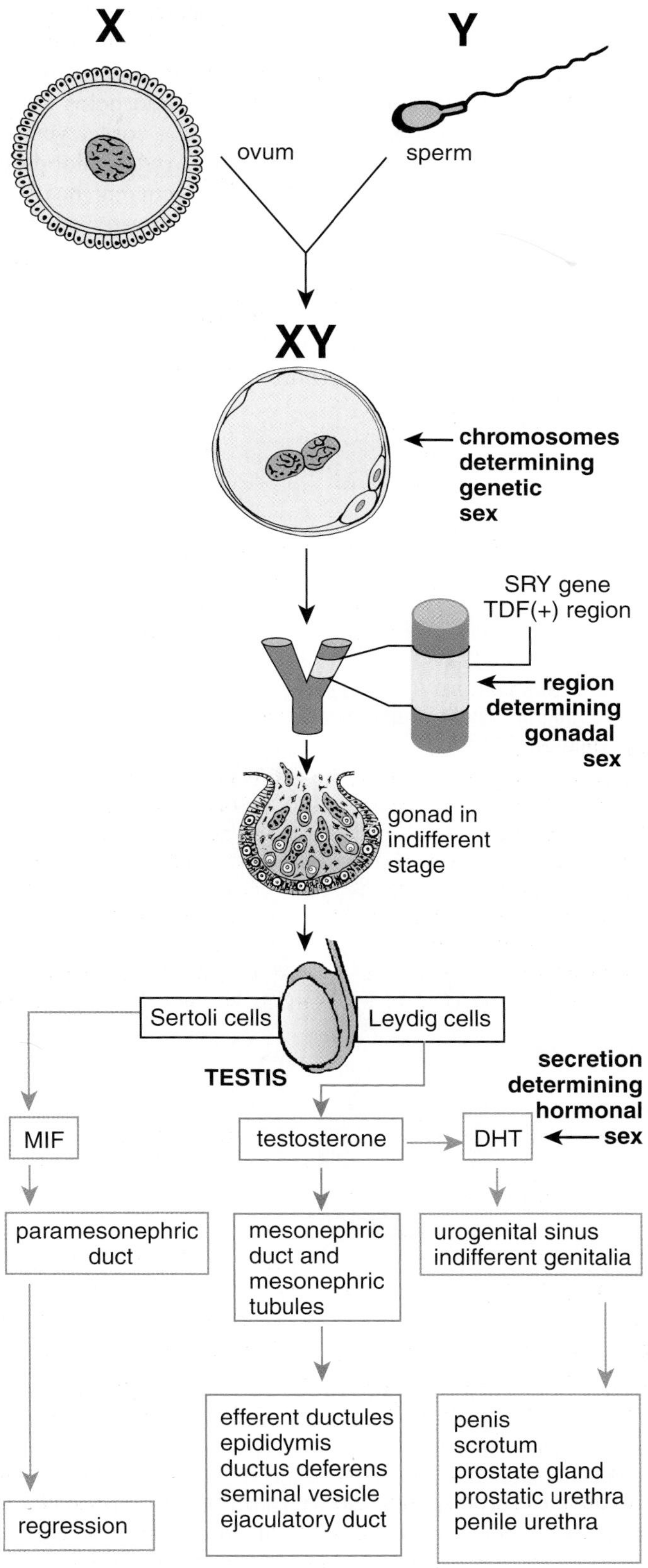

FIGURE 21.3
Schematic diagram of male sex development and hormonal influence on developing reproductive organs. This diagram illustrates three levels on which the sex of the developing embryo is determined. The genetic sex is determined at the time of fertilization; gonadal sex is determined by activation of the SRY gene located on the short arm of chromosome Y; and hormonal sex is determined by a hormone secreted by the developing gonad. The diagram shows the influence of Müllerian-inhibiting factor *(MIF)*, testosterone, and dihydrotestosterone *(DHT)* on the developing structures.

of fever) or if they fail to descend into the scrotum, sperm are not produced.

Each testis receives blood through a ***testicular artery,*** a direct branch of the abdominal aorta. It is highly convoluted near the testis, where it is surrounded by the ***pampiniform venous plexus,*** which carries blood from the testis to the abdominal veins. This arrangement allows heat exchange between the blood vessels and helps maintain the testes at a lower temperature. The cooler venous blood returning from the testis cools the arterial blood before it enters the testis through a countercurrent heat exchange mechanism. In addition, the ***cremaster muscle,*** whose fibers originate from the internal abdominal oblique muscle of the anterior abdominal wall, responds to changes in ambient temperature. Its contraction moves the testes closer to the abdominal wall, and its relaxation lowers the testes within the scrotum.

Structure of the Testis

The testes have an unusually thick connective tissue capsule, the tunica albuginea

An unusually thick, dense connective tissue capsule, the ***tunica albuginea,*** covers each testis (Fig. 21.4). The inner part of this capsule, the ***tunica vasculosa,*** is a loose connective tissue layer that contains blood vessels. Each testis is divided into approximately 250 lobules by incomplete connective tissue septa that project from the capsule.

Along the posterior surface of the testis, the tunica albuginea thickens and projects inward as the ***mediastinum testis.*** Blood vessels, lymphatic vessels, and the genital excurrent ducts pass through the mediastinum as they enter or leave the testis.

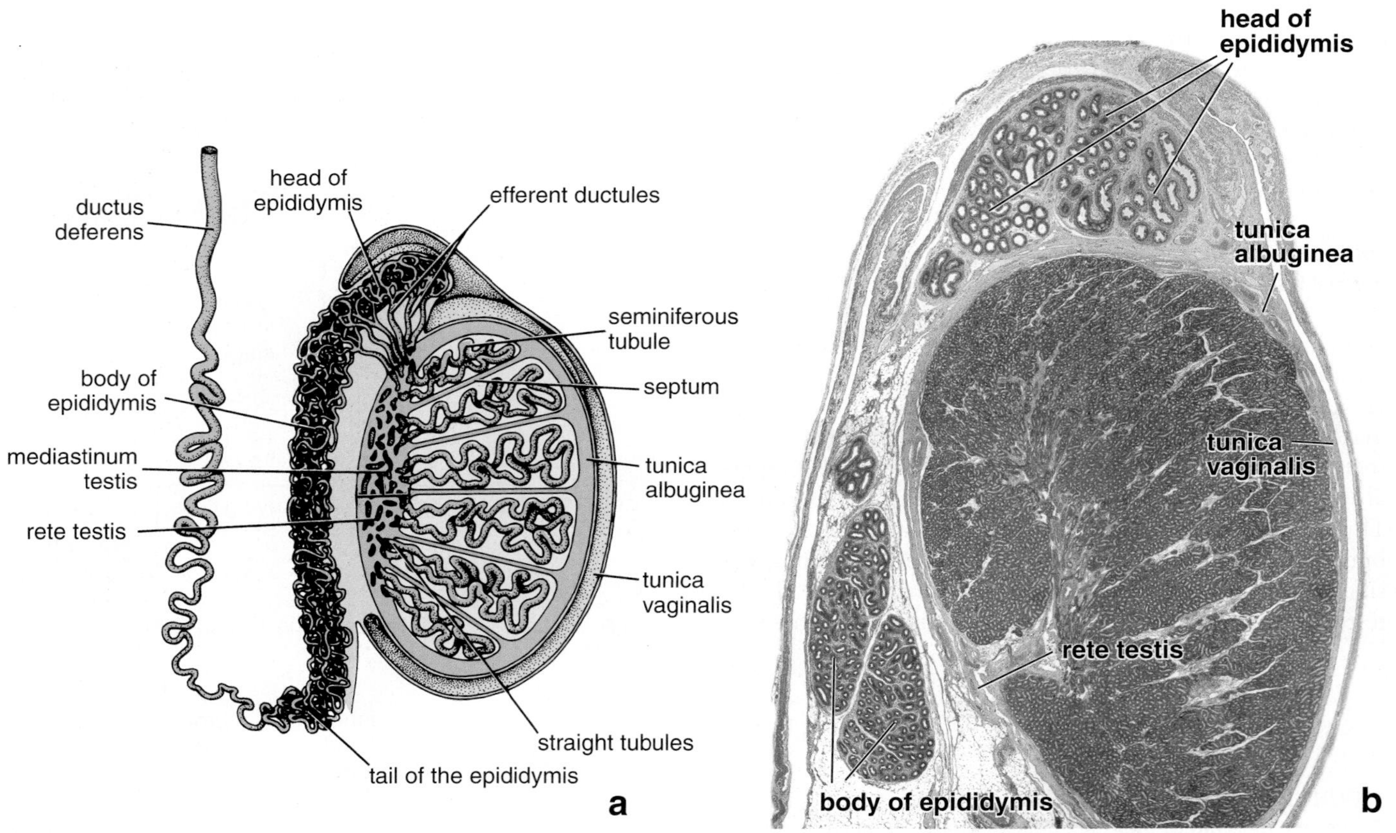

FIGURE 21.4
Sagittal section of the human testis. a. This schematic diagram shows a midsagittal section of the human testis. The genital duct system, which includes the tubuli recti, rete testis, efferent ducts, duct of the epididymis, and ductus deferens, is also shown. Note the thick connective tissue covering, the tunica albuginea, and the surrounding tunica vaginalis. (Modified from Dym M. In: Weiss L, ed. *Cell and Tissue Biology: A Textbook of Histology.* 6th ed. Baltimore: Urban & Schwarzenberg, 1988.) **b.** Sagittal section of a H&E–stained section of the testis and the head and body of the epididymis. Again note the surrounding tunica albuginea and tunica vaginalis. Only a small portion of the rete testis is visible in this section. Its connection with the excurrent duct system is not evident in the plane of this section. ×3.

Each lobule consists of several highly convoluted seminiferous tubules

Each lobule of the testis consists of 1 to 4 ***seminiferous tubules*** in which sperm are produced and a connective tissue stroma in which ***Leydig,*** or ***interstitial, cells*** are contained (Fig. 21.5). Each tubule within the lobule forms a loop and, because of its considerable length, is highly convoluted, actually folding on itself within the lobule. The ends of the loop are located near the ***mediastinum*** of the testis, where they assume a short straight course. This part of the seminiferous tubule is called the ***straight tubule (tubuli recti).*** It becomes continuous with the ***rete testis,*** an anastomosing channel system within the mediastinum.

The seminiferous tubules consist of a seminiferous epithelium surrounded by a tunica propria

Each seminiferous tubule is approximately 50 cm long (range, 30 to 80 cm) and 150 to 250 μm in diameter. The ***seminiferous epithelium*** is an unusual and complex stratified epithelium composed of two basic cell populations:

- ***Sertoli cells,*** also known as ***supporting,*** or ***sustentacular, cells.*** These cells do not replicate after puberty. Sertoli cells are columnar cells with extensive apical and lateral processes that surround the adjacent spermatogenic cells and occupy the spaces between them. However, this elaborate configuration of the Sertoli cells cannot be seen distinctly in routine hematoxylin and eosin (H&E) preparations. Sertoli cells give structural organization to the tubules as they extend through the full thickness of the seminiferous epithelium.
- ***Spermatogenic cells,*** which regularly replicate and differentiate into mature sperm. These cells are derived from primordial germ cells originating in the yolk sac that colonize the gonadal ridges during early development of the testis. Spermatogenic cells are organized in poorly defined layers of progressive development between adjacent Sertoli cells (Fig. 21.6). The most imma-

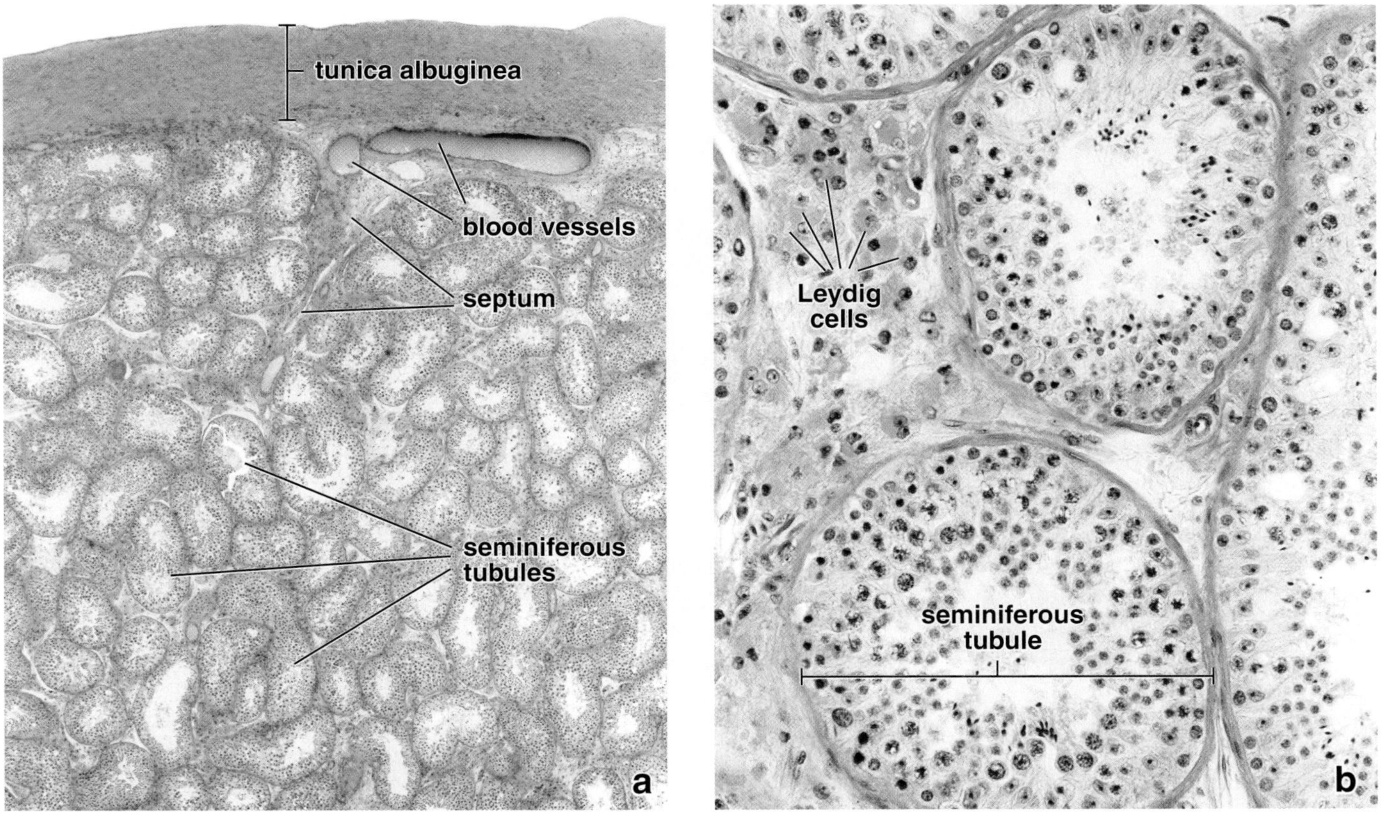

FIGURE 21.5
Photomicrographs of human testis. a. This low-magnification photomicrograph of a H&E–stained section of a human testis shows seminiferous tubules and the tunica albuginea. The larger blood vessels are present in the inner aspect of the tunica albuginea. The seminiferous tubules are highly convoluted; thus the profiles that they present in the section are variable in appearance. ×30. **b.** A higher magnification of the previous specimen shows several seminiferous tubules. Note the population of Leydig (interstitial) cells that occur in small clusters in the space between adjoining tubules. ×250.

ture spermatogenic cells, called ***spermatogonia,*** rest on the basal lamina. The most mature cells, called ***spermatids,*** are attached to the apical portion of the Sertoli cell, where they border the lumen of the tubule.

The ***tunica (lamina) propria,*** also called *peritubular tissue,* is a multilayered connective tissue that lacks typical fibroblasts. In man, it consists of three to five layers of ***myoid cells (peritubular contractile cells)*** and collagen fibrils, external to the basal lamina of the seminiferous epithelium (see Fig. 21.6). In rodents, the tunica propria consists of a single layer of squamous myoid cells in an epithelioid arrangement. At the ultrastructural level, myoid cells demonstrate features associated with smooth muscle cells, including a basal lamina and large numbers of actin filaments. They also exhibit a significant amount of rough endoplasmic reticulum (rER), a feature indicating their role in collagen synthesis in the absence of typical fibroblasts. Rhythmic contractions of the myoid cells create peristaltic waves that help move spermatozoa and testicular fluid through the seminiferous tubules to the excurrent duct system. Blood vessels and extensive lymphatic vasculature as well as Leydig cells are present external to the myoid layer.

As a normal consequence of aging, the tunica propria increases in thickness. This thickening is accompanied by a decreased rate of sperm production and an overall reduction in the size of the seminiferous tubules. Excessive thickening of the tunica propria earlier in life is associated with infertility.

Leydig Cells

Leydig cells (interstitial cells) are large, polygonal, eosinophilic cells that typically contain lipid droplets (Fig. 21.7). Lipofuscin pigment is also frequently present in these cells as well as distinctive, rod-shaped cytoplasmic crystals, the ***crystals of Reinke*** (Fig. 21.8). In routine histologic preparations, these crystals are refractile and measure approximately 3×20 μm Although their exact nature and function remain unknown, they probably represent a protein product of the cell.

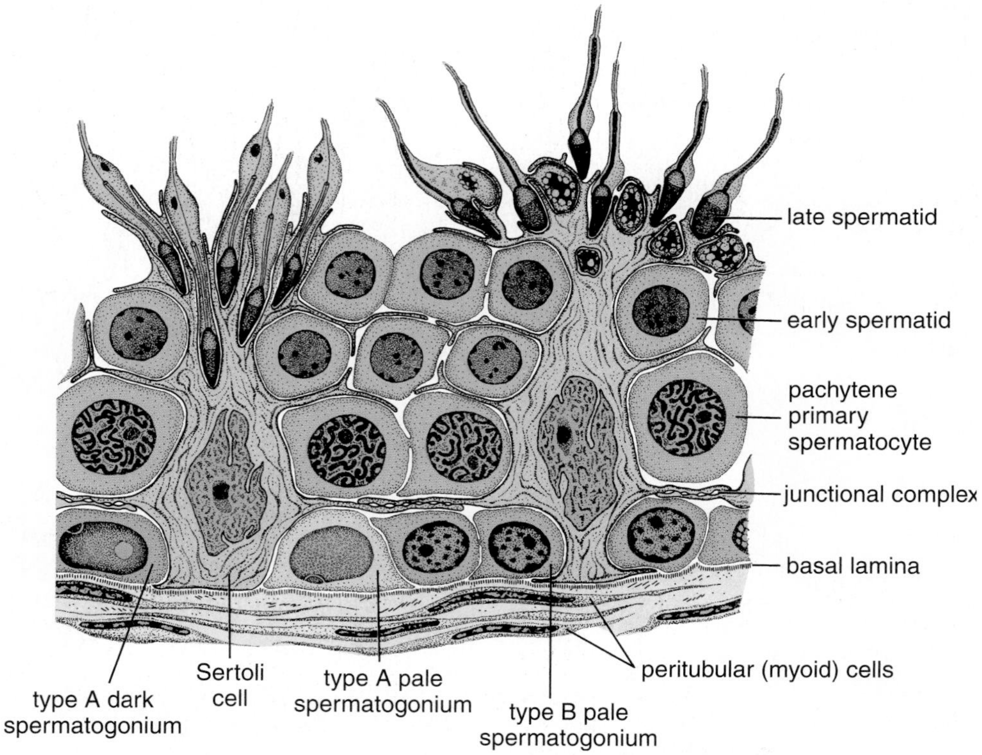

FIGURE 21.6
Schematic drawing of human seminiferous epithelium. This drawing shows the relationship of the Sertoli cells to the spermatogenic cells. The seminiferous epithelium rests on a basal lamina, and a layer of peritubular cells surrounds the seminiferous tubule. The spermatogonia–type A pale, type A dark, and type B pale–and preleptotene spermatocytes are located in the basal compartment of the seminiferous epithelium below the junctional complex, between adjacent Sertoli cells. Pachytene primary spermatocytes, early spermatids, and late spermatids, with partitioning residual cytoplasm that becomes the residual body, are seen above the junctional complex in the adluminal compartment. (Redrawn from Clermont Y. *Am J Anat* 1963;112:35.)

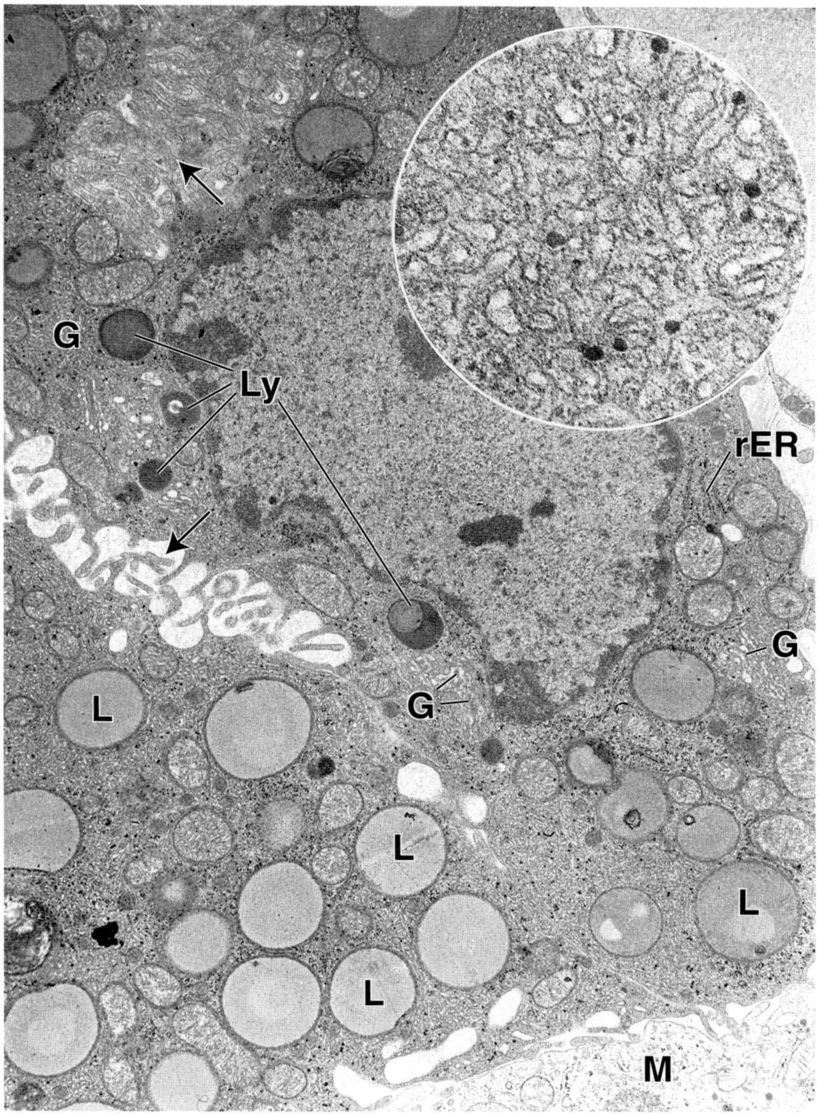

FIGURE 21.7
Electron micrograph of Leydig cells. This electron micrograph shows portions of several Leydig cells. The cytoplasm contains an abundance of sER, a characteristic of Leydig cells. Other features characteristic of the Leydig cell seen in the lower-power micrograph are the numerous lipid droplets *(L)*, the segmented profiles of the Golgi apparatus *(G)*, and the presence of variable numbers of lysosomes *(Ly)*. Occasional profiles of rER are also seen. Note also the presence of microvilli along portions of the cell surface *(arrows)*. *M*, cytoplasm of adjacent macrophage. ×10,000. **Inset.** sER at higher magnification. The very dense particles are glycogen. ×60,000

Like other steroid-secreting cells, Leydig cells have an elaborate smooth endoplasmic reticulum (sER), a feature that accounts for their eosinophilia (see Fig. 21.7). The enzymes necessary for the synthesis of testosterone from cholesterol are associated with the sER. Mitochondria with tubulovesicular cristae, another characteristic of steroid-secreting cells, are also present in Leydig cells.

Leydig cells differentiate and secrete testosterone during early fetal life. Secretion of testosterone is required during embryonic development, sexual maturation, and reproductive function:

- In the *embryo,* secretion of testosterone and other androgens is essential for the normal development of the gonads in the male fetus.
- At *puberty,* secretion of testosterone is responsible for the initiation of sperm production, accessory sex gland secretion, and development of secondary sex characteristics.
- In the *adult,* secretion of testosterone is essential for the maintenance of spermatogenesis and of secondary sex characteristics, genital excurrent ducts, and accessory sex glands.

The Leydig cells are active in the early differentiation of the male fetus and then undergo a period of inactivity beginning at about 5 months of fetal life. Inactive Leydig cells are difficult to distinguish from fibroblasts. When Leydig cells are exposed to gonadotropic stimulation at puberty, they again become androgen-secreting cells and remain active throughout life.

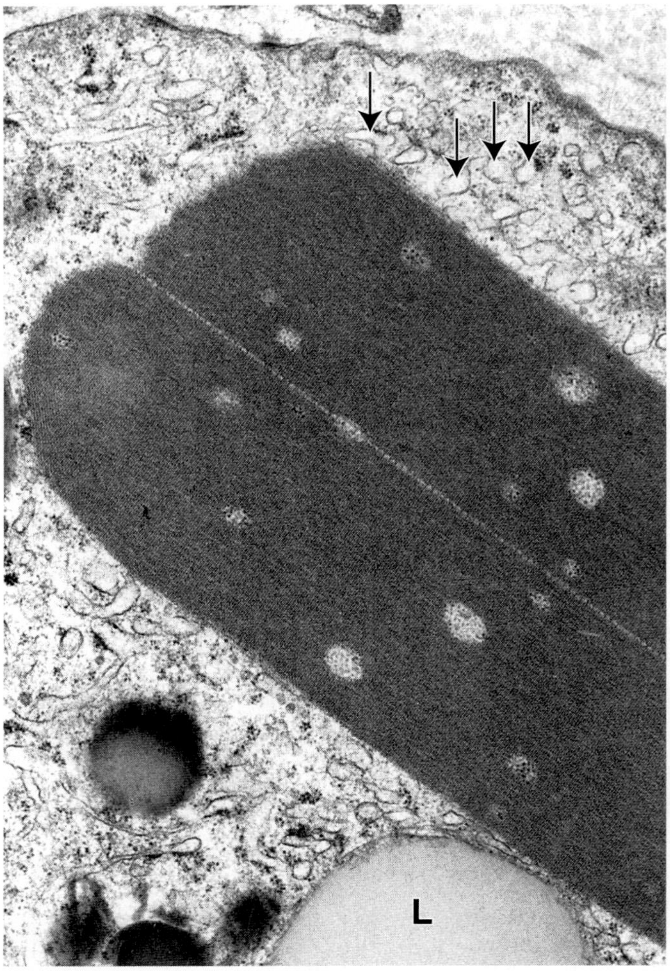

FIGURE 21.8
Electron micrograph of a Reinke crystal. This electron micrograph shows the internal structure of a Reinke crystal in the cytoplasm of a human Leydig cell. Also note the sER *(arrows)* and a lipid droplet *(L)* in the cytoplasm. ×16,000. (Courtesy of Dr. Don F. Cameron.)

BOX 21.1

Functional Considerations: Hormonal Regulation of Spermatogenesis

The endocrine function of the testis resides primarily in the Leydig cell population that synthesizes and secretes the principal circulating androgen, ***testosterone***. Nearly all of the testosterone is produced by the testis; less than 5% is produced by the adrenal glands. It is estimated in humans that the total Leydig cell population produces about 7 mg of testosterone per day. As the testosterone leaves the Leydig cells, it passes into blood and lymphatic capillaries and across the peritubular tissue to reach the seminiferous epithelium.

High local levels of testosterone within the testis (estimated to be as much as 200 times the circulating levels) are necessary for the proliferation and differentiation of spermatogenic cells. The lower peripheral level of testosterone influences

- Differentiation of the central nervous system (CNS) and the genital apparatus and genital excurrent duct system
- Growth and maintenance of secondary sexual characteristics (such as the beard, male distribution of pubic hair, and low-pitched voice)
- Growth and maintenance of the accessory sex glands (seminal vesicles, prostate, and bulbourethral glands), genital excurrent duct system, and the external genitalia (mainly by products of testosterone conversion to DHT)
- Anabolic and general metabolic processes, including skeletal growth, skeletal muscle growth, distribution of subcutaneous fat, and kidney function
- Behavior, including libido

The steroidogenic and spermatogenic activities of the testis are regulated by hormonal interaction among the hypothalamus, anterior lobe of the pituitary gland, and gonadal cells (i.e., Sertoli, spermatogenic, and Leydig cells). The anterior lobe of the pituitary gland produces three hormones involved in this process: luteinizing hormone (LH), which in the male is sometimes referred to as interstitial cell–stimulating hormone (ICSH); follicle-stimulating hormone (FSH); and prolactin (PRL). In response to LH release by the pituitary, Leydig cells produce increasing amounts of testosterone. PRL acts in combination with LH to increase the steroidogenic activity of the Leydig cells.

FSH and testosterone stimulate sperm production. Sertoli cells are the primary target for FSH and androgens. Therefore, Sertoli cells are the primary regulators of spermatogenesis.

SPERMATOGENESIS

Spermatogenesis is the process by which spermatogonia develop into sperm

Spermatogenesis, the process by which sperm are produced, involves a complex and unique series of events. It begins shortly before puberty, under the influence of rising levels of pituitary gonadotropins, and continues throughout life. For descriptive purposes, spermatogenesis is divided into three distinct phases:

- *Spermatogonial phase,* in which spermatogonia divide by mitosis to replace themselves as well as provide a population of committed spermatogonia that will eventually differentiate into ***primary spermatocytes***
- *Spermatocyte phase (meiosis),* in which primary spermatocytes undergo two meiotic divisions to reduce both the chromosome number and amount of DNA to produce haploid cells called ***spermatids***
- *Spermatid phase (spermiogenesis),* in which spermatids differentiate into mature ***sperm cells***

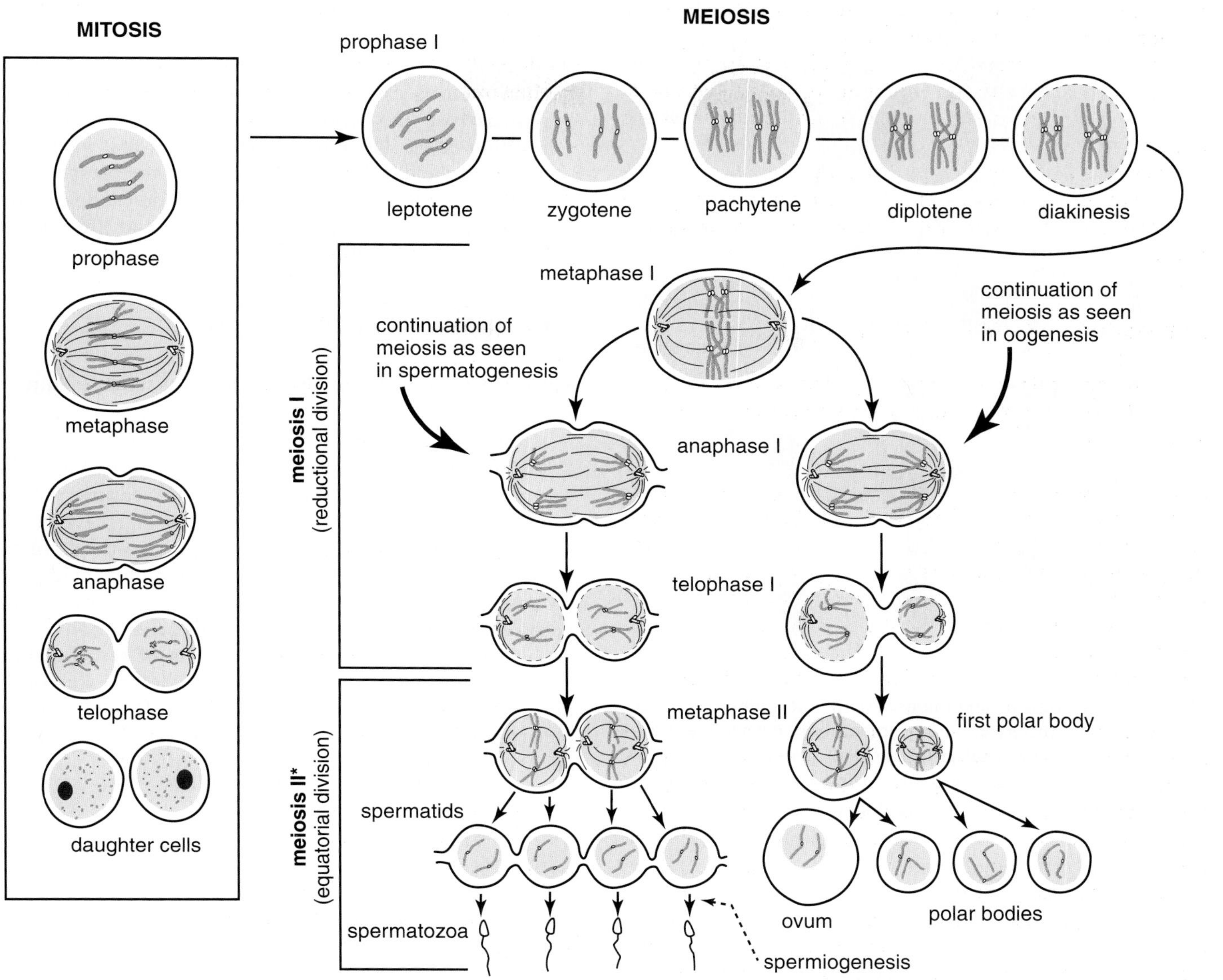

FIGURE 21.10

Comparison of mitosis and meiosis in a spermatogonial cell. The two pairs of chromosomes (2*n*) of maternal and paternal origin are depicted in *red* and *blue,* respectively. The mitotic division produces daughter cells that are genetically identical to the parental (2*n*) cell. The meiotic division, which has two components, a reductional division and an equatorial division, produces a cell that has only half the number of chomosomes *(n).* In addition, during the chromosome pairing in prophase I of meiosis, chromosome segments are exchanged, crossing-over, creating genetic diversity. In humans, the first polar body does not divide, but it does so in other species. *Note that prophase II, anaphase II, and telophase II are not shown.

nine peripheral microtubule doublets and two central microtubules that constitute the ***axoneme*** of the sperm tail (see page 92).

- ***Cap phase.*** In this phase, the acrosomal vesicle spreads over the anterior half of the nucleus. This reshaped structure is called the ***acrosomal cap.*** The portion of the nuclear envelope beneath the acrosomal cap loses its pores and becomes thicker. The nuclear contents also condense.
- ***Acrosome phase.*** In this phase, the spermatid reorients itself so that the head becomes deeply embedded in the Sertoli cell and points toward the basal lamina. The developing flagellum extends into the lumen of the seminiferous tubule. The condensed nucleus of the spermatid flattens and elongates, the nucleus and its overlying acrosome also move to a position immediately adjacent to the anterior plasma membrane, and the cytoplasm is displaced posteriorly. The cytoplasmic microtubules become organized into a cylindrical sheath, the ***manchette,*** which extends from the posterior rim of the acrosome toward the posterior pole of the spermatid.

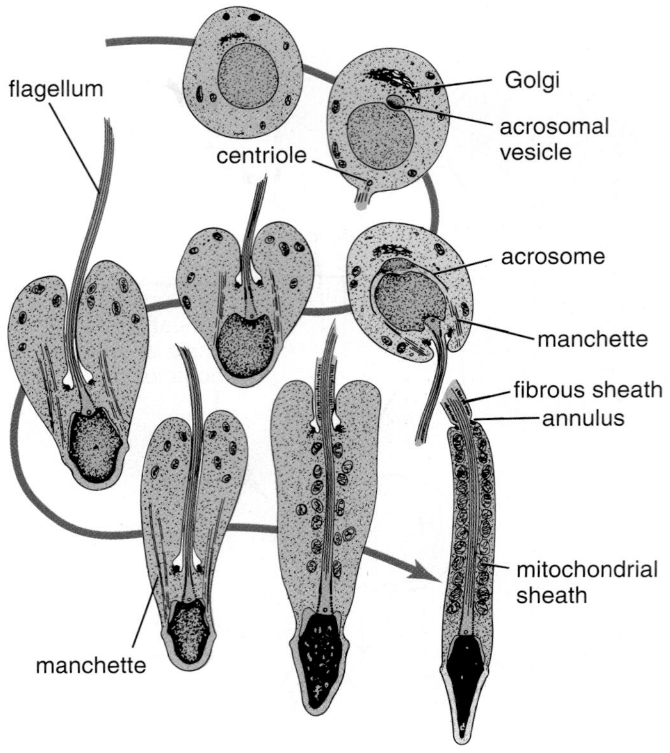

FIGURE 21.11
Schematic diagram of spermiogenesis in the human. The basic changes in the structure of the key organelles of the spermatid are illustrated (see text for detailed explanation). (Modified from Dym M. In: Weiss L, ed. *Cell and Tissue Biology: A Textbook of Histology.* 6th ed. Baltimore: Urban & Schwarzenberg, 1988.)

The centrioles, which had earlier initiated the development of the flagellum, now move back to the posterior surface of the nucleus where the immature centriole becomes attached to a shallow groove in the nucleus. They are then modified to form the ***connecting piece***, or ***neck region***, of the developing sperm. Nine coarse fibers develop from the centrioles attached to the nucleus and extend into the tail as the outer dense fibers peripheral to the microtubules of the axoneme. These fibers unite the nucleus with the flagellum, hence the name *connecting piece*.

As the plasma membrane moves posteriorly to cover the growing flagellum, the manchette disappears, and the mitochondria migrate from the rest of the cytoplasm to form a tight, helically wrapped sheath around the coarse fibers in the neck region and its immediate posterior extension (Fig. 21.12). This region is the ***middle piece*** of the tail of the sperm. Distal to the middle piece, a ***fibrous sheath*** consisting of two longitudinal columns and numerous connecting ribs surrounds the nine longitudinal fibers of the ***principal piece*** and extends nearly to the end of the flagellum. This short segment of the tail distal to the fibrous sheath is called the ***end piece***.

- ***Maturation phase.*** This last phase of spermatid remodeling reduces excess cytoplasm. The Sertoli cells then phagocytose this excess cytoplasm, also termed the ***residual body***. The intercellular bridges that have characterized the developing gametes since the prespermatocyte stages remain with the residual bodies. Spermatids are no longer attached to each other and are released from the Sertoli cells.

Structure of the Mature Sperm

The events of spermiogenesis result in a structurally unique cell

The mature human sperm is about 60 μm long. The sperm ***head*** is flattened and pointed and measures 4.5 μm long by 3 μm wide by 1 μm thick (see Fig. 21.12). The acrosomal cap that covers the anterior two-thirds of the nucleus contains hyaluronidase, neuraminidase, acid phosphatase, and a trypsin-like protease called acrosin. These acrosomal enzymes are essential for penetration of the zona pellucida of the ovum. The release of acrosomal enzymes as the sperm touches the egg is the first step in the ***acrosome reaction***. This complex process facilitates sperm penetration and subsequent fertilization and prevents the entry of additional sperm into the ovum.

BOX 21.2

Clinical Correlations: Factors Affecting Spermatogenesis

Spermatogenic cells are very sensitive to noxious agents. Degenerative changes, such as premature sloughing of the cells or formation of multinucleated giant cells, are readily apparent following exposure to such agents. Factors that affect spermatogenesis include

- Dietary deficiencies
- General or local infections
- Elevated testicular temperature
- Steroid hormones and related medications
- Toxic agents such as mutagens, drugs, antimetabolites, and pesticides (particularly short-chain halogenated hydrocarbons)
- Radiation

Proliferating cells are particularly sensitive to mutagenic agents and the absence of essential metabolites. Therefore, nondividing Sertoli cells, Leydig cells, and reserve stem cells, which demonstrate low mitotic activity, are much less vulnerable than actively dividing, differentiating spermatogenic cells.

Spermatogonial Phase

In the spermatogonial phase, stem cells divide to replace themselves and provide a population of committed spermatogonia

Spermatogonial stem cells undergo multiple divisions and produce spermatogonial progeny that display differences in nuclear appearance in routine H&E preparations. Human spermatogonia are classified into three types on the basis of the appearance of the nuclei in routine histologic preparations:

- ***Type A dark (Ad) spermatogonia*** have ovoid nuclei with intensely basophilic, finely granular chromatin. These spermatogonia are thought to be the stem cells of the seminiferous epithelium. They divide at irregular intervals to give rise to either a pair of type Ad spermatogonia that remain as stem cells or to a pair of type Ap spermatogonia (see below).
- ***Type A pale (Ap) spermatogonia*** have ovoid nuclei with lightly staining, finely granular chromatin. Ap spermatogonia are committed to the differentiation process that produces the sperm. They undergo several successive mitotic divisions, thereby increasing their number.
- ***Type B spermatogonia*** have generally spherical nuclei with chromatin that is condensed into large clumps along the nuclear envelope and around a central nucleolus (see Fig. 21.6).

An unusual feature of the division of an Ad spermatogonium into two type Ap spermatogonia is that the daughter cells remain connected by a thin cytoplasmic bridge. This same phenomenon occurs through each subsequent mitotic and meiotic division of the progeny of the original pair of Ap spermatogonia (Fig. 21.9). Thus, all of

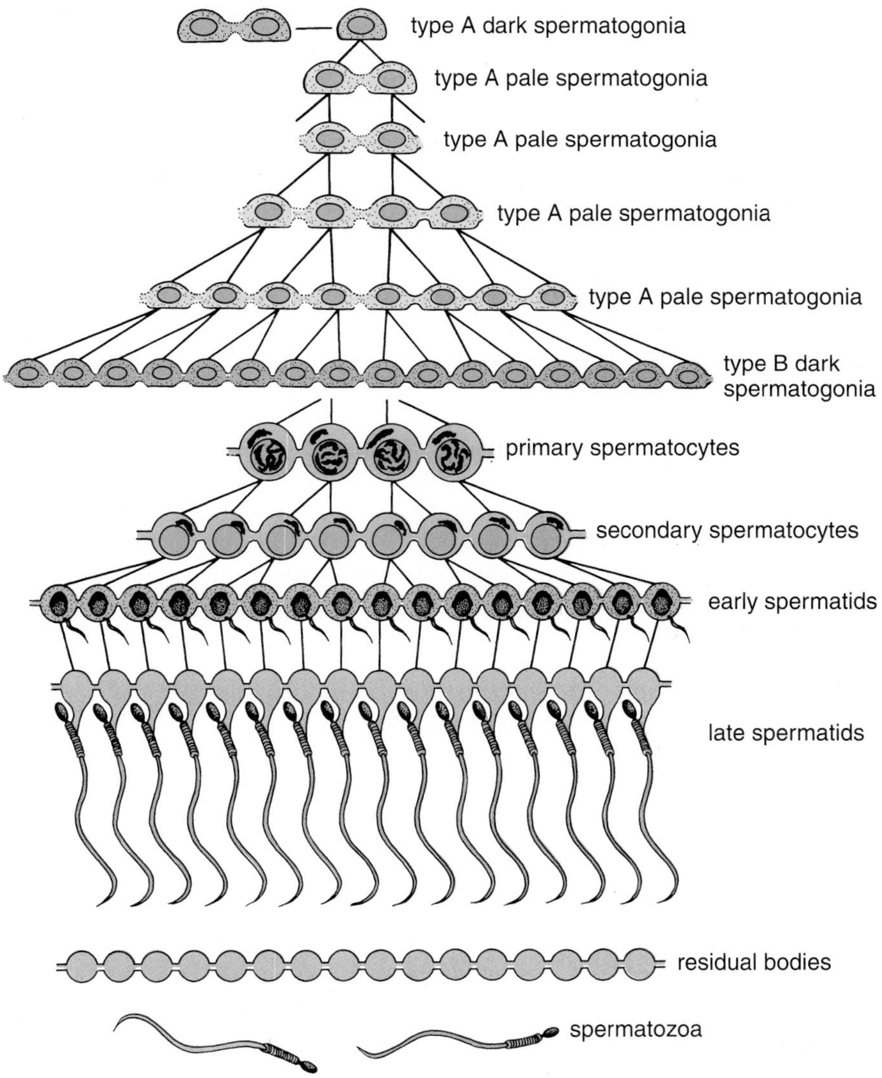

FIGURE 21.9
Schematic diagram illustrating the generations of spermatogenic cells. This diagram shows the clonal nature of the successive generations of spermatogenic cells. Cytoplasmic division is complete only in the primitive type A dark spermatogonia that serve as stem cells. All other spermatogenic cells remain connected by intercellular bridges as they undergo mitotic and meiotic division and differentiation of the spermatids. The cells separate into individual spermatozoa as they are released from the seminiferous epithelium. The residual bodies remain connected and are phagocytosed by the Sertoli cells. (From Dym M, Fawcett DW. *Biol Reprod* 1971;4:195–215.)

the progeny of an initial pair of Ap spermatogonia are connected, much like a strand of pearls. These cytoplasmic connections remain intact to the last stages of spermatid maturation and are essential for the synchronous development of each clone from an original pair of Ap cells.

After several divisions, type A spermatogonia differentiate into type B spermatogonia. The appearance of type B spermatogonia represents the last event in the spermatogonial phase.

Spermatocyte Phase (Meiosis)

In the spermatocyte phase, primary spermatocytes undergo meiosis to reduce both the chromosome number and the amount of DNA

The mitotic division of type B spermatogonia produces primary spermatocytes. They replicate their DNA shortly after they form and before meiosis begins, so that each primary spermatocyte contains twice the normal chromosomal number ($4n$) and double the amount of DNA.

Meiosis results in reduction of both the number of chromosomes and the amount of DNA to the haploid condition. Meiosis is described in detail in Chapter 2 (see page 69); a brief description of spermatocyte meiosis follows.

Prophase of the first meiotic division, during which the chromatin condenses into visible chromosomes, lasts up to 22 days in human primary spermatocytes. At the end of prophase, 44 autosomes and an X and a Y chromosome, each having two chromatin strands (chromatids), can be identified. Homologous chromosomes are paired as they line up on the metaphase plate.

The paired homologous chromosomes, called ***tetrads*** because they consist of four chromatids, exchange genetic material in a process called ***crossing-over.*** During this exchange, the four chromatids rearrange into a tripartite structure called a ***synaptonemal complex.*** This process ensures genetic diversity. Through genetic exchange, the four spermatids produced from each spermatocyte differ from each other and from every other spermatid. After crossing-over is complete, the homologous chromosomes separate and move to the opposite poles of the meiotic spindle. Thus, the tetrads, which have been modified by crossing-over, separate and become dyads again. The two chromatids of each original chromosome (although modified by crossing-over) remain together. This is just the opposite of what happens in mitosis, in which the paired chromatids—one representing "template" and the other, newly synthesized DNA—separate.

The movement of a particular chromosome of a homologous pair to either pole of the spindle is random; i.e., maternally derived chromosomes and paternally derived chromosomes do not sort themselves out at the metaphase plate. This random sorting is another source of genetic diversity in the resulting sperm.

The cells derived from the first meiotic division are called ***secondary spermatocytes.*** These cells immediately enter the prophase of the second meiotic division *without synthesizing new DNA* (i.e., without passing through an S phase; see page 69). Each secondary spermatocyte has 22 autosomes and an X or a Y chromosome. Each of these chromosomes consists of two sister chromatids. The secondary spermatocyte has the $2n$ (diploid) amount of DNA. During metaphase of the second meiotic division, the chromosomes line up at the metaphase plate, and the sister chromatids separate and move to opposite poles of the spindle. As the second meiotic division is completed and the nuclear membranes reform, two haploid ***spermatids,*** each containing 22 single-stranded chromosomes and the $1n$ amount of DNA, are formed from each secondary spermatocyte (Fig. 21.10).

Spermatid Phase (Spermiogenesis)

In the spermatid phase, spermatids undergo extensive cell remodeling as they differentiate into mature sperm

Each spermatid that results from the second meiotic division is haploid in DNA content and chromosome number (22 autosomes and an X or Y chromosome). No further division occurs. The haploid spermatids undergo a differentiation process that produces mature sperm, which are also haploid. The normal diploid condition is restored when a sperm fertilizes an oocyte.

The extensive cell remodeling that occurs during differentiation of the spermatid population into mature sperm (spermiogenesis) consists of four phases. These phases occur while the spermatids are physically attached to the Sertoli cell plasma membrane by specialized junctions. The morphologic changes in all four phases that occur during spermiogenesis are described below and summarized in Figure 21.11.

- ***Golgi phase.*** This phase is characterized by the presence of periodic acid–Schiff (PAS)-positive granules that accumulate in the multiple Golgi complexes of the spermatid. These ***proacrosomal granules,*** rich in glycoproteins, coalesce into a membrane-bounded vesicle, the ***acrosomal vesicle,*** adjacent to the nuclear envelope. The vesicle enlarges and its contents increase during this phase. The position of the acrosomal vesicle determines the anterior pole of the developing sperm. Also during this phase, the centrioles migrate from the juxtanuclear region to the posterior pole of the spermatid, where the mature centriole aligns at right angles to the plasma membrane. The centriole initiates the assembly of the

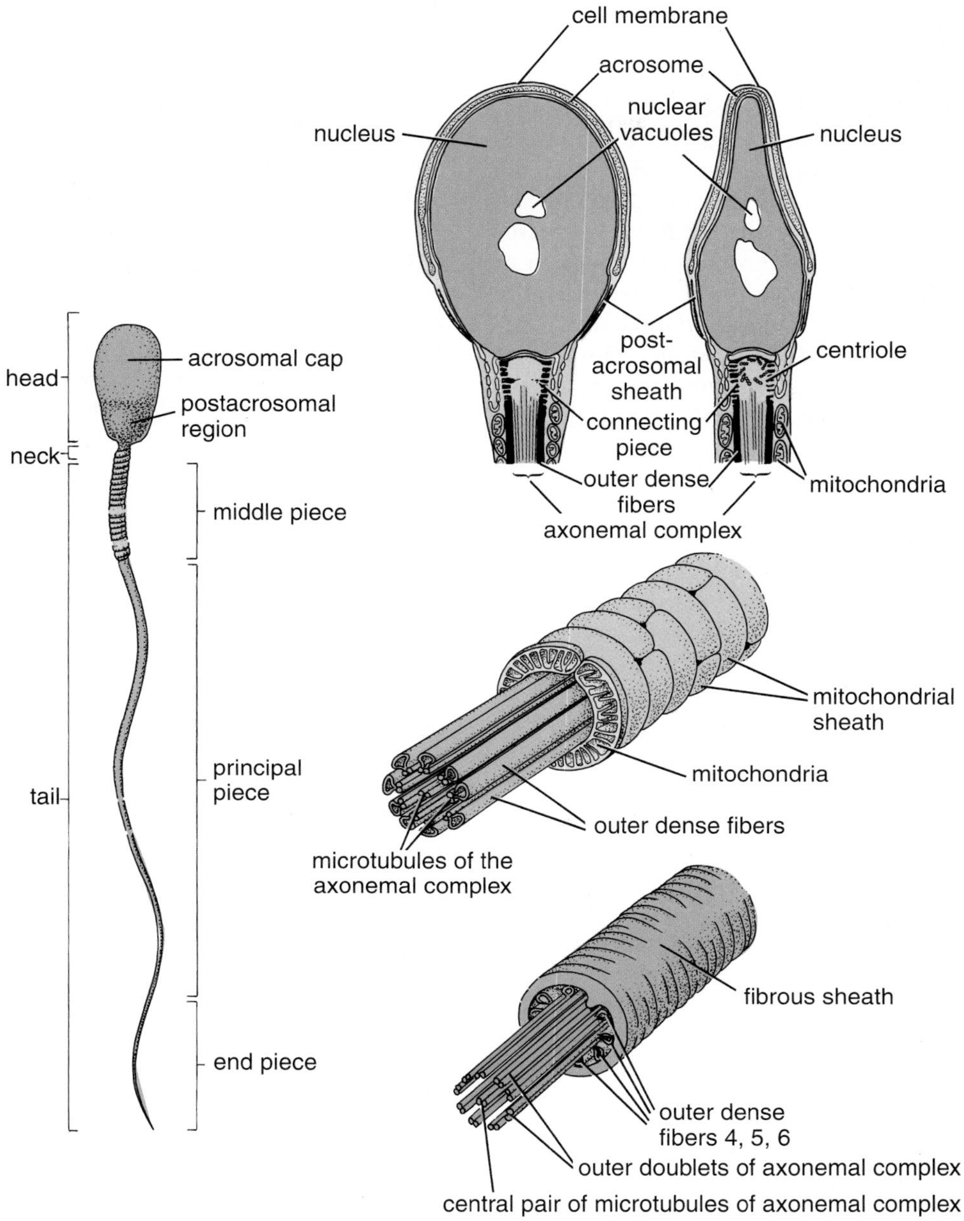

FIGURE 21.12
Diagram of a human spermatozoon. Regions of the spermatozoon are indicated on the left. Key structural features of the head (viewed in frontal and sagittal planes), the middle piece, and the principal piece of the spermatozoon are illustrated on the right. (Modified from Pederson PL, Fawcett DW. In: Hafez ESE, ed. *Human Semen and Fertility Regulation in the Male.* St. Louis: CV Mosby, 1976.)

The sperm ***tail*** is subdivided into the neck, the middle piece, the principal piece, and the end piece. The short neck contains the centrioles and the origin of the coarse fibers. The middle piece is approximately 7 μm long and contains the mitochondria, helically wrapped around the coarse fibers and the axonemal complex. These mitochondria provide the energy for movement of the tail and thus are responsible for the motility of the sperm. The principal piece is approximately 40 μm long and contains the fibrous sheath external to the coarse fibers and the axonemal complex. The end piece, approximately the last 5 μm of the flagellum in the mature sperm, contains only the axonemal complex.

Newly released sperm are nonmotile

Newly released sperm are carried from the seminiferous tubules in a fluid secreted by the Sertoli cells. The fluid and sperm flow through the seminiferous tubules, facilitated by peristaltic contractions of the peritubular contractile cells of the lamina propria. They then enter the ***straight tubules,***

a short segment of the seminiferous tubule where the epithelium consists only of Sertoli cells. At the mediastinum testis the fluid and sperm enter the ***rete testis,*** an anastomosing system of ducts lined by simple cuboidal epithelium. From the rete testis, they move into the extratesticular portion of the ***efferent ductules*** (ductuli efferentes), the first part of the excurrent duct system, and then into the proximal portion of the ***duct of the epididymis*** (ductus epididymis). As the sperm move through the 4 to 5 m of the highly coiled duct of the epididymis, they acquire motility. Contractions of the smooth muscle that surrounds the progressively distal and larger ducts continue to move the sperm by peristaltic action until they reach the distal portion of the duct of the epididymis where they are stored before ejaculation.

Sperm can *live* for several weeks in the male excurrent duct system, but they will *survive* only 2 to 3 days in the female reproductive tract. They acquire the ability to fertilize the ovum only after some time in the female tract. This process, which involves removal and replacement of glycocalyx components (glycoconjugates) on the sperm membrane, is called ***capacitation.***

▼ SEMINIFEROUS TUBULES

Cycle of the Seminiferous Epithelium

Differentiating spermatogenic cells are not arranged at random in the seminiferous epithelium; specific cell types are grouped together. These groupings or associations occur because intercellular bridges are present between the progeny of each pair of type Ap spermatogonia and because the synchronized cells spend specific times in each stage of maturation. All phases of differentiation occur sequentially at any given site in a seminiferous tubule as the progeny of stem cells remain connected by cytoplasmic bridges and undergo synchronous mitotic and meiotic divisions and maturation (see Fig. 21.10).

Each recognizable grouping, or ***cell association,*** is considered a ***stage*** in a cyclic process. The series of stages that appears between two successive occurrences of the same cell association pattern at any given site in the seminiferous tubule constitutes a ***cycle of the seminiferous epithelium.*** The cycle of the seminiferous epithelium has been most thoroughly studied in rats, in which 14 successive stages occur in linear sequence along the tubule. In man, 6 stages or cell associations are defined in the cycle of the seminiferous epithelium (Fig. 21.13). These stages are not as clearly delineated as those in rodents because in man the cellular associations occur in irregular patches that form a mosaic pattern.

Duration of spermatogenesis in humans is approximately 74 days

After injecting a pulse of tritiated thymidine, a specific generation of cells can be followed by sequential biopsies of the seminiferous tubules. In this way, the time required for the labeled cells to go through the various stages can be determined. Several generations of developing cells may be present in the thickness of the seminiferous epithelium at any given site and at any given time, which produces the characteristic cell associations. Autoradiographic studies have revealed that the duration of the cycle of the seminiferous epithelium is constant, lasting about 16 days in humans. In humans it would require about 4.6 cycles (each 16 days long), or approximately 74 days, for a spermatogonium produced by a stem cell to complete the process of spermatogenesis. It would then require approximately 12 days for the spermatozoon to pass through the epididymis. Approximately 300 million sperm cells are produced daily in the human testis. The length of the cycle and the time required for spermatogenesis are constant and specific in each species. Therefore, in any pharmacologic intervention (e.g., therapy for male infertility), if a drug is given that affects the initial phases of spermatogenesis, approximately 86 days are required to see the effect of that compound on sperm production.

Waves of the Seminiferous Epithelium

As indicated above, the cycle of the seminiferous epithelium describes changes that occur with time at any given site in the tubule. In addition, the ***wave of the seminiferous epithelium*** describes the distribution of patterns of cellular association (stages) along the length of the tubule. In rodents and other mammals that have been studied, including subhuman primates, each stage occupies a significant length of the seminiferous tubule, and the stages appear to occur sequentially along the length of the tubule. In the rat, there are approximately 12 waves in each tubule. A transverse section through the tubule usually reveals only one pattern of cell associations. There are no waves in the human seminiferous epithelium. Each pattern of cellular associations (stage of the cycle) has a patch-like distribution in the human seminiferous tubule (Fig. 21.14). Patches do not extend around the circumference of the tubule, nor are they in sequence. Therefore, a transverse section through a human seminiferous tubule may reveal as many as six different stages of the cycle arranged in a pie-wedge fashion around the circumference of the tubule.

Sertoli Cells

Sertoli cells constitute the true epithelium of the seminiferous epithelium

Sertoli cells ***(sustentacular cells)*** are tall, columnar, nonreplicating epithelial cells that rest on the thick, multilayered basal lamina of the seminiferous epithelium (Fig. 21.15). They are the supporting cells for the devel-

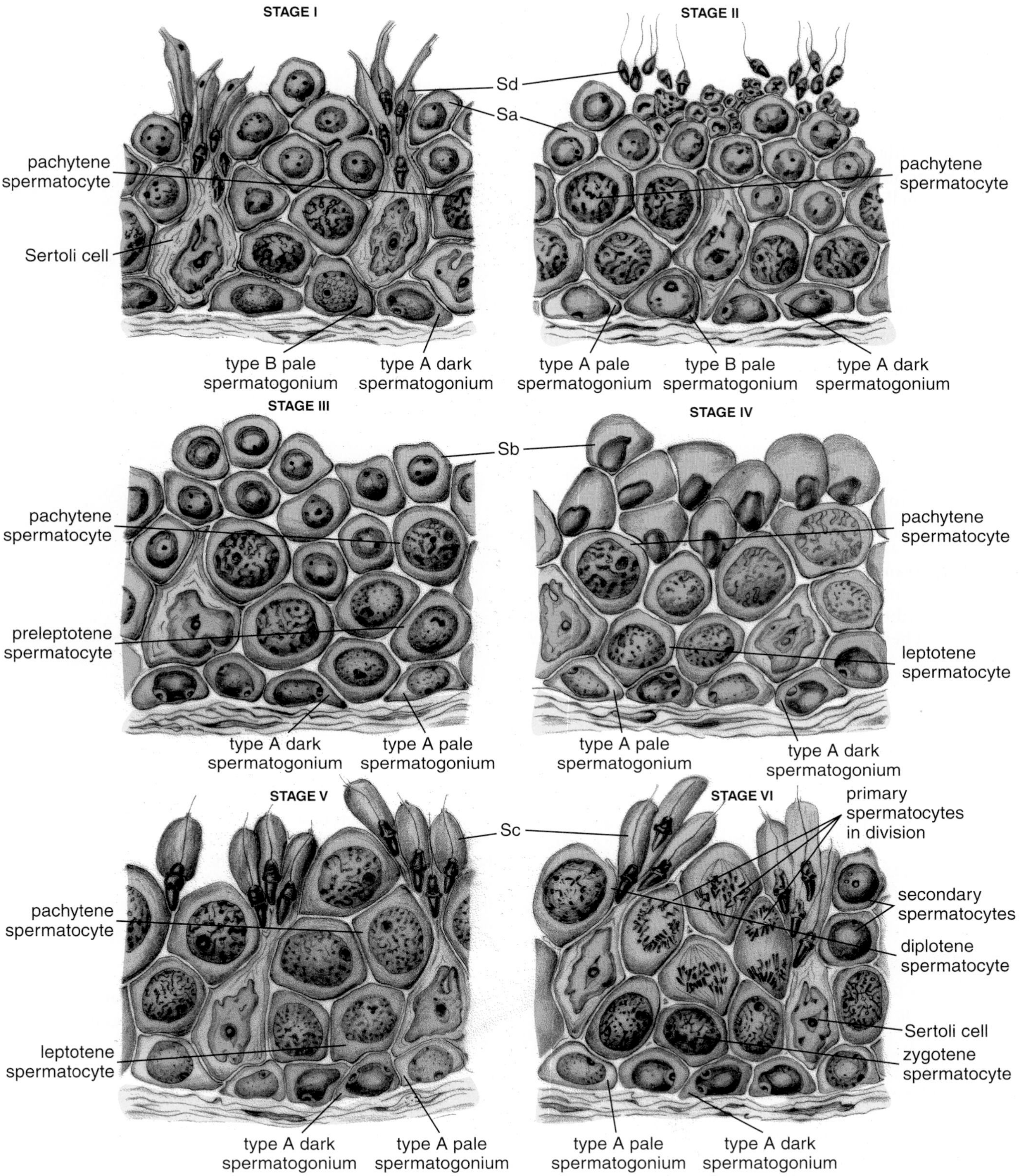

FIGURE 21.13
Schematic drawing of the stages of the human seminiferous epithelium. This diagram shows each of the six recognizable cell associations that occur in the cycle of the human seminiferous epithelium. *Sa, Sb, Sc,* and *Sd* indicate spermatids in various steps of differentiation. (Based on Clermont Y. *Am J Anat* 1963;112:50.)

oping sperm that attach to their surface after meiosis. Sertoli cells contain an extensive sER, a well-developed rER, and stacks of annulate lamellae. They have numerous spherical and elongated mitochondria; a well-developed Golgi apparatus; and varying numbers of microtubules, lysosomes, lipid droplets, vesicles, glycogen granules, and filaments. A sheath of 7- to 9-nm filaments surrounds the nucleus and separates it from other cytoplasmic organelles.

The euchromatic Sertoli cell nucleus, a reflection of this very active cell, is generally ovoid or triangular and may have one or more deep infoldings. Its shape and location vary. It may be flattened, lying in the basal portion of the cell near and parallel to the base of the cell, or it may be triangular or ovoid, lying near or some distance from the base of the cell. In some species, the Sertoli cell nucleus contains a unique tripartite structure that consists of a RNA-containing nucleolus flanked by a pair of DNA-containing bodies called ***karyosomes*** (Fig. 21.16).

In man, characteristic inclusion bodies (of Charcot-Böttcher) are found in the basal cytoplasm. These slender fusiform crystalloids measure 10 to 25 μm long by 1 μm wide and are visible in routine histologic preparations. With transmission electron microscopy, they are resolved as bundles of poorly ordered, parallel or converging, straight, dense 15-nm-diameter filaments (see Fig. 21.15). Their chemical composition and function are unknown

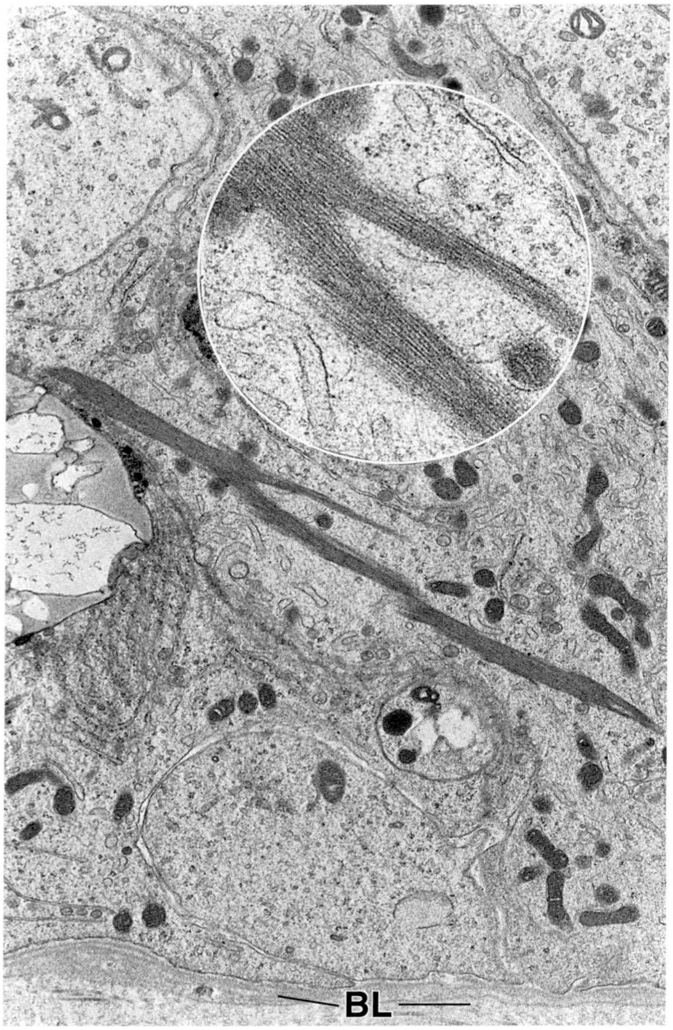

FIGURE 21.15
Electron micrograph of a human Sertoli cell. This electron micrograph shows characteristic crystalloid inclusion bodies of Charcot-Böttcher in the basal cytoplasm of the Sertoli cell. The basal lamina *(BL)* is indicated for orientation. ×9,000. **Inset.** This higher magnification shows filaments of the crystalloid. ×27,000. (Courtesy of Don F. Cameron.)

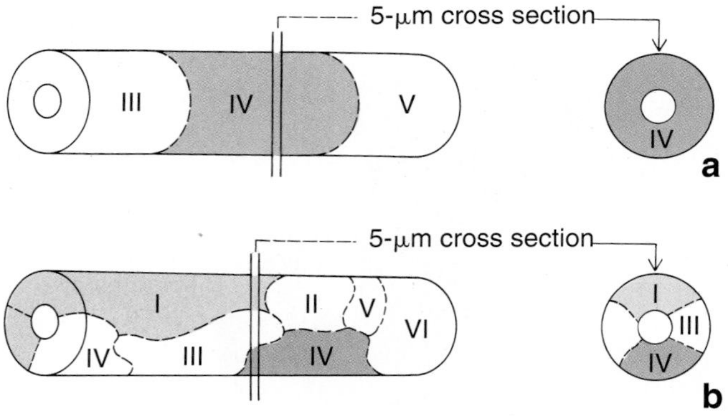

FIGURE 21.14
Diagram of organization of seminiferous epithelium in humans and other species. a. In subhuman species, a particular cellular association occupies varying lengths along the tubule. Therefore, in a typical cross section only a single cellular association is observed. **b.** In humans, cellular associations occur in irregularly shaped areas along the tubule, and therefore, a cross section typically shows two or more cellular associations. (Modified from Dym M. In: Weiss L, ed. *Cell and Tissue Biology: A Textbook of Histology.* 6th ed. Baltimore: Urban & Schwarzenberg, 1988.)

The Sertoli cell–to–Sertoli cell junctional complex consists of a structurally unique combination of membrane and cytoplasmic specializations

Sertoli cells are bound to one another by an unusual junctional complex (Fig. 21.17). This complex is characterized, in part, by an exceedingly tight junction (zonula occludens) that includes more than 50 parallel fusion lines in the adjacent membranes. In addition, two cytoplasmic components characterize this unique junctional complex:

- A *flattened cisterna of sER* lies parallel to the plasma membrane in the region of the junction in each cell.

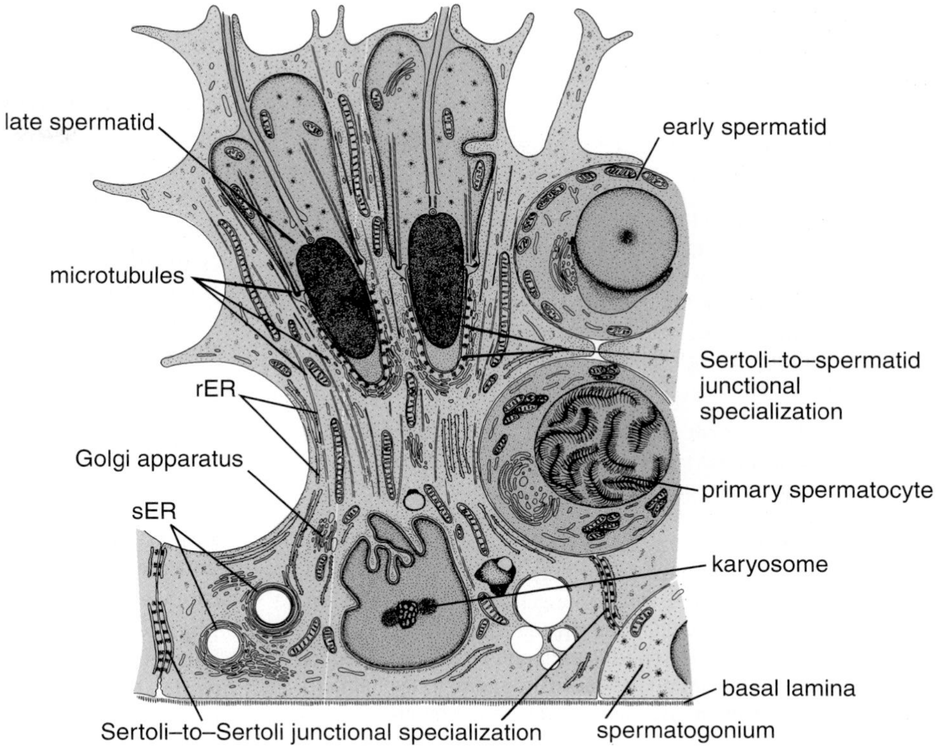

FIGURE 21.16
Schematic drawing of the Sertoli cell and its relationship to adjacent spermatogenic cells. This drawing shows the Sertoli–to–Sertoli junctional specialization between adjacent Sertoli cells and the Sertoli–to–spermatid junctional specialization between the Sertoli cell and late spermatids. The Sertoli–to–Sertoli junctional complex is an adhesion device that includes a tight junction that contributes to the blood–testis barrier. The junctional specialization between the Sertoli cell and late spermatids residing in deep recesses within the apical cytoplasm is an adhesion device only. Lateral processes of the Sertoli cells extend over the surface of the spermatocytes and spermatids. Note the ultrastructural features of the Sertoli cell, including the microtubule arrays and characteristic shape of the nucleus and its karyosome. (From Bloom W, Fawcett DW. *A Textbook of Histology.* Philadelphia: WB Saunders, 1975.)

- *Actin filament bundles*, hexagonally packed, are interposed between the sER cisternae and the plasma membranes.

A similar-appearing junctional complex in the Sertoli cell is also present at the site where the spermatids are attached. However, no tight junction is present, and the spermatid lacks flattened cisternae of sER and actin filament bundles (see Figs. 21.16 and 21.17). Other junc-

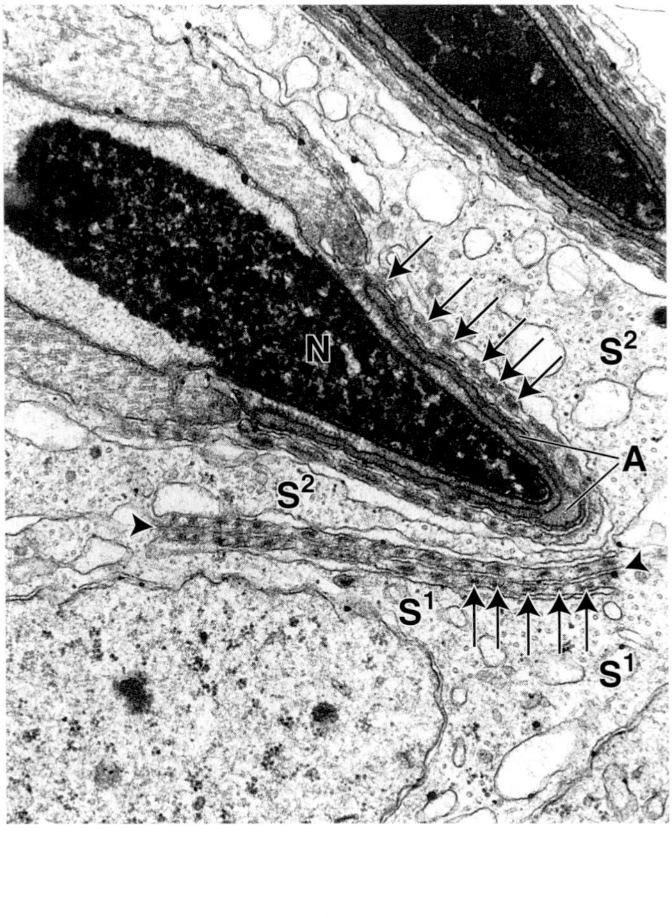

FIGURE 21.17
Electron micrograph of Sertoli cell junctions. This electron micrograph demonstrates a Sertoli–to–Sertoli junctional complex and, in close proximity, a Sertoli–to–spermatid junctional specialization. Condensation and shaping of the spermatid nucleus *(N)* are well advanced. The acrosome *(A)* of the spermatid appears as a V-shaped profile, and in close association with it is the Sertoli cell junctional specialization characterized by bundles of microfilaments that are cut in cross section *(arrows).* The associated profile of endoplasmic reticulum resides immediately adjacent to the microfilament bundles. The Sertoli–to–Sertoli junction lies below, joining one Sertoli cell *(S^1)* to the adjacent Sertoli cell *(S^2).* The *arrowheads* indicate the limits of the junction. Note that the junction here reveals the same elements, the microfilament bundles *(arrows)* and a profile of endoplasmic reticulum, as are seen in the Sertoli–to–spermatid junctional specialization. Not evident at this magnification is the tight junction associated with the Sertoli–to–Sertoli junctional complex. ×30,000.

BOX 21.3

Clinical Correlations: Sperm-Specific Antigens and the Immune Response

Two basic facts are well established about the immunologic importance of the blood–testis barrier:

- Spermatozoa and spermatogenic cells possess molecules that are unique to these cells and are recognized as "foreign" (not self) by the immune system.
- Spermatozoa are first produced at puberty, long after the individual has become immunocompetent, i.e., capable of recognizing foreign molecules and producing antibodies against them.

Failure of the spermatogenic cells and spermatozoa to remain isolated results in the production of sperm-specific antibodies. Such an immune response is sometimes seen after vasectomy and in some cases of infertility. After vasectomy, sperm-specific antibodies are produced as the cells of the immune system are exposed to the spermatozoa that may leak from the severed ductus deferens. Thus, sperm no longer remain isolated from the immune system within the reproductive tract. In some cases of infertility, sperm-specific antibodies have been found in the semen. These antibodies cause the sperm to agglutinate, preventing movement and interaction with the ovum.

tional specializations of the Sertoli cells include gap junctions between Sertoli cells, desmosome-like junctions between Sertoli cells and early-stage spermatogenic cells, and hemidesmosomes at the Sertoli cell–basal lamina interface.

The Sertoli cell–to–Sertoli cell junctional complex divides the seminiferous epithelium into basal and luminal compartments

The Sertoli cell–to–Sertoli cell junctions establish two epithelial compartments, a ***basal epithelial compartment*** and a ***luminal compartment.*** Spermatogonia and early primary spermatocytes are restricted to the basal compartment, i.e., between the Sertoli cell–to–Sertoli cell junctions and the basal lamina. More mature spermatocytes and spermatids are restricted to the luminal side of the Sertoli cell–to–Sertoli cell junctions. Early spermatocytes produced by mitotic division of type B spermatogonia must pass through the junctional complex to move from the basal compartment to the luminal compartment. This movement occurs via the formation of a new junctional complex between Sertoli cell processes that extend beneath the newly formed spermatocytes, followed by the breakdown of the junction above them. Thus, in the differentiation of the spermatogenic cells, the processes of meiosis and spermiogenesis occur in the luminal compartment.

In both compartments, spermatogenic cells are surrounded by complex processes of the Sertoli cells. Because of the unusually close relationships between Sertoli cells and differentiating spermatogenic cells, it has been suggested that Sertoli cells serve as "nurse," or supporting, cells, i.e., they function in the exchange of metabolic substrates and wastes between the developing spermatogenic cells and the circulatory system.

In addition, Sertoli cells phagocytose and break down the residual bodies formed in the last stage of spermiogenesis. They also phagocytose any spermatogenic cells that fail to differentiate completely.

The Sertoli cell–to–Sertoli cell junctional complex is the site of the blood–testis barrier

In addition to the physical compartmentalization described above, the Sertoli cell–to–Sertoli cell junctional complex also creates a permeability barrier called the ***blood–testis barrier.*** This barrier is essential in creating a physiologic compartmentalization within the seminiferous epithelium with respect to ionic, amino acid, carbohydrate, and protein composition. Therefore, the composition of the fluid in the seminiferous tubules and excurrent ducts differs considerably from the composition of the blood plasma and testicular lymph.

Plasma proteins and circulating antibodies are excluded from the lumen of the seminiferous tubules. The exocrine secretory products of the Sertoli cells, particularly 90-kDa ***androgen-binding protein (ABP)***, which has a high binding affinity for testosterone and DHT, are highly concentrated in the lumen of the seminiferous tubules and maintain a high concentration of testosterone, which provides a favorable microenvironment for the differentiating spermatogenic cells.

Most importantly, the blood–testis barrier isolates the genetically different and therefore antigenic haploid germ cells (secondary spermatocytes, spermatids, and sperm) from the immune system of the adult male. Antigens produced by, or specific to, the sperm are prevented from reaching the systemic circulation. Conversely, γ-globulins and specific sperm antibodies found in some individuals are prevented from reaching the developing spermatogenic cells in the seminiferous tubule.

Therefore, the blood–testis barrier serves an essential role in isolating the spermatogenic cells from the immune system.

Sertoli cells have both exocrine and endocrine secretory functions

In addition to secreting fluid that facilitates passage of the maturing sperm along the seminiferous tubules to the intratesticular ducts, Sertoli cells secrete ABP. ABP concentrates testosterone in the luminal compartment of the sem-

iniferous tubule, where high concentrations of testosterone are essential for normal maturation of the developing sperm.

Sertoli cells also secrete several endocrine substances such as ***inhibin***, a 32-kDa glycoprotein hormone involved in the feedback loop that inhibits FSH release from the anterior pituitary gland. Sertoli cells, themselves, are stimulated by both FSH and testosterone. In addition, Sertoli cells also synthesize ***plasminogen activator***, which converts plasminogen to the active proteolytic hormone plasmin) and ***transferrin*** (an iron-transporting protein). FSH receptors are believed to be present only on Sertoli cells and are essential for the secretion of ABP, inhibin, and plasminogen activator (Fig. 21.18).

INTRATESTICULAR DUCTS

At the end of each seminiferous tubule there is an abrupt transition to the ***straight tubules***, or ***tubuli recti***. This short terminal section of the seminiferous tubule is lined only by Sertoli cells. Near their termination, the straight tubules narrow, and their lining changes to a simple cuboidal epithelium.

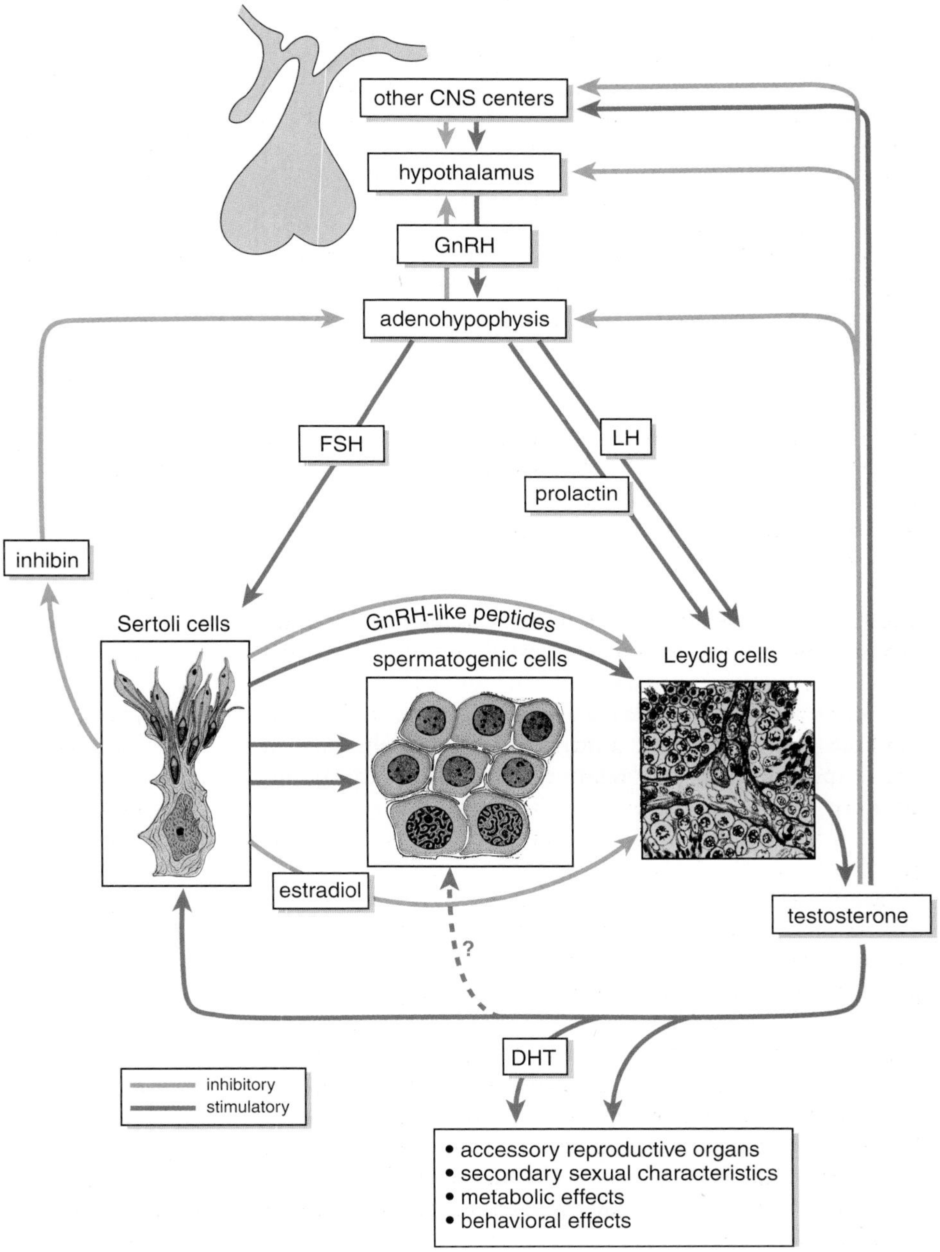

FIGURE 21.18
Diagram depicting the hormonal regulation of male reproductive function. *Blue arrows* indicate stimulatory action on the system; *red arrows* indicate inhibitory feedback. See text for explanation.

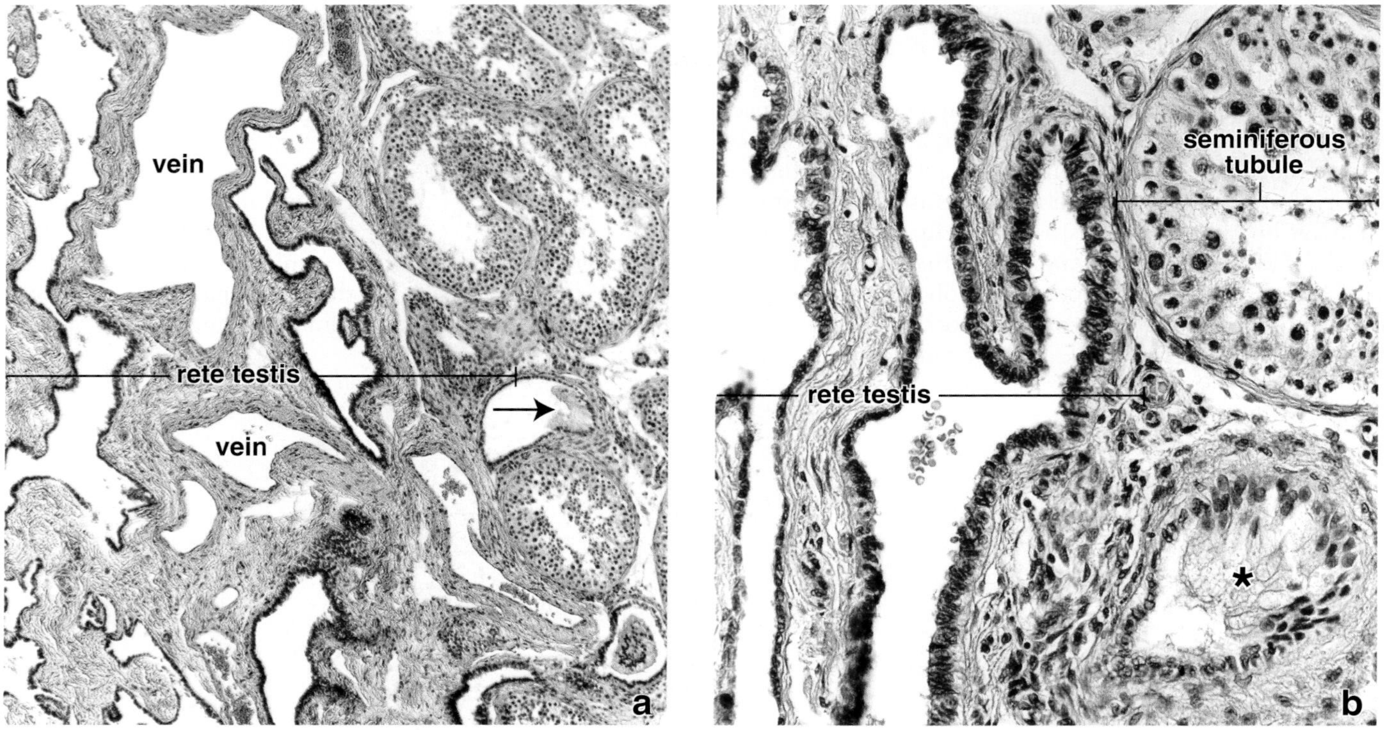

FIGURE 21.19
Photomicrograph of human testis. a. This H&E–stained specimen shows the site that includes the mediastinum of the testis. On the right are seminiferous tubules, and on the left are the anastomosing channels of the rete testis. The *arrow* indicates termination of a straight tubule that is lined only by Sertoli cells. It is at this site that the tubule content enters the rete testis and the channels are then lined by a simple cuboidal epithelium. ×70. **b.** This higher magnification from a slightly deeper section of the same specimen shows the rete testis (left), a cross section of a seminiferous tubule (upper right), and a terminating straight tubule *(asterisk)* where it is entering the rete testis. Note the abrupt change in the epithelial lining at this site. As noted, the lining epithelium of the rete testis is simple cuboidal. ×275.

The straight tubules empty into the ***rete testis***, a complex series of interconnecting channels within the highly vascular connective tissue of the mediastinum (Fig. 21.19). A simple cuboidal or low columnar epithelium lines the channels of the rete testis. These cells have a single apical cilium and relatively few short apical microvilli.

EXCURRENT DUCT SYSTEM

The excurrent duct system develops from the mesonephric (Wolffian) duct and mesonephric tubules

The initial development of Leydig cells and initiation of testosterone secretion stimulate the mesonephric (Wolffian) duct to differentiate into the excretory duct system for the developing testis (Fig. 21.20). The portion of the mesonephric duct adjacent to the developing testis becomes convoluted and differentiates into the ***duct of the epididymis.*** In addition, a number (about 20) of the remaining mesonephric tubules in this region make contact with the developing seminiferous cords and finally develop into the ***efferent ductules*** (Fig. 21.21). They connect the developing rete testis with the duct of the epididymis. The distal part of the mesonephric duct acquires a thick, smooth muscle coat and becomes the ***ductus deferens.*** The end of the distal mesonephric duct gives rise to the ***ejaculatory duct*** and ***seminal vesicles.***

The efferent ductules are lined with pseudostratified columnar epithelium

In man, approximately 20 ***efferent ductules*** connect the channels of the ***rete testis*** at the superior end of the mediastinum to the proximal portion of the ***duct of the epididymis.*** As the ***efferent ductules*** exit the testis, they become highly coiled and form 6 to 10 conical masses, the ***coni vasculosi,*** whose bases form part of the head of the epididymis. The coni vasculosi, each about 10 mm in length, contain the highly convoluted ducts that measure 15 to 20 cm in length. At the base of the cones, the efferent ducts open into a single channel, the duct of the epididymis (see Fig. 21.4).

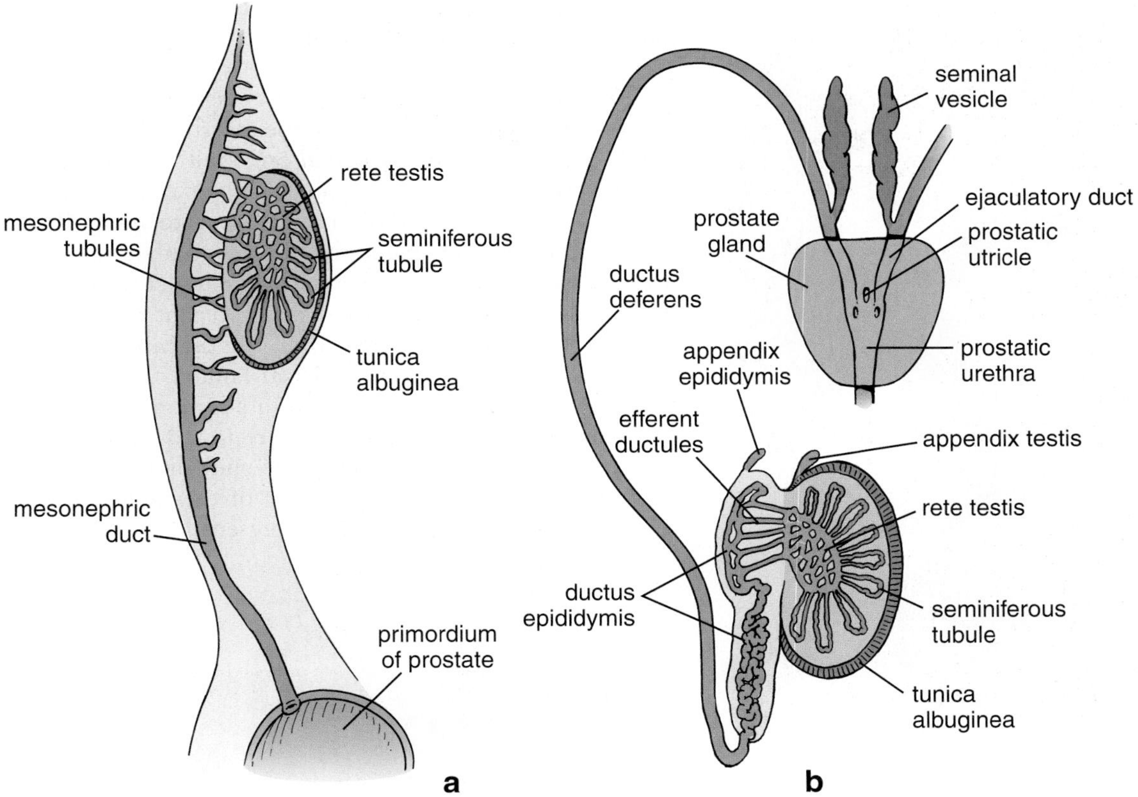

FIGURE 21.20
Schematic diagram of development of intratesticular and excurrent duct systems. a. This diagram shows the testis in the seventh week of development before it descends into the scrotal sac. Note that the mesonephric duct and its tubules give rise to the excurrent duct system for the developing testis. **b.** Sagittal section of a fully developed testis positioned within the scrotum. Note that the seminal vesicles, ejaculatory ducts, ductus deferens, epididymis, and efferent ductules are all developed from the mesonephric duct and tubules. The seminiferous tubules, straight tubules, and rete testis develop from the indifferent gonads. The prostate gland develops from the prostatic primordium that originates from the pelvic urethra.

The efferent ductules are lined with a pseudostratified columnar epithelium that contains clumps of tall and short cells, giving the luminal surface a sawtooth appearance (Fig. 21.21). Interspersed among the columnar cells are occasional basal cells that serve as epithelial stem cells. The tall columnar cells are ciliated. The short nonciliated cells have numerous microvilli and canalicular invaginations of the apical surface as well as numerous pinocytotic vesicles, membrane-bounded dense bodies, lysosomes, and other cytoplasmic structures associated with endocytotic activity. *Most of the fluid secreted in the seminiferous tubules is reabsorbed in the efferent ductules.*

A smooth muscle layer in the excurrent ducts first appears at the beginning of the efferent ductules. The smooth muscle cells form a layer several cells thick in which the cells are arrayed as a circular sheath in the wall of the ductule. Interspersed among the muscle cells are elastic fibers. Transport of the sperm in the efferent ductules is effected largely by both ciliary action and contraction of this fibromuscular layer.

Epididymis

The epididymis is an organ that contains the efferent ductules and the duct of the epididymis

The ***epididymis*** is a crescent-shaped structure that lies along the superior and posterior surfaces of the testis. It measures about 7.5 cm in length and consists of the ***efferent ductules*** and the ***duct of the epididymis*** and associated vessels, smooth muscles, and connective tissue coverings (Fig. 21.22). The duct of the epididymis is a highly coiled tube measuring 4 to 6 m in length. The epididymis is divided into a ***head***, a ***body***, and a ***tail*** (see Fig. 21.4). The efferent ductules occupy the head, and the duct of the epididymis occupies the body and tail. Newly produced sperm, which enter the epididymis from the testis, mature during their passage through the duct of the epididymis, acquiring motility and the ability to fertilize an oocyte. During this androgen-dependent maturation process, the head of the sperm is modified by the addition

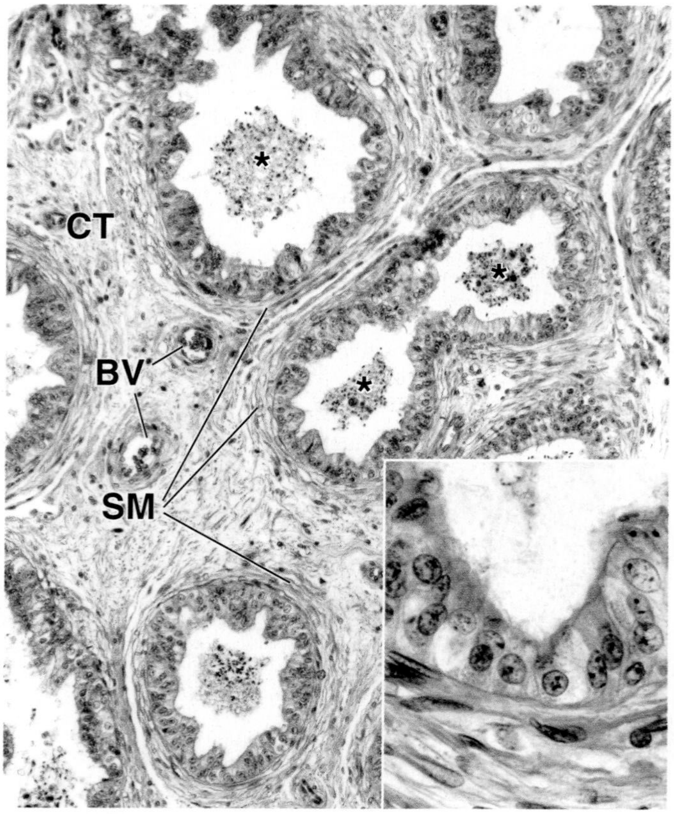

FIGURE 21.21
Photomicrograph of efferent ductules. The specimen in this photomicrograph was stained with picric acid and hematoxylin to better visualize the epithelial components of the efferent ductules. The efferent ductules are lined by pseudostratified columnar epithelium. The luminal surface has an uneven or wavy appearance because of the presence of alternating groups of tall columnar cells and cuboidal cells. The ductules are surrounded by several layers of circularly arranged smooth muscle *(SM)*. Within the ductule lumina are clumped spermatozoa (*asterisks*). Connective tissue *(CT)* makes up the stroma of the organ and contains blood vessels *(BV)* of various sizes. ×120. **Inset.** This higher magnification of the pseudostratified epithelium shows columnar and cuboidal cells that contain sparse cilia. ×500.

of ***surface-associated decapacitation factor*** containing epididymal fluid glycoconjugates. This process, called ***decapacitation,*** inhibits the fertilizing ability of the sperm in a reversible manner. The surface-associated decapacitation factor is later released during the ***capacitation process*** that occurs in the female reproductive tract just before fertilization. After maturation in the epididymis, sperm can transport their haploid content of DNA to the ovum; and after capacitation, they can bind to sperm receptors on the zona pellucida of the ovum. This binding triggers the acrosome reaction in which the sperm uses its acrosomal enzymes to penetrate the outer covering of the oocyte.

The principal cells in the pseudostratified epithelium of the epididymis are characterized by stereocilia

Like most of the excurrent duct system, the duct of the epididymis is also lined with a pseudostratified columnar epithelium. It contains ***principal cells*** (tall) and ***basal cells*** (short) (Fig. 21.23). The principal cells vary from about 80 μm in height in the head of the epididymis to about 40 μm in height in the tail. Numerous long, modified microvilli called ***stereocilia*** extend from the luminal surface of the principal cells. The stereocilia vary in height from 25 μm in the head to approximately 10 μm in the tail. The small, round basal cells rest on the basal lamina. They are the stem cells of the duct epithelium. In addition, intraepithelial lymphocytes called ***halo cells*** are found in the epithelium. Under normal conditions, the epithelium of the epididymis is the most proximal level of the excurrent duct system in which lymphocytes are present.

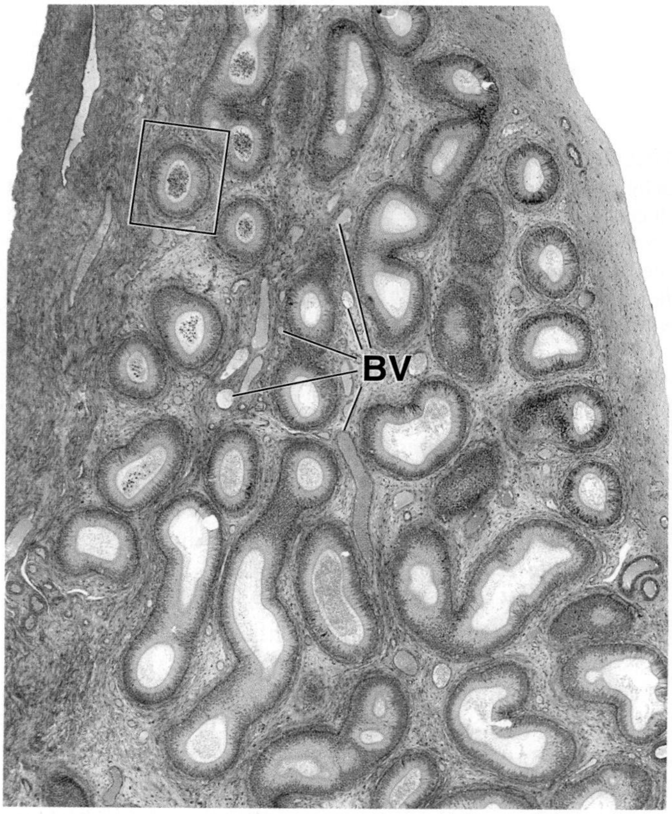

FIGURE 21.22
Photomicrograph of human epididymis. This photomicrograph of a H&E–stained section shows the highly coiled ductus epididymis. Its coiled nature is reflected in the variously shaped profiles of the duct. Within the connective tissue are numerous profiles of blood vessels *(BV)*. The vessels tend to follow the duct; thus they, too, reflect multiple profiles of several vessels. The section of the duct within the *rectangle* is shown at higher magnification in Figure 21.23. ×30.

Epididymal cells function in both absorption and secretion

Most of the fluid that is not reabsorbed by the efferent ductules is reabsorbed in the proximal portion of the epididymis. The epithelial cells also phagocytose any residual bodies not removed by the Sertoli cells as well as sperm that degenerate in the duct. The apical cytoplasm of the principal cells contains numerous invaginations at the bases of the stereocilia, along with coated vesicles, multivesicular bodies, and lysosomes (Fig. 21.24).

The principal cells secrete glycerophosphocholine, sialic acid, and glycoproteins, which, in addition to the glycocalyx and steroids, aid in the maturation of the sperm. They have numerous cisternae of rER surrounding the basally located nucleus and a remarkably large supranuclear Golgi apparatus. Profiles of sER and rER are also present in the apical cytoplasm.

The smooth muscle coat of the duct of the epididymis gradually increases in thickness to become three-layered in the tail

In the head of the epididymis and most of the body, the smooth muscle coat consists of a thin layer of circular smooth muscle resembling that of the efferent ductules. In the tail, inner and outer longitudinal layers are added. These three layers are then continuous with the three smooth muscle layers of the ductus deferens, the next component of the excurrent duct system.

Differences in smooth muscle function parallel these morphologic differences. In the head and body of the epididymis, spontaneous, rhythmic peristaltic contractions serve to move the sperm along the duct. Few peristaltic contractions occur in the tail of the epididymis, which serves as the principal reservoir for mature sperm. These sperm are forced into the ductus deferens by intense contractions of the three smooth muscle layers after appropriate neural stimulation associated with ejaculation.

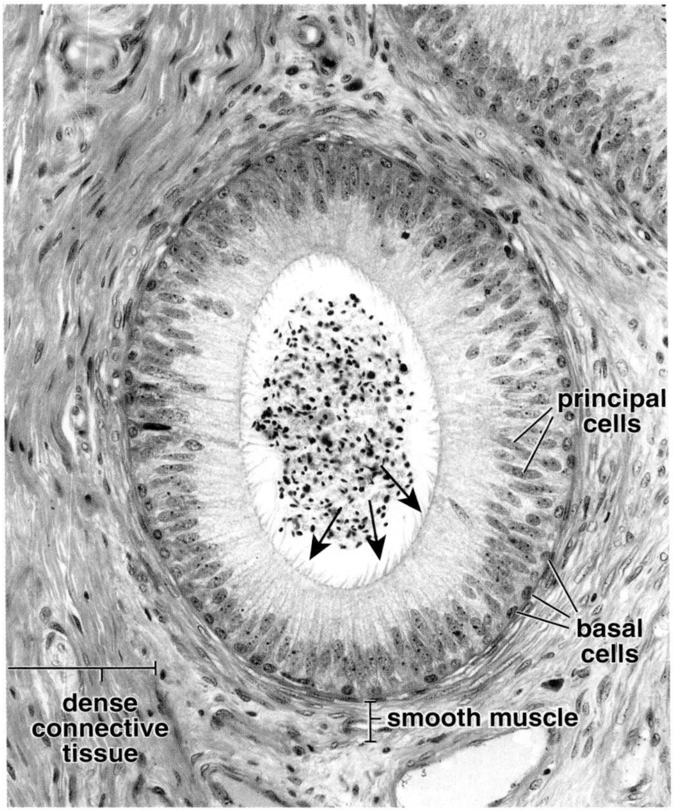

FIGURE 21.23
Photomicrograph of human ductus epididymis. This higher magnification of the *rectangular area* in Figure 21.22 reveals the two cell types of the epididymal epithelium, the principal cells and the basal cells. Stereocilia *(arrows)* extend from the apical surface of the principal cells. The nuclei of the basal cells are spherical and are located in close proximity to the basement membrane, whereas the nuclei of the principal cells are cylindrical and conform to the columnar shape of the cell. Surrounding the duct epithelium is a layer of circularly arranged smooth muscle cells. The duct lumen contains numerous sperm. ×250.

Ductus Deferens

The ductus deferens is the longest part of the excurrent duct system

The *ductus deferens (vas deferens)* is a direct continuation of the tail of the epididymis (see Fig. 21.1). It ascends along the posterior border of the testis, close to the testicular vessels and nerves. It then enters the abdomen as a component of the spermatic cord, by passing through the inguinal canal. The spermatic cord contains all of the structures that pass to and from the testis. In addition to the ductus deferens, the spermatic cord contains the testicular artery, small arteries to the ductus deferens and cremaster muscle, the pampiniform plexus, lymphatic vessels, sympathetic nerve fibers, and the genital branch of the genitofemoral nerve. All of these structures are surround by fascial coverings derived from the anterior abdominal wall. After leaving the spermatic cord, the ductus deferens descends in the pelvis to the level of the bladder, where its distal end enlarges to form the ***ampulla.*** The ampulla is joined there by the ***duct of the seminal vesicle*** and continues through the prostate gland to the urethra as the ***ejaculatory duct.***

The ductus deferens is lined with a pseudostratified columnar epithelium that closely resembles that of the epididymis. The tall columnar cells also have long microvilli that extend into the lumen. The rounded basal cells rest on the basal lamina. Unlike the epididymis, however, the lumen of the duct does not appear smooth. In histologic preparations (Fig. 21.25), it appears to be thrown into deep longitudinal folds throughout most of its length, probably because of contraction of the thick (1 to 1.5 mm) muscular coat of the duct during fixation.

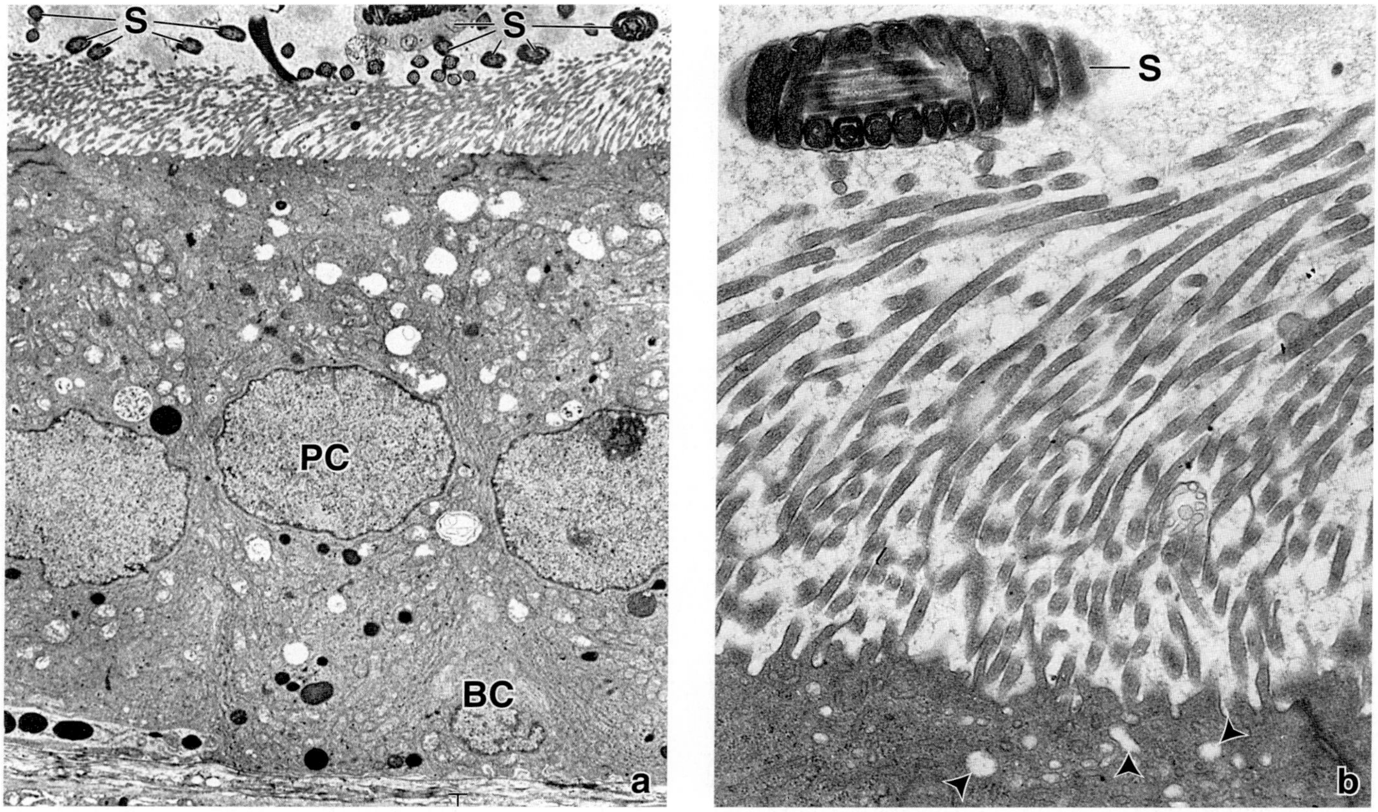

FIGURE 21.24
Electron micrograph of epididymis. a. Electron micrograph of the epididymal epithelium, showing principal cells *(PC)* extending to the lumen and a basal cell *(BC)* limited to the basal portion of the epithelium. Profiles of sperm *(S)* are seen in the lumen. The apical cytoplasm of the principal cells exhibits numerous long microvilli (stereocilia). ×3,000. **b.** Apical surface of the epithelial cell with its numerous long microvilli (stereocilia). The middle piece of a sperm *(S)* is evident in the lumen. The small, light circular profiles *(arrowheads)* are endocytotic vesicles. ×13,000.

The ***ampulla*** has taller, branched mucosal folds that often show glandular diverticula. The muscle coat surrounding the ampulla is thinner than that of the rest of the ductus deferens, and the longitudinal layers disappear near the origin of the ejaculatory duct. The epithelium of the ampulla and ejaculatory duct appears to have a secretory function. The cells contain large numbers of yellow pigment granules. The wall of the ejaculatory duct does not have a muscularis layer; the fibromuscular tissue of the prostate substitutes for it.

▼ ACCESSORY SEX GLANDS

The paired seminal vesicles secrete a fluid rich in fructose

The ***seminal vesicles*** are paired, elongate, and highly folded tubular glands located on the posterior wall of the urinary bladder, parallel to the ampulla of the ductus deferens. A short excretory duct from each seminal vesicle combines with the ampulla of the ductus deferens to form the ***ejaculatory duct.*** Seminal vesicles develop as evaginations of the mesonephric (Wolffian) ducts in the region of future ampullae. The wall of the seminal vesicles contains a mucosa, a thin layer of smooth muscle, and a fibrous coat (Fig. 21.26). The mucosa is thrown into numerous primary, secondary, and tertiary folds that increase the secretory surface area. All of the irregular chambers thus formed, however, communicate with the lumen.

The pseudostratified columnar epithelium contains tall, nonciliated columnar cells and short, round cells that rest on the basal lamina. The short cells appear identical to those of the rest of the excurrent duct system. They are the stem cells from which the columnar cells are derived. The columnar cells have the morphology of protein-secreting cells, with a well-developed rER and large secretory vacuoles in the apical cytoplasm.

The secretion of the seminal vesicles is a whitish yellow, viscous material. It contains fructose, which is the principal metabolic substrate for sperm, along with other simple sugars, amino acids, ascorbic acid, and prostaglandins. Al-

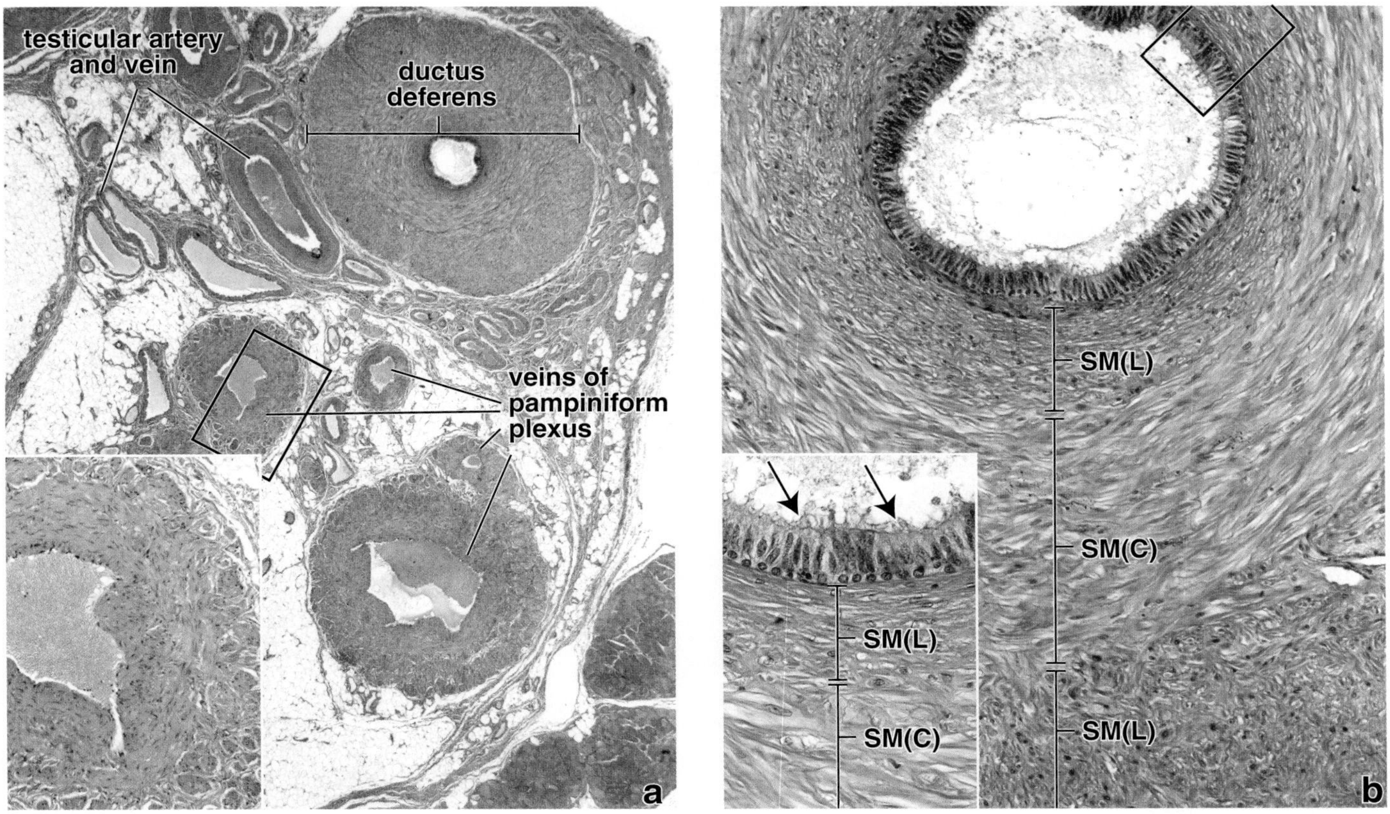

FIGURE 21.25
Photomicrograph of human spermatic cord. a. This low-magnification photomicrograph shows a cross section of the spermatic cord containing several structures. These include the ductus deferens, the accompanying testicular artery and vein, and veins of the pampiniform plexus. ×15. **Inset.** A higher magnification of a pampiniform vein. Note the bundles of longitudinal smooth muscles (cut in cross section) in the tunica adventitia and tunica intima. ×55. **b.** This cross section of the ductus deferens shows the thick muscular wall organized in three distinct smooth muscle layers: an inner longitudinal *(SM(L))*, middle circular *(SM(C))*, and outer longitudinal *(SM(L))*. ×100. **Inset.** A higher magnification shows the pseudostratified epithelium lining the ductus deferens. The tall principal cells possess long microvilli (stereocilia) *(arrows)*. The basal cells are in close proximity to the basement membrane and possess spherical nuclei. ×215.

though prostaglandins were first isolated from the prostate gland (hence the name), they are actually synthesized in large amounts in the seminal vesicles. Contraction of the smooth muscle coat of the seminal vesicles during ejaculation discharges their secretion into the ejaculatory ducts and helps to flush sperm out of the urethra. The secretory function and morphology of the seminal vesicles are under the control of testosterone.

Prostate Gland

The prostate, the largest accessory sex gland, is divided into several morphologic and functional zones

The *prostate* is the largest accessory sex gland of the male reproductive system. Its size and shape are commonly compared to those of a walnut. The gland is located in the pelvis, inferior to the bladder, where it surrounds the prostatic part of the urethra. It consists of 30 to 50 tubuloalveolar glands arranged in three concentric layers: an inner ***mucosal layer***, an intermediate ***submucosal layer***, and a peripheral layer containing the ***main prostatic glands*** (Fig. 21.27). The glands of the mucosal layer secrete directly into the urethra; the other two layers have ducts that open into the prostatic sinuses located on either side of the urethral crest on the posterior wall of the urethra.

The adult prostatic parenchyma is divided into four anatomically and clinically distinct zones:

- The ***peripheral zone*** corresponds to the main prostatic glands and constitutes 70% of the glandular tissue of the prostate. This zone is the most susceptible to inflammation. It is also the site of most prostatic carcinomas. The peripheral zone is palpable during digital examination of the rectum.

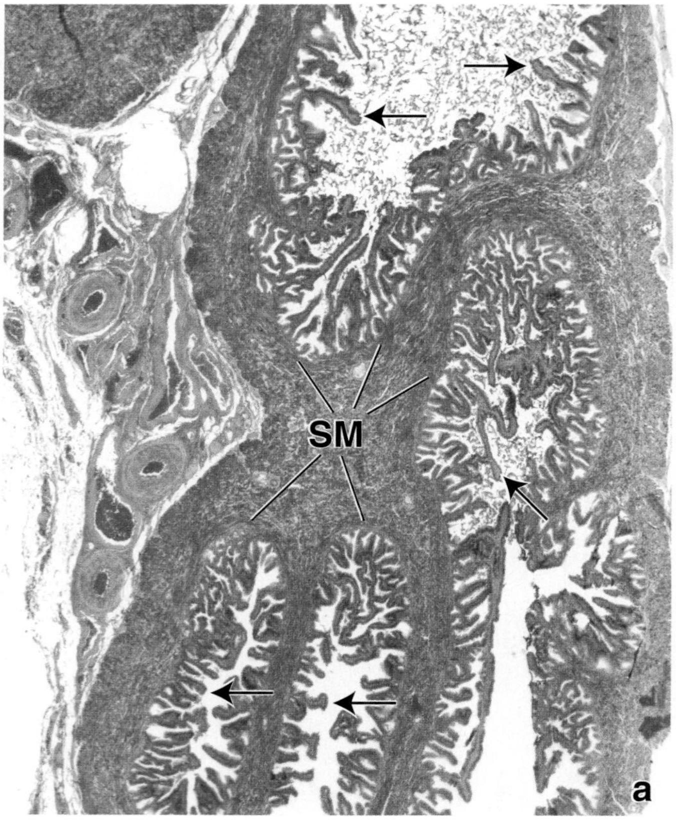

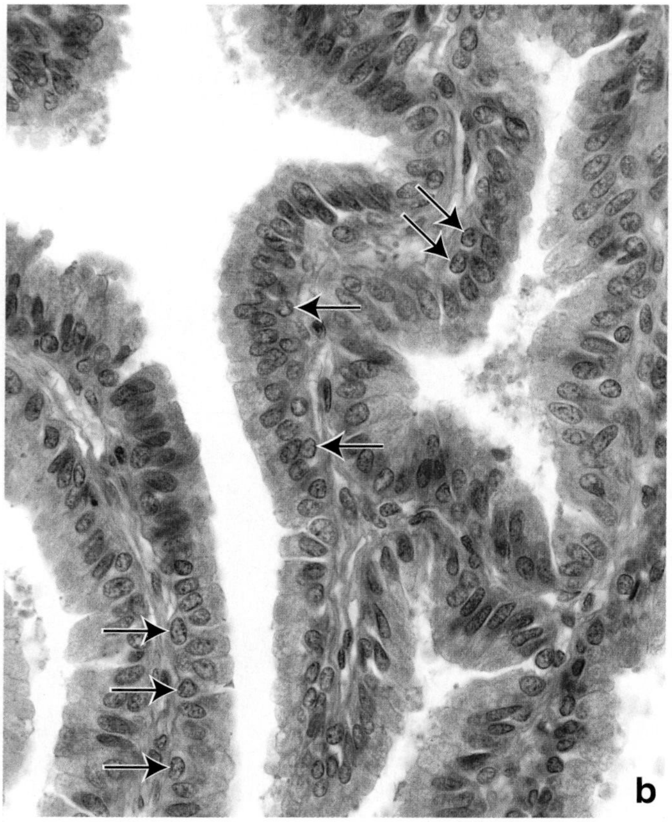

FIGURE 21.26
Photomicrograph of human seminal vesicle. a. This low-magnification photomicrograph shows part of a H&E–stained section of a human seminal vesicle. This gland is a tortuous tubular structure and in a section exhibits what appear to be a number of isolated lumina. In actuality, there is only one lumen. The mucosa is characterized by extensive folding. It rests on a thick smooth muscle *(SM)* investment that is organized in two layers: an inner circular layer and an outer longitudinal layer. ×20. **b.** This higher magnification shows the mucosal folds surfaced by a pseudostratified epithelium. *Arrows* indicate the basal cells. ×500.

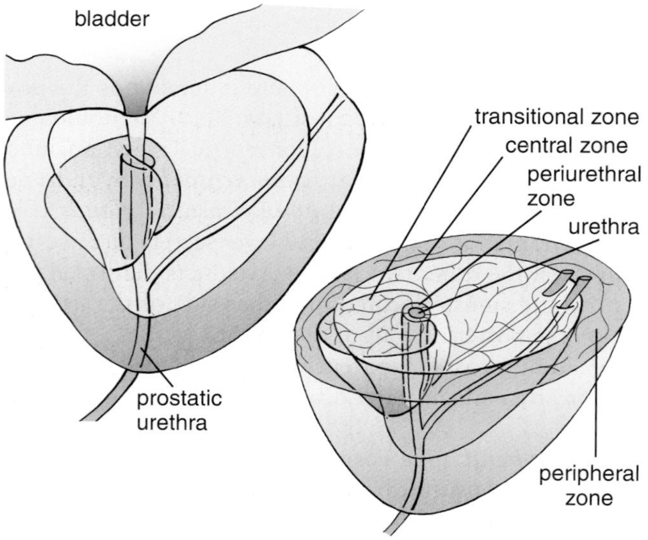

FIGURE 21.27
Schematic drawing of the zones of the human prostate gland. This drawing illustrates the relative location, by color, of the four zones of the prostate gland.

- The ***central zone*** contains about 25% of the glandular tissue and is resistant to both carcinoma and inflammation. In comparison to the other zones, cells in the central zone have distinctive morphologic features (more prominent and slightly basophilic cytoplasm and larger nuclei displaced at different levels in adjacent cells). Recent findings suggest that this zone originates embryologically from the inclusion of mesonephric duct cells into the developing prostate.
- The ***transitional zone*** contains the mucosal glands. In older individuals, the parenchymal cells of this zone frequently undergo extensive division (hyperplasia) and form nodular masses of epithelial cells. Because this zone is in close proximity to the prostatic urethra, these nodules can compress the prostatic urethra, causing difficulty in urination. This condition is known as ***benign prostatic hyperplasia (BPH)*** and is discussed in the clinical box (page 709).
- The ***periurethral zone*** contains mucosal and submucosal glands. In later stages of BPH this zone may undergo pathologic growth, but mainly from the stromal

BOX 21.4

Clinical Correlations: Benign Prostatic Hypertrophy and Prostatic Cancer

Benign prostatic hypertrophy (nodular hyperplasia, BPH) occurs almost exclusively in the transitional and periurethral zones, leading to partial or total obstruction of the urethra. A widely accepted theory of the pathogenesis of BPH is related to the action of DHT. DHT is synthesized in the stromal cells by conversion from circulating testosterone in the presence of 5α-reductase. Once synthesized, DHT acts as an autocrine agent on the stromal cells and as a paracrine hormone on the epithelial cells, causing them to proliferate. Clinical trials have shown that inhibitors of 5α-reductase reduce the DHT concentration and thus decrease the size of the prostate and reduce urethral obstruction. BHP is believed to occur to some extent in all men by age 80 years. It is routinely treated by the transurethral removal of prostatic parenchyma. This procedure is called transurethral prostatectomy (TURP).

Cancer of the prostate is one of the most common cancers in the male, affecting approximately 1 in 20. The incidence of prostatic cancer increases with age, and it is estimated that 70% of men between the ages of 70 and 80 will develop this disease. Tumors usually develop in the peripheral zone of the gland. In the past, early detection was uncommon, because the abnormal growth of the tumor did not impinge on the urethra to produce symptoms that demanded prompt attention. Therefore, prostatic cancer was often inoperable by the time it was discovered. However, beginning in the late 1980s, the introduction of PSA testing for prostate cancer has dramatically increased early diagnosis of this disease. The PSA test revolutionized the early detection, management, and follow-up of patients with prostate cancer and is considered one of the best biomedical markers currently available in the field of oncology. Its use with annual digital rectal examination in prostate cancer screening programs has significantly increased early detection of the disease. Treatment of the cancer is by surgery, radiotherapy, or both for patients with localized disease. Hormonal therapy is the treatment of choice for advanced cancer with metastases. Since prostatic cancer cells depend on androgens, the goal of the therapy is to deprive the cells of testosterone by performing orchiectomy (removal of the testis) or by administration of estrogens or gonadotropin-releasing hormone (GnRH) agonists to suppress testosterone production. Despite treatment, patients with metastasis have a poor prognosis.

components. Together with the glandular nodules of the transitional zone, this growth causes increased urethral compression and further retention of urine in the bladder.

The prostate gland secretes prostatic acid phosphatase (PAP), fibrinolysin, citric acid, and prostate-specific antigen (PSA)

Within each prostate zone the parenchymal epithelium is generally simple columnar, but there may be patches that are simple cuboidal, squamous, or occasionally pseudostratified (Fig. 21.28). The epithelium depends on testosterone for normal morphology and function. The alveoli of the prostatic glands, especially those in older men, often contain ***prostatic concretions (corpora amylacea)*** of varied shape and size, often up to 2 mm in diameter (see Fig. 21.28). They appear in sections as concentric lamellated bodies and are believed to be formed by precipitation of secretory material around cell fragments. They may become partially calcified.

The prostatic epithelial cells produce enzymes, particularly ***PAP, fibrinolysin,*** and ***citric acid.*** They also secrete ***serine protease,*** clinically known as ***PSA.*** This enzyme is secreted into the alveoli and is ultimately incorporated into seminal fluid. The alveolar secretion is pumped into the prostatic urethra during ejaculation by contraction of the fibromuscular tissue of the prostate. The fibrinolysin in the secretion serves to liquefy the semen.

Normal individuals have a low serum concentration of PSA. Circulating PSA is produced by the liver, not by the prostate gland, which in normal individuals releases PSA only into prostatic secretion. However, in prostate cancer, serum concentration of PSA increases. In this case, the additional PSA is produced and released into the circulation by the prostate gland. Therefore, the elevated levels of PSA are directly related to increased activity of the prostatic cancer cells. Increased blood levels of both PAP and PSA are used as markers of the presence and progression of the disease.

Bulbourethral Glands

The bulbourethral glands secrete preseminal fluid

The paired ***bulbourethral glands (Cowper's glands)*** are pea-sized structures located in the urogenital diaphragm (see Fig. 21.1). The duct of each gland passes through the inferior fascia of the urogenital diaphragm and joins the initial portion of the penile urethra. The glands are compound tubuloalveolar glands that structurally resemble mucus secretory glands (Fig. 21.29). The simple columnar epithelium, which varies considerably in height depending on the functional state of the gland, is under the control of testosterone.

The clear, mucus-like glandular secretion contains considerable amounts of galactose and galactosamine, galacturonic acid, sialic acid, and methylpentose. Sexual stimulation causes release of the secretion, which constitutes the major portion of the preseminal fluid and probably serves to lubricate the penile urethra.

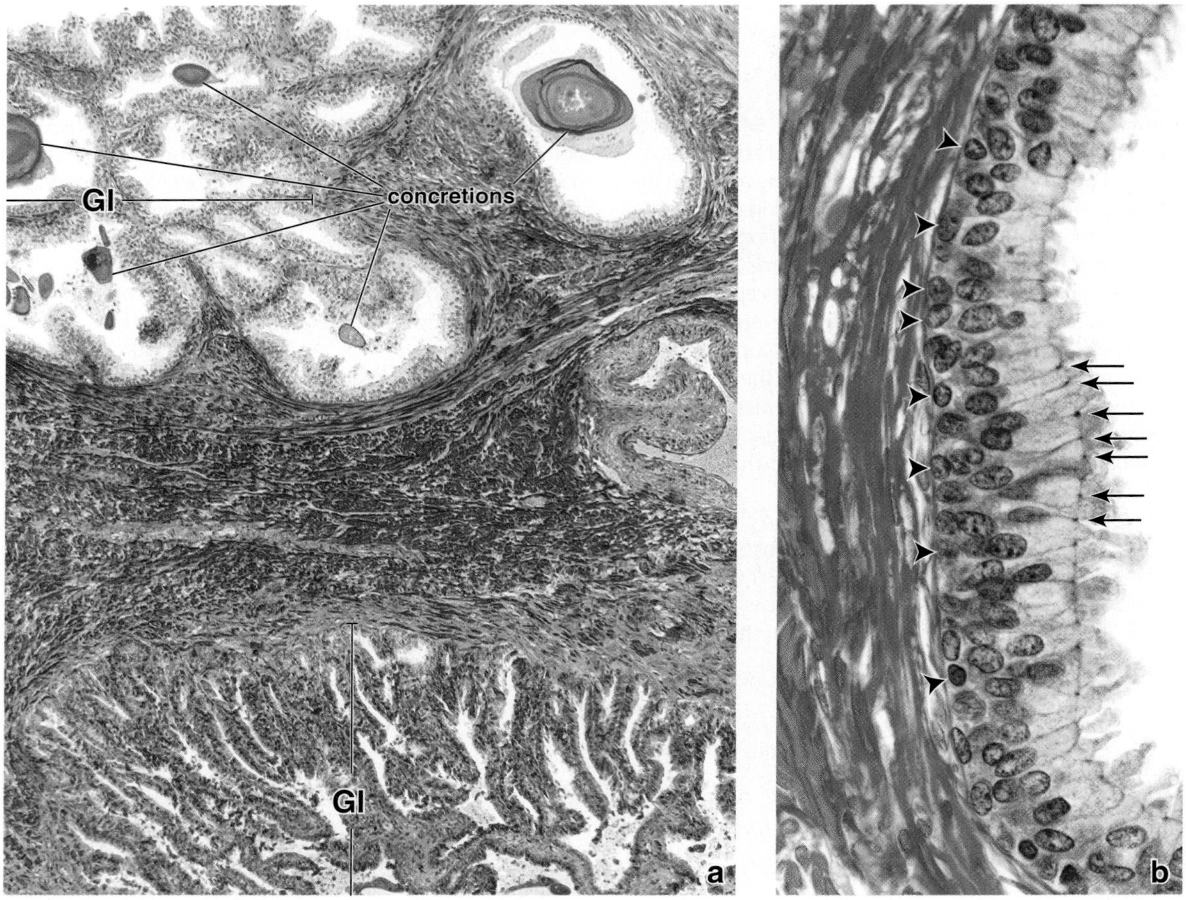

FIGURE 21.28
Photomicrograph of human prostate gland. a. This Mallory-azan–stained specimen shows the tubuloalveolar glands *(Gl)* and the fibromuscular tissue that forms the septa between glandular tissue. Within the lumina, various-sized prostatic concretions can be seen. The stain utilized for this specimen readily distinguishes the smooth muscle component (stained *red*) from the dense connective tissue component (stained *blue*) of the stroma. ×60. **b.** This higher magnification shows an area where the glandular epithelium is pseudostratified. The round nuclei adjacent to the connective tissue *(arrowheads)* belong to the basal cells. Those nuclei that are more elongate and further removed from the base of the epithelium belong to the secretory cells. Note the terminal bars *(arrows)* that are evident at the apical region of these cells. The red-stained sites within the dense connective tissue represent smooth muscle cells. ×635.

SEMEN

Semen contains fluids and sperm from the testis and secretory products from the epididymis, ductus deferens, prostate, seminal vesicles, and bulbourethral glands. It is alkaline and may help to neutralize the acid environment of the urethra and the vagina. Semen also contains prostaglandins that may influence sperm transit in both the male and female reproductive ducts and that may have a role in implantation of a fertilized ovum.

The average ejaculate of semen has a volume of about 3 mL and normally contains up to 100 million sperm per mL. It is estimated that 20% of the sperm in any ejaculate are morphologically abnormal and nearly 25% are immotile.

PENIS

Erection of the penis involves the filling of the vascular spaces of the corpora cavernosa and corpus spongiosum

The penis consists principally of two dorsal masses of erectile tissue, the ***corpora cavernosa***, and a ventral mass of erectile tissue, the ***corpus spongiosum***, in which the ***spongy part of the urethra*** is embedded. A dense, fibroelastic layer, the ***tunica albuginea***, binds the three together and forms a capsule around each (Fig. 21.30). The corpora cavernosa contain numerous wide, irregularly shaped vascular spaces lined with vascular endothelium. These spaces are surrounded by a thin layer of smooth muscle that forms trabeculae within the tunica albuginea interconnect-

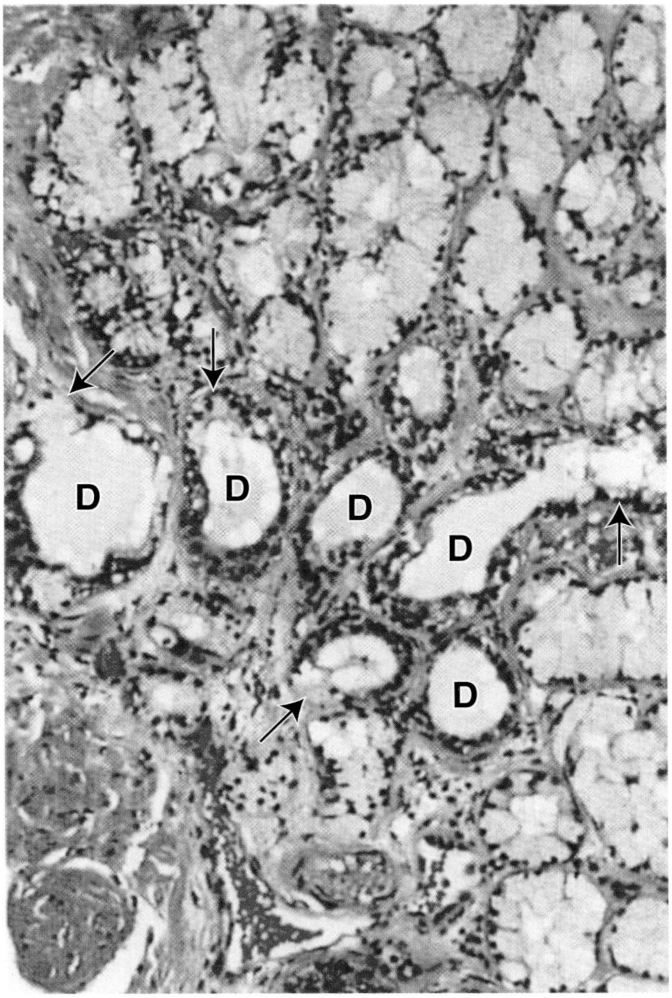

FIGURE 21.29
Photomicrograph of human bulbourethral gland. This photomicrograph shows a H&E–stained section of the compound tubuloalveolar bulbourethral gland. The epithelium consists of columnar mucus-secreting cells. The nuclei are displaced to the base of the cells by the accumulated secretory material that they contain. The cytoplasm has an appearance similar to typical mucus-secreting cells. Note several ducts *(D)* lined by a simple columnar epithelium. The ducts will merge to form a single excretory duct. In some sites the ducts contain mucus-secreting cells *(arrows)*. ×40.

ing and criss-crossing the corpus cavernosum. Irregular smooth muscle bundles are observed frequently as "subendothelial cushions" surrounding irregular vascular spaces (Fig. 21.31). The interstitial connective tissue contains many nerve endings and lymphatic vessels. The vascular spaces increase in size and rigidity by filling with blood, principally derived from the ***helicine arteries***. These arteries dilate during erection (see box) to increase the blood flow to the penis. An arteriovenous (AV) anastomosis exists between the deep artery of the penis and the peripheral venous system.

The skin of the penis is thin and loosely attached to the underlying loose connective tissue except at the ***glans***, where it is very thin and tightly attached. The skin of the glans is so thin that blood within its large, muscular anastomosing veins that drain the corpus spongiosum may give it a bluish color. There is no adipose tissue in the subcutaneous tissue. There is, however, a thin layer of smooth muscle that is continuous with the dartos layer of the scrotum. In uncircumcised males, the glans is covered with a fold of skin, the ***prepuce***, which resembles a mucous membrane on its inner aspect. Numerous sebaceous glands are present in the skin of the penis just proximal to the glans.

The penis is innervated by somatic, sympathetic, and parasympathetic nerves. Many sensory nerve endings are distributed throughout the tissue of the penis, and sympathetic and parasympathetic visceral motor fibers innervate the smooth muscle of the trabeculae of the tunica albuginea and the blood vessels. Both sensory and visceral motor fibers play essential roles in erectile and ejaculatory responses.

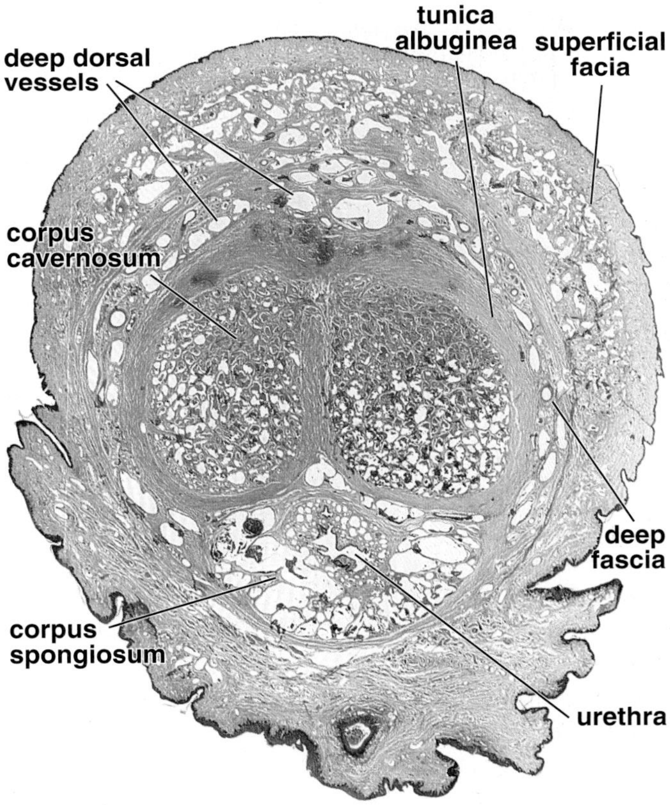

FIGURE 21.30
Photomicrograph of a histologic section of the penis. This photomicrograph shows a H&E–stained specimen of a cross section of the penis near the base of the organ. Note the arrangement of the corpora cavernosa and corpus spongiosum; the latter contains the urethra. ×3.

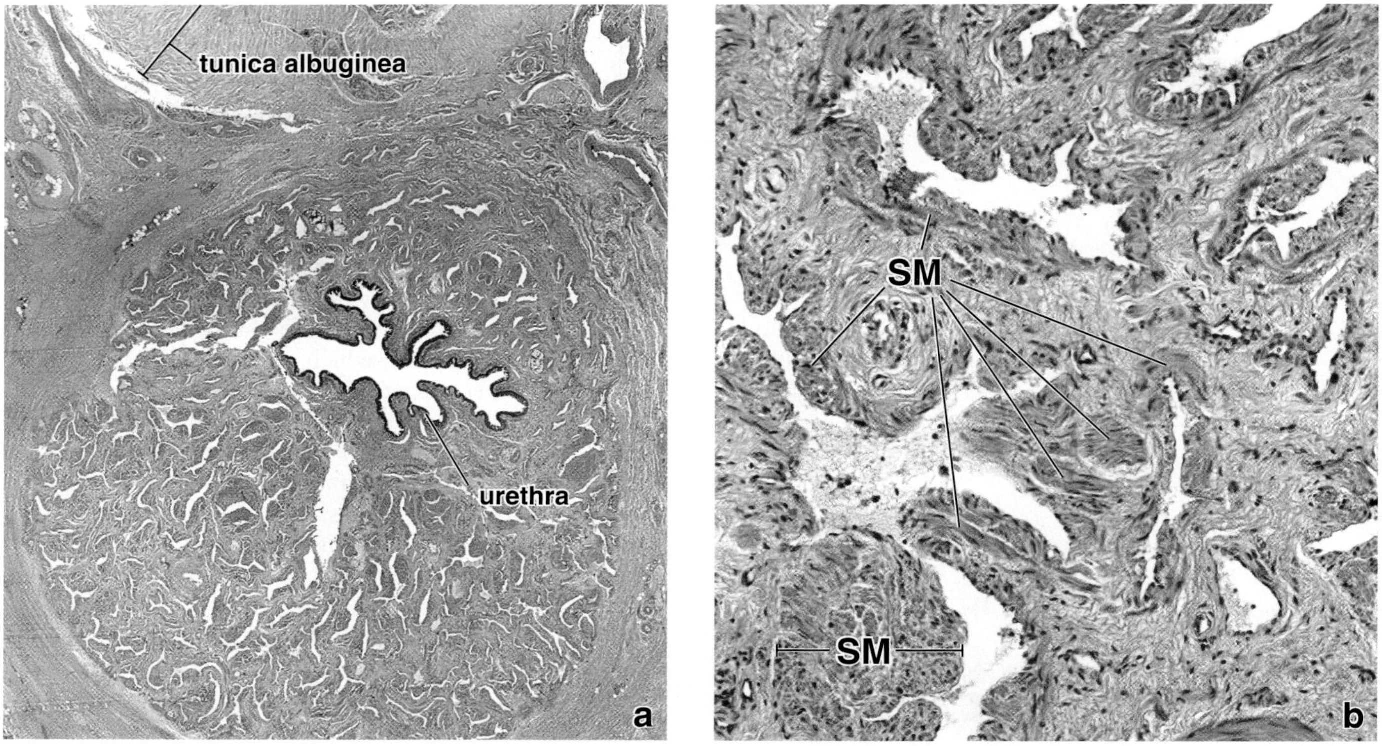

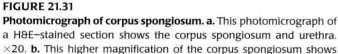

FIGURE 21.31
Photomicrograph of corpus spongiosum. a. This photomicrograph of a H&E–stained section shows the corpus spongiosum and urethra. ×20. **b.** This higher magnification of the corpus spongiosum shows the numerous irregularly shaped vascular spaces. Note the surrounding layer of smooth muscle (*SM*) forming the "subendothelial cushions." ×135.

BOX 21.5

Clinical Correlations: Mechanism of Erection and Erectile Dysfunction

Erection of the penis is a vascular event initiated by the CNS and maintained by complex interactions between vascular and neurologic events. The CNS responds to external and/or internal stimuli (sensory impulses, perception, desire, etc.) that involve the sympathetic and parasympathetic innervation of the penis.

Parasympathetic stimulation initiates erection by relaxation of the trabecular smooth muscle cells and dilation of the helicine arteries. This leads to expansion of the corpora cavernosa and, to a lesser degree, the corpus spongiosum. Arterial blood accumulates in these erectile tissues by compression of the venules against the nondistendible tunica albuginea. This process is referred to as the ***corporal veno-occlusive mechanism.*** The tunica albuginea also compresses the larger veins that drain blood from the corpora cavernosa so that venous outflow is also blocked, resulting in tumescence and rigidity of the penis.

Two neuromediators, acetylocholine and nitric oxide, are involved in the relaxation of smooth muscle during the initiation and maintenance of penile erection.

- ***Acetylcholine*** is released by the parasympathetic nerve endings and acts primarily on the endothelial cells that line the vascular spaces of the corpora cavernosa. This causes the release of vasoactive intestinal peptide (VIP) and, more importantly, nitric oxide.
- ***Nitric oxide (NO)*** activates guanylate cyclase in the trabecular smooth muscle cells to produce cyclic guanosine monophosphate (cGMP). cGMP causes the smooth muscle cells to relax.

Sympathetic stimulation terminates penile erection by causing contraction of the trabecular smooth muscle cells of the helicine arteries. These events decrease the flow of blood to the corpora cavernosa, reducing blood pressure in the erectile tissue to normal venous pressure. The lower pressure within the corpus cavernosum allows the veins leading from the corpora cavernosa to open and drain the excess blood.

Erectile dysfunction is an inability to achieve and maintain sufficient penile erection to complete satisfactory intercourse. Adequate arterial blood supply is critical for erection, therefore any disorder that decreases blood flow into the corpora cavernosa may cause erectile failure.

Many cases of erectile dysfunction that do not involve parasympathetic nerve damage can now be treated effectively with sildenafil citrate *(Viagra).* This compound enhances the relaxing effect of NO on smooth muscle cells of the corpora cavernosa by inhibiting phosphodiesterase, which is responsible for degradation of cGMP. As noted above, cGMP causes smooth muscle relaxation, which in turn allows inflow of blood into the corpus cavernosum to initiate erection. However, when parasympathetic nerve damage has occurred (e.g., as a complication of prostatic surgery), sildenafil citrate will have no effect because the event involving parasympathetic stimulation and release of acetylocholine cannot occur. Without acetylocholine, NO cannot produce cGMP. Without cGMP, smooth muscle cells cannot relax to allow inflow of blood to fill the erectile tissue.

PLATE 82. TESTIS I

The male reproductive system consists of the paired *testes, epididymides,* and *genital ducts,* as well as accessory reproductive glands and the penis. The functions of the testis are the production of *sperm* and the synthesis and secretion of *androgens,* especially *testosterone.* The events of cell division that lead to the mature sperm involve both normal cell division, *mitosis,* and reduction division, *meiosis,* to yield a haploid chromosome number and haploid DNA content. Androgen secretion by the testis begins early in fetal development and is essential for continued normal development of the male fetus. At puberty, androgen secretion resumes and is responsible for initiation and maintenance of sperm production *(spermatogenesis),* secretion by accessory sex glands (e.g., *prostate* and *seminal vesicle*), and development of secondary sex characteristics.

Figure 1, testis, monkey, H&E ×65.

This section of the testis shows the seminiferous tubules and the tunica albuginea *(TA),* the capsule of the organ. Extending from the very thick capsule are connective tissue septa *(S)* that divide the organ into compartments. Each compartment contains several seminiferous tubules and represents a lobule *(L).* Blood vessels *(BV)* are present within the inner portion of the capsule, the part referred to as the tunica vasculosa, and in the connective tissue septa.

The seminiferous tubules are convoluted; thus, the profiles they present in a section are variable in appearance. Not infrequently, the wall of a tubule is sectioned tangentially, thus obscuring the lumen and revealing what appears to be a solid mass of cells *(X).*

Figure 2, testis, monkey, H&E ×400.

Examination at higher magnification, as in this figure, reveals a population of interstitial cells that occur in small clusters and lie in the space between adjoining tubules. They consist mostly of Leydig cells *(LC),* the chief source of testosterone in the male. They are readily identified by virtue of their location and by their small round nucleus and eosinophilic cytoplasm. Macrophages are also found, in close association with the Leydig cells, but in lesser number. They are, however, difficult to identify in H&E sections.

A layer of closely apposed squamous cells forms a sheath-like investment around the tubule epithelium of each seminiferous tubule. In man, several layers of cells invest the tubule epithelium. The cells of this peritubular investment exhibit myoid features and account for the slow peristaltic activity of the tubules. Peripheral to the myoid layer is a broad lymphatic channel that occupies an extensive space between the tubules. In routine histologic sections, however, the lymphatic channels are usually collapsed and, thus, unrecognizable. The cellular elements that surround the tubule epithelium are generally referred to as a lamina propria *(LP)* or as a boundary tissue. As a lamina propria, it is atypical. It is not a loose connective tissue. Indeed, under normal circumstances, lymphocytes and other cell types related to the immune system are conspicuously absent.

Examination of the tubule epithelium reveals two kinds of cells: a proliferating population of spermatogenic cells and a nonproliferating population, the sustentacular, or Sertoli, cells. The Sertoli cells are considerably fewer and can be recognized by their elongate, pale-staining nuclei *(Sn)* and conspicuous nucleolus. The Sertoli cell cytoplasm extends from the periphery of the tubule to the lumen.

The spermatogenic cells consist of successive generations arranged in concentric layers. Thus, the spermatogonia *(Sg)* are found at the periphery. The spermatocytes *(Sc),* most of which have large round nuclei with a distinctive chromatin pattern (because of their chromatin material being reorganized), come to lie above the spermatogonia. The spermatid population *(Sp)* consists of one or two generations and occupies the site closest to the lumen. The tubules in this figure have been identified according to their stage of development. The tubule at the upper right can be identified as stage VI. At this stage, the mature population of spermatids (identified by their dark-blue heads and eosinophilic thread-like flagella protruding into the lumen) are in the process of being released (spermiogenesis). The younger generation of spermatids is composed of round cells and exhibits round nuclei. Moving clockwise, the tubule indicated as stage VII is slightly more advanced. The mature spermatids are now gone. Progressing to stage VIII, the tubule at the bottom of the micrograph reveals that the spermatid population is undergoing a change in nuclear shape. Note the tapered nuclei *(arrows).* Further maturation of the spermatids is reflected in the tubule at the top of the micrograph, stage XI. Finally, the tubule marked stage II, on the left, reveals slightly greater maturation of the luminal spermatids, and with the start of the new cycle (stage I), a newly formed spermatid population is now present. By examining the spermatid population and assessing the number of generations present (i.e., one or two) and the degree of maturation, it is possible with the aid of a chart to approximate the stage of a tubule.

KEY

BV, blood vessels
L, lobule
LC, Leydig cells
LP, lamina propria
S, connective tissue septa
Sc, spermatocytes
Sg, spermatogonia
Sn, Sertoli nuclei
Sp, spermatids
TA, tunica albuginea
X, tangential section of tubule with lumen obscured
arrows, spermatid nuclei displaying early shape change

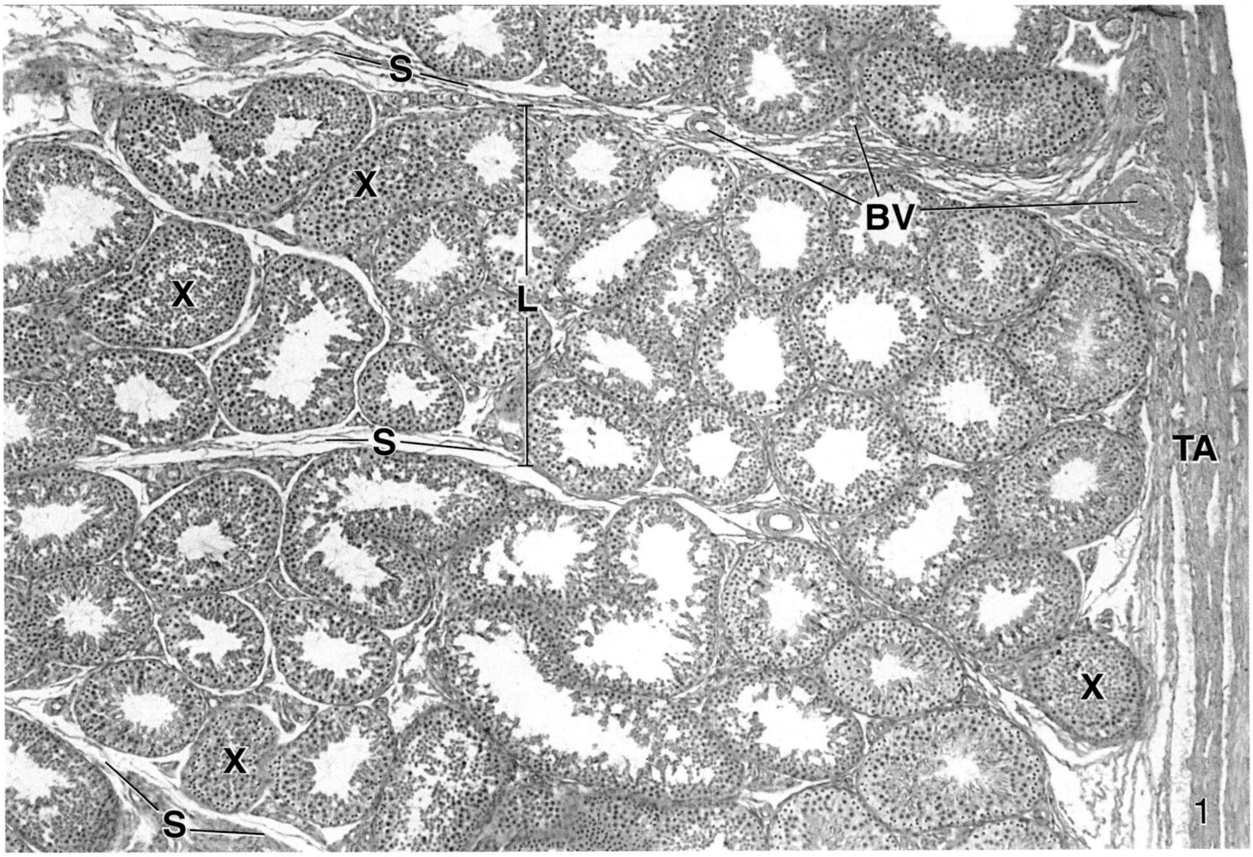
S
BV
X
L
S
TA
X
X
S
1

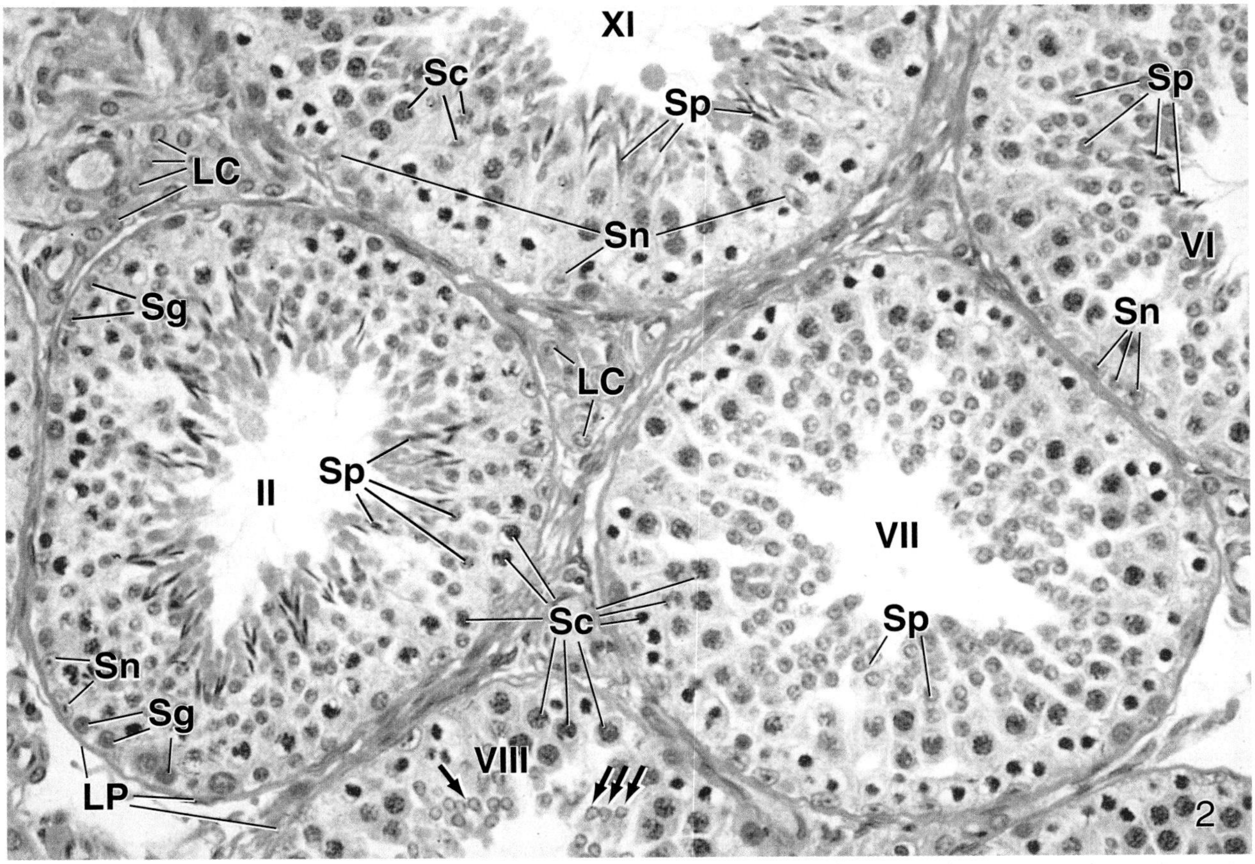
XI
Sc
Sp
Sp
LC
Sn
VI
Sg
Sn
LC
Sp
II
VII
Sc
Sp
Sn
Sg
VIII
LP
2

PLATE 83. TESTIS II

While the mature testis is characterized by seminiferous tubules, the immature testis is characterized by cords of cells consisting of an epithelium of *sustentacular (Sertoli) cells* surrounding occasional *gonocytes,* precursors of spermatogonia that are derived from the primordial germ cells that invaded the developing gonad in the embryo. At puberty, these cords become canalized, and the gonocytes begin the multiple divisions that give rise to the *spermatogonia* that, in turn, will divide and differentiate into the mature sperm. The seminiferous tubules terminate as *straight tubules (tubuli recti)* that are lined only by Sertoli cells. The tubuli recti lead to the *rete testis,* a complex series of anastomosing channels in the mediastinum testis that is the termination of the intratesticular tubule system.

Figure 1, testis, newborn human, H&E ×180; inset ×360.

Prepubertal testis. The various germ cell types representative of spermatogenesis in the mature seminiferous tubules are not present in the testis before puberty or in the postpubertal undescended testis. Instead, the "tubules" are represented by cords of cells in which a lumen is lacking. The seminiferous cords display the same tortuosity as in the adult; the tunica albuginea *(TA)* of the testis, though thinner, is of the same relative thickness.

The seminiferous cords are of considerably smaller diameter than the tubules of the adult and are composed of two cell types: the gonocyte, or first-generation spermatogonium, derived from the primordial germ cell that migrates from the yolk sac to the developing gonad in the embryo; and a cell that resembles the Sertoli cell of the adult. The latter cell type predominates and constitutes the bulk of the cord. The cells are columnar, and their nuclei are close to the basement membrane. The gonocytes *(G)* are the precursors of the definitive germ cells, or spermatogonia. They are round cells that have a centrally placed, spherical nucleus. The cytoplasm takes little stain and usually appears as a light ring around the nucleus. This gives the gonocyte a distinctive appearance in histologic sections **(inset).** Generally, the gonocytes are found at the periphery of the cord, but many are also found more centrally. The gonocytes give rise to spermatogonia that begin to proliferate in males between the ages of 10 and 13 years. The seminiferous epithelium then becomes populated with cells at various stages of spermatogenesis, as seen in the adult.

The epithelial cords are surrounded by one or two layers of cells with long processes and flat nuclei. They resemble fibroblasts at the ultrastructural level and give rise to the myoid peritubular cells of the adult.

The interstitial cells of Leydig are conspicuous in the newborn, a reflection of the residual effects of maternal hormones. Leydig cells, however, regress and do not become conspicuous again until puberty. In this preparation, the Leydig cells *(LC)* can be seen between the cords **(inset).** They are ovoid or polygonal and are closely grouped, so that adjacent cells are in contact with each other. Overall, they have the same appearance as the Leydig cells of the adult.

Figure 2, testis, H&E ×65.

Straight tubules and rete testes. In the posterior portion of the testis, the connective tissue of the tunica albuginea extends more deeply into the organ. This inward extension of connective tissue is called the mediastinum testis. It contains a network of anastomosing channels called the rete testis. Only a small portion of the mediastinum testis *(MT)* is evident in the figure. The area includes, however, a few seminiferous tubules *(ST)* in the upper portion of the micrograph and, fortuitously, the site where one of the seminiferous tubules terminates and joins the rete testis *(RT).* This can be recognized in the area delineated by the *rectangle,* which is shown at higher magnification in Figure 3. As noted above, the seminiferous tubules are arranged in the form of a loop, with each end joining the rete testis. The seminiferous tubules open into the rete testis by way of a straight tubule, or tubulus rectus. The tubuli recti are very short and are lined by Sertoli-like cells; no germ cell component is present.

Figure 3, testis, monkey, H&E ×400.

The tubulus rectus *(TR)* in this figure appears to end on one side before it ends on the other. This simply reflects the angle of section. When the straight tubule ends, however, the epithelial lining suddenly becomes cuboidal. This represents the rete testis, which constitutes an anastomosing system of channels that lead to the efferent ductules. The epithelial lining cells of the rete are sometimes more squamous than cuboidal or, occasionally, may be low columnar in appearance. Typically, they possess a single cilium; however, this is difficult to see in routine H&E preparations.

The connective tissue of the mediastinum is very dense but exhibits no other special features, nor is smooth muscle present. Adipose cells *(AC)* and blood vessels *(BV),* particularly veins of varying size, are present within the connective tissue.

KEY

AC, adipose cells
BV, blood vessels
G, gonocytes
LC, Leydig cells
MT, mediastinum testis
RT, rete testis
ST, seminiferous tubules
TA, tunica albuginea
TR, tubulus rectus

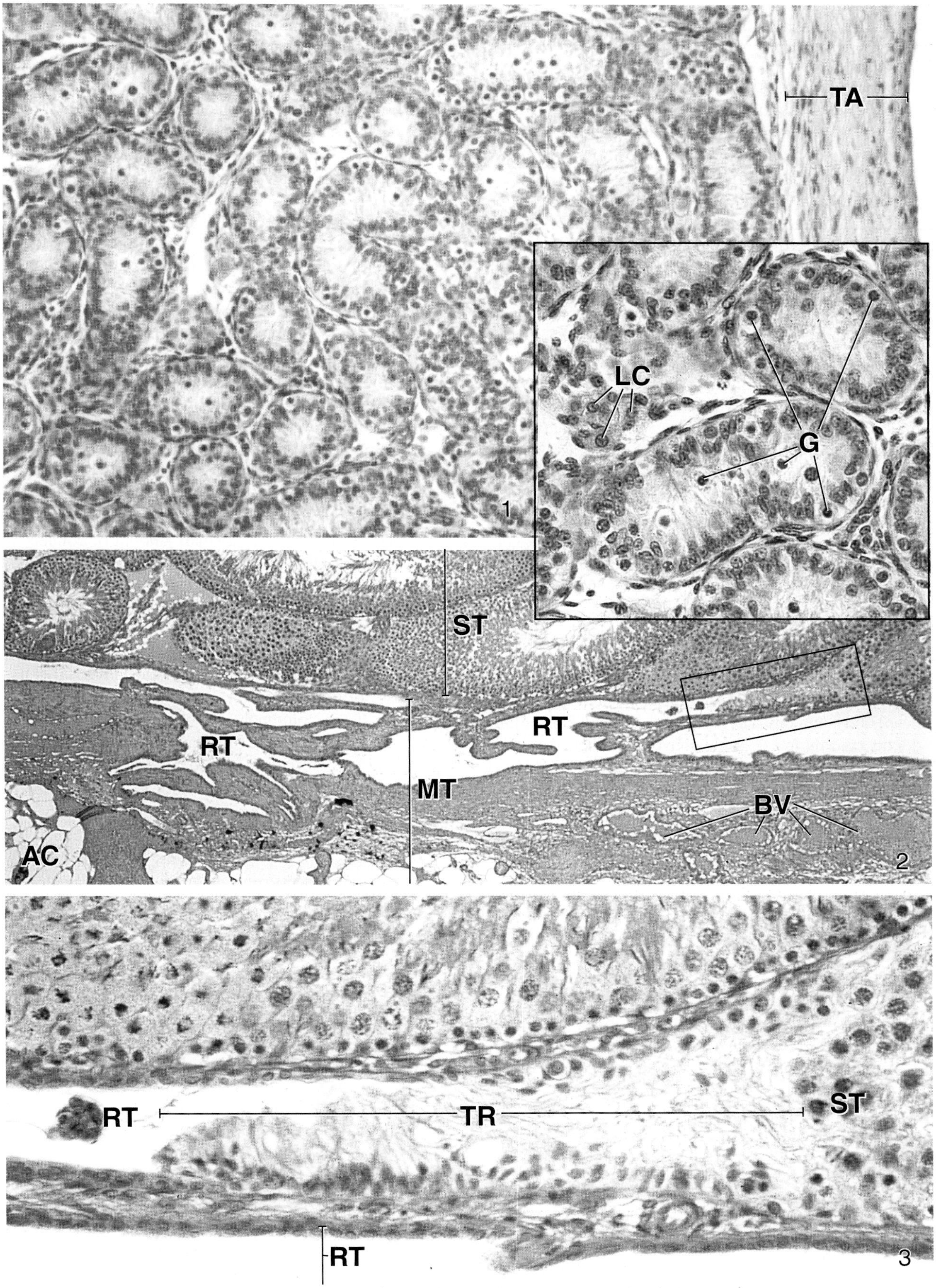
TA
LC
G
1
ST
RT
RT
MT
BV
AC
2
RT
TR
ST
RT
3

PLATE 84. DUCTULI EFFERENTES AND EPIDIDYMIS

The rete testis, in turn, is connected via ~20 *efferent ductules* (*ductuli efferentes;* remnants of nephrons of the fetal mesonephric kidney) to the *ductus epididymis*. These are the first elements of the excurrent duct system of the male genital system. Most of the fluid secreted in the seminiferous tubules is reabsorbed in the efferent ductules. The muscular coat characteristic of the excurrent duct system first appears at the beginning of the efferent ductules. The ductus epididymis is a highly coiled tube, 4 to 6 m long; sperm mature during their passage along its length, acquiring motility as well as the ability to fertilize an egg. This maturation is also androgen dependent and involves changes in the sperm plasma membrane and addition to the glycocalyx of glycoproteins secreted by the epididymal epithelial cells.

Figure 1, ductuli efferentes, monkey, H&E ×60; inset ×360.

About 12 to 20 efferent ductules leave the testis and serve as channels from the rete testis to the ductus epididymis. Each of the efferent ductules undergoes numerous spiral windings and convolutions to form a group of conical structures; together they constitute the initial part of the head of the epididymis. When examined in a tissue section, the ductules exhibit a variety of irregular profiles due to their twisting and turning. This is evident on the right side of this micrograph.

The epithelium that lines the efferent ductules is distinctive in that groups of tall columnar cells alternate with groups of cuboidal cells, giving the luminal surface an unevenly contoured appearance. Thus, small cup-like depressions are created where the epithelium contains groups of cuboidal or low columnar cells. Typically, these shorter cells exhibit a brush border-like apical surface because of the microvilli that they possess (*arrowhead,* **inset**). The basal surface of the ductule, in contrast, has a smooth contour (see Fig. 2 and **inset**). Some of the cells, generally the tall columnar cells, possess cilia *(C)* **(inset).** Whereas the ciliated cells aid in moving the contents of the tubule toward the epididymis, the cells with the microvilli are largely responsible for absorbing fluid from the lumen. In addition to the columnar and cuboidal cells, basal cells are also present; thus, the epithelium is designated pseudostratified columnar. The basal cells possess little cytoplasm and presumably serve as stem cells.

The efferent ductules possess a thin layer of circularly arranged smooth muscle cells (*SM,* **inset**). The muscle is close to the basal surface of the epithelial cells, being separated from it by only a small amount of connective tissue (*CT,* **inset**). Because of this close association, the smooth muscle may be overlooked or misidentified as connective tissue. Smooth muscle facilitates movement of luminal contents of the ductule to the ductus epididymis.

Figure 2, epididymis, monkey, H&E ×180.

The epididymis, by virtue of its shape, is divided into a head, body, and tail. The initial part of the head contains the ductus epididymis, a single convoluted duct into which the efferent ductules open. The duct is, at first, highly convoluted but becomes less tortuous in the body and tail. A section through the head of the epididymis, as shown in Figure 1, cuts the ductus epididymis in numerous places, and as in the efferent ductules, different-shaped profiles are observed.

The epithelium contains two distinguishable cell types: tall columnar cells and basal cells similar to those of the efferent ductules. The epithelium is, thus, also pseudostratified columnar. The columnar cells are tallest in the head of the epididymis and diminish in height as the tail is reached. The free surface of the cell possesses stereocilia *(SC).* These are extremely long, branching microvilli. They evidently adhere to each other during the preparation of the tissue to form the fine tapering structures that are characteristically seen with the light microscope. The nuclei of the columnar cells are elongated and are located a moderate distance from the base of the cell. They are readily distinguished from the spherical nuclei of the basal cells that lie close to the basement membrane. Other conspicuous features of the columnar cells include a very large supranuclear Golgi apparatus (not seen at the magnification offered here), pigment accumulations *(P),* and numerous lysosomes, demonstrable with appropriate techniques.

Because of the unusual height of the columnar cells and, again, the tortuosity of the duct, an uneven lumen appears in some sites; indeed, even "islands" of epithelium can be encountered in the lumen (see *arrows,* Fig. 1). Such profiles are accounted for by sharp turns in the duct where the epithelial wall on one side of the duct is partially cut. For example, a cut in the plane of the *double-headed arrow* indicated in this figure would create such an isolated epithelial island.

A thin layer of smooth muscle circumscribes the duct and appears similar to that associated with the efferent ductules. In the terminal portion of the epididymis, however, the smooth muscle acquires a greater thickness, and longitudinal fibers are also present. Beyond the smooth muscle coat there is a small amount of connective tissue *(CT)* that binds the loops of the duct together and carries the blood vessels *(BV)* and nerves.

KEY

AT, adipose tissue
BV, blood vessel
C, cilia
CT, connective tissue
P, pigment
SC, stereocilia
SM, smooth muscle
arrowhead (inset), brush border
arrows, "islands" of epithelium in the lumen

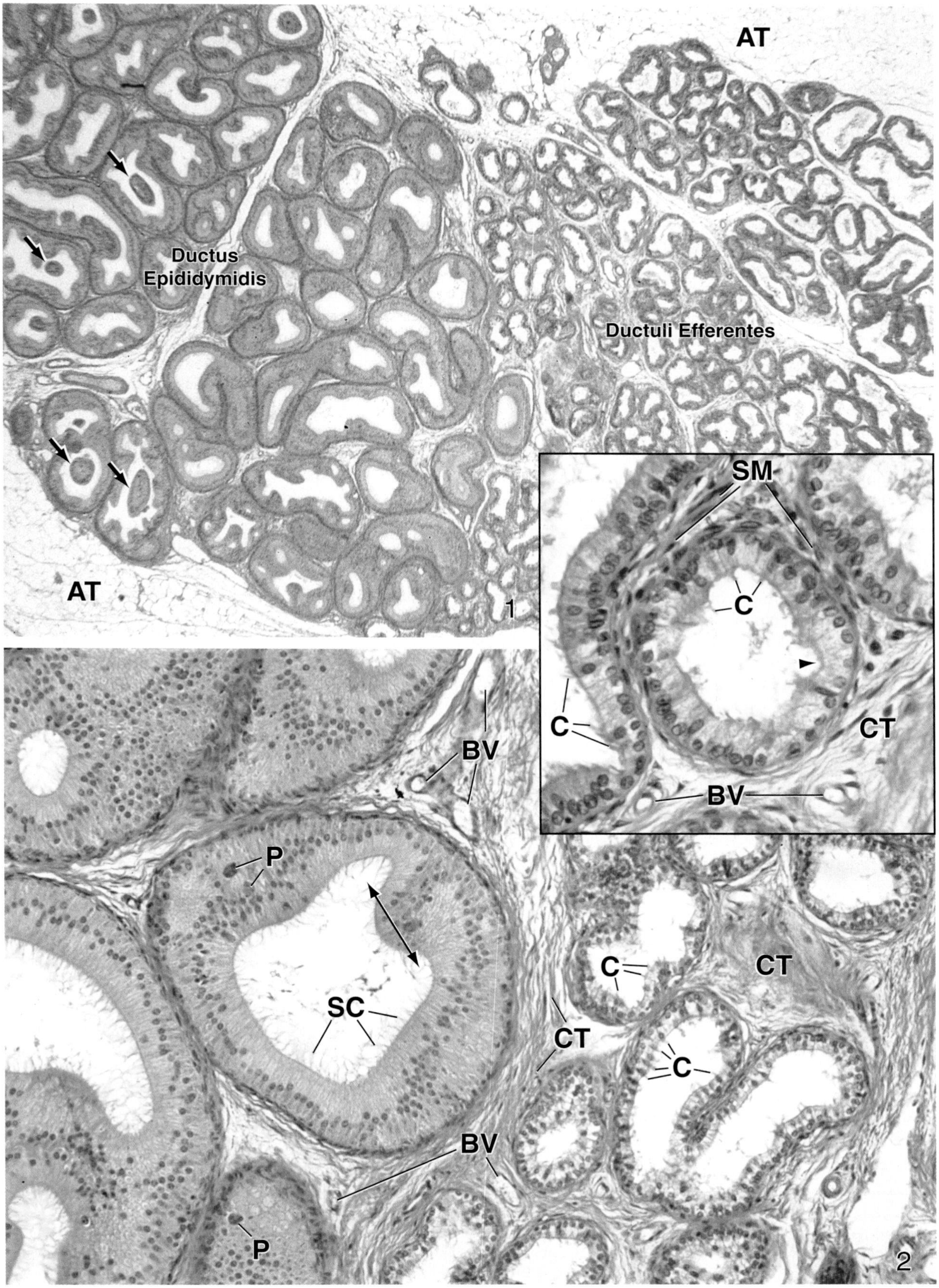
AT
Ductus Epididymidis
Ductuli Efferentes
AT
1
SM
C
C
CT
BV
BV
P
SC
C
CT
CT
C
BV
P
2

PLATE 85. SPERMATIC CORD AND DUCTUS DEFERENS

The ductus (vas) deferens continues from the duct of the epididymis as a thick-walled muscular tube that leaves the scrotum and passes through the inguinal canal as a component of the spermatic cord. At the deep inguinal ring, it continues into the pelvis and, behind the urinary bladder, joins with the seminal vesicle to form the ejaculatory duct. The ejaculatory duct then pierces the prostate gland and opens into the urethra.

Mature sperm are stored in the terminal portion (tail) of the ductus epididymis. These sperm are forced into the ductus deferens by intense contractions of the three smooth muscle layers of the ductus deferens following appropriate neural stimulation. Contraction of the smooth muscle of the ductus deferens continues the movement of the sperm through the ejaculatory duct into the urethra during the ejaculatory reflex. The seminal vesicles (see Plate 87) are not storage sites for sperm but, rather, secrete a fructose-rich fluid that becomes part of the ejaculated semen. Fructose is the principal metabolic substrate for sperm.

Figure 1, spermatic cord, human, H&E ×80.

A cross section through the ductus deferens and some of the vessels and nerves that accompany the duct in the spermatic cord are shown in this figure. The wall of the ductus deferens is extremely thick, mostly because of the presence of a large amount of smooth muscle. The muscle contracts when the tissue is removed, causing the mucosa to form longitudinal folds. For this reason, in histologic sections, the lumen *(L)* usually appears irregular in cross section.

The smooth muscle of the ductus deferens is arranged as a thick outer longitudinal layer *(SM(L))*, a thick middle circular layer *(SM(C))*, and a thinner inner longitudinal layer *(SM(L))*. Between the epithelium and the inner longitudinal smooth muscle layer there is a moderately thick cellular layer of loose connective tissue, the lamina propria *(LP)*. The connective tissue immediately surrounding the ductus deferens contains nerves and some of the smaller blood vessels that supply the duct. In fact, some of these vessels can be seen penetrating the outer longitudinal smooth muscle layer *(asterisks)*.

Figure 2, ductus deferens, human, H&E ×320; inset ×250.

The epithelial lining of the ductus deferens consists of pseudostratified columnar epithelium with stereocilia *(arrowheads)*. It resembles the epithelium of the epididymis, but the cells are not as tall. The elongated nuclei of the columnar cells are readily distinguished from the spherical nuclei of the basal cells *(arrows)*. The epithelium rests on a loose connective tissue that extends to the smooth muscle; no submucosa is described.

A unique feature of the spermatic cord is the presence of a plexus of atypical veins (pampiniform plexus) that arise from the spermatic veins. These vessels receive the blood from the testis. (The pampiniform plexus also receives tributaries from the epididymis.) The plexus is an anastomosing vascular network that constitutes the bulk of the spermatic cord. Portions of several of these veins *(BV)* are evident in the upper right of Figure 1 along with a number of nerves *(N)*. The unusual feature of the veins is their thick muscular wall that, at a glance, gives the appearance of an artery rather than a vein. Careful examination of these vessels **(inset)** shows that the bulk of the vessel wall is composed of two layers of smooth muscle—an outer circular layer *SM(C)* and an inner longitudinal layer *SM(L)*.

KEY

BV, blood vessels
CT, connective tissue
L, lumen of ductus deferens
LP, lamina propria
Lu, lumen of blood vessel
N, nerve
SM(C), circular layer of smooth muscle
SM(L), longitudinal layer of smooth muscle
arrowheads, stereocilia
arrows (Fig. 2), basal cell nucleus
asterisks (Fig. 1), small arteries supplying ductus deferens

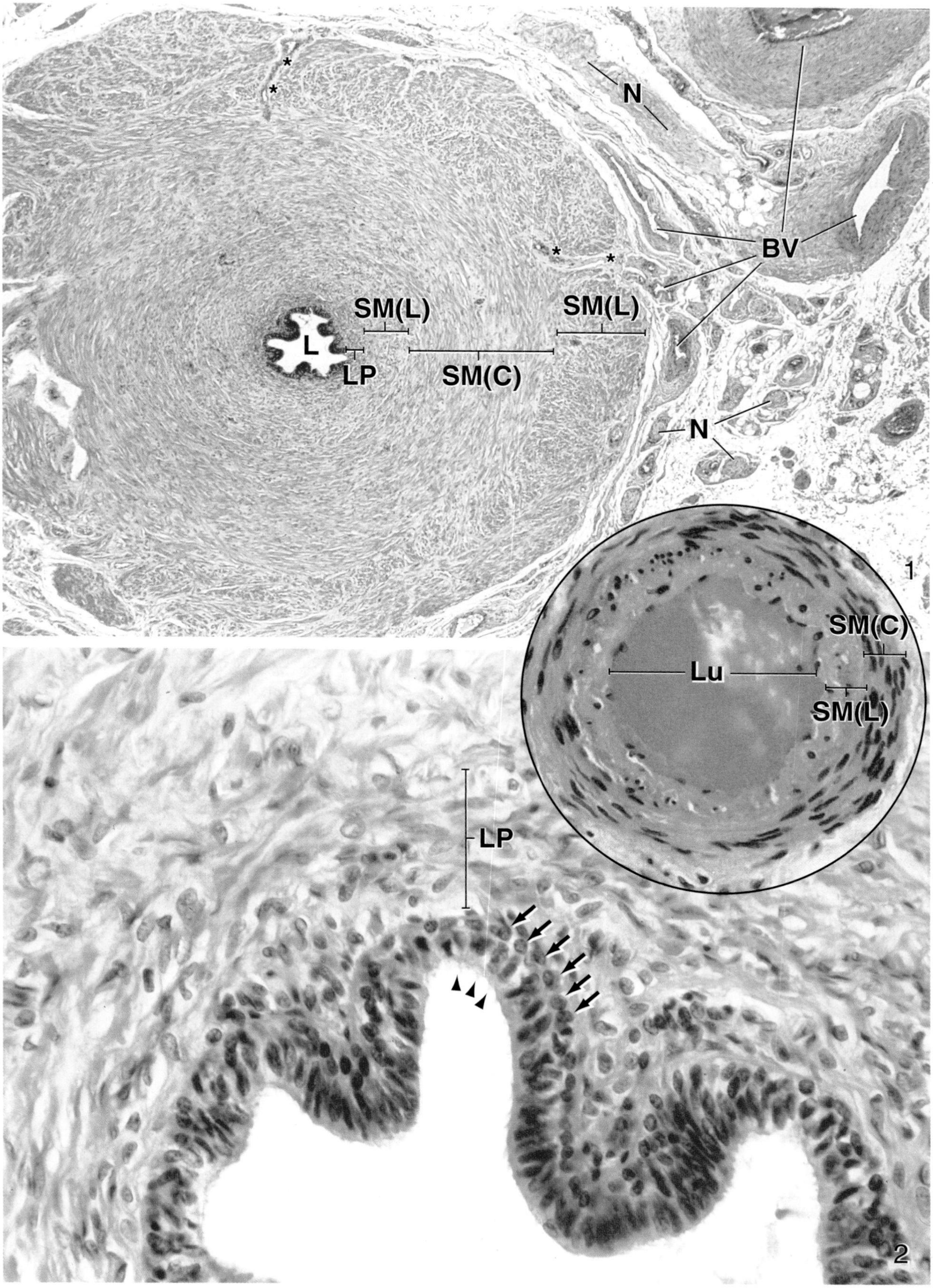
N
BV
SM(L)
SM(L)
L
LP
SM(C)
N
1
SM(C)
Lu
SM(L)
LP
2

PLATE 86. PROSTATE GLAND

The prostate gland is the largest accessory sex gland. It consists of 30 to 50 tubuloalveolar glands that surround the proximal urethra. Because of this relationship, a common condition in later life, benign prostatic hyperplasia, can result in partial or total obstruction of the urethra.

The prostatic glands are arranged in three concentric layers: a mucosal layer, a submucosal layer, and a peripheral layer containing the main prostatic glands. The mucosal glands secrete directly into the urethra; the other two sets of glands deliver their secretions through ducts that open into the prostatic sinuses on the posterior wall of the urethra. All of the glands are made up of a pseudostratified columnar epithelium that secretes several components of the semen, including acid phosphatase, citric acid (a nutrient for sperm), and fibrinolysin (which keeps the semen liquified). Aggregations of dead epithelial cells and precipitated secretory products form *concretions* in the alveoli of the glands; these are a characteristic feature that aids in recognition of the prostate.

The stroma is characterized by numerous small bundles of smooth muscle, so that it can also be described as a fibromuscular stroma. Contraction of this muscle occurs at ejaculation, forcing the secretion into the urethra. Surrounding the gland is a fibroelastic capsule that also contains small bundles of smooth muscle.

Figure 1, prostate, human H&E ×47.

A portion of the prostate gland in shown in this low-magnification micrograph. A small section of the capsule *(Cap)* of the gland is seen in the upper left corner. The rest of the field is filled with the glandular and stromal components of the prostate. The secretory tubuloalveoli of the prostate gland vary greatly in form, as is evident in the figure. They may appear as tubes, as isolated alveoli, as alveoli with branches, or as tubes with branches. Tangential sections through alveoli may even produce the appearance of "epithelial islands" *(arrowheads)* in the lumen of the alveoli. This is due to the extremely uneven contour of the epithelial surface. It should also be noted that many of the alveoli may appear rudimentary in structure *(arrows).* These are simply in an inactive state and are increasingly observed in older individuals. As noted above, aggregations of dead epithelial cells and precipitated secretions form prostatic concretions *(C)* in the lumina of the alveoli; these gradually increase in number and size with age. The concretions stain with eosin and may have a concentric lamellar appearance, as is clearly shown in the concretion in the lower right. With time, they may become impregnated with calcium salts and thus be easily recognized in x-rays of the lower abdomen.

Figure 2, prostate, human, H&E ×178; upper inset ×350; lower inset ×650.

In this higher magnification view of a portion of the prostate gland, the fibromuscular stroma is clearly seen both immediately subtending the secretory epithelium of the tubuloalveoli as well as in deeper, nonsecretory areas. In the **upper inset,** corresponding to the *larger rectangle,* the intensity of the staining of the smooth muscle *(SM)* clearly distinguishes it from the fibrous stromal connective tissue with which it is intimately intermingled. There are no clearly outlined bundles or layers of smooth muscle in the prostate; rather, it is randomly arrayed throughout the stroma. Concretions *(C)* are again evident in the lumina of alveoli, in one instance compressing the epithelium to a degree that makes it nearly unrecognizable. The **lower inset,** corresponding to the *smaller rectangle,* clearly demonstrates the pseudostratified columnar nature of the prostatic epithelium *(Ep).* Well-delineated basal cells *(arrowheads)* are seen along with the taller columnar secretory cells. A small blood vessel immediately subtending the epithelium is recognizable by the red blood cells in its lumen. A lymphocytic infiltration appears to fill the stroma along the lower border of Figure 2, suggesting an inflammatory process occurring in the prostate gland.

KEY

KEY
BV, blood vessel
C, prostatic concretion
Cap, capsule
Ep, epithelium
L, lymphocytes
SM, smooth muscle
arrows, inactive alveoli
arrowheads: Fig. 1, "epithelial islands"; Fig. 2, basal cells

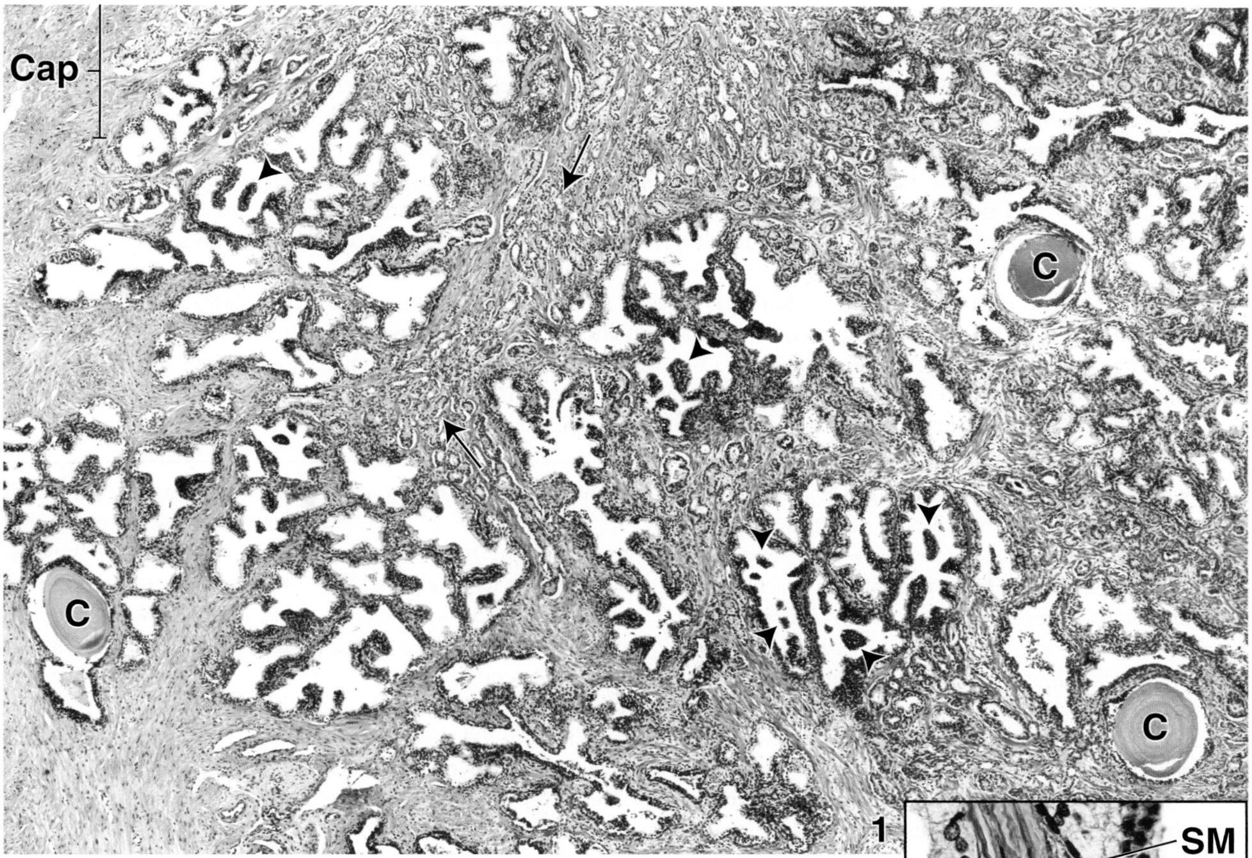
Cap
C
C
C
1

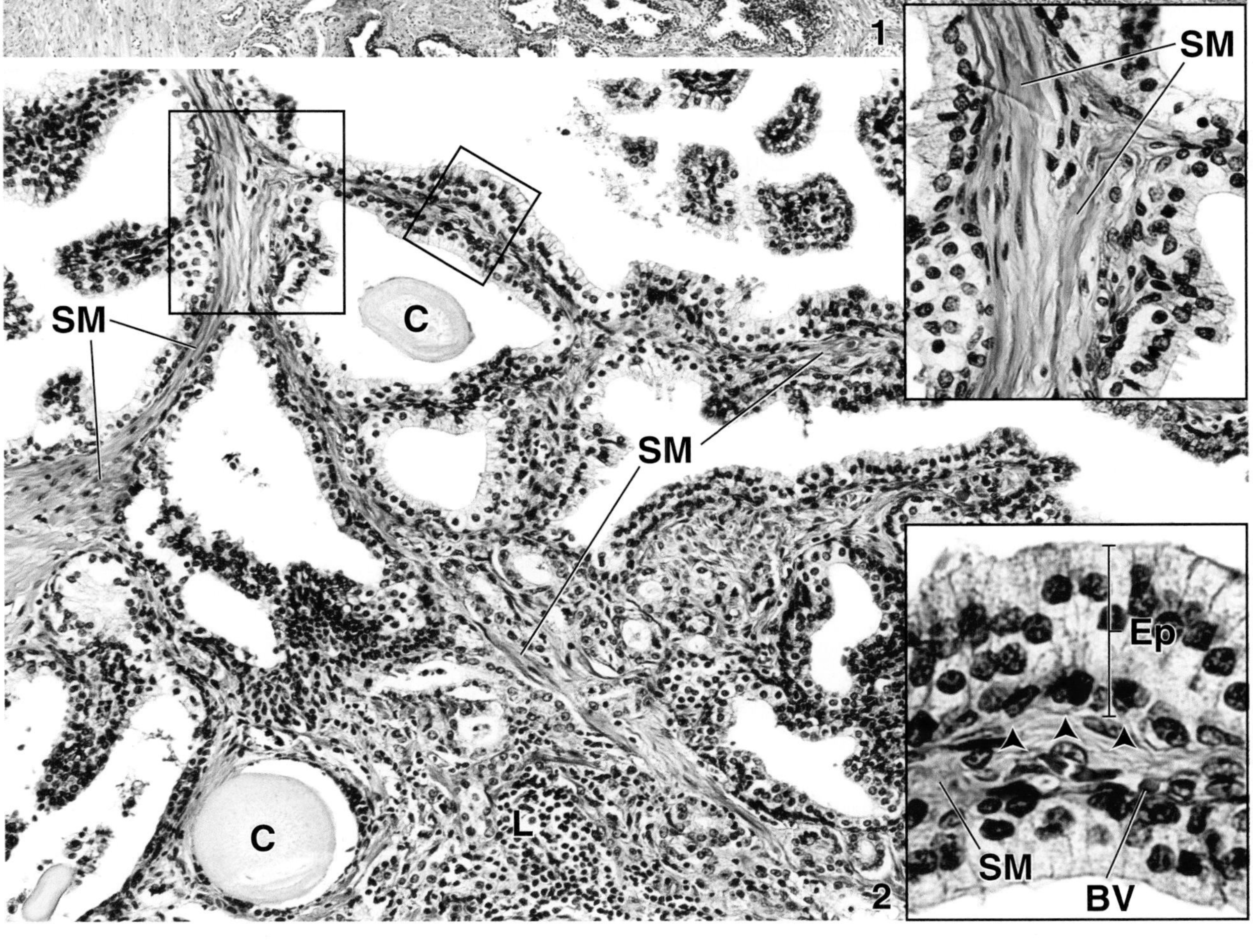
SM
SM
C
SM
SM
Ep
C
L
SM
BV
2

PLATE 87. SEMINAL VESICLE

The seminal vesicles are evaginations from the end of each ductus deferens that form tightly coiled tubes. Although sections through this structure may show many lumina, they are all profiles of a single continuous tubular lumen. The seminal vesicles are lined with a pseudostratified columnar epithelium that closely resembles that of the prostate gland.

The secretion of the seminal vesicles is a whitish yellow viscous material that contains fructose, other simple sugars, amino acids, ascorbic acid, and prostaglandins. Although prostaglandins were first isolated from the prostate gland (hence the name), they are actually synthesized in large amounts in the seminal vesicles. Fructose is the primary nutrient source for the sperm in the semen.

The mucosa rests on a thick layer of smooth muscle that is directly continuous with that of the ductus deferens, from which the seminal vesicle evaginates. The smooth muscle consists of an indistinct inner circular layer and an outer longitudinal layer (compare with the three layers of the ductus epididymis and the ductus deferens, Plate 84), which are difficult to distinguish. Contraction of the smooth muscle coat during ejaculation forces the secretions of the seminal vesicles into the ejaculatory ducts. Beyond the smooth muscle is the connective tissue of the adventitia.

Figure 1, seminal vesicle, human, H&E ×30.

This figure shows a cross section of a seminal vesicle. Because of the coiled nature of the vesicle, two almost distinct lumina, lying side by side, appear to be present. They are, however, connected so that, in effect, all of the internal spaces are continuous and what is seen here is actually a two-dimensional configuration reflecting coiling of the tube.

The mucosa of the seminal vesicles is characterized by being extensively folded or ridged. The ridges vary in size and typically branch and interconnect with one another. The larger ridges may form recesses that contain smaller ridges, and when cut obliquely, these appear as mucosal arches that enclose the smaller folds *(arrows)*. When the plane of section is normal to the surface, the mucosal ridges appear as "villi." In some areas, particularly the peripheral region of the lumen, the interconnecting folds of the mucosa appear as alveoli. Each of these chambers is, however, simply a pocket-like structure that is open and continuous with the lumen. The mucosa is subtended by a very cellular loose connective tissue *(CT)* that, in turn, is surrounded by smooth muscle *(SM)*.

The seminal vesicles are paired elongated sacs. Each vesicle consists of a single tube folded and coiled on itself with occasional diverticula in its wall. The upper extremity ends as a cul-de-sac; the lower extremity is constricted into a narrow straight duct that joins and empties into its corresponding ductus deferens.

Figure 2, seminal vesicle, human, H&E ×220.

This higher magnification of the mucosal folds reveals the epithelium *(Ep)* and the underlying loose connective tissue or lamina propria *(LP)*. The epithelium is described as pseudostratified. It is composed of low columnar or cuboidal cells and small, round basal cells. The latter are randomly interspersed between the larger principal cells, but they are relatively sparse. For this reason, the epithelium may not be readily recognized as pseudostratified. In some areas, the epithelium appears thick *(arrowhead)* and, based on the disposition of the nuclei, would seem to be multilayered. This is due to a tangential section of the epithelium and is not a true stratification. The lamina propria of the mucosa is composed of a very cellular connective tissue containing some smooth muscle cells and is rich in elastic fibers.

KEY

CT, connective tissue
Ep, epithelium
LP, lamina propria
SM, smooth muscle
arrowhead, oblique section of epithelium
arrows, mucosal arches

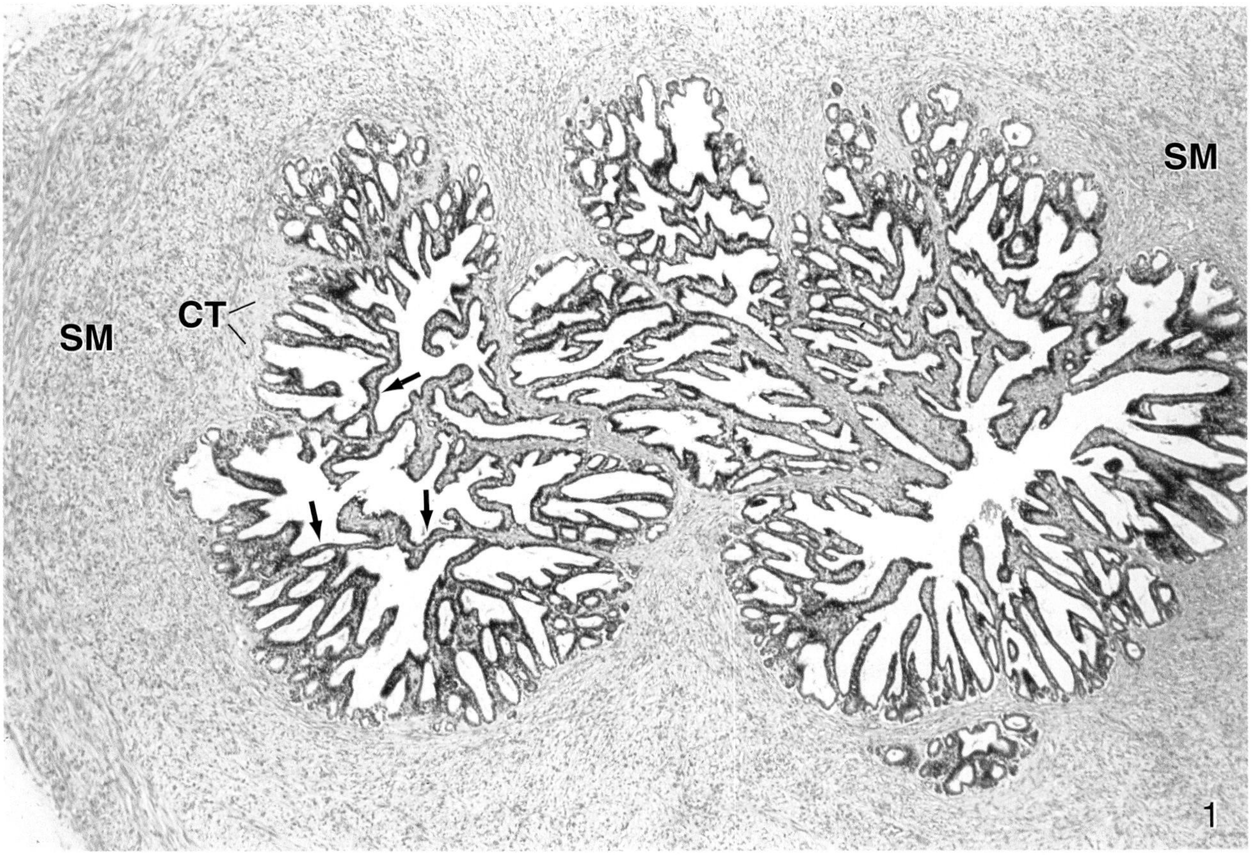
SM
SM
CT
1

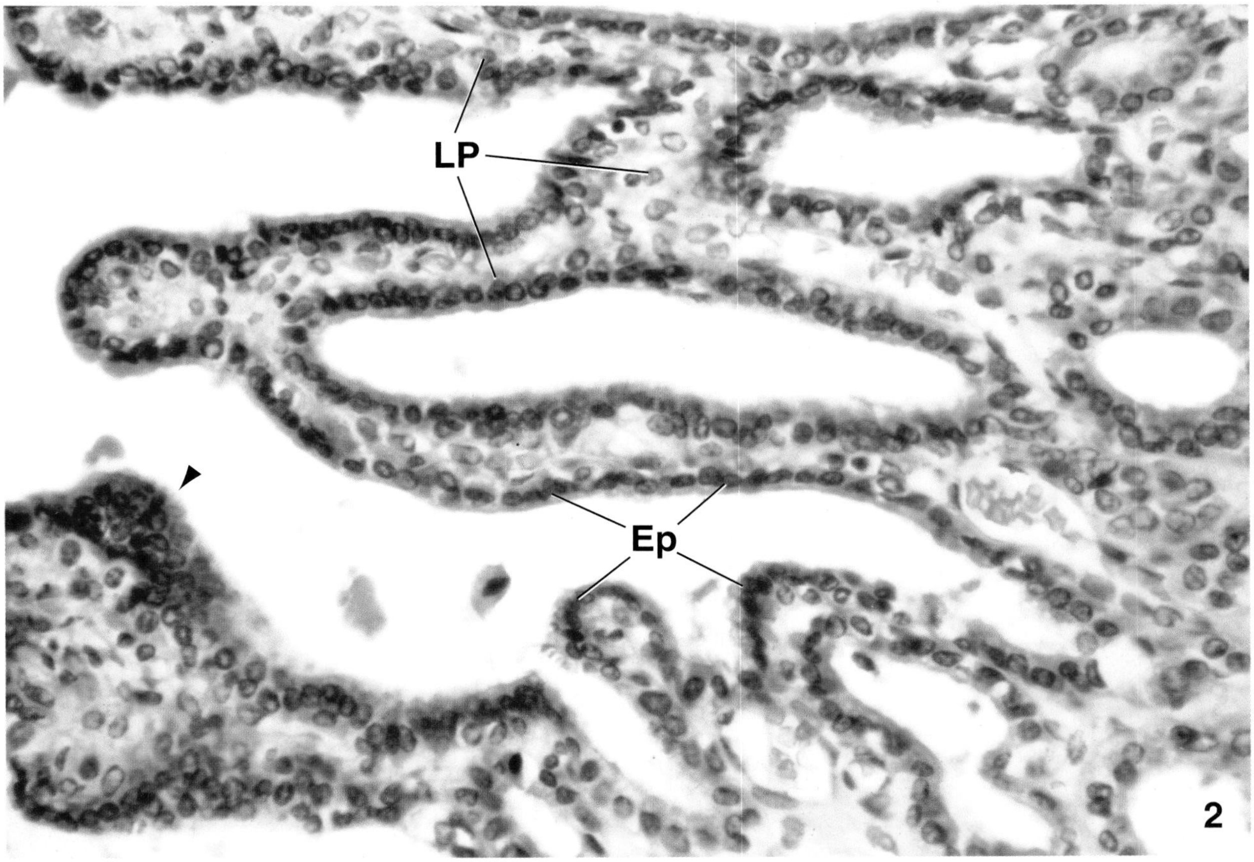
LP
Ep
2

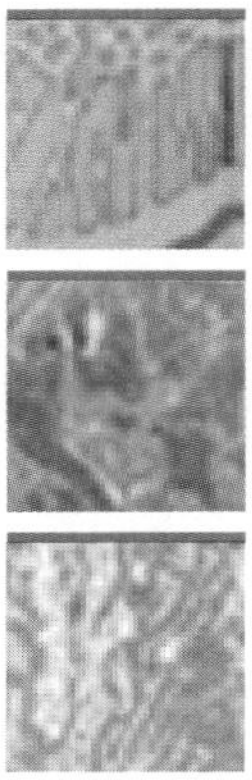

22

Female Reproductive System

▽ OVERVIEW OF THE FEMALE REPRODUCTIVE SYSTEM

The female reproductive system consists of internal sex organs and external genital structures

The internal female reproductive organs are located in the pelvis, and the external genital structures (external genitalia) are situated in the anterior part of the perineum known as the *vulva*.

- The internal organs are the ***ovaries, uterine tubes, uterus,*** and ***vagina*** (Fig. 22.1).
- The external genitalia include the ***mons pubis, labia majora*** and ***minora, clitoris, vestibule*** and ***opening of the vagina,*** and ***external urethral orifice.***

The mammary glands are included in this chapter because their development and functional state are directly related to the hormonal activity of the female reproductive system. Similarly, the placenta is included because of its functional and physical relationship to the uterus in pregnancy.

Female reproductive organs undergo regular cyclic changes from puberty to menopause

The ovaries, uterine tubes, and uterus of the sexually mature female undergo marked structural and functional changes related to neural activity and changes in hormone levels during each menstrual cycle and during pregnancy. These mechanisms also regulate the early development of the female reproductive system. The initiation of the menstrual cycle, referred to as the ***menarche,*** occurs in females between 9 and 14 years of age (average 13.5 years) and marks the end of puberty and the beginning of the reproductive lifespan. During this phase of life, the ***menstrual cycle*** averages about 28 to 30 days in length. Between 45 and 55 years of age, the menstrual cycle becomes infrequent and eventually ceases. This change in reproductive function is referred to as the ***menopause*** or climacterium (commonly called the "change of life"). The ovaries cease their reproductive function of producing oocytes and their endocrine function of producing hormones that regulate reproductive activity. Other organs, e.g., vagina and mammary glands, show varying degrees of reduced function, particularly secretory activity.

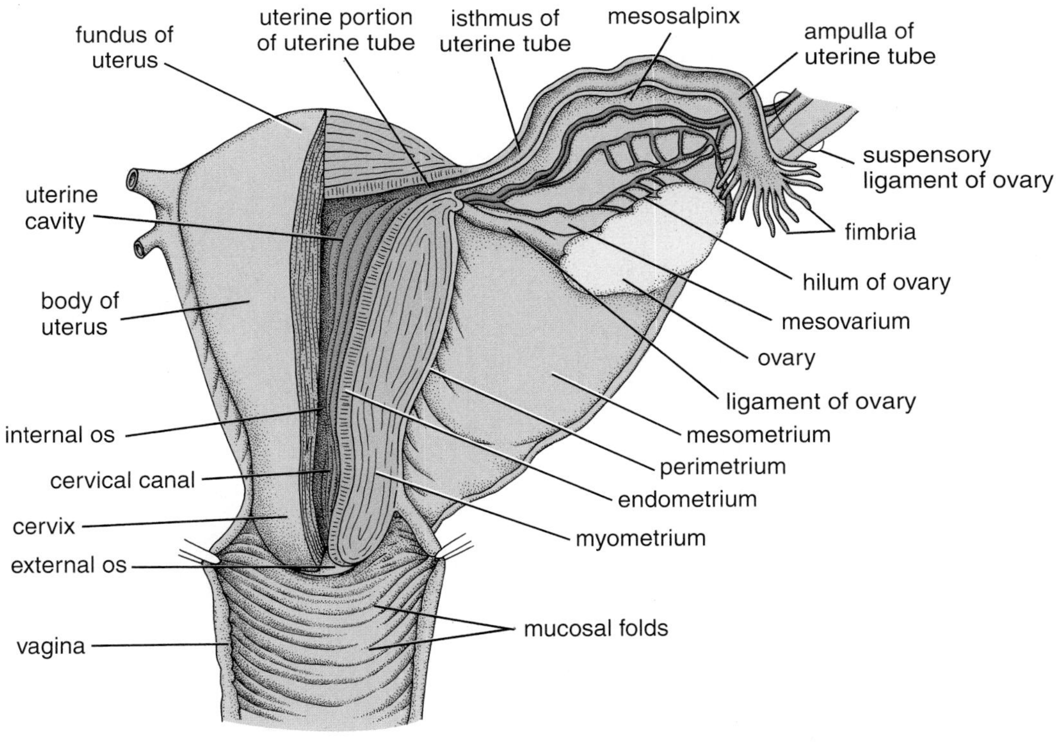

FIGURE 22.1
Schematic drawing of female internal sex organs. This drawing shows the posterior view of the female internal sex organs. Part of the wall of the uterus, uterine tube, and vagina has been removed to reveal their internal structure. Note the three distinct layers of the uterine wall: the inner layer, the endometrium lining the uterine cavity; the middle and thickest layer, the myometrium; and the outer layer, the perimetrium, which is the peritoneal covering of the uterus.

▼ OVARY

Production of gametes and steroid hormones are the two major functions of the ovary

The ovaries have two interrelated functions: the production of gametes *(gametogenesis)* and the production of steroids *(steroidogenesis)*. In the female, the production of gametes is called ***oogenesis***. Developing gametes are called ***oocytes;*** mature gametes are called ***ova***.

Two major groups of steroid hormones, estrogens and progestogens, are secreted by the ovaries:

- ***Estrogens*** promote growth and maturation of internal and external sex organs and are responsible for the female sex characteristics that develop at puberty. Estrogens also act on mammary glands to promote breast development by stimulating ductal and stromal growth and accumulation of adipose tissue.
- ***Progestogens*** prepare the internal sex organs, mainly the uterus, for pregnancy by promoting secretory changes in the endometrium (discussed in the section on cyclic changes in the endometrium). Progestogens also prepare the mammary gland for lactation by promoting lobular proliferation.

Both hormones play an important role in the menstrual cycle by preparing the uterus for implantation of a fertilized ovum. If implantation does not occur, the endometrium of the uterus degenerates and menstruation follows.

Ovarian Structure

In nulliparas (woman who have not borne children), the ovaries are paired, almond-shaped, pinkish white structures measuring about 3 cm in length, 1.5 cm in width, and 1 cm in thickness. Each ovary is attached to the posterior surface of the ***broad ligament*** by a peritoneal fold, the mesovarium (see Fig. 22.1). The ***superior (or tubal) pole*** of the ovary is attached to the pelvic wall by the ***suspensory ligament of the ovary***, which carries the ovarian vessels and nerves. The ***inferior (or uterine) pole*** is attached to the uterus by the ***ovarian ligament***. This ligament is a remnant of the ***gubernaculum***, the embryonic fibrous cord that attaches the developing gonad to the floor of the pelvis. Before puberty, the surface of the ovary is smooth, but during reproductive life it becomes progressively scarred and irregular due to repeated ovulations. In postmenopausal women, the ovaries are about one fourth the size observed during the reproductive period.

The ovary is composed of a cortex and a medulla

A section through the ovary reveals two distinct regions:

- ***Medulla*** or ***medullary region*** located in the central portion of the ovary. The medulla contains loose connective tissue, a mass of relatively large contorted blood vessels, lymphatic vessels, and nerves (Fig. 22.2).
- ***Cortex*** or ***cortical region*** found in the peripheral portion of the ovary surrounding the medulla. The cortex contains the ***ovarian follicles*** embedded in a richly cellular connective tissue. Scattered smooth muscle fibers are present in the stroma around the follicles. The boundary between the medulla and cortex is indistinct.

"Germinal epithelium" instead of mesothelium covers the ovary

The surface of the ovary is covered by a single layer of cuboidal and, in some parts, almost squamous cells. This cellular layer, known as the ***germinal epithelium***, is continuous with the mesothelium that covers the mesovarium. The term ***germinal epithelium*** is a carryover from the past when it was incorrectly thought to be the site of germ cell formation during embryonic development. It is now known that the ***primordial germ cells*** (both male and female) are of extragonadal origin and that they migrate from the embryonic yolk sac into the cortex of the embryonic gonad, where they differentiate and induce differentiation of the ovary. A dense connective tissue layer, the ***tunica albuginea***, lies between the germinal epithelium and the underlying cortex.

Ovarian follicles provide the microenvironment for the developing oocyte

Ovarian follicles of various sizes, each containing a single oocyte, are distributed in the stroma of the cortex. The

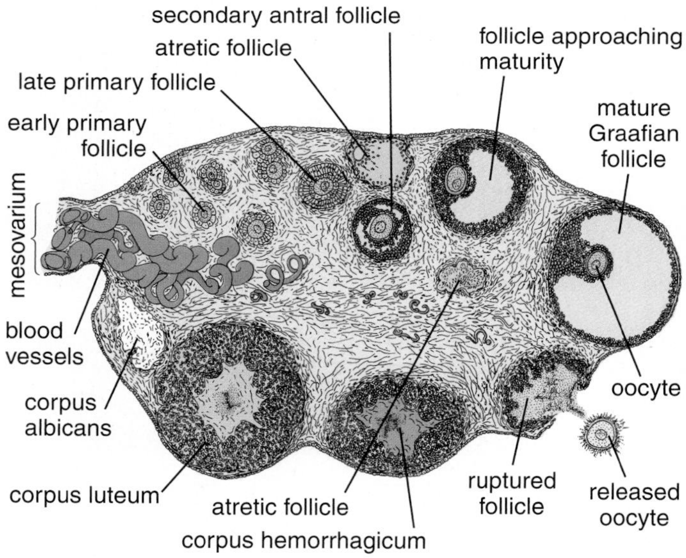

FIGURE 22.2
Schematic drawing of a section through the ovary. This section shows, in clockwise order, stages of follicular development from the early primary follicle to the mature (Graafian) follicle. Changes in the follicle after ovulation lead to development of the corpus luteum and eventually the corpus albicans. Note the highly coiled blood vessels in the hilum and medulla of the ovary.

size of a follicle indicates the developmental state of the oocyte. Early stages of oogenesis occur during fetal life when mitotic divisions massively increase the number of oogonia (see the section on oogenesis). The oocytes present at birth remain arrested in development at the first meiotic division (see page 69). During puberty, small groups of follicles undergo cyclic growth and maturation. The first ovulation generally does not take place for a year or more following menarche. A cyclic pattern of follicular maturation and ovulation is then established that continues in parallel with the menstrual cycle. Normally, only one oocyte reaches full maturity and is released from the ovary during each menstrual cycle. Obviously, the maturation and release of more than one egg at ovulation may lead to multiple zygotes. During the reproductive lifespan, a woman produces only about 400 mature ova. Most of the estimated 600,000 to 800,000 primary oocytes present at birth do not complete maturation and are gradually lost through *atresia*, the spontaneous death and subsequent resorption of immature oocytes. This process begins as early as the fifth month of fetal life and is mediated by apoptosis of cells surrounding the oocyte (see page 69). Atresia reduces the number of primary oocytes in a logarithmic fashion throughout life from as many as 5 million in the fetus to less than 20% of that number at birth. The oocytes that remain at menopause degenerate within a few years.

Follicle Development

Histologically, three basic types of ovarian follicles can be identified on the basis of developmental state:

- *Primordial follicles*
- *Growing follicles*
- *Mature* or *Graafian follicles*

Growing follicles are further subcategorized as ***primary*** and ***secondary (or antral) follicles.*** Some histologists identify additional stages in the continuum of follicular development. In the cycling ovary, follicles are found at all stages of development, but primordial follicles predominate.

The primordial follicle is the earliest stage of follicular development

Primordial follicles first appear in the ovaries during the third month of fetal development. Early growth of the primordial follicles is independent of gonadotropin stimulation. In the mature ovary, primordial follicles are found in the stroma of the cortex just beneath the tunica albuginea. A single layer of squamous follicle cells surrounds the oocyte (Fig. 22.3). The outer surface of the follicle cells is bounded by a basal lamina. At this stage, the oocyte and the surrounding follicle cells are closely apposed to one another. The oocyte in the follicle measures about 30 μm in

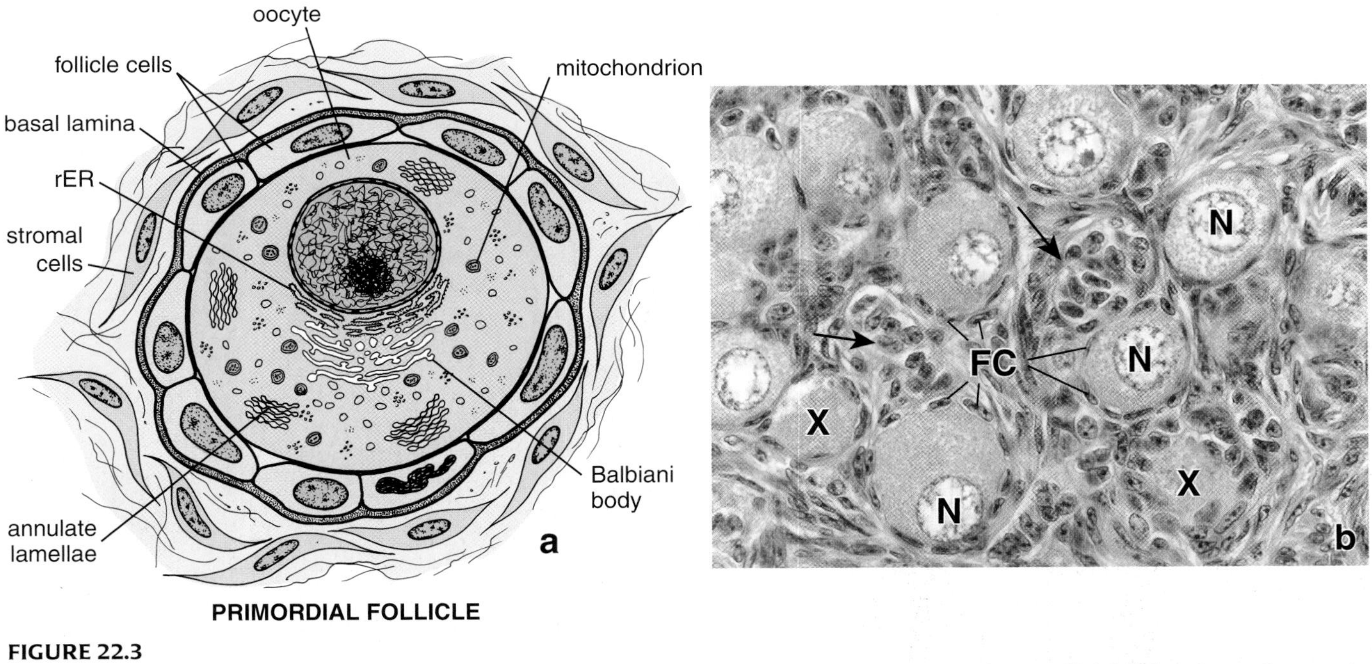

FIGURE 22.3
Primordial follicle. a. Schematic drawing of a primordial follicle shows the oocyte arrested in prophase of the first meiotic division. The oocyte is closely surrounded by a single layer of squamous follicle cells. The outer surface of these cells is separated from the connective tissue by a basal lamina. The ooplasm contains characteristic organelles, as seen with the electron microscope, including a Balbiani body, annulate lamellae, and small spherical mitochondria. **b.** This photomicrograph of primordial follicles shows the oocytes surrounded by a single layer of flattened follicle cells *(FC)*. Usually, the nucleus *(N)* of the oocyte is in an eccentric position. Two oocytes in which the nucleus is not included in the plane of section are indicated *(X)*. Similarly, there are two follicles *(arrows)* in which the follicle cells are revealed in face or tangential view and the enclosed oocytes are not included in the section. ×640.

diameter and has a large, eccentric nucleus that contains finely dispersed chromatin and one or more large nucleoli. The cytoplasm of the oocyte, referred to as ooplasm, contains a ***Balbiani body*** (Fig. 22.3a). At the ultrastructural level, the Balbiani body is revealed as a localized accumulation of Golgi membranes and vesicles, endoplasmic reticulum, numerous mitochondria, and lysosomes. In addition, human oocytes contain ***annulate lamellae,*** and numerous small vesicles are scattered throughout the cytoplasm along with small, spherical mitochondria. Annulate lamellae resemble a stack of nuclear envelope profiles. Each layer of the stack includes pore structures morphologically identical to nuclear pores.

The primary follicle is the first stage in the development of the growing follicle

As a primordial follicle develops into a growing follicle, changes occur in the oocyte, in the follicle cells, and in the adjacent stroma. Initially, the oocyte enlarges and the surrounding flattened follicle cells proliferate and become cuboidal. At this stage, i.e., when the follicle cells become cuboidal, the follicle is identified as a ***primary follicle.*** As the oocyte grows, a homogeneous, deeply staining, acidophilic refractile layer called the ***zona pellucida*** appears between the oocyte and the adjacent follicle cells (Fig. 22.4). The zona pellucida is first apparent in the light microscope when the oocyte, surrounded by a single layer of cuboidal or columnar follicle cells, has grown to a diameter of 50 to 80 μm. The growing oocyte secretes the gel-like zona pellucida, which is rich in glycosaminoglycans and glycoproteins and stains with the periodic acid–Schiff (PAS) reaction.

Follicle cells undergo stratification to form the granulosa layer of the primary follicle

Through rapid mitotic proliferation, the single layer of follicle cells gives rise to a stratified epithelium, the ***membrana granulosa (stratum granulosum),*** surrounding the oocyte. The follicle cells are now identified as ***granulosa cells.*** The basal lamina retains its position between the outermost layer of the follicle cells, which become columnar, and the connective tissue stroma.

During follicular growth, extensive gap junctions develop between granulosa cells. Unlike Sertoli cells in the testis, however, the basal layer of the granulosa cells does not possess elaborate tight junctions (zonulae occludentes), indicating the absence of a blood–follicle barrier. Movement of nutrients and small informational macromolecules from the blood into the follicular fluid is essential for normal development of the ovum and follicle.

Connective tissue cells form the theca layers of the primary follicle

As the granulosa cells proliferate, stromal cells immediately surrounding the follicle form a sheath of connective tissue cells, known as the ***theca folliculi,*** just external to

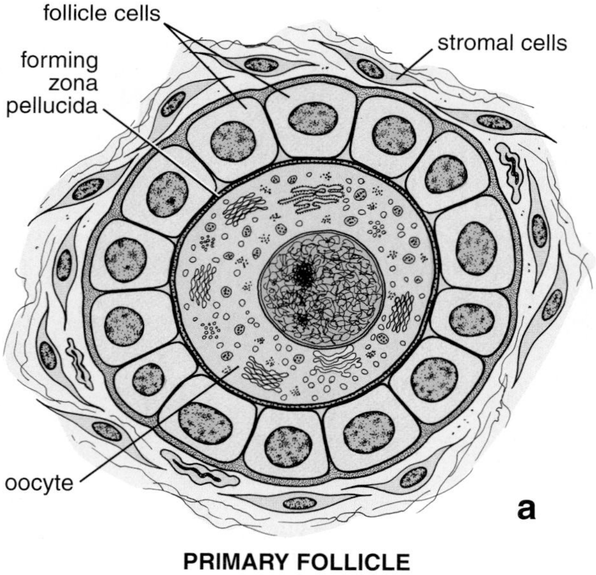

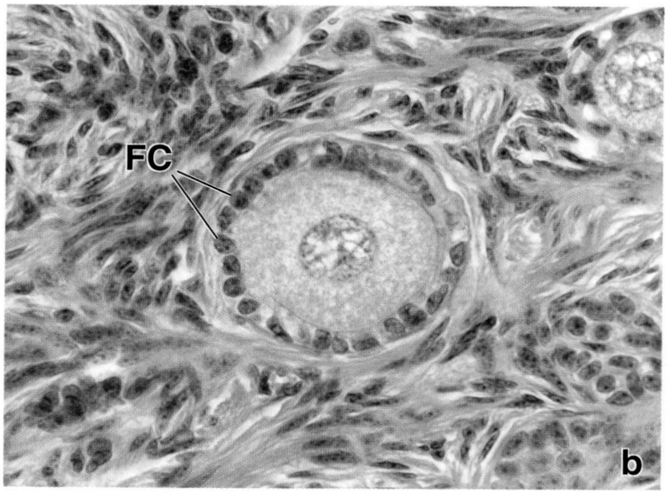

FIGURE 22.4
Early primary follicle. a. Schematic drawing of a primary follicle in an early stage of development. Note the formation of the zona pellucida between the oocyte and the adjacent follicle cells. A single layer of cuboidal follicle cells surrounds the growing oocyte. **b.** Photomicrograph of a primary follicle. Note the distinct layer of follicle cells *(FC)* surrounding the oocyte. ×640.

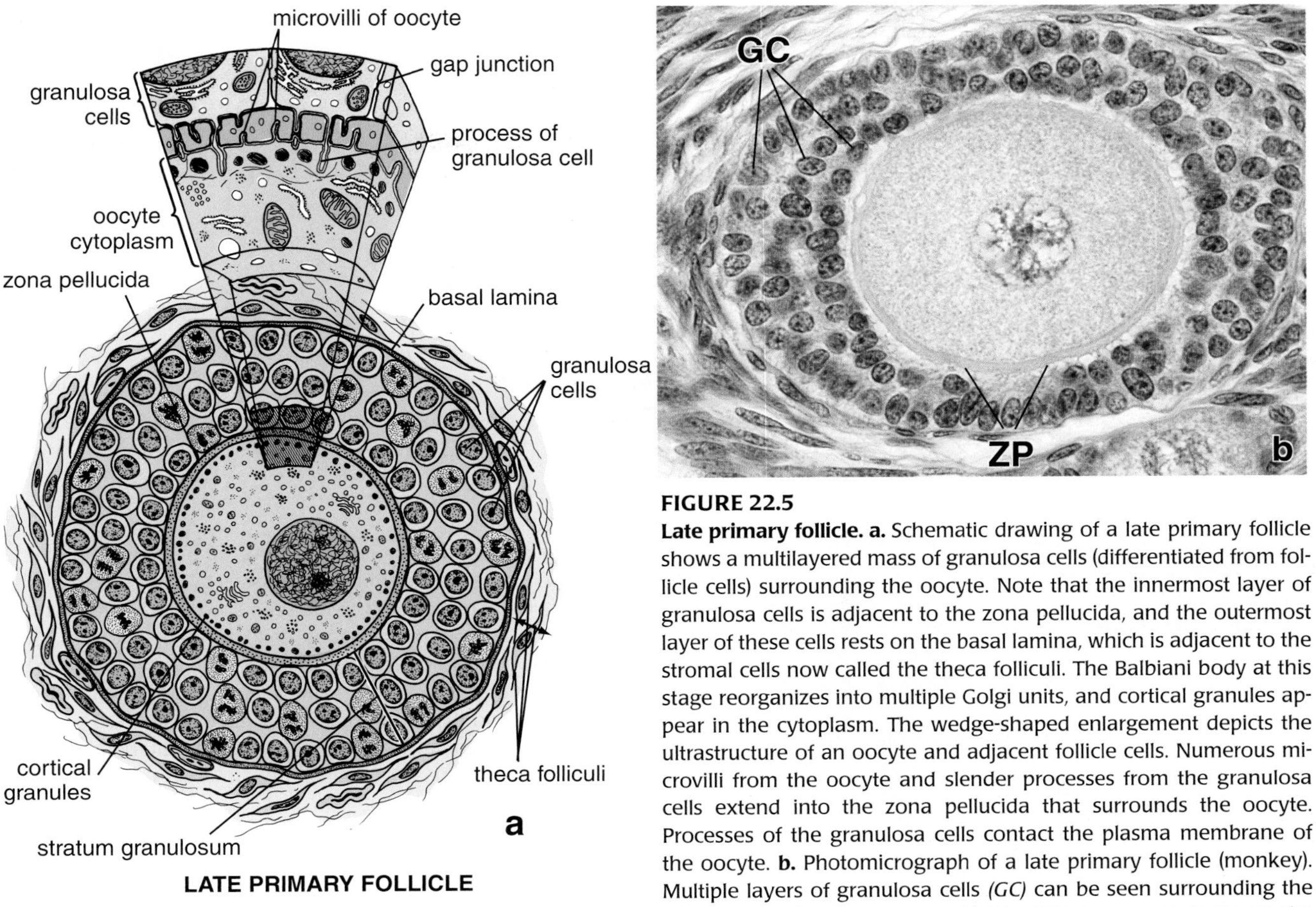

FIGURE 22.5
Late primary follicle. a. Schematic drawing of a late primary follicle shows a multilayered mass of granulosa cells (differentiated from follicle cells) surrounding the oocyte. Note that the innermost layer of granulosa cells is adjacent to the zona pellucida, and the outermost layer of these cells rests on the basal lamina, which is adjacent to the stromal cells now called the theca folliculi. The Balbiani body at this stage reorganizes into multiple Golgi units, and cortical granules appear in the cytoplasm. The wedge-shaped enlargement depicts the ultrastructure of an oocyte and adjacent follicle cells. Numerous microvilli from the oocyte and slender processes from the granulosa cells extend into the zona pellucida that surrounds the oocyte. Processes of the granulosa cells contact the plasma membrane of the oocyte. **b.** Photomicrograph of a late primary follicle (monkey). Multiple layers of granulosa cells *(GC)* can be seen surrounding the primary oocyte. The zona pellucida *(ZP)* is present between the oocyte and follicle cells. ×160.

the basal lamina (Fig. 22.5). The theca folliculi further differentiates into two layers:

- The ***theca interna*** is the inner, highly vascularized layer of cuboidal secretory cells. The fully differentiated cells of the theca interna possess ultrastructural features characteristic of steroid-producing cells. Cells of the theca interna possess a large number of luteinizing hormone (LH) receptors. In response to LH stimulation, they synthesize and secrete the androgens that are the precursors of estrogen. In addition to secretory cells, the theca interna contains fibroblasts, collagen bundles, and a rich network of small vessels typical of endocrine organs.
- The ***theca externa*** is the outer layer of connective tissue cells. It contains mainly smooth muscle cells and bundles of collagen fibers.

Boundaries between the thecal layers and between the theca externa and surrounding stroma are not distinct. However, the basal lamina between the granulosa layer and the theca interna establishes a distinct boundary between these layers. It separates the rich capillary bed of the theca interna from the granulosa layer, which is avascular during the period of follicular growth.

Maturation of the oocyte occurs in the primary follicle

The distribution of organelles changes as the oocyte matures. Multiple, dispersed Golgi elements derived from the single Balbiani body of the primordial oocyte become scattered in the cytoplasm. The number of free ribosomes, mitochondria, small vesicles, and multivesicular bodies and the amount of rough endoplasmic reticulum (rER) increase. Occasional lipid droplets and masses of lipochrome pigment may also be seen. The oocytes of many species, including mammals, exhibit specialized secretory vesicles known as ***cortical granules*** (see Fig. 22.5). They are located just beneath the plasma membrane ***(oolemma)***. The granules contain proteases that are released by exocytosis when the ovum is activated by the sperm (discussed in the section on fertilization).

Numerous irregular microvilli project from the oocyte into the ***perivitelline space*** between the oocyte and the sur-

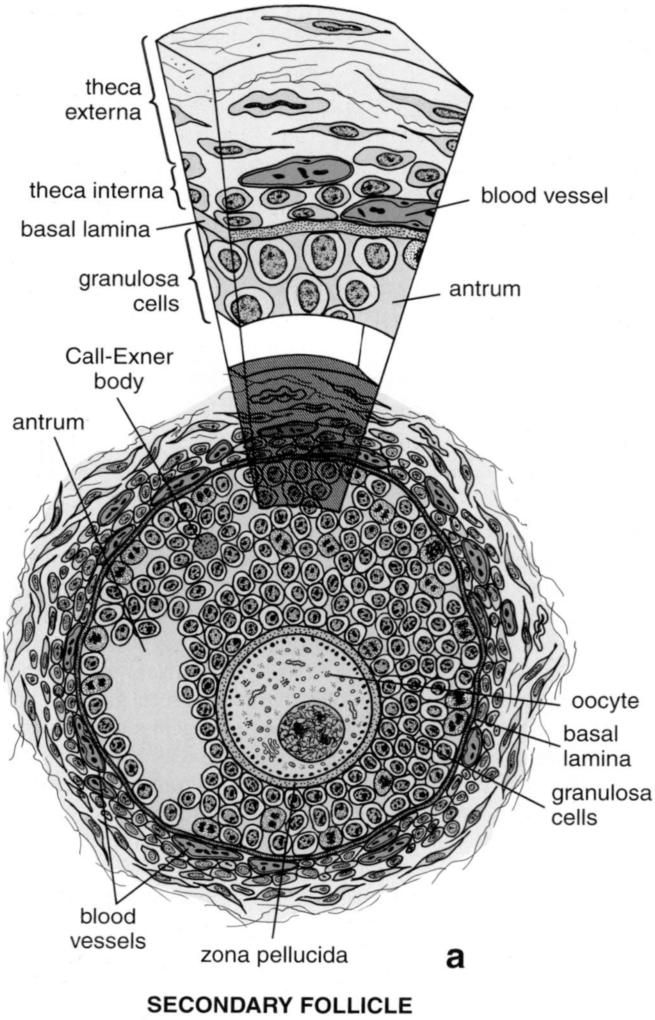

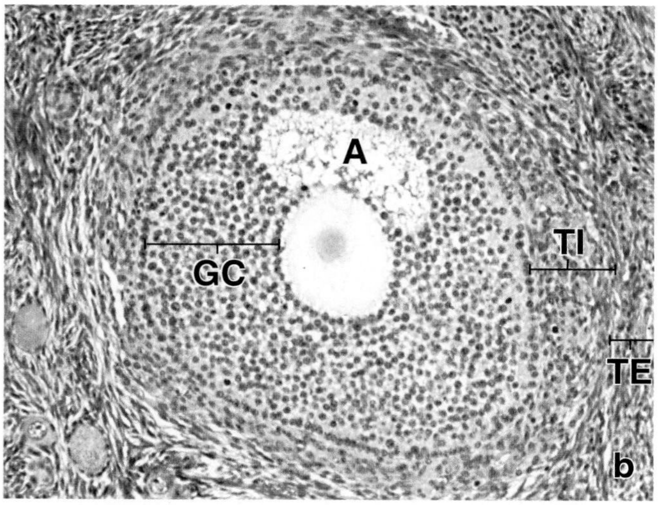

FIGURE 22.6
Secondary follicle. a. Schematic drawing of a secondary follicle showing the fluid-filled antrum, which arises by the coalescence of small fluid-filled cavities among the granulosa cells. Note that this actively growing follicle has many dividing granulosa cells. Call-Exner bodies appear at this stage. The *wedge-shaped enlargement* of the *shadowed area* depicts the relationship of the granulosa cells, basal lamina, and the theca interna and theca externa. The theca interna cells differentiate into highly vascularized, steroid-producing cells. The theca interna is surrounded by an outer layer of stromal cells called the theca externa. The basal lamina separates the granulosa cells from the theca interna. **b.** Photomicrograph of a secondary follicle. The antrum *(A),* filled with follicular fluid, is visible within the stratum granulosum *(GC).* Multiple layers of theca interna cells *(TI)* and theca externa cells *(TE)* can be seen outside the basal lamina of the secondary follicle. ×85.

rounding granulosa cells as the zona pellucida is deposited (see Fig. 22.5). At the same time, slender processes from the granulosa cells develop and project toward the oocyte, intermingling with oocyte microvilli and, occasionally, invaginating into the oocyte plasma membrane. The processes may contact the plasma membrane but do not establish cytoplasmic continuity between the cells.

The secondary follicle is characterized by a fluid-containing antrum

The primary follicle initially moves deeper into the cortical stroma as it increases in size, mostly through proliferation of the granulosa cells. Several factors are required for oocyte and follicular growth:

- *Follicle-stimulating hormone (FSH)*
- *Growth factors,* e.g., *epidermal growth factor, insulin-like growth factor I (IGF-I)*
- *Calcium ions* (Ca^{2+})

When the stratum granulosum reaches a thickness of 6 to 12 cell layers, fluid-filled cavities appear among the granulosa cells (Fig. 22.6). As the hyaluronic acid–rich fluid called ***liquor folliculi*** continues to accumulate among the granulosa cells, the cavities begin to coalesce, eventually forming a single, crescent-shaped cavity called the ***antrum.*** The follicle is now identified as a ***secondary*** or ***antral follicle.*** The eccentrically positioned oocyte, which has attained a diameter of about 125 μm, undergoes no further growth. The inhibition of growth is achieved by the presence of a small, 1- to 2-kDa peptide called ***oocyte maturation inhibitor (OMI),*** which is secreted by the granulosa cells into the antral fluid. A direct correlation is observed between the size of the secondary follicle and OMI concentration. The concentration is highest in small follicles and lowest in mature follicles. The follicle, which was 0.2 mm in diameter as an early secondary follicle when the fluid first appeared, continues to grow and reaches 10 mm or more in diameter.

Cells of the cumulus oophorus form a corona radiata around the secretory follicle oocyte

As the secondary follicle increases in size, the antrum, lined by several layers of granulosa cells, also enlarges (Fig. 22.7). The stratum granulosum has a relatively uniform thickness except for the region associated with the oocyte. Here, the granulosa cells form a thickened mound, the ***cumulus oophorus***, which projects into the antrum. The cells of the cumulus oophorus that immediately surround the oocyte and remain with it at ovulation are referred to as the ***corona radiata***. The corona radiata is composed of cumulus cells that send penetrating microvilli throughout the zona pellucida to communicate via gap junctions with microvilli of the oocyte. During follicular maturation, the number of surface microvilli of granulosa cells increases and is correlated with an increased number of LH receptors on the free antral surface. Extracellular, densely staining, PAS-positive material called ***Call-Exner bodies*** (see Fig. 22.6) may be seen between the granulosa cells. These bodies are secreted by granulosa cells and contain hyaluronic acid and proteoglycans.

The mature or Graafian follicle contains the mature secondary oocyte

The mature follicle, also known as a ***Graafian follicle***, has a diameter of 10 mm or more. Because of its large size, it extends through the full thickness of the ovarian cortex and causes a bulge on the surface of the ovary. As the follicle nears its maximum size, the mitotic activity of the granulosa cells decreases. The stratum granulosum appears to become thinner as the antrum increases in size. As the spaces between the granulosa cells continue to enlarge, the oocyte and cumulus cells are gradually loosened from the rest of the granulosa cells in preparation for ovulation. The cumulus cells immediately surrounding the oocyte now form a single layer of cells of the corona radiata. These cells and loosely attached cumulus cells remain with the oocyte at ovulation.

During this period of follicle maturation, the thecal layers become more prominent. Lipid droplets appear in the cytoplasm of the theca interna cells, and the cells demonstrate ultrastructural features associated with steroid-producing cells. In humans, LH stimulates the cells of the theca interna to secrete androgens, which serve as estro-

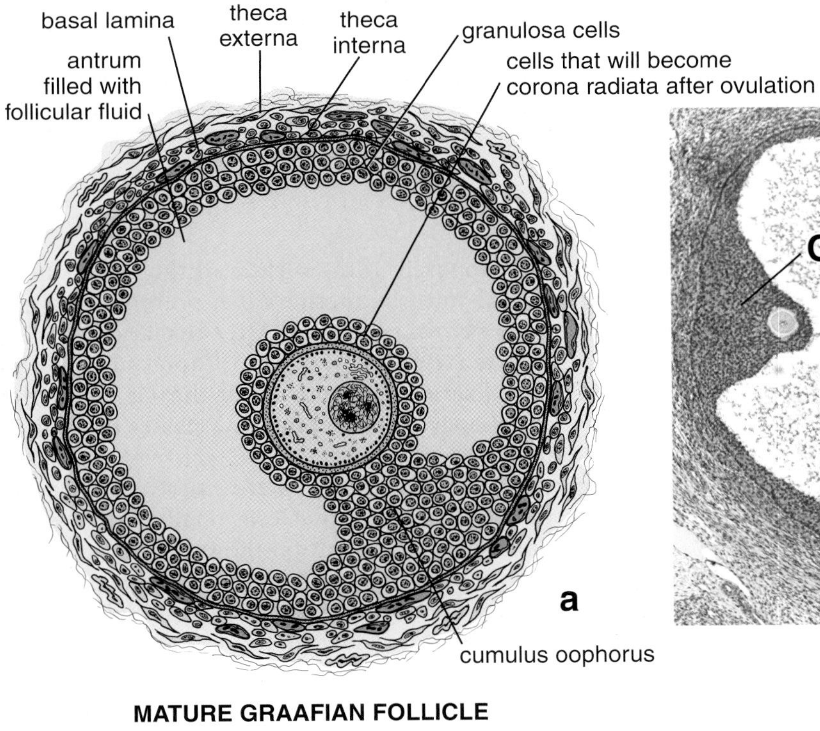

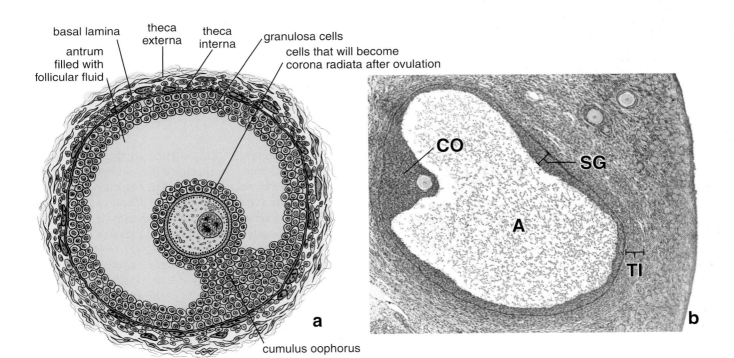

FIGURE 22.7
Secondary follicle in a late stage of development. a. Schematic drawing of a mature (Graafian) follicle with a large antrum containing an oocyte embedded within the cumulus oophorus. The cells of the cumulus oophorus immediately surrounding the oocyte remain with it after ovulation and are referred to as the corona radiata. **b.** Photomicrograph of a mature secondary follicle. Note the large fluid-filled antrum *(A)* and the cumulus oophorus *(CO)* containing the oocyte. The remaining cells that surround the lumen of the antrum make up the membrana granulosa (stratum granulosum, *SG*). The surface of the ovary is visible on the right. Note the presence of two primary follicles (upper right). *TI,* theca interna. ×45.

gen precursors. Some androgens are transported to the smooth endoplasmic reticulum (sER) in the granulosa cells. In response to FSH, the granulosa cells catalyze the conversion of androgens to estrogens, which in turn stimulate the granulosa cells to proliferate and thereby increase the size of the follicle. Increased estrogen levels from both follicular and systemic sources are correlated with increased sensitization of gonadotropes to gonadotropin-releasing hormone. A surge in the release of FSH and/or LH is induced in the adenohypophysis approximately 24 hours before ovulation. In response to the LH surge, LH receptors on granulosa cells are downregulated (desensitized), and granulosa cells no longer produce estrogens in response to LH. Triggered by this surge, the first meiotic division of the primary oocyte resumes. This event occurs between 12 and 24 hours after the LH surge, resulting in the formation of the secondary oocyte and the first polar body. The granulosa and thecal cells then undergo luteinization and produce progesterone (see page 736, on the corpus luteum).

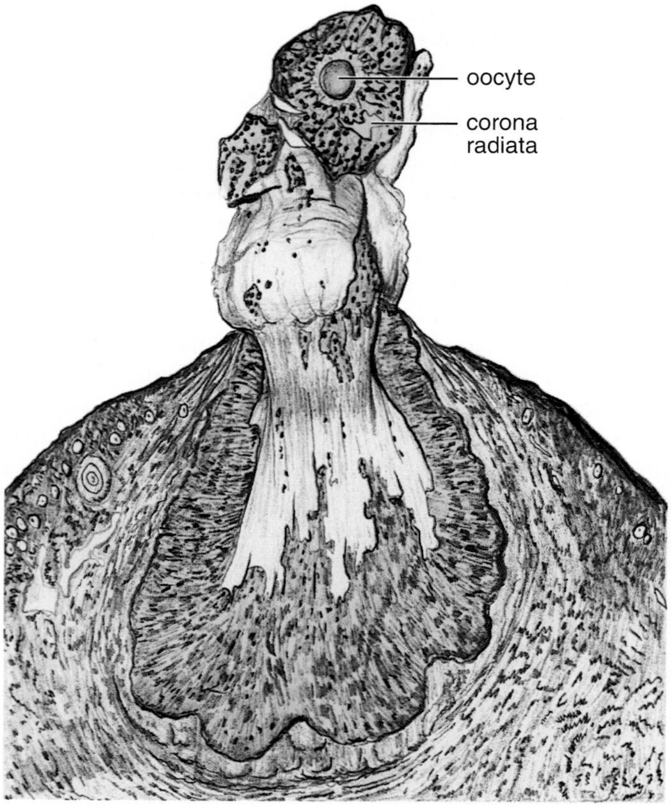

FIGURE 22.8
Ovulation. This drawing shows a rabbit oocyte, surrounded by the cumulus oophorus, being expelled from the ruptured ovarian follicle. (Based on Weiss L, Greep RO. *Histology.* 4th ed. New York: McGraw-Hill, 1977.)

Ovulation

Ovulation is a hormone-mediated process resulting in the release of the secondary oocyte

Ovulation is the process by which a secondary oocyte is released from the Graafian follicle. The follicle destined to ovulate in any menstrual cycle is recruited from a cohort of several primary follicles in the first few days of the cycle. During ovulation, the oocyte traverses the entire follicular wall, including the germinal epithelium.

A combination of hormonal changes and enzymatic effects is responsible for the actual release of the secondary oocyte in the middle of the menstrual cycle, i.e., on the 14th day of a 28-day cycle. These factors include:

- Increase in the volume and pressure of the follicular fluid
- Enzymatic proteolysis of the follicular wall by activated plasminogen
- Hormonally directed deposition of glycosaminoglycans between the oocyte–cumulus complex and the stratum granulosum
- Contraction of the smooth muscle fibers in the theca externa layer, triggered by prostaglandins

Just before ovulation, blood flow stops in a small area of the ovarian surface overlying the bulging follicle. This area of the germinal epithelium, known as the ***macula pellucida*** or ***stigma,*** becomes elevated and then ruptures. The oocyte, surrounded by the corona radiata and cells of the cumulus oophorus, is forcefully expelled from the ruptured follicle (Fig. 22.8). The oocyte is then transported into the abdominal ostium of the uterine tube. At the time of ovulation, the fimbriae of the uterine tube become closely apposed to the surface of the ovary and direct the oocyte into the uterine tube, preventing its passage into the peritoneal cavity. After ovulation, the secondary oocyte remains viable for approximately 24 hours. If fertilization does not occur during this period, the secondary oocyte degenerates as it passes through the uterine tube.

Oocytes that fail to enter the uterine tube usually degenerate in the peritoneal cavity. Occasionally, however, one may be fertilized and implant on the surface of the ovary or intestine or inside the rectouterine (Douglas) pouch. Such ***ectopic implantations*** usually do not develop beyond early fetal stages but may have to be removed surgically for the health of the mother.

Normally, only one follicle completes maturation in each cycle and ruptures to release its secondary oocyte. Rarely, oocytes are released from other follicles that have reached full maturity during the same cycle, leading to the possibility of multiple zygotes. Drugs, such as clomiphene citrate (Serophene) or human menopausal gonadotropins, which stimulate ovarian activity, greatly increase the pos-

BOX 22.1

Clinical Correlations: Polycystic Ovarian Disease

Polycystic ovarian disease is characterized by bilaterally enlarged ovaries with numerous follicular cysts. (When associated with oligomenorrhea, scanty menstruation, the clinical term Stein-Leventhal syndrome is used.) The individual is infertile due to lack of ovulation. Morphologically, the ovaries resemble a small, white balloon filled with tightly packed marbles. Affected ovaries, often called oyster ovaries, have a smooth, pearl-white surface but do not show surface scarring, as no ovulations have occurred. The condition is due to the large number of fluid-filled follicular cysts and atrophic secondary follicles that lie beneath an unusually thick tunica albuginea. The pathogenesis is not clear but seems to be related to a defect in the regulation of androgen biosynthesis that causes production of excessive amounts of androgens that are converted to estrogens. The selection process of the follicles that undergo maturation also seems to be disturbed. The individual has an anovulatory cycle characterized by only estrogenic stimulation of the endometrium because of the inhibition of progesterone production. Progesterone inhibition is caused by failure of the Graafian follicle to transform into a progesterone-producing corpus luteum. The treatment of choice is hormonal to stabilize and reconstruct the estrogen-to-progesterone ratio, but in some cases, surgical intervention is necessary. A wedge-shaped incision is made into the ovary to expose the cortex, thus allowing the ova, following hormonal treatment, to leave the ovary without physical restrictions created by the preexisting thickened tunica albuginea (Fig. 22.9).

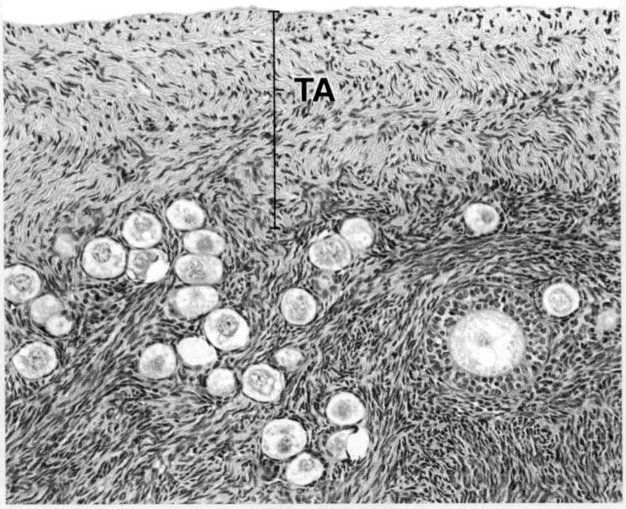

FIGURE 22.9
Polycystic ovarian disease. This photomicrograph shows a section through the cortex of the ovary from an individual with polycystic ovarian disease. Note the unusually thick tunica albuginea (*TA*) that overlies numerous follicles. The thickness of the tunica albuginea prevents ovulation of the mature (Graafian) follicles. Note that one of the follicles has developed to the primary follicle stage. ×45.

sibility of multiple births by causing simultaneous maturation of several follicles.

The primary oocyte is arrested for 12 to 50 years in the diplotene stage of prophase of the first meiotic division

The primary oocytes within the primordial follicles begin the first meiotic division in the embryo, but the process is arrested at the diplotene stage of meiotic prophase (see the section on meiosis in Chapter 2). The first meiotic prophase is not completed until just before ovulation. Therefore, primary oocytes remain arrested in the first meiotic prophase for 12 to 50 years. This long period of meiotic arrest exposes the primary oocyte to adverse environmental influences and may contribute to errors in meiotic division, such as nondisjunction. Such errors result in anomalies such as trisomy of chromosome 21 (Down syndrome).

As the first meiotic division (reduction division) is completed in the mature follicle (Fig. 22.10), each daughter cell of the ***primary oocyte*** receives an equal share of chromatin, but one daughter cell receives most of the cytoplasm and becomes the ***secondary oocyte***. It measures 150 μm in diameter. The other daughter cell receives a minimal amount of cytoplasm and becomes the ***first polar body***.

The secondary oocyte is arrested at metaphase in the second meiotic division just before ovulation

As soon as the first meiotic division is completed, the secondary oocyte begins the second meiotic division. As the secondary oocyte surrounded by the cells of the corona radiata leaves the follicle at ovulation, the second meiotic division (equatorial division) is in progress. This division is arrested at metaphase and is completed only if the secondary oocyte is penetrated by a spermatozoon. If fertilization occurs, the secondary oocyte completes the second meiotic division and forms a mature ***ovum*** with the ***maternal pronucleus*** containing a set of 23 chromosomes. The other cell produced at this division is a ***second polar body***. In humans, the first polar body does not divide; therefore, the fertilized egg can be recognized by the presence nearby of the second polar body. The polar bodies, which are not capable of further development, degenerate.

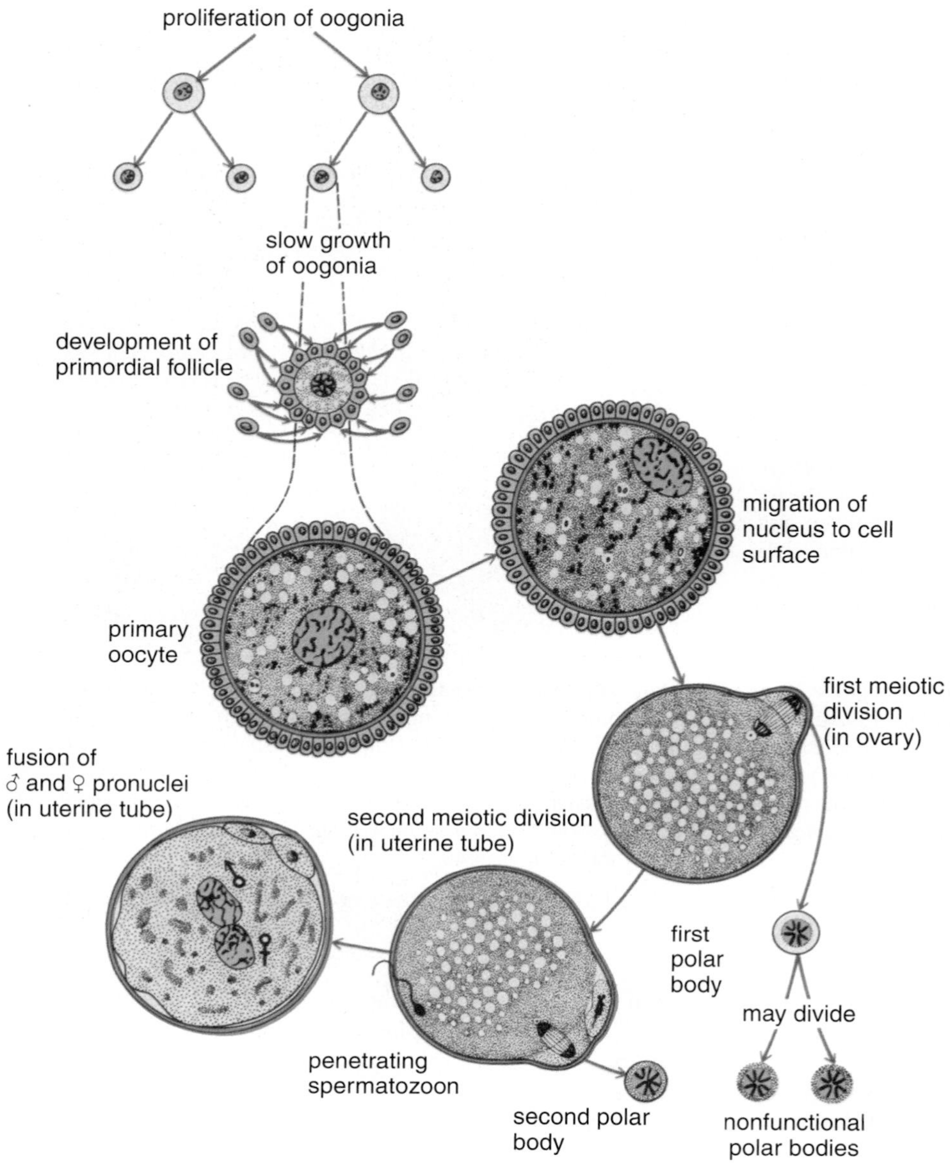

FIGURE 22.10
Diagram illustrating changes that occur during growth, maturation, and fertilization of the oocyte. In the initial development of the primordial follicle, stromal cells migrate to the oogonium and form a surrounding layer. The oogonium then enlarges to form the primary oocyte. Note that the primary oocyte remains arrested in prophase I of meiosis. The first meiotic or reductional division is completed only after the oocyte progresses to ovulation. The second meiotic or equatorial division is not completed unless the secondary oocyte is penetrated by a spermatozoon. (Courtesy of Dr. Clark E. Corliss.)

CORPUS LUTEUM

The collapsed follicle undergoes reorganization into the corpus luteum after ovulation

At ovulation, the follicular wall, composed of the remaining granulosa and thecal cells, is thrown into deep folds as the follicle collapses and is transformed into the ***corpus luteum*** (yellow body), or ***luteal gland*** (Fig. 22.11a). At first, bleeding from the capillaries in the theca interna into the follicular lumen leads to formation of the ***corpus hemorrhagicum*** with a central clot. Connective tissue from the stroma then invades the former follicular cavity. Cells of the granulosa and theca interna layers then undergo dramatic morphologic changes. These luteal cells increase in size and become filled with lipid droplets (Fig. 22.11b). A lipid-soluble pigment, lipochrome, in the cytoplasm of the cells gives them a yellow appearance in fresh preparations. At the ultrastructural level, the cells demonstrate features associated with steroid-secreting cells, namely, abundant sER and mitochondria with tubular cristae (Fig. 22.12).

Two types of luteal cells are identified:

- ***Granulosa lutein cells,*** large (about 30 μm in diameter), centrally located cells derived from the granulosa cells
- ***Theca lutein cells,*** smaller (about 15 μm), more deeply staining, peripherally located cells derived from the cells of the theca interna layer

As the corpus luteum begins to form, blood and lymphatic vessels from the theca interna rapidly grow into the granulosa layer. A rich vascular network is established within the corpus luteum. This highly vascularized structure located in the cortex of the ovary secretes proges-

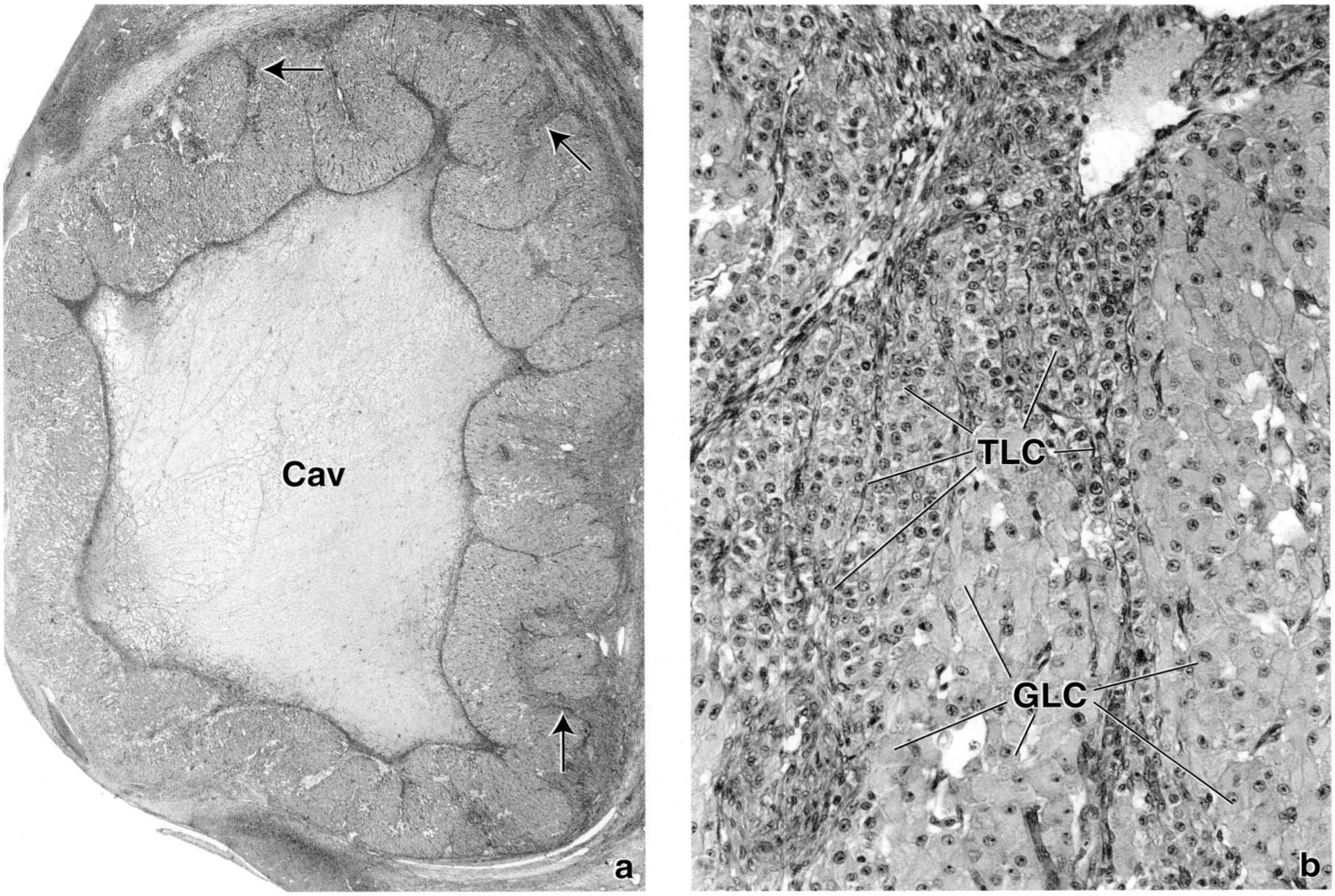

FIGURE 22.11
Photomicrograph of human corpus luteum. a. The corpus luteum is formed from the collapsed follicle wall that contains the granulosa and theca cells. The granulosa lutein cells form a thick, folded layer around the former follicular cavity *(Cav)*. Within the folds are cells of the theca interna *(arrows)*. ×12. **b.** This photomicrograph shows the wall of the corpus luteum at higher magnification. The main cell mass is composed of granulosa lutein cells *(GLC)*. These cells have a large spherical nucleus and a large amount of cytoplasm. The theca lutein cells *(TLC)* also have a spherical nucleus, but the cells are considerably smaller than the granulosa lutein cells. ×240.

terone and estrogens. These hormones stimulate the growth and secretory activity of the lining of the uterus, the ***endometrium***, to prepare it for the implantation of the developing zygote in the event that fertilization occurs.

The corpus luteum of menstruation is formed in the absence of fertilization

If fertilization and implantation do not occur, the corpus luteum remains active only for 14 days; in this case it is called the ***corpus luteum of menstruation***. In the absence of human chorionic gonadotropin (hCG) and other luteotropins, the rate of secretion of progestogens and estrogens declines, and the corpus luteum begins to degenerate about 10 to 12 days after ovulation.

The corpus luteum degenerates and undergoes a slow involution after pregnancy or menstruation. The cells become loaded with lipid, decrease in size, and undergo autolysis. A white scar, the ***corpus albicans***, is formed as intercellular hyaline material accumulates among the degenerating cells of the former corpus luteum (Fig. 22.13). The corpus albicans sinks deeper into the ovarian cortex as it slowly disappears over a period of several months.

Fertilization

Fertilization normally occurs in the ampulla of the uterine tube

Usually, only a few hundred of the millions of spermatozoa in an ejaculate reach the site of fertilization, typically the ampulla of the uterine tube. On arrival, the spermatozoon penetrates the corona radiata, where the final steps of ***capacitation*** occur. Capacitation involves the release of the epididymal fluid glycoconjugate from the surface of the head of the spermatozoon. These surface glycosides added

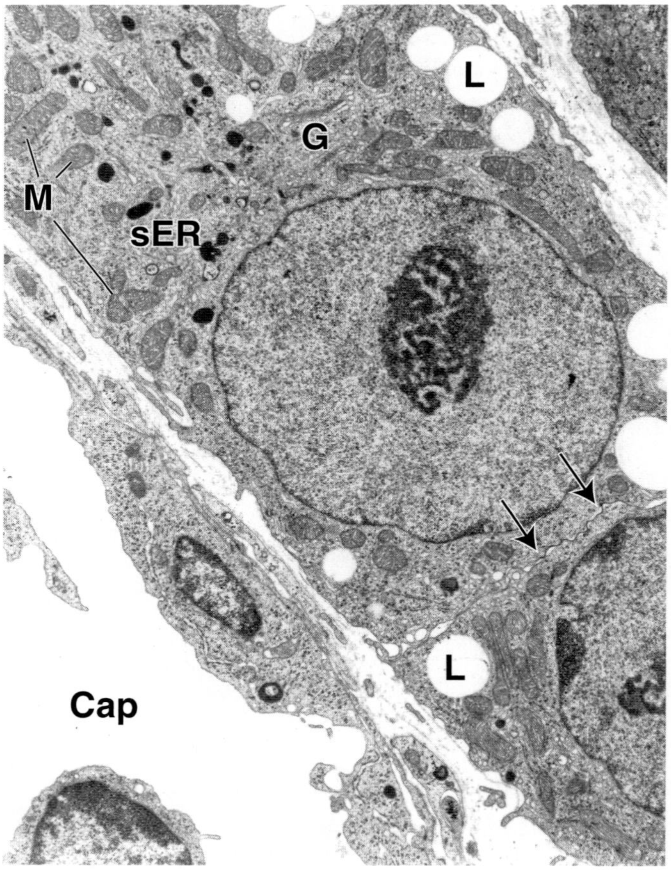

FIGURE 22.12
Electron micrograph of theca lutein cells from the corpus luteum of a monkey. At this early implantation stage (day 10.5 of gestation), membrane-bounded dense bodies are clustered near the Golgi apparatus *(G)*; most of the cytoplasm is packed with tubules of smooth endoplasmic reticulum *(sER)*, lipid droplets *(L)*, and mitochondria *(M)*. Note the capillary *(Cap)* and the closely apposed cell membranes of the theca lutein cells *(arrows)*. ×10,000. (Courtesy of Dr. Carolynn B. Booher.)

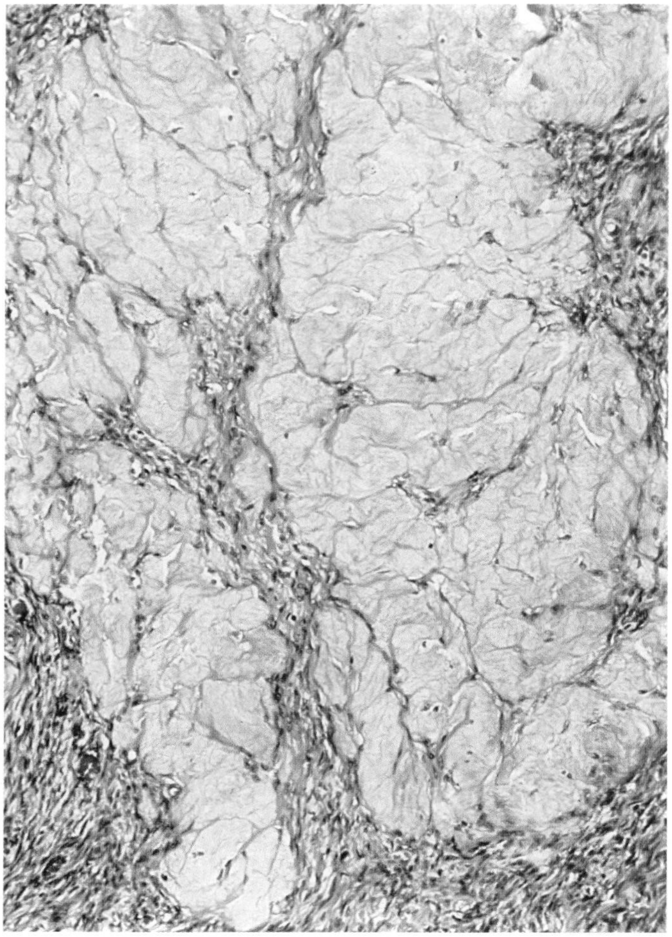

FIGURE 22.13
Photomicrograph of the corpus albicans of a human ovary. Large amounts of hyaline material can be seen among the degenerating cells of the former corpus luteum. The corpus albicans is surrounded by ovarian stroma. ×125.

during sperm maturation in the epididymis inhibit binding to the zona pellucida receptor. After capacitation, the spermatozoon can bind to the zona pellucida receptors. Binding to the receptors on the zona pellucida triggers the ***acrosome reaction*** in which enzymes released from the acrosome enable the spermatozoon to penetrate the zona pellucida. Penetration is accomplished by limited proteolysis of the zona pellucida in front of the advancing spermatozoon.

The nucleus of the sperm head that enters the secondary oocyte forms the ***male pronucleus*** containing 23 paternal chromosomes. After the fusion of the two pronuclei, the resulting ***zygote,*** with its diploid ($2n$) complement of 46 chromosomes, undergoes a mitotic division or first cleavage. This two-cell stage marks the beginning of embryonic development.

Several spermatozoa may penetrate the zona pellucida, but only one spermatozoon completes the fertilization process

As the fertilizing spermatozoon penetrates the ooplasm, at least three types of postfusion reactions occur to prevent other spermatozoa from entering the secondary oocyte (polyspermy). These events include

- ***Fast block to polyspermy.*** A large and long-lasting (up to 1 minute) depolarization of the oolemma creates a transient electrical block to polyspermy.
- ***Cortical reaction.*** Changes in the polarity of the oolemma then trigger release of Ca^{2+} from the ooplasmic stores. The Ca^{2+} propagates a cortical reaction wave, in which cortical granules move to the surface and fuse with the oolemma, leading to a transient increase in

BOX 22.2

Clinical Correlations: In Vitro Fertilization

There are several indications for in vitro fertilization (IVF), but the primary one is infertility due to surgically uncorrectable damage to, or absence of, the uterine tubes. To induce multiple follicle development and maturation, women selected for an IVF procedure undergo controlled hyperstimulation of the ovaries. Hyperstimulation is achieved by different hormonal therapies using human menopausal gonadotropins and clomiphene citrate (Serophene), with or without FSH.

Mature preovulatory oocytes are collected from the Graafian follicles by either laparoscopic or ultrasound-guided percutaneous aspiration or transvaginal aspiration. Prior to insemination, the oocytes are preincubated in a specialized medium with serum complements for a time determined by their stage of maturity.

The collected semen is placed in a special medium. The oocytes are then added to the medium containing the collected semen for fertilization. Twelve to 16 hours later, the oocytes are examined with the differential interference contrast microscope to determine the presence of female and male pronuclei, the indication of successful fertilization. Generally, 80% of mature oocytes cultured in vitro are fertilized.

At this point the embryo is transferred to a special growth medium for 24 to 48 hours, where it is allowed to grow to the stage of four to six cells. Several embryos are then transferred into the uterus via the vagina and cervical canal on the third or fourth day after the initial aspiration of the oocyte. Prior to embryo transfer, the uterus has been prepared to receive the embryo by administration of appropriate hormones. Embryos are therefore placed into a hormonally prepared uterus under conditions equivalent to those in normal implantation (see page 748). Intensive progesterone treatment is usually begun just after the transfer, to mimic the function of the corpus luteum of pregnancy.

In recent years, existing treatment protocols have been optimized to such extent that successful pregnancy and delivery with IVF programs have reached over 30% per embryo transfer. Further improvements in pregnancy rates may be achieved by the introduction of new drugs, such as recombinant FSH or gonadotropin-releasing hormone (GnRH) antagonists that provide individualized hormonal treatment. On the other hand, the occurrence of multiple pregnancies, which is the main complication of IVF, may be limited by reducing the number of transferred embryos.

surface area of the ovum and reorganization of the membrane. The contents of the cortical granules are released into the perivitelline space.

- ***Zona reaction.*** The released enzymes (proteases) of the cortical granules not only degrade the glycoprotein oocyte plasma membrane receptors for sperm binding but also form the ***perivitelline barrier*** by cross-linking proteins on the surface of the zona pellucida. This event creates the final and permanent block to polyspermy.

The corpus luteum of pregnancy is formed after fertilization and implantation

If fertilization and implantation occur, the corpus luteum increases in size to form the ***corpus luteum of pregnancy.*** The existence and function of the corpus luteum depends on a combination of paracrine and endocrine secretions, collectively described as ***luteotropins.***

Paracrine luteotropins are locally produced by the ovary. They include

- *Estrogens*
- *IGF-I and IGF-II*

Endocrine luteotropins are produced at a distance from their target organ, the corpus luteum. They include

- *hCG,* secreted by the trophoblast of the chorion, which stimulates the corpus luteum and prevents its degeneration
- *LH* and ***prolactin,*** both secreted by the pituitary gland
- ***Insulin,*** produced by the pancreas

High levels of progesterone, produced from cholesterol by the corpus luteum, block the cyclic development of ovarian follicles. In early pregnancy, the corpus luteum measures 2 to 3 cm, thus filling most of the ovary. Its function begins to decline gradually after 8 weeks of pregnancy, although it persists throughout pregnancy. Although the corpus luteum remains active, the placenta produces sufficient amounts of estrogens and progestogens from maternal and fetal precursors to take over the function of the corpus luteum after 6 weeks of pregnancy. hCG can be detected in the serum as early as 6 days after conception and in the urine as early as 10 to 14 days of pregnancy. Detection of hCG in the urine forms the basis of most pregnancy tests.

Atresia

Most ovarian follicles are lost by atresia mediated by apoptosis of granulosa cells

As stated, very few of the ovarian follicles that begin their differentiation in the embryonic ovary are destined to complete their maturation. Most of the follicles degenerate and disappear through a process called ***ovarian follicular atresia.*** Atresia is mediated by apoptosis of granulosa cells. Large numbers of follicles undergo atresia during fetal development, early postnatal life, and puberty. After puberty, groups of follicles begin to mature during each menstrual cycle; normally, only one follicle completes its maturation. Atresia is now thought to be a mechanism whereby a few follicles are stimulated to maintain their development through the programmed death of the other follicles. Thus, at any stage of its maturation a follicle may undergo atre-

sia. The process becomes more complex as the follicle progresses toward maturation.

In atresia of primordial and small, growing follicles, the immature oocyte becomes smaller and degenerates; similar changes occur in the granulosa cells. Atretic follicles shrink and eventually disappear from the stroma of the ovary as a result of repeated apoptosis and phagocytosis by granulosa cells. As the cells are reabsorbed and disappear, the surrounding stromal cells migrate into the space previously occupied by the follicle, leaving no trace of its existence.

In atresia of large, growing follicles, the degeneration of the mature oocyte is delayed and appears to occur secondary to degenerative changes in the follicular wall. This delay indicates that once the oocyte has achieved its maturity and competence, it is no longer sensitive to the same stimuli that initiate the atresia in granulosa cells. The follicular changes include the following sequential events:

- Initiation of apoptosis within the granulosa cells, indicated by cessation of mitosis and expression of endonucleases and other hydrolytic enzymes within the granulosa cells
- Invasion of the granulosa layer by neutrophils and macrophages
- Invasion of the granulosa layer by strands of vascularized connective tissue
- Sloughing of the granulosa cells into the antrum of the follicle
- Hypertrophy of the theca interna cells
- Collapse of the follicle as degeneration continues
- Invasion of connective tissue into the cavity of the follicle

Recent studies indicate that several gene products regulate the process of follicular atresia. One of these products is the gonadotropin-induced ***neural apoptosis inhibitory protein (NAIP)***, which inhibits and delays apoptotic changes in the granulosa cell. NAIP gene expression is present in all stages of the growing follicle but absent in follicles undergoing atresia. A high level of gonadotropins inhibits apoptosis in ovarian follicles by increasing expression of NAIP in the ovaries.

The oocyte undergoes typical changes associated with degeneration and autolysis, and the remnants are phagocytosed by invading macrophages. The zona pellucida, which is resistant to the autolytic changes occurring in the cells associated with it, becomes folded and collapses as it is slowly broken down within the cavity of the follicle. Macrophages in the connective tissue are involved in the phagocytosis of the zona pellucida and the remnants of the degenerating cells. The basement membrane between the follicle cells from the theca interna may separate from the follicle cells and increase in thickness, forming a wavy hyaline layer called the ***glassy membrane***. This structure is characteristic of follicles in late stages of atresia.

Enlargement of the cells of the theca interna occurs in some atretic follicles. These cells are similar to theca lutein cells and become organized into radially arranged strands separated by connective tissue. A rich capillary network develops in the connective tissue. These atretic follicles, which resemble an old corpus luteum, are called ***corpora lutea atretica***.

The interstitial gland arises from the theca interna of the atretic follicle

As atretic follicles continue to degenerate, a scar with hyaline streaks develops in the center of the cell mass, giving it the appearance of a small corpus albicans. This structure eventually disappears as the ovarian stroma invades the degenerating follicle. In the ovaries of a number of mammals the strands of luteal cells do not degenerate immediately but become broken up and scattered in the stroma. These cords of cells contribute to the ***interstitial gland*** of the ovary and produce steroid hormones. The development of the interstitial gland is most extensive in animal species that have large litters.

In the human ovary, there are relatively few interstitial cells. They occur in the largest numbers in the first year of life and during the early phases of puberty, corresponding to times of increased follicular atresia. At menarche, involution of the interstitial cells occurs; therefore, few are present during the reproductive lifespan and menopause. It has been suggested that in humans the interstitial cells are an important source of the estrogens that influence growth and development of the secondary sex organs during the early phases of puberty. In other species, the interstitial cells have been shown to produce progesterone.

In humans, cells called ***ovarian hilar cells*** are found in the hilum of the ovary in association with vascular spaces and nonmyelinated nerve fibers. These cells, which appear to be structurally related to the interstitial cells of the testis, contain ***Reinke crystalloids***. The hilar cells appear to respond to hormonal changes during pregnancy and at the onset of menopause. Research suggests that the hilar cells secrete androgens; hyperplasia or tumors associated with these cells usually lead to masculinization.

Blood Supply and Lymphatics

Blood supply to the ovaries comes from two different sources: ovarian and uterine arteries

The ***ovarian arteries*** are the branches of the abdominal aorta that pass to the ovaries through the suspensory ligaments and provide the principal arterial supply to the ovaries and uterine tubes. These arteries anastomose with the second blood source to the ovary, the ***ovarian branches of the uterine arteries***, which arise from the internal iliac arteries. Relatively large vessels arising from this region of anastomosis pass through the mesovarium and enter the hilum of the ovary. These large arteries are called ***helicine***

BOX 22.3

Functional Considerations: Summary of Hormonal Regulation of the Ovarian Cycle

During each menstrual cycle, the ovary undergoes cyclic changes that involve two phases:

- ***Follicular phase***
- ***Luteal phase***

Ovulation occurs between the two phases (Fig. 22.14).

The ***follicular phase*** begins with the development of a small number of primary follicles (10 to 20) under the influence of FSH and LH. During the first 8 to 10 days of the cycle, FSH is the principal hormone influencing the growth of the follicles. It stimulates the granulosa and thecal cells, which begin to secrete steroid hormones, principally estrogens, into the follicular lumen. Late in the follicular phase, before ovulation, progesterone levels begin to rise under the influence of LH. Estrogens continue to accumulate in the follicular lumen, finally reaching a level that makes the follicle independent of FSH for its continued growth and development. The amount of estrogens in the circulating blood inhibits further production of FSH by the adenohypophysis. Ovulation is induced by a surge in the LH level, which occurs concomitantly with a smaller increase in the FSH level.

The ***luteal phase*** begins immediately after ovulation, as the granulosa and thecal cells of the ruptured follicle undergo rapid morphologic transformation to form the corpus luteum. Estrogens and large amounts of progesterone are secreted by the corpus luteum. Under the influence of both hormones, but primarily progesterone, the endometrium begins its secretory phase, which is essential for the preparation of the uterus for implantation in the event that the egg is fertilized. LH appears to be responsible for the development and maintenance of the corpus luteum during the menstrual cycle. If fertilization does not occur, the corpus luteum degenerates within a few days as the hormonal levels drop. If fertilization does occur, the corpus luteum is maintained and continues to secrete progesterone and estrogens. hCG, which is initially produced by the embryo and later by the placenta, stimulates the corpus luteum and is responsible for its maintenance during pregnancy.

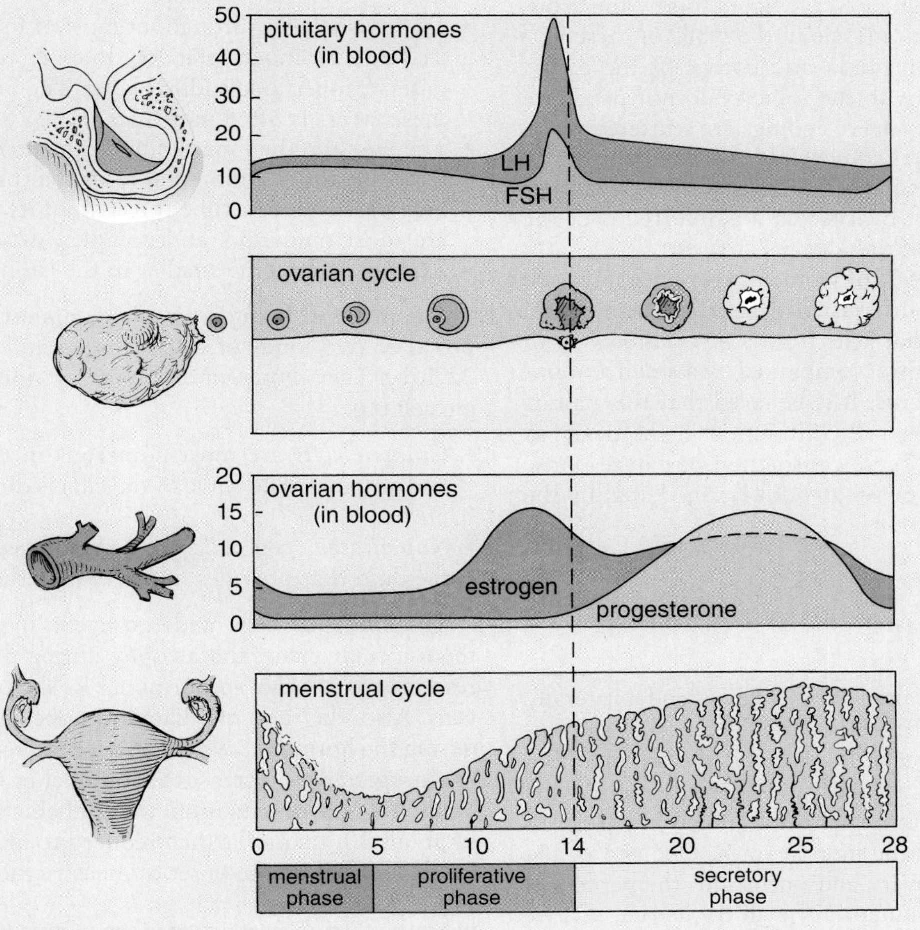

FIGURE 22.14
Relationship of morphologic and physiologic events that occur in the menstrual cycle. This diagram illustrates the relation of the morphologic changes in the endometrium and ovary to the pituitary and ovarian blood hormone levels that occur during the menstrual cycle. The pituitary and ovarian hormones and their plasma concentrations are indicated in arbitrary units. *LH,* luteinizing hormone; *FSH,* follicle-stimulating hormone.

arteries because they branch and become highly coiled as they pass into the ovarian medulla (see Fig. 22.2).

Veins accompany the arteries and form a plexus, called the ***pampiniform plexus***, as they emerge from the hilum. The ovarian vein is formed from the plexus.

In the cortical region of the ovary, networks of lymphatic vessels in the thecal layers surround the large developing and atretic follicles and corpora lutea. The lymphatic vessels follow the course of the ovarian arteries as they ascend to paraaortic lymph nodes in the lumbar region.

Innervation

Ovaries are innervated by the autonomic ovarian plexus

Sensory and autonomic nerve fibers that supply the ovary are conveyed mainly by the ovarian plexus. Although it is clear that the ovary receives both sympathetic and parasympathetic fibers, little is known about their actual distribution. Groups of parasympathetic ganglion cells are scattered in the medulla. Nerve fibers follow the arteries, supplying the smooth muscle in the walls of these vessels, as they pass into medulla and cortex of the ovary. Nerve fibers associated with the follicles do not penetrate the basal lamina. Sensory nerve endings are scattered in the stroma. The sensory fibers convey impulses via the ovarian plexus and reach the dorsal root ganglia of the first lumbar spinal nerves. Therefore, ovarian pain is referred over the cutaneous distribution of these spinal nerves.

At ovulation, about 45% of women experience midcycle pain ("mittelschmerz"). It is usually described as a sharp, lower abdominal pain that lasts from a few minutes up to 24 hours and is frequently accompanied by a small amount of bleeding from the uterus. It is believed that this pain is related to smooth muscle cell contraction in the ovary as well as in its ligaments. These contractions are in response to an increased level of prostaglandin $F_{2\alpha}$ mediated by the surge of LH.

▼ UTERINE TUBES

The ***uterine tubes*** are paired tubes that extend bilaterally from the uterus toward the ovaries (see Fig. 22.1). Also commonly referred to as the ***Fallopian tubes***, the uterine tubes transport the ovum from the ovary to the uterus and provide the necessary environment for fertilization and initial development of the zygote to the morula stage. One end of the tube is adjacent to the ovary and opens into the peritoneal cavity; the other end communicates with the uterine cavity.

Each uterine tube is approximately 10 to 12 cm long and can be divided into four segments by gross inspection:

- The ***infundibulum*** is the funnel-shaped segment of the tube adjacent to the ovary. At the distal end, it opens into the peritoneal cavity. The proximal end communicates with the ampulla. Fringed extensions, or ***fimbriae***, extend from the mouth of the infundibulum toward the ovary.
- The ***ampulla*** is the longest segment of the tube, constituting about two thirds of the total length, and is the site of fertilization.
- The ***isthmus*** is the narrow, medial segment of the uterine tube adjacent to the uterus.
- The ***uterine*** or ***intramural*** part, measuring about 1 cm in length, lies within the uterine wall and opens into the cavity of the uterus.

The wall of the uterine tube is composed of three layers

The uterine tube wall resembles the wall of other hollow viscera, consisting of an external serosal layer, an intermediate muscular layer, and an internal mucosal layer. However, there is no submucosa.

- The ***serosa*** or peritoneum is the outermost layer of the uterine tube and is composed of mesothelium and a thin layer of connective tissue.
- The ***muscularis***, throughout most of its length, is organized into an inner, relatively thick circular layer and an outer, thinner longitudinal layer. The boundary between these layers is often indistinct.
- The ***mucosa***, the inner lining of the uterine tube exhibits relatively thin longitudinal folds that project into the lumen of the uterine tube throughout its length. The folds are most numerous and complex in the ampulla (Fig. 22.15) and become smaller in the isthmus.

The mucosal lining is simple columnar epithelium composed of two kinds of cells, ciliated and nonciliated (Fig. 22.15b). They represent different functional states of a single cell type.

- ***Ciliated cells*** are most numerous in the infundibulum and ampulla. The wave of the cilia is directed toward the uterus.
- ***Nonciliated, peg cells*** are secretory cells that produce the fluid that provides nutritive material for the ovum.

The epithelial cells undergo cyclic hypertrophy during the follicular phase and atrophy during the luteal phase in response to changes in hormonal levels, particularly estrogens. Also, the ratio of ciliated to nonciliated cells changes during the hormonal cycle. Estrogen stimulates ciliogenesis, and progesterone increases the number of secretory cells. At about the time of ovulation, the epithelium reaches a height of about 30 μm and is then reduced to about one half that height just before the onset of menstruation.

Bidirectional transport occurs in the uterine tube

The uterine tube demonstrates active movements just before ovulation as the fimbriae become closely apposed to the ovary and localize over the region of the ovarian

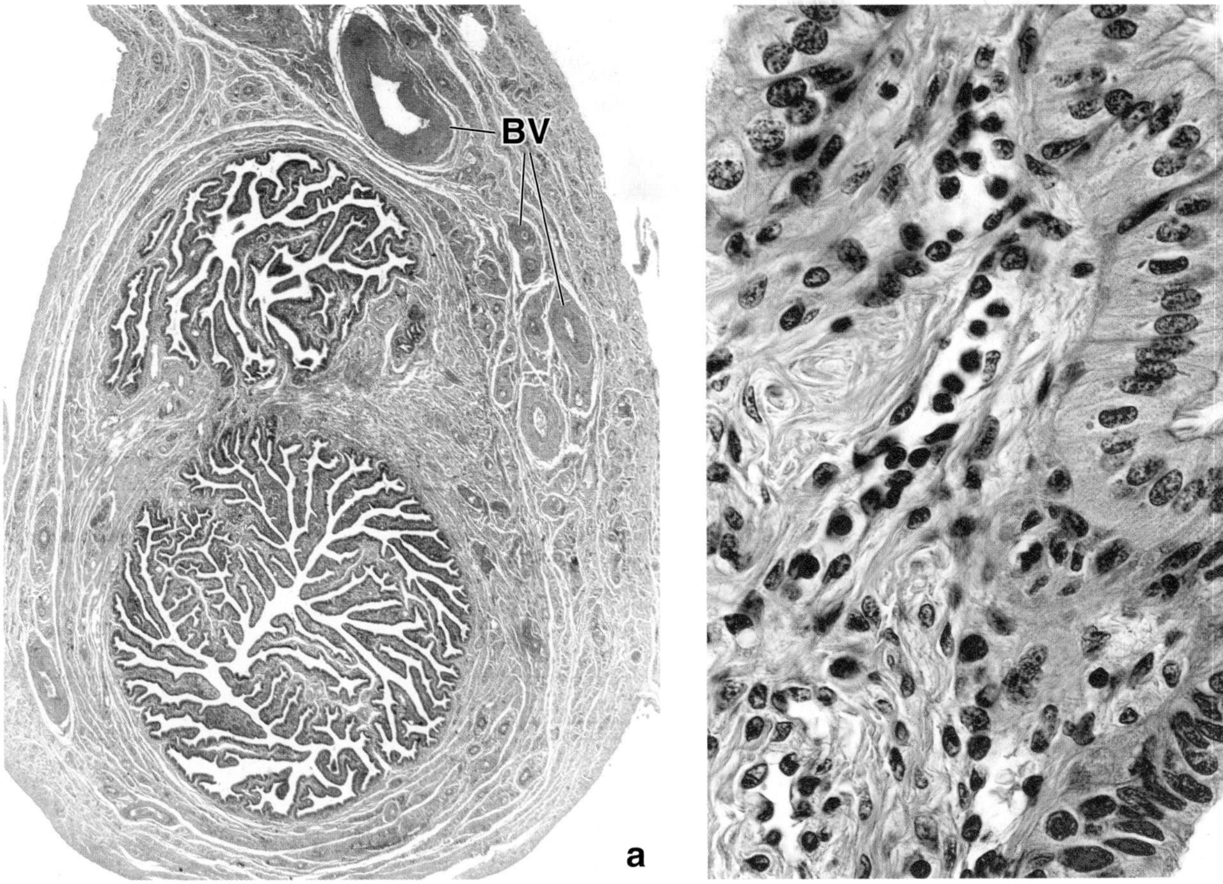

FIGURE 22.15
Photomicrograph of a human uterine tube. a. This cross section is near the ampulla region of the uterine tube. The mucosa is thrown into extensive folds that project into the lumen of the tube. The muscularis is composed of a thick inner layer of circularly arranged fibers and an outer layer of longitudinal fibers. Note several branches of the uterine and ovarian arteries *(BV)* that travel along the uterine tube. ×16. **b.** The lumen of the tube is lined by a simple columnar epithelium composed of ciliated cells (above the point of the *arrow*) and nonciliated cells (below the point of the *arrow*). ×640.

surface where rupture will occur. As the oocyte is released, the ciliated cells in the infundibulum sweep it toward the opening of the uterine tube and thus prevent it from entering the peritoneal cavity. The oocyte is transported along the uterine tube by peristaltic contractions. The mechanisms by which spermatozoa and the oocyte are transported from opposite ends of the uterine tube are not fully understood. Research suggests that both ciliary movements and peristaltic muscular activity are involved in the movements of the oocyte. The movement of the spermatozoa is much too rapid, however, to be accounted for by intrinsic motility. Fertilization usually occurs in the ampulla, near its junction with the isthmus. The ovum remains in the uterine tube for about 3 days before it enters the uterine cavity. Several conditions that may alter the integrity of the tubal transport system (inflammation, use of intrauterine devices, surgical manipulation, tubal ligation) may cause ectopic pregnancies and are thus clinically important.

▼ UTERUS

The uterus receives the rapidly developing morula from the uterine tube. All subsequent embryonic and fetal development occurs within the uterus, which undergoes dramatic increases in size and development. The human uterus is a hollow, pear-shaped organ located in the pelvis between the bladder and rectum. In a nulliparous woman, it weighs 30 to 40 g and measures 7.5 cm in length, 5 cm in width at its superior aspect, and is 2.5 cm thick. Its lumen, which is also flattened, is continuous with the uterine tubes and the vagina.

Anatomically, the uterus is divided into two regions:

- The ***body*** is the large upper portion of the uterus. The anterior surface is almost flat; the posterior surface is convex. The upper, rounded part of the body that expands above the attachment of the uterine tubes is termed the ***fundus***.

- The ***cervix*** is the lower, barrel-shaped part of the uterus separated from the body by the ***isthmus*** (see Fig. 22.1). The lumen of the cervix, the ***cervical canal,*** has a constricted opening or ***os*** at each end. The ***internal os*** communicates with the cavity of the uterus; the ***external os,*** with the vagina.

The uterine wall is composed of three layers (Fig. 22.16). From the lumen outward they are

- ***Endometrium,*** the mucosa of the uterus.
- ***Myometrium,*** the thick muscular layer. It is continuous with the muscle layer of the uterine tube and vagina. The smooth muscle fibers also extend into the ligaments connected to the uterus.
- ***Perimetrium,*** the outer serous layer or visceral peritoneal covering of the uterus. The perimetrium is continuous with the pelvic and abdominal peritoneum and consists of a mesothelium and a thin layer of loose connective tissue. Beneath the mesothelium, a layer of elastic tissue is usually prominent. The perimetrium covers the entire posterior surface of the uterus but only part of the anterior surface. The remaining part of the anterior surface consists of connective tissue or adventitia.

Both myometrium and endometrium undergo cyclic changes each month to prepare the uterus for implantation of an embryo. These changes constitute the menstrual cycle. If an embryo implants, the cycle stops, and both layers undergo considerable growth and differentiation during pregnancy (described below).

The myometrium forms a structural and functional syncytium

The myometrium is the thickest layer of the uterine wall. It is composed of three indistinctly defined layers of smooth muscle:

- The ***middle muscle layer*** contains numerous large blood vessels (venous plexuses) and lymphatics and is called the ***stratum vasculare.*** It is the thickest layer and has interlaced smooth muscle bundles oriented in a circular or spiral pattern.
- The smooth muscle bundles in the ***inner and outer layers*** are predominantly oriented parallel to the long axis of the uterus.

As in most bulb-shaped hollow organs, such as the gallbladder and urinary bladder, muscular orientation is not distinctive. The muscle bundles seen in routine histologic sections appear to be randomly arrayed. During uterine contraction, all three layers of the myometrium work together as a functional syncytium expelling the contents of the lumen through a narrow orifice.

In the nonpregnant uterus, the smooth muscle cells are about 50 μm long. During pregnancy, the uterus undergoes enormous enlargement. The growth is primarily due to the hypertrophy of existing smooth muscle cells, which may reach more than 500 μm in length, and secondarily due to the development of new fibers through the division of existing muscle cells and the differentiation of undifferentiated mesenchymal cells. The amount of connective tissue also increases. As pregnancy proceeds, the uterine wall becomes progressively thinner as it stretches because of the growth of the fetus. After parturition, the uterus returns to almost its original size. Some muscle fibers degenerate, but most return to their original size. The collagen produced during pregnancy to strengthen the myometrium is then enzymatically degraded by the cells that secreted it. The uter-

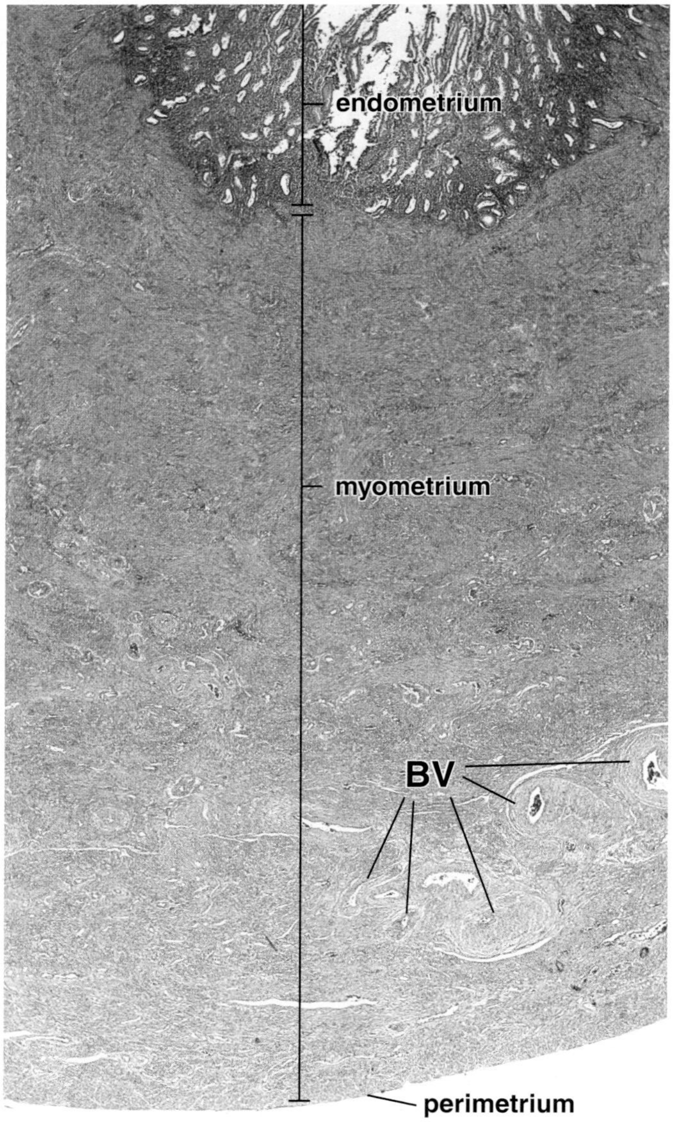

FIGURE 22.16
Photomicrograph of a sagittal section of a human uterus. This section shows the three layers of the uterine wall: the endometrium, the innermost layer that lines the uterine cavity; the myometrium, the middle layer of smooth muscle; and the perimetrium, the very thin layer of peritoneum that covers the exterior surface of the uterus. The deep portion of the myometrium contains the larger blood vessels *(BV)* that supply the uterus. ×8.

ine cavity remains larger and the muscular wall remains thicker than before pregnancy.

Compared with the body of the uterus, the cervix has more connective tissue and less smooth muscle. Elastic fibers are abundant in the cervix but are found in appreciable quantities only in the outer layer of the myometrium of the body of the uterus.

The endometrium proliferates and then degenerates during a menstrual cycle

Throughout the reproductive lifespan, the endometrium undergoes cyclic changes each month that prepare it for the implantation of the embryo and the subsequent events of embryonic and fetal development. Changes in the secretory activity of the endometrium during the cycle are correlated with the maturation of the ovarian follicles (see Fig. 22.14). The end of each cycle is characterized by the partial destruction and sloughing of the endometrium, accompanied by bleeding from the mucosal vessels. The discharge of tissue and blood from the vagina, which usually continues for 3 to 5 days, is referred to as ***menstruation*** or ***menstrual flow***. The ***menstrual cycle*** is defined as beginning on the day when menstrual flow begins.

During reproductive life, the endometrium consists of two layers or zones that differ in structure and function (Fig. 22.17):

- ***Stratum functionale*** or ***functional layer***. This layer is the thick part of the endometrium, which is sloughed off at menstruation.
- ***Stratum basale*** or ***basal layer***. This layer is retained during menstruation and serves as the source for the regeneration of the stratum functionale.

The stratum functionale is the layer that proliferates and degenerates during the menstrual cycle

During the phases of the menstrual cycle, the endometrium varies from 1 to 6 mm in thickness. It is lined by a simple columnar epithelium with a mixture of secretory and ciliated cells. The surface epithelium invaginates into the underlying lamina propria, the ***endometrial stroma***, forming the ***uterine glands***. These simple tubular glands, containing fewer ciliated cells, occasionally branch in the deeper aspect of the endometrium. The endometrial stroma, which resembles mesenchyme, is highly cellular and contains abundant intercellular ground substance. As in the uterine tube, no submucosa separates the endometrium from the myometrium.

The vasculature of the endometrium also proliferates and degenerates during each menstrual cycle

The endometrium contains a unique system of blood vessels (see Fig. 22.17). The uterine artery gives off 6 to 10 arcuate arteries that anastomose in the myometrium. Branches from these arteries, the ***radial arteries***, enter the basal layer of the endometrium where they give off ***small straight arteries*** that supply this region of the endometrium. The main branch of the radial artery continues upward and becomes highly coiled; it is therefore called the ***spiral artery***. Spiral arteries give off numerous arterioles that often anastomose as they supply a rich capillary bed. The capillary bed includes thin-walled dilated segments called ***lacunae***. Lacunae may also occur in the venous system that drains the endometrium. The straight arteries and the proximal part of the spiral arteries do not change during the menstrual cycle. The distal portion of the spiral arteries, under the influence of estrogens and

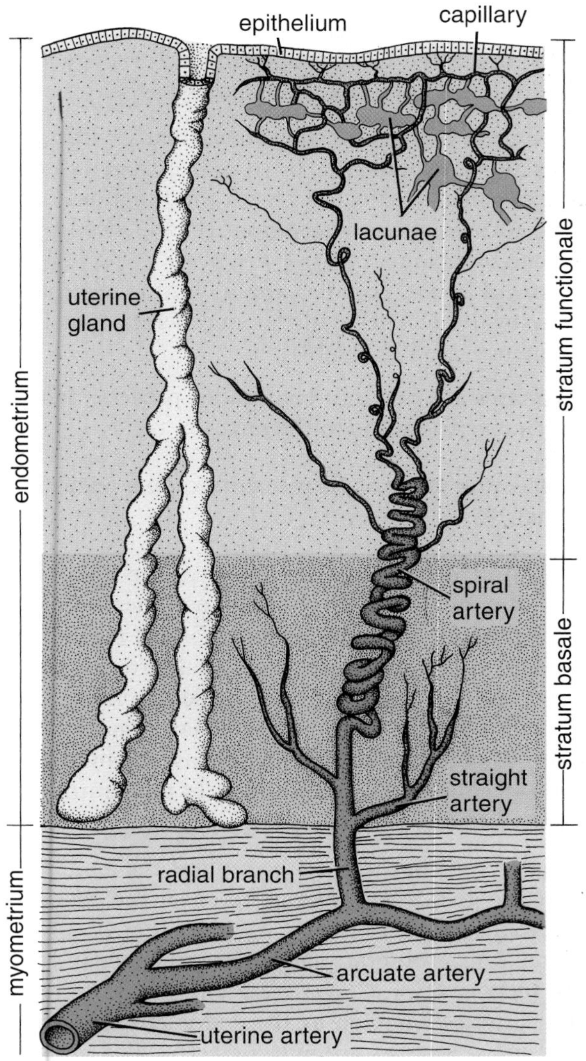

FIGURE 22.17

Schematic diagram illustrating arterial blood supply to the endometrium of the uterus. The two layers of the endometrium, the stratum basale and stratum functionale, are supplied by branches of the uterine artery. The spiral arteries located at the interface between these two layers degenerate and regenerate during the menstrual cycle under the influence of estrogens and progesterone. (Based on Weiss L, ed. *Cell and Tissue Biology: A Textbook of Histology.* 6th ed. Baltimore: Urban & Schwarzenberg, 1988.)

progesterone, undergoes degeneration and regeneration with each menstrual cycle.

Cyclic Changes During the Menstrual Cycle

Cyclic changes of the endometrium during the menstrual cycle are represented by the proliferative, secretory, and menstrual phases

The menstrual cycle is a continuum of developmental stages in the functional layer of the endometrium. It is ultimately controlled by gonadotropins secreted by the pars distalis of the pituitary gland that regulate the steroid secretions of the ovary. The cycle normally repeats every 28 days, during which the endometrium passes through a sequence of morphologic and functional changes. It is convenient to describe the cycle as having three successive phases:

- *Proliferative phase,* occurring concurrently with follicular maturation and influenced by ovarian estrogen secretion
- *Secretory phase,* coinciding with the functional activity of the corpus luteum and primarily influenced by progesterone secretion
- *Menstrual phase,* commencing as hormone production by the ovary declines with the degeneration of the corpus luteum (see Fig. 22.14)

The phases are part of a continuous process; there is no abrupt change from one to the next.

The proliferative phase of the menstrual cycle is regulated by estrogens

At the end of the menstrual phase, the endometrium consists of a thin band of connective tissue, about 1 mm thick, containing the basal portions of the uterine glands and the lower portions of the spiral arteries (see Fig. 22.17). This layer is the stratum basale; the layer that was sloughed off was the stratum functionale. Under the influence of estrogens, the proliferative phase is initiated. Stromal, endothelial, and epithelial cells in the stratum basale proliferate rapidly, and the following changes can be seen:

- Epithelial cells in the basal portion of the glands reconstitute the glands and migrate to cover the denuded endometrial surface.
- Stromal cells proliferate and secrete collagen and ground substance.
- Spiral arteries lengthen as the endometrium is reestablished; these arteries are only slightly coiled and do not extend into the upper third of the endometrium.

The proliferative phase continues until 1 day after ovulation, which occurs at about day 14 of a 28-day cycle. At the end of this phase, the endometrium has reached a thickness of about 3 mm. The glands have narrow lumina and are relatively straight but have a slightly wavy appearance (Fig. 22.18a). Accumulations of glycogen are present in the basal portions of the epithelial cells. In routine histologic preparations, extraction of the glycogen gives an empty appearance to the basal cytoplasm.

The secretory phase of the menstrual cycle is regulated by progesterone

Under the influence of progesterone, dramatic changes occur in the stratum functionale, beginning a day or two after ovulation. The endometrium becomes edematous and may eventually reach a thickness of 5 to 6 mm. The glands enlarge and become corkscrew shaped, and their lumina become sacculated as they fill with secretory products (Fig. 22.18b). The mucoid fluid produced by the gland epithelium is rich in nutrients, particularly glycogen, required to support development if implantation occurs. Mitoses are now rare. The growth seen at this stage results from hypertrophy of the epithelial cells, an increase in vascularity, and edema of the endometrium. The spiral arteries, however, lengthen and become more coiled. They extend nearly to the surface of the endometrium.

The sequential influence of estrogens and progesterone on the *stromal cells* enables their transformation into ***decidual cells.*** The stimulus for transformation is the implantation of the blastocyst. Large, pale cells rich in glycogen result from this transformation. Although the precise function of these cells is not known, it is clear that they provide a favorable environment for the nourishment of the embryo and that they create a specialized layer that facilitates the separation of the placenta from the uterine wall at the termination of pregnancy.

The menstrual phase results from a decline in the ovarian secretion of progesterone and estrogen

The corpus luteum actively produces hormones for about 10 days if fertilization does not occur. As hormone levels rapidly decline, changes occur in the blood supply to the stratum functionale. Initially, periodic contractions of the walls of the spiral arteries, lasting for several hours, cause the stratum functionale to become ischemic. The glands stop secreting, and the endometrium shrinks in height as the stroma becomes less edematous. After about 2 days, extended periods of arterial contraction, with only brief periods of blood flow, cause disruption of the surface epithelium and rupture of the blood vessels. When the spiral arteries close off, blood flows into the stratum basale but not into the stratum functionale. Blood, uterine fluid, and sloughing stromal and epithelial cells from the stratum functionale constitute the vaginal discharge. As patches of tissue separate from the endometrium, the torn ends of veins, arteries, and glands are exposed (Fig. 22.18c). The desquamation continues until only the stratum basale remains. Clotting of blood is inhibited during this period of menstrual flow. Arterial blood flow is restricted except for the brief periods of relaxation of the walls of the spiral arteries. Blood continually seeps from the open ends of the veins. The period of menstrual flow normally lasts about 5

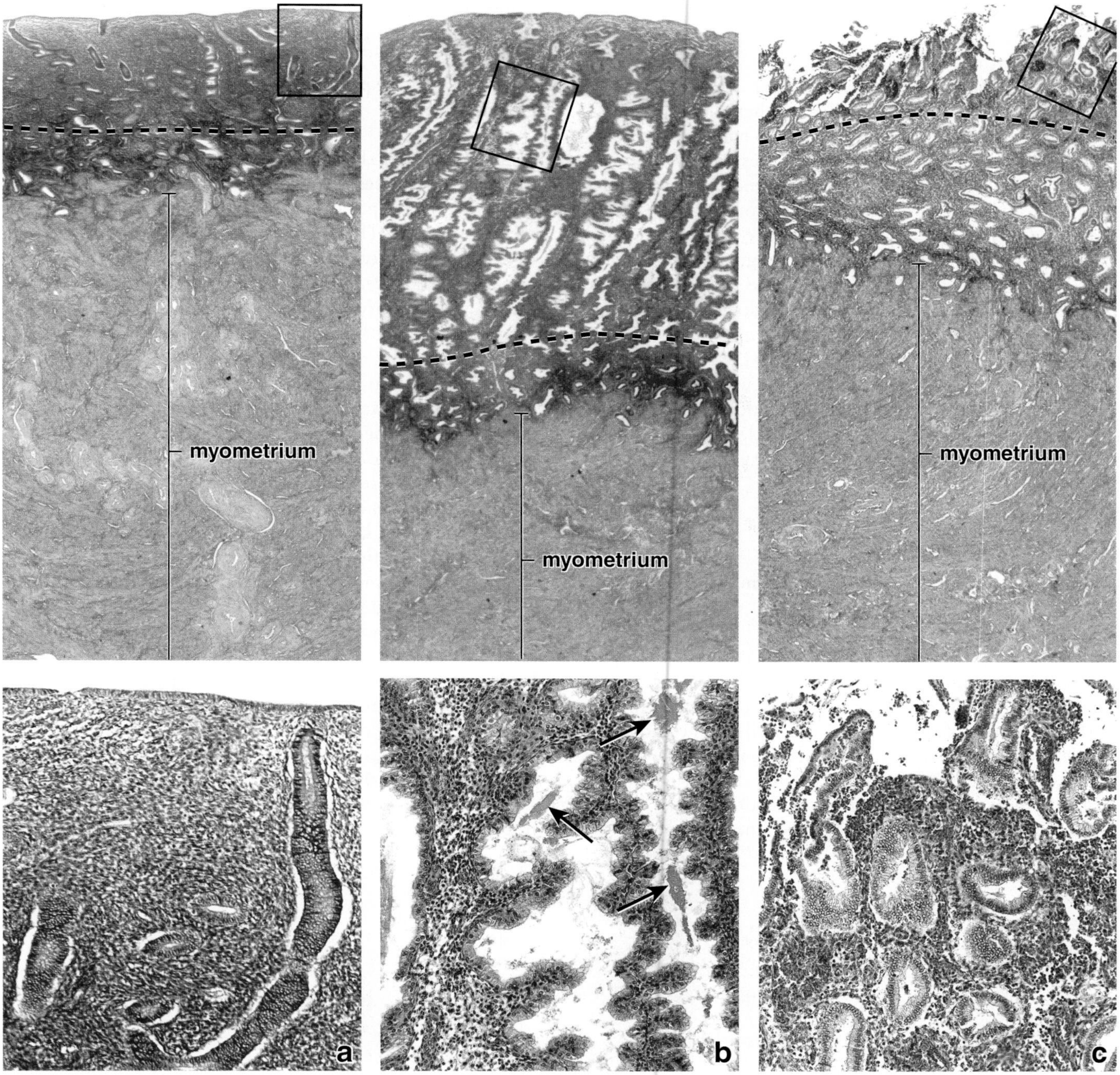

FIGURE 22.18

Photomicrographs of the uterine lining in proliferative, secretory, and menstrual phases of the menstrual cycle. a. The *upper panel* shows the endometrium at the proliferative phase of the cycle. During this phase the stratum functionale (separated by the *dashed line* from the stratum basale) greatly thickens. ×15. The *lower panel* shows at higher magnification the endometrial glands that extend from the stratum basale to the surface. ×55. **b.** The *upper panel* shows the endometrium at the secretory phase of the cycle. The glands have acquired a corkscrew shape as the endometrium increases further in thickness. The stratum basale (below the *dashed line*) exhibits less dramatic changes in morphology. ×20. The *lower panel* shows uterine glands that have been cut in a plane that is close to their long axes. Note the pronounced corkscrew shape of the glands and mucous secretion *(arrows).* ×60. **c.** The *upper panel* shows the stratum functionale *(above the dashed line).* Much of the stratum functionale has degenerated and sloughed away. ×15. The *lower panel* shows the extravasated blood and necrosis of the stratum functionale. ×55.

days. The average blood loss in the menstrual phase is 35 to 50 mL. Blood flow through the straight arteries maintains the stratum basale.

As noted, this process is cyclic. Figure 22.14 shows a single cycle of the endometrium and then demonstrates a gravid state as it is established at the end of a secretory phase. In the absence of fertilization, cessation of bleeding would accompany the growth and maturation of new ovarian follicles. The epithelial cells would rapidly proliferate and migrate to restore the surface epithelium as the proliferative phase of the next cycle begins.

In the absence of ovulation (a cycle referred to as an ***anovulatory cycle***), a corpus luteum does not form, and progesterone is not produced. In the absence of progesterone, the endometrium does not enter the secretory phase and continues in the proliferative phase until menstruation. In cases of infertility, biopsies of the endometrium can be used to diagnose such anovulatory cycles as well as other disorders of the ovary and endometrium.

Implantation

If fertilization and implantation occur, a gravid phase replaces the menstrual phase of the cycle

If fertilization and subsequent implantation occur, decline of the endometrium is delayed until after parturition. As the blastocyst becomes embedded in the uterine mucosa in the early part of the second week, cells in the chorion of the developing placenta begin to secrete hCG and other luteotropins. These hormones maintain the corpus luteum and stimulate it to continue the production of progesterone and estrogens. Thus, the decline of the endometrium is prevented, and the endometrium undergoes further development during the first few weeks of pregnancy.

Implantation is the process by which the blastocyst settles into the endometrium

The fertilized human ovum undergoes a series of changes as it passes through the uterine tube into the uterine cavity in preparation for becoming embedded in the uterine mucosa. The zygote undergoes cleavage, followed by a series of mitotic divisions without cell growth, resulting in a rapid increase in the number of cells in the embryo. Initially, the embryo is under the control of maternal informational macromolecules that have accumulated in the cytoplasm of the ovum during oogenesis. Later development depends on activation of the embryonic genome, which encodes various growth factors, cell junction components, and other macromolecules required for normal progression to the blastocyst stage.

The cell mass resulting from the series of mitotic divisions is known as a ***morula*** *[L. morum, mulberry]*, and the individual cells are known as ***blastomeres***. During the third day after fertilization, the morula, which has reached a 12- to 16-cell stage and is still surrounded by the zona pellucida, enters the uterine cavity. The morula remains free in the uterus for about a day while continued cell division and development occur. The early embryo gives rise to a blastocyst, a hollow sphere of cells with a centrally located clump of cells. This ***inner cell mass*** will give rise to the tissues of the embryo proper; the surrounding layer of cells, the ***outer cell mass***, will form the trophoblast and then the ***placenta*** (Fig. 22.19).

Fluid passes inward through the zona pellucida during this process, forming a fluid-filled cavity, the ***blastocyst***

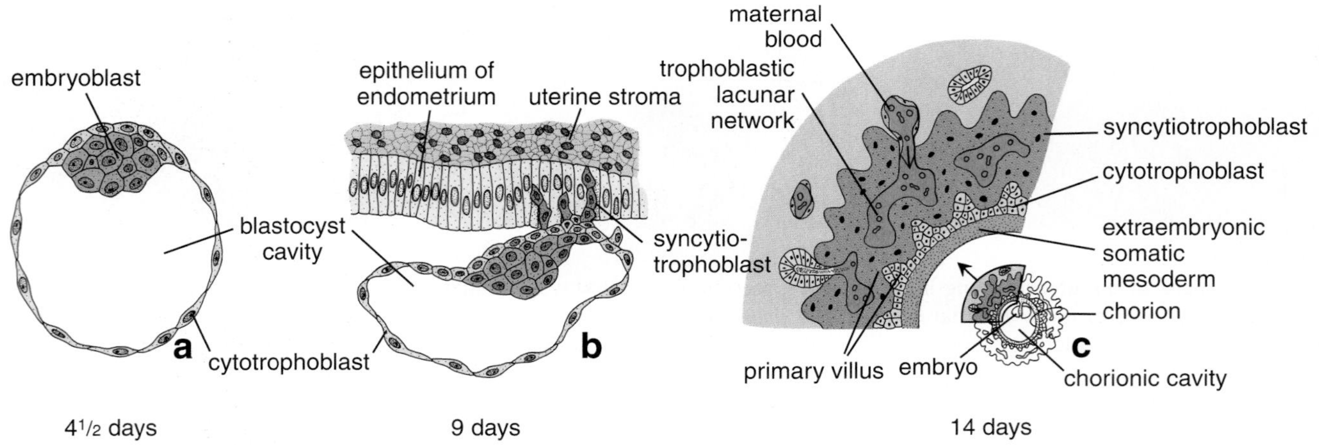

FIGURE 22.19
Schematic diagrams of sectioned blastocysts. a. A human blastocyst at about 4.5 days of development showing formation of the inner cell mass. **b.** A monkey blastocyst at about 9 days of development. The trophoblastic cells of the monkey blastocyst have begun to invade the epithelial cells of the endometrium. In humans, the blastocyst begins to invade the endometrium at about the fifth or sixth day of development. **c.** A human blastocyst at 14 days of development. The *small diagram* shows the relationship of the embryo to the chorionic sac. At this stage, the trophoblast cells have differentiated into syncytiotrophoblasts and cytotrophoblasts. (Based on Sadler TW. *Langman's Medical Embryology.* 8th ed. Baltimore: Lippincott Williams & Wilkins, 2000.)

cavity. This event defines the beginning of the ***blastocyst***. As the blastocyst remains free in the uterine lumen for 1 or 2 days and undergoes further mitotic divisions, the zona pellucida disappears. The outer cell mass is now called the ***trophoblast***, and the inner cell mass is referred to as the ***embryoblast***.

Implantation occurs during a short period known as the implantation window

The attachment of the blastocyst to the endometrial epithelium occurs during the ***implantation window***, the period that the uterus is receptive for implantation of the blastocyst. This short period results from a series of programmed actions of progesterone and estrogens on the endometrium. Antiprogesterone drugs, such as Mifepristone (RU 486) and its derivatives, compete for the receptors in the endometrial epithelium, thus blocking hormone binding. The failure of progesterone to gain access to its receptors prevents implantation, thus effectively closing the window. In the human, the implantation window begins on day 6 after the LH surge and is completed by day 10.

As contact is made with the uterine wall by the trophoblastic cells over the embryoblast pole, the trophoblast rapidly proliferates and begins to invade the endometrium. The invading trophoblast differentiates into the ***syncytiotrophoblast*** and the ***cytotrophoblast***.

- The ***cytotrophoblast*** is a mitotically active inner cell layer producing cells that fuse with the syncytiotrophoblast, the outer erosive layer.
- The ***syncytiotrophoblast*** is not mitotically active and consists of a multinucleate cytoplasmic mass; it actively invades the epithelium and underlying stroma of the endometrium.

Through the activity of the trophoblast, the blastocyst is entirely embedded within the endometrium on about the 11th day of development (further development of the syncytiotrophoblast and cytotrophoblast is described in the section on the placenta).

The syncytiotrophoblast has well-developed Golgi complexes, abundant sER and rER, numerous mitochondria, and relatively large numbers of lipid droplets. These features are consistent with the secretion of progesterone, estrogens, hCG, and lactogens by this layer. Recent evidence indicates that cytotrophoblast cells may also be a source of steroid hormones and hCG.

After implantation, the endometrium undergoes decidualization

During pregnancy, the portion of the endometrium that undergoes morphologic changes is called the ***decidua*** or ***decidua graviditas***. As its name implies, this layer is shed with the placenta at parturition. The decidua includes all but the deepest layer of the endometrium. The stromal cells differentiate into large, rounded decidual cells (see page 745). The uterine glands enlarge and become more coiled during the early part of pregnancy and then become thin and flattened as the growing fetus fills the uterine lumen.

Three different regions of the decidua are identified by their relationship to the site of implantation (Fig. 22.20):

- The ***decidua basalis*** is the portion of the endometrium that underlies the implantation site.

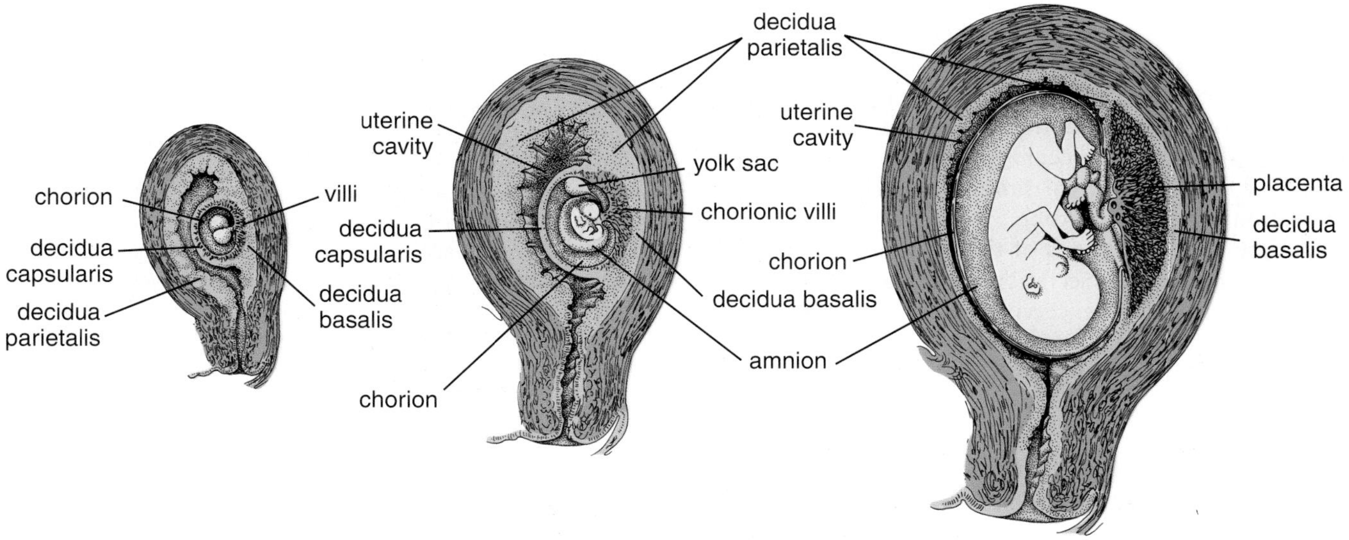

FIGURE 22.20
Development of the placenta. This schematic drawing shows growth of the uterus during human pregnancy and development of the placenta and its membranes. Note that there is a gradual obliteration of the uterine lumen and disappearance of the decidua capsularis as the definitive placenta is established. (Modified from Williams J. *Am J Obstet Gynecol* 1927;13:1.)

- The *decidua capsularis* is a thin portion of endometrium that lies between the implantation site and the uterine lumen.
- The *decidua parietalis* includes the remaining endometrium of the uterus.

By the end of the third month, the fetus grows to the point that the overlying decidua capsularis fuses with the decidua parietalis of the opposite wall, thereby obliterating the uterine cavity.

By the 13th day of development, an extraembryonic space, the ***chorionic cavity,*** has been established (see Fig. 22.19c). The cell layers that form the outer boundary of this cavity, i.e., the syncytiotrophoblast, cytotrophoblast, and extraembryonic somatic mesoderm, are collectively referred to as the ***chorion.*** The innermost membranes enveloping the embryo are called the ***amnion*** (Fig. 22.20).

Cervix

The endometrium of the cervix differs from the rest of the uterus

The cervical mucosa measures about 2 to 3 mm in thickness and differs dramatically from the rest of the uterine endometrium in that it contains large, branched glands (Fig. 22.21). It also lacks spiral arteries. The cervical mucosa undergoes little change in thickness during the menstrual cycle and is not sloughed during the period of menstruation. During each menstrual cycle, however, the cervical glands undergo important functional changes that are related to the transport of spermatozoa within the cervical canal. The amount and properties of the mucus secreted by the gland cells vary during the menstrual cycle under the influence of the ovarian hormones. At midcycle, the amount of mucus produced increases 10-fold. This mucus is less viscous and appears to provide a more favorable environment for sperm migration. The cervical mucus at other times in the cycle restricts the passage of sperm into the uterus. Thus, hormonal mechanisms ensure that ovulation and changes in the cervical mucus are coordinated, thereby increasing the possibility that fertilization will occur if freshly ejaculated spermatozoa and the ovum arrive simultaneously at the site of fertilization in the uterine tube.

Blockage of the openings of the mucosal glands results in the retention of their secretions, leading to formation of dilated cysts within the cervix, called ***Nabothian cysts.*** Nabothian cysts develop frequently but are clinically important only if numerous cysts produce marked enlargement of the cervix.

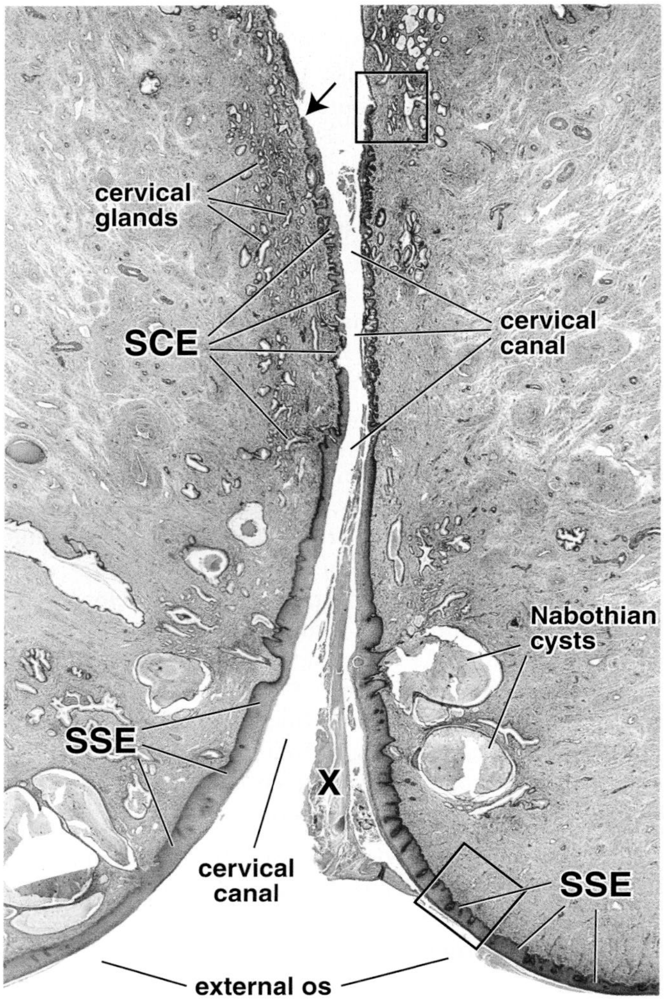

FIGURE 22.21
Photomicrograph of a human cervix. This H&E–stained specimen is from a postmenopausal woman. Its lower portion projects into the upper vagina where an opening, the external os, leads to the uterus through the cervical canal. The surface of the cervix is covered by stratified squamous epithelium *(SSE)* that is continuous with the epithelial lining of the vagina. An abrupt transition from stratified squamous epithelium to simple columnar epithelium *(SCE)* occurs at the entry to the cervical canal. In this specimen, the stratified epithelium has extended into the canal, an event that occurs with aging. Mucus-secreting cervical glands are seen along the cervical canal. These are simple branched tubular glands that arise as invaginations of the epithelium lining the canal. Frequently, the glands develop into Nabothian cysts as a result of retention of mucous secretion by blockage of the gland opening. The material marked by the *X* is mucus secreted from the cervical glands. ×10.

The transformation zone is the site of transition between vaginal stratified squamous epithelium and cervical simple columnar epithelium

The portion of the cervix that projects into the vagina, the vaginal part, the ***ectocervix,*** is covered with a stratified squamous epithelium (Fig. 22.22). An abrupt transition between this squamous epithelium and the mucus-secreting columnar epithelium of the cervical canal, the ***endocervix,*** occurs in the ***transformation zone*** that during the reproductive age of the woman is located just outside the external os. Before puberty and after menopause the transfor-

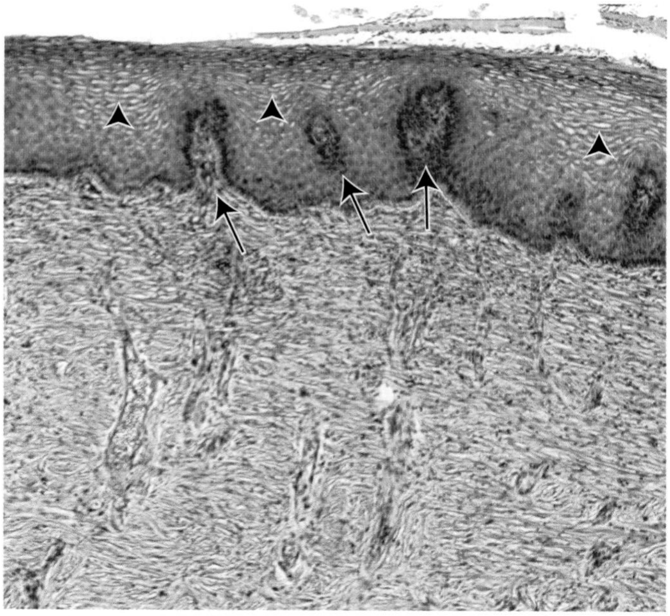

FIGURE 22.22
Stratified squamous epithelium of the ectocervix. The stratified squamous epithelium and underlying fibrous connective tissue within the *lower rectangle* in Figure 22.21 is shown here at higher magnification. The more mature epithelial cells have a clear cytoplasm *(arrowheads)*, a reflection of their high glycogen content. Also, note the connective tissue papillae protruding into the epithelium *(arrows)*. The bulk of the cervix is made up of dense, fibrous connective tissue with relatively little smooth muscle. ×120.

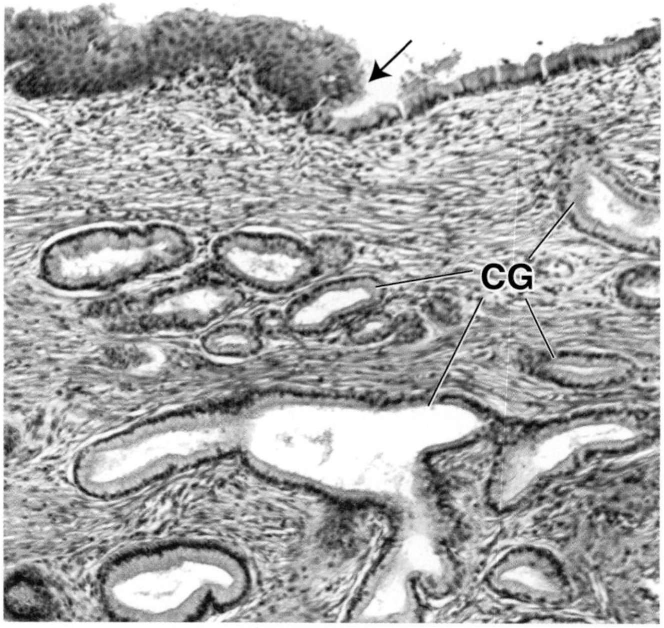

FIGURE 22.23
Transformation zone of the cervix. The site of the squamocolumnar junction from the *upper rectangle* in Figure 22.21 is shown here at higher magnification. Note the abrupt change from stratified squamous epithelium to simple columnar epithelium *(arrow)*. Neoplastic changes leading to development of cervical cancer most frequently begin in this transformation zone. Within the connective tissue are the branched, mucus-secreting cervical glands *(CG)* composed of a simple columnar epithelium that is continuous with the lining epithelium of the cervical canal. ×120.

mation zone resides in the cervical canal (Fig. 22.23). Metaplastic changes in this transition zone constitute precancerous lesions of the cervix. The cervical epithelial cells are constantly exfoliated into the vagina. Stained preparations of the cervical cells (Papanicolaou [Pap] smears) are used routinely for screening and diagnosis of precancerous and cancerous lesions of the cervix.

PLACENTA

The developing fetus is maintained by the placenta, which develops from fetal and maternal tissues

The placenta consists of a fetal portion, formed by the chorion, and a maternal portion, formed by the decidua basalis. The two parts are involved in physiologic exchange of substances between the maternal and fetal circulation.

The ***uteroplacental circulatory system*** begins to develop around day 9, with development of vascular spaces called ***trophoblastic lacunae*** within the syncytiotrophoblast. Maternal sinusoids, which develop from capillaries of the maternal side, anastomose with the trophoblastic lacunae (Fig. 22.24). The differential pressure between the arterial and venous channels that communicate with the lacunae establishes directional flow from the arteries into the veins, thereby establishing a primitive uteroplacental circulation. Numerous pinocytotic vessels present in the syncytiotrophoblast indicate the transfer of nutrients from the maternal vessels to the embryo.

Proliferation of the cytotrophoblast, growth of chorionic mesoderm, and blood vessel development successively give rise to

- ***Primary chorionic villi***, which are formed by the rapidly proliferating cytotrophoblast. It sends cords or masses of cells into the blood-filled trophoblastic lacunae in the syncytiotrophoblast (see Fig. 22.19b). The primary villi appear between days 11 and 13 of development.
- ***Secondary chorionic villi***, which are composed of a central core of mesenchyme, surrounded by an inner layer of cytotrophoblast and an outer layer of syncytiotrophoblast. They develop at about day 16, when the primary chorionic villi become invaded by loose connective tissue from chorionic mesenchyme. The secondary villi cover the entire surface of the chorionic sac (Fig. 22.24a).
- ***Tertiary chorionic villi*** are formed by the end of the third week as the secondary villi become vascularized by

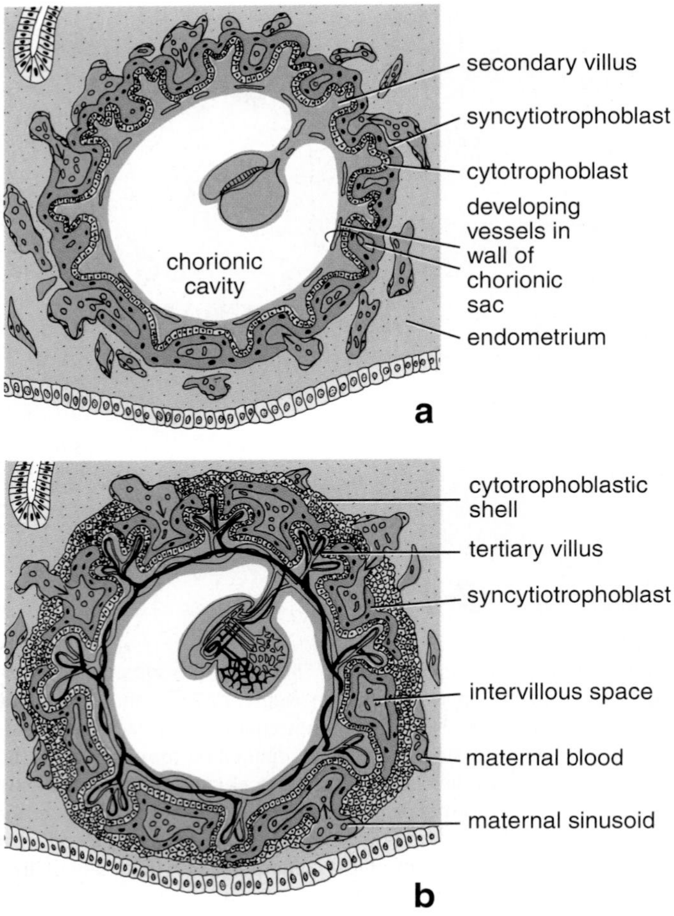

FIGURE 22.24
Schematic diagrams of sections through a developing human embryo. a. This drawing shows the chorionic sac and placenta at 16 days of development. **b.** The same embryo at 21 days of development. The diagrams illustrate the separation of the fetal and maternal blood vessels by the placental membrane, which is composed of the endothelium of the capillaries, mesenchyme, cytotrophoblast, and syncytiotrophoblast. (Based on Moore KL, Persaud TVN. *The Developing Human, Clinically Oriented Embryology.* Philadelphia: WB Saunders, 1993.)

blood vessels that have developed in their connective tissue cores (Fig. 22.24b)

As the tertiary villi are forming, cytotrophoblastic cells in the villi continue to grow out through the syncytiotrophoblast. When they meet the maternal endometrium, they grow laterally and meet similar processes growing from neighboring villi. Thus, a thin layer of cytotrophoblastic cells, called the ***trophoblastic shell,*** is formed around the syncytiotrophoblast. The trophoblastic shell is interrupted only at sites where maternal vessels communicate with the intervillous spaces. Future growth of the placenta is accomplished by interstitial growth of the trophoblastic shell.

Two types of cells are recognized in the connective tissue stroma of the villi: mesenchymal cells and ***Hofbauer cells*** (Fig. 22.25). Hofbauer cells are more common in the early placenta. They appear to be macrophages. The vacuoles in these cells contain lipids, glycosaminoglycans, and glycoproteins. Recent studies of HIV-infected placentas indicate that HIV is primarily localized within Hofbauer cells as well as in the syncytiotrophoblast.

Early in development, the blood vessels of the villi become connected with vessels from the embryo

Blood begins to circulate through the embryonic cardiovascular system and the villi at about 21 days. The intervillous spaces provide the site of exchange of nutrients, metabolic products and intermediates, and wastes between the maternal and fetal circulatory systems.

During the first 8 weeks, villi cover the entire chorionic surface, but as growth continues, villi on the decidua capsularis begin to degenerate, producing a smooth, relatively avascular surface called the ***chorion laeve.*** The villi adjacent to the decidua basalis rapidly increase in size and number and become highly branched. This region of the chorion, which is the fetal component of the placenta, is called the ***chorion frondosum*** or ***villous chorion.*** The layer of the placenta from which the villi project is called the ***chorionic plate.***

During the period of rapid growth of the chorion frondosum, at about the fourth to fifth month of gestation, the fetal part of the placenta is divided by the ***placental (decidual) septa*** into 15 to 25 areas called ***cotyledons.*** Wedge-like placental septa form the boundaries of the cotyledons, and because they do not fuse with the chorionic plate, maternal blood can circulate easily between them. Cotyledons are visible as the bulging areas on the maternal side of the basal plate.

The decidua basalis forms a compact layer, known as the ***basal plate,*** which is the maternal component of the placenta. Vessels within this part of the endometrium supply blood to the intervillous spaces. Except for relatively rare rupturing of capillary walls, which is more common at delivery, fetal blood and maternal blood do not mix.

Fetal and maternal blood are separated by the placental barrier

Separation of the fetal and maternal blood, referred to as the ***placental barrier,*** is maintained primarily by the layers of fetal tissue. Starting at the fourth month, these layers become very thin to facilitate the exchange of products across the placental barrier. The thinning of the wall of the villus is due in part to the degeneration of the inner cytotrophoblast layer.

At its thinnest, the placental barrier consists of the

- Syncytiotrophoblast
- Discontinuous inner cytotrophoblast layer

- Basal lamina of the trophoblast
- Connective (mesenchymal) tissue of the villus
- Basal lamina of the endothelium
- Endothelium of the fetal placental capillary in the tertiary villus

This barrier bears a strong resemblance to the air–blood barrier of the lung, with which it has an important parallel function, namely, the exchange of oxygen and carbon dioxide, in this case between the maternal blood and the fetal blood. It also resembles the air–blood barrier by having a particular type of macrophage in its connective tissue, in this instance, the Hofbauer cell.

The placenta is the site of exchange of gases and metabolites between the maternal and fetal circulation

Fetal blood enters the placenta through a pair of ***umbilical arteries*** (Fig. 22.26). As they pass into the placenta, these arteries branch into several radially disposed vessels that give numerous branches in the chorionic plate. Branches from these vessels pass into the villi, forming extensive capillary networks in close association with the intervillous spaces. Gases and metabolic products are exchanged across the thin fetal layers that separate the two bloodstreams at this level. Antibodies can also cross this layer and enter the fetal circulation to provide passive immunity against a variety of infectious agents, e.g., those of diphtheria, smallpox, and measles. Fetal blood returns through a system of veins that parallel the arteries except that they converge on a single ***umbilical vein.***

Maternal blood is supplied to the placenta through 80 to 100 spiral endometrial arteries that penetrate the basal plate. Blood from these spiral arteries flows into the base

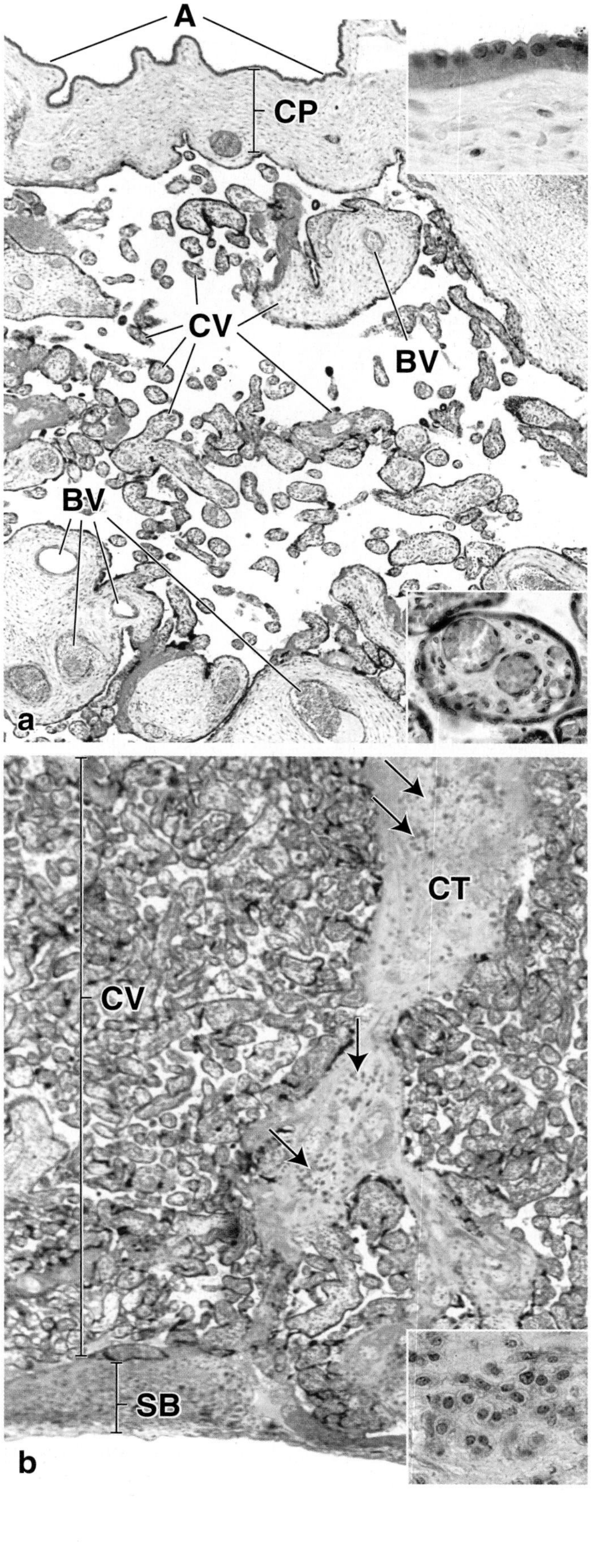

FIGURE 22.25
Photomicrographs of a human placenta. a. This H&E–stained specimen shows the amniotic surface *(A),* the chorionic plate *(CP),* and, below, the various-sized profiles of the chorionic villi *(CV).* These villi emerge from the chorionic plate as large stem villi and branch into the increasingly smaller villi. Blood vessels *(BV)* are evident in the larger villi. The smallest villi contain capillaries where exchange takes place. ×60. **Upper inset.** This higher magnification shows the simple cuboidal epithelium of the amnion and the underlying connective tissue. ×200. **Lower inset.** This higher magnification shows a cross-sectioned villus containing several larger blood vessels and its thin surface syncytiotrophoblast layer. ×200. **b.** This H&E–stained specimen shows the maternal side of the placenta. The stratum basale *(SB),* the part of the uterus to which some of the chorionic villi *(CV)* anchor, is seen at the *bottom* of the micrograph. Also evident is a stromal connective tissue *(CT)* component, part of the stratum basale, to which many of the chorionic villi are also attached. Within the stratum basale and the connective tissue stroma are clusters of cells, the decidual cells *(arrows),* which arose from connective tissue cells. ×60. **Inset.** Decidual cells seen at higher magnification. ×200.

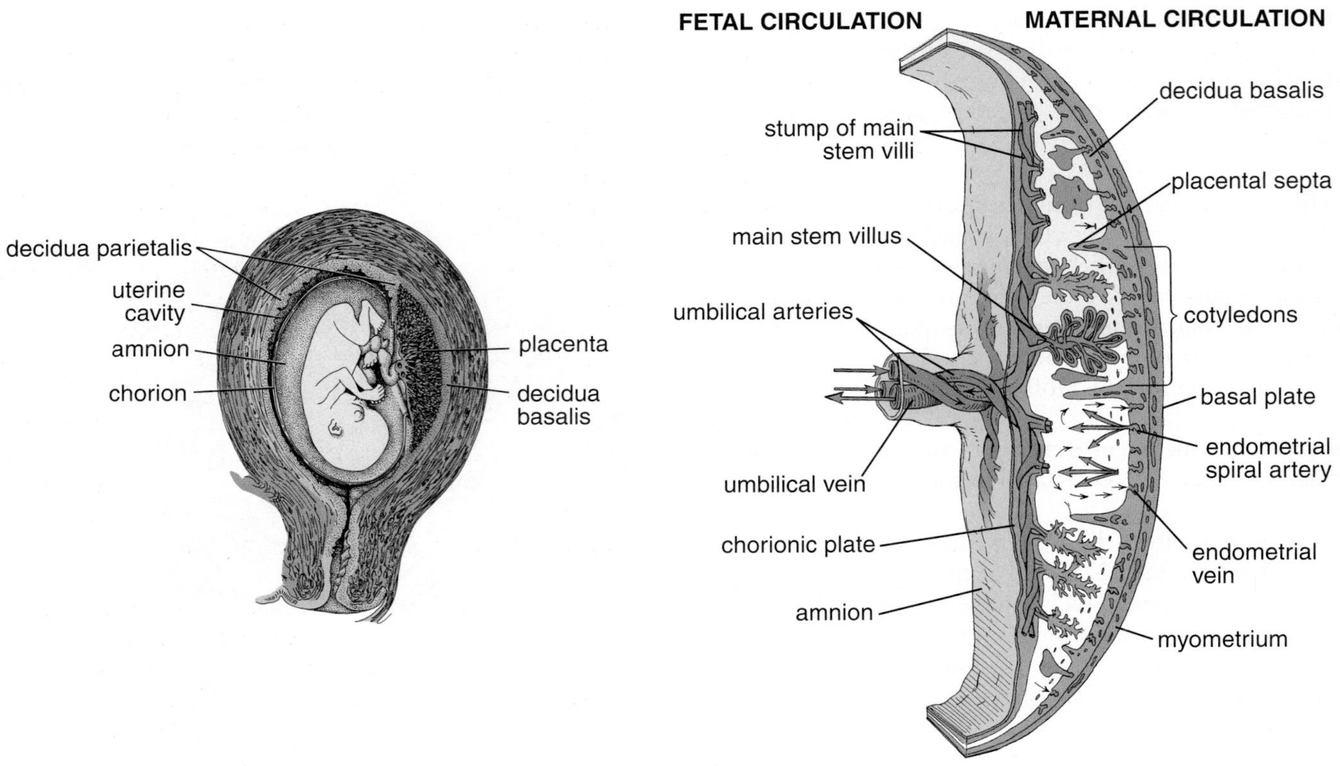

FIGURE 22.26
Schematic diagram of mature human placenta. The sagittal section of the uterus (*left*) with the developing embryo shows the most common location of the placenta. The mature placenta (*right*) is divided into cotyledons by placental septa that are formed by outgrowths of the decidua basalis. Maternal blood enters the placenta through numerous endometrial spiral arteries that penetrate the basal plate. As the blood enters the cotyledon, it is directed deep into the intervillous spaces (*red arrows*). It then passes over the surface of the villi, where exchange of gases and metabolic products occurs. The maternal blood finally leaves the intervillous space (*black arrows*) through endometrial veins. The fetal blood enters the placenta through the umbilical arteries that divide into a series of radially disposed arteries within the chorionic plate. Branches from the vessels pass into the main stem villi and there form extensive capillary networks. The veins within the villi then carry the blood back through a system of veins that parallels the fetal arteries.

of the intervillous spaces, which contain about 150 mL of maternal blood that is exchanged 3 to 4 times per minute. The blood pressure in the spiral arteries is much higher than that in the intervillous spaces. As blood is injected into these spaces at each pulse, it is directed deep into the spaces. As the pressure decreases, the blood flows back over the surfaces of the villi and eventually enters endometrial veins also located in the base of the spaces.

Exchange of gases and metabolic products occurs as the blood passes over the villi. Normally, water, carbon dioxide, metabolic waste products, and hormones are transferred from the fetal blood to the maternal blood; water, oxygen, metabolites, electrolytes, vitamins, hormones, and some antibodies pass in the opposite direction. The placental barrier does not exclude many potentially dangerous agents, such as alcohol, nicotine, viruses, drugs, exogenous hormones, and heavy metals. Therefore, during pregnancy, exposure to or ingestion of such agents should be avoided to reduce the risk of injury to the embryo or fetus.

Before the establishment of blood flow through the placenta, the growth of the embryo is supported in part by metabolic products that are synthesized by or transported through the trophoblast. The syncytiotrophoblast synthesizes glycogen, cholesterol, and fatty acids, as well as other nutrients used by the embryo.

The placenta is a major endocrine organ producing steroid and protein hormones

The placenta also functions as an endocrine organ, producing steroid and peptide hormones as well as prostaglandins that play an important role in the onset of labor. Immunocytochemical studies indicate that the syncytiotrophoblast is the site of synthesis of these hormones.

The steroid hormones, progesterone and estrogen, have essential roles in the maintenance of pregnancy. As pregnancy proceeds, the placenta takes over the major role in the secretion of these steroids from the corpus luteum. The

placenta produces enough progesterone by the end of the eighth week to maintain pregnancy if the corpus luteum is surgically removed or fails to function. In the production of placental estrogen, the *fetal adrenal cortex* plays an essential role, providing the precursors needed for estrogen synthesis. Because the placenta lacks the enzymes needed for the production of estrogen precursors, a cooperative ***fetoplacental (endocrine) unit*** is established. Clinically, the monitoring of estrogen production during pregnancy can be used as an index of fetal development.

The following peptide hormones are secreted by the placenta:

- ***hCG,*** the synthesis of which begins around day 6, even before syncytiotrophoblast formation. hCG exhibits marked homology to pituitary thyroid-stimulating hormone (TSH) and stimulates the maternal thyroid gland to increase secretion of tetraiodothyronine (T_4). It also maintains the corpus luteum during early pregnancy. Measurement of hCG is used to detect pregnancy and assess early embryonic development.
- ***Human chorionic somatomammotropin (hCS),*** also known as human placental lactogen (hPL), is closely related to human growth hormone. Synthesized in the syncytiotrophoblast, it promotes general growth, regulates glucose metabolism, and stimulates mammary duct proliferation in the maternal breast. hCS effects on maternal metabolism are significant, but the role of this hormone in fetal development remains unknown.

BOX 22.4

Clinical Correlations: Fate of Mature Placenta at Birth

The mature placenta measures about 15 to 20 cm in diameter and 2 to 3 cm in thickness, covers 25 to 30% of the uterine surface, and weighs 500 to 600 g at term. The surface area of the villi in the human placenta is estimated to be about 10 m². The microvilli on the syncytiotrophoblast increase the effective area for metabolic exchange to more than 90 m². After birth, the uterus continues to contract, reducing the luminal surface and inducing placental separation from the uterine wall. The entire fetal portion of the placenta, fetal membranes, and the intervening projections of decidual tissue are released. During uncomplicated labor, the placenta is delivered approximately 30 minutes after birth.

After delivery of the placenta, the endometrial glands and stroma of the decidua basalis regenerates. Endometrial regeneration is completed by the end of the third week postpartum except at the placental site, where regeneration usually extends through the next 3 weeks. During the first week after delivery, remnants of the decidua are shed and constitute the blood-tinged uterine discharge known as the ***lochia rubra***.

- ***IGF-I and IGF-II*** are produced by and stimulate proliferation and differentiation of the cytotrophoblast.
- ***Endothelial growth factor (EGF)*** exhibits an age-dependent dual action on the early placenta. In the 4- to 5-week-old placenta, EGF is synthesized by the cytotrophoblast and stimulates proliferation of the trophoblast. In the 6- to 12-week-old placenta, synthesis of EGF is shifted to the syncytiotrophoblast; it then stimulates and maintains the function of the differentiated trophoblast.
- ***Relaxin*** is synthesized by decidual cells and is involved in the "softening" of the cervix and the pelvic ligaments in preparation for parturition.
- ***Leptin*** is synthesized by syncytiotrophoblast, particularly during the last month of gestation. Leptin appears to regulate maternal nutrient storage to the nutrient requirements of the fetus. It is also involved in transporting nutrients across the placental barrier from mother to the fetus.
- ***Other growth factors*** stimulate cytotrophoblastic growth (e.g., fibroblast growth factor, colony-stimulating factor [CSF-1], platelet-derived growth factor, and interleukins [IL-1 and IL-3]) or inhibit trophoblast growth and proliferation (e.g., tumor necrosis factor).

VAGINA

The vagina is a fibromuscular tube that joins internal reproductive organs to the external environment

The vagina is a fibromuscular sheath extending from the cervix to the vestibule, which is the area between the labia minora. In a virgin, the opening into the vagina may be surrounded by the ***hymen,*** folds of mucous membrane extending into the vaginal lumen. The hymen or its remnants are derived from the endodermal membrane that separated the developing vagina from the cavity of the definitive urogenital sinus in the embryo.

The vaginal wall (Fig. 22.27) consists of an

- Inner ***mucosal layer,*** which has numerous transverse folds or rugae (see Fig. 22.1) and is lined with stratified squamous epithelium (Fig. 22.28). Connective tissue papillae from the underlying lamina propria project into the epithelial layer. In humans and other primates, keratohyalin granules may be present in the epithelial cells, but under normal conditions, keratinization does not occur. Therefore, nuclei can be seen in epithelial cells throughout the thickness of the epithelium.
- Intermediate ***muscular layer,*** which is organized into two sometimes indistinct, intermingling smooth muscle layers, an outer longitudinal layer and an inner circular layer. The outer layer is continuous with the corresponding layer in the uterus and is much thicker than the inner layer. Striated muscle fibers of the bulbospongiosus muscle are present at the vaginal opening.

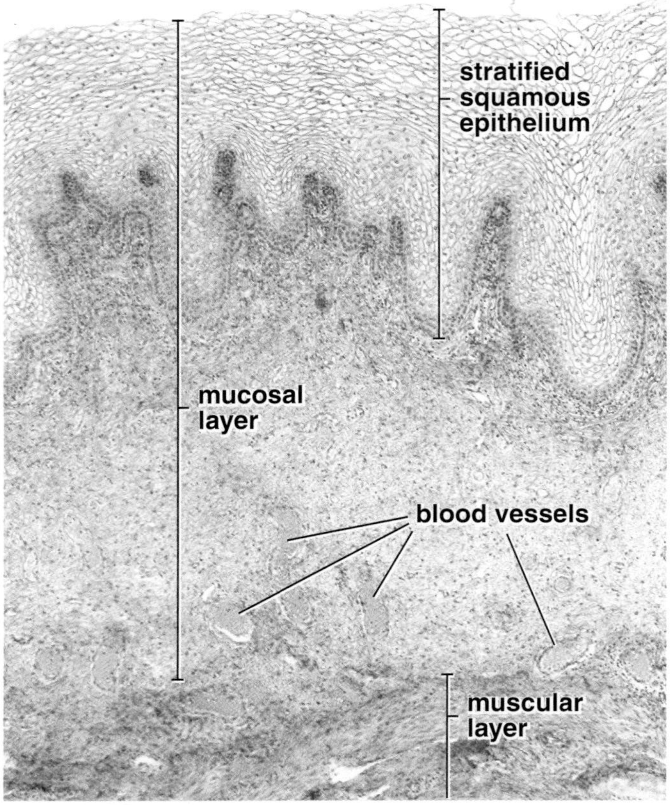

FIGURE 22.27
Photomicrograph of a human vagina. This low-magnification H&E–stained specimen of the vaginal wall shows two of three layers of the vagina: the mucosal layer and the muscular layer (the outer layer, the adventitia, is not included). The mucosal layer consists of a stratified squamous epithelium and the underlying connective tissue. The epithelial connective tissue boundary is typically very irregular, with prominent papillae projecting into the undersurface of the epithelium. The muscular layer is seen only in part; it consists of irregularly arranged bundles of smooth muscle cells. Also, the deep region of the connective tissue contains a rich supply of blood vessels that supply the various layers of the vaginal wall. ×40.

- Outer ***adventitial layer,*** which is organized into an inner dense connective tissue layer adjacent to the muscularis and an outer loose connective tissue layer that blends with the adventitia of the surrounding structures. The inner layer contains numerous elastic fibers that contribute to the elasticity and strength of the vaginal wall. The outer layer contains numerous blood and lymphatic vessels and nerves.

The vagina possesses a stratified, squamous nonkeratinized epithelium and lacks glands

The lumen of vagina is lined by stratified squamous, nonkeratinized epithelium. Its surface is lubricated mainly by mucus produced by the cervical glands. The greater and lesser vestibular glands located in the wall of the vaginal vestibule produce additional mucus that lubricates the vagina. Glands are not present in the wall of the vagina. The epithelium of the vagina undergoes cyclic changes during the menstrual cycle. Under the influence of estrogens, during the follicular phase, the epithelial cells synthesize and accumulate glycogen as they migrate toward the surface. Cells are continuously desquamated, but near or during the menstrual phase, the superficial layer of the vaginal epithelium may be shed.

The lamina propria exhibits two distinct regions. The outer region immediately below the epithelium is a highly cellular loose connective tissue. The deeper region, adjacent to the muscular layer, is denser and may be considered a submucosa. The deeper region contains many thin-walled veins that simulate erectile tissue during sexual arousal. Numerous elastic fibers are present immediately below the epithelium, and some of the fibers extend into the muscular layer. Many lymphocytes and leukocytes

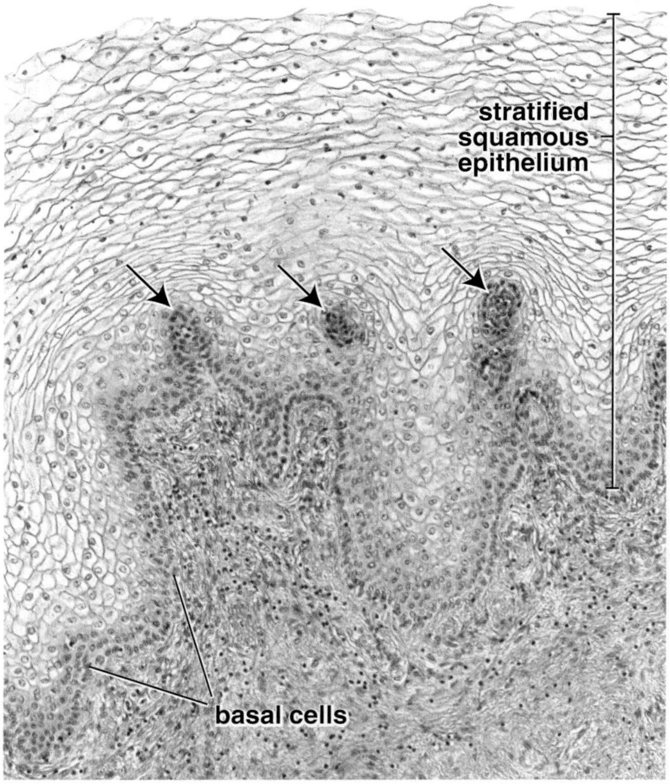

FIGURE 22.28
Photomicrograph of the vaginal mucosa. This micrograph, a higher magnification of Figure 22.27, shows the stratified squamous epithelium and mature cells with small pyknotic nuclei. Note a single layer of basal cells and two or three layers of cells undergoing differentiation (with eosinophilic cytoplasm). Projections of the connective tissue papillae into the epithelium give the connective tissue–epithelial junction an uneven appearance. The tips of these projections often appear as isolated structures surrounded by epithelium *(arrows).* ×180.

BOX 22.5

Clinical Correlations: Cytologic Pap Smears

The examination of Pap smears is a valuable diagnostic tool in evaluating the vaginal and cervical mucosae (Fig. 22.29). The superficial epithelial cells are scraped from the mucosa, spread on a glass slide, fixed, and then stained with the Papanicolaou stain (a combination of hematoxylin, orange G, and eosin azure). Examination of the Pap smear provides valuable diagnostic information about the epithelium regarding pathologic changes, response to hormonal changes during the menstrual cycle, and the microbial environment of the vagina.

The synthesis and release of glycogen by the epithelial cells of the uterus and vagina are directly related to changes in the pH of vaginal fluid. The pH of the fluid, which is normally low, around pH 4, becomes more acid near midcycle as *Lactobacillus acidophilus,* a lactic acid–forming bacterium in the vagina, metabolizes the secreted glycogen. An alkaline environment can favor the growth of infectious agents such as staphylococci, *Corynebacterium vaginale, Trichomonas vaginalis,* and *Candida albicans,* causing an abnormal increase in vaginal transexudates and inflammation of the vaginal mucosa and vulvar skin known as ***vulvovaginitis***. These pathologic conditions are readily diagnosed with Pap smears. Specific antimicrobial agents (antibiotics, sulfonamides) are used together with nonspecific therapy (acidified 0.1% hexetidine gel) to restore the normal low pH in the vagina and thus prevent the growth of these agents.

In addition, cervicovaginal Pap smears are widely used for diagnosis of early cervical cancer as well as endometrial carcinoma. Because cervical lesions may exist in a noninvasive stage for as long as 20 years, the abnormal cells shed from the epithelium are easily detected with a Pap smear examination. Microscopic examination of these cells permits differentiation between normal and abnormal cells, determines their site of origin, and allows classifying cellular changes related to the spread of the disease. The Pap smear is an extremely effective and inexpensive screening method in preventing cervical cancer. Most of the cell abnormalities detected by Pap smears are in the precancerous stage, which allows the clinician to implement appropriate therapy.

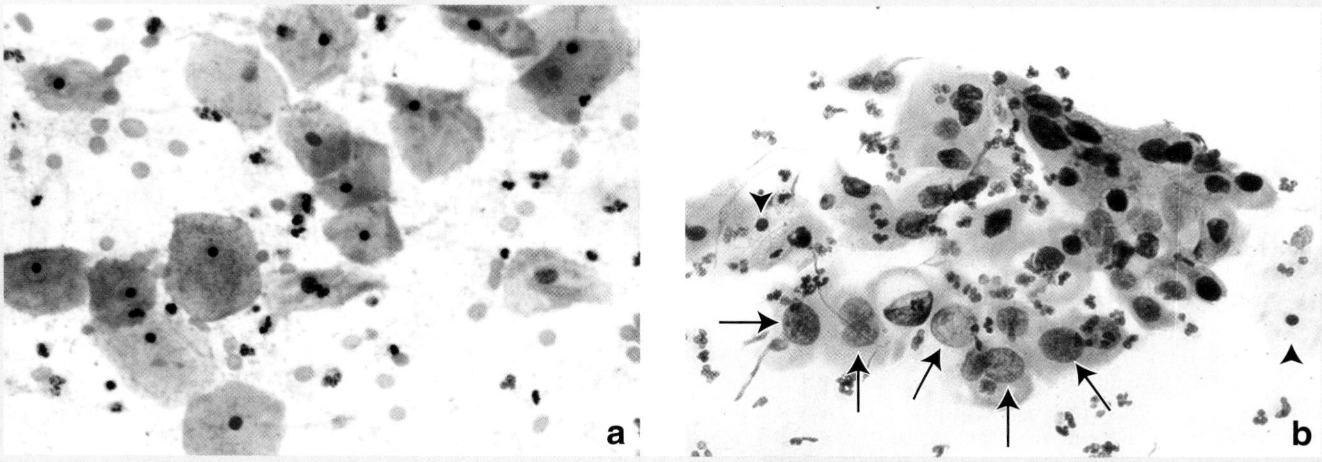

FIGURE 22.29
Photomicrographs of cervical smears. a. Negative cervical smear. The surface squamous cells reveal small pyknotic nuclei and abundant cytoplasm. Other cells in the micrograph include red blood cells and neutrophils. ×600. **b.** Abnormal smear. Many of the cells in this specimen contain large nuclei with no evidence of pyknosis *(arrows).* The cytoplasm is relatively scant. Other cells exhibit a more normal appearance with pyknotic nuclei and more surrounding cytoplasm *(arrowheads).* Neutrophils are also present. ×600.

(particularly neutrophils) are found in the lamina propria and migrate into the epithelium. Solitary lymphatic nodules may also be present. The number of lymphocytes and leukocytes in the mucosa and vaginal lumen dramatically increases around the time of menstrual flow. The vagina has few general sensory nerve endings. The sensory nerve endings that are more plentiful in the lower third of the vagina are probably associated primarily with pain and stretch sensations.

EXTERNAL GENITALIA

The female external genitalia consist of the following parts, which are collectively referred to as the ***vulva*** and have a stratified squamous epithelium:

- ***Mons pubis.*** The mons pubis is the rounded prominence over the pubic symphysis, formed by subcutaneous adipose tissue.

- ***Labia majora.*** The labia majora are two large longitudinal folds of skin, homologous to the skin of the scrotum, that extend from the mons pubis and form the lateral boundaries of the urogenital cleft. They contain a thin layer of smooth muscle that resembles the dartos muscle of the scrotum and a large amount of subcutaneous adipose tissue. The outer surface, like that of the mons pubis, is covered with pubic hair. The inner surface is smooth and devoid of hair. Sebaceous and sweat glands are present on both surfaces (Fig. 22.30).
- ***Labia minora.*** The labia minora are paired, hairless folds of skin that border the vestibule and are homologous to the skin of the penis. Abundant melanin pigment is present in the deep cells of the epithelium. The core of connective tissue within each fold is devoid of fat but does contain numerous blood vessels and fine elastic fibers. Large sebaceous glands are present in the stroma.
- ***Clitoris.*** The clitoris is an erectile structure that is homologous to the penis. Its body is composed of two small erectile bodies, the ***corpora cavernosa;*** the ***glans clitoris*** is a small, rounded tubercle of erectile tissue. The skin over the glans is very thin, forms the prepuce of the clitoris, and contains numerous sensory nerve endings.
- ***Vestibule.*** The vestibule is lined with stratified squamous epithelium. Numerous small mucous glands, the ***lesser vestibular glands*** (also called ***Skene's glands***), are present primarily near the clitoris and around the external urethral orifice. The large, paired ***greater vestibular glands*** (also called ***Bartholin's glands***) are homologous to the male bulbourethral glands. These tuboalveolar glands are about 1 cm in diameter and are located in the lateral wall of the vestibule posterior to the bulb of the vestibule. The greater vestibular glands secrete lubricating mucus. The ducts of these glands open into the vestibule near the vaginal opening.

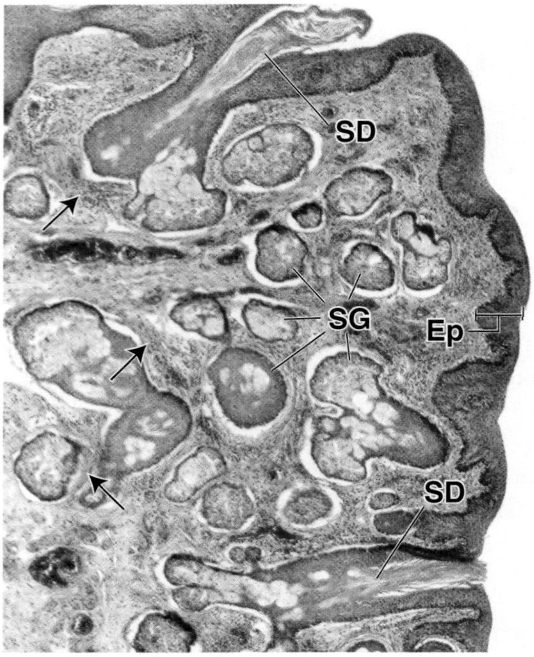

FIGURE 22.30
Photomicrograph of the inner surface of the labia majora. This low-power H&E–stained specimen of the labia majora's inner surface shows its nonkeratinized epithelium *(Ep)* and abundant sebaceous glands *(SG)*. Two sebaceous ducts *(SD)* are also evident. Note the continuity of the duct epithelium with the epithelium of the skin and the sebaceous gland epithelium. At this magnification, several smooth muscle bundles can be just barely discerned *(arrows)*.

Numerous sensory nerve endings are present in the external genitalia:

- ***Meissner's corpuscles*** are particularly abundant in the skin over the mons pubis and labia majora.
- ***Pacinian corpuscles*** are distributed in the deeper layers of the connective tissue and are found in the labia majora and in association with the erectile tissue. The sensory impulses from these nerve endings play an important role in the physiologic response during sexual arousal.
- ***Free nerve endings*** are present in large numbers and are equally distributed in the skin of the external genitalia.

MAMMARY GLANDS

The mammary glands, or breasts, are a distinguishing feature of mammals. During embryologic development, growth and development of breast tissue occur in both sexes. Multiple glands develop along paired epidermal thickenings, called ***mammary ridges (milk lines),*** which extend from the developing axilla to the developing inguinal region. In humans, normally only one group of cells develops into a breast on each side. An extra breast (polymastia) or nipple (polythelia) may occur as an inheritable condition in about 1% of the female population. These relatively rare conditions may also occur in males.

In males, little additional development of the mammary glands normally occurs in postnatal life, and the glands remain rudimentary. In females, the mammary glands undergo further development under hormonal influence. They are also influenced by changes in ovarian hormone levels during each menstrual cycle. The actual initiation of milk secretion is induced by prolactin secreted by the adenohypophysis. The ejection of the milk from the breast is stimulated by oxytocin released from the neurohypophysis. With the change in the hormonal environment at menopause, the glandular component of the breast regresses or involutes and is replaced by fat and connective tissue.

Mammary glands are modified apocrine sweat glands that develop under the influence of sex hormones

The inactive adult mammary gland is composed of 15 to 20 irregular lobes of branched tubuloalveolar glands (Fig.

22.31). The lobes, separated by fibrous bands of connective tissue, radiate from the ***mammary papilla***, or ***nipple***, and are further subdivided into numerous lobules. Some of the fibrous bands, called ***suspensory*** or ***Cooper's ligaments***, connect with the dermis. Abundant adipose tissue is present in the dense connective tissue of the interlobular spaces. The intralobular connective tissue is much less dense and contains little fat.

The epidermis of the adult nipple and areola is highly pigmented and somewhat wrinkled and has long dermal papillae invading into its deep surface (Fig. 22.32). It is covered by keratinized stratified squamous epithelium. The pigmentation of the nipple increases at puberty, and the nipple becomes more prominent. During pregnancy, the areola becomes larger and the degree of pigmentation increases further. Deep to the areola and nipple, bundles of smooth muscle fibers are arranged radially and circumferentially in the dense connective tissue and longitudinally along the lactiferous ducts. These muscle fibers allow the nipple to become erect in response to various stimuli.

The areola contains sebaceous glands, sweat glands, and modified mammary glands (glands of Montgomery). These glands, have a structure intermediate between sweat glands and true mammary glands, and produce small elevations on the surface of the areola. Numerous sensory nerve endings are present in the nipple; the areola contains fewer sensory nerve endings. The tubuloalveolar glands, derived from modified sweat glands in the epidermis, lie in the subcutaneous tissue. Each gland

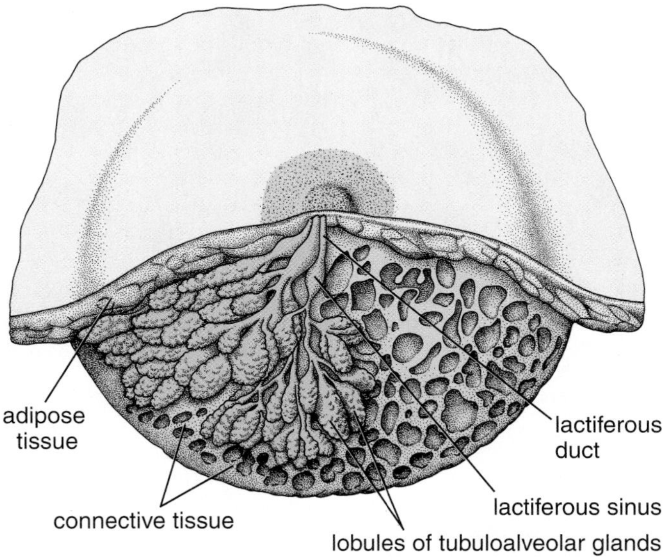

FIGURE 22.31
Schematic drawing of the human breast as seen during lactation. The breast is composed largely of branched tubuloalveolar glands contained within an extensive connective tissue stroma and variable amounts of adipose tissue. (Modified from Warwick R, Williams PL, eds. *Gray's Anatomy.* 35th ed. Edinburgh: Churchill Livingstone, 1973.)

ends in a ***lactiferous duct*** that opens through a constricted orifice onto the nipple. Beneath the ***areola***, the pigmented area surrounding the nipple, each duct has a dilated portion, the ***lactiferous sinus***. Near their openings, the lactiferous ducts are lined with stratified squamous epithelium. The epithelial lining of the duct shows a gradual transition from stratified squamous to two layers of cuboidal cells in the lactiferous sinus and finally to a single layer of columnar or cuboidal cells through the remainder of the duct system. Myoepithelial cells of ectodermal origin lie within the epithelium between the surface epithelial cells and the basal lamina. These cells, arranged in a basket-like network, are present in the secretory portion of the gland but are more apparent in the larger ducts.

The morphology of the secretory portion of the mammary gland varies with the menstrual cycle

In the *inactive gland,* the glandular component is sparse and consists chiefly of duct elements (Fig. 22.33). During the menstrual cycle, the inactive breast undergoes slight cyclic changes. Early in the cycle, the ducts appear as cords with little or no lumen. Under estrogen stimulation, at about the time of ovulation, the secretory cells increase in height, lumina appear in the ducts as small amounts of secretions accumulate, and fluid accumulates in the connective tissue.

Mammary glands undergo dramatic proliferation and development during pregnancy

The mammary glands exhibit a number of changes in preparation for lactation. The changes in the glandular tissue are accompanied by a decrease in the amount of connective tissue and adipose tissue. Plasma cells, lymphocytes, and eosinophils infiltrate the fibrous component of the connective tissue as the breast develops. The development of the glandular tissue is not uniform, and variation in the degree of development is seen even within a single lobule. The cells vary in shape from flattened to low columnar. As the cells proliferate by mitotic division, the ducts branch and alveoli begin to develop. In the later stages of pregnancy, alveolar development becomes more prominent (Fig. 22.34). The actual proliferation of the stromal cells declines, and subsequent enlargement of the breast occurs through hypertrophy of the secretory cells and accumulation of secretory product in the alveoli.

Both merocrine and apocrine secretion are involved in production of milk

The secreting cells contain abundant granular endoplasmic reticulum, a moderate number of large mitochondria, a supranuclear Golgi apparatus, and a number of

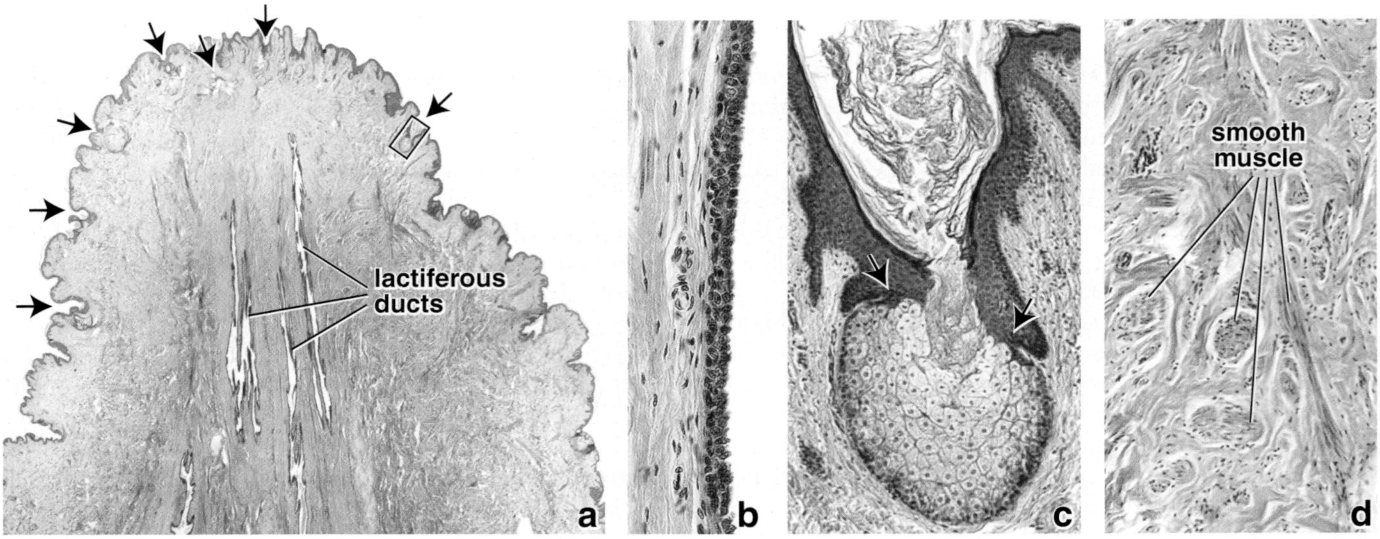

FIGURE 22.32

Photomicrographs of a section through the female nipple. a. This low-magnification micrograph of a H&E–stained sagittal section through the nipple shows the wrinkled surface contour, a thin stratified squamous epithelium, and associated sebaceous glands *(arrows)*. The core of the nipple consists of dense connective tissue, smooth muscle bundles, and the lactiferous ducts that open at the nipple surface. ×6. **b.** The wall of one of the lactiferous ducts is shown here at higher magnification. Its epithelium is stratified cuboidal, consisting of two cell layers. As it approaches the tip of the nipple it changes to a stratified squamous epithelium and becomes continuous with the epidermis. ×175. **c.** A higher magnification of the sebaceous gland from the *rectangle* in *a*. Note how the glandular epithelium is continuous with the epidermis *(arrows)* and the sebum is being secreted onto the epidermal surface. ×90. **d.** A higher magnification showing bundles of smooth muscle in longitudinal and cross-sectional profiles. ×350.

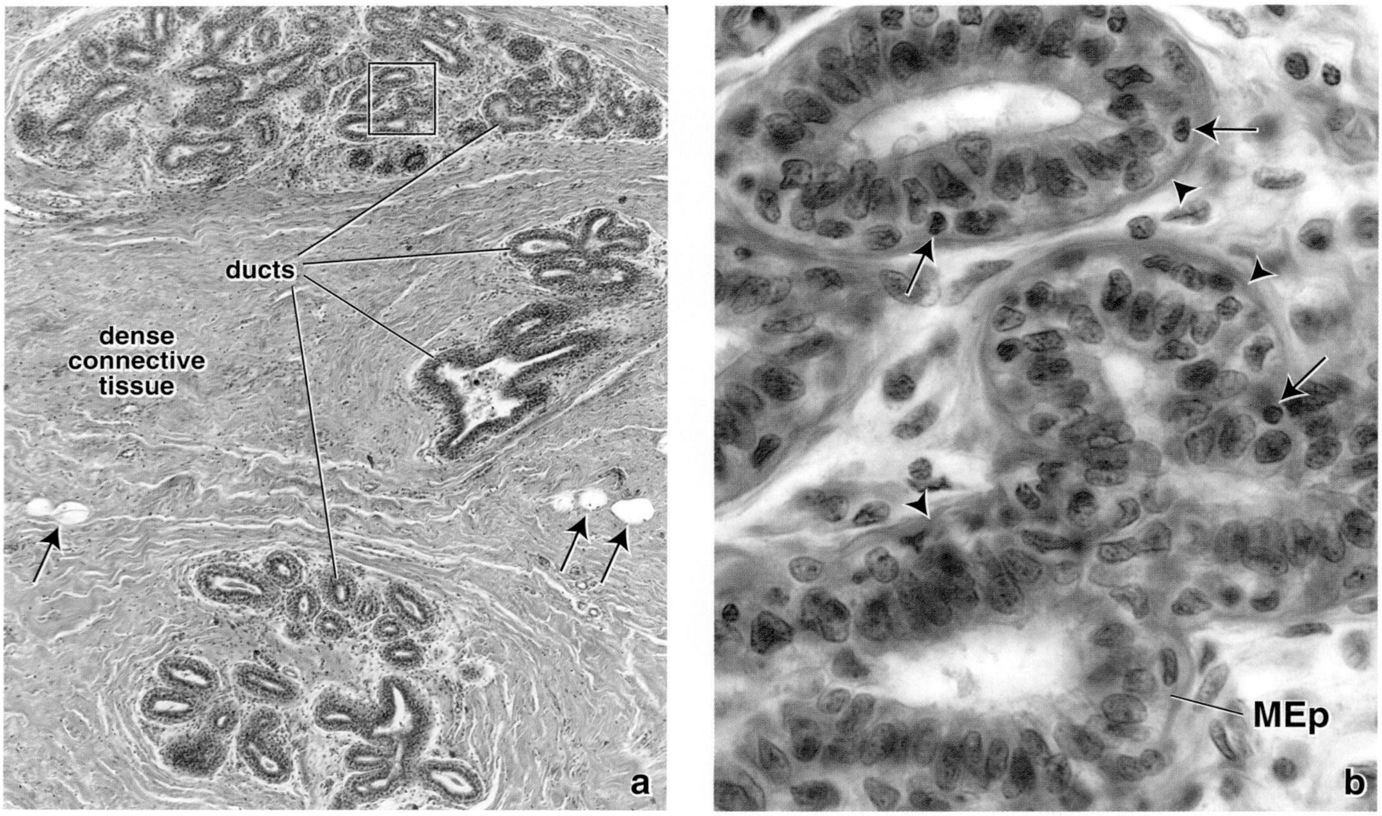

FIGURE 22.33

Photomicrograph of an inactive mammary gland. a. This low-magnification H&E–stained specimen shows several lobules within the dense connective tissue of the breast. The epithelial component consists of a branching duct system that makes up the lobule. The clear areas *(arrows)* are adipose cells. ×60. **b.** A higher magnification of the area in the *rectangle* of *a*. The epithelial cells of the ducts are columnar and exhibit interspersed lymphocytes *(arrows)* that have entered the epithelium. The surrounding stained material *(arrowheads)* represents the myoepithelial cells *(MEp)* and collagen bundles in the adjacent connective tissue. ×700.

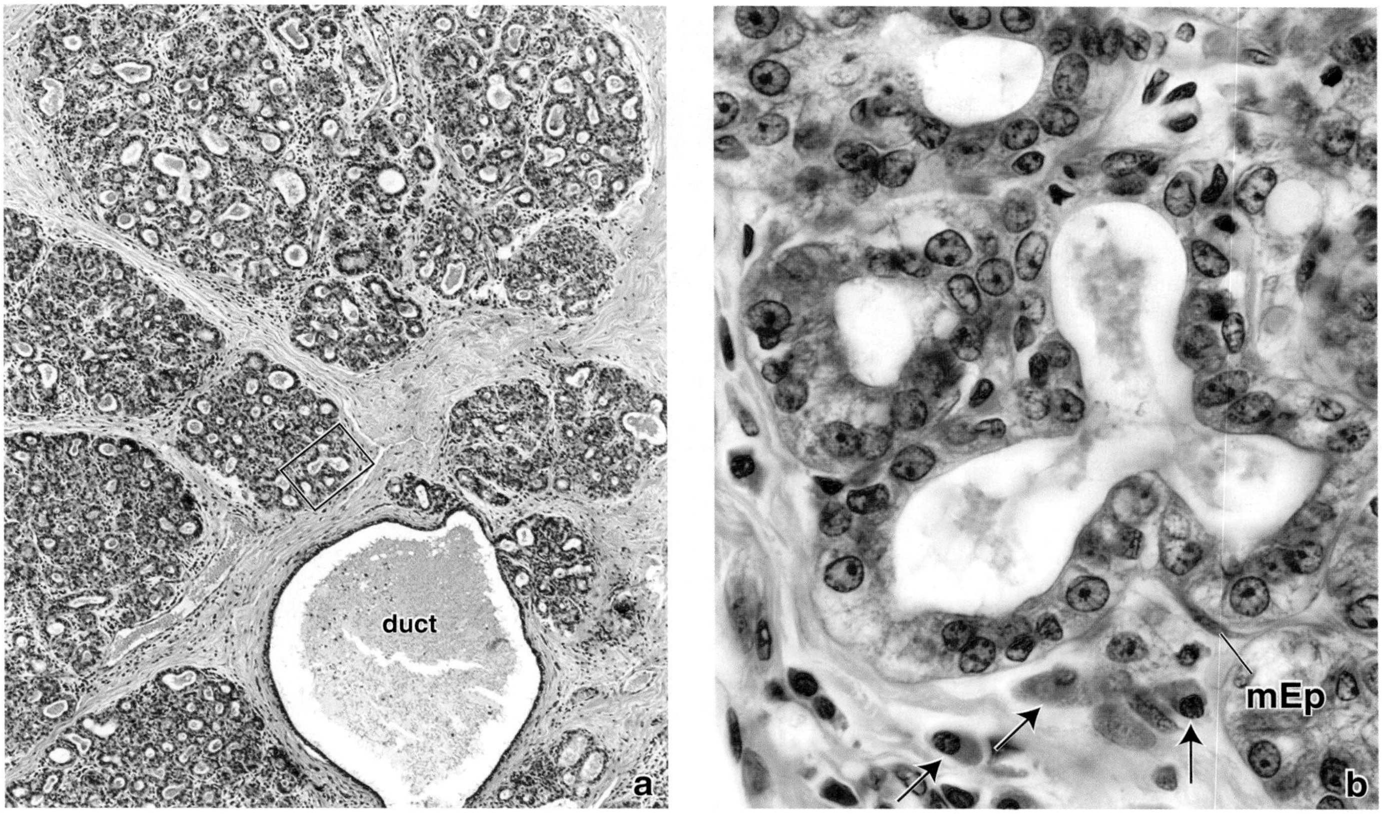

FIGURE 22.34
Photomicrograph of an active mammary gland during late pregnancy. a. This low-magnification H&E–stained specimen shows the marked proliferation of the duct system, giving rise to the secretory alveoli that constitute the major portion of the lobules. The intralobular ducts are difficult to identify, as their epithelium also secretes. Outside the lobules is a large excretory duct. ×60. **b.** A higher magnification of an area in *a*. The secretory alveolar cells are mostly cuboidal here. A myoepithelial cell *(mEp)* as well as a number of plasma cells *(arrows)* can be identified in the adjacent loose connective tissue. ×700.

dense lysosomes (Fig. 22.35). Depending on the secretory state, large lipid droplets and secretory vesicles may be present in the apical cytoplasm. The secretory cells produce two distinct products that are released by different mechanisms:

- *Merocrine secretion.* The protein component of the milk is synthesized in the rER, packaged into membrane-limited secretory vesicles for transport in the Golgi apparatus, and released from the cell by fusion of the vesicle's limiting membrane with the plasma membrane.
- *Apocrine secretion.* The fatty or lipid component of the milk arises as lipid droplets free in the cytoplasm. The lipid coalesces to form large droplets that pass to the apical region of the cell and project into the lumen of the acinus. The droplets are invested with an envelope of plasma membrane as they are released. A thin layer of cytoplasm is trapped between the plasma membrane and lipid droplet and is released with the lipid, but the *cytoplasmic loss in this process is minimal.*

The secretion released in the first few days after childbirth is known as ***colostrum***. This premilk is an alkaline, yellowish secretion with a higher protein, vitamin A, sodium, and chloride content and a lower lipid, carbohydrate, and potassium content than milk. It contains considerable amounts of antibodies that provide the newborn with some degree of passive immunity. The antibodies in the colostrum are believed to be produced by the lymphocytes and plasma cells that infiltrate the loose connective tissue of the breast during its proliferation and development and are secreted across the glandular cells as in salivary glands and intestine. As these wandering cells decrease in number after parturition, the production of colostrum stops, and lipid-rich milk is produced.

Hormonal Regulation of the Mammary Gland

The initial growth and development of the mammary gland at puberty occur under the influence of estrogens and progesterone produced by the maturing ovary. Sub-

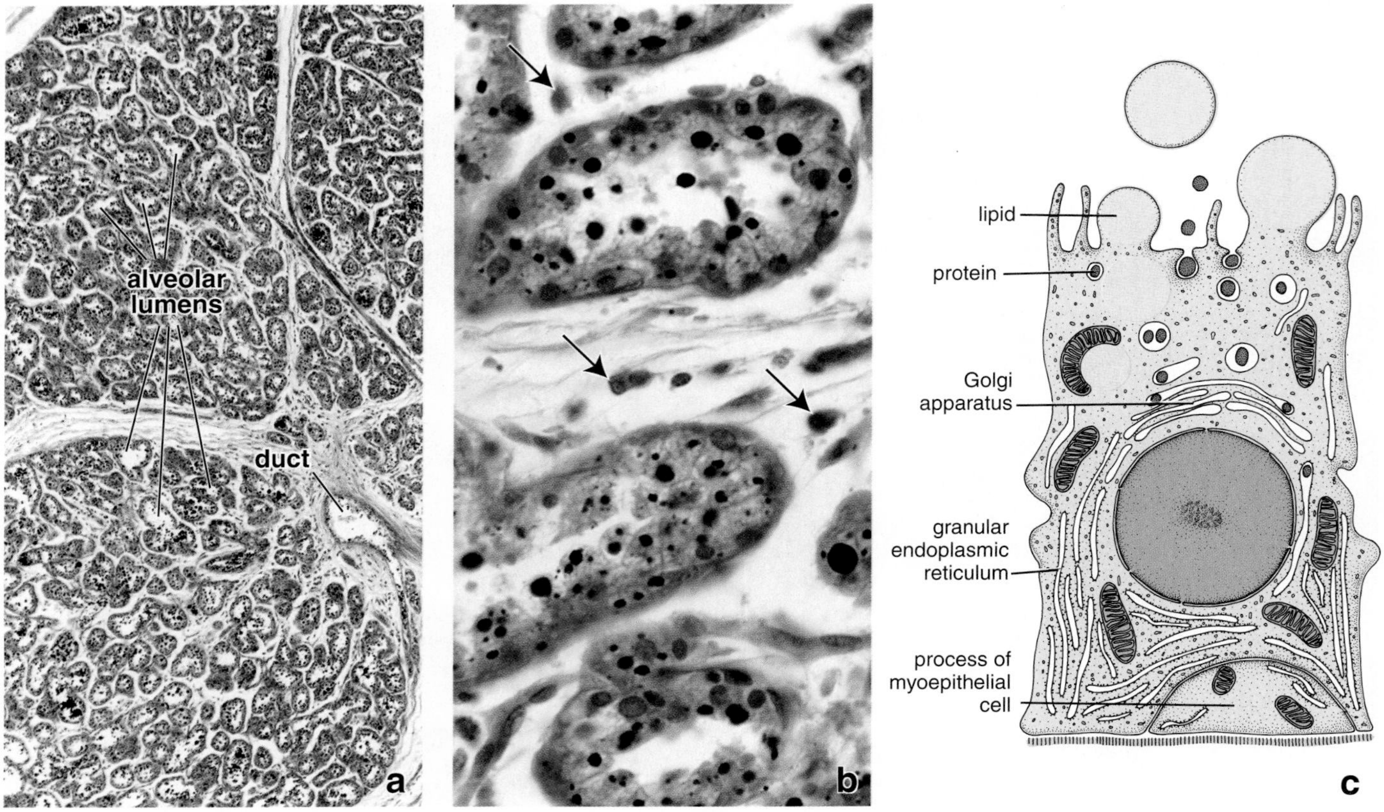

FIGURE 22.35

Photomicrographs and diagram of a lactating mammary gland. **a.** Low-magnification micrograph of a fast green-osmium–stained section of a lactating mammary gland. Portions of several large lobules and an excretory duct are seen. Many of the alveoli exhibit a prominent lumen, even at this magnification. ×60. **b.** A higher magnification of an area in *a* shows lipid droplets *(black circular profiles)* within the secretory cells of the alveoli as well as in the alveolar lumina. The *arrows* indicate plasma cells within the interstitial spaces. ×480. **c.** Diagram of a lactating mammary gland epithelial cell. (Redrawn after Bloom W, Fawcett DW. *A Textbook of Histology.* 10th ed. Philadelphia: WB Saunders, 1975.)

sequent to this initial development, slight changes in the morphology of the glandular tissue occur during each ovarian cycle. During pregnancy, the corpus luteum and placenta continuously produce estrogens and progesterone. Estrogen present in the circulation stimulates proliferation of the lactiferous duct components, and progesterone stimulates growth of alveoli. It is now believed that the growth of the mammary glands also depends on the presence of prolactin, produced by the adenohypophysis; hCS, produced by the placenta; and adrenal glucocorticoids.

Lactation is under the neurohormonal control of the adenohypophysis and hypothalamus

Although estrogen and progesterone are essential for the physical development of the breast during pregnancy, both of these hormones also suppress the effects of prolactin and hCS, the levels of which increase as pregnancy progresses. Immediately after birth, however, the sudden loss of estrogen and progesterone secretion from the placenta and corpus luteum allows the prolactin to assume its lactogenic role. Production of milk also requires adequate secretion of growth hormone, adrenal glucocorticoids, and parathyroid hormones.

The act of suckling during breast-feeding initiates sensory impulses from receptors in the nipple to the hypothalamus. The impulses inhibit the release of prolactin-inhibiting factor, and prolactin is then released from the adenohypophysis. The sensory impulses also cause the release of oxytocin in the neurohypophysis. Oxytocin stimulates the myoepithelial cells that surround the base of the alveolar secretory cells and the base of the cells in the larger ducts, causing them to contract and eject the milk from the alveoli and the ducts. In the absence of suckling, secretion of milk ceases, and the mammary glands begin to regress. The glandular tissue then returns to an inactive condition.

Involution of the Mammary Gland

The mammary gland atrophies or involutes after menopause. In the absence of ovarian hormone stimulation, the secretory cells of the alveoli degenerate and disappear, but some ducts may remain. The connective tissue also demonstrates degenerative changes, marked by a decrease in the number of fibroblasts and collagen fibers, and loss of elastic fibers.

Blood Supply and Lymphatics

The arteries that supply the breast are derived from the thoracic branches of the axillary artery, the internal thoracic (internal mammary) artery, and anterior intercostal arteries. Branches of the vessels pass primarily along the path of the alveolar ducts as they reach capillary beds surrounding the alveoli. Veins basically follow the path of the arteries as they return to the axillary and internal thoracic veins.

Lymphatic capillaries are located in the connective tissue surrounding the alveoli. The larger lymphatic vessels drain into axillary, supraclavicular, or parasternal lymph nodes.

BOX 22.6

Functional Considerations: Lactation and Infertility

Almost 50% of fully breast-feeding women exhibit ***lactational amenorrhea*** (lack of menstruation during lactation) and infertility. This effect is due to high levels of serum prolactin, which suppress secretion of LH. Ovulation usually resumes after 6 months or earlier with a decrease in suckling frequency. In cultures in which breast-feeding may continue for 2 to 3 years, lactational amenorrhea is the principal means of birth control.

Innervation

The nerves that supply the breast are anterior and lateral cutaneous branches from the second to sixth intercostal nerves. The nerves convey afferent and sympathetic fibers to and from the breast. The secretory function is primarily under hormonal control, but afferent impulses associated with suckling are involved in the reflex secretion of prolactin and oxytocin.

PLATE 88. OVARY I

The ovaries are small, paired, ovoid structures that exhibit a cortex and medulla when sectioned. On one side is a hilum for the transit of neurovascular structures; on this same side is a *mesovarium* that joins the ovary to the *broad ligament.* The functions of the ovary are the production of *ova* and the synthesis and secretion of *estrogen* and *progesterone.*

In the cortex are numerous *primordial follicles* that are present at the time of birth and that remain unchanged until sexual maturation. The oogonia in these follicles are arrested in prophase of the first meiotic division. At puberty, under the influence of pituitary *gonadotropins,* the ovaries begin to undergo the cyclical changes designated the *ovarian cycle.* During each cycle, the ovaries normally produce a single oocyte that is ready for fertilization.

At the beginning of the ovarian cycle, under the influence of pituitary *follicle-stimulating hormone* (*FSH*), some of the primordial follicles begin to undergo changes that lead to the development of a mature (*Graafian*) follicle. These changes include a proliferation of follicular cells and enlargement of the follicle. Although several primordial follicles begin these developmental changes, usually only one reaches maturity and yields an oocyte. Occasionally, two follicles will mature and ovulate, leading to the possibility of dizygotic twin development. The discharge of the oocyte and its adherent cells is called *ovulation.* At ovulation, the oocyte completes the first meiotic division. Only if fertilization occurs does the oocyte complete the second meiotic division. Whether or not fertilization occurs, the other follicles that began to proliferate in the same cycle degenerate, a process referred to as *atresia.*

Figure 1, ovary, monkey, H&E ×120.

The cortex of an ovary from a sexually mature individual is shown here. On the surface, there is a single layer of epithelial cells designated the germinal epithelium *(GEp).* This epithelium is continuous with the serosa (peritoneum) of the mesovarium. Contrary to its name, the epithelium does not give rise to the germ cells. The germinal epithelium covers a dense fibrous connective tissue layer, the tunica albuginea *(TA);* under the tunica albuginea are the primordial follicles *(PF).* It is not unusual to see follicles at various stages of development or atresia in the ovary. In this figure, along with the large number of primordial follicles, there are four growing follicles *(SF),* an atretic follicle *(AF),* and part of a large follicle on the right. The region of the large follicle shown in the figure includes the theca interna *(TI),* granulosa cells *(GC),* and part of the antrum *(A).*

Figure 2, ovary, monkey, H&E ×450.

When a *primordial* follicle begins the changes leading to the formation of a mature follicle, the layer of squamous follicular cells becomes cuboidal, as in this figure. In addition, the follicular cells proliferate and become multilayered. A follicle undergoing these early changes is called a *primary* follicle. Thus, an early primary follicle may still be unilaminar, but it is surrounded by cuboidal cells, and this distinguishes it from the more numerous unilaminar primordial follicles that are surrounded by squamous cells.

Figure 3, ovary, monkey, H&E ×450.

This figure shows several primordial follicles at higher magnification. Each follicle consists of an oocyte surrounded by a single layer of squamous follicular cells *(F).* The nucleus *(N)* of the oocyte is typically large, but the oocyte itself is so large that the nucleus is often not included in the plane of section, as in the oocyte marked *X.* The group of epithelioid-appearing cells *(arrowhead)* are follicular cells of a primordial follicle that has been sectioned in a plane that just grazes the follicular surface. In this case, the follicular cells are seen en face.

Figure 4, ovary, monkey, H&E ×450.

The primary follicle in this figure shows a multilayered mass of follicular cells *(FC)* surrounding the oocyte. The innermost layer of follicular cells is adjacent to a thick eosinophilic layer of extracellular homogeneous material called the zona pellucida *(ZP).* At this stage of development, the oocyte has also enlarged slightly. The entire structure surrounded by the zona pellucida is actually the oocyte.

Surrounding the follicles are elongate cells of the highly cellular connective tissue, referred to as stromal cells. The stromal cells surrounding a secondary follicle become disposed into two layers designated the theca interna and the theca externa. As seen in Figure 1, stromal cells become epithelioid in the cell-rich theca interna *(TI).*

KEY

A, antrum
AF, atretic follicle
F, follicle cells, primordial
FC, follicle cells
GEp, germinal epithelium
N, nucleus of oocyte
PF, primordial follicles
SF, growing follicles
TA, tunica albuginea
TI, theca interna
X, oocyte showing only cytoplasm
ZP, zona pellucida
arrowhead, follicle cells seen en face

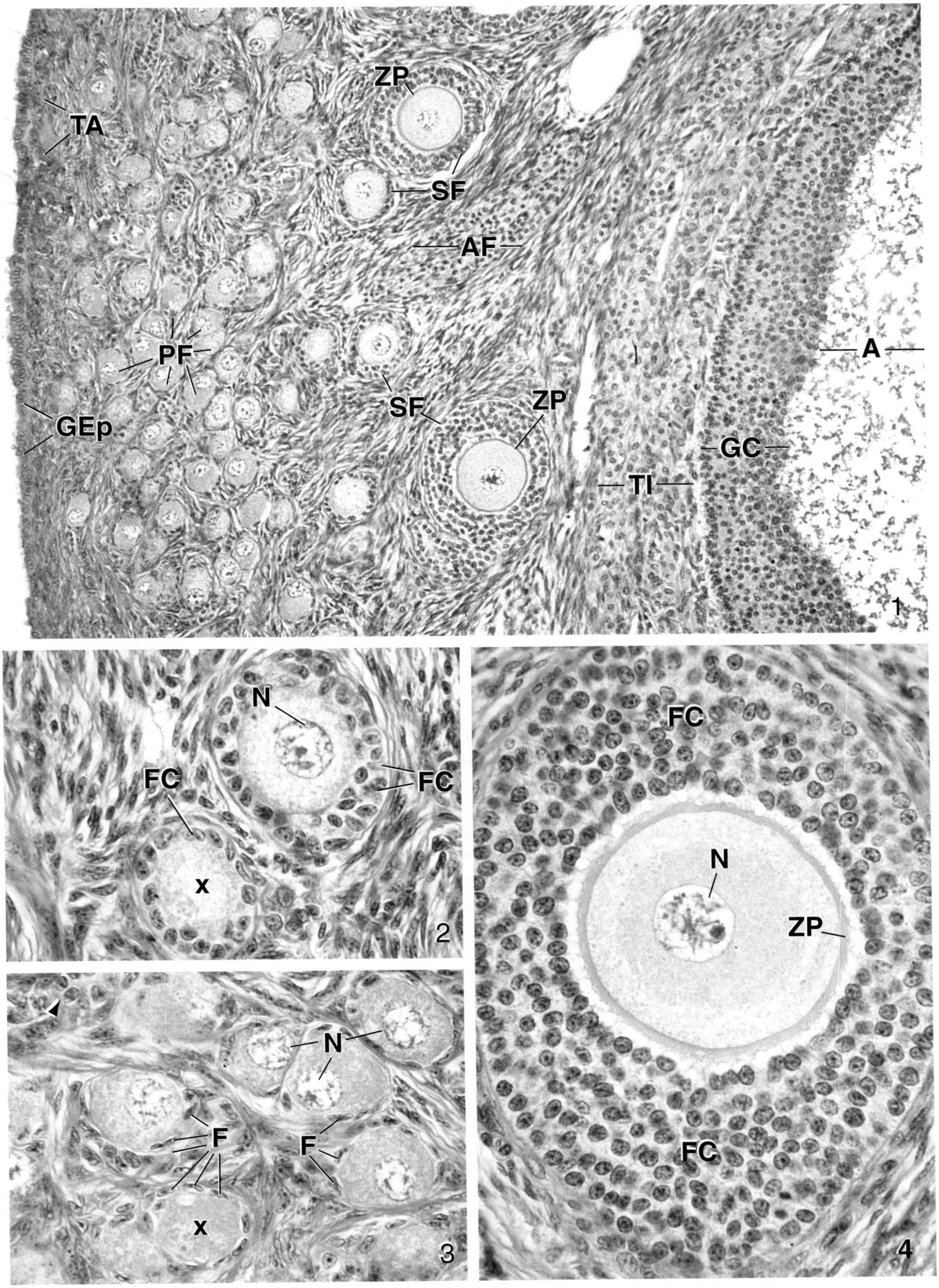

ZP
TA
SF
AF
PF
A
SF
ZP
GEp
GC
TI
1
N
FC
FC
x
2
N
F
F
x
3
FC
N
ZP
FC
4

PLATE 89. OVARY II

Atresia of follicles is a regular event in the ovary, beginning in embryonic life. In any section through the postpubertal ovary, follicles of various stages can be seen undergoing atresia. In atresia, the initial changes involve *pyknosis* of the nuclei of the follicular cells and dissolution of their cytoplasm. The follicle is then invaded by macrophages and other connective tissue cells. The oocyte degenerates, leaving behind the prominent *zona pellucida.* This may fold inward or collapse, but it usually retains its thickness and staining characteristics. When included in the plane of section, a distorted zona pellucida serves as a reliable diagnostic feature of an atretic follicle.

In atresia of large, nearly mature follicles, cells of the *theca interna* remain to form clusters of epithelioid cells in the ovarian cortex. These are referred to collectively as *interstitial glands* and continue to secrete steroid hormones.

Figures 1 and 2, ovary, monkey, H&E ×120.

Two follicles growing under the influence of FSH are shown in Figure 1. The more advanced follicle is a secondary follicle. The oocyte in this follicle is surrounded by several layers of follicular cells *(FC)* that, at this stage, are identified as granulosa cells. At a slightly earlier time, small lakes of fluid formed between the follicular cells, and these lakes have now fused into a well-defined larger cavity called the follicular antrum *(FA),* which is evident in the figure. The antrum is also filled with fluid and stains with the periodic acid–Schiff (PAS) reaction, although only lightly. The substance that stains with the PAS reaction has been retained as an eosinophilic precipitate in the antra of the secondary follicles shown here and in Figure 2. Immediately above the obvious secondary follicle is a slightly smaller follicle. Because no antral spaces are evident between the follicular cells, it is appropriate to classify it as a primary follicle. In both follicles, but particularly in the larger follicle with the antrum, the surrounding stromal cells have become altered to form two distinctive layers designated theca interna *(TI)* and theca externa *(TE).* The theca interna is a more cellular layer, and the cells are epithelioid. When seen with the electron microscope, they display the characteristics of endocrine cells, particularly steroid-secreting cells. In contrast, the theca externa is a connective tissue layer. Its cells are more or less spindle shaped.

In Figure 2, a later stage in the growth of the secondary follicle is shown. The antrum *(FA)* is larger, and the oocyte is off to one side, surrounded by a mound of follicular cells called the cumulus oophorus. The remaining follicular cells that surround the antral cavity are referred to as the membrana granulosa *(MG),* or simply granulosa cells.

Figure 3, ovary, monkey, H&E ×65.

Atretic follicles *(AF)* are shown here and at higher magnification in Figure 4. The two smaller atretic follicles can be identified by virtue of the retained zona pellucida *(ZP)* (see Fig. 4). The two larger, more advanced follicles do not display the remains of a zona pellucida, but they do display other features of follicular atresia.

Figure 4, ovary, monkey, H&E ×120.

In atresia of a more advanced follicle, the follicular cells tend to degenerate more rapidly than the cells of the theca interna, and the basement membrane separating the two becomes thickened to form a hyalinized membrane, the glassy membrane. Thus, the glassy membrane *(arrows)* separates an outer layer of remaining theca interna cells from the degenerating inner follicular cells. The remaining theca interna cells may show cytologic integrity *(RTI);* these intact theca cells remain temporarily functional in steroid secretion.

Figure 5, ovary, monkey, H&E ×120.

Additional atretic follicles *(AF)* are shown here. Again, some show remnants of a zona pellucida *(ZP),* and two show a glassy membrane *(arrows).* Note that even though the atresia in these follicles is well advanced, some of the cells external to one of the glassy membranes still retain their epithelioid character *(arrowhead).* These are persisting theca interna cells.

KEY

AF, atretic follicle
FA, antrum of follicle
FC, follicle cells
MG, membrana granulosa
RTI, remaining theca interna cells
TE, theca externa
TI, theca interna
ZP, zona pellucida
arrowhead, persisting theca interna cells
arrows, glassy membrane

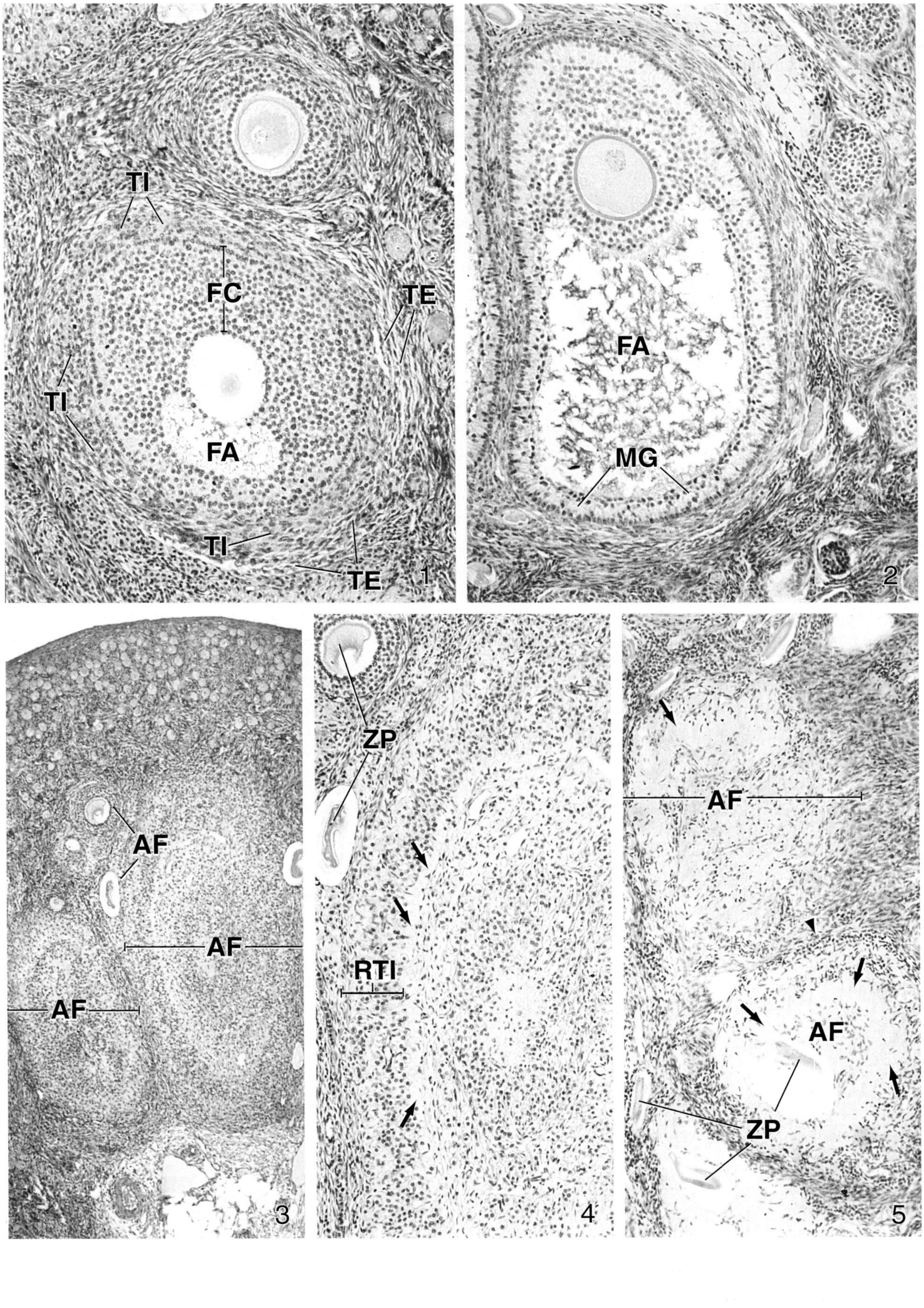
TI
FC
TE
TI
FA
TI
TE
1
FA
MG
2
AF
AF
AF
3
ZP
RTI
4
AF
AF
ZP
5

PLATE 90. CORPUS LUTEUM

After the oocyte and its immediately surrounding cells (i.e., the cells of the *cumulus oophorus*) are discharged from the mature ovarian follicle (ovulation), the remaining follicle cells *(membrana granulosa)* and the adjacent *theca interna* cells differentiate into a new functional unit, the *corpus luteum.*

The cells of the corpus luteum, *luteal cells,* rapidly increase in size and become filled with lipid droplets. A lipid-soluble pigment in the cytoplasm of the cells, *lipochrome,* gives them their yellow appearance in fresh tissue. Electron micrographs of the luteal cells demonstrate that they have features typical of steroid-secreting cells, namely, abundant smooth endoplasmic reticulum and mitochondria with tubular cristae. Two types of luteal cells are identified: Large, centrally located *granulosa lutein cells* are derived from the granulosa cells; smaller, peripherally located *theca lutein cells* are derived from the theca interna. A rich vascular network is established in the corpus luteum into which progesterone and estrogen are secreted by the lutein cells. These hormones stimulate growth and differentiation of the uterine endometrium to prepare it for implantation of a fertilized ovum.

Figure 1, corpus luteum, human, H&E ×20.

This figure shows ovarian cortex shortly after ovulation. The *arrowhead* points toward the surface of the ovary at the site of ovulation. The cavity *(FC)* of the former follicle has been invaded by connective tissue *(CT).* The membrana granulosa has become plicated, and the granulosa cells, now transforming into cells of the corpus luteum, are called granulosa lutein cells *(TC).* The plication of the membrana granulosa begins just before ovulation and continues as the corpus luteum develops. As the corpus luteum becomes more plicated, the former follicular cavity becomes reduced in size. At the same time, blood vessels *(BV)* from the theca of the follicle invade the former cavity and the transforming membrana granulosa cells. Cells of the theca interna follow the blood vessels into the outermost depressions of the plicated structure. These theca interna cells become transformed into cells of the corpus luteum called theca lutein cells.

Figure 2, corpus luteum, human, H&E ×20.

A portion of a fully formed corpus luteum is shown here. Most endocrine cells are the granulosa lutein cells *(GLC).* These form a folded cell mass that surrounds the remains of the former follicular cavity *(FC).* External to the corpus luteum is the connective tissue of the ovary *(CT).* Keep in mind that the theca interna was derived from the connective tissue stroma of the ovary. The location of theca lutein cells reflects this origin, and these cells *(TLC)* can be found in the deep outer recesses of the glandular mass, adjacent to the surrounding connective tissue.

Figures 3 and 4, corpus luteum, human, H&E ×65 (Fig. 3) and ×240 (Fig. 4).

A segment of the plicated corpus luteum is shown in Figure 3 at higher magnification. As noted above, the main cell mass is composed of granulosa lutein cells *(GLC).* On one side of this cell mass is the connective tissue *(CT)* within the former follicular cavity; on the other side are the theca lutein cells. The granulosa lutein cells contain a large spherical nucleus (see, also, *GLC,* Fig. 4) and a large amount of cytoplasm. The cytoplasm contains yellow pigment (usually not evident in routine H&E sections), hence the name, corpus luteum. Theca lutein cells also contain a spherical nucleus *(TLC),* but the cells are smaller than the granulosa lutein cells. Thus, when identifying the two cell types, aside from location, note that the nuclei of adjacent theca lutein cells generally appear to be closer to each other than nuclei of adjacent granulosa lutein cells. The connective tissue *(CT)* and small blood vessels that invaded the mass of granulosa lutein cells can be identified as the flattened and elongated components between the granulosa lutein cells.

The changes whereby the ruptured ovarian follicle is transformed into a corpus luteum occur under the influence of pituitary luteinizing hormone. In turn, the corpus luteum itself secretes progesterone, which has a profound effect on the estrogen-primed uterus. If pregnancy occurs, the corpus luteum remains functional; if pregnancy does not occur, the corpus luteum regresses after having reached a point of peak development, roughly 2 weeks after ovulation. The regressing cellular components of the corpus luteum are replaced by fibrous connective tissue, and the structure is then called a corpus albicans.

KEY

BV, blood vessels
CT, connective tissue
FC, former follicular cavity
GLC, granulosa lutein cells
TC, granulosa cells transforming into corpus luteum cells
TLC, theca lutein cells

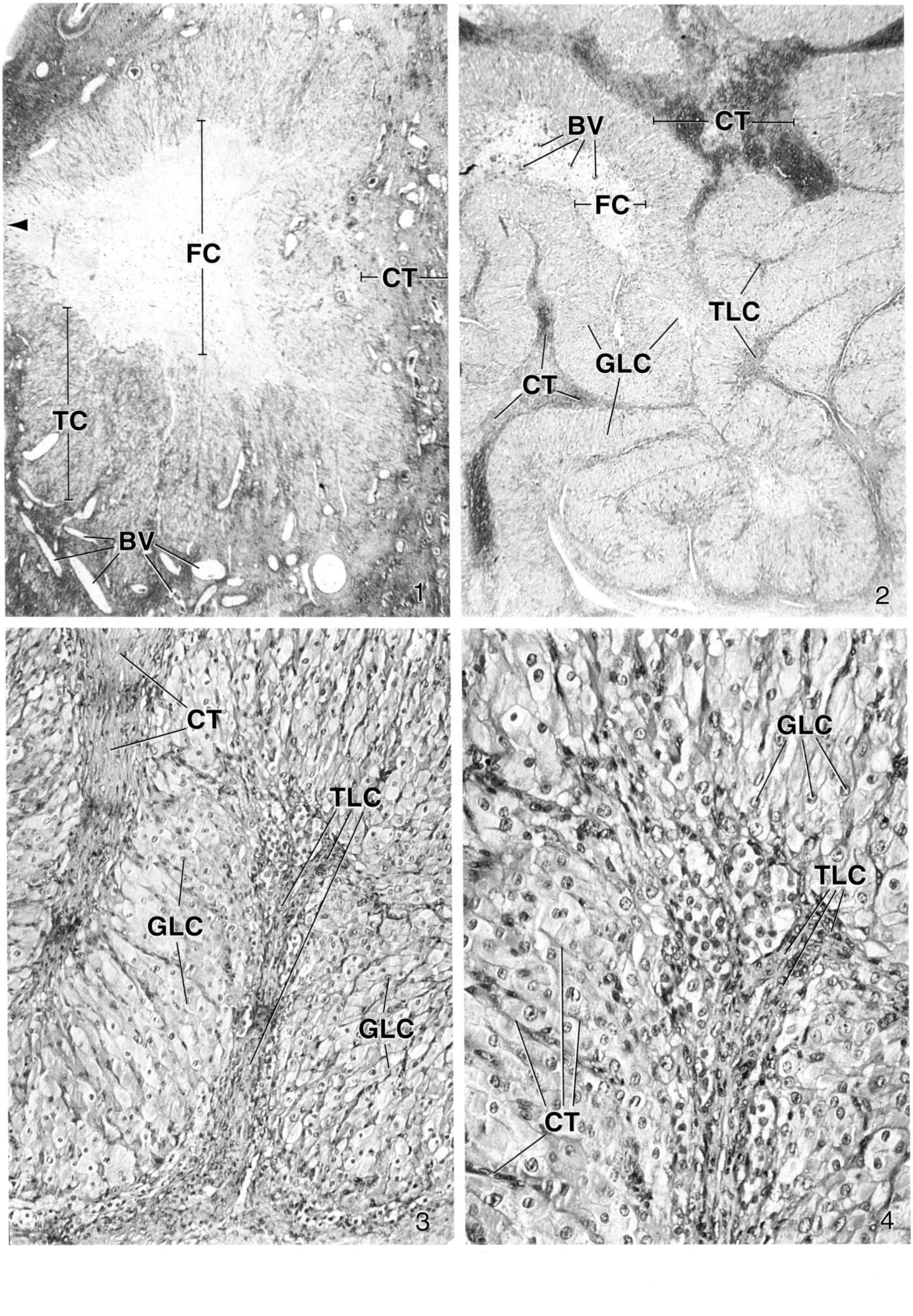
FC
CT
TC
BV
1
BV
CT
FC
TLC
GLC
CT
2
CT
TLC
GLC
GLC
3
GLC
TLC
CT
4

PLATE 91. OVIDUCT-UTERINE TUBE

The *oviducts* (uterine tubes, Fallopian tubes) are joined to the uterus and extend to the ovaries, where they present an open flared end (abdominal ostium) for entry of the ovum at ovulation. The oviduct undergoes cyclical changes along with those of the uterus, but these are not nearly as pronounced. The epithelial cells increase in height during the middle of the cycle, just about the time the ovum will be passing through the tube, and become reduced during the premenstrual period. Some of the epithelial cells are ciliated. The epithelial cells depend on the ovaries for their viability. Not only does the number of ciliated cells increase during the follicular phase of the ovarian cycle, but also removal of the ovaries leads to atrophy of the epithelium and loss of ciliated cells.

The uterine tube varies in size and degree of mucosal folding along its length. The mucosal folds are evident in its distal portion, the infundibulum, as it nears the open end. Near the opening, the tube flares outward and is called the *infundibulum.* It has fringed folded edges called *fimbria.* The infundibulum leads proximally to the *ampulla,* which constitutes about two thirds of the length of the oviduct, has the most numerous and complex mucosal folds, and is the site of fertilization. Mucosal folds are least numerous at the proximal end of the oviduct, near the uterus, where the tube is narrow and referred to as the *isthmus.* A *uterine* or *intramural* portion measures about 1 cm in length and passes through the uterine wall to empty into the uterine cavity.

Fertilization of the ovum usually occurs in the distal portion of the ampulla. For the first several days of development, as it navigates the complex pathway created by the mucosal folds, the embryo is transported proximally by the beating of the cilia of the ciliated epithelial cells and by peristaltic contractions of the well-developed muscularis layer that underlies the mucosa.

Figure 1, oviduct, human, H&E ×40.
A cross section through the ampulla of the tube is shown here. Many mucosal folds project into the lumen *(L),* and the complicated nature of the folds is evident by the variety of profiles that is seen. In addition to the mucosa *(Muc),* the remainder of the wall consists of a muscularis *(Mus)* and connective tissue.

The muscularis consists of smooth muscle that forms a relatively thick layer of circular fibers and a thinner outer layer of longitudinal fibers. The layers are not clearly delineated, and no sharp boundary separates them.

Figure 2, oviduct, human, H&E ×160; inset ×320.
The area enclosed by the *rectangle* in Figure 1 is shown here at higher magnification. The specimen shows a longitudinal section through a lymphatic vessel *(Lym).* In other planes of section, the lymphatic vessels are difficult to identify. The fortuitously sectioned lymphatic vessel is seen in the core of the mucosal fold, along with a highly cellular connective tissue *(CT)* and the blood vessels *(BV)* within the connective tissue. The epithelium lining the mucosa is shown in the **inset.** The ciliated cells are readily identified by the presence of well-formed cilia *(C).* Nonciliated cells, also called peg cells *(PC),* are readily identified by the absence of cilia; moreover, they have elongate nuclei and sometimes appear to be squeezed between the ciliated cells. The connective tissue *(CT)* contains cells whose nuclei are arranged typically in a random manner. They vary in shape, being elongated, oval, or round. Their cytoplasm cannot be distinguished from the intercellular material **(inset).** The character of the connective tissue is essentially the same from the epithelium to the muscularis, and for this reason, no submucosa is described.

KEY

BV, blood vessels
C, cilia
CT, connective tissue
Ep, epithelium
L, lumen
Lym, lymphatic vessel
Muc, mucosa
Mus, muscularis
PC, peg cells

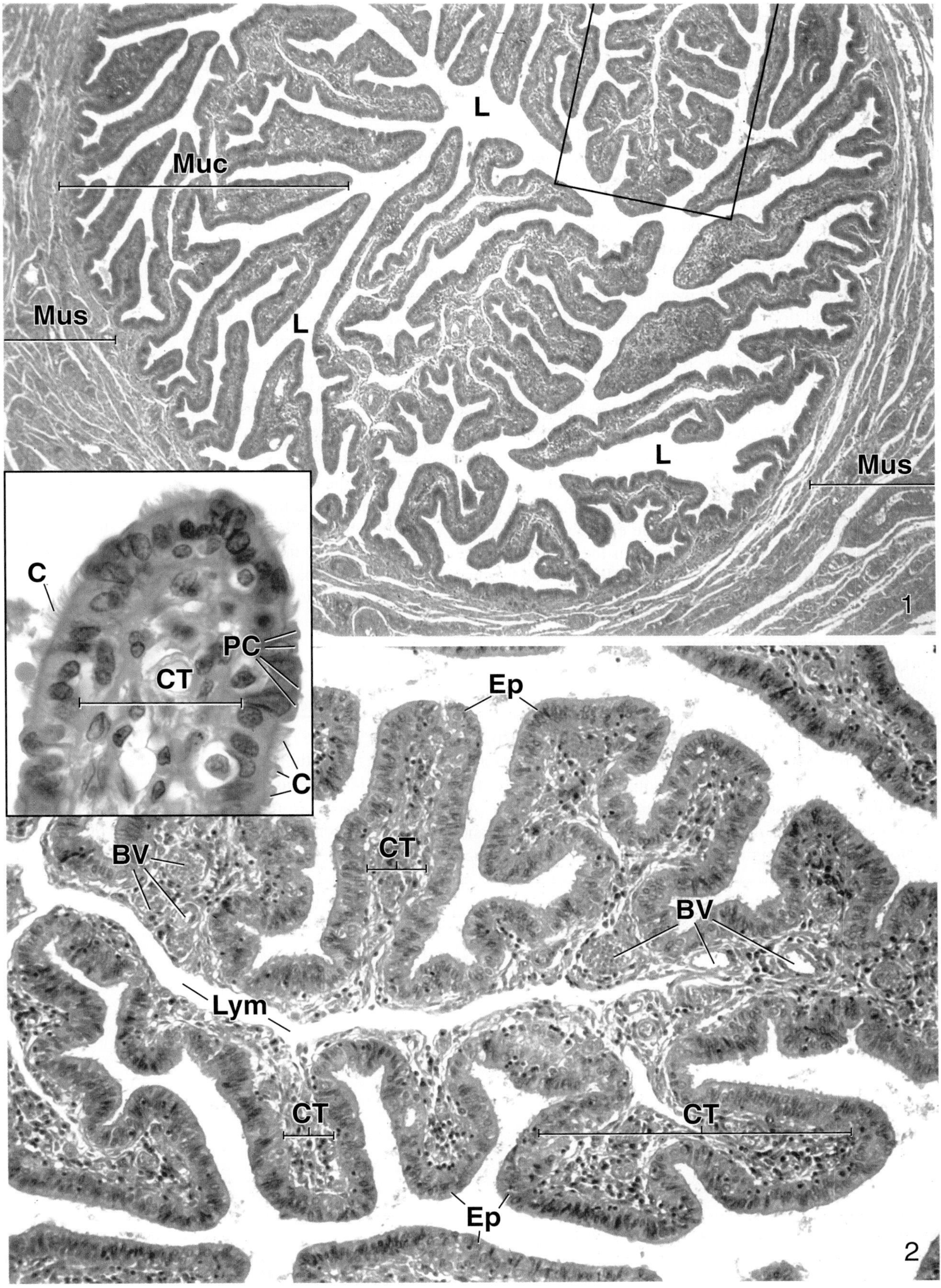
L
Muc
Mus
L
L
Mus
1
C
PC
CT
C
C
Ep
CT
BV
BV
Lym
CT
CT
Ep
2

PLATE 92. UTERUS I

The uterus is a hollow, pear-shaped organ with a thick wall and, in the nonpregnant state, a narrow cavity. The uterine wall is composed of a mucosa, referred to as the *endometrium;* a muscularis, referred to as a *myometrium;* and, externally, a serosal cover, the *perimetrium.* The myometrium consists of smooth muscle and connective tissue and contains the large blood vessels that give rise to the vessels that supply the endometrium.

The uterus undergoes cyclical changes that are largely manifested by changes that occur in the endometrium. If implantation of an ovum does not occur after preparation for this event, the state of readiness is not maintained, and much of the endometrium degenerates and is sloughed off, constituting the menstrual flow. The part of the endometrium that is lost is referred to as the *stratum functionale;* the part that is retained is called the *stratum basale.* The stratum basale is the deeper part of the endometrium and adjoins the myometrium.

The myometrium also undergoes changes associated with implantation of a zygote. In the nonpregnant uterus, the smooth muscle cells are about 50 μm in length; during pregnancy, they undergo enormous hypertrophy, often reaching more than 500 μm in length. In addition, new muscle fibers develop after division of existing muscle cells and division and differentiation of undifferentiated mesenchymal cells. The connective tissue also increases to strengthen the uterine wall. Fibroblasts increase by division and secrete additional collagen and elastic fibers. After parturition, the uterus nearly returns to its normal size. Most muscle fibers return to their normal size, and some degenerate. Collagen secreted during pregnancy is digested by the very cells that secreted it, the fibroblasts. Similar, but less pronounced, proliferation and degeneration of fibroblasts and collagen occur in each menstrual cycle.

Figure 1, uterus, human, H&E ×25; inset ×120.

After the stratum functionale *(SF)* is sloughed off, resurfacing of the raw tissue occurs. The epithelial resurfacing comes from the glands that remain in the stratum basale *(SB).* The gland epithelium simply proliferates and grows over the surface. This figure shows the endometrium as it appears when resurfacing is complete. The area inscribed in the *upper small rectangle* is shown at higher magnification in the **inset** on the right. Note the simple columnar epithelium *(SEp)* that covers the endometrial surface and its similarity to the glandular epithelium *(Gl).* The endometrium is relatively thin at this stage, and over half of it consists of the stratum basale. The area inscribed by the *lower small rectangle,* located in the region of the stratum basale, is shown at higher magnification in the **inset** in Figure 2. The glandular epithelium of the deep portion of the glands is similar to that of the endometrial surface. Below the endometrium is the myometrium *(M),* in which a number of large blood vessels *(BV)* are present.

Figure 2, uterus, human, H&E ×25; inset ×120.

Under the influence of estrogen, the various components of the endometrium proliferate (proliferative stage), so that the total thickness of the endometrium is increased. As shown in this figure, the glands *(Gl)* become rather long and follow a fairly straight course within the stratum functionale *(SF)* to reach the surface. The stratum basale *(SB)* remains essentially unaffected by the estrogen and appears much the same as in Figure 1. In this figure, the stratum functionale *(SF),* on the other hand, has increased in thickness and constitutes about four fifths of the endometrial thickness.

KEY

BV, blood vessels
Gl, glands
M, myometrium
SB, stratum basale
SEp (inset, Fig. 1), surface epithelium
SF, stratum functionale

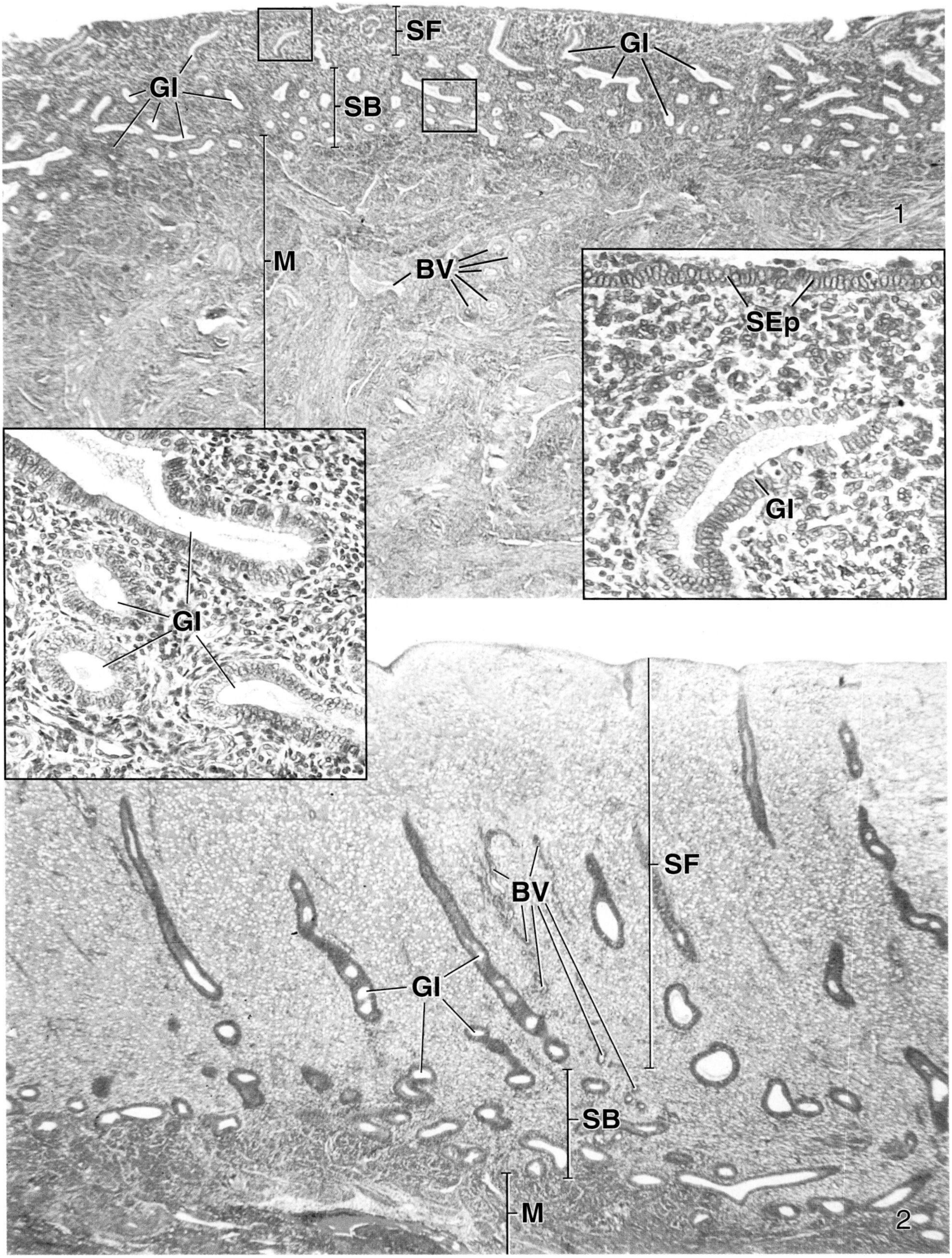
SF
Gl
Gl
SB
M
BV
1
SEp
Gl
Gl
BV
SF
Gl
SB
M
2

PLATE 93. UTERUS II

After *estrogen* brings about the uterine events designated the proliferative stage, another hormone, *progesterone,* influences additional uterine changes that constitute the secretory stage of the uterine cycle. This hormone brings the endometrium to a state of readiness for implantation, and as a consequence of its actions, the thickness of the endometrium increases further. There are conspicuous changes in the glands, primarily in the stratum functionale, where the glands take on a more pronounced corkscrew shape and secrete mucus that accumulates in sacculations along their length.

The vasculature of the endometrium also proliferates and degenerates in each menstrual cycle. *Radial arteries* enter the stratum basale of the endometrium from the myometrium and give rise to small, straight arteries that supply the stratum basale and continue into the endometrium to become the highly coiled *spiral arteries.* Arterioles derived from the spiral arteries supply the stratum functionale. The distal portion of the spiral arteries and the arterioles are sloughed with the stratum functionale during menstruation. Alternating contraction and relaxation of the basal portions of the spiral arteries prevent excessive blood loss during menstruation.

Figure 1, uterus, human, H&E ×25.

This view of the endometrium in the secretory stage shows the stratum functionale *(SF),* the stratum basale *(SB),* and, in the lower left of the photomicrograph, a small amount of the myometrium *(M).* The uterine glands have been cut in a plane that is close to their long axes, and one gland *(arrow)* is seen opening at the uterine surface. Except for a few glands near the center of the figure that resemble those of the proliferative stage, most of the glands *(Gl)* in this figure, including those that are labeled, show numerous shallow sacculations that give the profile of the glandular epithelium a serrated appearance. This is one of the distinctive features of the secretory stage. It is seen most advantageously in areas where the plane of section is close to the long axis of the gland. In contrast to the characteristic sinuous course of the glands in the stratum functionale, glands of the stratum basale more closely resemble those in the proliferative stage. They are not oriented in any noticeable relationship to the uterine surface, and many of their long profiles are even parallel to the plane of the surface.

Figure 2, uterus, human, H&E ×30; inset ×120.

This slightly higher magnification view of the stratum functionale shows essentially the same characteristics of the glands *(Gl)* described above; it also shows other modifications that occur during the secretory stage. One of these is that the endometrium becomes edematous. The increase in endometrial thickness because of edema is reflected by the presence of empty spaces between cells and other formed elements. Thus, many areas of this figure, especially the area within and near the *rectangle,* show histologic signs of edema.

In addition, in this stage the glandular epithelial cells begin to secrete a mucoid fluid that is rich in glycogen. This product is secreted into the lumen of the glands, causing them to dilate. Typically, the glands of the secretory endometrium are more dilated than those of the proliferative endometrium.

The *rectangle* in this figure highlights two glands that are shown at higher magnification in the **inset.** Each of these glands contains some substance within the lumen. The mucoid character of the substance within one of the glands can be surmised from its blue staining. Although not evident in routine H&E paraffin sections, the epithelial cells also contain glycogen during the secretory stage, and as mentioned above, this becomes part of the secretion. The *arrowheads* indicate stromal cells; some of these cells undergo enlargement late in the secretory stage. These modified stromal cells, called decidual cells, play a role in implantation.

KEY

Gl, glands	**SB,** stratum basale	**arrow,** glandular opening at uterine surface
M, myometrium	**SF,** stratum functionale	**arrowheads,** stromal cells

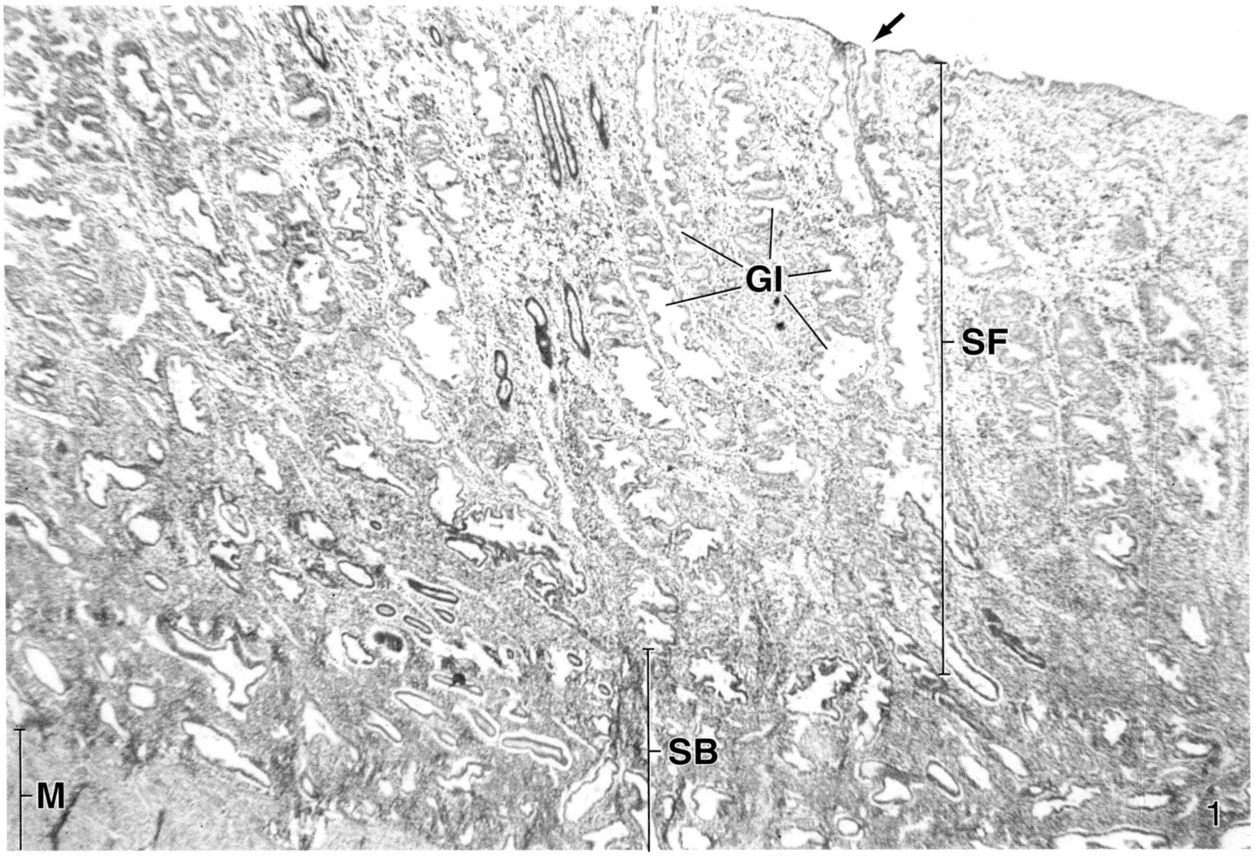
GI
SF
SB
M
1

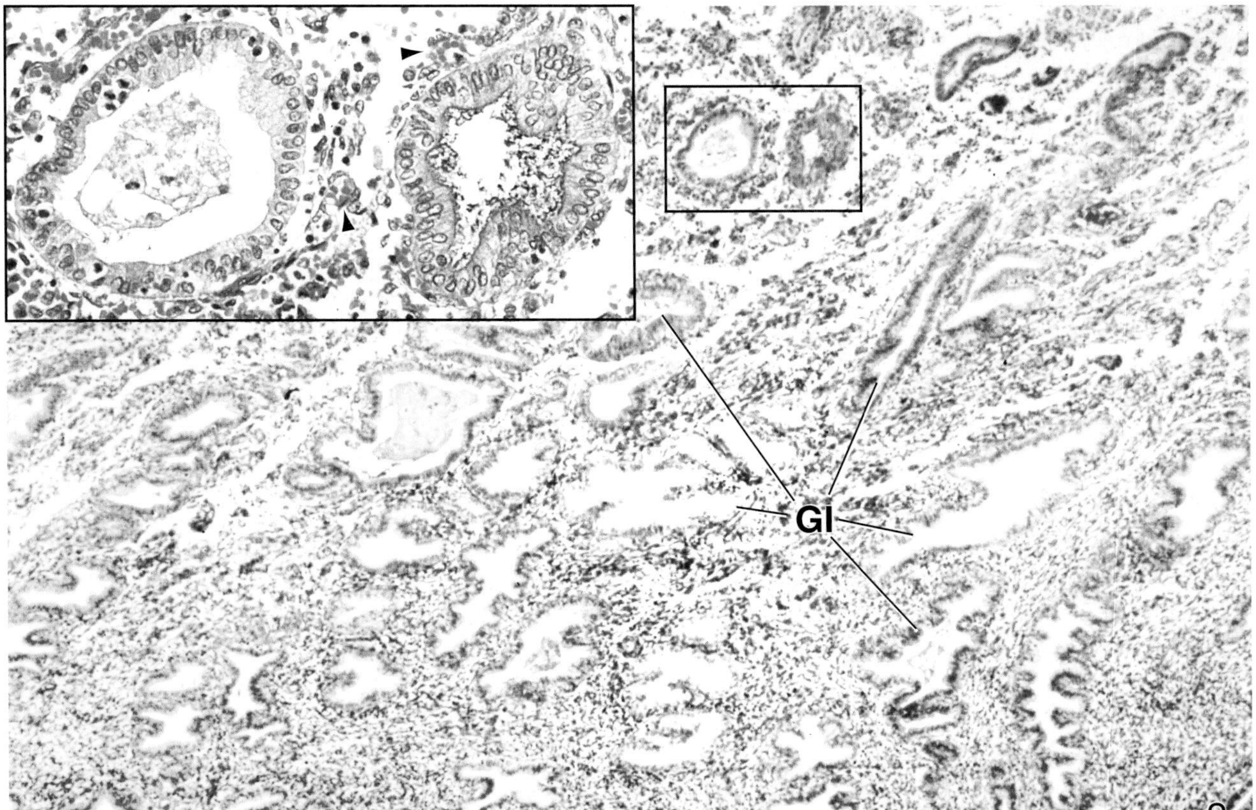
GI
2

PLATE 94. CERVIX

The *cervix* is the narrow or constricted inferior portion of the uterus, part of which projects into the vagina. The cervical canal traverses the cervix and provides a channel connecting the vagina and the uterine cavity. The structure of the cervix resembles the rest of the uterus in that it consists of a mucosa (endometrium) and a myometrium. There are, however, some important differences in the mucosa.

The endometrium of the cervix does not undergo the cyclical growth and loss of tissue that is characteristic of the body and fundus of the uterus. Rather, the amount and character of the mucous secretion of its simple columnar epithelium vary at different times in the uterine cycle under the influence of the ovarian hormones. At midcycle, there is a 10-fold increase in the amount of mucus produced; this mucus is less viscous and provides a favorable environment for sperm migration. At other times in the cycle, the mucus restricts the passage of sperm into the uterus.

The myometrium forms the major thickness of the cervix. It consists of interweaving bundles of smooth muscle cells in an extensive, continuous network of fibrous connective tissue.

Figures 1 and 2, cervix, human, H&E ×15.

The portion of the cervix that projects into the vagina, the portio vaginalis, is represented by the upper two thirds of Figure 1. The lower third of the micrograph reveals the supravaginal portion of the cervix (portio supravaginalis). Figure 2 shows the supravaginal cervix at a slightly higher level than in Figure 1. The plane of section in both figures passes through the long axis of the cervical canal. The cervical canal *(CC)* is narrowed and cone shaped at its two ends. The upper end, the ***internal os***, communicates with the uterine cavity, and the lower end, the ***external os*** *(Os)*, communicates with the vagina. (For purposes of orientation, realize that only one side of the longitudinal section of the cervix is shown in these figures and that the actual specimen, as seen in a section, would present a similar image on the other side of the cervical canal.)

The mucosa *(Muc)* of the cervix differs according to the cavity it faces. The *two rectangles* in Figure 1 delineate representative areas of the mucosa that are shown at higher magnification in Figures 3 and 4, respectively.

Figure 2 emphasizes the nature of the cervical glands *(Gl)*. The glands differ from those of the uterus in that they branch extensively. They secrete a mucous substance into the cervical canal that serves to lubricate the vagina.

Figure 3, cervix, human, H&E ×240.

The surface of the portio vaginalis is stratified squamous epithelium *(SSEp)*. The epithelium–connective tissue junction presents a relatively even contour in contrast to the irregular profile seen in the vagina. In other respects, the epithelium has the same general features as the vaginal epithelium. Another similarity is that the epithelial surface of the portio vaginalis undergoes cyclical changes similar to those of the vagina in response to ovarian hormones. The mucosa of the portio vaginalis, like that of the vagina, is devoid of glands.

Figure 4, cervix, human, H&E ×240.

The mucosa of the cervical canal is covered with columnar epithelium. An abrupt change from stratified squamous epithelium *(SSEp)* to simple columnar epithelium *(CEp)* occurs at the opening of the cervical canal (external os). The *lower rectangle* in Figure 1 marks this site, known as the transition zone, which is shown at higher magnification here. Note the abrupt change in the epithelium at the point indicated by the *diamond-shaped marker,* as well as the large number of lymphocytes present in this region (compare with Fig. 3).

Figure 5, cervix, human, H&E ×500.

Figure 5 shows, at high magnification, portions of the gland identified in the *rectangle* in Figure 2. Note the tall epithelial cells and the lightly staining supranuclear cytoplasm, a reflection of the mucin dissolved out of the cell during tissue preparation. The crowding and the change in shape of the nuclei *(asterisk)* seen at the upper part of one of the glands in this figure are due to a tangential cut through the wall of the gland as it passed out of the plane of section. (It is not uncommon for cervical glands to develop into cysts as a result of obstruction in the duct. Such cysts are referred to as Nabothian cysts.)

KEY

BV, blood vessels
CC, cervical canal
CEp, columnar epithelium
Gl, cervical glands
Muc, mucosa
Os, ostium of the uterus
SSEp, stratified squamous epithelium
asterisk (Fig. 5), tangential cut of the epithelial surface

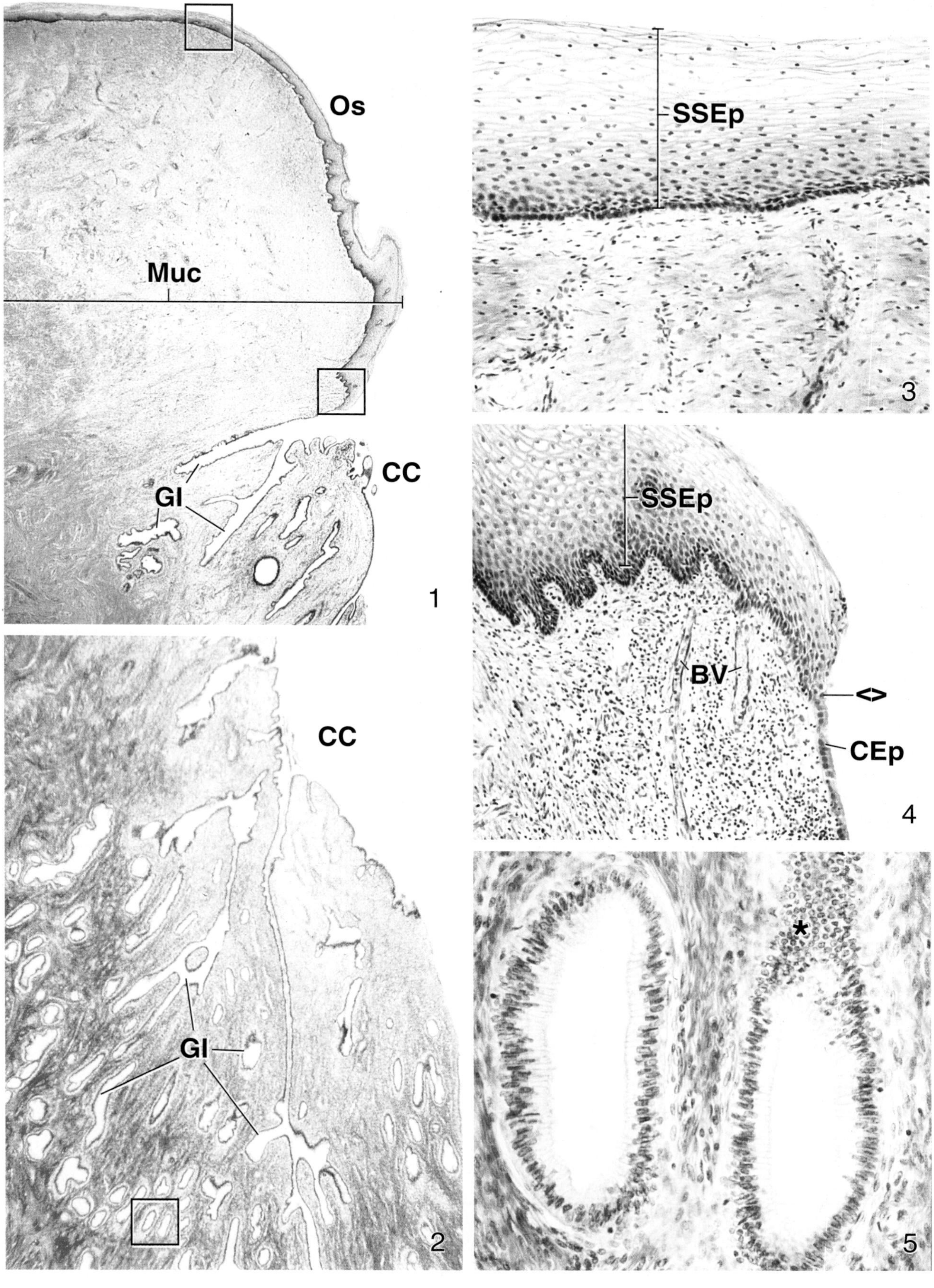
Os
Muc
CC
Gl
1
CC
Gl
2
SSEp
3
SSEp
BV
<>
CEp
4
*
5

PLATE 95. PLACENTA I

The *placenta* is a disk-shaped organ that serves for the exchange of materials between the fetal and maternal circulations during pregnancy. It develops primarily from embryonic tissue, the *chorion frondosum.* One side of the placenta is embedded in the uterine wall at the basal plate. The other side faces the amniotic cavity that contains the fetus. After birth, the placenta separates from the wall of the uterus and is discharged along with the contiguous membranes of the amniotic cavity.

The *umbilical cord* connects the fetus to the placenta. It contains two arteries that carry blood from the fetus to the placenta and a vein that returns blood from the placenta to the fetus. The umbilical arteries have thick muscular walls. These are arranged as two layers, an inner longitudinal layer and an outer circular layer. Elastic lamellae are poorly developed in these vessels and, indeed, may be absent. The umbilical vein is similar to the arteries, also having a thick muscular wall arranged as an inner longitudinal and an outer circular layer.

Figure 1, placenta, human, H&E ×16.

A section extending from the amniotic surface into the substance of the placenta is shown here. This includes the amnion *(A),* the chorionic plate *(CP),* and the chorionic villi *(CV).* The amnion consists of a layer of simple cuboidal epithelium and an underlying layer of connective tissue. The connective tissue of the amnion is continuous with the connective tissue of the chorionic plate as a result of their fusion at an earlier time. The plane of fusion, however, is not evident in H&E sections; the separation *(asterisks)* in parts of this figure in the vicinity of the fusion is an artifact.

The chorionic plate is a thick connective tissue mass that contains the ramifications of the umbilical arteries and vein. These vessels *(BVp)* do not have the distinct organizational features characteristic of arteries and veins; rather, they resemble the vessels of the umbilical cord. Although their identification as blood vessels is relatively simple, it is difficult to distinguish which vessels are branches of an umbilical artery and which are tributaries of the vein.

The main substance of the placenta consists of chorionic villi of different sizes (see Plate 96). These emerge from the chorionic plate as large stem villi that branch into increasingly smaller villi. Branches of the umbilical arteries and vein *(BVv,* Fig. 2*)* enter the stem villi and ramify through the branching villous network. Some villi extend from the chorionic plate to the material side of the placenta and make contact with the maternal tissue; these are called ***anchoring villi.*** Other villi, the ***free villi,*** simply arborize within the substance of the placenta without anchoring onto the maternal side.

Figure 2, placenta, human, H&E ×70; inset ×370.

The maternal side of the placenta is shown in this figure. The basal plate, or ***stratum basale*** *(SB),* is on the right side of the illustration. This is the part of the uterus to which the chorionic villi anchor. Along with the usual connective tissue elements, the basal plate contains specialized cells called ***decidual cells*** *(DC).* The same cells are shown at higher magnification in the **inset.** Decidual cells are usually found in clusters and have an epithelial appearance. Because of these features, they are easily identified.

Septa from the basal plate extend into the portion of the placenta that contains the chorionic villi. The septa do not contain the branches of the umbilical vessels and, on this basis, can frequently be distinguished from stem villi or their branches.

KEY

A, amnion
BVp, blood vessels in chorionic plate
BVv, blood vessels in chorionic villi
CP, chorionic plate
CV, chorionic villi
DC, decidual cells
SB, stratum basale
asterisk, separation that is actually an artifact

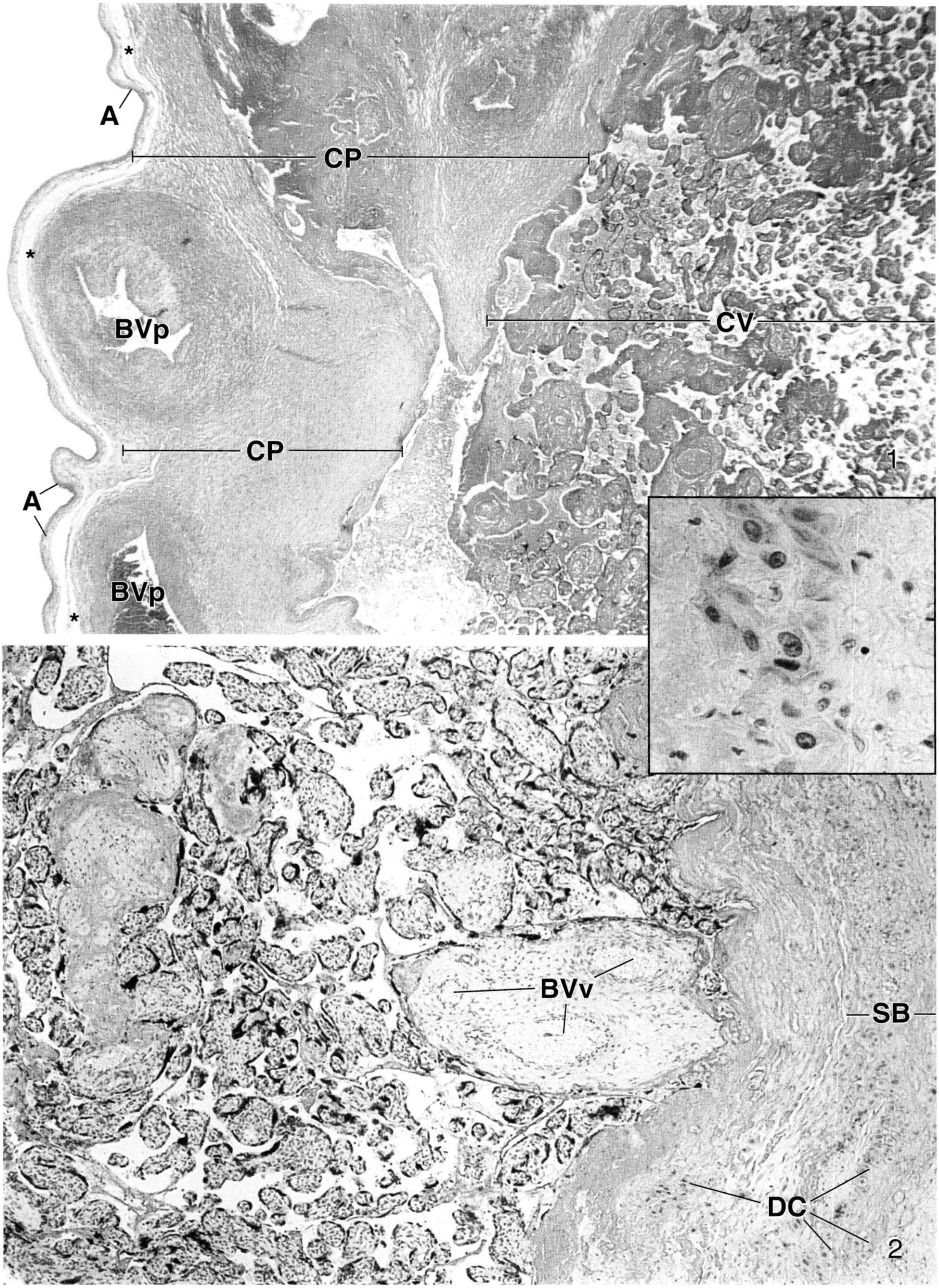
*
A
CP
*
BVp
CV
CP
1
A
BVp
*
BVv
SB
DC
2

PLATE 96. PLACENTA II

Chorionic villi, which constitute the functional tissue of the placenta, consist of a connective tissue core and a two-layered epithelial cellular covering. The outermost layer consists of *syncytiotrophoblasts.* Immediately under this is a layer of cells, referred to as *cytotrophoblasts,* from which the syncytiotrophoblast derives. Thus, cytotrophoblasts are numerous in the early placenta but relatively sparse in the placenta of late pregnancy.

The syncytiotrophoblast not only covers the surface of the chorionic villi but also extends from the anchoring villi onto the surface of the basal plate and onto the placental septa. As a consequence, the entire compartment in which maternal blood is contained is walled by syncytiotrophoblasts.

Except for relatively rare rupturing of capillary walls, which is more common at delivery, fetal and maternal blood do not mix. This separation of the fetal and maternal blood, referred to as the *placental barrier,* is maintained primarily by the layers of fetal tissue. Starting at the fourth month, these layers become very thin to facilitate the exchange of products across the placental barrier. The thinning of the wall of the villus is due to the loss of the inner cytotrophoblastic layer. At its thinnest, the placental barrier consists of the syncytiotrophoblast, a sparse discontinuous inner cytotrophoblast layer, basal lamina of the trophoblast, connective tissue of the villus, basal lamina of the endothelium, and endothelium of the fetal placental capillary in the tertiary villus. Thus, this barrier bears a strong resemblance to the air–blood barrier of the lung, with which it has an important parallel function, namely, the exchange of oxygen and carbon dioxide, in this case between the maternal blood and the fetal blood. In addition, metabolic substrates and products, hormones and other regulatory molecules, and antibodies that confer passive immunity on the fetus also routinely cross the placental barrier. Unfortunately, so too do potentially dangerous agents such as alcohol, nicotine, drugs, viruses, exogenous hormones, and heavy metals that can harm the embryo or fetus.

Figure, placenta, human, H&E ×280.

A section through the substance of a full-term placenta shows chorionic villi *(CV)* of different sizes and the surrounding intervillous space *(IS).* The connective tissue of the villi contains branches and tributaries of the umbilical arteries and vein *(BV).* The smallest villi contain only capillaries; larger villi contain correspondingly larger blood vessels. The intervillous space contains maternal blood. Maternal blood was drained from the specimen before its preparation, and therefore, few maternal blood cells are seen in the section.

The nuclei of the syncytiotrophoblast may be more or less evenly distributed, giving this layer an appearance (in H&E sections) similar to that of cuboidal epithelium. There are, however, sites where the nuclei are gathered in clusters *(arrowheads),* as well as regions of syncytium relatively free of nuclei *(arrows).* These stretches of syncytium may be so attenuated as to give the impression that the villous surface is devoid of a covering. It is thought that the nuclear clusters and the adjacent cytoplasm may separate from the villus and enter the maternal blood pool.

The syncytiotrophoblast contains microvilli that project into the intervillous space. These may appear as a striated border in paraffin sections, but they are not always adequately preserved and may not be evident.

In earlier placentas, the cytotrophoblasts form an almost complete layer of cells immediately deep to the syncytiotrophoblast. Cytotrophoblasts are the source of the syncytiotrophoblast. Cell division occurs in the cytotrophoblast layer, and the newly formed cells become incorporated into the syncytial layer. In this full-term placenta, only occasional cytotrophoblasts *(Cy)* can be discerned.

Most of the cells within the core of the villus are typical connective tissue fibroblasts. The nuclei of these cells stain well with hematoxylin, but the cytoplasm cannot be distinguished from the delicate intercellular fibrous material. Other cells have a recognizable amount of cytoplasm surrounding the nucleus. These are considered to be phagocytotic and are named Hofbauer cells. The Hofbauer cells *(HC)* shown in the figure do not contain any distinctive cytoplasmic inclusions.

KEY

BV, blood vessels
CV, chorionic villi
Cy, cytotrophoblasts
HC, Hofbauer cells
IS, intervillous space
arrowheads, clusters of syncytial trophoblast nuclei
arrows, attenuated syncytial cytoplasm
asterisk, tangentially sectioned villus

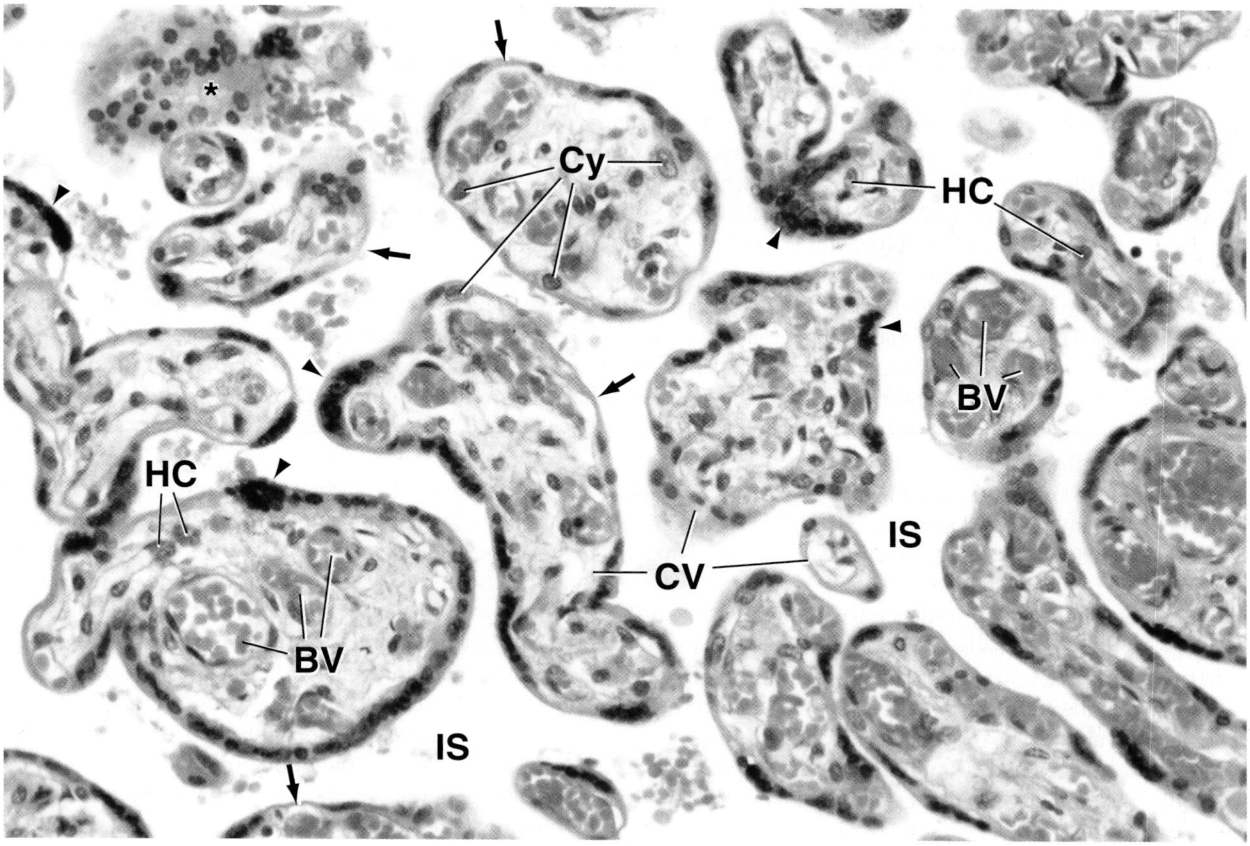
*
Cy
HC
BV
HC
CV
IS
BV
IS

PLATE 97. VAGINA

The *vagina* is the fibromuscular tube of the female reproductive tract that leads to the exterior of the body. The wall of the vagina consists of three layers: a *mucosa,* a *muscularis,* and an *adventitia.* The epithelium of the mucosa is nonkeratinized stratified squamous. It undergoes changes that correspond to the ovarian cycle. The amount of glycogen stored in the epithelial cells increases under the influence of *estrogen,* whereas the rate of desquamation increases under the influence of *progesterone.* The glycogen liberated from the desquamated cells is fermented by *lactobacilli vaginalis,* producing lactic acid that acidifies the vaginal surface and inhibits colonization by yeasts and potentially harmful bacteria.

The vagina has certain histologic similarities to the proximal portion of the alimentary canal but is distinguished by the following features: The epithelium does not keratinize, and except for the deepest layers, the cells appear to be empty in routine H&E sections; the mucosa contains neither glands nor a muscularis mucosae; the muscle is smooth and not well ordered. This should be contrasted with the oral cavity, pharynx, and upper part of the esophagus in which the muscle is striated. The more distal portion of the esophagus, which contains smooth muscle, can be distinguished easily from the vagina because it has a muscularis mucosae.

Figure 1, vagina, human, H&E ×90.
The mucosa of the vagina consists of a stratified squamous epithelium *(Ep)* and an underlying fibrous connective tissue *(CT)* that often appears more cellular than other fibrous connective tissue. The boundary between the two is readily identified because of the conspicuous staining of the closely packed small cells of the basal layer *(B)* of the epithelium. Connective tissue papillae project into the underside of the epithelium, giving the epithelial–connective tissue junction an uneven appearance. The papillae may be cut obliquely or in cross section and thus may appear as connective tissue islands *(arrows)* within the lower portion of the epithelium. The epithelium is characteristically thick and although keratohyaline granules may be found in the superficial cells, keratinization does not occur in human vaginal epithelium. Thus, nuclei can be observed throughout the entire thickness of the epithelium despite the fact that the cytoplasm of most of the cells above the basal layers appears empty. These cells are normally filled with large deposits of glycogen that is lost in the processes of fixation and embedding of the tissue. The *rectangle* outlines a portion of the epithelium and connective tissue papillae that is examined at higher magnification in Figure 2. The muscular layer of the vaginal wall consists of smooth muscle arranged in two ill-defined layers. The outer layer is generally said to be longitudinally arranged *(SML),* and the inner layer is generally said to be circularly arranged *(SMC),* but the fibers are more usually organized as interlacing bundles surrounded by connective tissue. Many blood vessels *(BV)* are seen in the connective tissue.

Figure 2, vagina, human H&E ×110.
This is a higher magnification of the epithelium that includes the area outlined by the *rectangle* in Figure 1 (turned 90°). The obliquely cut and cross-sectioned portions of connective tissue papillae that appear as connective tissue islands in the epithelium are more clearly seen here *(arrows),* in some instances outlined by the surrounding closely packed cells of the basal epithelial cell layer. Note, again, that the epithelial cells even at the surface still retain their nuclei and there is no evidence of keratinization.

Figure 3, vagina, human H&E ×225.
This is higher-magnification micrograph of the basal portion of the epithelium *(Ep)* between connective tissue papillae. Note the regularity and dense packing of the basal epithelial cells. They are the stem cells for the stratified squamous epithelium. Daughter cells of these cells migrate toward the surface and begin to accumulate glycogen and become less regularly arranged as they move towards the surface. The highly cellular connective *(CT)* tissue immediately beneath the basal layer *(B)* of the epithelium typically contains many lymphocytes *(L).* The number of lymphocytes varies with the stage of the ovarian cycle. Lymphocytes invade the epithelium around the time of menstruation and appear along with the epithelial cells in vaginal smears.

Figure 4, vagina, human, H&E ×125.
This higher-magnification micrograph of the smooth muscle of the vaginal wall emphasizes the irregularity of the arrangement of the muscle bundles. At the right edge of the figure is a bundle of smooth muscle cut in a longitudinal section *(SML).* Adjacent to this is a bundle of smooth muscle cut in cross section *(SMC).* This bundle abuts on a longitudinally sectioned lymphatic vessel *(LV).* To the left of the lymphatic vessel is another longitudinal bundle of smooth muscle *(SML).* A valve *(Va)* is seen in the lymphatic vessel. A small vein *(V)* is present in the circular smooth muscle close to the lymphatic.

KEY

B, basal layer of vaginal epithelium
BV, blood vessels
CT, connective tissue
Ep, epithelium
L, lymphocytes
LV, lymphatic vessel
SMC, smooth muscle, cross section
SML, smooth muscle, longitudinal section
V, vein
Va, valve in lymphatic vessel
arrows, connective tissue islands in epithelium

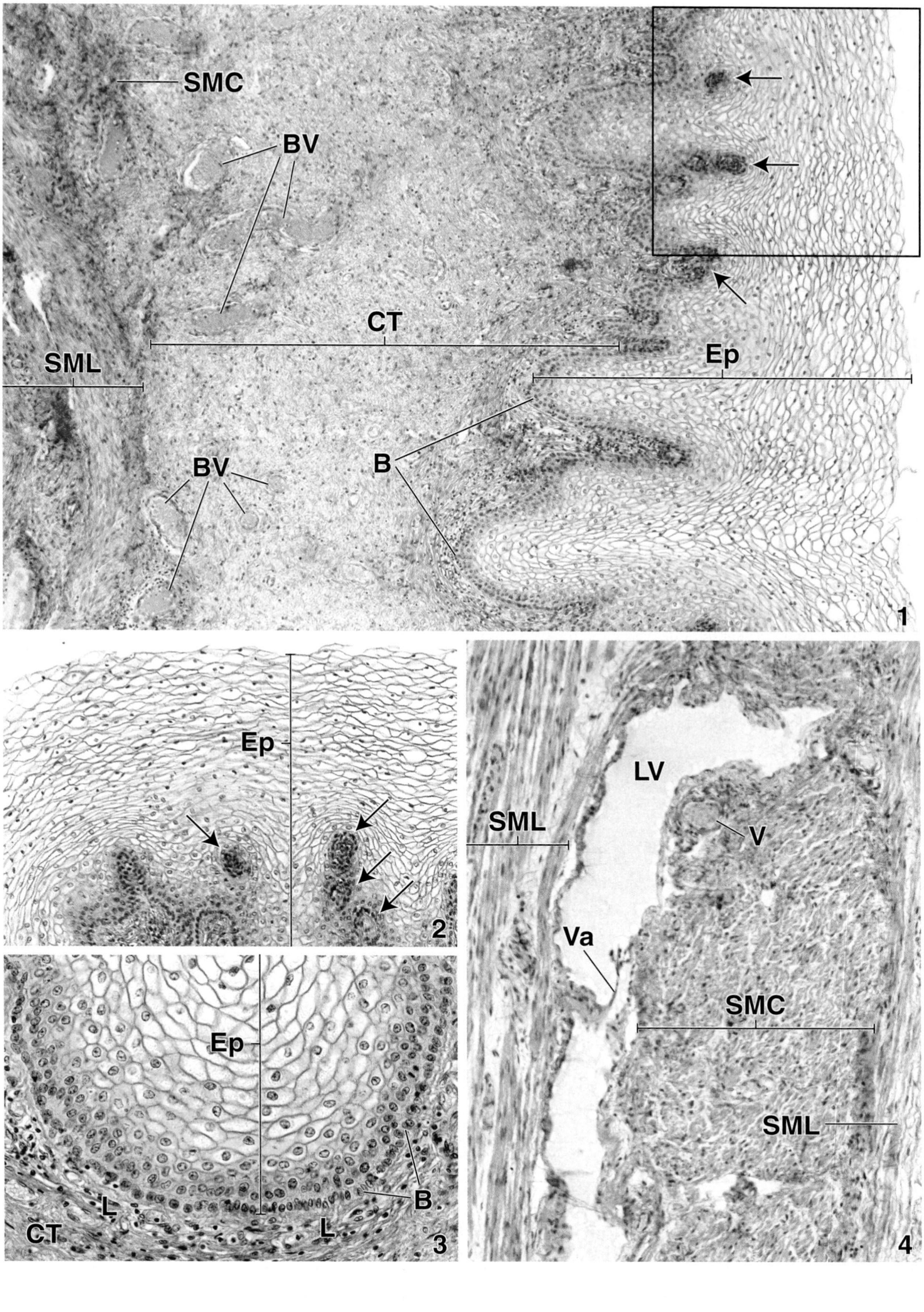
SMC
BV
CT
SML
Ep
B
BV
1
Ep
2
Ep
B
L
CT
L
3
LV
SML
V
Va
SMC
SML
4

PLATE 98. MAMMARY GLANDS

The mammary glands are branched tubuloalveolar glands that develop from epidermis and come to lie in the subcutaneous tissue (superficial fascia). They begin to develop at puberty in the female but do not reach a fully functional state until after pregnancy. The glands also develop in the male at puberty; the development is limited, however, and the glands usually remain in a stabilized state.

Figure 1, mammary gland, human, H&E ×80.
This figure is a section through an inactive gland. The parenchyma is sparse and consists mainly of duct elements. Several ducts *(D)* are shown in the center of the field. A small lumen can be seen in each. The ducts are surrounded by a loose connective tissue (see *CT(L),* Fig. 2), and together, the ducts and surrounding connective tissue constitute a lobule. Two lobules *(L)* are bracketed in this figure. Beyond the lobule, the connective tissue is more dense *(CT(D))*. The two types of connective tissues can be distinguished at the low magnification of this figure.

Figure 2, mammary gland, human, H&E ×200; inset ×400.
Additional details are evident at higher magnification. In distinguishing between the loose and dense connective tissue, recall that both extracellular and cellular features show differences that are evident in both the figure and the **inset.** Note the thicker collagenous fibers in the dense connective tissue in contrast to the much thinner fibers of the loose connective tissue. The loose connective tissue contains far more cells per unit area and a greater variety of cell types. This figure shows a cluster of lymphocytes *(L)* and, at still higher magnification **(inset),** plasma cells *(P)* and individual lymphocytes *(L).* Both plasma cells and lymphocytes are cells with a rounded shape, but plasma cells are larger and show more cytoplasm. In addition, regions of plasma cell cytoplasm display basophilia. Elongate nuclei in spindle-shaped cells belong to fibroblasts. In contrast, although the cell types in the dense connective tissue may also be diverse, a simple examination of equal areas of loose and dense connective tissue will, by far, show fewer cells in the dense connective tissue. Characteristically, the dense connective tissue contains numerous aggregates of adipocytes *(A).*

The epithelial cells within the resting lobule are regarded as being chiefly duct elements. Usually, alveoli are not found; their precursors, however, are represented as cellular thickenings of the duct wall. The epithelium of the resting lobule is cuboidal; in addition, myoepithelial cells are present. Reexamination of the **inset** shows a thickening of the epithelium in one location, presumably the precursor of an alveolus, and myoepithelial cells *(M)* at the base of the epithelium. As elsewhere, the myoepithelial cells are on the epithelial side of the basement membrane. During pregnancy, the glands begin to proliferate. This can be thought of as a dual process in which ducts proliferate and alveoli grow from the ducts.

KEY

A, adipocytes
CT(D), dense connective tissue
CT(L), loose connective tissue
D, ducts
L: Fig. 1, lobules; Fig. 2 and inset, lymphocytes
M, myoepithelial cells
P, plasma cells

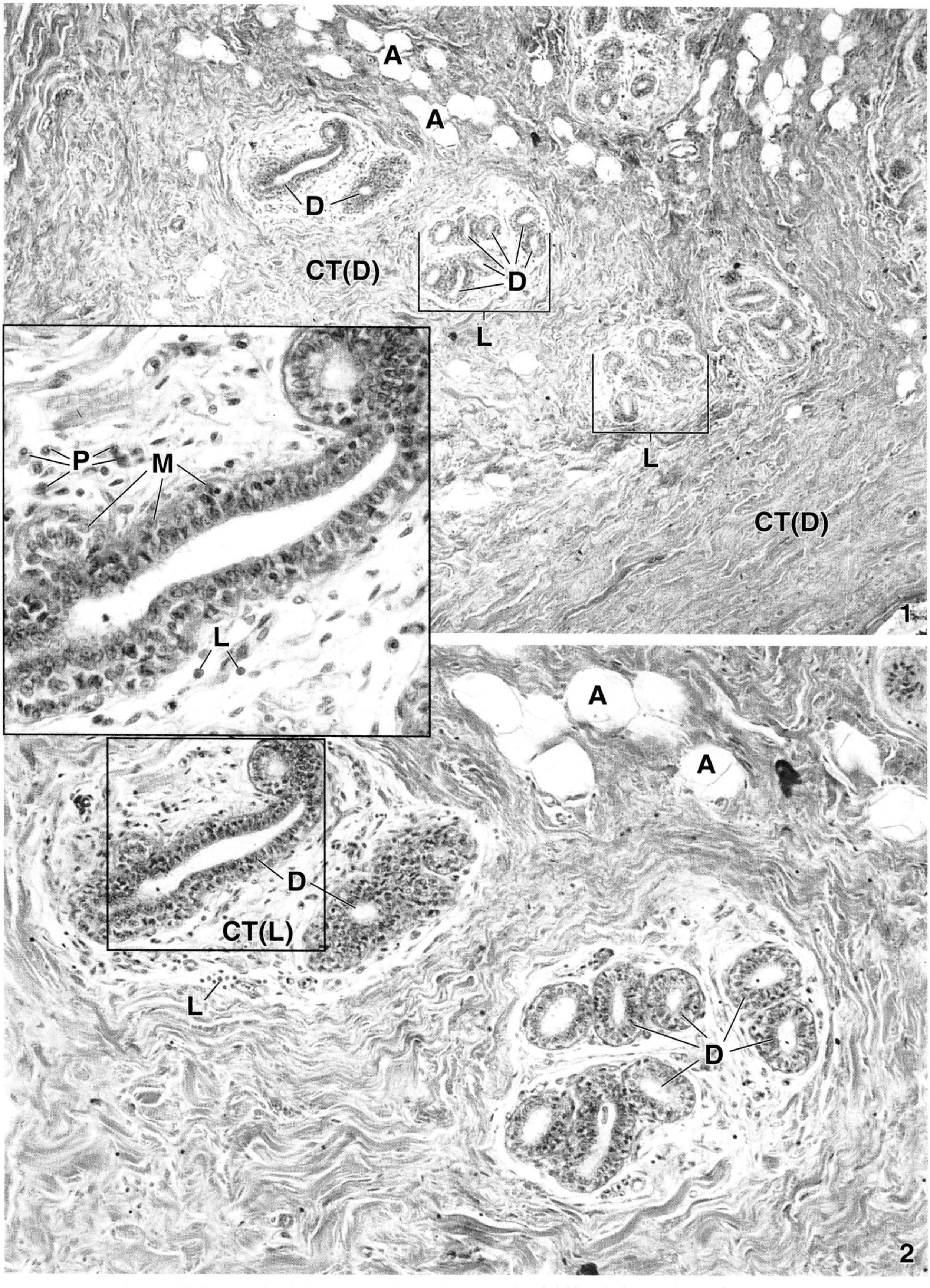
A
A
D
CT(D)
D
L
L
CT(D)
1
P
M
L
A
A
D
CT(L)
L
D
2

PLATE 99. MAMMARY GLAND, LATE PROLIFERATIVE AND LACTATING

Mammary glands exhibit a number of changes during pregnancy in preparation for lactation. Lymphocytes and plasma cells infiltrate the loose connective tissue as the glandular tissue develops. As the cells of the glandular portion proliferate by mitotic division, the ducts branch and alveoli begin to develop at their growing ends. Alveolar development becomes most prominent in the later stages of pregnancy, and accumulation of secretory product takes place in the alveoli. At the same time, lymphocytes and plasma cells become prominent in the loose connective tissue of the developing lobules. Myoepithelial cells proliferate between the base of the epithelial cells and the basal lamina in both the alveolar and the ductal portion of the glands. They are most prominent in the larger ducts.

Both merocrine and apocrine secretion are involved in the production of milk. The protein component is synthesized, concentrated, and secreted by exocytosis in a manner typical for protein secretion. The lipid component begins as droplets in the cytoplasm that coalesce into large droplets in the apical cytoplasm of the alveolar cells and cause the apical plasma membrane to bulge into the alveolar lumen. The droplets are surrounded by a thin layer of cytoplasm and are enveloped in plasma membrane as they are released.

The initial secretion in the first days after birth is called *colostrum.* This premilk is an alkaline secretion with a higher protein, vitamin A, sodium, and chloride content than milk and a lower lipid, carbohydrate, and potassium content. Considerable amounts of antibodies are contained in colostrum, and these provide the newborn with passive immunity to many antigens. The antibodies are produced by the plasma cells in the stroma of the breast and are carried across the glandular cells in a manner similar to that for secretory IgA in the salivary glands and intestine. A few days after parturition, the secretion of colostrum stops and lipid-rich milk is produced.

Figure 1, mammary gland, late proliferative stage, human, H&E ×90; inset ×560.

Whereas the development of the duct elements in the mammary gland occurs during the early proliferative stage, the development of the alveolar elements becomes conspicuous in the late proliferative stage. This figure shows the lobules *(L)* at the late proliferative stage. Individual lobules are separated by narrow dense connective tissue septa *(S).* The connective tissue within the lobule is a typical loose connective tissue that is now more cellular, containing mostly plasma cells and lymphocytes. The alveoli are well developed, and many exhibit precipitated secretory product. Each of the alveoli is joined to a duct, although that relationship can be difficult to identify. The epithelium of the intralobular ducts is similar in appearance to the alveolar epithelium. The cells of both components are secretory. The alveoli as well as the intralobular ducts consist of a single layer of cuboidal epithelial cells subtended by myoepithelial cells. Often, what appear to be several alveoli are seen merging with one another *(asterisks).* Such profiles represent alveolar units opening into a duct. Interlobular ducts *(D)* are easy to identify as they are surrounded by dense connective tissue. In one instance, an intralobular duct can be seen emptying into an interlobular duct *(arrow).* The **inset** shows the secretory epithelium at a much higher magnification. Note that it is a simple columnar epithelium. The nucleus of a myoepithelial cell *(M)* is seen at the base of the epithelium. Generally, these cells are difficult to recognize. Also, as noted above, numerous plasma cells *(P)* and lymphocytes *(Ly)* are present in the loose connective tissue of the lobule.

Figure 2, mammary gland, lactating, human, methyl green-osmium ×90; inset ×700.

The specimen shown here is from a lactating mammary gland. It is similar in appearance to the gland at the late proliferative stage but differs mainly to the extent that the alveoli are more uniform in appearance and their lumina are larger. As in the late proliferative stage, several alveoli can be seen merging with one another *(asterisks).* The use of osmium in this specimen stains the lipid component of the secretion. The **inset** reveals the lipid droplets within the epithelial cell cytoplasm as well as lipid that has been secreted into the lumen of the alveolus. The lipid first appears as small droplets within the epithelial cells. These droplets become larger and ultimately are secreted into the alveolar lumen along with milk proteins. The milk proteins are present in small vacuoles in the apical part of the cell but cannot be seen by light microscopic methods. They are secreted by exocytosis. The lipid droplets, in contrast, are large and surrounded by the apical cell membrane as they are pinched off to enter the lumen; thus it is an apocrine secretion. Several interlobular ducts *(D)* are evident. One of these ducts reveals a small branch, an ending intralobular duct *(arrows)* joining the interlobular duct.

KEY

D, interlobular duct
L, lobule
Ly, lymphocyte
M, myoepithelial cell
P, plasma cell
S, connective tissue septa
arrow, union of intralobular duct with interlobular duct
asterisks, sites of merging alveoli

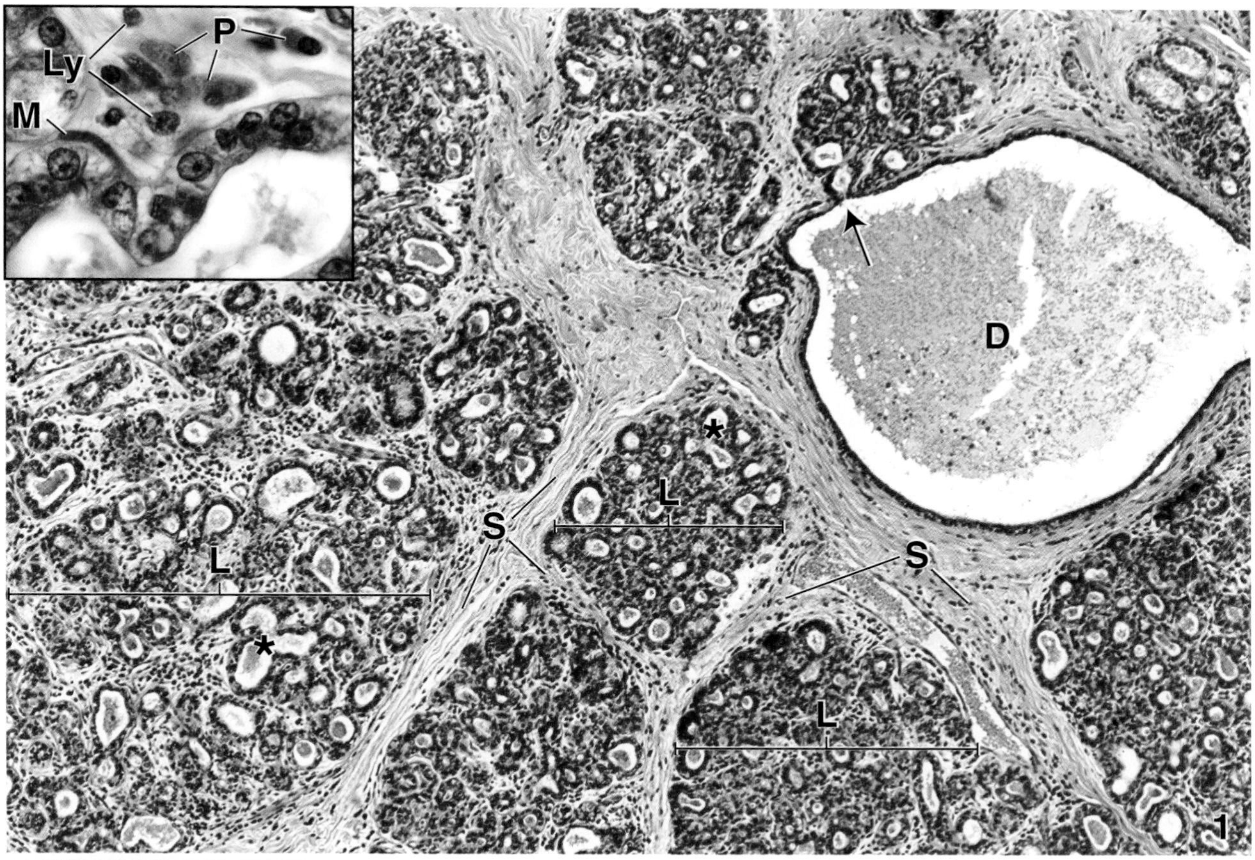
P
Ly
M
D
L
S
S
L
L
1

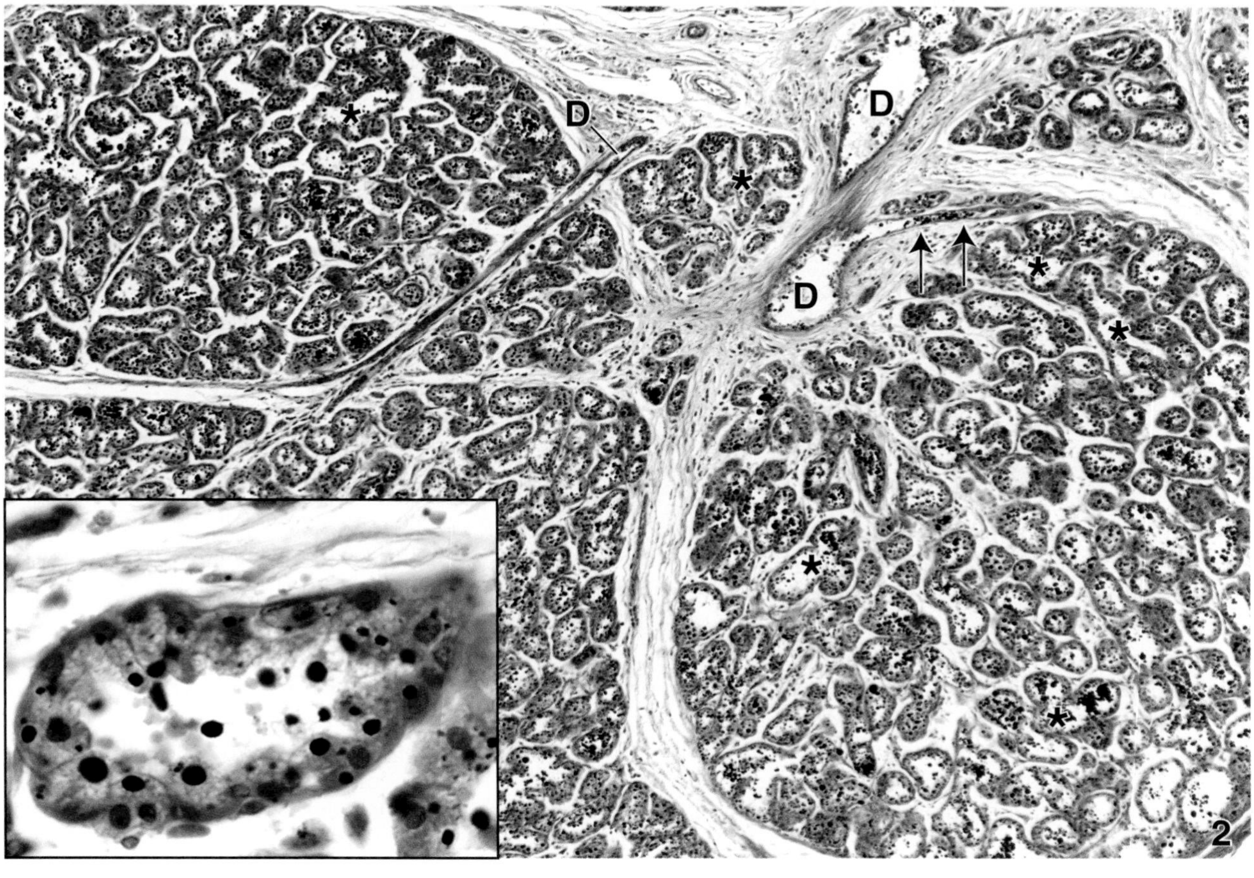
D
D
D
2

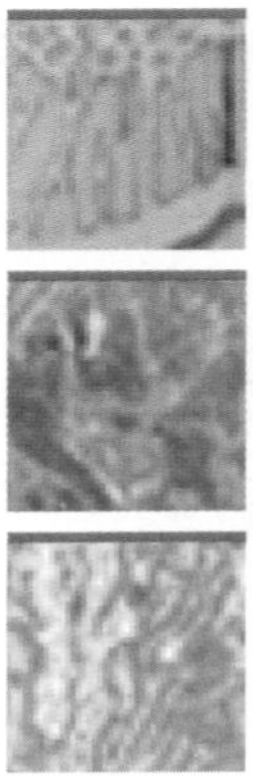

23

Eye

▼ OVERVIEW OF THE EYE

The eye is a complex sensory organ that provides the sense of sight. In many ways, the eye is similar to a digital camera. Like the optical system of a camera, the cornea and lens of the eye capture and focus light. The light detector in a digital camera, called the charge-coupled device (CCD), consists of closely spaced photodiodes that capture, collect, and convert the light image into a series of electrical impulses. Similarly, the ***photoreceptors*** in the ***retina*** of the eye detect light intensity and color and encode these parameters into electrical impulses for transmission to the brain via the ***optic nerve.***

Because the eyes are paired, two somewhat different and overlapping images (visual fields) are sent to the brain. Complex neural mechanisms coordinate eye movements and interpret the slightly different images. Binocular vision enables us to perceive depth and distance to achieve a three-dimensional image.

▼ GENERAL STRUCTURE OF THE EYE

The eye measures approximately 25 mm in diameter. It is suspended in the bony orbital socket by six extrinsic muscles that control its movement. A thick layer of adipose tissue partially surrounds and cushions the eye as it moves

within the orbit. The extraocular muscles are coordinated so that the eyes move symmetrically about their own central axes.

Layers of the Eye

The wall of the eye consists of three concentric layers or coats

The eyeball is composed of three structural layers (Fig. 23.1):

- *Corneoscleral coat,* the outer or *fibrous layer,* which includes the *sclera,* the white portion, and the *cornea,* the transparent portion
- *Vascular coat,* the middle layer or ***uvea,*** which includes the ***choroid*** and the stroma of the ***ciliary body*** and ***iris***
- *Retina,* the inner layer, which includes an outer pigment epithelium, the inner neural retina, and the epithelium of the ciliary body and iris

On the anterior aspect of the eye the layers are modified to admit and regulate the passage of light. The neural retina is continuous with the central nervous system through the ***optic nerve.*** The internal cavity of the eye is filled with a transparent gel, the ***vitreous body,*** which helps to maintain shape.

The corneoscleral coat consists of the transparent cornea and the white opaque sclera

The *cornea* covers the anterior one sixth of the eye (Fig. 23.1a). In this window-like region, the surface of the eye has a prominence or convexity. The cornea is continuous with the ***sclera*** *(Gr. skleros, hard).* The sclera is composed of dense fibrous connective tissue that provides attachment for the extrinsic muscles of the eye. The sclera constitutes the "white" of the eye but has a slightly blue tint in children because of its thinness and is yellow in the elderly because of the accumulation of lipofuscin in its stromal cells. The corneoscleral coat encloses the inner two layers except where it is penetrated by the optic nerve.

The uvea consists principally of the choroid, the vascular layer that provides nutrients to the retina

Blood vessels and melanin pigment give the ***choroid*** an intense dark-brown color. The pigment absorbs scattered and reflected light to minimize glare within the eye. The choroid contains many venous plexuses and layers of capillaries and is firmly attached to the retina (Fig. 23.1b). The anterior rim of the uveal layer continues forward, where it forms the stroma of the ***ciliary body*** and ***iris.***

The ***ciliary body*** is a ring-like thickening that extends inward just posterior to the level of the corneoscleral junction. Within the ciliary body is the ***ciliary muscle,*** a smooth muscle that is responsible for ***lens accommodation.*** Contraction of the ciliary muscle changes the shape of the lens, which enables it to bring light rays from different distances to focus on the retina.

The ***iris*** is a contractile diaphragm that extends over the anterior surface of the lens. It also contains smooth muscle and melanin-containing pigment cells scattered in the connective tissue. The ***pupil*** is the central circular aperture of

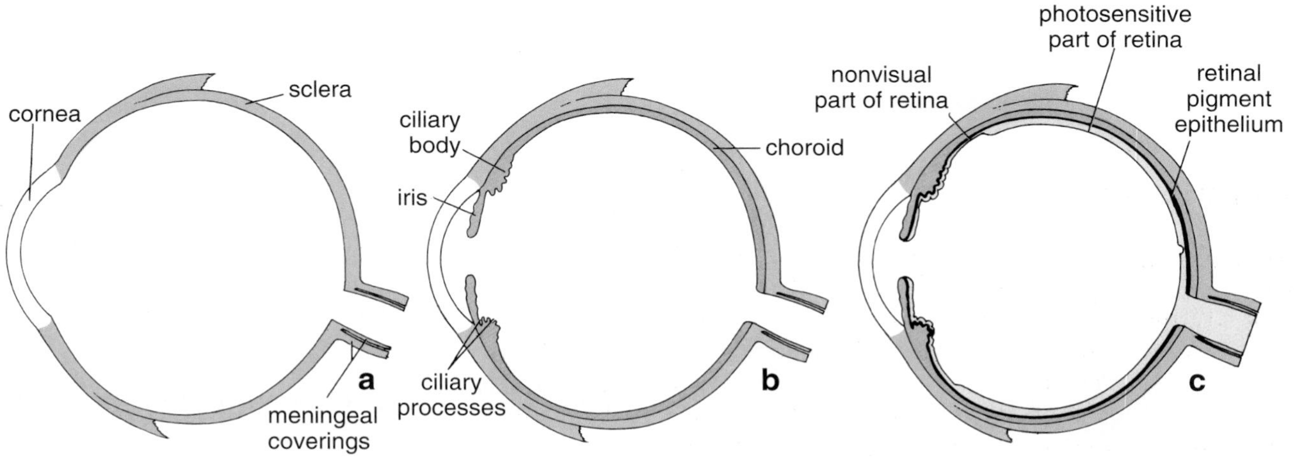

FIGURE 23.1
Schematic diagram of the layers of the eye. The wall of the eyeball is organized in three separate concentric layers: **(a)** an outer supporting layer, the corneoscleral coat (*clear* and *blue*); **(b)** a middle vascular coat or uvea *(pink)*; and **(c)** an inner photosensitive layer, the retina *(yellow)*.

the iris. It appears black because one looks through the lens toward the heavily pigmented back of the eye. In the process of ***adaptation,*** the pupil changes in size to control the amount of light that passes through the lens to reach the retina.

The retina consists of two components, the neural retina and pigment epithelium

The ***retina*** is a thin, delicate layer (Fig. 23.1c) consisting of two components:

- ***Neural retina,*** an inner layer that contains light-sensitive receptors and complex neuronal networks
- ***Retinal pigment epithelium (RPE),*** an outer layer composed of simple cuboidal melanin-containing cells

Externally, the retina rests on the choroid; internally, it is associated with the vitreous body. The neural retina consists largely of ***photoreceptor cells,*** called retinal ***rods*** and ***cones,*** and interneurons. Visual information encoded by the rods and cones is sent to the brain via impulses conveyed along the optic nerve.

Chambers of the Eye

The layers of the eye and the lens serve as boundaries for three chambers within the eye

The chambers of the eye are

- ***Anterior chamber,*** the space between the cornea and the iris
- ***Posterior chamber,*** the space between the posterior surface of the iris and the anterior surface of the lens
- ***Vitreous chamber,*** the space between the posterior surface of the lens and the neural retina (Fig. 23.2). The cornea, the anterior and posterior chambers, and their contents constitute the anterior segment of the eye; the vitreous chamber, visual retina, RPE, posterior sclera, and uvea constitute the posterior segment.

The refractile media components of the eye alter the light path to focus it on the retina

As light rays pass through the components of the eye, they are refracted. Refraction focuses the light rays on the photoreceptors of the retina. Four transparent components of the eye, called the ***refractile (or dioptric) media,*** alter the path of the light rays:

- ***Cornea,*** the anterior window of the eye
- ***Aqueous humor,*** the watery fluid located in the anterior and posterior chambers
- ***Lens,*** a transparent, crystalline, biconcave structure suspended from the inner surface of the ciliary body by a ring of radially oriented fibers, the ***zonule of Zinn***
- ***Vitreous body,*** composed of a transparent gel substance that fills the vitreous chamber. It contains hyaluronic acid, widely dispersed collagen fibrils, and other proteins and glycoproteins. The fluid component of the vitreous body is called the ***vitrous humor.***

The cornea is the chief refractive element of the eye. It has a refractive index of 1.376 (air has a refractive index of 1.0). The lens is second in importance to the cornea in the refraction of light rays. Because of its elasticity, the shape of the lens can undergo slight changes in response to the tension of the ciliary muscle. These changes are important in ***accommodation*** for proper focusing on near ob-

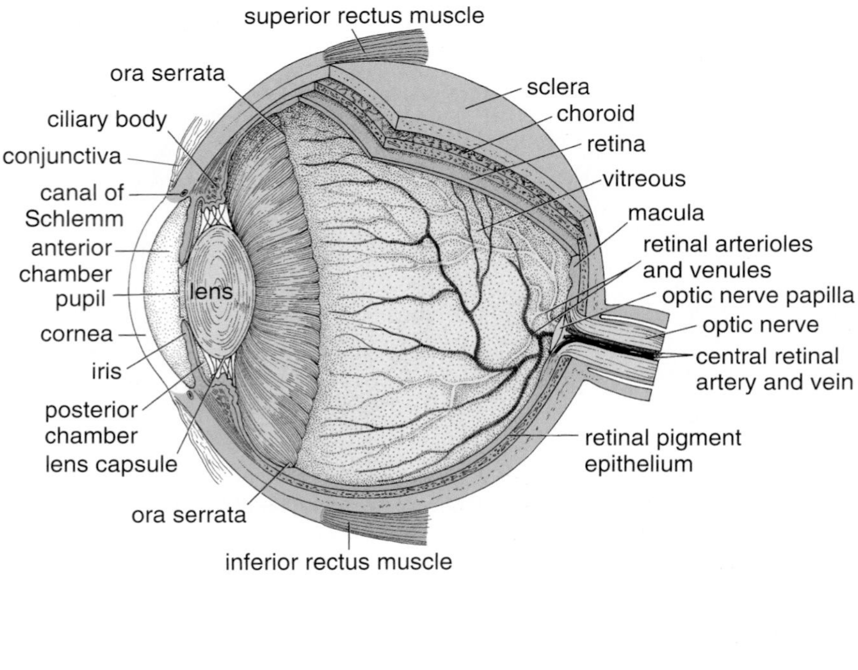

FIGURE 23.2
Schematic diagram illustrating the internal structures of the human eye. The retina consists of photosensitive and nonphotosensitive regions that differ in their function. Note that the photosensitive region of the retina occupies the posterior part of the eye and terminates anteriorly along the ora serrata. The nonphotosensitive region of the retina is located anterior to the ora serrata and lines the inner aspect of the ciliary body and the posterior surface of the iris. The other layers of the eyeball as well as the attachment of two of the extraocular muscles to the sclera are also shown.

jects. The aqueous humor and vitreous body have only minor roles in refraction. However, the aqueous humor plays an important role in providing nutrients to two avascular structures, the lens and cornea. In addition to transmitting light, the vitreous body helps maintain the position of the lens and helps keep the neural retina in contact with the RPE.

Development of the Eye

To appreciate the unusual structural and functional relationships in the eye, it is helpful to understand how it forms in the embryo.

The tissues of the eye are derived from neuroectoderm, surface ectoderm, and mesoderm

By the 22nd day of development, the eyes are evident as shallow grooves, the ***optic sulci*** or ***grooves,*** in the neural folds at the cranial end of the human embryo. As the neural tube closes, the paired grooves form outpocketings called ***optic vesicles*** (Fig. 23.3a). As each optic vesicle grows laterally, the connection to the forebrain becomes constricted into an optic stalk, and the overlying surface ectoderm thickens and forms a ***lens placode.*** These events are followed by concomitant invagination of the optic vesicles and the lens placodes. The invagination of the optic vesicle results in the formation of a double-layered ***optic cup*** (Fig. 23.3b). The inner layer becomes the neural retina. The outer layer becomes the RPE.

Invagination of the central region of each lens placode results in the formation of the ***lens vesicles.*** By the fifth week of development, the lens vesicle loses contact with the surface ectoderm and comes to lie in the mouth of the optic cup. After the lens vesicle detaches from the surface ectoderm, this same site again thickens to form the corneal epithelium. Mesenchymal cells from the periphery then give rise to the corneal endothelium and the corneal stroma.

Grooves containing blood vessels derived from mesenchyme develop along the inferior surface of each optic cup and stalk. Called the ***choroid fissures,*** the grooves enable the hyaloid artery to reach the inner chamber of the eye. This artery and its branches supply the inner chamber of the optic cup, lens vesicle, and mesenchyme within the optic cup. The hyaloid vein returns blood from these structures. The distal portions of the hyaloid vessels degenerate, but the proximal portions remain as the ***central artery*** and ***vein.*** By the end of the seventh week, the edges of the choroid fissure fuse, and a round opening, the future pupil, is formed over the lens vesicle.

The outer layer of the optic cup forms a single layer of pigmented cells (Fig. 23.3c) Pigmentation begins at the end of the fifth week. The inner layer undergoes a complex differentiation into the nine layers of the neural retina. The photoreceptor (rod and cone) cells as well as the bipolar, amacrine, and ganglion cells and nerve fibers are present by the seventh month. The macular depression begins to develop during the eighth month and is not complete until about 6 months after birth.

During the third month, growth of the optic cup gives rise to the ciliary body and the future iris, which forms a double row of epithelium in front of the lens. The mesoderm located external to this region becomes the stroma of the ciliary body and iris. Both epithelial layers of the iris become pigmented. In the ciliary body, however, only the outer layer is pigmented. At birth, the iris is light blue in fair-skinned people because pigment is usually not present. The dilator and sphincter pupillary muscles develop during

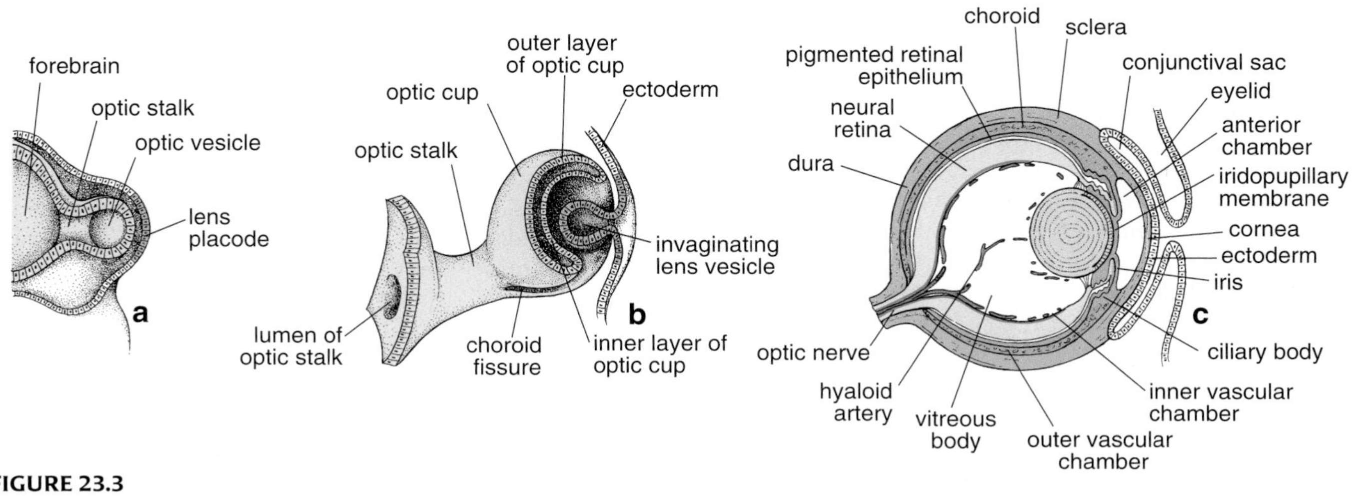

FIGURE 23.3

Schematic drawing illustrating the development of the eye. a. Forebrain and developing optic vesicles as seen in a 4-mm embryo. **b.** Bilayered optic cup and invaginating lens vesicle as seen in a 7.5-mm embryo. The optic stalk connects the developing eye to the brain. **c.** The eye as seen in a 15-week fetus. All the layers of the eye are established, and the hyaloid artery traverses the vitreous body from the optic disc to the posterior surface of the lens. (Modified from Mann IC. *The Development of the Human Eye.* New York: Grune & Stratton, 1974.)

TABLE 23.1. **Embryonic Origins of the Individual Structures of the Eye**

Source	Derivative
Surface ectoderm	Lens Epithelium of the cornea, conjunctiva, and lacrimal gland and its drainage system
Neural ectoderm	Vitreous body (derived partly from neural ectoderm of the optic cup and partly from mesenchyme) Epithelium of the retina, iris, and ciliary body Sphincter pupillae and dilator pupillae muscles Optic nerve
Mesoderm	Sclera Stroma of the cornea, ciliary body, iris, and choroid Extraocular muscles Eyelids (except epithelium and conjunctiva) Hyaloid system (most of which degenerates before birth) Coverings of the optic nerve Connective tissue and blood vessels of the eye, bony orbit, and vitreous body

the sixth month as derivatives of the neuroectoderm of the outer layer of the optic cup.

The embryonic origins of the individual eye structures are summarized in Table 23.1.

MICROSCOPIC STRUCTURE OF THE EYE

Corneoscleral Coat

The cornea consists of five layers: three cellular layers and two noncellular layers

The transparent cornea (see Figs. 23.1 and 23.2) is only 0.5 mm thick at its center and about 1 mm thick peripherally. It consists of three cellular layers that are distinct in both appearance and origin. These layers are separated by two important membranes that appear homogeneous when viewed in the light microscope. Thus, the five layers of the cornea seen in a transverse section are

- *Corneal epithelium*
- *Bowman's membrane (anterior basement membrane)*
- *Corneal stroma*
- *Descemet's membrane (posterior basement membrane)*
- *Corneal endothelium*

The corneal epithelium is a nonkeratinized stratified squamous epithelium

The *corneal epithelium* (Fig. 23.4) consists of approximately five layers of nonkeratinized cells and measures about 50 μm in average thickness. It is continuous with the conjunctival epithelium that overlies the adjacent sclera. The epithelial cells adhere to neighboring cells via desmosomes that are present on short interdigitating processes. Like other stratified epithelium, such as that of the skin, the cells proliferate from a basal layer and become squamous at the surface. The basal cells are low columnar with round, ovoid nuclei; the surface cells acquire a squamous or discoid shape and their nuclei are flattened and pyknotic (see Fig. 23.4b). As the cells migrate to the surface, the cytoplasmic organelles gradually disappear, indicating a progressive decline in metabolic activity. The cornea has a remarkable regenerative capacity with a turnover time of approximately 7 days.

The actual stem cells for the corneal epithelium reside at the *corneoscleral limbus*, the junction of the cornea and sclera. The microenvironment of the limbus is important in maintaining the population of stem cells that also act as a "barrier" to conjunctival epithelial cells and normally prevent their migration to the corneal surface. The corneal epithelial stem cells may be partially or totally depleted by disease or extensive injury, resulting in abnormalities of the corneal surface that lead to "conjunctivalization" of the cornea, characterized by vascularization, appearance of goblet cells, and an irregular and unstable epithelium. These changes cause ocular discomfort and reduced vision. Minor injuries of the corneal surface heal rapidly by inducing stem cell proliferation and migration of cells from the corneoscleral limbus to fill the defect.

Numerous free nerve endings in the corneal epithelium provide it with extreme sensitivity to touch. Stimulation of these nerves, e.g., by small foreign bodies, elicits blinking of the eyelids, flow of tears, and, sometimes, severe pain. Microvilli present on the surface epithelial cells help retain the tear film over the entire corneal surface. Drying of the corneal surface may cause ulceration.

DNA in corneal epithelial cells is protected from UV light damage by nuclear ferritin

Despite constant exposure of the corneal epithelium to UV light, cancer of this epithelium is extremely rare. Unlike the epidermis, which is also exposed to UV light, melanin is not present as a defense mechanism in corneal epithelium. The presence of melanin in the cornea would

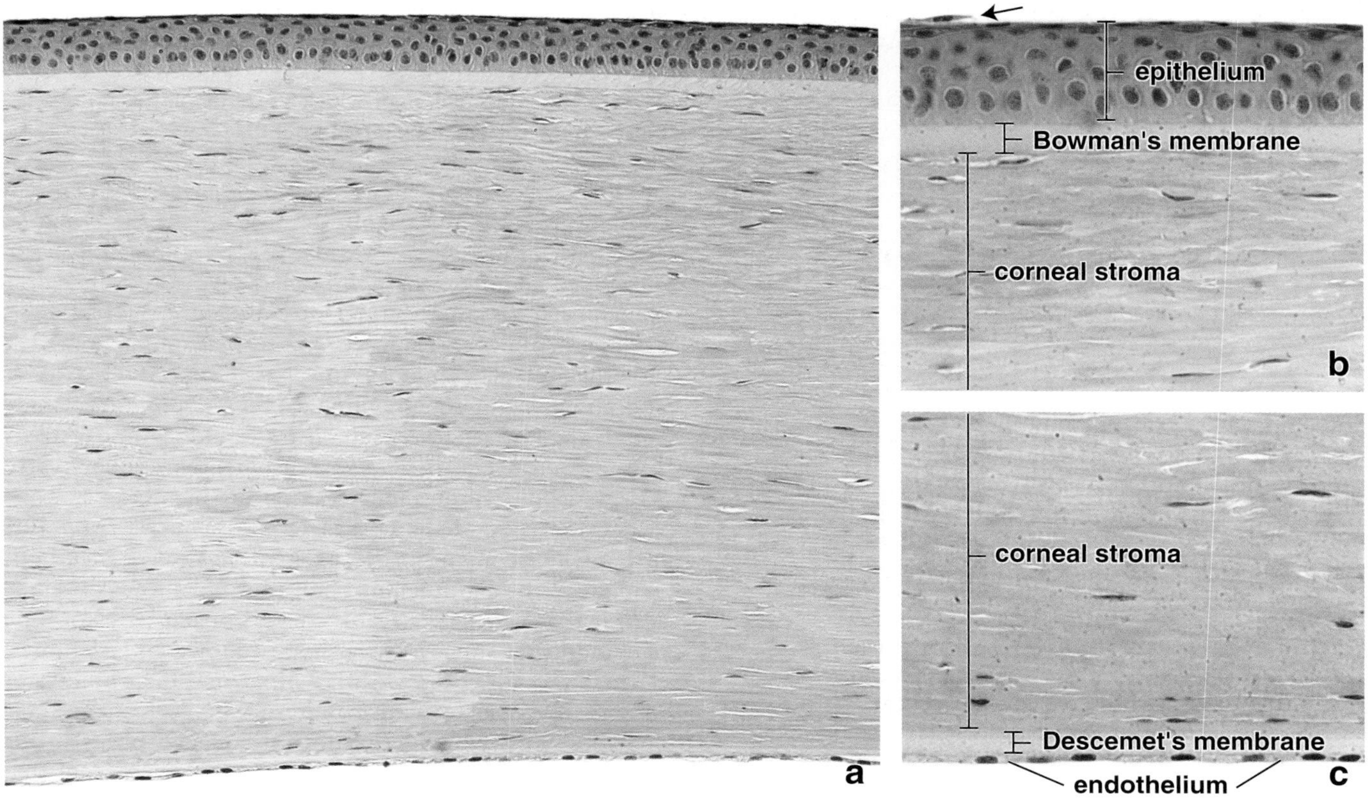

FIGURE 23.4
Photomicrograph of the cornea. a. This photomicrograph of a section through the full thickness of the cornea shows the corneal stroma and the two corneal surfaces covered by different types of epithelia. The corneal stroma does not contain blood or lymphatic vessels. ×140. **b.** A higher magnification of the anterior surface of the cornea showing the corneal stroma covered by a stratified squamous (corneal) epithelium. The basal cells that rest on Bowman's membrane, which is a homogenous condensed layer of corneal stroma, are low columnar in contrast to the squamous surface cells. Note that one of the surface cells is in the process of desquamation *(arrow)*. ×280. **c.** A higher-magnification photomicrograph of the posterior surface of the cornea covered by a thin layer of simple squamous epithelium (corneal endothelium). These cells are in direct contact with the aqueous humor of the anterior chamber of the eye. Note the very thick Descemet's membrane (basal lamina) of the corneal endothelial cells. ×280.

diminish light transmission. Instead, it has recently been shown that corneal epithelial cell nuclei contain ***ferritin,*** an iron-storage protein. Experimental studies with avian corneas have shown that nuclear ferritin protects the DNA in the corneal epithelial cells from free radical damage due to UV light exposure.

Bowman's membrane is a homogeneous-appearing layer on which the corneal epithelium rests

Bowman's membrane (anterior basement membrane) is a homogeneous, faintly fibrillar lamina that is approximately 8 to 10 μm thick. It lies between the corneal epithelium and the underlying corneal stroma and ends abruptly at the corneoscleral limbus. The collagen fibrils of Bowman's membrane have a diameter of about 18 nm and are randomly oriented. Bowman's membrane imparts some strength to the cornea, but more significantly, it acts as a barrier to the spread of infections. It does not regenerate. Therefore, if damaged, an opaque scar forms that may impair vision. In addition, changes in Bowman's membrane are associated with ***recurrent corneal erosions.***

The corneal stroma constitutes 90% of the corneal thickness

The corneal ***stroma,*** also called ***substantia propria,*** is composed of about 60 thin lamellae. Each lamella consists of parallel bundles of collagen fibrils. Located between lamellae are nearly complete sheets of slender, flattened fibroblasts. The fibrils measure approximately 23 nm in diameter and up to 1 cm in length. The collagen fibrils in each lamella are arranged at approximate right angles to those in the adjacent lamellae (Fig. 23.5). The ground substance contains ***corneal proteoglycans*** (lumican), which are sulfated glycosaminoglycans (chiefly, keratan sulfate and chondroitin sulfate) covalently bound to protein (decorin).

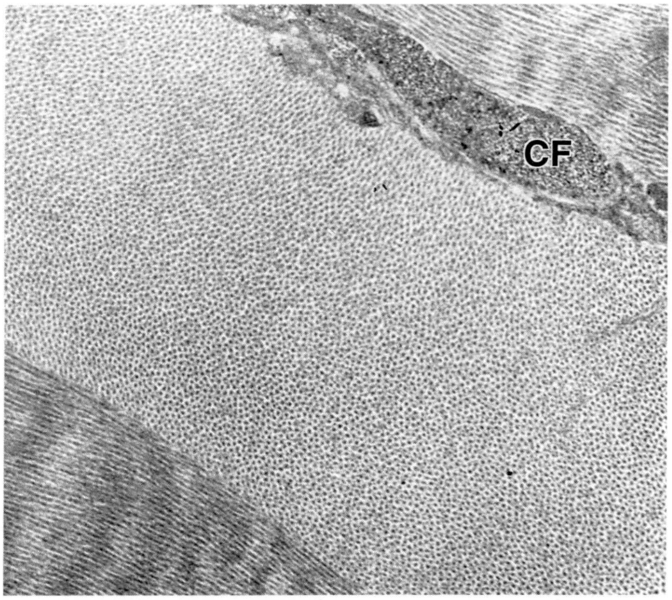

FIGURE 23.5
Electron micrograph of the corneal stroma. This electron micrograph shows parts of three lamellae and a portion of a corneal fibroblast *(CF)* between two of the lamellae. Note that the collagen fibrils in adjacent lamellae are oriented at right angles to one another. ×16,700.

It is believed that the uniform spacing of collagen fibrils and lamellae, as well as the ***orthogonal array*** of the lamellae (alternating layers at right angles), is responsible for the transparency of the cornea. Proteoglycans, along with collagen type V, regulate the precise diameter and spacing of the collagen fibrils. Swelling of the cornea following injury to the epithelium or endothelium disrupts this precise array and leads to translucency or opacity of the cornea.

Normally, the cornea contains no blood vessels or pigments. During an inflammatory response involving the cornea, large numbers of neutrophilic leukocytes and lymphocytes migrate from blood vessels of the corneoscleral limbus and penetrate between the stromal lamellae.

Descemet's membrane is an unusually thick basal lamina

Descemet's membrane (posterior basement membrane) is the basal lamina of corneal endothelial cells. It is intensely periodic acid–Schiff positive and can be as much as 10 μm thick. Descemet's membrane has a felt-like appearance and consists of an interwoven meshwork of fibers and pores.

It separates the corneal endothelium from the adjacent corneal stroma. Unlike Bowman's membrane, Descemet's membrane readily regenerates after injury. It also slowly thickens with age.

Descemet's membrane extends peripherally beneath the sclera as a meshwork called the ***pectinate ligament.*** Strands from the pectinate ligament penetrate the ciliary muscle and sclera and may help to maintain the normal curvature of the cornea by exerting tension on Descemet's membrane.

The corneal endothelium provides for metabolic exchange between the cornea and aqueous humor

The corneal endothelium is a single layer of squamous cells covering the surface of the cornea that faces the anterior chamber (see Fig. 23.4). The cells are joined by well-developed zonulae adherentes, relatively leaky zonulae occludentes, and desmosomes. Virtually all of the metabolic exchanges of the cornea occur across the endothelium. The endothelial cells contain many mitochondria and vesicles and an extensive rough endoplasmic reticulum (rER) and Golgi apparatus. They demonstrate endocytotic activity and are engaged in active transport. Na^+/K^+-activated ATPase is located on the lateral plasma membrane.

Transparency of the cornea requires precise regulation of the water content of the stroma. Physical or metabolic damage to the endothelium leads to rapid corneal swelling and, if the damage is severe, corneal opacity. Restoration of endothelial integrity is usually followed by deturgescence, although corneas can swell beyond their ability for self-repair. Such swelling can result in permanent focal opacities caused by aggregation of collagen fibrils in the swollen cornea. Essential sulfated glycosaminoglycans that normally separate the corneal collagen fibers are extracted from the swollen cornea.

Human corneal endothelium has a limited proliferative capacity. Severely damaged endothelium can only be repaired by transplantation of a donor cornea. Recent studies indicate that the periphery of the cornea represents a regenerative zone of the corneal endothelial cells. However, soon after corneal transplantation, endothelial cells exhibit contact inhibition when exposed to the extracellular matrix of Descemet's membrane. This finding that inhibitory factors released by Descemet's membrane prevent proliferation of endothelial cells has focused some current corneal research on reversal or prevention of this inhibition with exogenous growth factors.

The sclera is an opaque layer that consists predominantly of dense connective tissue

The sclera is a thick fibrous layer containing flat collagen bundles that pass in various directions and in planes parallel to its surface. Both the collagen bundles and fibrils that form them are irregular in diameter and arrangement. Interspersed between the collagen bundles are fine networks of elastic fibers and a moderate amount of ground substance. Fibroblasts are scattered among these fibers.

The opacity of the sclera, like that of other dense connective tissues, is primarily due to the irregularity of its structure. The sclera is pierced by blood vessels, nerves, and the optic nerve (see Fig. 23.2). It is 1 mm thick posteriorly, 0.3 to 0.4 mm thick at its equator, and 0.7 mm thick at the corneoscleral margin or "limbus."

The sclera is divided into three rather ill-defined layers:

- ***Episcleral layer (episclera),*** the external layer, is the loose connective tissue adjacent to the periorbital fat.
- ***Substantia propria*** (***sclera proper,*** also called ***Tenon's capsule***), the investing fascia of the eye, is composed of a dense network of thick collagen fibers.
- ***Suprachorioid lamina (lamina fusca),*** the inner aspect of the sclera, is located adjacent to the choroid and contains thinner collagen fibers and elastic fibers as well as fibroblasts, melanocytes, macrophages, and other connective tissue cells.

Episcleral space (Tenon's space) is located between the episcleral layer and substantia propria of the sclera. This space and the surrounding periorbital fat allow the eye to rotate freely within the orbit. The tendons of the extraocular muscles attach to the substantia propria of the sclera.

The corneoscleral limbus is the transitional zone between the cornea and sclera

At the junction of the cornea and sclera (Fig. 23.6), Bowman's membrane ends abruptly. The overlying epithelium at this site thickens from the 5 cell layers of the cornea to the 10 to 12 cell layers of the conjunctiva. The surface of the limbus is composed of two distinct types of epithelial cells: one type constitutes the conjunctival cells and the other corneal epithelial cells.

At this junction, the corneal lamellae become less regular as they merge with the oblique bundles of collagen fibers of the sclera. An abrupt transition from the avascular cornea to the well-vascularized sclera also occurs here.

The limbus region, specifically, the ***iridocorneal angle,*** contains the apparatus for the outflow of aqueous humor (Fig. 23.7). In the stromal layer, endothelium-lined channels called the ***trabecular meshwork*** (or ***spaces of Fontana***) merge to form the ***scleral venous sinus (canal of Schlemm).*** This sinus encircles the eye (Figs. 23.6 and 23.7). The aqueous humor is produced by the ciliary processes that border the lens in the posterior chamber of the eye. The fluid passes from the posterior chamber into the anterior chamber through the valve-like potential opening between the iris and lens. The fluid then passes through the openings in the trabecular meshwork in the limbus region as it continues its course to enter the scleral

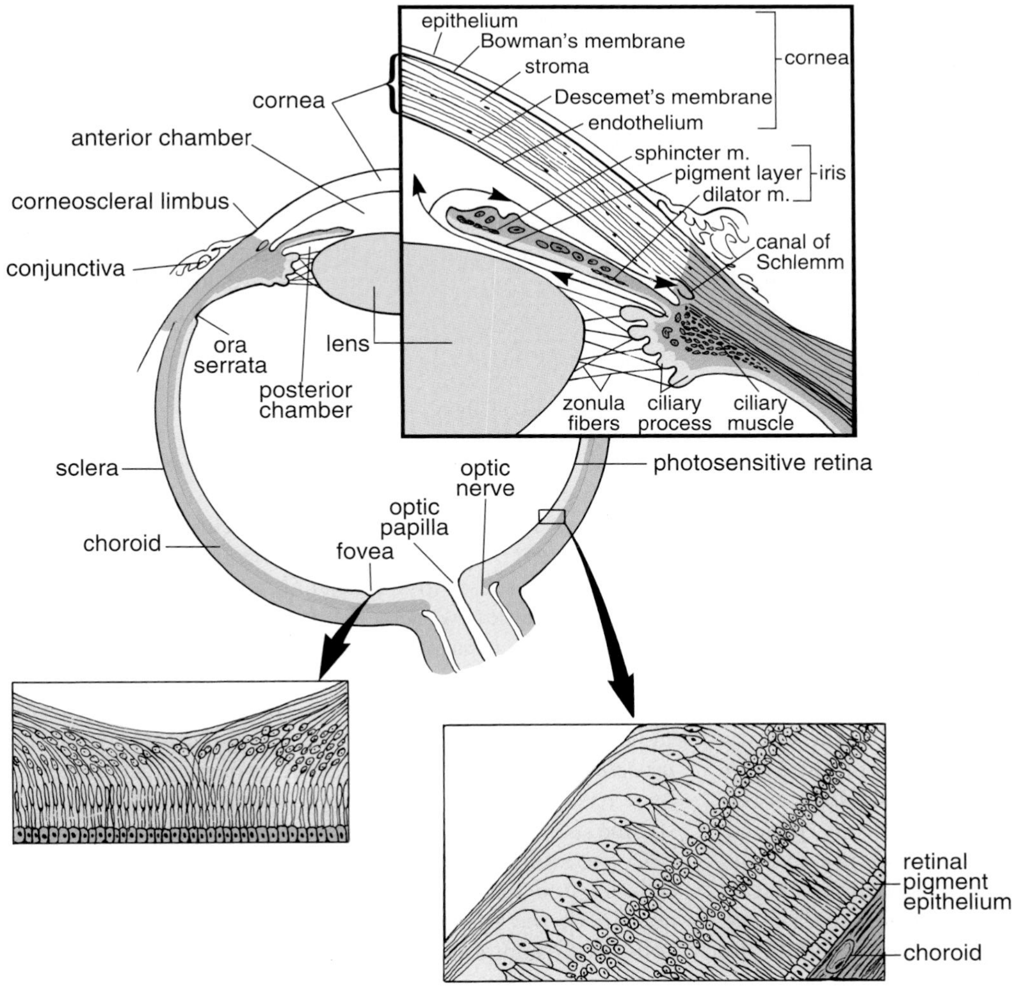

FIGURE 23.6
Schematic diagram of the structure of the eye. This drawing shows a horizontal section of the eyeball with color-coded layers of its wall. **Upper inset.** Enlargement of the anterior and posterior chambers shown in more detail. Note the direction of the flow of aqueous humor *(arrows),* which is drained by the scleral venous sinus (canal of Schlemm) at the iridocorneal angle. **Lower insets.** Typical organization of the cells and nerve fibers of the fovea centralis *(left)* and the retina *(right).*

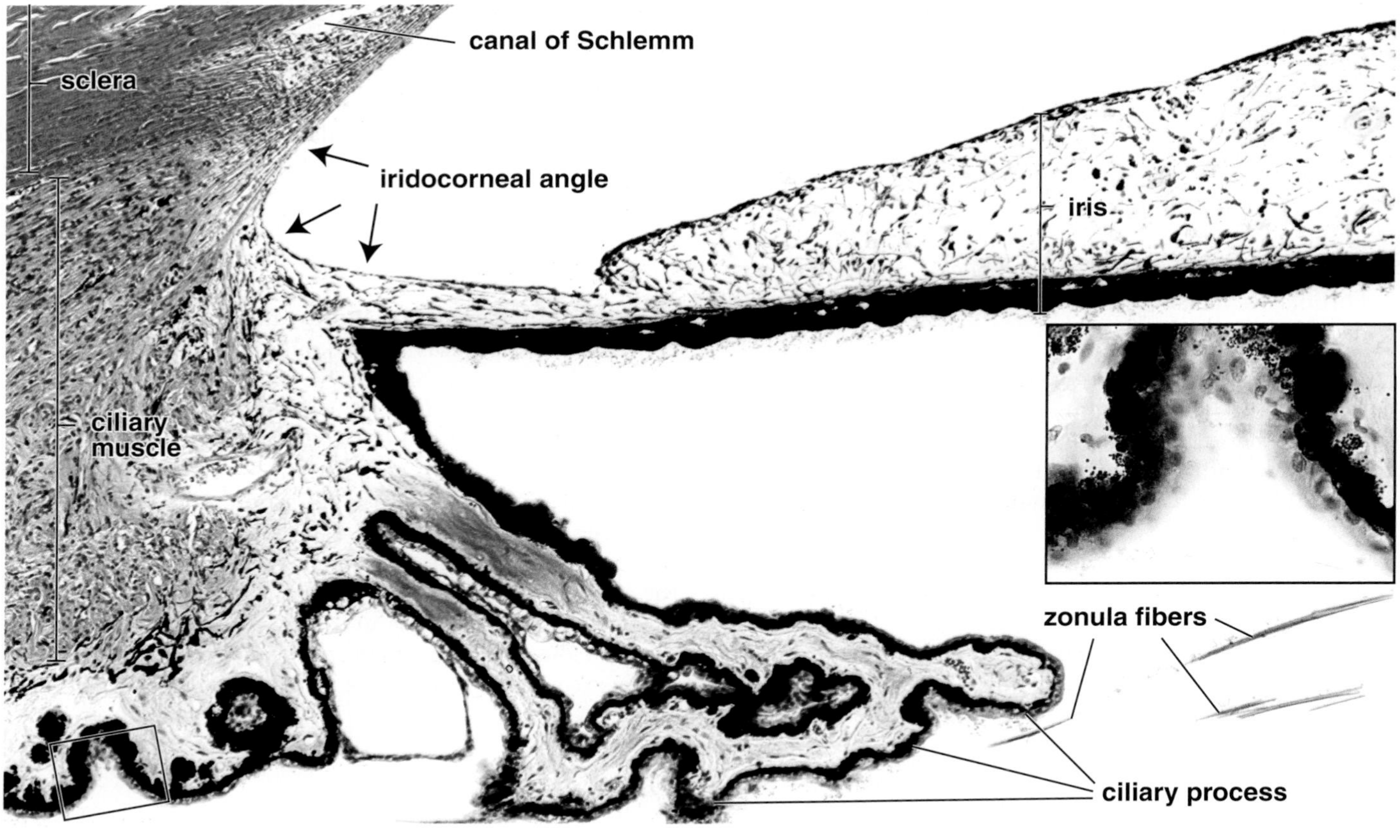

FIGURE 23.7
Photomicrograph of the ciliary body and iridocorneal angle. This photomicrograph of the human eye shows the anterior portion of the ciliary body and parts of the iris and sclera. The inner surface of the ciliary body forms radially arranged, ridge-shaped elevations, the ciliary processes, to which the zonular fibers are anchored. The ciliary body contains the ciliary muscle, connective tissue with blood vessels of the vascular coat, and the ciliary epithelium, which is responsible for the production of aqueous humor. Anterior to the ciliary body, between the iris and the cornea, is the iridocorneal angle. The scleral venous sinus (canal of Schlemm) located in close proximity to this angle drains the aqueous humor to regulate intraocular pressure. ×120. The **inset** shows that the ciliary epithelium consists of two layers, the outer pigmented layer and the inner nonpigmented layer. ×480.

venous sinus. Collecting vessels in the sclera, called ***aqueous veins*** because they convey aqueous humor instead of blood, transport the aqueous humor to (blood) veins located in the sclera.

Vascular Coat (Uvea)

The iris, the most anterior part of the vascular coat, forms a contractile diaphragm in front of the lens

The ***iris*** arises from the anterior border of the ciliary body (Fig. 23.7) and is attached to the sclera about 2 mm posterior to the corneoscleral junction. The ***pupil*** is the central aperture of this thin disc. The iris is pushed slightly forward as it changes in size in response to light intensity. It consists of highly vascularized connective tissue stroma that is covered on its posterior surface by highly pigmented cells, the ***posterior pigment epithelium*** (Fig. 23.8). The basal lamina of these cells faces the posterior chamber of the eye. The degree of pigmentation is so great that neither the nucleus nor character of the cytoplasm can be seen in the light microscope. Located beneath this layer is a layer of myoepithelial cells, the ***anterior pigment myoepithelium.*** The apical (posterior) portions of these myoepithelial cells are laden with melanin granules, which effectively obscure their boundaries with the adjacent posterior pigment epithelial cells. The basal (anterior) portions of myoepithelial cells possess processes containing contractile elements that extend radially and collectively make up the ***dilator pupillae muscle*** of the iris. The contractile processes are enclosed by a basal lamina that separates them from the adjacent stroma.

Constriction of the pupil is produced by smooth muscle cells located in the stroma of the iris near the pupillary margin of the iris. These circumferentially oriented cells collectively compose the ***constrictor pupillae muscle.***

The anterior surface of the iris reveals numerous ridges and groves, which can be seen in clinical examination with the ophthalmoscope. When this surface is examined in the light microscope it appears as a discontinuous layer of fibroblasts and melanocytes. The number of melanocytes in the stroma is responsible for variation in eye color. The function of these pigment-containing cells in the iris is to absorb light rays. If there are few melanocytes in the stroma, eye color is derived from light reflected from the pigment present in the cells of the posterior surface of the iris, giving it a blue appearance. As the amount of pigment present in the stroma increases, the color changes from blue to shades of greenish blue, gray, and, finally, brown.

The sphincter pupillae is innervated by parasympathetic nerves; the dilator pupillae muscle is under sympathetic nerve control

The size of the pupil is controlled by contraction of the sphincter pupillae and dilator pupillae muscles. The process of **adaptation** (increasing or decreasing the size of the pupil) ensures that only the appropriate amount of light enters the eye. Two muscles actively involved in adaptation are

- ***Sphincter pupillae muscle,*** a circular band of smooth muscle cells. This muscle is innervated by parasympathetic nerves carried in the oculomotor nerve (cranial nerve III) and is responsible for reducing pupillary size in response to bright light (see Fig. 12.8). Failure of the pupil to respond when light is shined into the eye—"pupil fixed and dilated"—is an important clinical sign of the lack of nerve or brain function.
- ***Dilator pupillae muscle,*** a thin sheet of radially oriented pigmented myoepithelial cells constituting the anterior pigment epithelium of the iris. This muscle is innervated by sympathetic nerves from the superior cervical ganglion and is responsible for increasing pupillary size in response to dim light.

The ciliary body is the thickened anterior portion of the vascular coat and is located between the iris and choroid

The ***ciliary body*** extends about 6 mm from the root of the iris posterolaterally to the ***ora serrata*** (see Fig. 23.2). As

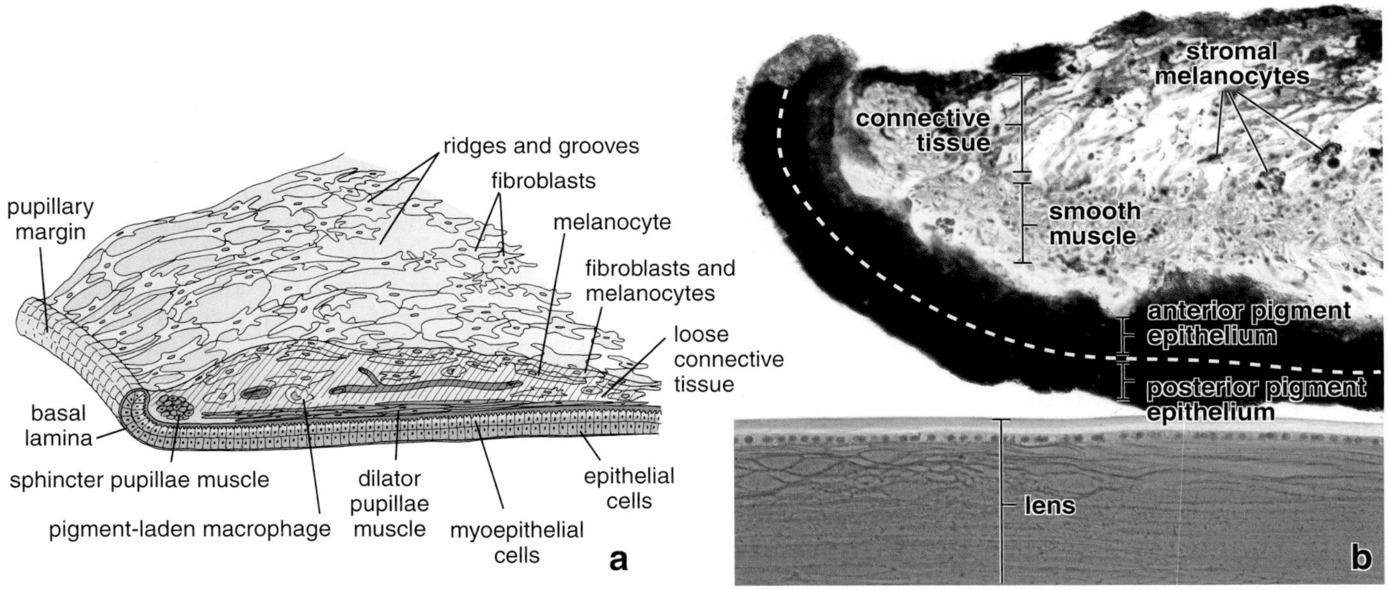

FIGURE 23.8
Structure of the iris. a. This schematic diagram shows the layers of the iris. Note that the pigmented epithelial cells are reflected as occurs at the pupillary margin of the iris. The two layers of pigmented epithelial cells are in contact with the dilator pupillae muscle. The incomplete layer of fibroblasts and stromal melanocytes is indicated on the anterior surface of the iris. **b.** Photomicrograph of the iris showing the histologic features of this structure. The lens, which lies posterior to the iris, is included for orientation. The iris is composed of a connective tissue stroma covered on its posterior surface by the posterior pigment epithelium. The basal lamina (not visible) faces the posterior chamber of the eye. Because of intense pigmentation, the histologic features of these cells are not discernable. Just anterior to these cells is the anterior pigment myoepithelium layer (the *dashed line* separates the two layers). Note that the posterior portion of the myoepithelial cells contains melanin, whereas the anterior portion contains contractile elements forming the dilator pupillae muscle of the iris. The constrictor pupillae muscle is evident in the stroma. The color of the iris depends on the number of stromal melanocytes scattered throughout the connective tissue stroma. At the bottom, note the presence of the lens. ×570.

seen from behind, the lateral edge of the ora serrata bears 17 to 34 grooves or crenulations. These grooves mark the anterior limit of both the retina and the choroid. The anterior third of the ciliary body has about 75 radial ridges or ***ciliary processes*** (see Fig. 23.7). The fibers of the zonule arise from the grooves between the ciliary processes.

The layers of the ciliary body are similar to those of the iris and consist of a stroma and an epithelium. The stroma is divided into two layers:

- An outer layer of smooth muscle, the ***ciliary muscle,*** which makes up the bulk of the ciliary body
- An inner vascular region that extends into the ciliary processes

The epithelial layer covering the internal surface of the ciliary body is a direct continuation of the two layers of the retinal epithelium (see Fig. 23.1).

The ciliary muscle is organized into three functional portions or groups of smooth muscle fibers

The smooth muscle of the ciliary body has its origin in the scleral spur, a ridge-like projection on the inner surface of the sclera at the corneoscleral junction. The muscle fibers spread out in several directions and are classified into three functional groups on the basis of their direction and insertion:

- ***Meridional (or longitudinal) portion*** consists of the outer muscle fibers that pass posteriorly into the stroma of the choroid. These fibers function chiefly in stretching the choroid. It also may help open the iridocorneal angle and facilitate drainage of the aqueous humor.
- ***Radial (or oblique) portion*** consists of deeper muscle fiber bundles that radiate in a fan-like fashion to insert in the ciliary body. Its contraction causes the lens to flatten and thus focus for distant vision.
- ***Circular (or sphincteric) portion*** consists of inner muscle fiber bundles oriented in a circular pattern forming a sphincter. It reduces the tension on the lens, causing the lens to accommodate for near vision.

Examination of a histologic preparation does not clearly reveal the arrangement of the muscle fibers. Rather, the organizational grouping is based on microdissection techniques.

Ciliary processes are ridge-like extensions of the ciliary body from which zonular fibers emerge and extend to the lens

Ciliary processes are thickenings of the inner vascular region of the ciliary body. They are continuous with the vascular layers of the choroid. Scattered macrophages containing melanin pigment granules and elastic fibers are present in these processes. The processes and the ciliary body are covered by a double layer of columnar epithelial cells, the ***ciliary epithelium,*** that was originally derived from the two layers of the optic cup. The ciliary epithelium has three principal functions:

- Secretion of aqueous humor
- Participation in the ***blood–aqueous barrier*** (part of the ***blood–ocular barrier,*** see below)
- Secretion and anchoring of the ***zonular fibers*** that form the ***suspensory ligament of the lens***

The inner cell layer of the ciliary epithelium has a basal lamina facing the posterior and vitreous chambers. The cells in this layer are nonpigmented. The cell layer that has its basal lamina facing the connective tissue stroma of the ciliary body is heavily pigmented and is directly continuous with the pigmented epithelial layer of the retina. The double-layered ciliary epithelium continues over the iris where it becomes the posterior pigmented epithelium and anterior pigmented myoepithelium. The zonular fibers extend from the basal lamina of the nonpigmented epithelial cells of the ciliary processes and insert into the lens capsule (the thickened basal lamina of the lens).

The cells of the nonpigmented layer have all the characteristics of a fluid-transporting epithelium, including complex cell-to-cell junctions with a well-developed zonular occludens, extensive lateral and basal plications, and localization of Na^+/K^+-ATPase in the lateral plasma membrane. In addition, they have an elaborate rER and Golgi complex consistent with their role in secreting the zonular fibers. The cells of the pigmented layer have a less developed junctional zone and often exhibit large, irregular lateral intercellular spaces. The apical surfaces of the two cell layers are held together by both desmosomes and gap junctions, creating discontinuous "luminal" spaces called ***ciliary channels.***

The ***aqueous humor*** is similar in ionic composition to plasma but contains less than 0.1% protein (compared with 7% protein in plasma). The aqueous humor passes from the ciliary body toward the lens, then between the iris and lens, before it reaches the anterior chamber of the eye (see Fig. 23.6). In the anterior chamber of the eye, the aqueous humor passes laterally to the angle formed between the cornea and iris. Here, it penetrates the tissues of the limbus as it enters the labyrinthine spaces and finally reaches the canal of Schlemm, which communicates with the veins of the sclera.

The choroid is the portion of the vascular coat that lies deep to the retina

The ***choroid*** is a dark-brown vascular sheet only 0.25 mm thick posteriorly and 0.1 mm thick anteriorly. It lies between the sclera and retina (see Fig. 23.1).

Two layers can be identified in the choroid:

- ***Choriocapillary layer,*** an inner vascular layer
- ***Bruch's membrane,*** a thin, amorphous hyaline membrane

The choroid is attached firmly to the sclera at the margin of the optic nerve. A potential space, the ***perichoroidal space*** (between the sclera and retina), is traversed by thin ***lamellae*** or strands that pass from the sclera to the choroid. These lamellae originate from the suprachoroid lamina (lamina fusca) and consist of large, flat melanocytes scattered between connective tissue elements including collagen and elastic fibers, fibroblasts, macrophages, lymphocytes, plasma cells, and mast cells. The lamellae pass inward to surround the vessels in the remainder of the choroid layer. Free smooth muscle cells, not associated with blood vessels, are present in this tissue. Lymphatic channels called ***epichoroid lymph spaces,*** long and short posterior ciliary vessels, and nerves on their way to the front of the eye are also present in the suprachoroid lamina.

Most of the blood vessels decrease in size as they approach the retina. The largest vessels continue forward beyond the ora serrata into the ciliary body. These vessels can be seen with an ophthalmoscope. The large vessels are mostly veins that course in whorls before passing obliquely through the sclera as vortex veins. The inner layer of vessels, arranged in a single plane, is called the ***choriocapillary layer.*** The vessels of this layer provide nutrients to the cells of the retina. The fenestrated capillaries have lumina that are large and irregular in shape. In the region of the fovea, the choriocapillary layer is thicker, and the capillary network is denser. This layer ends at the ora serrata.

Bruch's membrane measures 1 to 4 μm in thickness and lies between the choriocapillary layer and the pigment epithelium of the retina. It is a thin, amorphous refractile layer, also called the ***lamina vitrea.*** With the transmission electron microscope (TEM), five different layers are identified in Bruch's membrane:

- The basal lamina of the endothelial cells of the choriocapillary layer
- A layer of collagen fibers approximately 0.5 μm thick
- A layer of elastic fibers approximately 2 μm thick
- A second layer of collagen fibers (thus forming a "sandwich" around the intervening elastic tissue layer)
- The basal lamina of the retinal epithelial cells

Retina

The retina represents the innermost layer of the eye

The retina, derived from the inner and outer layers of the optic cup, is the innermost of the three concentric layers of the eye (see Fig. 23.1c). It consists of two basic layers:

- ***Neural retina*** or ***retina proper,*** the inner layer that contains the photoreceptors
- ***RPE,*** the outer layer that rests on and is firmly attached to the choriocapillary layer of the choroid

A potential space exists between the two layers of the retina. The two layers may be separated mechanically in the preparation of histologic specimens. Separation of the layers, "retinal detachment" (see Box 23.2), also occurs in the living state as a result of eye disease or trauma.

In the neural retina, two regions or portions that differ in function are recognized:

- The ***nonphotosensitive region (nonvisual part),*** located anterior to the ora serrata, which lines the inner aspect of the ciliary body and the posterior surface of the iris (this portion of the retina is described in the sections on the iris and ciliary body)
- The ***photosensitive region (optic part),*** which lines the inner surface of the eye posterior to the ora serrata except where it is pierced by the optic nerve (see Fig. 23.1)

The site where the optic nerve joins the retina is called the ***optic papilla*** or ***disc.*** Because the optic papilla is devoid of photoreceptors, it is a blind spot in the visual field. The ***fovea centralis*** is a shallow depression located about 2.5 mm lateral to the optic disc. It is the area of greatest visual acuity. The visual axis of the eye passes through the fovea. A yellow-pigmented zone called the ***macula lutea*** surrounds the fovea. In relative terms, the fovea is the re-

BOX 23.1

Clinical Correlations: Glaucoma

Glaucoma is a clinical condition resulting from increased intraocular pressure. It can be caused by excessive secretion of aqueous humor or impedance of the drainage of aqueous humor from the anterior chamber. The internal tissues of the eye, particularly the retina, are nourished by the diffusion of oxygen and nutrients from the intraocular vessels. Blood flows normally through these vessels (including the capillaries and veins), when the hydrostatic pressure within the vessels exceeds the intraocular pressure. If the drainage of the aqueous humor is impeded, the intraocular pressure increases because the layers of the eye do not allow the wall to expand. This increased pressure interferes with normal retinal nourishment and function. Visual deficits associated with glaucoma include blurring of vision and impaired dark adaptation (symptoms that indicate loss of normal retinal function) and halos around lights (a symptom indicating corneal endothelial damage). If the condition is not treated, the retina will be permanently damaged and blindness will occur. Treatments are directed toward lowering the intraocular pressure by decreasing the rate of production of aqueous humor or eliminating the cause of the obstruction of normal drainage. Recently, ***carbonic anhydrase*** inhibitors that specifically inhibit carbonic anhydrase isoenzyme CA-II, which plays an important role in the production of aqueous humor in humans, are used as the pharmacologic treatment of choice. Dorzolamide and brinzolamide are two carbonic anhydrase inhibitors that are currently available as eyedrops to treat glaucoma.

gion of the retina that contains the highest concentration and most precisely ordered arrangement of the visual elements.

LAYERS OF THE RETINA

Ten layers of cells and their processes constitute the neural retina

Before discussing the ten layers of the retina, it is important to identify the types of cells found there. This identification will aid in understanding the functional relationships of the cells. Studies of the retina in primates have identified at least 15 types of neurons that form at least 38 different types of synapses. For convenience, neurons and supporting cells can be classified into four groups of cells (Fig. 23.9):

- ***Photoreceptors***—the retinal ***rods*** and ***cones***
- ***Conducting neurons—bipolar*** and ***ganglion cells***
- ***Association*** and other ***neurons—horizontal, centrifugal,*** and ***amacrine***
- ***Supporting cells—Müller's cells*** and ***neuroglial cells***

The specific arrangement and associations of the nuclei and processes of these cells result in the retina being organized in ten layers that are seen with the light microscope. The ten layers of the retina, from outside inward, are (Figs. 23.9 and 23.10)

1. ***Pigment epithelium***—the outer layer of the retina, actually not part of the neural retina but intimately associated with it
2. ***Layer of rods and cones***—contains the outer and inner segments of photoreceptor cells
3. ***Outer limiting membrane***—the apical boundary of Müller's cells
4. ***Outer nuclear layer***—contains the cell bodies (nuclei) of retinal rods and cones

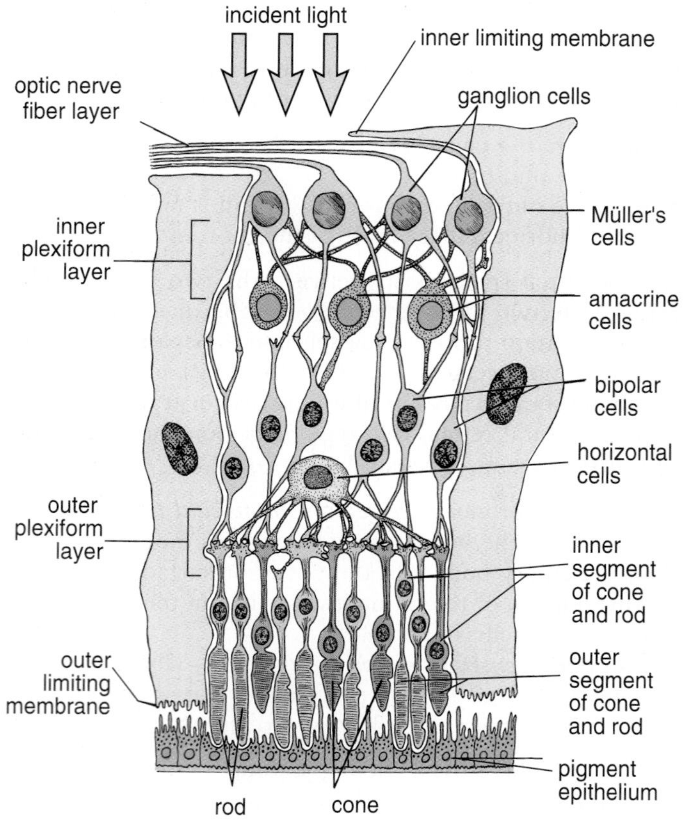

FIGURE 23.9
Schematic drawing of the layers of the retina. The interrelationship of the neurons is indicated. Light enters the retina and passes through the inner layers of the retina before reaching the photoreceptors of the rods and cones that are closely associated with the pigment epithelium.

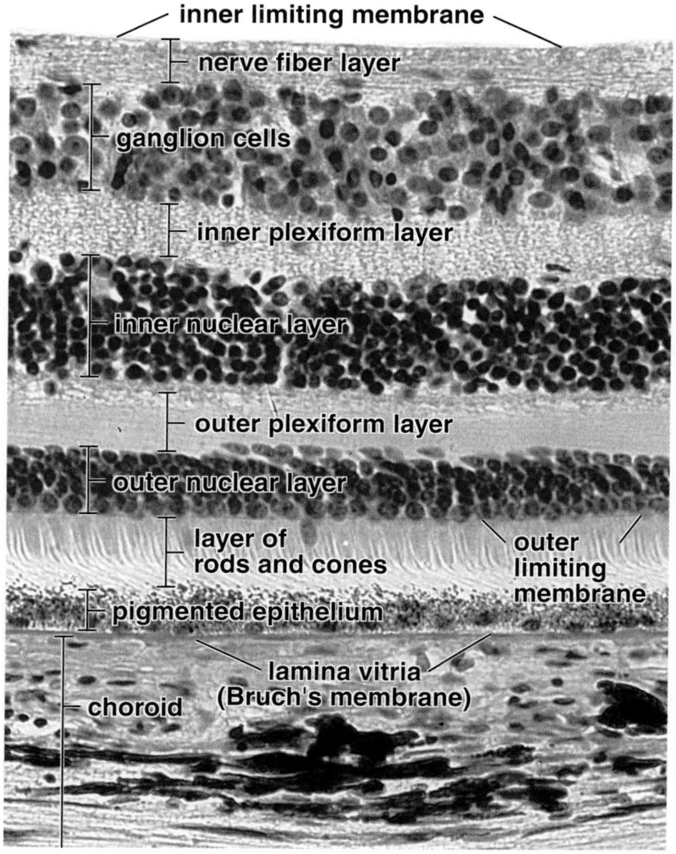

FIGURE 23.10
Photomicrograph of a human retina. On the basis of histologic features that are evident in this micrograph, the retina can be divided into ten layers as indicated on this photomicrograph. Note that Bruch's membrane (lamina vitria) separates the inner layer of the vascular coat (chorioid) from the pigment epithelium. ×440.

5. ***Outer plexiform layer***—contains the processes of retinal rods and cones and processes of the horizontal, amacrine, and bipolar cells that connect to them
6. ***Inner nuclear layer***—contains the cell bodies (nuclei) of horizontal, amacrine, bipolar, and Müller's cells
7. ***Inner plexiform layer***—contains the processes of horizontal, amacrine, bipolar, and ganglion cells that connect to each other
8. ***Ganglion cell layer***—contains the cell bodies (nuclei) of ganglion cells
9. ***Layer of optic nerve fibers***—contains processes of ganglion cells that lead from the retina to the brain
10. ***Inner limiting membrane***—composed of the basal lamina of Müller's cells

Each of the layers is more fully described in the following sections (see corresponding numbers).

The cells of the RPE (layer 1) have extensions that surround the processes of the rods and cones

The ***RPE*** is a single layer of cuboidal cells about 14 μm wide and 10 to 14 μm tall. The cells rest on Bruch's membrane of the choroid layer. The pigment cells are tallest in the fovea and adjacent regions, which accounts for the darker color of this region.

Adjacent RPE cells are connected by a junctional complex consisting of gap junctions and elaborate zonulae occludentes and adherentes. This junctional complex is the site of the "***blood–retina barrier.***"

The pigment cells have cylindrical sheaths on their apical surface that are associated with, but do not directly contact, the tip of the photoreceptor processes of the adjacent rod and cone cells. Complex cytoplasmic processes project for a short distance between the photoreceptors of the rods and cones. Numerous elongated melanin granules, unlike those found elsewhere in the eye, are present in many of these processes. They aggregate on the side of the cell nearest the rods and cones and are the most prominent feature of the cells. The nucleus with its many convoluted infoldings is located near the basal plasma membrane adjacent to Bruch's membrane. The cells also contain material phagocytosed from the processes of the photoreceptors in the form of lamellar debris contained in residual bodies or phagosomes. A supranuclear Golgi apparatus and an extensive network of smooth endoplasmic reticulum (sER) surround the melanin granules and residual bodies that are present in the cytoplasm.

The RPE serves several important functions including

- ***Absorption of light*** passing through the neural retina to prevent reflection and resultant glare.
- ***Isolation of the retinal cells*** from blood-borne substances. It serves as a major component of the ***blood–retina barrier*** via tight junctions between RPE cells.
- Participation in ***restoration of photosensitivity*** to visual pigments that were dissociated in response to light. The metabolic apparatus for visual pigment resynthesis is present in the RPE cells.
- ***Phagocytosis and disposal*** of membranous discs from the rods and cones of the retinal photoreceptor cells.

The rods and cones of the photoreceptor cell (layer 2) extend from the outer layer of the neural retina to the pigment epithelium

The ***rods*** and ***cones*** are the outer segments of photoreceptor cells whose nuclei form the outer nuclear layer of the retina (Figs. 23.10 and 23.11). *The light that reaches the photoreceptors must first pass through all of the internal layers of the neural retina.* The rods and cones are arranged in a palisade manner; therefore, in the light microscope, they appear as vertical striations.

The retina contains approximately 120 million rods and 7 million cones. The rods are about 2 μm thick and 50 μm long (ranging from about 60 μm at the fovea to 40 μm peripherally). The cones vary in length from 85 μm at the fovea to 25 μm at the periphery of the retina.

Functionally, the rods are more sensitive to light and are the receptors used during periods of low light intensity (e.g., at dusk or at night). The visual image provided is one composed of gray tones ("a black and white picture"). In contrast, the cones exist in three classes: L, M, and S (long-, middle-, and short-wavelength sensitive, respectively) that cannot be distinguished morphologically. They are less sensitive to low light and have maximal sensitivity to the red, green, or blue region of the visual spectrum. They provide a visual image composed of color, which is believed to permit better visual acuity. The specificity of the cones provides a functional basis to explain color blindness that is believed to result from the lack of red-, green-, or (much less commonly) blue-sensitive cones.

BOX 23.2

Clinical Correlations: Retinal Detachment

A potential space exists in the retina as a vestige of the space between the apical surfaces of the two epithelial layers of the optic cup. If this space expands, the neural retina separates from the pigment epithelium. This condition is called ***retinal detachment***. If not corrected, blindness results. More commonly, as the vitreous body ages (in the sixth and seventh decades of life), it tends to shrink and pull away from the neural retina, which causes single or multiple tears in the neural retina. Retinal detachment is repaired by cryosurgery or laser surgery to prevent visual loss.

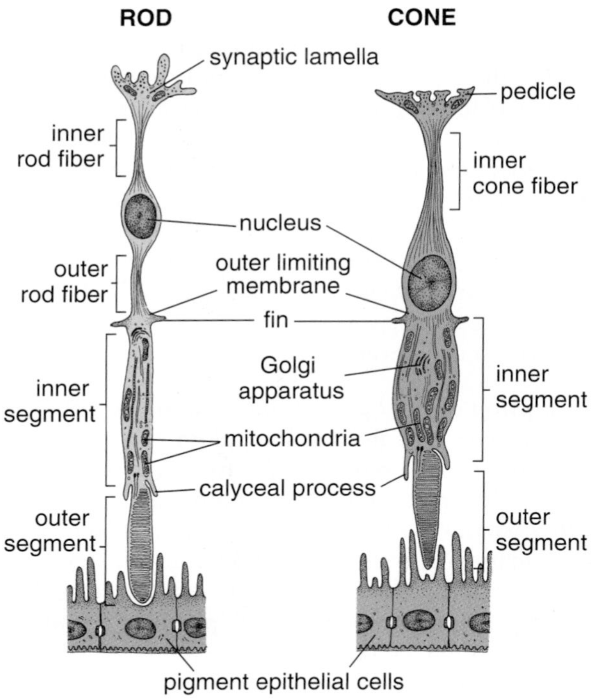

FIGURE 23.11
Schematic diagram of the ultrastructure of rod and cone cells. The outer segments of the rods and cones are closely associated with the adjacent pigment epithelium.

Each rod and cone photoreceptor consists of three parts:

- ***Outer segment*** of the photoreceptor is roughly cylindrical or conical (hence, the descriptive name *rod* or *cone*). This portion of the photoreceptor is intimately related to microvilli projecting from the adjacent pigment epithelial cells.
- ***Connecting stalk*** contains a cilium composed of nine peripheral microtubule doublets extending from a basal body. The connecting stalk appears as the constricted region of the cell that joins the inner to the outer segment. In this region, a thin, tapering process called the ***calyceal process*** extends from the distal end of the inner segment to surround the proximal portion of the outer segment (see Fig. 23.11).
- ***Inner segment*** is divided into an outer ***ellipsoid*** and an inner ***myoid*** portion. This segment contains a typical complement of organelles associated with a cell actively synthesizing proteins. A prominent Golgi apparatus, rER, and free ribosomes are concentrated in the myoid region. Mitochondria are most numerous in the ellipsoid region. Microtubules are distributed throughout the inner segment. In the outer ellipsoid portion, cross-striated fibrous rootlets may extend from the basal body among the mitochondria.

The outer segment is the site of photosensitivity, and the inner segment contains the metabolic machinery that supports the activity of the photoreceptors. The outer segment is considered to be a highly modified cilium because it is joined to the inner segment by a short connecting stalk containing a basal body (Fig. 23.12a).

With the TEM, 600 to 1000 regularly spaced horizontal discs are seen in the outer segment (Fig. 23.12). In rods, these discs are membrane-bounded structures measuring about 2 μm in diameter. They are enclosed within the plasma membrane of the outer segment (Fig. 23.12a). The parallel membranes of the discs are about 6 nm thick and are continuous at their ends. The central enclosed space is about 8 nm across. In both rods and cones, the membranous discs are formed from repetitive transverse infolding of the plasma membrane in the region of the outer segment near the cilium. Autoradiographic studies have demonstrated that rods form new discs by infolding of the plasma membrane throughout their lifespan. Discs are formed in cones in a similar manner but are not replaced on a regular basis.

Rod discs lose their continuity with the plasma membrane from which they are derived soon after they are formed. They then pass like a stack of plates, proximally to distally, along the length of the cylindrical portion of the outer segment until they are eventually shed and phagocytosed by the pigment epithelial cells. Thus, each rod disc is a membrane-enclosed compartment within the cytoplasm. Discs within the cones retain their continuity with the plasma membrane (Fig. 23.12b).

Rod cells contain the visual pigment rhodopsin; cone cells contain the visual pigment iodopsin

Rhodopsin (visual purple) in rod cells initiates the visual stimulus when it is bleached by light. Rhodopsin is present in globular form on the outer surface of the lipid bilayer (on the cytoplasmic side) of the membranous discs. In the cone cells, the visual pigment on the membranous discs is the photopigment ***iodopsin***. Each cone cell is specialized to respond maximally to one of three colors: red, green, or blue. Both rhodopsin and iodopsin, contain a membrane-bound subunit called an ***opsin*** and a second component called a ***chromophore***. The opsin of rods is ***scotopsin;*** the opsins of cones are ***photopsins***. The chromophore of rods is a vitamin A–derived carotenoid called ***retinal***. Thus, an adequate intake of vitamin A is essential for normal vision. Prolonged dietary deficiency of vitamin A leads to the inability to see in dim light ("night blindness").

The interior of the discs of cones is continuous with the extracellular space

The basic difference in the structure of the rod and cone discs, i.e., continuity with the plasma membrane, is correlated with the slightly different means by which the visual pigments are renewed in rods and cones. Newly synthesized rhodopsin is incorporated into the membrane of the rod disc as the disc is being formed at the base of the outer segment.

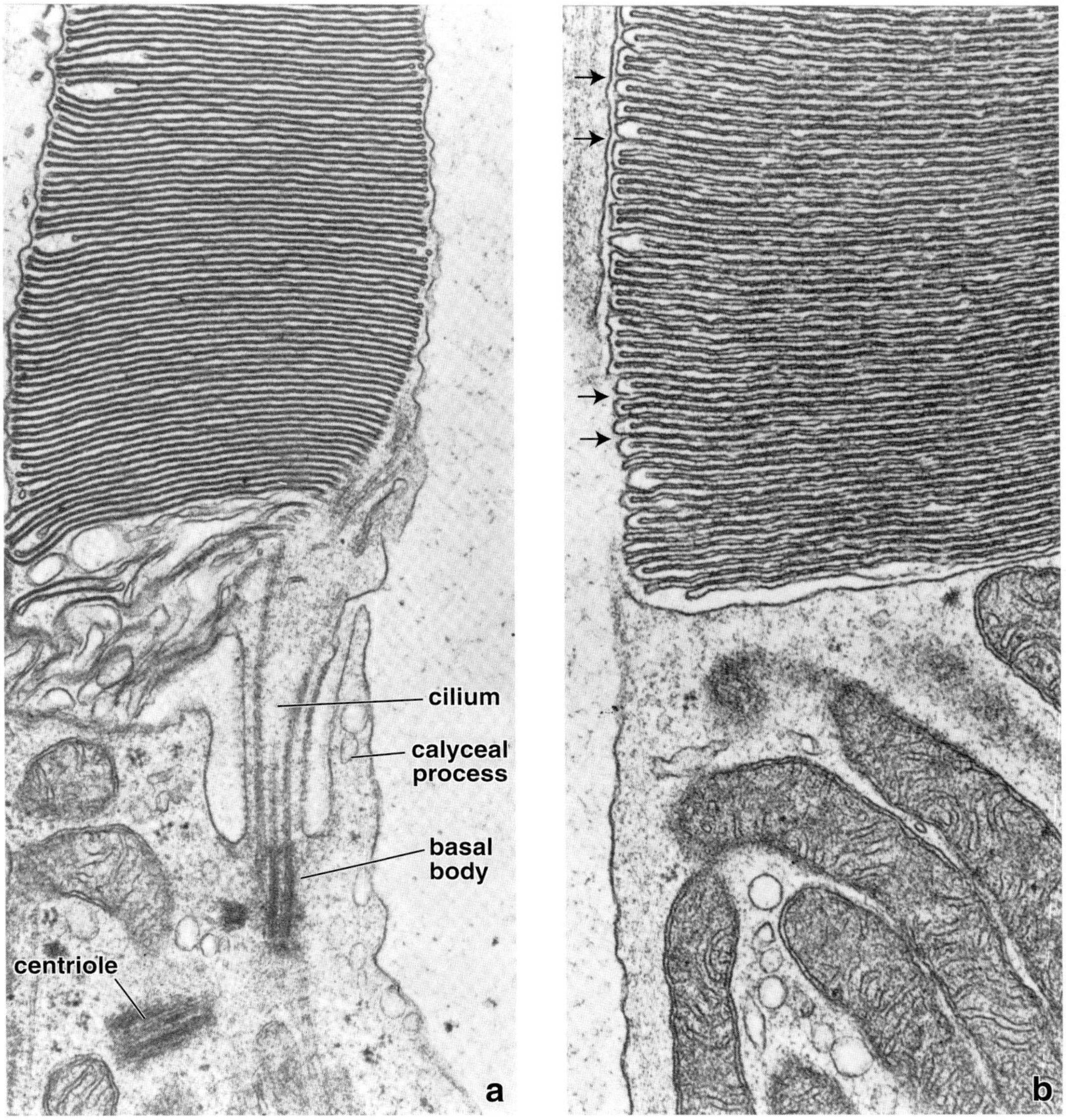

FIGURE 23.12
Electron micrographs of portions of the inner and outer segments of cones and rods. a. This electron micrograph shows the junction between the inner and outer segments of the rod cell. The outer segments contain the horizontally flattened discs. The plane of this section passes through the connecting stalk and cilium. A centriole, a cilium and its basal body, and a calyceal process are identified. ×32,000. **b.** Another electron micrograph shows a similar section of a cone cell. The interior of the discs in the outer segment of the cone is continuous with the extracellular space *(arrows).* × 32,000. (Courtesy of Dr. Toichiro Kuwabara.)

It then takes several days for the disc to reach the tip of the outer segment. In contrast, although visual proteins are constantly produced in retinal cones, the proteins are incorporated into cone discs located anywhere in the outer segment.

Vision is a process by which light striking the retina is converted into electrical impulses that are transmitted to the brain

The impulses produced by light reaching the photoreceptors are conveyed to the brain by an elaborate network of nerves. The conversion of the incident light into nerve impulses is called ***transduction*** and involves two basic steps:

- **Step 1** is a photochemical reaction that occurs in the outer segment of the rod and cone receptors as absorbed light energy causes *conformational changes in the chromophores.*
- **Step 2** consists of *changes in the concentration of internal transmitters* within the cytoplasm of the inner segment of the photoreceptors. These changes influence the

ionic permeability of the plasma membrane and cause the photoreceptor to become hyperpolarized, thus initiating impulses that are conveyed to the brain.

In rods, absorbed light energy causes conformational changes in retinal, converting it to retinol

The conversion of retinal to retinol results in its release from scotopsin (a reaction called "bleaching"). The cell becomes hyperpolarized as calcium diffuses from the receptor cell and reduces its permeability to sodium. The visual pigment is then reassembled, and calcium is transported back into the cell. The energy for this process is provided by the mitochondria located in the inner segment. Müller's cells and pigment epithelial cells also participate in the interconversion of retinal and retinol and the reactions necessary for the resynthesis of rhodopsin.

During normal functioning of the photoreceptors, the membranous discs of the outer segment are shed and phagocytosed by the pigment epithelial cells (Fig. 23.13). It is estimated that each of these cells is capable of phagocytosing and disposing of about 7500 discs/day. The discs are constantly turning over, and the production of new discs must equal the rate of disc shedding.

Discs are shed from both rods and cones

In rods, after a period of sleep, a burst of disc shedding occurs as light first enters the eye. The time of disc shedding in cones is more variable. The shedding of discs in cones also enables the receptors to eliminate superfluous membrane. Although not fully understood, the shedding process in cones also alters the size of the discs, so that the conical form is maintained as discs are released from the distal end of the cone.

The outer limiting membrane (layer 3) is formed by a row of zonulae adherentes between Müller's cells

The outer limiting membrane is not a true membrane. It is a row of zonulae adherentes that attaches the apical ends of Müller's cells (i.e., the end that faces the pigment epithelium) to each other and to the rods and cones (see Fig. 23.10). Because Müller's cells end at the base of the inner segments of the receptors, they mark the location of this layer. Thus, the supporting processes of Müller's cells on which the rods and cones rest are pierced by the inner and outer segments of the photoreceptors.

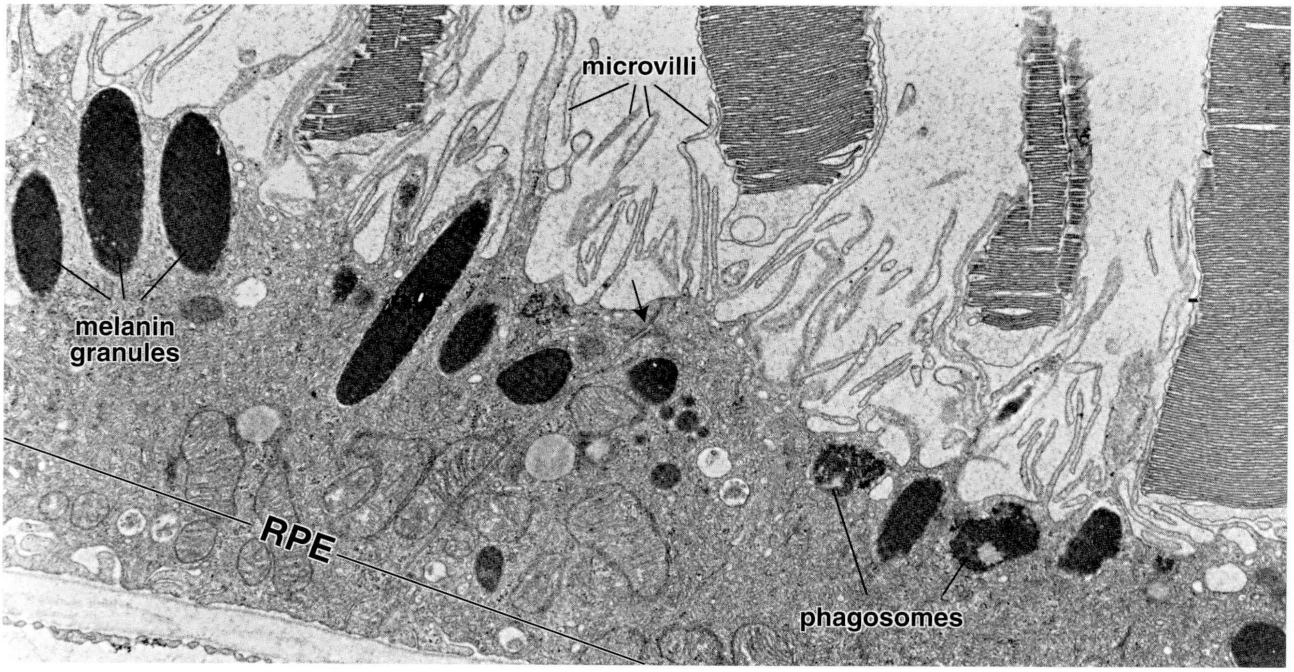

FIGURE 23.13
Electron micrograph of the retinal pigment epithelium in association with the outer segments of rods and cones. Retinal pigment epithelial cells *(RPE)* contain numerous elongated melanin granules that are aggregated in the apical portion of the cell, where the microvilli extend from the surface toward the outer segments of the rod and cone cells. The retinal pigment epithelial cells contain numerous mitochondria and phagosomes. The *arrow* indicates the location of the junctional complex between two adjacent cells. ×20,000. (Courtesy of Dr. Toichiro Kuwabara.)

The outer nuclear layer (4) contains the nuclei of the retinal rods and cones

The region of the rod cytoplasm that contains the nucleus is separated from the inner segment by a tapering process of the cytoplasm. In cones, the nuclei are located close to the outer segments, and no tapering is seen. The cone nuclei stain lightly and are larger and more oval than rod nuclei. Rod nuclei are surrounded by only a thin rim of cytoplasm. In contrast, a relatively thick investment of cytoplasm surrounds the cone nuclei (see Fig. 23.11).

The outer plexiform layer (5) is formed by the processes of the photoreceptor cells and neurons

The outer plexiform layer is formed by the processes of retinal rods and cones and the processes of horizontal, amacrine, and bipolar cells. The processes allow the electrical coupling of photoreceptor cells to these specialized interneurons via synapses. A thin process extends from the region of the nucleus of each rod or cone to an inner expanded portion with several lateral processes. The expanded portion is called a ***spherule*** in a rod and a ***pedicle*** in a cone. Normally, many photoreceptors converge onto one bipolar cell and form interconnecting neural networks. Cones located in the fovea, however, synapse with a single bipolar cell. The fovea is also unique in that the compactness of the inner neural layers of the retina causes the photoreceptors to be oriented obliquely. Horizontal cell dendritic processes synapse with photoreceptors throughout the retina and further contribute to the elaborate neuronal connections in this layer.

The inner nuclear layer (6) consists of the nuclei of horizontal, amacrine, bipolar, and Müller's cells

Müller's cells form the scaffolding for the entire retina. Their processes invest the other cells of the retina so completely that they fill most of the extracellular space. The basal and apical ends of Müller's cells form the inner and outer limiting membranes, respectively. Microvilli extending from their apical border lie between the photoreceptors of the rods and cones. Capillaries from the retinal vessels extend only to this layer. The rods and cones carry out their metabolic exchanges with extracellular fluids transported across the blood-retina barrier of the RPE.

The three types of conducting cells—***bipolar, horizontal,*** and ***amacrine***—found in this layer have distinct orientations (see Fig. 23.9). The processes of ***bipolar cells*** extend to both the inner and outer plexiform layer. Through these connections, the bipolar cells establish synaptic connections with multiple cells in each layer except in the fovea, where the number of interconnected cells is reduced to provide greater visual acuity. The processes of ***horizontal cells*** extend to the outer plexiform layer where they intermingle with processes of bipolar cells. The cells have synaptic connections with rod spherules, cone pedicles, and bipolar cells. This electrical coupling of cells is thought to affect the functional threshold between rods and cones and bipolar cells. The processes of ***amacrine cells*** branch extensively to provide sites of synaptic connections with axonal endings of bipolar cells and dendrites of ganglion cells.

In the peripheral regions of the retina, the axons of bipolar cells pass to the inner plexiform layer where they synapse with several ganglion cells. In the fovea, they may synapse with a single ganglion cell, again reflecting the greater visual acuity in this region. Amacrine cell processes pass inward, contributing to a complex interconnection of cells. They synapse in the inner plexiform layer with bipolar, ganglion, and other amacrine cells (see Fig. 23.9).

The inner plexiform layer (7) consists of a complex array of intermingled neuronal cell processes

The inner plexiform layer consists of a complex intermingling of the processes of the amacrine, bipolar, and ganglion cells. The course of these processes is parallel to the inner limiting membrane, thus giving the appearance of horizontal striations to this layer (see Fig. 23.10).

The ganglion cell layer (8) consists of the cell bodies of large multipolar neurons

The cell bodies of large multipolar nerve cells, measuring up to 30 μm in diameter, constitute the ganglion cell layer. These nerve cells have lightly staining round nuclei with prominent nucleoli and have Nissl bodies in their cytoplasm. An axonal process emerges from the rounded cell body, passes into the nerve fiber layer, and then goes into the optic nerve. The dendrites extend from the opposite end of the cell to ramify in the inner plexiform layer. In the peripheral regions of the retina, a single ganglion cell may synapse with a hundred bipolar cells. In marked contrast, in the macular region surrounding the fovea, the bipolar cells are smaller (some authors refer to them as "midget" bipolar cells), and they tend to make one-to-one connections with ganglion cells. Over most of the retina, the ganglion cells are only a single layer of cells. At the macula, however, they are piled up to eight deep, although they are absent over the fovea itself. Scattered among the ganglion cells are small neuroglial cells with densely staining nuclei (see Fig. 23.10).

The layer of optic nerve fibers (9) contains axons of the ganglion cells

The axonal processes of the ganglion cells form a flattened layer running parallel to the retinal surface. This layer increases in depth as the axons converge at the optic disc. The axons are thin, nonmyelinated processes measuring up to 5 μm in diameter (see Fig. 23.10).

BOX 23.3

Clinical Correlations: Age-Related Macular Degeneration (ARMD)

Age-related macular degeneration (ARMD) is the most common cause of blindness in older individuals. Although the etiology of this disease is still unknown, evidence suggests both genetic and environmental (UV irradiation, drugs) components. The disease causes loss of central vision, while peripheral vision remains unaffected. Two forms of ARMD are recognized: a dry (atrophic, nonexudative) form and a wet (exudative, neovascular) form. The latter is considered a complication of the first. Dry ARMD is the most common form (90% of all cases) and involves degenerative lesions localized in the area of the macula lutea. The degenerative lesions include a focal thickening of Bruch's membrane called "drusen," atrophy and depigmentation of RPE, and obliteration of capillaries in the underlying chorioid layer. These changes lead to deterioration of the overlying photosensitive retina, resulting in the formation of "blind spots" in the visual field (Fig. 23.14). Wet ARMD is a complication of dry ARMD caused by neovascularization of "blind spots" of the retina in the large drusen. These newly formed, thin, fragile vessels frequently leak and produce exudates and hemorrhages in the space just beneath the retina, resulting in fibrosis and scarring. These changes are responsible for the progressive loss of central vision over a short time. The treatment of wet ARMD includes conventional laser treatment therapy; however, new surgical methods such as macular translocation have been recently introduced. In this procedure, the retina is detached, translocated, and reattached in a new location, away from the chorioid neovascular tissue. Conventional laser treatment is then applied to destroy pathologic vessels without destroying central vision.

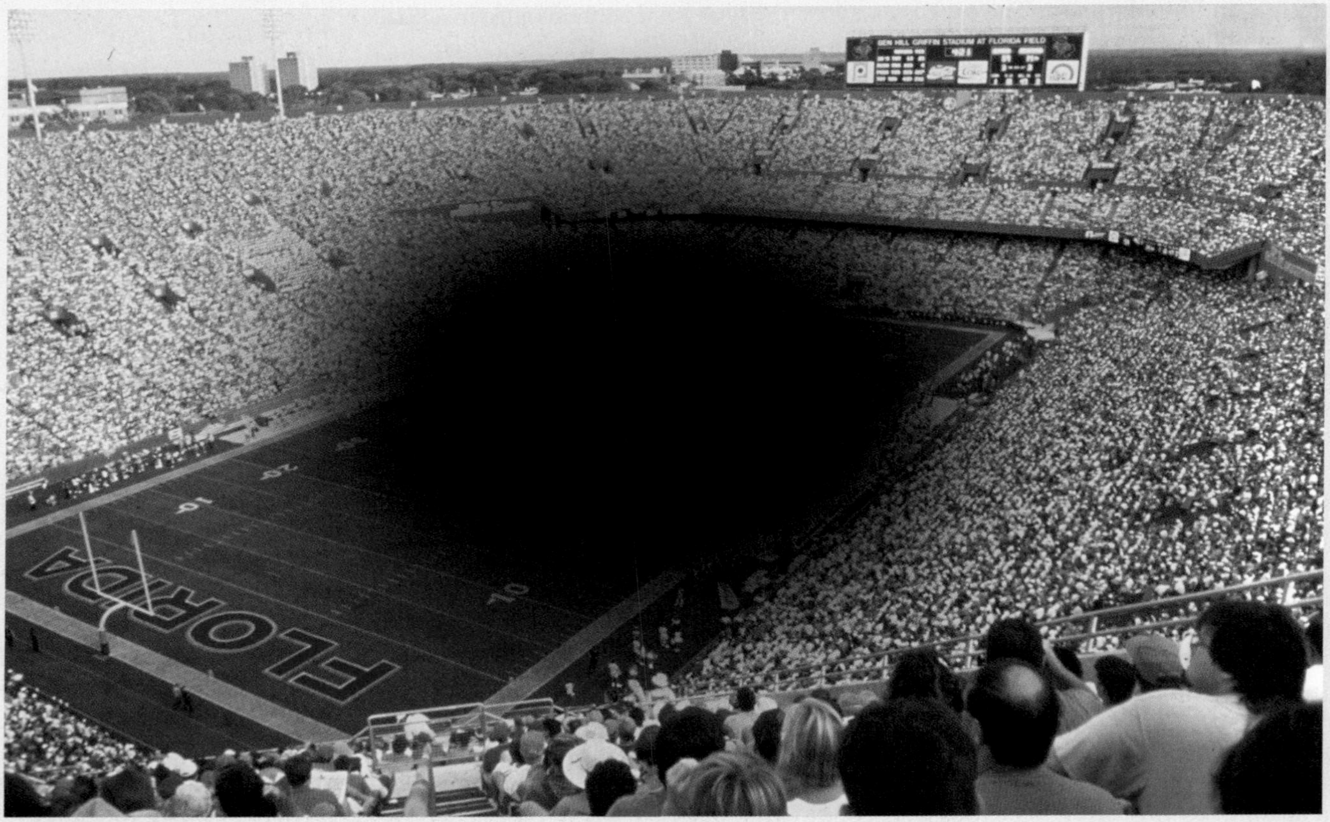

FIGURE 23.14
Photograph depicting the visual field in individuals with age-related macular degeneration. Note that central vision is absent because of the changes in the macula region of the retina. To maximize their remaining vision, individuals with this condition are instructed to use eccentric fixation of their eyes.

The inner limiting membrane (layer 10) consists of a basal lamina separating the retina from the vitreous body

The inner limiting membrane is the basal lamina of Müller's cells (see Fig. 23.10).

SPECIALIZED REGIONS OF THE RETINA

The *fovea* appears as a shallow depression located at the posterior pole of the optical axis of the eye. Its central region, known as the *fovea centralis*, is about 200 μm in di-

ameter. Except for the photoreceptor layer, most of the layers of the retina are markedly reduced or absent in this region (see Fig. 23.6). Here, the photoreceptor is composed entirely of cones that are longer and more slender and rod-like than they are elsewhere. The adjacent pigment epithelial cells and choriocapillaris are also thickened in this region.

The ***macula lutea*** is the area surrounding the fovea. It is yellowish due to the presence of yellow pigment (xanthophyll). Retinal vessels are absent in this region. Here, the retinal cells and their processes, especially the ganglion cells, are heaped up on the sides of the fovea so that light may pass unimpeded to this most sensitive area of the retina.

VESSELS OF THE RETINA

The ***central retinal artery*** and ***vein***, the vessels that can be seen and assessed with an ophthalmoscope, pass through the center of the optic nerve to enter the bulb of the eye at the optic disc (see Fig. 23.2 and pages 791 to 792, the section on the developing eye). The artery branches immediately into upper and lower branches, each of which divides again. Veins undergo a similar pattern of branching. The vessels initially lie between the vitreous body and inner limiting membrane. As the vessels pass laterally, they pass deeper within the inner retinal layers. Branches from these vessels form a capillary plexus that does not extend beyond the inner nuclear layer. The branches of the central retinal artery do not anastomose and therefore are classified as anatomic end arteries. Evaluation of the retinal vessels and optic disc during the physical examination of a patient not only provides important information on the state of the eye but also provides early clinical signs of a number of conditions, including elevated intracranial pressure, hypertension, glaucoma, and diabetes.

Crystalline Lens

The lens is a transparent, avascular, biconvex structure. It is suspended between the edges of the ciliary body by the ***zonular fibers***. The pull of the zonular fibers keeps the lens in a flattened condition. Release of tension causes the lens to fatten or ***accommodate*** to bend light rays originating close to the eye so that they focus on the retina.

The lens has three principal components (Fig. 23.15):

- ***Lens capsule***, a thick basal lamina measuring approximately 10 to 20 μm, produced by the anterior lens cells
- ***Subcapsular epithelium***, a cuboidal layer of cells present only on the anterior surface of the lens
- ***Lens fibers***, structures derived from subcapsular epithelial cells

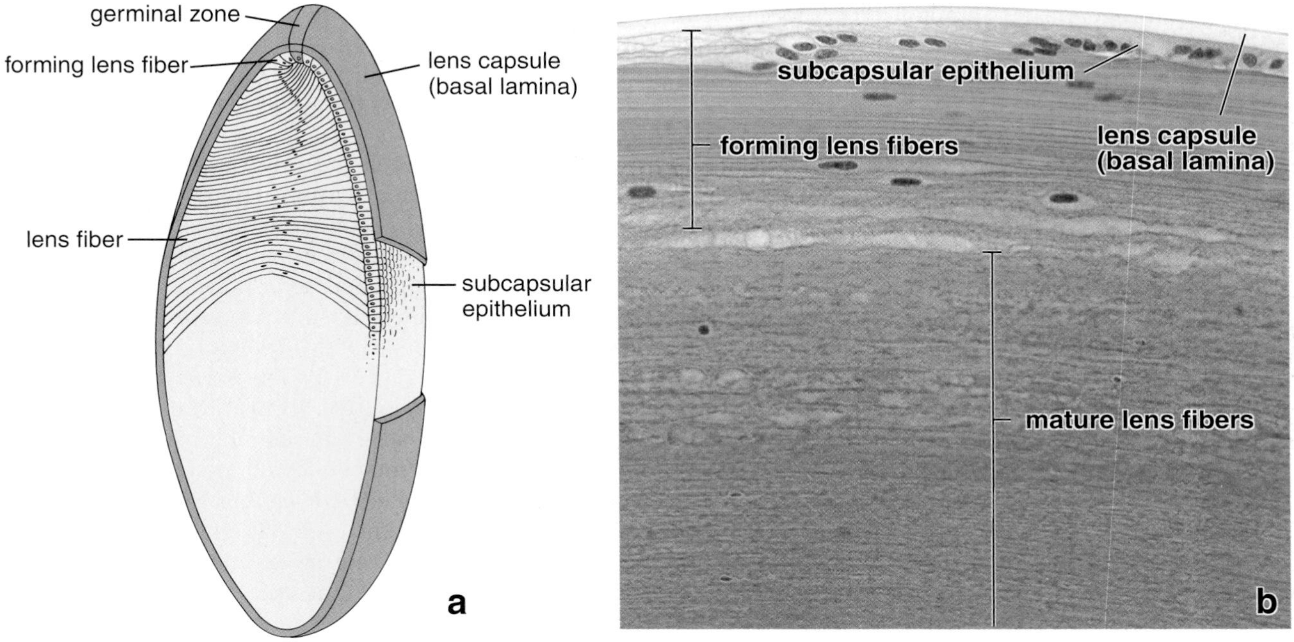

FIGURE 23.15
Structure of the lens. a. This schematic drawing of the lens indicates its structural components. Note that the capsule of the lens is formed by the basal lamina of the lens fibers and the subcapsular epithelium located on the anterior surface of the lens. Also note the location of the germinal zone at the equatorial area of the lens. **b.** This high-magnification photomicrograph of the germinal zone of the lens (near its equator) shows the active process of lens fibers formation from the subcapsular epithelium. Note the thick lens capsule and the underlying layer of nuclei of lens fibers during their differentiation. The mature lens fibers do not possess nuclei. ×570.

The ***lens capsule,*** composed primarily of type IV collagen and proteoglycans, is elastic. It is thickest at the equator where the fibers of the zonule attach to it.

Gap junctions connect the cuboidal cells of the subcapsular epithelium. They have few cytoplasmic organelles and stain faintly. The apical region of the cell is directed toward the internal aspect of the lens and the ***lens fibers*** with which they form junctional complexes. The lens increases in size during normal growth and then continues to produce new ***lens fibers*** at an ever-decreasing rate throughout life. The new lens fibers develop from the subcapsular epithelial cells located near the equator (see Fig. 23.15). Cells in this region increase in height and then differentiate into lens fibers.

As the lens fibers develop, they become highly elongated and appear as thin, flattened structures. They lose their nuclei and other organelles as they become filled with proteins called ***crystallins.*** Mature lens fibers attain a length of 7 to 10 mm, a width of 8 to 10 μm, and a thickness of 2 μm. Near the center of the lens, in the nucleus, the fibers are compressed and condensed to such a degree that individual fibers are impossible to recognize. Despite its density and protein content, the lens is normally transparent (see Fig. 23.15). The high density of lens fibers makes it difficult to obtain routine histologic sections of the lens that are free from artifacts.

Changes in the lens are associated with aging

With increasing age, the lens gradually loses its elasticity and ability to accommodate. This condition, called ***presbyopia,*** usually occurs in the fourth decade of life. It is easily corrected by wearing reading glasses or using a magnifying lens.

Loss of transparency of the lens or its capsule is also a relatively common condition associated with aging. This condition, called ***cataract,*** may be due to conformational changes or cross-linking of proteins. The development of a cataract may also be related to disease processes, metabolic or hereditary conditions, trauma, or exposure to a deleterious agent (such as ultraviolet radiation). Cataracts that significantly impair vision can usually be corrected surgically by removing the lens and replacing it with a plastic lens implanted in the posterior chamber.

Vitreous Body

The vitreous body is the transparent jelly-like substance that fills the vitreous chamber in the posterior segment of the eye

The vitreous body is loosely attached to the surrounding structures, including the inner limiting membrane of the retina. The main portion of the vitreous body is a homogeneous gel containing approximately 99% water (the vitreous humor), collagen, glycosaminoglycans (principally hyaluronic acid), and a small population of cells called ***hyalocytes.*** These cells are believed to be responsible for synthesis of collagen fibrils and glycosaminoglycans. Hyalocytes in routine hematoxylin and eosin (H&E) preparation are difficult to visualize. Often, they exhibit a well-developed rER and Golgi apparatus. Fibroblasts and tissue macrophages are sometimes seen in the periphery of the vitreous body. The ***hyaloid canal*** (or ***Cloquet's canal***), which is not always visible, runs through the center of the vitreous body from the optic disc to the posterior lens capsule. It is the remnant of the pathway of the hyaloid artery of the developing eye.

Accessory Structures of the Eye

The conjunctiva lines the space between the inner surface of the eyelids and the anterior surface of the eye lateral to the cornea

The ***conjunctiva*** is a thin, transparent mucous membrane that extends from the corneoscleral limbus located on the lateral margin of the cornea across the sclera ***(bulbar conjunctiva)*** and covers the internal surface of the eyelids ***(palpebral conjunctiva).*** It consists of a stratified columnar epithelium containing numerous goblet cells and rests on a lamina propria composed of loose connective tissue. The goblet cell secretion is a component of the tears that bathe the eye.

The primary function of the eyelids is to protect the eye

The skin of the eyelids is loose and elastic to accommodate their movement. Within each eyelid is a flexible support, the ***tarsal plate,*** consisting of dense fibrous and elastic tissue. Its lower free margin extends to the lid margin, and its superior border serves for the attachment of smooth muscle fibers of the ***superior tarsal muscle (of Müller).*** The undersurface of the tarsal plate is covered by the conjunctiva (Fig. 23.16). The ***orbicularis oculi muscle,*** a facial expression muscle, forms a thin oval sheet of circularly oriented skeletal muscle fibers overlying the tarsal plate. In addition, the connective tissue of the eyelid contains tendon fibers of the ***levator palpebrae superioris muscle,*** which open the eyelid (see Fig. 23.16)

In addition to eccrine sweat glands, which discharge their secretions directly onto the skin, the eyelid contains four other major types of glands (see Fig. 23.16):

- *Tarsal glands (Meibomian glands),* long sebaceous glands embedded in the tarsal plates that appear as vertical yellow streaks in the tissue deep to the conjunctiva. About 25 tarsal glands are present in the upper eyelid, and 20 are present in the lower eyelid. The sebaceous se-

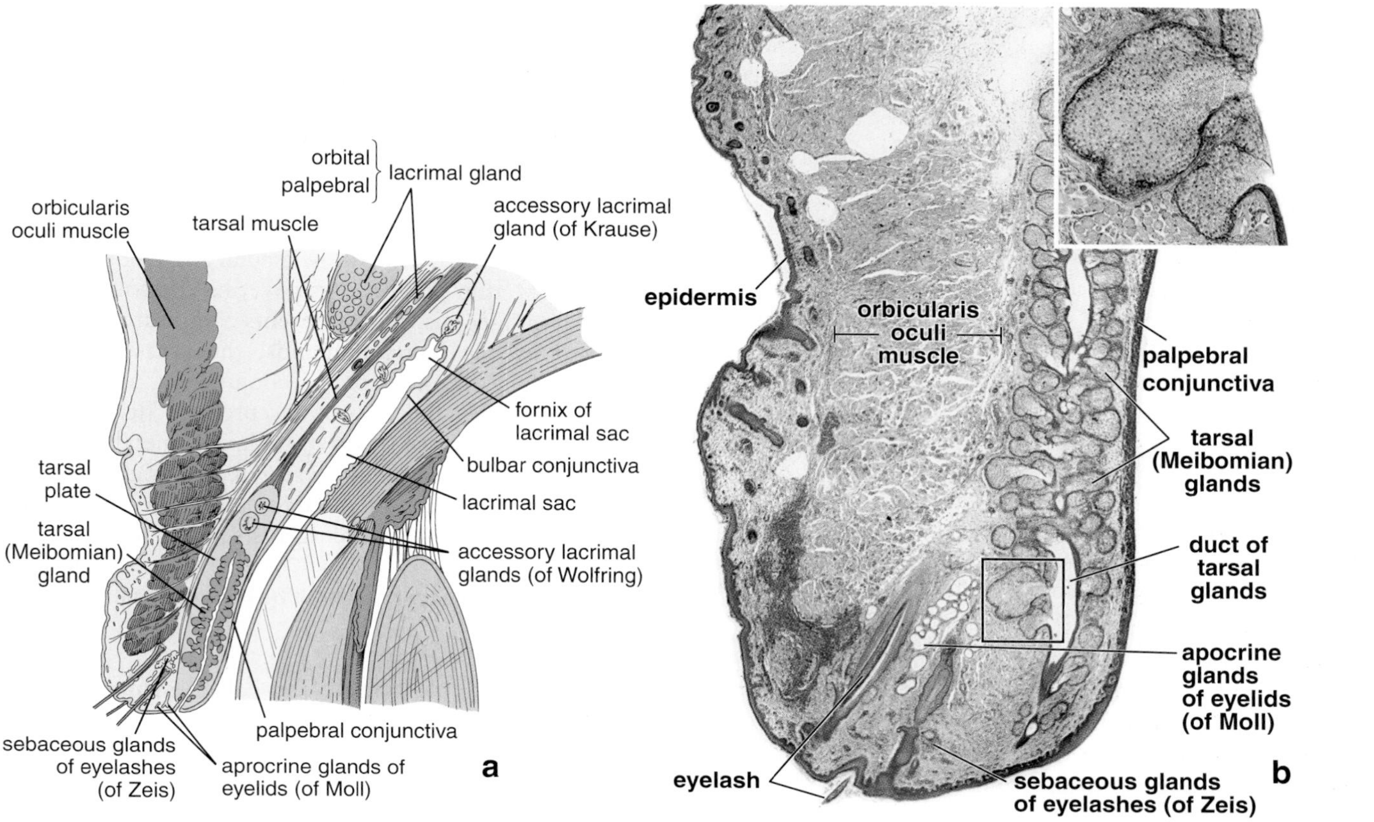

FIGURE 23.16
Structure of the eyelid. a. This schematic drawing of the eyelid shows the skin, associated skin appendages, muscles, tendons, connective tissue, and conjunctiva. Note the distribution of multiple small glands associated with the eyelid and observe the reflection of the palpebral conjunctiva in the fornix of the lacrimal sac to become the bulbar conjunctiva. **b.** Photomicrograph of a sagittal section of the eyelid stained with picric acid for better visualization of epithelial components of the skin and the numerous glands. In this preparation, muscle tissue (i.e., orbicularis oculi muscle) stains yellow, and the epithelial cells of skin, conjunctiva, and glandular epithelium are green. Note the presence of the numerous glands within the eyelid. The tarsal (Meibomian) gland is the largest gland, and it is located within the dense connective tissue of the tarsal plates. This sebaceous gland secretes into ducts opening onto the eyelids. ×20. **Inset.** Higher magnification of a tarsal gland from the *boxed area,* showing the typical structure of a holocrine gland. ×60.

cretion of the tarsal glands produces an oily layer on the surface of the tear film that retards the evaporation of the normal tear layer.

- *Sebaceous glands of eyelashes (glands of Zeis),* small, modified sebaceous glands that are connected with and empty their secretion into the follicles of the eyelashes
- *Apocrine glands of eyelashes (glands of Moll),* small sweat glands with unbranched sinuous tubules that begin as a simple spiral
- *Accessory lacrimal glands,* compound serous tubuloalveolar glands that have distended lumina. They are located on the inner surface of the upper eyelids *(glands of Wolfring)* and in the *fornix of the lacrimal sac (glands of Krause).*

All glands of the human eyelid are innervated by neurons of the autonomic nerve system, and their secretion is synchronized with the lacrimal glands by a common neurotransmitter, vasoactive intestinal polypeptide (VIP).

The *eyelashes* emerge from the most anterior edge of the lid margin, in front of the openings of the Meibomian glands. The lashes are short, stiff, curved hairs and may occur in double or triple rows. The lashes on the same eyelid margin may have different lengths and diameters.

The lacrimal gland produces tears that moisten the cornea and pass to the nasolacrimal duct

Tears are produced by the lacrimal glands and to lesser degree by the accessory lacrimal glands. The lacrimal gland is located beneath the conjunctiva on the upper lateral side of the orbit (Fig. 23.17). The lacrimal gland consists of several separate lobules of tubuloacinar serous glands. The acini have large lumina lined with columnar

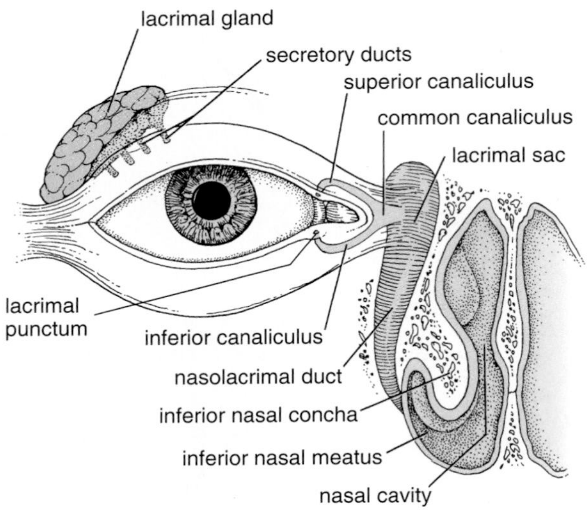

FIGURE 23.17
Schematic diagram of the eye and lacrimal apparatus. This drawing shows the location of the lacrimal gland and components of the lacrimal apparatus, which drains the lacrimal fluid into the nasal cavity.

cells. Myoepithelial cells, located below the epithelial cells within the basal lamina, aid in the release of tears. Approximately 12 ducts drain from the lacrimal gland into the reflection of conjunctiva just beneath the upper eyelid, known as the fornix of the lacrimal sac.

Tears drain from the eye through ***lacrimal puncta***, the small openings of the ***lacrimal canaliculi***, located at the medial angle. The upper and lower canaliculi join to form the ***common canaliculus*** that opens into the lacrimal sac. The sac is continuous with the ***nasolacrimal duct*** that opens into the nasal cavity below the inferior turbinate. A pseudostratified ciliated epithelium lines the lacrimal sac and the nasolacrimal duct.

Tears protect the corneal epithelium and contain antibacterial and ultraviolet-protective agents

Tears keep the conjunctiva and corneal epithelium moist and wash foreign material from the eye as they flow across the corneal surface toward the medial angle of the eye (Fig. 23.17). The thin film of tears covering the corneal surface is not homogenous, but represents a mixture of products secreted by the lacrimal glands, the accessory lacrimal glands, the goblet cells of the conjunctiva, and the tarsal glands of the eyelid. It contains proteins (tear albumins, lactoferrin), enzymes (lysozyme), lipids, metabolites, electrolytes, and drugs, the latter secreted during therapy.

The tear cationic protein lactoferrin increases the activity of various antimicrobial agents such as lysozyme.

The eye is moved within the orbit by the extraocular muscles

Six muscles of the eyeball (also called ***extraocular*** or ***extrinsic muscles***) attach to each eye. These are the medial, lateral, superior, and inferior rectus muscles and the superior and inferior oblique muscles. The ***superior oblique muscle*** is innervated by the ***trochlear nerve (cranial nerve IV)***. The ***lateral rectus muscle*** is innervated by the ***abducens nerve (cranial nerve VI)***. All of the remaining extraocular muscles are innervated by the ***oculomotor nerve (cranial nerve III)***. The combined, precisely controlled action of these muscles allows vertical, lateral, and rotational movement of the eye. Normally, the actions of the muscles of both eyes are coordinated so that the eyes move in parallel ***(conjugate gaze)***.

PLATE 100. EYE I

The human eye is a complex sensory organ that provides sight. The wall of the eye consists of three concentric layers or coats: the *retina,* the inner layer; the *uvea,* the middle or vascular layer; and the *corneosclera,* the outer fibrous layer. The eye is often compared to a simple camera with a lens to capture and focus light, a diaphragm to regulate the amount of light, and film to record the image. In the eye, the *cornea* and *lens* concentrate and focus light on the *retina.* The *iris,* located between the cornea and lens, regulates the size of the pupil through which light enters the eye. *Photoreceptor cells (rods and cones)* in the retina detect the intensity (rods) and color (cones) of the light that reaches them and encode the various parameters for transmission to the brain via the optic nerve (cranial nerve II).

The eye measures ~25 mm in diameter. It is suspended in the bony orbit by six extrinsic striated muscles that control its movement. The extraocular muscles are coordinated so that both eyes move synchronously, with each moving symmetrically around its own central axis. A thick layer of adipose tissue partially surrounds and cushions the eye as it moves within the orbit.

Modified drawing of human eye, meridional perspective by E. Sobotta.

The innermost layer is the retina *(R),* which consists of several layers of cells. Among these are receptor cells (rods and cones), neurons (e.g., bipolar and ganglion cells), supporting cells, and a pigment epithelium (see Plate 101). The receptor components of the retina are situated in the posterior three fifths of the eyeball. At the anterior boundary of the receptor layer, the ora serrata *(OS),* the retina becomes reduced in thickness, and nonreceptor components of the retina continue forward to cover the posterior or inner surface of the ciliary body *(CB)* and the iris *(I).* This anterior nonreceptor extension of the inner layer is highly pigmented, and the pigment (melanin) is evident as the black inner border of these structures.

The uvea, the middle layer of the eyeball, consists of the choroid, the ciliary body, and the iris. The choroid is a vascular layer; it is relatively thin and difficult to distinguish in the accompanying figure except by location. On this basis, the choroid *(Ch)* is identified as being just external to the pigmented layer of the retina. It is also highly pigmented; the choroidal pigment is evident as a discrete layer in several parts of the section.

Anterior to the ora serrata, the uvea is thickened; here, it is called the *ciliary body (CB).* This contains the ciliary muscle (see Plate 102), which brings about adjustments of the lens to focus light. The ciliary body also contains processes to which the zonular fibers are attached. These fibers function as suspensory ligaments of the lens *(L).* The iris *(I)* is the most anterior component of the uvea and contains a central opening, the pupil.

The outermost layer of the eyeball, the fibrous layer, consists of the sclera *(S)* and the cornea *(C).* Both of these contain collagenous fibers as their main structural element; however, the cornea is transparent, and the sclera is opaque. The extrinsic muscles of the eye insert into the sclera and effect movements of the eyeball. These are not included in the preparation except for two small pieces of a muscle insertion *(arrows)* in the lower left and top center of the illustration. Posteriorly, the sclera is pierced by the emerging optic nerve *(ON).* A deep depression in the neural retina lateral to the optic nerve (above the *ON* in this figure) is the fovea centralis *(FC),* the thinnest and most sensitive portion of the neural retina.

The lens is considered in Plate 103. Just posterior to the lens is the large cavity of the eye, the vitreous cavity *(V),* which is filled with a thick jelly-like material, the vitreous humor or body. Anterior to the lens are two additional, fluid-filled chambers of the eye, the anterior *(AC)* and posterior chambers *(PC),* separated by the iris.

KEY

AC, anterior chamber
C, cornea
CB, ciliary body
Ch, choroid
FC, fovea centralis
I, iris
L, lens
ON, optic nerve
OS, ora serrata
PC, posterior chamber
R, retina
S, sclera
V, vitreous cavity
arrows, muscle insertions

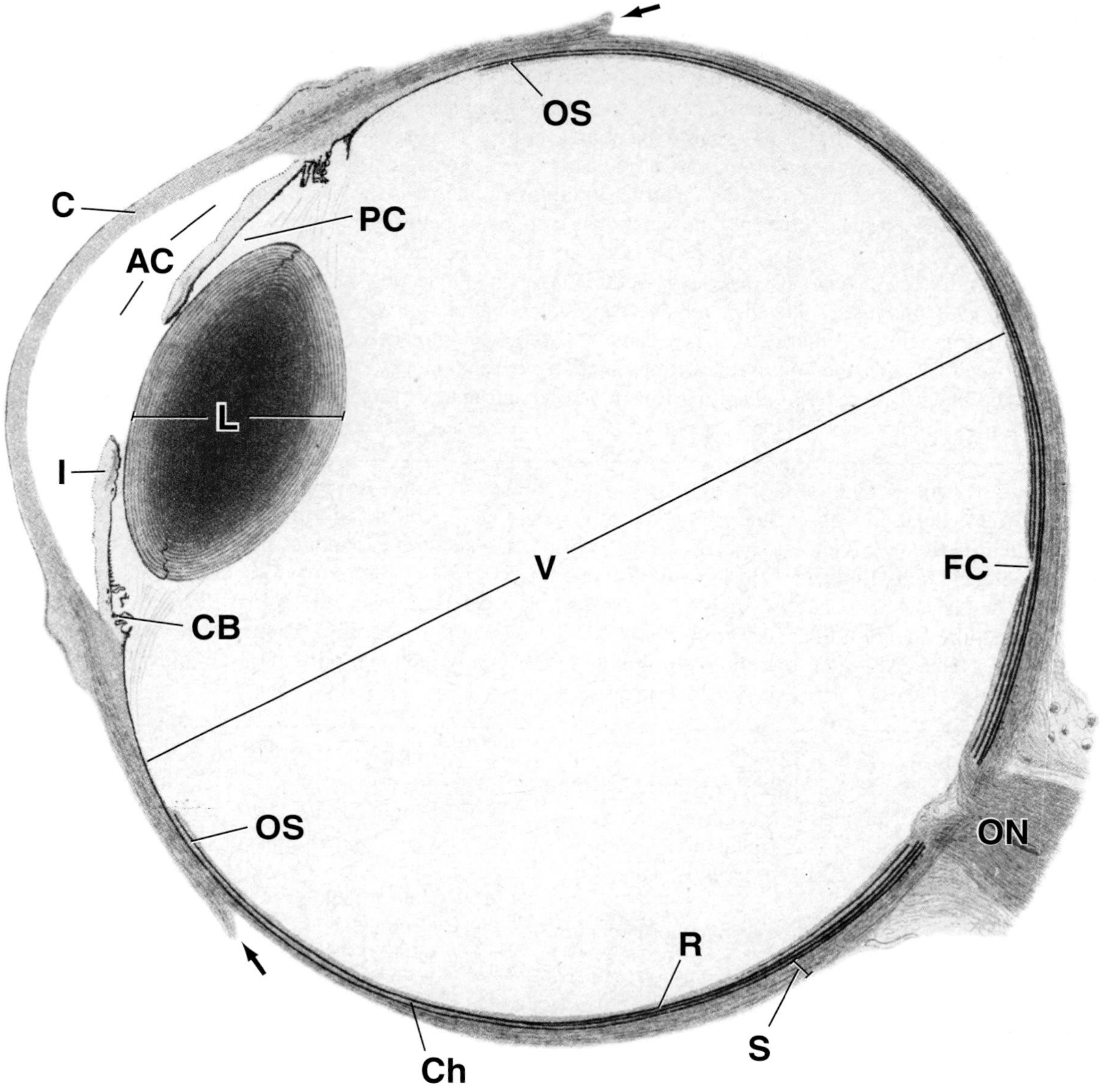
OS
C
PC
AC
L
I
V
FC
CB
OS
ON
R
S
Ch

PLATE 101. EYE II: RETINA

The *retina* and *optic nerve* are projections of the brain. The fibrous cover of the optic nerve is an extension of the meninges of the brain. The neural retina is a multilayered structure consisting of neurons, some of which are specialized as photoreceptors, and supporting cells (*Müller's cells*). External to the neural retina is a layer of simple columnar *pigment epithelium.* The Müller's cells are comparable to neuroglia in the rest of the central nervous system. Processes of Müller's cells ramify virtually through the entire thickness of the retina. The internal limiting membrane is the basal lamina of these cells; the external limiting membrane is actually a line formed by the junctional complexes between processes of these cells and the *photoreceptor cells.*

The neurons of the retina are arranged sequentially in three layers: (1) a deep layer of rods and cones; (2) an intermediate layer of *bipolar, horizontal,* and *amacrine* cells; and (3) a superficial layer of *ganglion* cells. Nerve impulses originating in the rods and cones are transmitted to the intermediate layer and then to the ganglion cells. Synaptic connections occur in the *outer plexiform layer* (between the rods and cones and the intermediate neuronal layer) and the *inner plexiform layer* (between the intermediate layer and the ganglion cells), resulting in summation and neuronal integration. Finally, the ganglion cells send their axons to the brain as components of the optic nerve.

Figure 1, eye, human, H&E ×65.

The site where the optic nerve leaves the eyeball is called the *optic disc (OD).* It is characteristically marked by a depression, evident here. Receptor cells are not present at the optic disc, and because it is not sensitive to light stimulation, it is sometimes referred to as the *blind spot.*

The fibers that give rise to the optic nerve originate in the retina, more specifically, in the ganglion cell layer (see below). They traverse the sclera through a number of openings *(arrows)* to form the optic nerve *(ON).* The region of the sclera that contains these openings is called the *lamina cribrosa (LC)* or cribriform plate. The optic nerve contains a central artery and vein (not seen here) that also traverse the lamina cribrosa. Branches of these blood vessels *(BV)* supply the inner portion of the retina.

Figure 2, eye, human, H&E ×325.

On the basis of structural features that are evident in histologic sections, the retina is divided into ten layers, from posterior to anterior, as listed below and labeled in this figure:

1. Pigment epithelium *(PEp),* the outermost layer of the retina
2. Layer of rods and cones *(R&C),* the photoreceptor layer of the retina
3. External limiting membrane *(ELM),* a line formed by the junctional complexes of the photoreceptor cells
4. Outer nuclear layer *(ONL),* containing nuclei of rod and cone cells
5. Outer plexiform layer *(OPL),* containing neural processes and synapses of rod and cone cells with bipolar, amacrine, and horizontal cells
6. Inner nuclear layer *(INL),* containing nuclei of bipolar, horizontal, amacrine, and Müller's cells
7. Inner plexiform layer *(IPL),* containing processes and synapses of bipolar, horizontal, amacrine, and ganglion cells
8. Layer of ganglion cells *(GC),* containing cell bodies and nuclei of ganglion cells
9. Nerve fiber layer *(NFL),* containing axons of ganglion cells
10. Internal limiting membrane *(ILM),* consisting of the external (basal) lamina of Müller's cells

This figure also shows the innermost layer of the choroid *(Ch),* a cell-free membrane, the lamina vitrea *(LV),* also called *Bruch's membrane.* Electron micrographs reveal that it corresponds to the basement membrane of the pigment epithelium. Immediately external to the lamina vitrea is the capillary layer of the choroid (lamina choriocapillaris). These vessels supply the outer part of the retina.

KEY

BV, blood vessels
Ch, choroid
ELM, external limiting membrane
GC, layer of ganglion cells
ILM, internal limiting membrane
INL, inner nuclear layer (nuclei of bipolar, horizontal, amacrine, and Müller's cells)
IPL, inner plexiform layer
LC, lamina cribrosa
LV, lamina vitrea
NFL, nerve fiber layer
OD, optic disc
ON, optic nerve
ONL, outer nuclear layer (nuclei of rod and cone cells)
OPL, outer plexiform layer
PEp, pigment epithelium
R&C, layer of rods and cones
arrows, openings in sclera (lamina cribrosa)

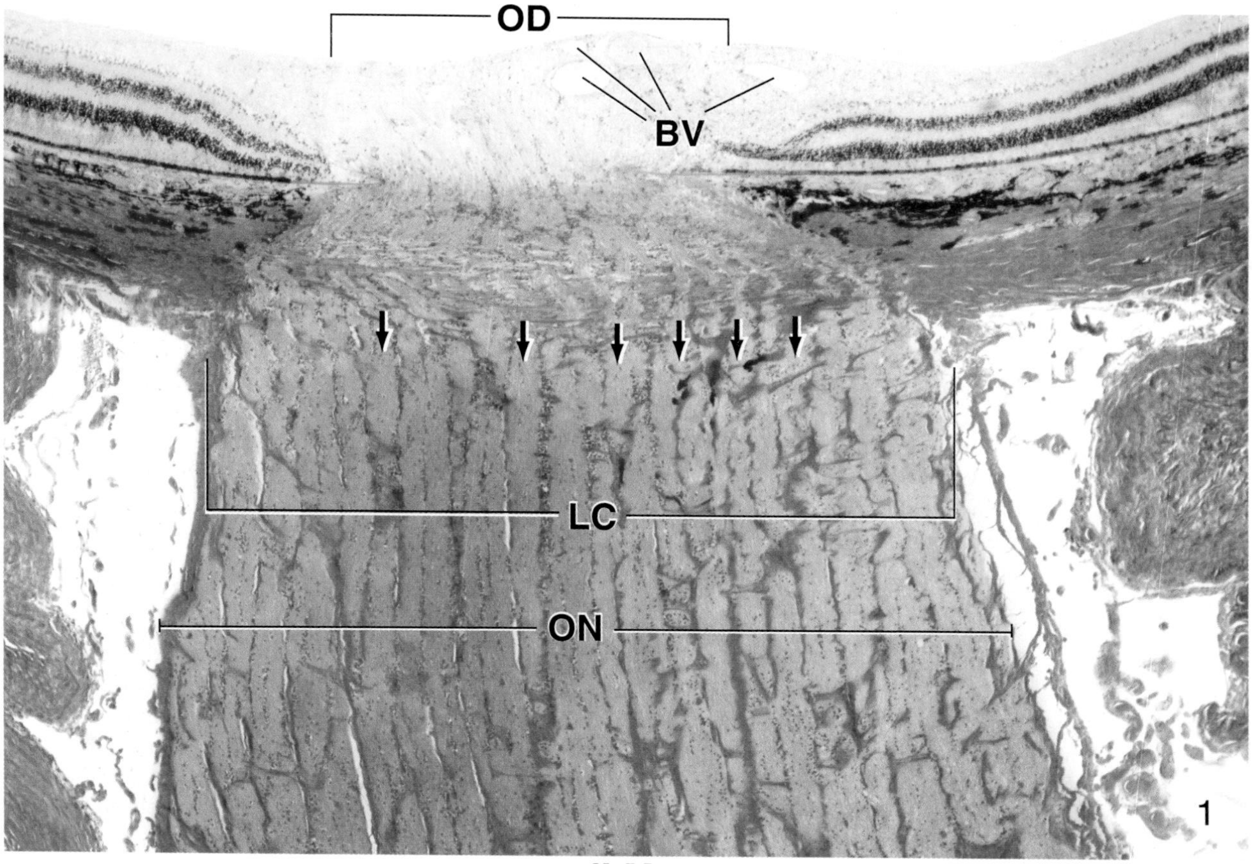
OD
BV
LC
ON
1

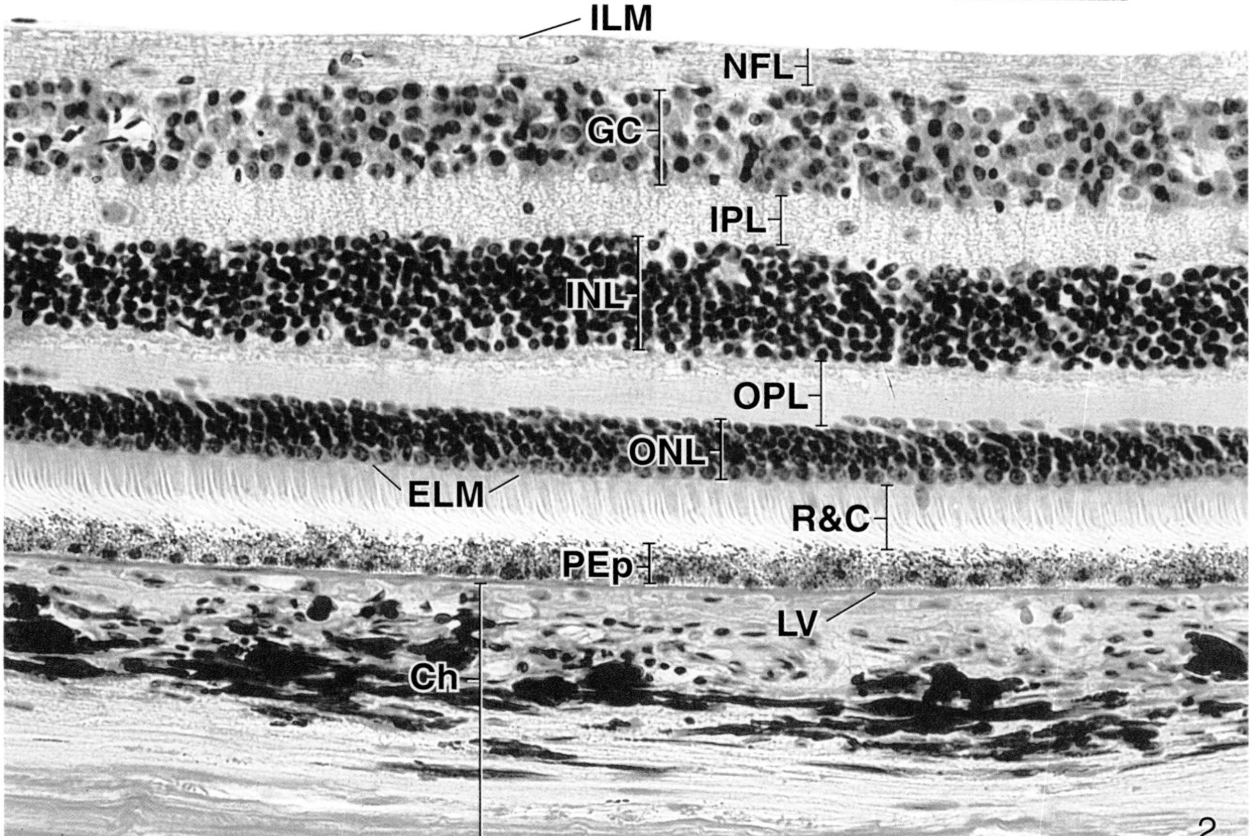
ILM
NFL
GC
IPL
INL
OPL
ONL
ELM
R&C
PEp
LV
Ch
2

PLATE 102. EYE III: ANTERIOR SEGMENT

The *anterior segment* is that part of the eye anterior to the *ora serrata,* the most anterior extension of the neural retina, and includes the *anterior* and *posterior chambers* and the structures that define them. These include the cornea and sclera, the iris, the lens, the ciliary body, and the connections between the basal lamina of the ciliary processes and the lens capsule (thick basal lamina of the lens epithelium) that form the suspensory ligament of the lens, the *zonular fibers.* The posterior chamber is bounded posteriorly by the anterior surface of the lens and anteriorly by the posterior surface of the iris. The ciliary body forms the lateral boundary. Aqueous humor flows through the pupil into the anterior chamber, which occupies the space between the cornea and the iris, and drains into the *canal of Schlemm.*

Figure 1, eye, human, H&E ×45; inset ×75.

A portion of the anterior segment of the eye, shown in this figure, includes parts of the cornea *(C),* sclera *(S),* iris *(I),* ciliary body *(CB),* anterior chamber *(AC),* posterior chamber *(PC),* lens *(L),* and zonular fibers *(ZF).*

The relationship of the cornea to the sclera is illustrated to advantage here. The junction between the two *(arrows)* is marked by a change in staining, with the substance of the cornea appearing lighter than that of the sclera. The corneal epithelium *(CEp)* is continuous with the conjunctival epithelium *(CjEp)* that covers the sclera. Note that the epithelium thickens considerably at the corneoscleral junction and resembles that of the oral mucosa. The conjunctival epithelium is separated from the dense fibrous component of the sclera by a loose vascular connective tissue. Together, this connective tissue and the epithelium constitute the conjunctiva *(Cj).* The epithelial-connective tissue junction of the conjunctiva is irregular; in contrast, the undersurface of the corneal epithelium presents an even profile.

Just lateral to the junction of the cornea and sclera is the canal of Schlemm (*CS;* see also Fig. 2). This canal takes a circular route about the perimeter of the cornea. It communicates with the anterior chamber through a loose trabecular meshwork of tissue, the spaces of Fontana. The canal of Schlemm also communicates with episcleral veins. By means of its communications, the canal of Schlemm provides a route for the fluid in the anterior and posterior chambers to reach the bloodstream.

The **inset** shows the tip of the iris. Note the heavy pigmentation on the posterior surface of the iris, which is covered by the same double-layered epithelium as the ciliary body and ciliary processes. In the ciliary epithelium, the outer layer is pigmented and the inner layer is nonpigmented. In the iris, both layers of the iridial epithelium *(IEp)* are heavily pigmented. A portion of the iridial constrictor muscle *(M)* is seen beneath the epithelium.

Figure 2, eye, human, H&E ×90; inset ×350.

Immediately internal to the anterior margin of the sclera *(S)* is the ciliary body *(CB).* The inner surface of this forms radially arranged, ridge-shaped elevations, the ciliary processes *(CP),* to which the zonular fibers *(ZF)* are anchored. From the outside in, the components of the ciliary body are the ciliary muscle *(CM),* the connective tissue (vascular) layer *(VL)* representing the choroid coat in the ciliary body, the lamina vitrea (*LV,* **inset**), and the ciliary epithelium (*CiEp,* **inset**). The ciliary epithelium consists of two layers **(inset),** the pigmented layer *(PE)* and the nonpigmented layer *(npE).* The lamina vitrea is a continuation of the same layer of the choroid; it is the basement membrane of the pigmented ciliary epithelial cells.

The ciliary muscle is arranged in three patterns. The outer layer is immediately deep to the sclera. These are the meridionally arranged fibers of Brücke. The outermost of these continues more posteriorly into the choroid and is referred to as the *tensor muscle of the choroid.* The middle layer is the radial group. It radiates from the region of the sclerocorneal junction into the ciliary body. The innermost layer of muscle cells is circularly arranged. These are seen in cross section. The circular artery (*CA;* barely discernable) and vein *(CV)* for the iris, also cut in cross section, are just anterior to the circular group of muscle cells.

KEY

A, artery
AC, anterior chamber
C, cornea
CA, circular artery
CB, ciliary body
CEp, corneal epithelium
Ch, choroid
CiEp, ciliary epithelium
Cj, conjunctiva
CjEp, conjunctival epithelium
CM, ciliary muscle
CP, ciliary processes
CS, canal of Schlemm
CV, circular vein
I, iris
IEp, iridial epithelium
L, lens
LV, lamina vitrea
M, iridial constrictor muscle
npE, nonpigmented layer of ciliary epithelium
PC, posterior chamber
PE, pigmented layer of ciliary epithelium
S, sclera
V, vein
VL, vascular layer (of ciliary body)
ZF, zonular fibers
arrows, junction between cornea and sclera

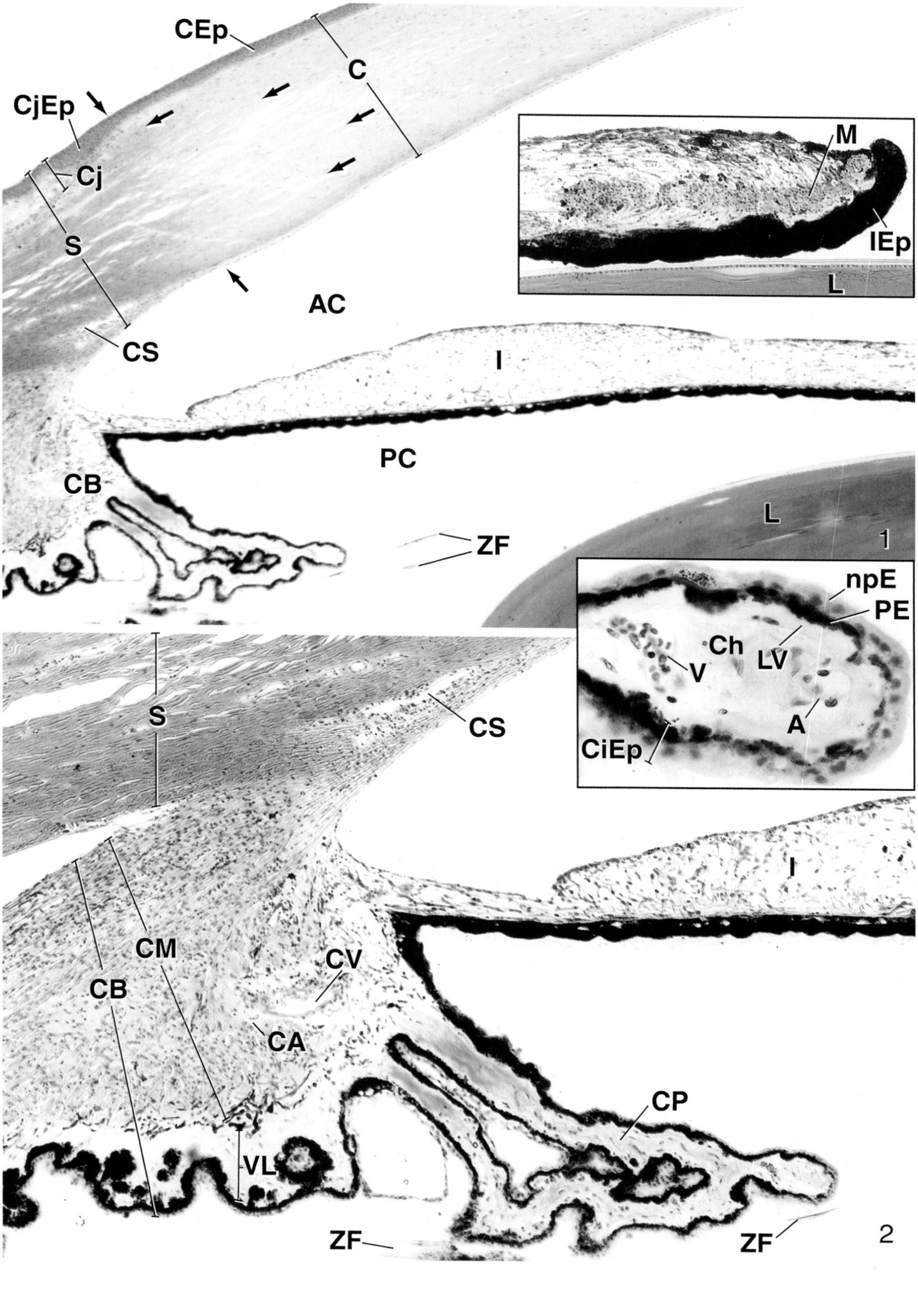
CEp
C
CjEp
Cj
S
AC
CS
M
IEp
L
I
PC
CB
L
ZF
1
npE
PE
Ch
LV
V
A
CiEp
S
CS
I
CM
CV
CB
CA
CP
VL
ZF
ZF
2

PLATE 103. EYE IV: SCLERA, CORNEA, AND LENS

The transparent *cornea* is the primary dioptric (refractive element) of the eye and is covered with nonkeratinized, stratified squamous epithelium. Its stroma consists of alternating lamellae of collagen fibrils and fibroblasts (*keratocytes*). The fibrils in each lamella are extremely uniform in diameter and uniformly spaced; fibrils in adjacent lamellae are arranged at approximately right angles to each other. This orthogonal array of highly regular fibrils is responsible for the transparency of the cornea. The posterior surface is covered with a single layer of low cuboidal cells, the *corneal endothelium,* which rest on a thickened basal lamina called *Descemet's membrane.* Nearly all of the metabolic exchanges of the avascular cornea occur across the endothelium. Damage to this layer leads to corneal swelling and can produce temporary or permanent loss of transparency.

The *lens* is a transparent, avascular, biconvex epithelial structure suspended by the zonular fibers. Tension on these fibers keeps the lens flattened; reduced tension allows it to fatten or *accommodate* to bend light rays originating close to the eye to focus them on the retina.

Figure 1, sclera, human, H&E ×130.

This low-magnification micrograph shows the full thickness of the sclera just lateral to the corneoscleral junction or limbus. To the left of the *arrow* is sclera; to the right is a small amount of corneal tissue. The conjunctival epithelium *(CjEp)* is irregular in thickness and rests on a loose vascular connective tissue. Together, this epithelium and underlying connective tissue represents the conjunctiva *(Cj).* The white opaque appearance of the sclera is due to the irregular dense arrangement of the collagen fibers that make up the stroma *(S).* The canal of Schlemm *(CS)* is seen at the left close to the inner surface of the sclera.

Figures 2 and 3, sclera, human, H&E ×360.

Figure 2 is a higher-magnification micrograph showing the transition from the corneal epithelium *(CEp)* to the irregular and thicker conjunctival epithelium *(CjEp)* covering the sclera. Note that Bowman's membrane *(B),* lying under the corneal epithelium, is just perceptible but disappears beneath the conjunctival epithelium. Figure 3 shows at higher magnification of the canal of Schlemm *(CS)* than does Figure 1. That the space shown here is not an artifact is evidenced by the endothelial lining cells *(En)* that face the lumen.

Figure 4, cornea, human, H&E ×175.

This low-magnification micrograph shows the full thickness of the cornea *(C)* and can be compared with the sclera shown in Figure 1. The corneal epithelium *(CEp)* presents a uniform thickness and the underlying stroma *(S)* has a more homogeneous appearance than the stroma of the sclera (the white spaces seen here and in Figure 1 are artifacts). Nuclei *(N)* of the keratocytes of the stroma lie between lamellae. The corneal epithelium rests on a thickened anterior basement membrane called Bowman's membrane *(B).* The posterior surface of the cornea is lined by a simple squamous epithelium called the corneal endothelium *(CEn);* its thick posterior basement membrane is called Descemet's membrane *(D).*

Figures 5 and 6, cornea, human, H&E ×360.

Figure 5 is a higher magnification showing the corneal epithelium *(CEp)* with its squamous surface cells, the very thick homogeneous-appearing Bowman's membrane *(B),* and the underlying stroma *(S).* Note that the stromal tissue has a homogeneous appearance, a reflection of the dense packing of its collagen fibrils. The flattened nuclei belong to the keratocytes. Figure 6 shows the posterior surface of the cornea. Note the thick homogeneous Descemet's membrane *(D)* and the underlying corneal endothelium *(CEn).*

Figure 7, lens, human, H&E ×360.

This micrograph shows a portion of the lens near its equator. The lens consists entirely of epithelial cells surrounded by a homogeneous-appearing lens capsule *(LC)* to which the zonula fibers attach. The lens capsule is a very thick basal lamina of the epithelial cells. Simple cuboidal lens epithelial cells are present on the anterior surface of the lens, but at the lateral margin they become extremely elongated and form layers that extend toward the center of the lens. These elongated columns of epithelial cytoplasm are referred to as lens fibers *(LF).* New cells are produced at the margin of the lens and displace the older cells inwardly. Eventually, the older cells lose their nuclei, as evidenced by the deeper portion of the cornea in this micrograph.

KEY

AC, anterior chamber
B, Bowman's membrane
BV, blood vessels
C, cornea
CEn, corneal endothelium
CEp, corneal epithelium
Cj, conjunctiva
CjEp, conjunctival epithelium
CS, canal of Schlemm
D, Descemet's membrane
En, endothelial lining cells
LC, lens capsule
LF, lens fibers
N, nuclei
S, stroma

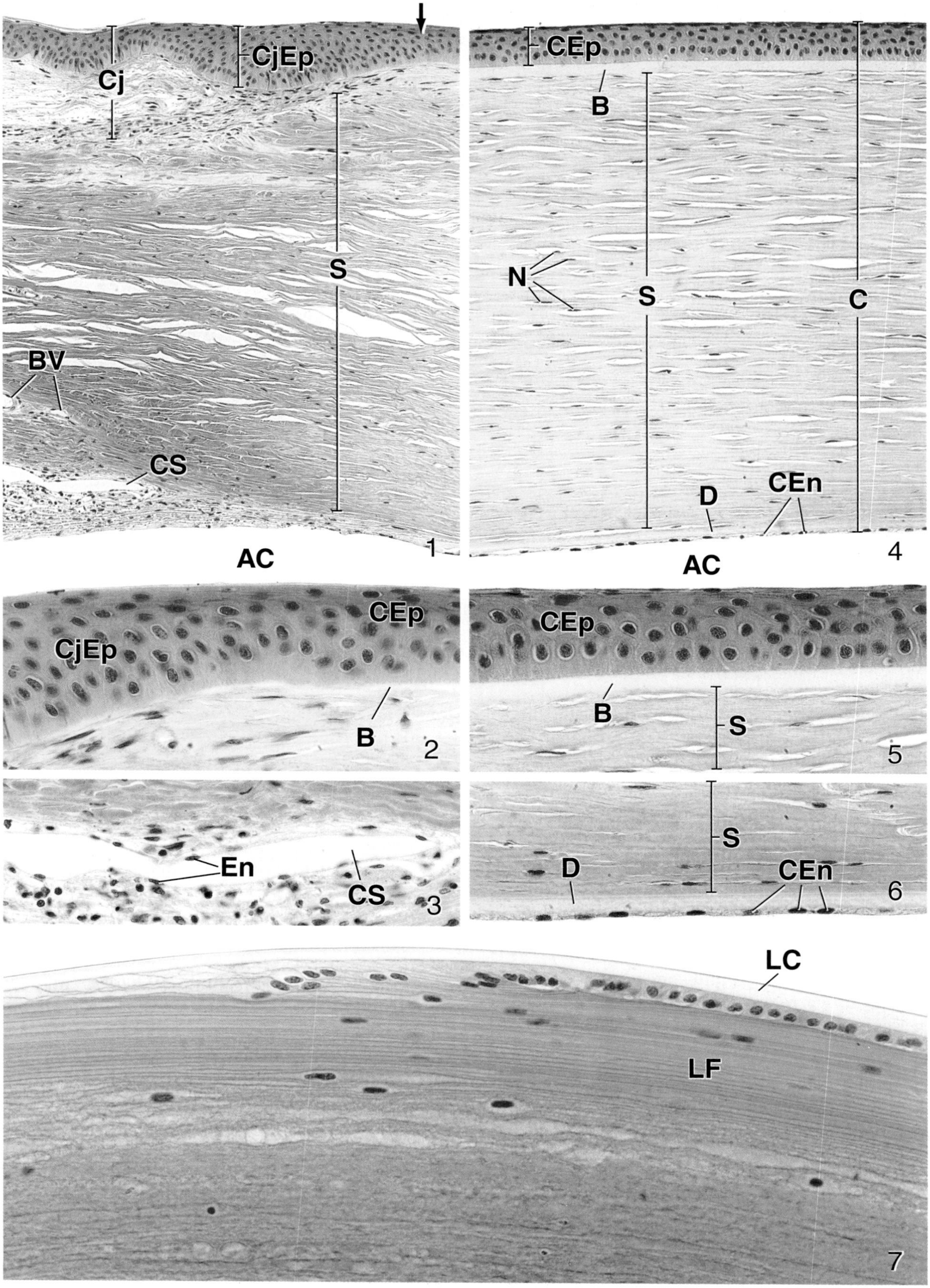
CjEp
Cj
S
BV
CS
1
AC
CEp
B
N
S
C
D
CEn
4
AC
CEp
CjEp
B
2
CEp
B
S
5
En
CS
3
S
D
CEn
6
LC
LF
7

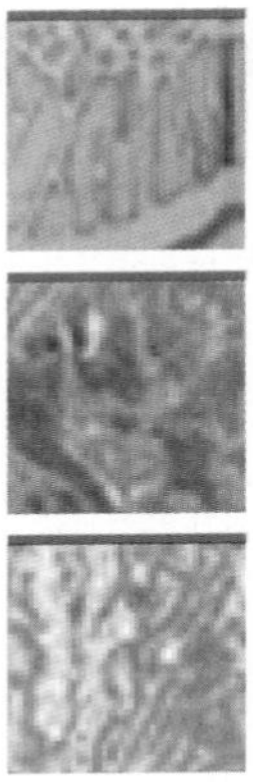

24

Ear

OVERVIEW OF THE EAR

The ear is a three-chambered sensory organ that functions as an ***auditory system*** for sound perception and as a ***vestibular system*** for balance. Each of the three divisions of the ear, the ***external ear***, ***middle ear***, and ***internal ear***, is an essential part of the auditory system (Fig. 24.1). The external and middle ear collect and conduct sound energy to the internal ear, where auditory sensory receptors convert that energy into electrical impulses. The sensory receptors of the vestibular system are also located in the internal ear. These receptors respond to gravity and movement of the head.

The ear develops from surface ectoderm and components of the first and second pharyngeal arch

Embryologically, the functions of the ear, hearing and balance, are elaborated from an invagination of surface ectoderm that appears on each side of the myelencephalon. This invagination forms the *octic vesicle (otocyst)*, which sinks deep to the surface ectoderm into the underlying mesenchyme (Fig. 24.2). The otic vesicle serves as a primordium for development of the epithelia that line the membranous labyrinth of the internal ear. Later, development of the first and part of the second pharyngeal arch provides structures that augment hearing. The endodermal component of the first pouch gives rise to the ***tubotympanic recess***, which ultimately develops into the ***auditory tube (Eustachian tube)*** and the ***middle ear*** and its epithelial lining. The corresponding ectodermal outgrowth of the ***first pharyngeal groove*** gives rise to the ***external acoustic meatus*** and its epithelial lining (see Fig. 24.2). The connective tissue part of the pharyngeal arches produces the ossicles. The ***malleus*** and ***incus*** develop from the first pharyngeal arch, and the ***stapes*** from the second pharyngeal arch. The sensory epithelia of the membranous labyrinth that originates from the otic vesicle link with cranial nerve VIII, which is an outgrowth of the central nervous system. The cartilaginous, bony, and muscular structures of the ear develop from the mesenchyme surrounding these early epithelia.

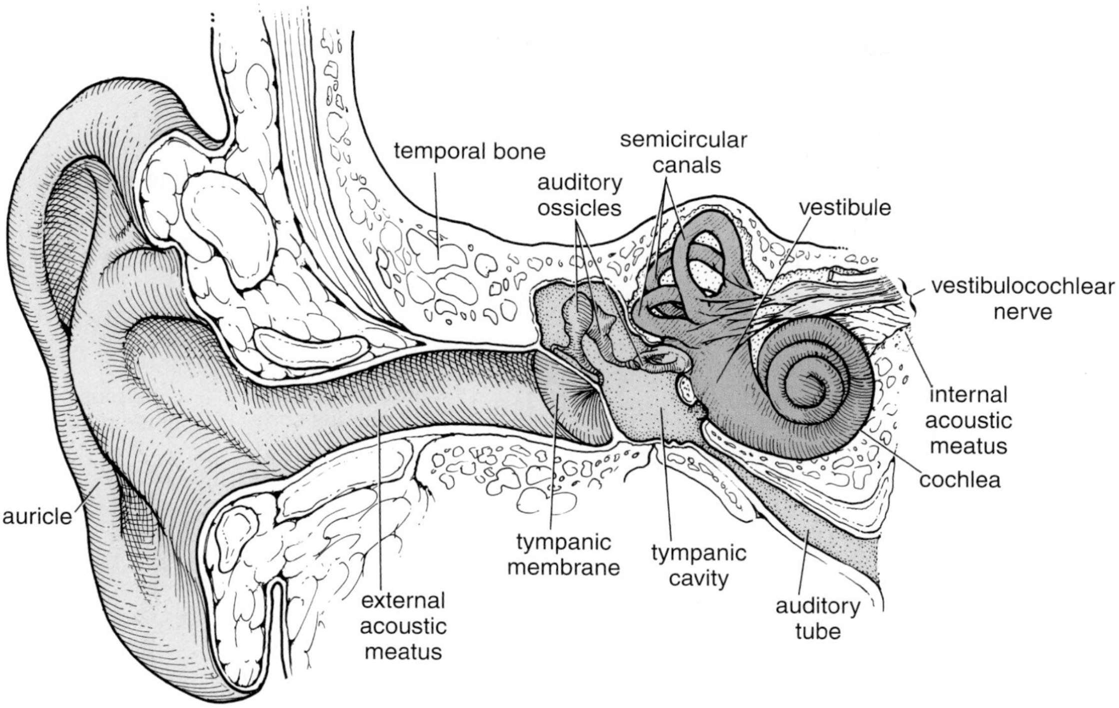

FIGURE 24.1
Three divisions of the ear. The three divisions of the ear are represented by different colors and consist of the external ear (auricle and external acoustic meatus) *(flesh tone)*, the middle ear (tympanic cavity, auditory ossicles, tympanic membrane, and auditory tube) *(pink)*, and the internal ear containing the bony labyrinth (semicircular canals, vestibule, and cochlea) *(blue)* and the membranous labyrinth (not visible).

EXTERNAL EAR

The auricle is the external component of the ear that collects and amplifies sound

The *auricle (pinna)* is the oval appendage that projects from the lateral surface of the head. The characteristic shape of the auricle is determined by an internal supporting structure of elastic cartilage. Thin skin with hair follicles, sweat glands, and sebaceous glands covers the auricle. The auricle is considered a nearly vestigial structure in humans, compared with its development and role in other animals. However, it is an essential component in sound localization and amplification.

The external acoustic meatus conducts sounds to the tympanic membrane

The *external acoustic meatus* is an air-filled tubular space that follows a slightly S-shaped course for about 25 mm to the *tympanic membrane (eardrum)*. The wall of the canal is continuous externally with the auricle. The wall of the lateral one third of the canal is cartilaginous and is continuous with the elastic cartilage of the auricle. The medial two thirds of the canal is contained within the temporal bone.

The lateral part of the canal is lined by skin that contains hair follicles, sebaceous glands, and ***ceruminous glands***, but no eccrine sweat glands. The coiled tubular ceruminous glands closely resemble the apocrine glands found in the axillary region. Their secretion mixes with that of the sebaceous glands and desquamated cells to form ***cerumen***, or ***earwax***. The cerumen lubricates the skin and coats the meatal hairs to impede the entry of foreign particles into the ear. Excessive accumulation of cerumen can plug the meatus, however, resulting in conductive hearing loss. The medial part of the canal located within the temporal bone has thinner skin and fewer hairs and glands.

MIDDLE EAR

The middle ear is an air-filled space that contains three small bones, the ossicles

The middle ear is located in an air-filled space, called the ***tympanic cavity***, within the temporal bone (Fig. 24.3). It is spanned by three small bones, the ***auditory ossicles***, that

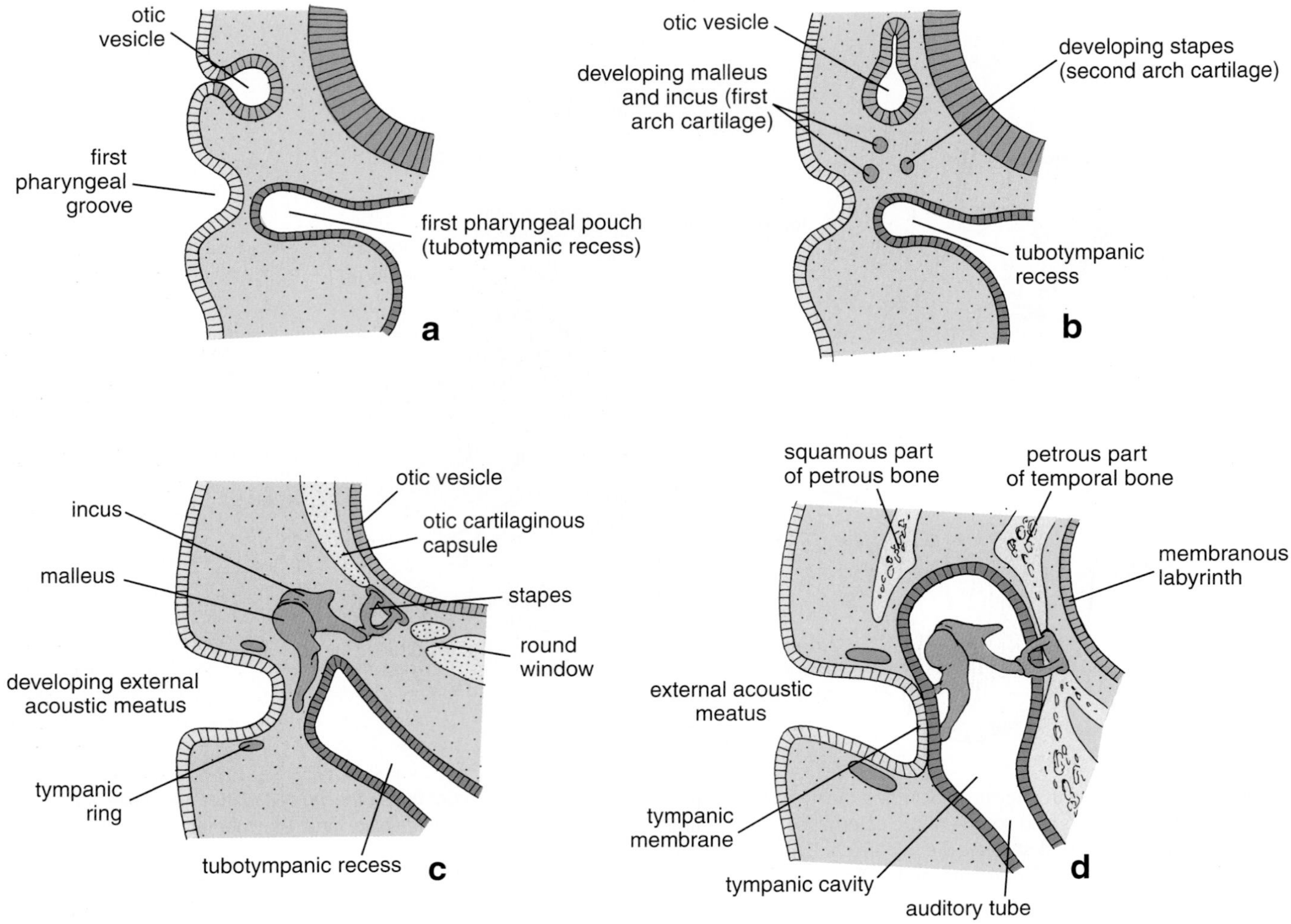

FIGURE 24.2
Schematic drawings showing development of the ear. a. This drawing shows the relationship of the surface ectoderm-derived otic vesicle to the first pharyngeal arch during the fourth week of development. **b.** The otic vesicle sinks deep into the mesenchymal tissue and develops into the membranous labyrinth. Note the development of the tubotympanic recess lined by endoderm into the future middle-ear cavity and auditory tube. In addition, accumulation of mesenchyme from the first and second pharyngeal arches gives rise to the auditory ossicles. **c.** At this later stage of development, the first pharyngeal groove grows toward the developing tubotympanic recess. The auditory ossicles assume a location inside the tympanic cavity. **d.** This final stage of development shows how the tympanic membrane develops from all three germ layers: surface ectoderm, mesoderm, and endoderm. Note that the wall of the otic vesicle develops into the membranous labyrinth.

are connected by two movable joints. The middle ear also contains the ***auditory tube (Eustachian tube)*** as well as the muscles that move the ossicles. The middle ear is bounded anteriorly by the auditory tube and posteriorly by the spongy bone of the ***mastoid process,*** which contains the mastoid antrum and other, smaller air-filled spaces called mastoid cells. Laterally, the middle ear is bounded by the ***tympanic membrane*** and medially by the bony wall of the internal ear.

The primary function of the middle ear is to convert sound waves (air vibrations) arriving from the external acoustic meatus into mechanical vibrations that are transmitted to the internal ear. Two openings in the medial wall of the middle ear, the ***oval (vestibular) window*** and the ***round (cochlear) window,*** are essential components in this conversion process.

The tympanic membrane separates the external acoustic meatus from the middle ear

The tympanic membrane (eardrum) is the medial boundary of the external acoustic meatus and the lateral wall of

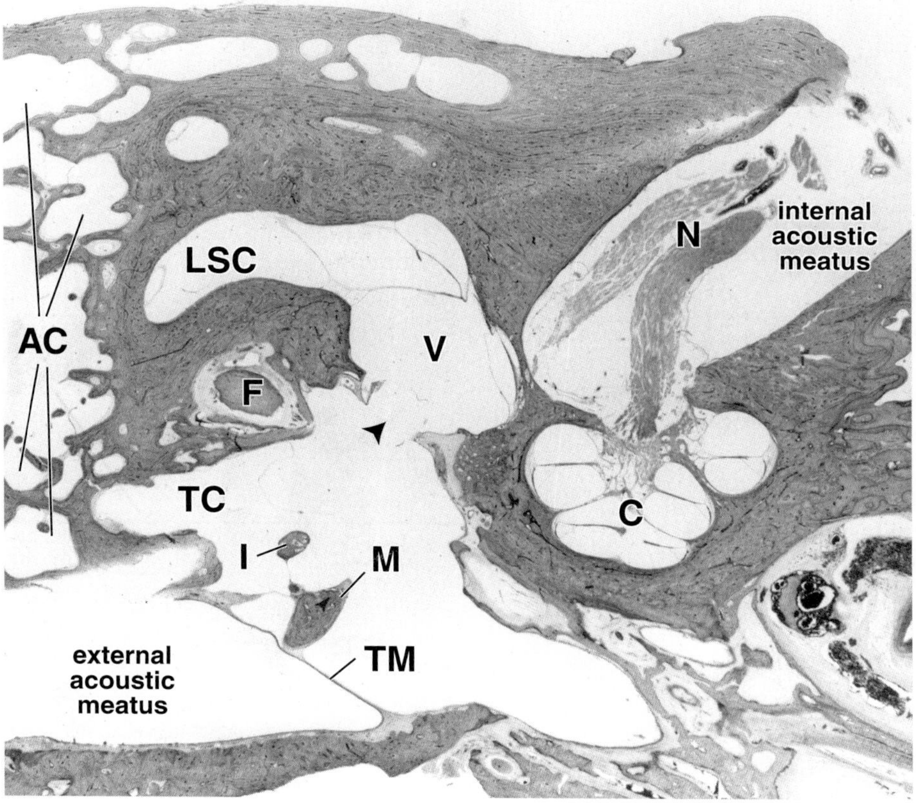

FIGURE 24.3
Horizontal section of a human temporal bone. The relationships of the three divisions of the ear within the temporal bone are shown. The tympanic membrane *(TM)* separates the external acoustic meatus from the tympanic cavity *(TC)*. Within the tympanic cavity, sections of the malleus *(M)* and incus *(I)* can be seen. The posterior wall of the tympanic cavity is associated with the mastoid air cells *(AC)*. The lateral wall of the cavity is formed principally by the tympanic membrane. The opening to the internal ear or oval window *(arrowhead)* is seen in the medial wall of the cavity (the stapes has been removed). The facial nerve *(F)* can be observed near the oval window. The cochlea *(C)*, the vestibule *(V)*, and a portion of the lateral semicircular canal *(LSC)* of the bony labyrinth are identified. The cochlear and vestibular divisions of cranial nerve VIII *(N)* can also be observed within the internal acoustic meatus. ×65.

the middle ear (Fig. 24.4). The layers of the tympanic membrane from outside to inside are

- The skin of the external acoustic meatus
- A core of radially and circularly arranged collagen fibers
- The mucous membrane of the middle ear

One of the auditory ossicles, the ***malleus,*** is attached to the tympanic membrane (see Fig. 24.1). Sound in the form of airwaves causes the tympanic membrane to vibrate, and these vibrations are transmitted to the attached auditory ossicles that link the external ear to the internal ear. Perforation of the tympanic membrane may cause transient or permanent hearing impairment.

The auditory ossicles connect the tympanic membrane to the oval window

The three small ossicles, or bones, the ***malleus,*** the ***incus,*** and the ***stapes,*** cross the space of the middle ear in series (Fig. 24.5) and connect the tympanic membrane to the oval window. These bones help to convert sound waves (i.e., vibrations in air) to mechanical (hydraulic) vibrations in tissues and fluid-filled chambers. Movable joints connect the bones, which are named according to their approximate shape:

- ***Malleus (hammer),*** attached to the tympanic membrane
- ***Stapes (stirrup),*** whose footplate fits into the oval window
- ***Incus (anvil),*** linking the malleus to the stapes

Two muscles attach to the ossicles and affect their movement

The ***tensor tympani muscle*** lies in a bony canal above the auditory tube; its tendon inserts on the malleus. Contraction of this muscle increases tension on the tympanic membrane. The ***stapedius muscle*** lies in a bony eminence on the posterior wall of the middle ear; its tendon inserts on the stapes. Contraction of the stapedius tends to dampen the movement of the stapes at the oval window. The stapedius is only a few millimeters long and is the smallest skeletal muscle.

The two muscles of the middle ear are responsible for a protective reflex called the ***attenuation reflex.*** Contraction of the muscles makes the chain of ossicles more rigid, thus reducing the transmission of vibrations to the internal ear. This reflex protects the internal ear from the damaging effects of very loud sound.

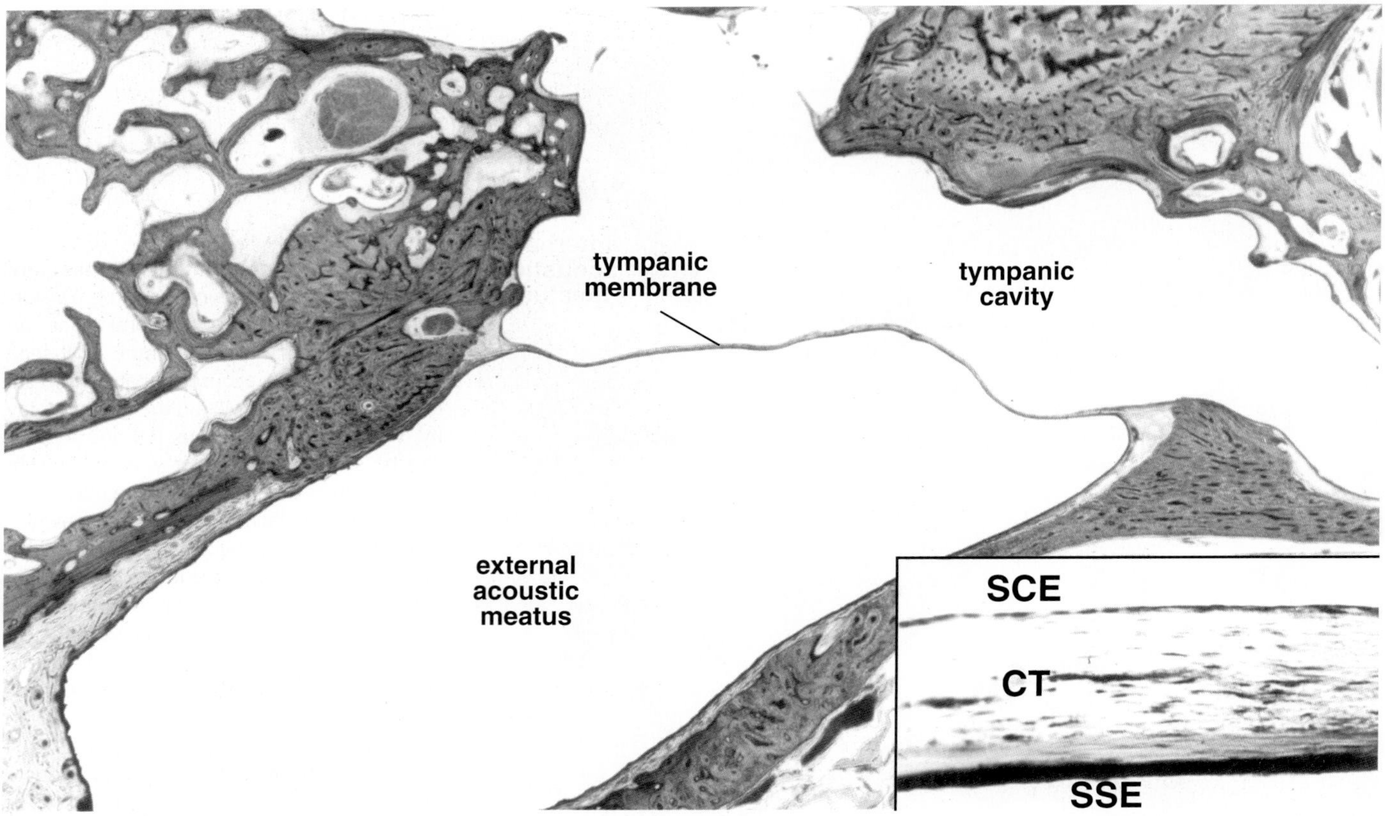

FIGURE 24.4
Cross section through a human tympanic membrane. This photomicrograph shows the tympanic membrane, external acoustic meatus, and tympanic cavity. ×9. **Inset.** Higher magnification of the tympanic membrane. The outer epithelial layer of the membrane consists of stratified squamous epithelium *(SSE),* and the inner epithelial layer of the membrane consists of low simple cuboidal epithelium *(SCE).* A middle layer of connective tissue *(CT)* lies between the two epithelial layers. ×190.

The auditory tube connects the middle ear to the nasopharynx

The auditory (Eustachian) tube is a narrow flattened channel approximately 3.5 cm long. This tube is lined with ciliated pseudostratified columnar epithelium, about one fifth of which is composed of goblet cells. It vents the middle ear, equalizing the pressure of the middle ear with atmospheric pressure. The walls of the tube are normally pressed together but separate during yawning and swallowing. It is common for infections to spread from the pharynx to the middle ear via the auditory tube (causing ***otitis media***). A small mass of lymphatic tissue, the ***tubal tonsil,*** is often found at the pharyngeal orifice of the auditory tube.

The mastoid air cells extend from the middle ear into the temporal bone

A system of air cells projects into the mastoid portion of the temporal bone from the middle ear. The epithelial lining of these air cells is continuous with that of the tympanic cavity and rests on periosteum. This continuity allows infections in the middle ear to spread into these cells, causing ***mastoiditis.*** Before the development of antibiotics, repeated episodes of otitis media and mastoiditis usually led to deafness.

▼ INTERNAL EAR

The internal ear consists of two labyrinthine compartments, one contained within the other

The ***bony labyrinth*** is a complex system of interconnected cavities and canals in the petrous part of the temporal bone. The ***membranous labyrinth*** lies within the bony labyrinth and consists of a complex system of small sacs and tubules that also form a continuous space enclosed within a wall of epithelium and connective tissue.

There are three fluid-filled spaces in the internal ear:

- ***Endolymphatic spaces,*** contained within the membranous labyrinth. The ***endolymph*** of the membranous labyrinth is similar in composition to ***intra***cellular

fluid (it has a high K^+ concentration and low Na^+ concentration).

- *Perilymphatic space,* lying between the wall of the bony labyrinth and the wall of the membranous labyrinth. The ***perilymph*** is similar in composition to ***extra***cellular fluid (it has a low K^+ concentration and a high Na^+ concentration).
- *Cortilymphatic space,* lying within the organ of Corti. It is a true intercellular space. The cells surrounding the space loosely resemble an absorptive epithelium. The cortilymphatic space is filled with ***cortilymph,*** which has a composition similar to that of ***extra***cellular fluid.

The bony labyrinth consists of three connected spaces within the temporal bone

The three spaces of the bony labyrinth, as illustrated in Figure 24.6, are

- *Semicircular canals*
- *Vestibule*
- *Cochlea*

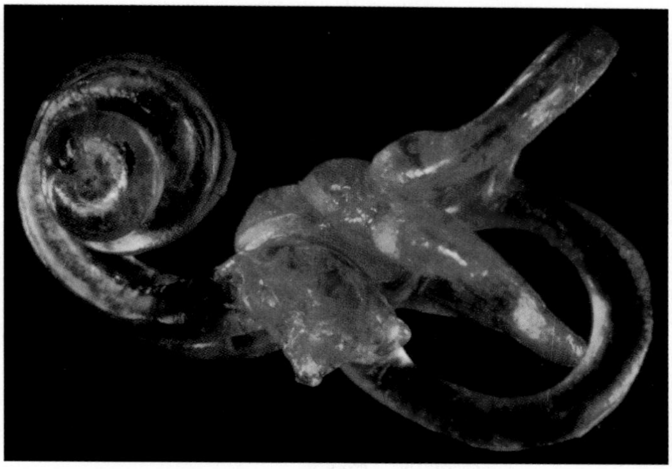

FIGURE 24.6
Photograph of a cast of the bony labyrinth of the internal ear. The cochlear portion of the bony labyrinth appears blue-green; the vestibule and semicircular canals appear orange-red. (Courtesy of Dr. Merle Lawrence.)

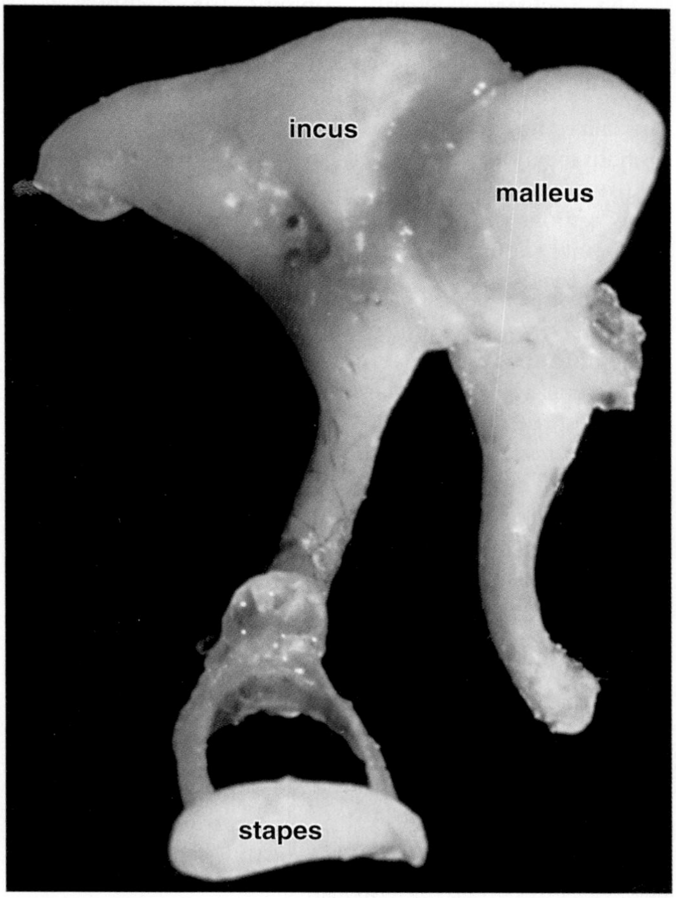

FIGURE 24.5
Photograph of the three articulated human auditory ossicles. The three ossicles are the malleus, the incus, and the stapes. ×30.

The vestibule is the central space that contains the utricle and saccule of the membranous labyrinth

The vestibule is the small oval chamber located in the center of the bony labyrinth. The ***utricle*** and ***saccule*** of the membranous labyrinth lie in elliptical and spherical recesses, respectively. The ***semicircular canals*** extend from the vestibule posteriorly, and the ***cochlea*** extends from the vestibule anteriorly. The oval window into which the footplate of the stapes inserts lies in the lateral wall of the vestibule.

The semicircular canals are tubes within the temporal bone that lie at right angles to each other

Three semicircular canals, each forming about three quarters of a circle, extend from the wall of the vestibule and return to it. The semicircular canals are identified as anterior, posterior, and lateral and lie within the temporal bone at approximately right angles to each other. They occupy three planes in space, sagittal, frontal, and horizontal. The end of each semicircular canal closest to the vestibule is expanded to form the ***ampulla*** (Fig. 24.7a). The three canals open into the vestibule through five orifices; the anterior and posterior semicircular canals join at one end to form the ***common bony limb*** (Fig. 24.7a).

The cochlea is a cone-shaped helix connected to the vestibule

The lumen of the cochlea, like that of the semicircular canals, is continuous with that of the vestibule. It connects to the vestibule on the side opposite the semicircular canals. Between its base and the apex, the cochlea

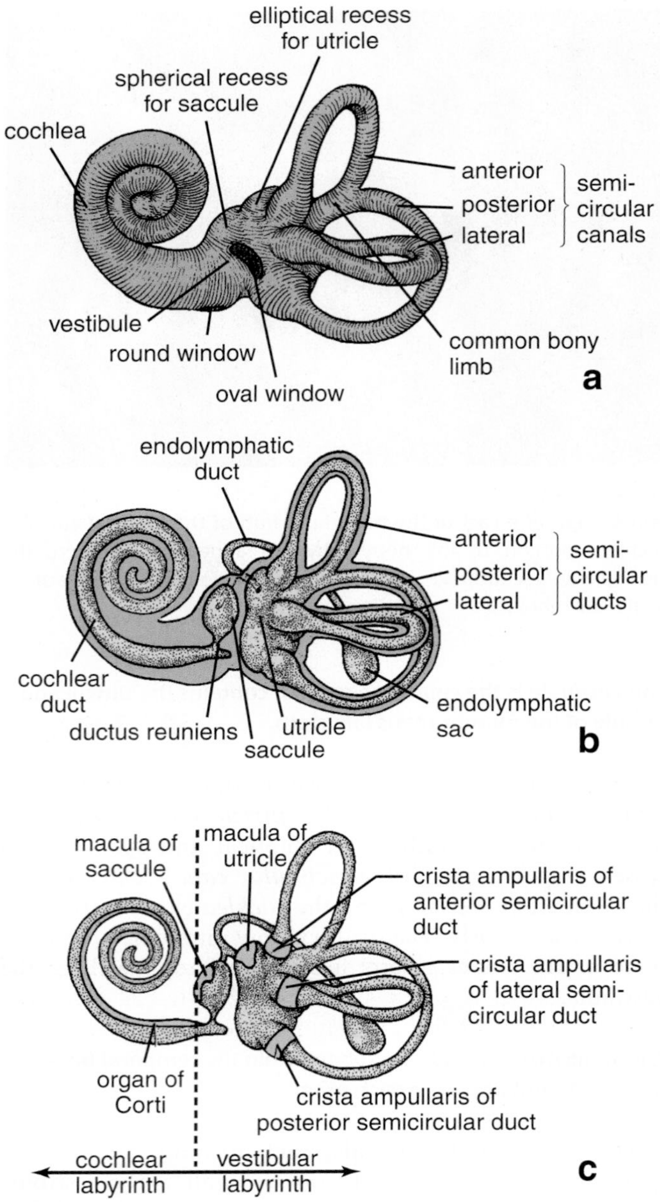

FIGURE 24.7
Diagrams of the human internal ear. a. This lateral view of the left bony labyrinth shows its divisions: the vestibule, cochlea, and three semicircular canals. The openings of the oval window and the round window can be observed. **b.** Diagram of the membranous labyrinth of the internal ear lying within the bony labyrinth. The cochlear duct can be seen spiraling within the bony cochlea. The saccule and utricle are positioned within the vestibule, and the three semicircular ducts are lying within their respective canals. This view of the left membranous labyrinth allows the endolymphatic duct and sac to be observed. **c.** This view of the left membranous labyrinth shows the sensory regions of the internal ear for equilibrium and hearing. These regions are the macula of the saccule and macula of the utricle, the cristae ampullaris of the three semicircular ducts, and the spiral organ of Corti of the cochlear duct.

makes about $2\frac{3}{4}$ turns around a central core of spongy bone called the ***modiolus.*** A sensory ganglion, the ***spiral ganglion,*** lies in the modiolus. One opening of the canal, the round window on its inferior surface near the base, is covered by a thin membrane *(the secondary tympanic membrane).*

The membranous labyrinth contains the endolymph and is suspended within the bony labyrinth

The membranous labyrinth consists of series of communicating sacs and ducts containing endolymph. It is suspended within the bony labyrinth (Fig. 24.7b), and the remaining space is filled with perilymph. The membranous labyrinth is composed of two divisions: the ***cochlear labyrinth*** and the ***vestibular labyrinth*** (Fig. 24.7c).

The vestibular labyrinth contains

- Three ***semicircular ducts,*** which lie within the semicircular canals and are continuous with the utricle
- ***Utricle*** and ***saccule,*** which are contained in recesses in the vestibule and are connected by the membranous ***utriculosaccular duct***

The cochlear labyrinth contains the ***cochlear duct,*** which is contained within the cochlea and is continuous with the saccule (see Fig. 24.7b and c).

Specialized sensory cells are located in six regions in the membranous labyrinth

Six regions of sensory receptors project from the wall of the membranous labyrinth into the endolymphatic space in each internal ear (see Fig. 24.7c):

- Three ***cristae ampullaris (ampullary crest)*** located in the membranous ampullae of the semicircular ducts. They are sensitive to angular acceleration of the head (i.e., turning the head).
- Two ***maculae,*** one in the utricle ***(macula of utricle)*** and the other in the saccule ***(macula of saccule).*** They sense the position of the head and its linear movement.
- The ***spiral organ of Corti,*** which projects into the endolymph of the cochlear duct. It functions as the sound receptor.

Hair cells are epithelial mechanoreceptors of the vestibular and cochlear labyrinth

The hair cells of the vestibular and cochlear labyrinths function as ***transducers;*** i.e., they convert mechanical energy into electrical energy that is then transmitted via the vestibulocochlear nerve to the brain. They possess numerous stereocilia, actually modified microvilli, called ***sensory hairs*** (Fig. 24.8). In the vestibular system, each hair cell possesses a single true cilium called a ***kinocil-***

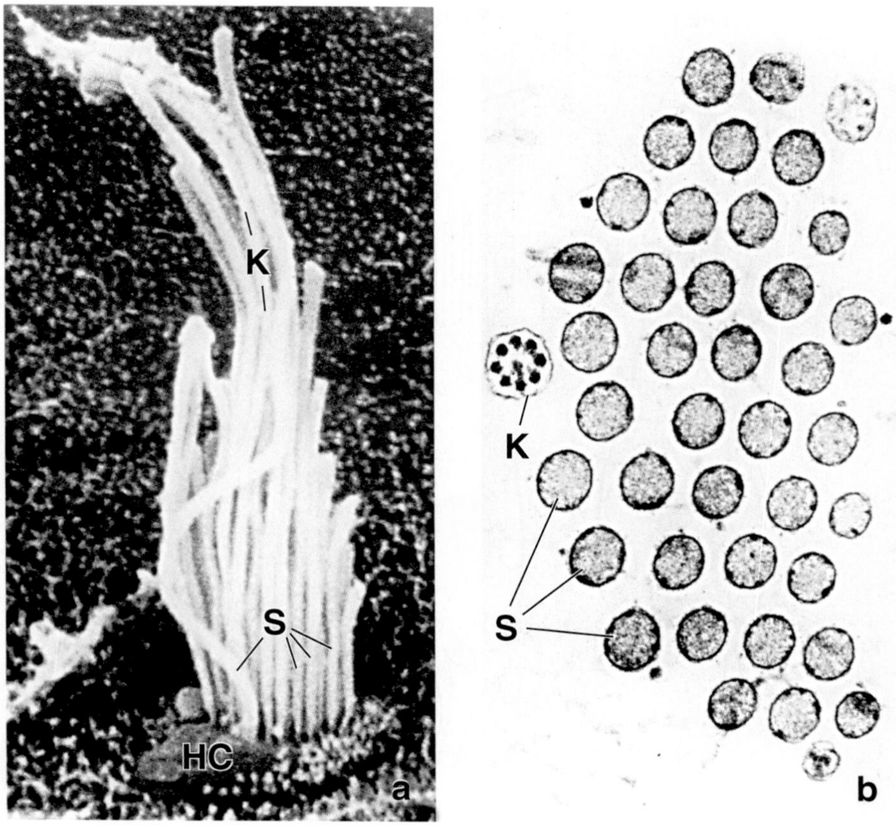

FIGURE 24.8
Electron micrographs of the kinocilium and stereocilia of a vestibular sensory hair cell. **a.** Scanning electron micrograph of the apical surface of a sensory hair cell *(HC)* from the macula of the utricle. Note the relationship of the kinocilium *(K)* to the stereocilia *(S)*. ×47,500. **b.** Transmission electron micrograph of the kinocilium *(K)* and stereocilia *(S)* of a vestibular hair cell in cross section. The kinocilium has a larger diameter than the stereocilia. ×47,500. (From Hunter-Duvar IM, Hinojosa R. Vestibule: sensory epithelia. In: Friedmann I, Ballantyne J, eds. *Ultrastructural Atlas of the Inner Ear.* London: Butterworths, 1984.)

ium. In the auditory system, the hair cells lose their cilium during development but retain the ***basal body.*** Each hair cell is associated with both ***afferent*** and ***efferent nerve endings.***

Two types of hair cells and associated nerve endings are present in the vestibular labyrinth (Fig. 24.9). ***Type I hair cells*** are flask-shaped with a rounded base and thin neck and are surrounded by an afferent nerve chalice and a few efferent nerve fibers. ***Type II hair cells*** are cylindrical and have afferent and efferent bouton nerve endings at the base of the cell (Fig. 24.9).

All hair cells have a common basis of receptor cell function

All hair cells of the internal ear appear to function by bending or flexing their stereocilia. The means by which stereocilia are bent varies from receptor to receptor and is discussed in the section on each specific receptor area. Stretching of the plasma membrane caused by bending of the stereocilia generates transmembrane potential changes in the receptor cell that are conveyed to the afferent nerve ending(s) associated with each hair cell. When a kinocilium is present, its location relative to the bending of the stereocilia is important. Stereocilia that bend away from the kinocilium cause hyperpolarization of the receptor cell; stereocilia that bend toward the kinocilium cause depolarization of the receptor cell and consequent generation of an action potential.

Cristae ampullaris are sensors of angular movements of the head

Each ampulla of the semicircular duct contains a crista ampullaris, which is a sensory receptor for angular movements of the head. (see Figs. 24.7c and 24.10). The crista ampullaris is a thickened transverse epithelial ridge that is oriented perpendicular to the long axis of the semicircular canal and consists of the epithelial hair cells and supporting cells.

A gelatinous protein–polysaccharide mass, known as the ***cupula,*** is attached to the hair cells of each crista (see Fig. 24.10). The cupula projects into the lumen and is surrounded by endolymph. During rotational movement of the head, the walls of the semicircular canal and the membranous semicircular ducts move, but the endolymph contained within the ducts tends to lag behind because of inertia. The cupula, projecting into the endolymph, is swayed by the movement differential between the crista

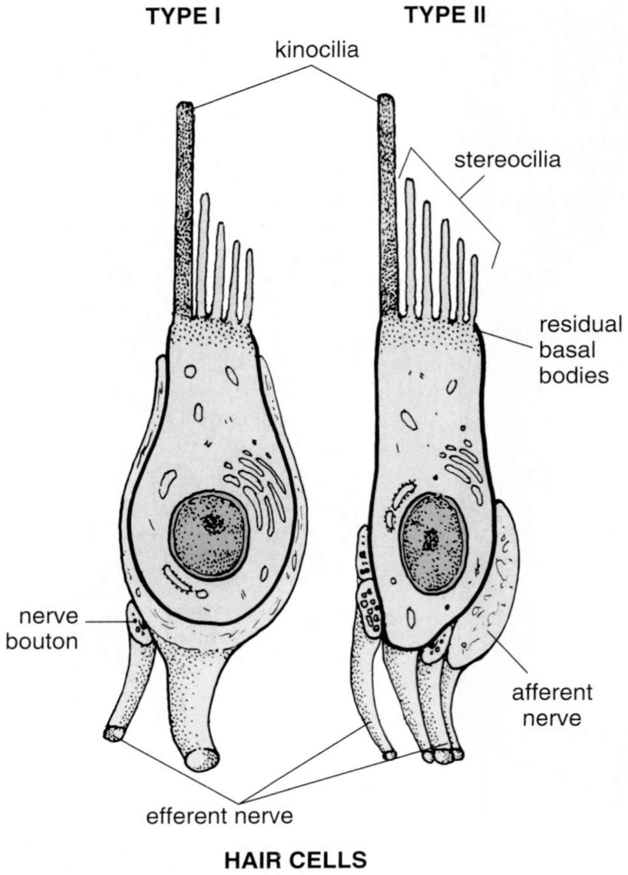

FIGURE 24.9
Diagram of two types of sensory hair cells in the sensory areas of the membranous labyrinth. The type I hair cell has a flask-shaped structure with a rounded base. The base is enclosed in a chalice-like afferent nerve ending that has several synaptic boutons for efferent nerve endings. Note the apical surface specializations of this cell, which include a kinocilium and several stereocilia. The apical cytoplasm contains residual basal bodies. The type II hair cell is cylindrical and possesses several nerve terminals at its base for both afferent and efferent nerve fibers. The apical surface specializations are identical with those of the type I cell.

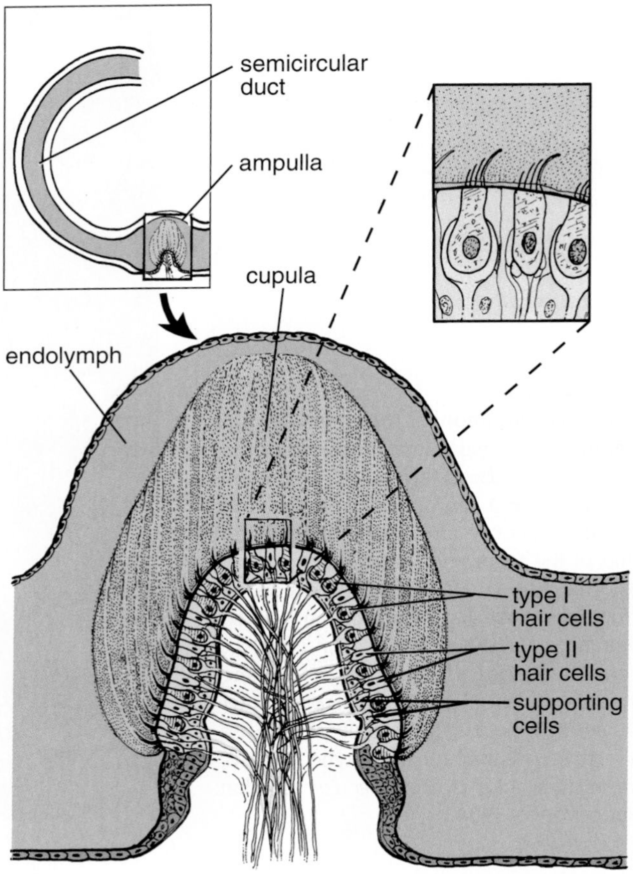

FIGURE 24.10
Diagram of the crista ampullaris within a semicircular duct. The cellular organization of the crista ampullaris of a semicircular duct is shown in the *large diagram* and the *enlarged rectangle.* The crista ampullaris is composed of both type I and type II sensory hair cells and supporting cells. The stereocilia and kinocilium of each hair are embedded in the cupula that projects toward the nonsensory wall of the ampulla.

fixed to the wall of the duct and the endolymph. Bending of the stereocilia in the narrow space between the hair calls and the cupula generates nerve impulses in the associated nerve endings.

The maculae of the saccule and utricle are sensors of gravity and linear acceleration

The maculae of the saccule and the utricle are innervated sensory thickenings of the epithelium that face the endolymph of the saccule and utricle (see Fig. 24.7c). As in the cristae, each macula consists of type I and type II hair cells, supporting cells, and nerve endings associated with the hair cells. The maculae of the utricle and saccule are oriented at right angles to one another. When a person is standing, the macula of the utricle is in a horizontal plane, and the macula of the saccule is in a vertical plane.

The gelatinous polysaccharide material that overlies the maculae is called the ***otolithic membrane*** (Fig. 24.11). Its outer surface contains 3- to 5-μm crystalline bodies of calcium carbonate and a protein (Fig. 24.12). Otoliths are heavier than the endolymph. The outer surface of the otolithic membrane lies opposite the surface in which the stereocilia of the hair cells are embedded. The otolithic membrane moves on the macula in a manner analogous to that by which the cupula moves on the crista. Stereocilia of the hair cells are bent by gravity in the stationary individual when the otolithic membrane and its otoliths pull on the stereocilia. They are also bent during linear movement when the individual is moving in a straight line and the otolithic membrane drags on the stereocilia because of in-

ertia. In both cases, movement of the otolithic membrane triggers an action potential.

The spiral organ of Corti is the sensor of sound vibrations

The cochlear duct divides the cochlear canal into three parallel compartments or ***scalae:***

- ***Scala media,*** the middle compartment in the cochlear canal
- ***Scala vestibuli***
- ***Scala tympani***

The cochlear duct itself is the scala media (Figs. 24.13 and 24.14). The scala vestibuli and scala tympani are the spaces above and below, respectively, the scala media. The scala media is an endolymph-containing space that is continuous with the lumen of the saccule and contains the spiral organ of Corti, which rests on its lower wall (see Fig. 24.14).

The scala vestibuli and the scala tympani are perilymph-containing spaces that communicate with each other at the apex of the cochlea through a small channel called the ***helicotrema*** (see Fig. 24.13). The scala vestibuli begins at the

BOX 24.1

Clinical Correlations: Vertigo

The sense of rotation without equilibrium (dizziness, vertigo) signifies dysfunction of the vestibular system. Causes of vertigo include viral infections, certain drugs, and tumors such as acoustic neuroma. Acoustic neuromas develop in or near the internal acoustic meatus and exert pressure on the vestibular division of cranial nerve VIII or branches of the labyrinthine artery. Also, vertigo can be produced normally in individuals by excessive stimulation of the semicircular ducts. Similarly, excessive stimulation of the utricle can produce motion sickness (seasickness, carsickness, or airsickness) in some individuals.

Some diseases of the internal ear affect both hearing and equilibrium. For example, people with Ménière's syndrome initially complain of episodes of dizziness and tinnitus (ringing) and later develop a low-frequency hearing loss. The causes of Ménière's syndrome are related to blockage of the cochlear aqueduct, which drains excess endolymph from the membranous labyrinth. Blockage of this duct causes an increase in endolymphatic pressure and distension of the membranous labyrinth (endolymphatic hydrops).

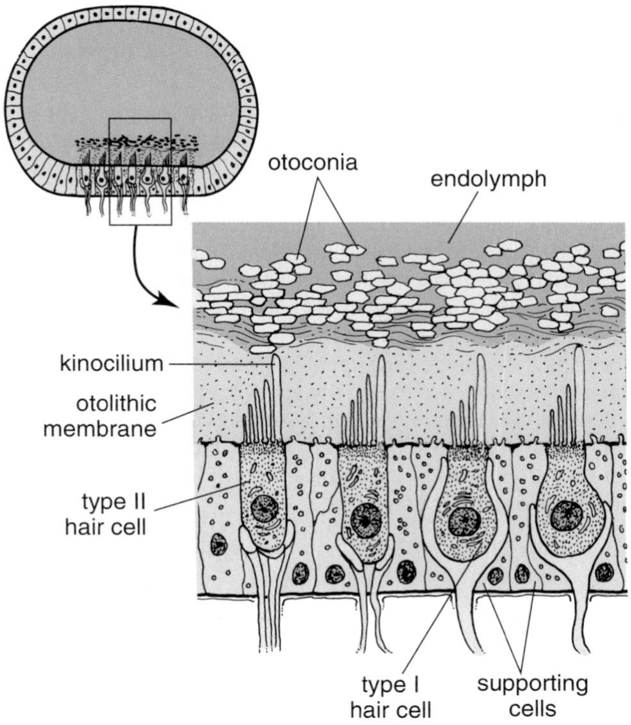

FIGURE 24.11
Diagram of a macula within the utricle. A more detailed diagram of the cellular organization of the macula of the utricle is shown in the *enlarged rectangle.* Supporting cells can be seen lying between the two principal types of sensory hair cells (types I and II). The stereocilia and kinocilium of each sensory hair cell are embedded in the otolithic membrane on which otoconia lie.

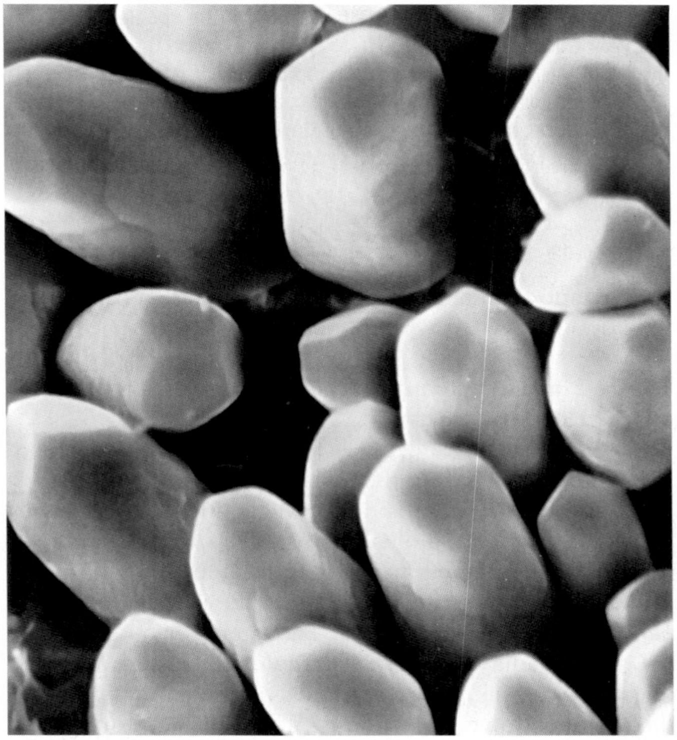

FIGURE 24.12
Scanning electron micrograph of human otoconia. Each otoconium has a long cylindrical body with a three-headed facet on each end. ×5,000.

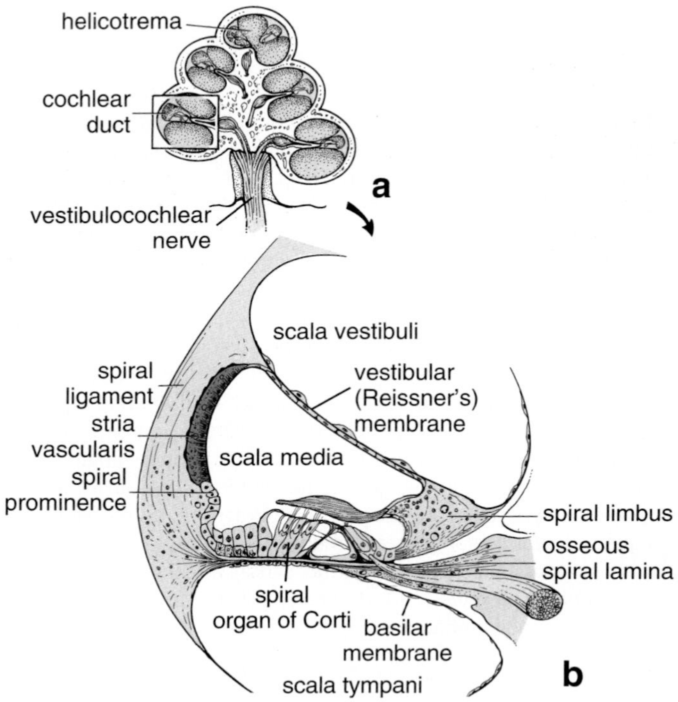

FIGURE 24.13
Schematic diagram of the cochlea. a. Schematic diagram of a mid-modiolar section of the cochlea that illustrates the position of the cochlear duct within the $2\frac{3}{4}$ turns of the bony cochlea. Observe that the scala vestibuli and scala tympani are continuous apically (helicotrema). **b.** Cross section of the basal turn of the cochlear duct. The cochlear duct and the osseous spiral lamina divide the cochlea into the scala vestibuli and the scala tympani, which contain perilymph. The scala media (the space within the cochlear duct) is filled with endolymph and contains the organ of Corti. (Modified from Goodhill V. *Ear, Diseases, Deafness, and Dizziness.* Hagerstown, MD: Harper & Row, 1979.)

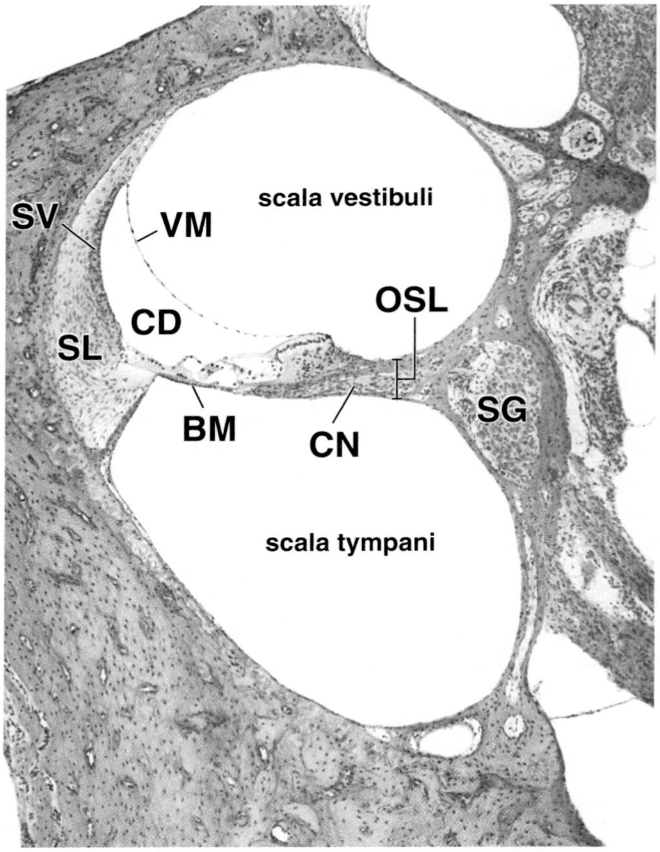

FIGURE 24.14
Photomicrograph of cochlear canal. This photomicrograph shows a section of the basal turn of the cochlear canal. The osseous spiral lamina *(OSL)* and its membranous continuation, the basilar membrane *(BM),* as well as the vestibular membrane *(VM)* divide the cochlear canal into three parallel compartments: the scala vestibuli, the cochlear duct *(CD),* and the scala tympani. Both the scala vestibuli and the scala tympani are filled with perilymph, whereas the cochlear canal is filled with endolymph. Note the three walls of the cochlear canal, which are formed by the basilar membrane inferiorly, the stria vascularis *(SV)* and underlying spiral ligament *(SL)* laterally, and the vestibular membrane superiorly. The spiral organ of Corti resides on the inferior wall of the cochlear canal. Dendrites of the cochlear nerve *(CN)* fibers that originate in the spiral ganglion *(SG)* enter the spiral organ of Corti. The axons of the cochlear nerve form the cochlear part of the vestibulocochlear nerve. ×65.

oval window, and the scala tympani ends at the round window.

The scala media is a triangular space with its acute angle attached to the modiolus

In transverse section, the scala media appears as a triangular space with its most acute angle attached to a bony extension of the modiolus, the ***osseous spiral lamina*** (see Fig. 24.14). The upper wall of the scala media, which separates it from the scala vestibuli, is the ***vestibular (Reissner's) membrane*** (Fig. 24.15). The lateral or outer wall of the scala media is the ***stria vascularis*** (Fig. 24.16). It is lined with a thick, pseudostratified epithelium that may be the site of endolymph synthesis. The lower wall or floor of the scala media is the ***basilar membrane.*** The spiral organ of Corti rests on the basilar membrane and is overlain by the ***tectorial membrane.***

The spiral organ of Corti is composed of hair cells, phalangeal cells, and pillar cells

The spiral organ of Corti is a complex epithelial layer on the floor of the scala media (Fig. 24.17). It is formed by

- ***Inner*** (close to the spiral lamina) and ***outer*** (farther from the spiral lamina) ***hair cells***
- ***Inner*** and ***outer phalangeal (supporting) cells***
- ***Pillar cells***

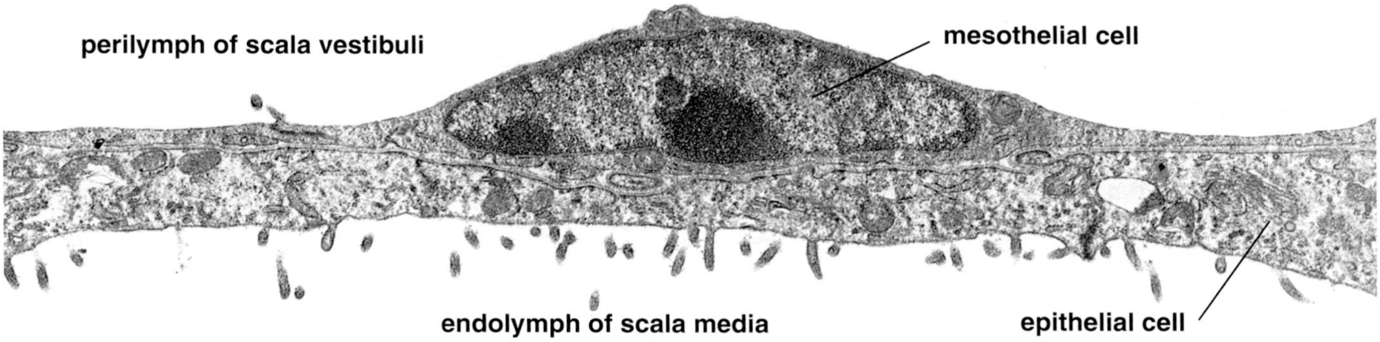

FIGURE 24.15
Transmission electron micrograph of the vestibular (Reissner's) membrane. Two cell types can be observed: a mesothelial cell, which faces the scala vestibuli and is bathed by perilymph, and an epithelial cell, which faces the scala media and is bathed by endolymph. ×8,400.

Several other named cell types of unknown function are also present in the spiral organ. Interested readers should consult specialized texts for more-detailed descriptions.

The hair cells are arranged in an inner and an outer row of cells

The inner hair cells form a single row of cells throughout all 2¾ turns of the cochlear duct. The number of cells forming the width of the continuous row of outer hair cells is variable. Three ranks of hair cells are found in the basal part of the coil (Fig. 24.18). The width of the row gradually increases to five ranks of cells at the apex of the cochlea.

The phalangeal and pillar cells provide support for the hair cells

Phalangeal cells are supporting cells for both rows of hair cells. The phalangeal cells associated with the inner hair cells surround the cells completely (Fig. 24.19a). The phalangeal cells associated with the outer hair cells surround only the basal portion of the hair cell completely and send apical processes toward the endolymphatic space (Fig. 24.19b). These processes flatten near the apical ends of the hair cells and collectively form a complete plate surrounding each hair cell (Fig. 24.20).

The apical ends of the phalangeal cells are tightly bound to one another and to the hair cells by elaborate tight junctions. These junctions form the ***reticular lamina*** that seals the endolymphatic compartment from the true intercellular spaces of the organ of Corti (Figs. 24.17 and 24.19b). The extracellular fluid in this intercellular space is ***cortilymph.*** Its composition is similar to that of other extracellular fluids and to perilymph.

Pillar cells have broad apical and basal surfaces that form plates and a narrowed cytoplasm. The inner pillar

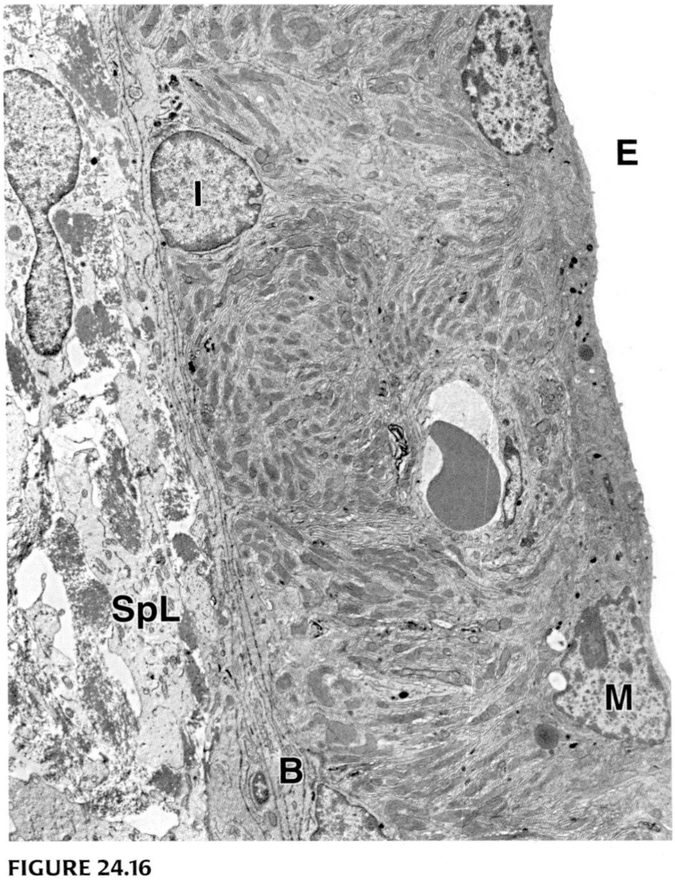

FIGURE 24.16
Transmission electron micrograph of the stria vascularis. The apical surfaces of the marginal cells *(M)* of the stria are bathed by endolymph *(E)* of the scala media. Intermediate cells *(I)* are positioned between the marginal cells and the basal cells *(B)*. The basal cells separate the other cells of the stria vascularis from the spiral ligament *(SpL)*. ×4,700.

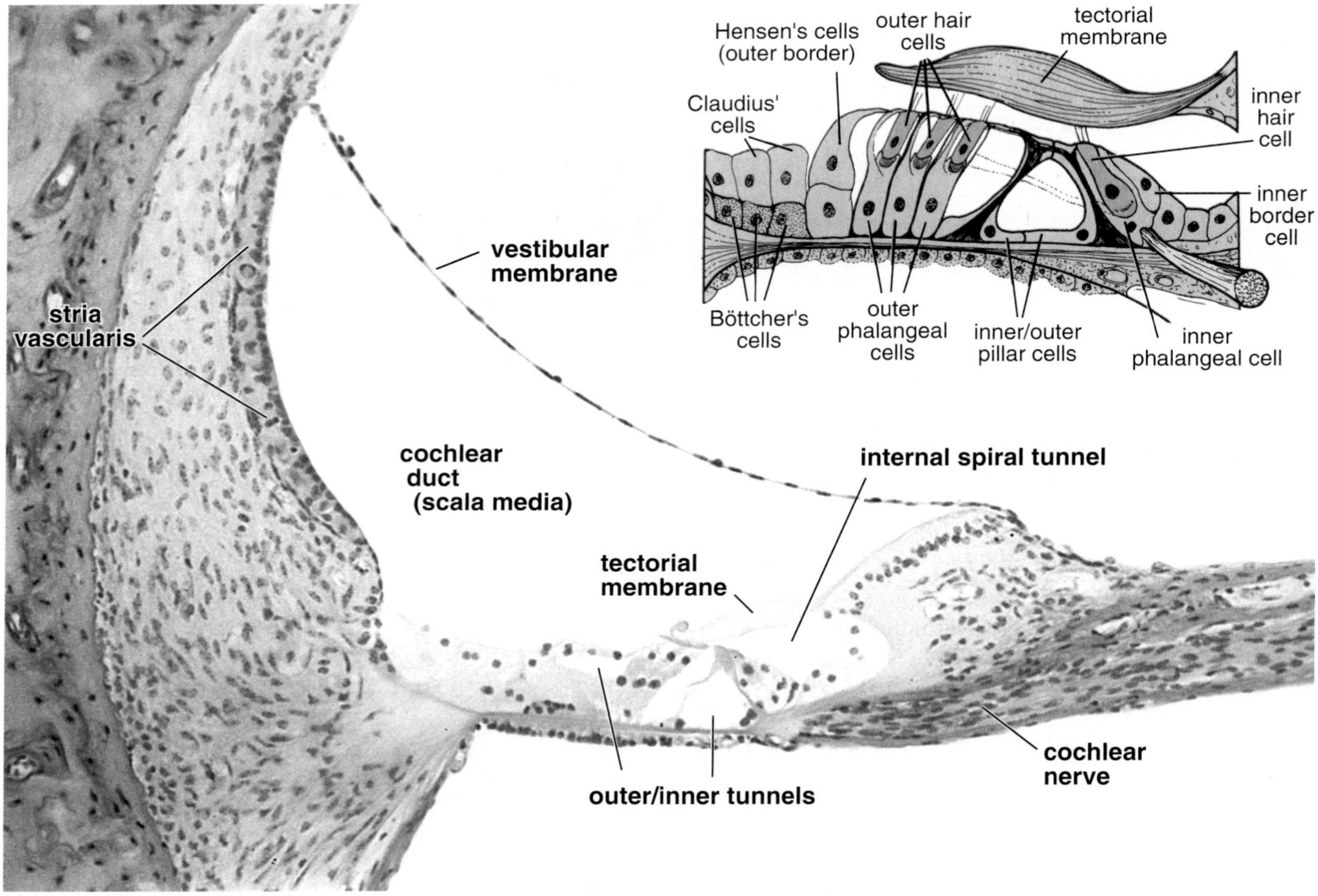

FIGURE 24.17

Photomicrograph of the vestibular duct and spiral organ of Corti. This higher-magnification photomicrograph of the cochlear duct shows the structure of the spiral organ of Corti. Relate this structure to the *inset,* which labels the structural features of the spiral organ. ×180. **Inset.** Diagram of the sensory and supporting cells of the spiral organ of Corti. The sensory cells are divided into an inner row of sensory hair cells and three rows of outer sensory hair cells. The supporting cells are the inner and outer pillar cells, inner and outer (Deiters') phalangeal cells, outer border cells (Hensen's cells), inner border cells, Claudius' cells, and Böttcher's cells. (Modified from Goodhill V. *Ear, Diseases, Deafness, and Dizziness.* Hagerstown, MD: Harper & Row, 1979.)

BOX 24.2

Clinical Correlations: Hearing Loss—Vestibular Dysfunction

Several types of disorders can affect the auditory and vestibular system, resulting in deafness, dizziness (vertigo), or both. Auditory disorders are classified as either conductive or sensorineural in nature. ***Conductive hearing loss*** results when sound waves are mechanically impeded from reaching the auditory sensory receptors within the internal ear. This type of hearing loss principally involves the external ear or structures of the middle ear. One example of a conductive hearing loss is otosclerosis, a disease characterized by the growth of new spongy bone within the bony labyrinth near the oval window. This spongy bone growth can cause the fixation of the base of the stapes (ankylosis) in the oval window, decreasing the efficiency of sound conduction to the internal ear.

Sensorineural hearing impairment may also occur after injury to the auditory sensory hair cells within the internal ear or to the cochlear division of cranial nerve VIII. Such hearing losses may be congenital or acquired. Causes of acquired sensorineural hearing loss include infections of the membranous labyrinth (e.g., meningitis, chronic otitis media), acoustic trauma (i.e., prolonged exposure to excessive noise), and administration of certain classes of antibiotics and diuretics.

Another example of sensorineural hearing loss often occurs as a result of aging. A loss of the sensory hair cells or associated nerve fibers begins in the basal turn of the cochlea and progresses apically over time. The characteristic impairment is a high-frequency hearing loss termed ***presbycusis*** (see presbyopia, page 808).

In selected patients the use of a ***cochlear implant*** can partially restore some hearing function. The cochlear implant is an electronic device consisting of an external microphone, amplifier, and speech processor linked to a receiver implanted under the skin of the mastoid region. The receiver is connected to the multielectrode intracochlear implant inserted along the wall of the cochlear canal. After considerable training and tuning of the speech processor, the patient's hearing can be partially restored to various degrees ranging from recognition of critical sounds to the ability to converse.

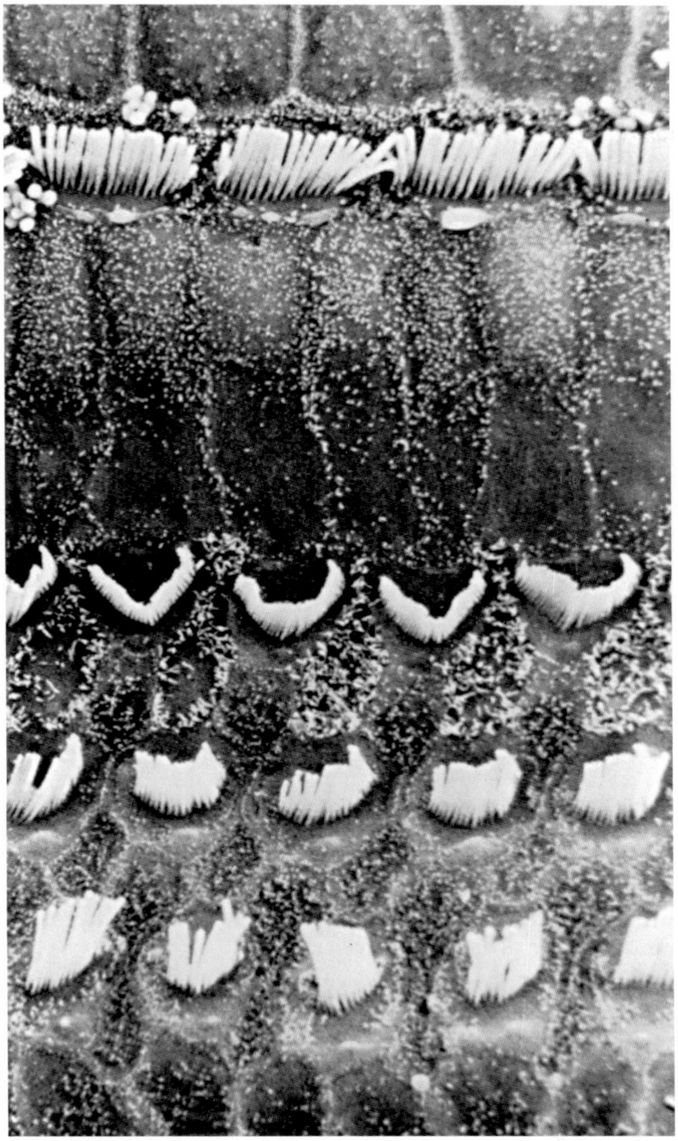

FIGURE 24.18
Scanning electron micrograph of the spiral organ of Corti. This electron micrograph illustrates the configuration of stereocilia on the apical surfaces of the inner row and three outer rows of the cochlear sensory hair cells. ×3,250.

cells rest on the tympanic lip of the spiral lamina; the outer pillar cells rest on the basilar membrane. Between them, they form a triangular tunnel, the ***inner spiral tunnel*** (see Fig. 24.17).

The tectorial membrane extends from the spiral limbus over the cells of the spiral organ of Corti

The tectorial membrane is attached medially to the modiolus. Its lateral free edge projects over and attaches to the organ of Corti by the stereocilia of the hair cells. It is described as a keratin-like layer containing fibrils embedded in a dense amorphous ground substance.

Sound Perception

As described on page 822, sound waves striking the tympanic membrane are translated into simple mechanical vibrations. The ossicles of the middle ear convey these vibrations to the cochlea.

In the internal ear the vibrations of the ossicles are transformed into waves in the perilymph

Movement of the stapes in the oval window of the vestibule sets up vibrations or traveling waves in the perilymph of the scala vestibuli. The vibrations are transmitted through the vestibular membrane to the scala media (cochlear duct), which contains endolymph, and are also propagated to the perilymph of the scala tympani. Pressure changes in this closed perilymphatic–endolymphatic system are reflected in movements of the membrane that covers the round window in the base of the cochlea.

As a result of sound vibrations entering the internal ear, a traveling wave is set up in the basilar membrane (Fig. 24.21). A sound of specified frequency causes displacement of a relatively long segment of the basilar membrane, but the region of maximal displacement is narrow. The point of maximal displacement of the basilar membrane is specified for a given frequency of sound and is the morphologic basis of frequency discrimination. High-frequency sounds cause maximal vibration of the basilar membrane near the base of the cochlea; low-frequency sounds cause maximal displacement nearer the apex. Amplitude discrimination, i.e., perception of sound intensity or loudness, depends on the degree of displacement of the basilar membrane at any given frequency range.

Movement of the stereocilia of the hair cells in the cochlea initiates neuronal transduction

Hair cells are attached through the phalangeal cells to the basilar membrane, which vibrates during sound reception. The stereocilia of these hair cells are in turn attached to the tectorial membrane, which also vibrates. However, the tectorial membrane and the basilar membrane are hinged at different points. Thus, a shearing effect occurs between the basilar membrane (and the cells attached to it) and the tectorial membrane when sound vibrations impinge on the internal ear.

Because they are inserted into the tectorial membrane, the stereocilia of the hair cells are the only structures that connect the basilar membrane and its complex epithelial layer to the tectorial membrane. The shearing effect between the basilar membrane and the tectorial membrane distorts the stereocilia and thus the apical portion of the hair cells. This distortion generates membrane potentials that are conveyed to the brain via the ***cochlear nerve (cochlear division of the vestibulocochlear nerve, cranial nerve VIII)***.

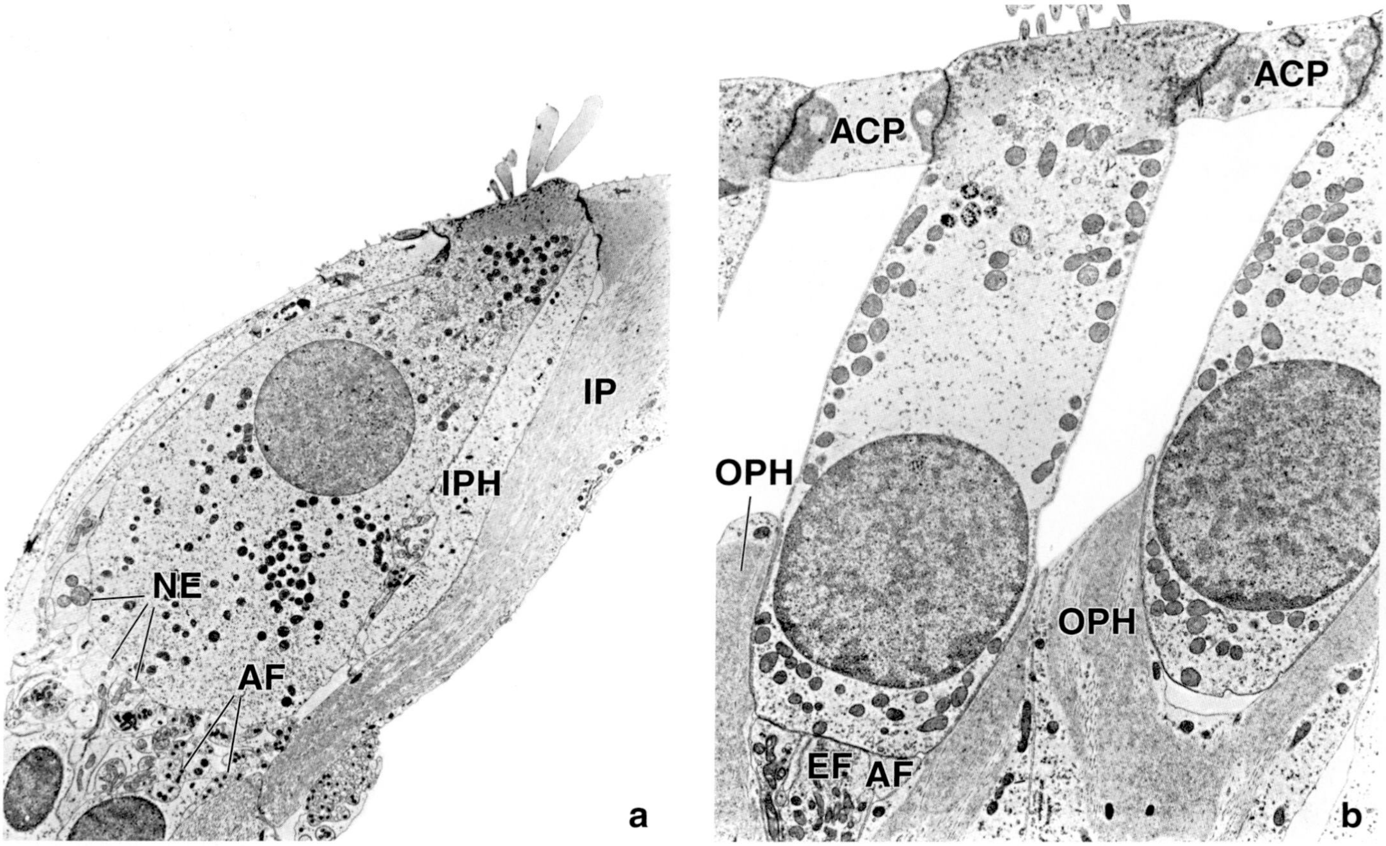

FIGURE 24.19

Electron micrograph of an inner and outer hair cell. a. Observe the rounded base and constricted neck of the inner hair cell. Nerve endings *(NE)* from afferent nerve fibers *(AF)* to the inner hair cells are seen basally. *IP,* inner pillar cell; *IPH,* inner phalangeal cell. ×6,300. **b.** Afferent *(AF)* and efferent *(EF)* nerve fiber endings on the base of an outer sensory hair cell are evident. Outer phalangeal cells *(OPH)* surround the outer hair cells basally. Their apical projections form the apical cuticular plate *(ACP).* Note that the lateral domains in the middle third of the outer hair cells are not surrounded by supporting cells. ×6,300. (From Kimura RS. Sensory and accessory epithelia of the cochlea. In: Friedmann I, Ballantyne J, eds. *Ultrastructural Atlas of the Inner Ear.* London: Butterworths, 1984.)

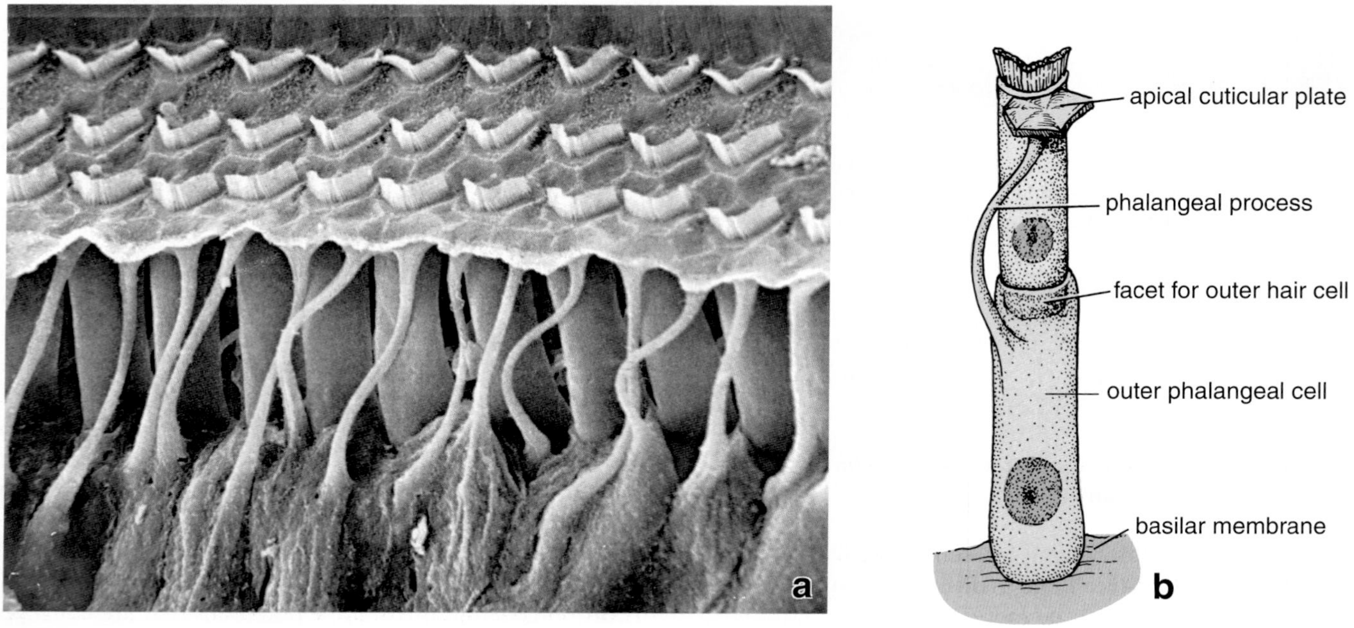

FIGURE 24.20

Structure of the outer phalangeal cell. a. This scanning electron micrograph illustrates the architecture of the outer phalangeal (Deiters') cells. Each phalangeal cell cups the basal surface of an outer sensory hair cell and extends its phalangeal process apically to form an apical cuticular plate that supports the outer sensory hair cells. ×2,400. **b.** Schematic drawing showing the relationship of an outer phalangeal cell to an outer sensory hair cell.

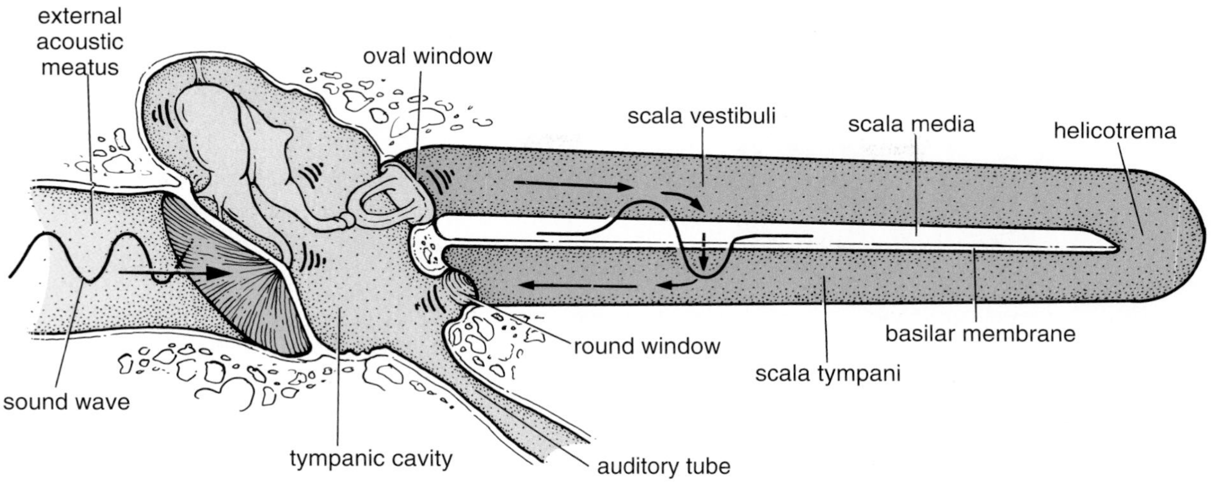

FIGURE 24.21
Schematic diagram illustrating the dynamics of the three divisions of the ear. The cochlear duct is shown here as if straightened. Sound waves are collected and transmitted from the external ear to the middle ear, where they are converted into mechanical vibrations. The mechanical vibrations are then converted at the oval window into fluid vibrations within the internal ear. Fluid vibrations cause displacement of the basilar membrane on which rest the auditory sensory hair cells. Such displacement leads to stimulation of the hair cells and a discharge of neural impulses from them. (Modified from Karmody CS. *Textbook of Otolaryngology.* Philadelphia: Lea & Febiger, 1983.)

Innervation of the Internal Ear

The vestibular nerve innervates the sensory receptors associated with the vestibular labyrinth

The vestibulocochlear nerve (cranial nerve VIII) is divided into a vestibular nerve, which innervates the sensory receptors associated with the vestibular labyrinth, and a cochlear nerve, which innervates the sensory receptors associated with the cochlear labyrinth (Fig. 24.22). The vestibular nerve innervates the cristae ampullaris of the three semicircular ducts, the macula of the utricle, and the macula of the saccule.

The cell bodies of the bipolar neurons of the ***vestibular nerve*** are located in the ***vestibular ganglion (of Scarpa)*** in the internal acoustic meatus. Dendritic processes of the vestibular nerve fibers synapse at the base of the vestibular sensory hair cells, either as a chalice around a type I hair cell or as a bouton associated with a type II hair cell. The axons of the vestibular nerve fibers enter the brainstem and terminate in the vestibular nuclei. Some secondary neuronal fibers travel to the cerebellum and to the nuclei of cranial nerves III, IV, and VI, which innervate the muscles of the eye.

The cochlear nerve innervates the sensory receptors of the spiral organ of Corti

Nerve fibers of the ***cochlear nerve*** division enter the bony cochlea through the modiolus from the internal acoustic meatus (see Fig. 24.22). Neurons of the cochlear nerve fibers are also bipolar, and their cell bodies are located in the ***spiral ganglion*** within the modiolus. Dendritic processes of the afferent cochlear nerve fibers exit the modiolus through foramina nervosa and enter the spiral organ. The axons of the cochlear nerve enter the brainstem and terminate in the cochlear nuclei of the medulla. Nerve fibers from these nuclei pass to the geniculate nucleus of the thalamus and then to the auditory cortex of the temporal lobe.

Efferent fibers conveying impulses from the brain pass parallel to the ascending afferent nerve fibers of the vestibulocochlear nerve (cochlear efferents of Rasmussen). Efferent nerve fibers from the brainstem pass through the vestibular nerve. They synapse either on afferent endings of the inner hair cell or on the basal aspect of an outer hair cell. Efferent fibers are thought to effect control of auditory and vestibular input to the central nervous system, presumably by enhancing some afferent signals while suppressing other signals.

Blood Vessels of the Membranous Labyrinth

Arterial blood is supplied to the membranous labyrinth by the labyrinthine artery; venous blood drainage is to the venous dural sinuses

The blood supply to the external ear, middle ear, and bony labyrinth of the internal ear is derived from vessels associated with the external carotid arteries. The arterial

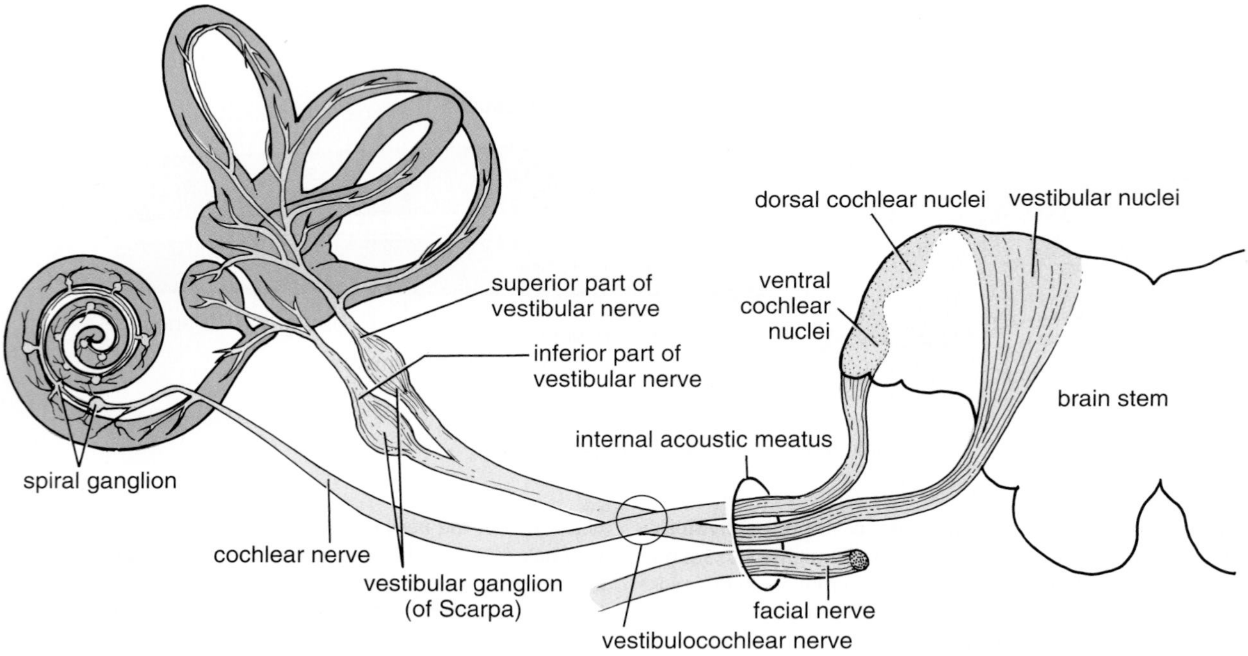

FIGURE 24.22
Diagram illustrating the innervation of the sensory regions of the membranous labyrinth. Note the two parts of the vestibulocochlear nerve. The cochlear nerve carries the hearing impulses from the cochlear duct; the vestibular nerve carries balance information from the semicircular canals. The cell bodies of these sensory fibers are located in the spiral ganglion (for hearing) and vestibular ganglion (for equilibrium). (Modified from Hawke M, Keene M, Alberti PW. *Clinical Otoscopy: A Text and Colour Atlas.* Edinburgh: Churchill Livingstone, 1984.)

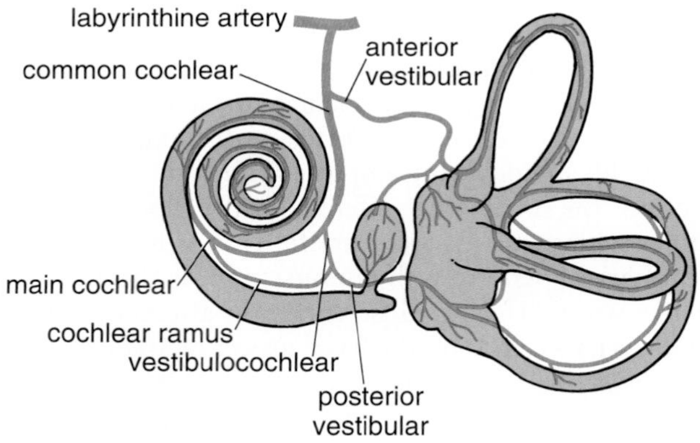

FIGURE 24.23
Diagram of the arterial supply of the membranous labyrinth of the internal ear. The blood supply to the membranous labyrinth of the internal ear is derived from the labyrinthine artery, a branch of the anterior inferior cerebellar or basilar artery. (Modified from Schuknecht HF. *Pathology of the Ear.* Cambridge, MA: Harvard University Press, 1974.)

blood supply to tissues of the membranous labyrinth of the internal ear is derived intracranially from the labyrinthine artery, a common branch of the anterior inferior cerebellar or basilar artery (Fig. 24.23). The labyrinthine artery is a terminal artery, in that it has no anastomoses with other surrounding arteries. Branches of this artery exactly parallel the distribution of the superior and inferior parts of the vestibular nerve.

Venous drainage from the cochlear labyrinth is via the posterior and anterior spiral modiolar veins that form the common modiolar vein. The common modiolar vein and the vestibulocochlear vein form the ***vein of the cochlear aqueduct***, which empties into the ***inferior petrosal sinus***. Venous drainage from the vestibular labyrinth is via vestibular veins that join the vein of the cochlear aqueduct and by the ***vein of vestibular aqueduct***, which drains into the ***sigmoid sinus***.

PLATE 104. EAR

The inner ear, located in the temporal bone, consists of a system of chambers and canals that contain a network of membranous channels. These are referred to, respectively, as the *bony labyrinth* and *membranous labyrinth.* In places, the membranous labyrinth forms the lining of the bony labyrinth; in other places, there is a separation of the two. Within the space lined by the membranous labyrinth is a watery fluid called *endolymph.* External to the membranous labyrinth, i.e., between the membranous and bony labyrinths, is additional fluid called *perilymph.*

The bony labyrinth is divided into three parts: *cochlea, semicircular canals,* and *vestibule*. The cochlea and semicircular canals contain membranous counterparts of the same shape; however, the membranous components of the vestibule are more complex in form, being composed of ducts and two chambers, the *utricle* and *saccule.* The cochlea contains the receptors for hearing, i.e., the *organ of Corti,* the semicircular canals contain the receptors for movement of the head, and the utricle and saccule contain receptors for position of the head.

Figure 1, ear, guinea pig, H&E ×20.

In this section through the inner ear, bone surrounds the entire inner ear cavity. Because of its labyrinthine character, sections of the inner ear appear as a number of separate chambers and ducts. These, however, are all interconnected (except that the perilymphatic and endolymphatic spaces remain separate). The largest chamber is the vestibule *(V).* The left side of this chamber *(black arrow)* leads into the cochlea *(C).* Just below the *black arrow* and to the right is the oval ligament *(OL)* surrounding the base of the stapes *(S).* Both structures have been cut obliquely and are not seen in their entirety. The facial nerve *(FN)* is in an osseous tunnel to the left of the oval ligament. The communication of the vestibule with one of the semicircular canals is marked by the *white arrow.* At the upper right are cross sections of the membranous labyrinth passing through components of the semicircular duct system *(DS).*

The cochlea is a spiral structure having the general shape of a cone. The specimen illustrated here makes $3\frac{1}{2}$ turns (in humans, there are $2\frac{3}{4}$ turns). The section goes through the central axis of the cochlea. This consists of a bony stem called the modiolus *(M).* It contains the beginning of the cochlear nerve *(CN)* and the spiral ganglion *(SG).* Because of the plane of section and the spiral arrangement of the cochlear tunnel, the tunnel is cut crosswise in seven places (note $3^1/_2$ turns). A more detailed examination of the cochlea and the organ of Corti is provided in Plate 105.

Figure 2, ear, guinea pig, H&E ×225.

A higher magnification of one of the semicircular canals and of the crista ampullaris *(CA)* within the canal seen in the lower right of Figure 1 is provided here. The receptor for movement, the crista ampullaris (note its relationships in Fig. 1), is present in each of the semicircular canals. The epithelial *(EP)* surface of the crista consists of two cell types, sustentacular (supporting) cells and hair (receptor) cells. (Two types of hair cells are distinguished with the electron microscope.) It is difficult to identify the hair and sustentacular cells on the basis of specific characteristics; they can, however, be distinguished on the basis of location (see **inset**), as the hair cells *(HC)* are situated in a more superficial location than the sustentacular cells *(SC).* A gelatinous mass, the cupula *(Cu),* surmounts the epithelium of the crista ampullaris. Each receptor cell sends a hair-like projection deep into the substance of the cupula.

The epithelium rests on a loose, cellular connective tissue *(CT)* that also contains the nerve fibers associated with the receptor cells. The nerve fibers are difficult to identify because they are not organized into a discrete bundle.

KEY

C, cochlea
CA, crista ampullaris
CN, cochlear nerve
CT, connective tissue
Cu, cupula
DS, duct system (of membranous labyrinth)
EP, epithelium
FN, facial nerve
HC, hair cell
M, modiolus
OL, oval ligament
S, stapes
SC, sustentacular cell
SG, spiral ganglion
V, vestibule
black arrow, entry to cochlea
white arrow, entry to semicircular canal

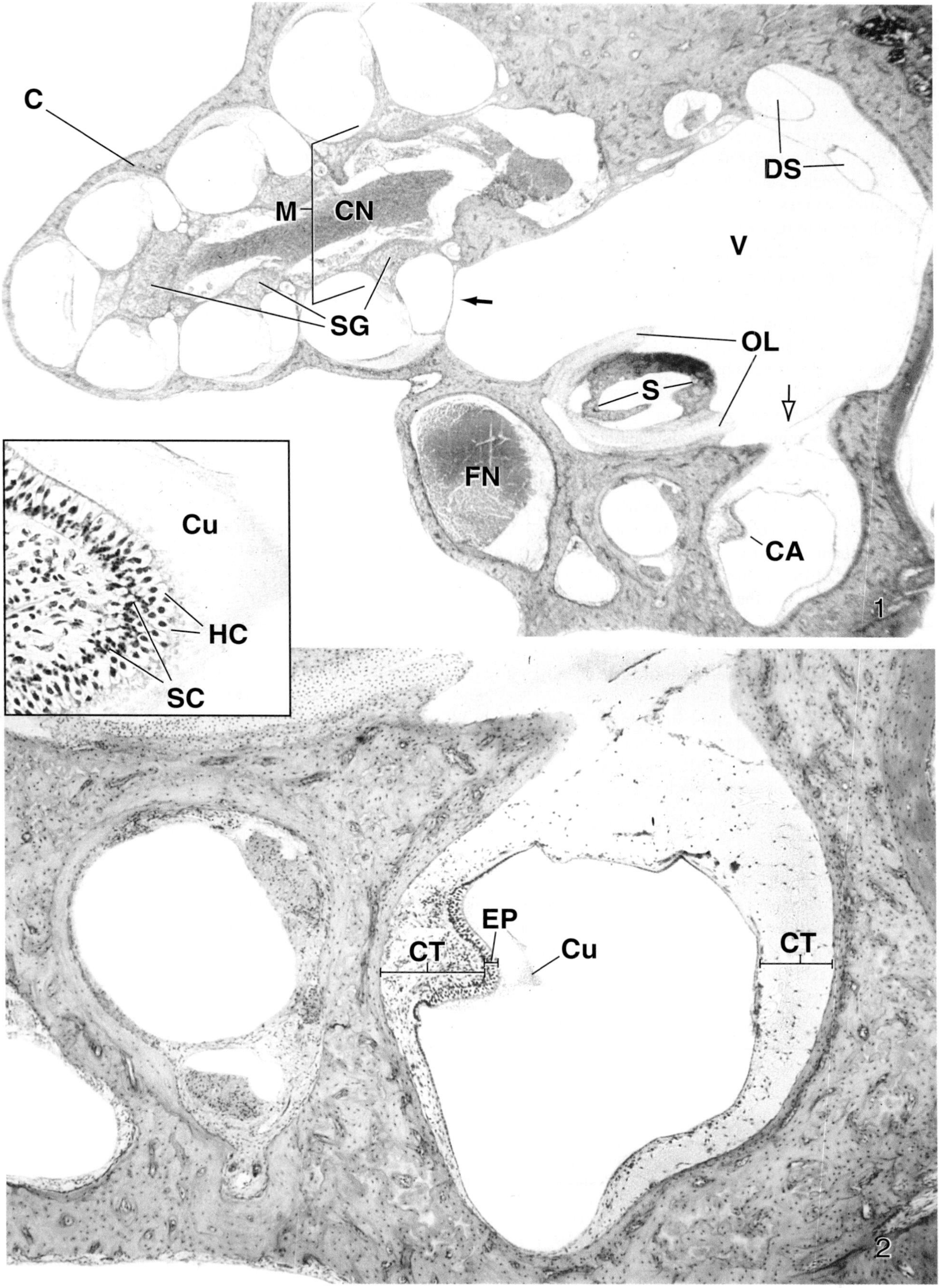
C
M
CN
SG
DS
V
OL
S
FN
CA
1
Cu
HC
SC
EP
CT
Cu
CT
2

PLATE 105. ORGAN OF CORTI

The *hair cell,* a nonneuronal mechanoreceptor, is the common receptor cell of the vestibulocochlear system. Hair cells are epithelial cells that possess numerous *stereocilia,* modified microvilli also called *sensory hairs.* They convert mechanical energy to electrical energy that is transmitted via the vestibulocochlear nerve (cranial nerve VIII) to the brain. Hair cells are associated with afferent, as well as efferent, nerve endings. All hair cells have a common basis of receptor cell function that involves bending or flexing of their stereocilia. The specific means by which the stereocilia are bent varies from receptor to receptor, but in each case, stretching of the plasma membrane caused by the bending of the stereocilia generates transmembrane potential changes that are transmitted to the afferent nerve endings associated with each cell. Efferent nerve endings on the hair cells serve to regulate their sensitivity.

Figure 1, ear, guinea pig, H&E ×65; inset ×380.

A section through one of the turns of the cochlea is shown here. The most important functional component of the cochlea is the organ of Corti, enclosed by the *rectangle* and shown at higher magnification in Figure 2. Other structures are included in this figure. The spiral ligament *(SL)* is a thickening of the periosteum on the outer part of the tunnel. Two membranes, the basilar membrane *(BM)* and the vestibular membrane *(VM),* join with the spiral ligament and divide the cochlear tunnel into three parallel canals, namely, the scala vestibuli *(SV),* the scala tympani *(ST),* and the cochlear duct *(CD).* Both the scala vestibuli and the scala tympani are perilymphatic spaces; these communicate at the apex of the cochlea. The cochlear duct, on the other hand, is the space of the membranous labyrinth and is filled with endolymph. It is thought that the endolymph is formed by the portion of the spiral ligament that faces the cochlear duct, the stria vascularis *(StV).* This is highly vascularized and contains specialized "secretory" cells.

A shelf of bone, the osseous spiral lamina *(OSL),* extends from the modiolus to the basilar membrane. Branches of the cochlear nerve *(CN)* travel along the spiral lamina to the modiolus, where the main trunk of the nerve is formed. The components of the cochlear nerve are bipolar neurons whose cell bodies constitute the spiral ganglion *(SG).* These cell bodies are shown at higher magnification in the **inset** (upper right). The spiral lamina supports an elevation of cells, the limbus spiralis *(LS).* The surface of the limbus is composed of columnar cells.

Figure 2, ear, guinea pig, H&E ×180; inset ×380.

The components of the organ of Corti, beginning at the limbus spiralis *(LS),* are as follows: inner border cells *(IBC);* inner phalangeal and hair cells *(IP&HC);* inner pillar cells *(IPC);* (the sequence continues, repeating itself in reverse) outer pillar cells *(OPC);* hair and outer phalangeal cells *(HC&OP);* and outer border cells or cells of Hensen *(CH).* Hair cells are receptor cells; the other cells are collectively referred to as *supporting cells.* The hair and outer phalangeal cells can be distinguished in this figure by their location (see **inset**) and because their nuclei are well aligned. Because the hair cells rest on the phalangeal cells, it can be concluded that the upper three nuclei belong to outer hair cells, whereas the lower three nuclei belong to outer phalangeal cells.

The supporting cells extend from the basilar membrane *(BM)* to the surface of the organ of Corti (this is not evident here but can be seen in the **inset**), where they form a reticular membrane *(RM).* The free surface of the receptor cells fits into openings in the reticular membrane, and the "hairs" of these cells project toward, and make contact with, the tectorial membrane *(TM).* The latter is a cuticular extension from the columnar cells of the limbus spiralis. In ideal preparations, nerve fibers can be traced from the hair cells to the cochlear nerve *(CN).*

In their course from the basilar membrane to the reticular membrane, groups of supporting cells are separated from other groups by spaces that form spiral tunnels. These tunnels are named the inner tunnel *(IT),* the outer tunnel *(OT),* and the internal spiral tunnel *(IST).* Beyond the supporting cells are two additional groups of cells, the cells of Claudius *(CC)* and the cells of Böttcher *(CB).*

KEY

BM, basilar membrane
CB, cells of Böttcher
CC, cells of Claudius
CD, cochlear duct
CH, cells of Hensen
CN, cochlear nerve
HC&OP, hair and outer phalangeal cells
IBC, inner border cells
IP&HC, inner phalangeal and hair cells
IPC, inner pillar cells
IST, internal spiral tunnel
IT, inner tunnel
LS, limbus spiralis
OPC, outer pillar cells
OSL, osseous spiral lamina
OT, outer tunnel
RM, reticular membrane
SG, spiral ganglion
SL, spiral ligament
ST, scala tympani
StV, stria vascularis
SV, scala vestibuli
TM, tectorial membrane
VM, vestibular membrane

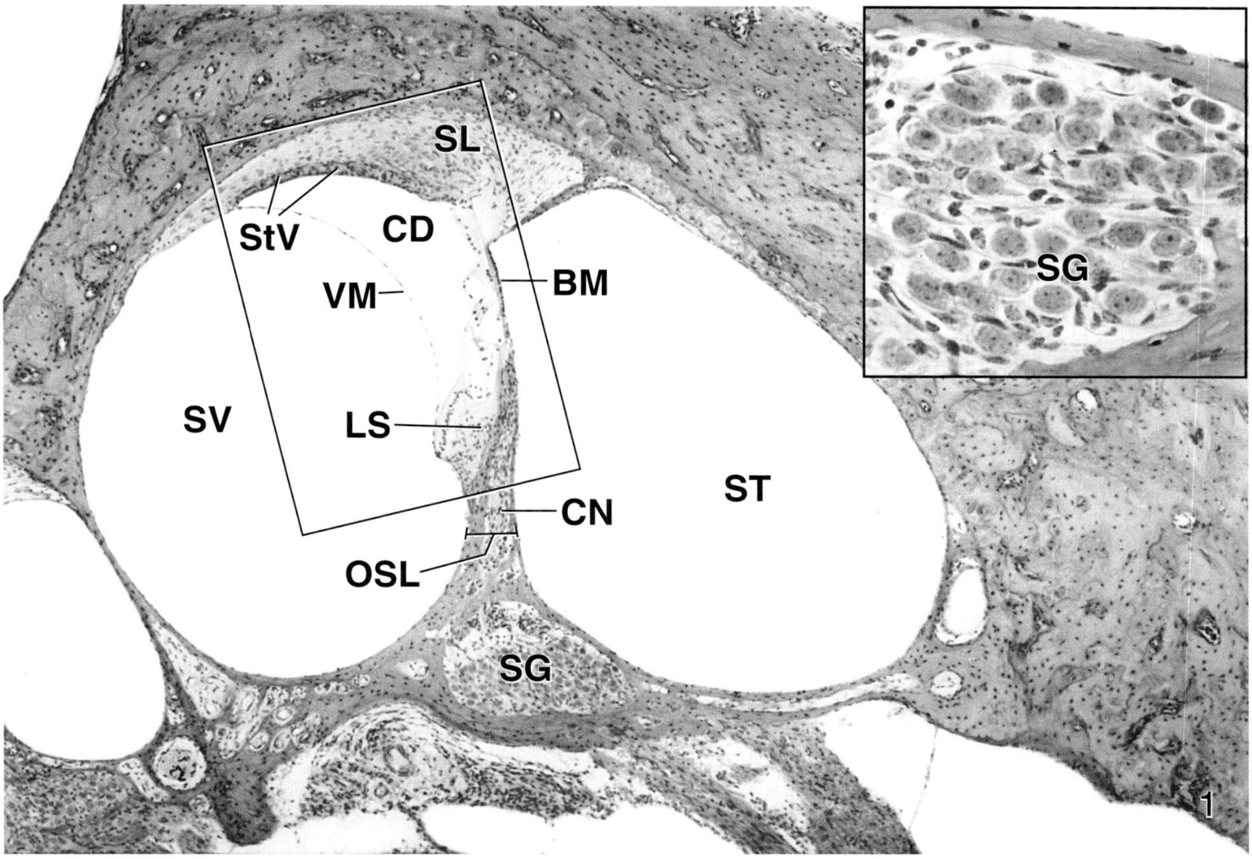
SL
StV
CD
VM
BM
SV
LS
ST
CN
OSL
SG
SG
1

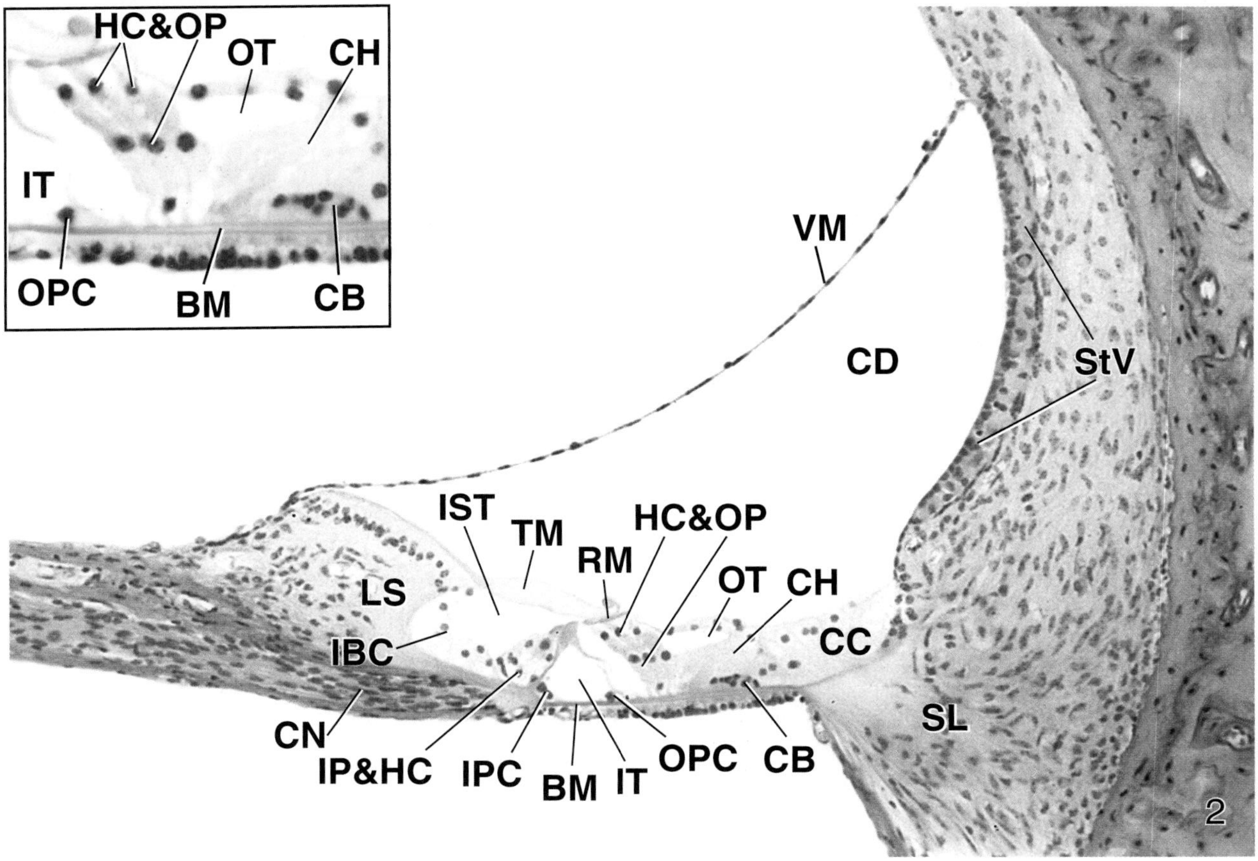
HC&OP
OT
CH
IT
OPC
BM
CB
VM
CD
StV
IST
TM
HC&OP
RM
OT
CH
LS
CC
IBC
SL
CN
IP&HC
IPC
BM
IT
OPC
CB
2

INDEX

In this index, page numbers in *italics* designate figures; page numbers followed by *b* designate boxes; page numbe
page numbers followed by *t* designate tables; and page numbers followed by *n* designate footnotes. Cross-referenc
ignate related topics or more detailed lists of subtopics.

C

D

M

T